SEVENTH EDITION
VOLUME 1

Moss and Adams'
HEART DISEASE IN INFANTS, CHILDREN, AND ADOLESCENTS

INCLUDING THE FETUS AND YOUNG ADULT

Editors

Hugh D. Allen, MD, ScD (Hon)
Vice Chair for Academic Affairs, Department
    of Pediatrics
Professor of Pediatrics and Medicine
The Ohio State University College of
    Medicine
Columbus, Ohio
Staff Cardiologist
Heart Center at Columbus
    Children's Hospital

David J. Driscoll, MD
Professor, Department of Pediatrics
Mayo Clinic College of Medicine
Mayo Clinic
Rochester, Minnesota

Robert E. Shaddy, MD
Professor of Pediatrics
Division Chief, Pediatric Cardiology
The Children's Hospital of Philadelphia
University of Pennsylvania School of
    Medicine
Philadelphia, Pennsylvania

Timothy F. Feltes, MD
Professor of Pediatrics
Division Chief, Pediatric Cardiology
The Ohio State University College of
    Medicine
Codirector, Heart Center at Columbus
    Children's Hospital
Columbus, Ohio

 Wolters Kluwer | Lippincott Williams & Wilkins
Health
Philadelphia · Baltimore · New York · London
Buenos Aires · Hong Kong · Sydney · Tokyo

Acquisitions Editor: Frances R. DeStefano
Developmental Editor: Julia Seto
Managing Editor: Chris Potash
Project Manager: Rosanne Hallowell
Manufacturing Manager: Benjamin Rivera
Marketing Manager: Kim Schonberger
Design Coordinator: Teresa Mallon
Cover Designer: Joseph DePinho
Production Services: Aptara, Inc.

7th Edition
© 2008 by Lippincott Williams & Wilkins, a Wolters Kluwer business
530 Walnut Street
Philadelphia, PA 19106
LWW.com

© 2008 by Lippincott Williams & Wilkins

Printed in India.

Library of Congress Cataloging-in-Publication Data

Moss and Adams' heart disease in infants, children, and adolescents : including the fetus and young adult.—7th ed. / editors Hugh D. Allen . . . [et al.].
      p. ; cm.
   Includes bibliographical references.
   ISBN-13: 978-0-7817-8684-3 (case)
   ISBN-10: 0-7817-8684-3 (case)
   1. Heart—Diseases.   2. Pediatric cardiology.   I. Moss, Arthur J.   II. Allen, Hugh D.   III. Title: Heart disease in infants, children, and adolescents.
   [DNLM: 1. Heart Diseases.   2. Child.   3. Embryonic Development.   4. Fetal Development.   5. Fetal Diseases.   6. Fetal Heart—abnormalities.   WS 290 M9128 2008]
   RJ421.H38 2008
   618.92'12—dc22

                                                                                    2007023954

Moss and Adams'

HEART DISEASE IN INFANTS, CHILDREN, AND ADOLESCENTS

INCLUDING THE FETUS AND YOUNG ADULT

■ CONTENTS

VOLUME ONE

PART I ■ STRUCTURE AND FUNCTION OF THE CARDIOVASCULAR SYSTEM

PART II ■ DIAGNOSTIC METHODS

PART VII ■ CONGENITAL CARDIOVASCULAR MALFORMATIONS

CONTRIBUTING AUTHORS

Hugh D. Allen, MD, ScD (Hon)
Professor
Department of Pediatrics and Medicine
Vice Chair for Academic Affairs, Department of Pediatrics
Ohio State University College of Medicine
Staff Cardiologist, The Heart Center
Columbus Children's Hospital
Columbus, Ohio

Joseph Atallah, MD, FRCP(c)
Pediatric Cardiology Fellow
Department of Pediatrics
University of Alberta
Stollery Children's Hospital
Edmonton, Alberta, Canada

David E. Atkinson, MD
Assistant Professor
Department of Pediatrics, Division of Cardiology
University California Los Angeles
Assistant Professor
Department of Pediatrics, Cardiology Division
Los Angeles County Harbor/UCLA Medical Center
Torrance, California

H. Scott Baldwin, MD
Professor
Department of Pediatrics
Vanderbilt University Medical Center
Chief, Pediatric Cardiology
Vanderbilt University School of Medicine
Nashville, Tennessee

Yaniv Bar-Cohen, MD
Assistant Professor
Department of Pediatrics
University of Southern California
Pediatric Electrophsyiologist
Division of Cardiology
Children's Hospital Los Angeles
Los Angeles, California

Robyn J. Barst, MD
Professor of Pediatrics
Department of Pediatric Cardiology
Columbia University College of Physicians and Surgeons
Attending Pediatrician
Department of Pediatric Cardiology
Morgan Stanley Children's Hospital
New York Presbyterian Medical Center
Columbia University Medical Center
New York, New York

Barry G. Baylen, MD
Clinical Professor
Department of Pediatrics
University California Los Angeles
Chief, Division of Pediatric Cardiology
Clinical Professor of Pediatrics
Los Angeles County Harbor UCLA Medical Center
Torrance, California

Robert H. Beekman III, MD
Professor
Department of Pediatrics
University of Cincinnati
Professor
Division of Cardiology
Children's Hospital Medical Center
Cincinnati, Ohio

Stuart Berger, MD
Professor of Pediatrics
Department of Pediatrics
Medical Director, The Heart Center
Department of Pediatric Cardiology
Milwaukee, Wisconsin

Elizabeth D. Blume, MD
Assistant Professor of Pediatrics
Harvard Medical School
Medical Director, Heart Failure/Transplant Program
Department of Cardiology
Children's Hospital Boston
Boston, Massachusetts

Lorenzo D. Botto, MD
Division of Medical Genetics
Department of Pediatrics
Assistant Professor
University of Utah and Utah Birth Defect Network
Salt Lake City, Utah

Mark M. Boucek, MD
Clinical Professor of Pediatric Cardiology
Department of Pediatrics
University of Colorado Health Sciences Center
Denver, Colorado
Director of Cardiovascular Services
Department of Pediatrics
Joe DiMaggio Children's Hospital
Hollywood, Florida

Harisios Boudoulas, MD
Center for Clinical Research
Foundation of Biomedical Research
Academy of Athens
Athens, Greece

Michael M. Brook, MD
Professor
Department of Pediatrics
University of California, San Francisco
Director of Pediatric Echocardiography
Department of Pediatric Cardiology
UCSF Children's Hospital
San Francisco, California

Allison K. Cabalka, MD
Associate Professor
Department of Pediatrics
Mayo Clinic College of Medicine
Rochester, Minnesota

Steven C. Cassidy, MD
Associate Professor
Department of Pediatrics
Ohio State University College of Medicine
Director, Inpatient Services
Heart Center
Children's Hospital
Columbus, Ohio

Frank Cetta, MD
Professor
Department of Pediatrics and Medicine
Mayo Clinic College of Medicine
Chair, Division of Pediatric Cardiology
Mayo Clinic
Rochester, Minnesota

David P. Chan, MD
Clinical Associate Professor
Department of Pediatrics
Ohio State University
Director of Electrophysiology
Department of Pediatrics
Columbus Children's Hospital
Columbus, Ohio

Anthony C. Chang, MD, MBA
Associate Professor of Pediatric Cardiology
Chief, Critical Care Cardiology
Director, Cardiac Intensive Care Service
Houston, Texas

John P. Cheatham, MD
Professor of Pediatrics
Division of Cardiology, The Ohio State University
    College of Medicine
Director, Cardiac Catheterization and Interventional Therapy
Columbus Children's Hospital
Columbus, Ohio

Jack M. Colman, MD
Associate Professor
Department of Medicine
University of Toronto
Staff Cardiologist
University Health Network and Mount Sinai Hospital
Toronto, Ontario, Canada

Stephen C. Cook, MD
Assistant Professor
Department of Internal Medicine
    and Pediatrics
Ohio State University
The Ross Heart Hospital
Director, Non-Invasive Imaging/Research
The Heart Center
Columbus Children's Hospital
Columbus, Ohio

James J. Corrigan, Jr., MD
Professor of Pediatrics
Chief, Section of Pediatric Hematology-Oncology
University of Arizona
Health Sciences Center
Tucson, Arizona

Curt J. Daniels, MD
Assistant Professor of Clinical Internal
    Medicine/Pediatrics
Ohio State University
Director, Adolescent/Adult Congenital Heart
    Disease and Pulmonary Hypertension Programs
The Heart Center at Columbus
    Children's Hospital
Columbus, Ohio

Stephen R. Daniels, MD, PhD
Chairman
Department of Pediatrics
University of Colorado at Denver Health
    Sciences Center
Pediatrician-in-Chief
Department of Pediatrics
The Children's Hospital
Denver, Colorado

Joseph A. Dearani, MD
Associate Professor
Department of Cardiovascular Surgery
Mayo Clinic College of Medicine
Rochester, Minnesota

Susan W. Denfield, MD
Clinical Associate Professor of Pediatrics
Department of Pediatric Cardiology
Baylor College of Medicine
Clinical Associate Professor of Pediatrics
Department Cardiology
Texas Children's Hospital
Houston, Texas

David J. Driscoll, MD
Professor
Department of Pediatrics
Mayo Clinic College of Medicine
Rochester, Minnesota

Anne M. Dubin, MD
Associate Professor of Pediatrics
Stanford University School of Medicine
Director, Pediatric Electrophysiology
    Laboratory
Lucile Packard Children's Hospital
Palo Alto, California

John D. Dyck, MD, FRCP(c)
Professor
Director, Pediatric Cardiology
Division of Cardiology
Department of Pediatrics
Stollery Children's Hospital
University of Alberta
Edmonton, Alberta, Canada

Hugo Ector, MD, PhD
Professor
Department of Cardiology
Catholic University of Leuven
Kliniekhoofd
Department of Cardiology
University Hospital Gasthuisberg
Leuven, Belgium

William D. Edwards, MD
Professor
Department of Laboratory Medicine and Pathology
Mayo Clinic College of Medicine
Consultant in Anatomic Pathology
Department of Laboratory Medicine and Pathology
Mayo Clinic
Rochester, Minnesota

Joachim G. Eichhorn, MD
Head of the Working Group "Cardiac Imaging in Children"
Department of Pediatric Cardiology
Ruprechts Karls University of Heidelberg
Pediatric Cardiologist
Department of Pediatric Cardiology
University Children's Hospital
Heidelberg, Germany

Michael L. Epstein, MD
Affiliate Professor
Department of Pediatrics
University of South Florida College of Medicine
Tampa, Florida
Senior Vice President of Medical Affairs
All Children's Hospital
St. Petersburg, Florida

Francine G. Erenberg, MD
Assistant Professor
Department of Pediatrics
Case Western Reserve University, School of Medicine
Pediatric Cardiologist
Department of Pediatric Cardiology
Rainbow Babies and Children's Hospital
Cleveland, Ohio

Timothy F. Feltes, MD
Professor of Pediatrics
Division Chief, Pediatric Cardiology
The Ohio State University College of
  Medicine
Codirector, Heart Center at Columbus
  Children's Hospital
Columbus, Ohio

Jeffrey R. Fineman, MD
Professor, Department of Pediatrics
University of California, San Francisco
San Francisco, California

Frank A. Fish, MD
Associate Professor
Department of Pediatrics and Medicine
Vanderbilt University
Director, Pediatric Electrophysiology
Monroe Carell Jr. Children's Hospital at Vanderbilt
Nashville, Tennessee

Michele A. Frommelt, MD
Associate Professor
Department of Pediatrics
Medical College of Wisconsin
Staff Physician
Department of Pediatric Cardiology
Children's Hospital of Wisconsin
Milwaukee, Wisconsin

Tal Geva, MD
Professor of Pediatrics
Department of Pediatrics
Harvard Medical School
Chief, Division of Noninvasive Imaging
Department of Cardiology
Children's Hospital Boston
Boston, Massachusetts

Michael H. Gewitz, MD
Director of Pediatrics
Westchester Medical Center
Valhalla, New York

Nancy S. Ghanayem, MD
Associate Professor
Department of Pediatrics (Critical Care Section)
Medical College of Wisconsin
Clinical Director
Cardiac Critical Care
Children's Hospital of Wisconsin
Milwaukee, Wisconsin

Julie S. Glickstein, MD
Associate Professor of Clinical Pediatrics
Department of Pediatrics
Columbia University
Pediatric Cardiologist
Department of Pediatrics
Morgan Stanley Children's Hospital of Presbyterian
New York, New York

Elizabeth Goldmuntz, MD
Associate Professor
Department of Pediatrics
University of Pennsylvania School of Medicine
Associate Physician
Division of Cardiology, Pediatrics
The Children's Hospital of Philadelphia
Philadelphia, Pennsylvania

Ronald G. Grifka, MD
Professor
Department of Pediatrics
Michigan State University College of Human Medicine
East Lansing, Michigan
Chief, Cardiology Division
Helen DeVos Children's Hospital
Grand Rapids, Michigan

Howard P. Gutgesell, MD
Professor
Department of Pediatrics
University of Virginia Medical School
Physician
Department of Pediatrics
University of Virginia Hospital
Charlottesville, Virginia

Donald J. Hagler, MD
Professor of Pediatrics
Pediatric Cardiology and Cardiovascular Diseases
Mayo Clinic College of Medicine
Rochester, Minnesota

Michael A. Heymann, MD
Professor Emeritus
Department of Pediatrics
University of California-San Francisco
San Francisco, California

George M. Hoffman, MD
Professor, Anesthesiology and Pediatrics
Medical College of Wisconsin
Medical Director and Chief, Pediatric Anesthesiology
Associate Director, Pediatric Intensive Care
Children's Hospital of Wisconsin
Milwaukee, Wisconsin

Timothy M. Hoffman, MD
Associate Professor of Pediatrics
The Ohio State University College of Medicine
Medical Director, Heart Transplant and Heart Failure
    Program
Department of Pediatrics, Division of Pediatric Cardiology
Columbus Children's Hospital
Columbus, Ohio

Ralf J. Holzer, MD, MSc
Assistant Professor of Pediatrics
Cardiology Division
The Ohio State University
Assistant Director
Cardiac Catheterization and Interventional Therapy
The Heart Center
Columbus Children's Hospital
Columbus, Ohio

Paul R. Julsrud, MD
Professor of Radiology
Mayo School of Graduate Medical Education
Physician
Department of Radiology
Mayo Clinic
Rochester, Minnesota

Prince J. Kannankeril, MD, MSCI
Assistant Professor
Department of Pediatrics
Vanderbilt University School of Medicine
Assistant Professor
Division of Pediatric Cardiology
Vanderbilt Children's Hospital
Nashville, Tennessee

Thomas R. Kimball, MD
Professor
Department of Pediatrics
University of Cincinnati College of Medicine
Director
Cardiac Ultrasound and Cardiovascular Imaging Core
Research Laboratory
Cincinnati Children's Hospital
Cincinnati, Ohio

Charles S. Kleinman, MD
Professor of Clinical Pediatrics in Obstetrics and Gynecology
Columbia University College of Physicians and Surgeons
Weill Medical College of Cornell University
Division of Pediatric Cardiology
Morgan Stanley Children's Hospital of New York—Presbyterian
New York, New York

John D. Kugler, MD
Chief, University of Nebraska and
    Creighton University Joint Division of Pediatric
    Cardiology at Children's Hospital
D.B. and Paula Varner Professor of Pediatrics
University of Nebraska College of Medicine
Director of Cardiology
Children's Hospital
Omaha, Nebraska

Larry A. Latson, MD
Professor
Department of Pediatrics
Cleveland Clinic College of Medicine
Case Western Reserve University
Staff Physician
Department of Pediatric Cardiology
Cleveland Clinic Foundation
Cleveland, Ohio

Peter C. Laussen, MBBS
Associate Professor
Department of Anesthesia
Harvard Medical School
Chief, Division Cardiac Critical Care
Department of Cardiology
Children's Hospital
Boston, Massachusetts

D. Scott Lim, MD
Assistant Professor
Departments of Pediatrics and Internal Medicine
University of Virginia
Director, Cardiac Catheterization
University of Virginia Medical Center
Charlottesville, Virginia

Angela E. Lin, MD
Associate Clinical Professor
Department of Pediatrics
Harvard Medical School
Clinical Geneticist
Genetics Unit
MassGeneral Hospital for Children
Boston, Massachusetts

Frederick R. Long, MD
Clinical Professor
Department of Radiology
Ohio State University College of Medicine
  and Public Health
Section Chief, Body CT and MRI Imaging
Department of Radiology
Columbus Children's Hospital
Columbus, Ohio

Lynn Mahony, MD
Professor
Department of Pediatrics
University of Texas Southwestern Medical Center
Staff Physician
Department of Cardiology
Children's Medical Center of Dallas
Dallas, Texas

Barry J. Maron, MD
Director, Hypertrophic Cardiomyopathy Center
Minneapolis Heart Institute Foundation
Minneapolis, Minnesota

Gerald R. Marx, MD
Associate Professor
Department of Pediatrics
Harvard Medical School
Senior Associate
Department of Cardiology
Boston Children's Hospital
Boston, Massachusetts

G. Paul Matherne, MD
J. Francis Dammann Professor
Department of Pediatrics
University of Virginia
Division Head Pediatric Cardiology
University of Virginia Children's Hospital
University of Virginia Health System
Charlottesville, Virginia

Nancy L. McDaniel, MD
Associate Professor
Department of Pediatrics
University of Virginia
Medical Director
University of Virginia
Children's Hospital
Charlottesville, Virginia

Timothy C. McQuinn, MD
Assistant Professor
Department of Pediatrics
Cardiac Intensive Care Unit
The Children's Heart Center
Charleston, South Carolina

Jerry R. Mendell, MD
Professor
Departments of Pediatrics and Neurology
College of Medicine
Director, Center for Gene Therapy
Columbus Children's Research Institute
Columbus, Ohio

Erik C. Michelfelder, MD
Associate Professor
Department of Pediatrics
University of Cincinnati College of Medicine
Director of Fetal Cardiology
Division of Cardiology
Cincinnati Children's Hospital Medical Center
Cincinnati, Ohio

L. LuAnn Minich, MD
Professor of Pediatrics
Department of Pediatric Cardiology
University of Utah
Professor of Pediatrics
Department of Pediatric Cardiology
Primary Children's Medical Center
Salt Lake City, Utah

John W. Moore, MD, MPH
Professor of Pediatrics
Chief, Section of Cardiology
Department of Pediatrics, UCSD School of Medicine
Director, Division of Cardiology
Children's Specialists of San Diego
San Diego, CA

Phillip Moore, MD, MBA
Professor of Clinical Pediatrics
Department of Pediatrics
University of California San Francisco
Director, Interventional Catheterization Laboratory
Department of Pediatrics
University of California San Francisco
San Francisco, California

Adrian M. Moran, MD
Clinical Associate Professor
University of Vermont
Burlington, Vermont
Attending Cardiologist Maine Medical Center
Department of Pediatrics
Portland, Maine

Charles E. Mullins, MD
Professor Emeritus
Department of Pediatrics
Baylor College of Medicine
Director Emeritus, Cardiac Catheterization Laboratory
Department of Pediatric Cardiology
Texas Children's Hospital
Houston, Texas

Kathleen A. Mussatto, RN, PhDc
Research Manager
Herma Heart Center
Children's Hospital of Wisconsin
Milwaukee, Wisconsin

Jane W. Newburger, MD, MPH
Professor of Pediatrics
Department of Pediatrics
Harvard Medical School
Associate Chief for Academic Affairs
Department of Cardiology
Children's Hospital Boston
Boston, Massachusetts

David G. Nykanen, MD
Director, Cardiology and Cardiac Catheterization
Department of Pediatrics
Congenital Heart Institute
Arnold Palmer Medical Center
Orlando, Florida

Patrick W. O'Leary, MD, FACC, FASE
Associate Professor
Department of Pediatrics
Mayo Clinic College of Medicine
Consultant, Division of Pediatric Cardiology
Director, Pediatric Echocardiography
Mayo Clinic
Rochester, Minnesota

Timothy M. Olson, MD
Associate Professor
Department of Medicine and Pediatrics
Mayo Clinic College of Medicine
Rochester, Minnesota

Francesco Parisi, MD
Medical Director
Thoracic Transplant Unit
Department of Pediatric Cardiology and Cardiac Surgery
Bambino Gesù Pediatric Hospital and Research Institute
Rome, Italy

John R. Phillips, MD
Pediatric Cardiologist
West Virginia University
The Heart Institute
Morgantown, West Virginia

Paolo T. Pianosi, MD
Associate Professor
Department of Pediatrics and Adolescent Medicine
Mayo Clinic College of Medicine
Rochester, Minnesota

Arthur S. Pickoff, MD
Professor and Chair
Department of Pediatrics
Wright State University Boonshoft School of Medicine
The Children's Medical Center
Dayton, Ohio

Co-Burn J. Porter, MD
Professor of Pediatrics
Department of Pediatrics and Adolescent Medicine
Mayo Clinic College of Medicine
Rochester, Minnesota

Andrew J. Powell, MD
Assistant Professor of Pediatrics
Department of Pediatrics
Harvard Medical School
Director, Cardiovascular MR
Department of Cardiology
Children's Hospital Boston
Boston, Massachusetts

Tamar J. Preminger, MD
Pediatric Cardiologist
Cleveland Clinic Foundation
Children's Hospital Cleveland
Cleveland, Ohio

Lourdes R. Prieto, MD
Staff Physician
Department of Pediatric Cardiology
Cleveland Clinic Foundation
Cleveland, Ohio

Francisco J. Puga, MD
Professor
Department of Surgery
Mayo Clinic College of Medicine
Rochester, Minnesota

Marlene Rabinovitch, MD
Dwight and Vera Dunlevie Professor
Department of Pediatrics
Stanford University School of Medicine
Staff Cardiologist
Department of Pediatrics
Lucile Packard Children's Hospital
Stanford, California

Subha V. Raman, MD, MSEE, FACC
Assistant Professor
Department of Internal Medicine/
   Cardiovascular Medicine
Ohio State University College of Medicine
Medical Director
Department of Cardiac MR/CT
Ohio State University Hospitals
Columbus, Ohio

Chitra Ravishankar, MBBS
Assistant Professor
Department of Pediatrics
University of Pennsylvania
Staff Cardiologist
Department of Pediatrics
The Children's Hospital of Philadelphia
Philadelphia, Pennsylvania

Andrew N. Redington, MD, FRCS
Professor of Pediatrics
Department of Medicine
University of Toronto
Head, Division of Cardiology
Hospital for Sick Children
Toronto, Ontario, Canada

Robert M. Rennebohm, MD
Associate Professor
Department of Pediatrics
Ohio State University College of Medicine
Pediatric Rheumatologist
Columbus Children's Hospital
Columbus, Ohio

Tony Reybrouck, PhD
Professor
Department of Rehabilitation Sciences
University of Leuven
Cardiovascular Rehabilitation Specialist
Department Cardiovascular Rehabilitation
Gasthuisberg University Hospital
Leuven, Belgium

Karen S. Rheuban, MD
Professor
Department of Pediatrics
University of Virginia
Medical Director
Office of Telemedicine
University of Virginia
UVA Health System
Charlottesville, Virginia

Albert P. Rocchini, MD
Professor
Department of Pediatrics
University of Michigan
University of Michigan Health Center
Director of Pediatric Cardiology
Department of Pediatrics
C.S. Mott Children's Hospital
University of Michigan
Ann Arbor, Michigan

Erika B. Rosenzweig, MD
Assistant Professor of Clinical Pediatrics
    in Medicine
Department of Pediatrics
Columbia University College of Physicians
    and Surgeons
Assistant Attending of Clinical Pediatrics in Medicine
Department of Pediatrics
Columbia Presbyterian Children's Hospital of New York
New York, New York

J. Philip Saul, MD
Professor
Department of Pediatrics
Medical University of South Carolina
Chief, Pediatric Cardiology
Medical Director, MUSC Children's Hospital
Department of Pediatrics
Medical University of South Carolina
Charleston, South Carolina

Douglas J. Schneider, MD
Clinical Associate Professor of Pediatrics
University of Illinois College of Medicine at Peoria
Director, Cardiac Catheterization Laboratory
Children's Hospital of Illinois
Peoria, Illinois

Robert E. Shaddy, MD
Professor of Pediatrics
Division Chief, Pediatric Cardiology
The Children's Hospital of Philadelphia
University of Pennsylvania School of Medicine
Philadelphia, Pennsylvania

Roxana Shaw, MD
Columbia University College of
    Physicians and Surgeons
Weill Medical College of Cornell University
Center for Prenatal Pediatrics
Division of Pediatric Cardiology
Department of Pediatrics
Morgan Stanley Children's Hospital of
    New York—Presbyterian
New York, New York

Michael J. Silka, MD
Professor
Department of Pediatrics
University of Southern California
Chief, Division of Cardiology
Children's Hospital Los Angeles
Los Angeles, California

Candice K. Silversides, MD, SM
Assistant Professor
Department of Medicine
University of Toronto
Staff Cardiologist
University Health Network and
    Mount Signal Hospital
Toronto, Ontario, Canada

Samuel C. Siu, MD, SM
Professor
Department of Medicine
University of Toronto
Staff Cardiologist, Director of Echocardiography
University Health Network and
    Mount Sinai Hospital
Toronto, Ontario, Canada

Ernest S. Siwik, MD
Assistant Professor
Department of Pediatrics
Case University
Director, Cardiac Catheterization Laboratory
Department of Pediatrics
Rainbow Babies and Children's Hospital
Cleveland, Ohio

Gary A. Smith, MD, DrPH
Associate Professor
Department of Pediatrics
Ohio State University College of Medicine
Director
Center for Injury Research and Policy
Children's Hospital
Columbus, Ohio

Elizabeth Sparks, RN, MS, CNP, APNG
Clinical Assistant Professor of
    Internal Medicine
The Ohio State University College of Medicine
Coordinator, Adolescent/Adult Congenital
    Heart Disease
The Heart Center
Columbus Children's Hospital
Columbus, Ohio

Deepak Srivastava, MD
Professor and Director, Gladstone Institute of Cardiovascular
  Disease
Wilma and Adeline Pirag Distinguished Chair in Pediatric
  Developmental Cardiology
Department of Pediatrics, Biochemistry, and Biophysics
University of California San Francisco
Attending Physician
UCSF Children's Hospital
San Francisco, California

Masato Takahashi, MD
Professor of Pediatrics Emeritus
Department of Pediatrics
University of Southern California
Keck School of Medicine
Attending Cardiologist
Department of Pediatrics
Children's Hospital, Los Angeles
Los Angeles, California

Lloyd Y. Tani, MD
Professor of Pediatrics
Department of Pediatrics
University of Utah School of Medicine
Associate Director
Division of Pediatric Cardiology
Primary Children's Medical Center
Salt Lake City, Utah

Kathryn A. Taubert, PhD
Adjunct Professor
Department of Physiology
University of Texas Southwestern Medical School
Senior Scientist
Department of Science
American Heart Association
Dallas, Texas

David F. Teitel, MD
Professor of Pediatrics
Chief of Pediatric Cardiology
University of California, San Francisco
Director, Pediatric Heart Center
UCSF Children's Hospital
San Francisco, California

Jeffrey A. Towbin, MD
Professor
Department of Pediatrics
Baylor College of Medicine
Chief, Pediatric Cardiology
Department of Pediatric Cardiology
Texas Children's Hospital
Houston, Texas

James S. Tweddell, MD
Professor of Surgery and Pediatrics
Chair, Division of Cardiothoracic Surgery
Department of Surgery
Medical College of Wisconsin
S. Bert Litwin Chair
Department of Cardiothoracic Surgery
Children's Hospital of Wisconsin
Milwaukee, Wisconsin

George F. Van Hare, MD
Professor of Pediatrics
Department of Pediatric Cardiology
Stanford University School of Medicine
Director
Pediatric Arrhythmia Center at UCSF and Stanford
Lucile Packard Children's Hospital
Palo Alto, California

Stella Van Praagh, MD
Pediatric Cardiologist
Harvard Medical School
Children's Hospital Boston
Boston, Massachusetts

Paul M. Weinberg, MD
Professor of Pediatrics and Pediatric Pathology and
  Laboratory Medicine
Associate Professor of Radiology
Departments of Pediatrics, Pediatric Pathology and
  Laboratory Medicine, Radiology
University of Pennsylvania School of Medicine
Senior Cardiologist, Consultant in Pathology (Cardiac)
Consultant in Radiology (MRI)
Division of Cardiology
Departments of Pathology and Radiology
The Children's Hospital of Philadelphia
Philadelphia, Pennsylvania

Stephen E. Welty, MD
Associate Professor
Department of Pediatrics
The Ohio State University College of Medicine
Chief, Division of Neonatology
Department of Pediatrics
Columbus Children's Research Institute
Columbus Children's Hospital
Columbus, Ohio

Gil Wernovsky, MD
Professor of Pediatrics
University of Pennsylvania School of Medicine
Staff Cardiologist, CICU
Director of Program Development
The Cardiac Center
The Children's Hospital of Philadelphia
Philadelphia, Pennsylvania

David L. Wessel, MD
Professor of Pediatrics (Anesthesia)
Harvard Medical School
Senior Associate in Cardiology and Anesthesia
Children's Hospital Boston
Boston, Massachusetts

John J. Wheller, MD
Assistant Professor
Department of Pediatrics
The Ohio State University College of Medicine
Staff Cardiologist
The Heart Center
Columbus Children's Hospital
Columbus, Ohio

Charles F. Wooley, MD
Professor of Medicine
The Heart Center at The Ohio State University College
  of Medicine
Columbus, Ohio

Kenneth G. Zahka, MD
Professor of Pediatrics
Department of Pediatric Cardiology
Case Western Reserve University School of Medicine
Rainbow Babies and Children's Hospital
Cleveland, Ohio

■ PREFACE

This 7th edition of *Moss and Adam's Heart Disease in Infants, Children, and Adolescents* represents a major revision of the 6th edition, undertaken in response to our ever-advancing discipline, to comments from readers of the 6th edition, and to reviews of the 6th edition—especially the very thoughtful and considered suggestions offered by Drs. Welton Gersony and David Sahn.

Genetic information regarding congenital heart disease is rapidly expanding. We have tried to include basic genetic information and as much new information as possible. The reader should understand that these ongoing data advance rapidly and will continue to progress.

New sections and chapters in the text include:

■ An ICU section with chapters on neonatal care, cardiac intensive care, mechanical support, and interactions between the ventricles as well as cardiopulmonary interactions
■ An expanded young adult section with attention to the natural history, therapeutic catheterization information specific to this population, cardiac imaging techniques specific to the young adult, lesion-based management pathways, and challenges for the future
■ Congestive heart failure, a chapter that was dropped from the 6th edition and which is clearly needed
■ Sports screening and participation, an issue that we all face daily
■ The heart in muscular dystrophy, an increasingly important topic as newer therapies emerge
■ Ischemia, a topic that is increasingly important to pediatric cardiologists

Updated information is provided on genetics and epidemiology in every lesion-specific chapter. Some chapters and appendices have been deleted because of the electronic availability of up-to-date information on such topics as drug preparations, doses, and side effects.

As with all textbooks, new authors emerge. We wish to thank all previous contributors, many of whom are pioneers of our field, for their mentorship, guidance, and information. In the last text we committed an egregious error by not including Dr. William Friedman as co-author of the aortic stenosis chapter, much of which was information from his initial contribution. We subsequently corrected this and again apologize to him and his memory. Likewise, many other original contributors deserve credit, including Drs. George Veasy, William Strong, Thomas Graham, Julien I. E. Hoffman, Amnon Rosenthal, James R. Zuberbuhler, Milton Paul, Russell V. Lucas, Jr., Douglas Mair, Robert Feldt, Robert Freedom, Elia Ayoub, Syamar Sanyal, Leon Chameides, Ehud Krongrad, Richard M. Schieken, Michael R. Nihill, Robert R. Wolfe, Norman S. Talner, and Thomas A. Riemenschneider. We also wish to recognize the important contributions by two previous editors of the 6th edition, Howard P. Gutgesell and Edward B. Clark. We apologize in advance to any not named in the above list. We also pause to offer respect to the many on this list who have died. Our discipline would not be where it is without the contributions of all of you.

We hope that this new edition provides you important and new useful information that enhances your understanding of our discipline. Any success in this regard should be credited to the authors.

Acknowledgments The editors most of all thank the authors of the chapters in this revised textbook. Their many long hours, attention to detail, and expertise make the book what it is.

We thank our support staff, Mary Lou Naftzger and Megan Krueger (HDA), Tina Erickson (DJD), Randi Holdridge (RES), and Lisa Johnson (TFF), who have helped organize, file, mail, set up calls and meetings, and juggle these tasks with our daily schedules without complaint.

Again, Dr. George Emmanoulidies remains a close and respected friend and counselor.

The staff at Lippincott Williams & Wilkins have been instrumental in keeping the project (and editors) on track. We especially thank Frances DeStefano, Chris Potash, and Julia Seto for their enthusiasm and support.

Hugh D. Allen, MD
David J. Driscoll, MD
Robert E. Shaddy, MD
Timothy F. Feltes, MD

THE DEVELOPMENT OF PEDIATRIC CARDIOLOGY: HISTORICAL MILESTONES

Pediatric cardiology as a subspecialty owes its origin to pediatrics and medical cardiology. The main impetus for its development has been the unprecedented progress made in the past 50 years in the diagnosis and the medical and surgical treatment of congenital heart disease. There is no doubt that the advent of cardiac surgery and the rapid development of cardiac surgical techniques in conjunction with the advances in medical technology were responsible for this progress. Clinicians interested in cardiovascular disease together with physiologists and radiologists began to study circulatory hemodynamics and produce *in vivo* images of a number of cardiac malformations using cardiac catheterization and angiocardiography. By applying fundamental laws of rheology and hydraulics for the first time, it became possible to establish the scientific basis of the pathogenesis and significance of clinical signs and symptoms associated with each cardiac defect.

Early on, pediatric cardiologists recognized that major efforts should be directed toward the infant under 1 year of age, where morbidity and mortality from congenital heart disease were the greatest. It was this realization that made obvious the need for specially trained pediatricians to meet this challenge. Consequently, the subspecialty of pediatric cardiology was formally established in 1961, when the first qualifying examination was instituted by the Sub-Board of Pediatric Cardiology. Special requirements included a prior formal training in general pediatrics, followed by 2 additional years of training in pediatric cardiology at an approved center. Even before the formal establishment of the subspecialty, pediatric cardiologists saw the need to establish their own professional organizations, such as the Section on Cardiology of the American Academy of Pediatrics (1957), or special groups within the context of larger cardiology organizations, such as the Council on Cardiovascular Disease of the Young of the American Heart Association, which had its roots as the Council on Rheumatic Fever (1945), with subsequent expansion of its name to include Congenital Heart Disease (1950).

Following the advent of coronary angiography and coronary bypass surgery—and, more recently, coronary angioplasty—medical cardiologists primarily concentrated their efforts on the much larger problem of coronary artery disease and its sequelae. Pediatric cardiologists, at the same time, continued their own way, exploring the problems associated with congenital heart diseases. Arrhythmias, cardiomyopathies, and rheumatic heart disease continued to be the link between the two subspecialties.

Thus, an unavoidable dichotomy between the two specialties developed, dictated by the nature of their interests and subjects. Presently, graduates of medical cardiology training programs know very little about the intricacies of congenital heart disease and its sequelae, whereas pediatric cardiology trainees have minimal, if any, exposure to the current issues related to coronary heart disease.

With continuous improvement of surgical techniques and with the infant operative mortality having decreased from 50% to less than 15%, a large number of individuals with "mended" heart, with long-term predictable or as yet unknown sequelae and residua, pose a major health problem. It has been estimated that presently in the United States, over 1 million individuals have surgically or medically palliated or "corrected" forms of congenital heart disease. The majority of them are in need of careful continued periodic evaluation. Because of the unavailability of health insurance ("preexisting condition"), a large number of these patients, as they enter adulthood, are left either without specialized medical care or with suboptimal care, offered by specialists unfamiliar with their unique cardiac problems. Alternatively, if pediatric cardiologists continue to provide such care to these individuals, they may not be capable of dealing with their other needs and problems inherent to adulthood. In a recent conference on this subject, it was suggested that pediatric cardiologists and medical cardiologists interested in congenital heart disease establish special clinics associated with major medical centers for the care of these older patients. Such clinics already exist in a few medical centers and function quite successfully. It is hoped that in the near future, such clinics combining the expertise of several types of professionals besides cardiologists and cardiovascular surgeons will be created to meet the needs of this increasing patient population.

The following discussion pertains to some of the milestones in the development of pediatric cardiology, for the benefit of our younger colleagues and other interested readers.

The modern era of pediatric cardiology can be traced to the turn of this century and the work of Dr. Maude E. Abbott, a Canadian physician. Her important contributions over a number of years culminated in 1936 in the classic *Atlas of Congenital Heart Disease*. In this monumental book, she meticulously described her findings based on 1,000 pathologic cardiac specimens and provided an orderly classification of the anomalies including invaluable information on their natural history. Additionally, she reviewed the development and comparative anatomy of reptilian, amphibian, and mammalian hearts.

Although anatomopathologic descriptions of congenital malformations of the heart had been made by a number of observers during the last three centuries, serious attempts to correlate symptoms and signs to specific anatomic entities only began to appear during the 19th century. Several monographs and compendia on congenital cardiac defects were published during the first half of that century. Two books that appeared in the latter half of the century, by Peacock and Rokitansky, added considerably to the existing knowledge on the subject. Although the malformation now coined as tetralogy of Fallot had been described previously by many authors, Fallot, in 1888, was the first to emphasize its clinical features and make an accurate premortem diagnosis. However, all of these pathologic and clinical descriptions were strictly of academic interest since there was no available treatment. The study of congenital malformations was ignored by the bulk of medical practitioners at the time, whose role was limited to matters of general advice and prognosis. This is clearly reflected in the first textbook on pediatrics, by Dr. Thomas Morgan Roch in 1896, where only 7 of 1,100 pages were devoted to congenital diseases of the heart, although rheumatic heart disease could be diagnosed quite readily in any child with fever and a heart murmur. Subsequently, many clinicians, stimulated by Abbott's contributions, began to clinically diagnose specific congenital heart defects with greater frequency. In 1939, a modern clinical text, *Congenital Heart Disease*, was published by J. W. Brown in England, but it was somewhat premature and not widely read.

In 1938, the first successful ductus arteriosus ligation was accomplished in Boston by Robert Gross in a 7½-year-old girl. With the encouragement of J. P. Hubbard, a pediatrician (and without the permission of his chief, who was on leave), Gross, a junior pediatric surgeon, made medical history. In 1945, Crafoort and Nylin, in Sweden, and Gross and Hufnagel, in the United States, reported successful repair of coarctation of the aorta by surgical resection. At about the same time (1944), Blalock, Thomas, and Taussig demonstrated that subclavian artery-to-pulmonary artery anastomosis considerably improved the oxygenation of the cyanotic patient by providing more blood flow to the lungs. These three "vascular" operations, two corrective for acyanotic and one palliative for cyanotic patients, provided a great stimulus to clinicians, pediatricians, internists, and cardiologists to attempt to make accurate diagnoses. The decade of the 1940s marked the beginning of the modern era of pediatric cardiology. Precise diagnostic techniques such as cardiac catheterization and angiocardiography have been added to the diagnostic armamentarium of clinicians which, until then, relied on physical examination, electrocardiography, and chest fluoroscopy and roentgenography.

A number of physicians were attracted to this budding subspecialty and sought advanced training. A major force in the development of pediatric cardiology at that time was Dr. Helen B. Taussig, Director of the Children's Cardiac Clinic at Johns Hopkins University. Over the years, Taussig made unique clinical observations relating to the diagnosis, pathophysiology, and natural history of practically all congenital malformations of the heart. She was particularly intrigued by those cyanotic patients with decreased pulmonary blood flow and suggested the subclavian-pulmonary artery shunt as a means of surgical palliation. Because of her reputation, she attracted physicians from all over the world to study with her. She developed an unusual ability to arrive at a correct clinical diagnosis by meticulously gathering all the facts pertaining to the patient. Her observations were detailed in her classic first edition of the book *Congenital Malformations of the Heart* (1947). A number of prominent pediatric cardiologists from the United States and abroad studied with her. For all her original contributions, she is rightfully considered the founder of clinical pediatric cardiology.

The application of cardiac catheterization in the study of congenital heart disease began approximately during the same period. In 1929, Forssmann in Germany was the first to show that the heart can be approached *in vivo* by insertion of a tube into the vein of an arm. He used a ureteral catheter, and after a cutdown exposure of his own left antecubital vein, he advanced the catheter 30 cm. He walked down a flight of stairs, after having restrained his nurse, and under fluoroscopy he advanced the catheter to 60 cm and took a chest radiograph to prove that the catheter's tip was in his heart! Ten years later, adopting Forssmann's catheterization technique, Cournand and Richards of New York City began studying patients who were in shock. It was not long before the same technique was used in the diagnosis of congenital heart disease. In 1956, these three physicians received the Nobel Prize in physiology and medicine. With the introduction of angiocardiography and improvements in cardiac catheterization techniques and equipment, complete exploration of cardiac chambers and vessels became possible. Cardiac hemodynamics and ventricular function could be easily measured and correlated with clinical signs and symptoms.

The possibility that virtually all congenital cardiac defects as well as certain acquired valvar problems could be corrected or palliated, challenged some of the more aggressive cardiac surgeons and cardiologists. A necessary prerequisite for such treatment was to open the heart. Consequently, closed-heart techniques (without the use of cardiopulmonary bypass) were developed to relieve pulmonary stenosis (Brock, 1948) and rheumatic mitral stenosis (Bailey, 1949) and to repair atrial septal defects. Banding of the pulmonary artery was introduced as a means of reducing excessive pulmonary blood flow due to large left-to-right ventricular shunt (Muller, 1952). All these heroic attempts were made before the clinical application of cardiopulmonary bypass.

The first successful repair of an atrial septal defect using cardiopulmonary bypass and a pump-oxygenator was performed in 1953 by Gibbon. He had been experimenting for many years in the development of this device. However, Lillehei and associates were the first to successfully repair ventricular septal defects using the open technique. The initial operations were performed by employing cross-circulation between humans (1954). Subsequently, both Lillehei et al. and Kirklin et al. reported "total" correction of cyanotic lesions such as tetralogy and pentalogy of Fallot and pulmonary atresia. The successful "open-heart" surgical repairs of a number of congenital and acquired cardiac lesions resulted in widespread interest in their diagnosis and management and the creation of a number of research and training programs throughout America and Europe. In the late 1950s, three new textbooks on the subject emerged from Boston, Stockholm, and Toronto. The following decades witnessed further advancement in diagnostic and surgical techniques. In the late 1960s, the use of deep hypothermia and circulatory arrest, developed initially in Japan by Dr. Mori and perfected in New Zealand by Dr. Brian Barratt-Boyes and his group, made possible primary repair of congenital cardiac defects in early infancy without the need of prior palliative operations. During the 1970s, further refinements of the deep hypothermia approach, by providing low-level body perfusion and improvements in myocardial preservation by cardioplegia, made possible safe primary reparative or palliative surgery of smaller and younger infants with more complex cardiac malformations.

One of the most challenging and difficult-to-treat cyanotic cardiac malformations has been transposition of the great arteries with intact ventricular septum. This defect is invariably lethal unless a native intraatrial communication exists or is created surgically. It took the imagination and persistence of the late Dr. William Rashkind of Philadelphia to develop the lifesaving technique of "balloon atrial septostomy" (Rashkind procedure). Introduced in the mid-1960s, this emergency procedure enabled a large number of neonates with this malformation to survive the immediate newborn period, rendering them candidates for subsequent intraatrial switch operations (i.e., Senning or Mustard procedures). The evolution in the medical and surgical treatment of transposition of the great arteries is a prime example of the dynamic and evolving nature of pediatric cardiology and pediatric cardiovascular surgery. In the past 10 years or so, the majority of newborns with d-transposition of the great arteries have been treated with arterial rather than intraatrial "switch" operations, and in some instances without the performance of balloon atrial septostomy. Although long-term results of the arterial switch operation are not available as yet, without question, the frequently encountered and, at times, serious atrial arrhythmias and late right ventricular dysfunction associated with the intraatrial switch operation will be eliminated. It remains to be seen if coronary perfusion abnormalities, neo-aortic valve regurgitation, or supravalvar great vessel stenosis will develop with time in patients subjected to this operation.

Dr. Rashkind continued to develop appropriate devices, introduced intravascularly, to nonsurgically treat lesions such as patent ductus arteriosus and secundum atrial septal defect. Successful closure of these defects was accomplished in the cardiac catheterization laboratory. At present, his techniques are being explored in several centers, where new and improved devices are being developed and used in patients with various shunting lesions. For his pioneering work, Dr. Rashkind should be considered the father of therapeutic interventional pediatric cardiology.

In the late 1970s, the introduction of prostaglandin E_1 for the treatment of ductus-dependent pulmonary or systemic circulation provided a means of securing adequate oxygenation or systemic perfusion in a number of neonates. As a result, pediatric cardiologists and pediatric cardiovascular surgeons are not obliged to perform emergency diagnostic cardiac catheterizations or palliative or reparative operations in very ill, severely hypoxemic, and acidotic infants. The majority of these infants now do not need prolonged invasive diagnostic studies because of the availability of two-dimensional echocardiography and Doppler technology.

During the last 15 years, the development and application of two-dimensional Doppler echocardiography revolutionized the diagnostic approach and management of infants and children with congenital heart disease. The heart and great vessels could be viewed and blood flows and cardiac function assessed noninvasively by this technique with remarkable clarity and safety. As more information was obtained with this technique and correlated with clinical, hemodynamic, and angiocardiographic findings, senior pediatric cardiologists acquired more confidence in the images they were seeing, and younger cardiologists were unable to function without them! The new generation of pediatric cardiologists is undoubtedly fortunate to be able to rely completely on diagnoses made by the echo-Doppler study. Consequently, there is concern that clinical diagnostic abilities based on auscultation of the patient will diminish as more reliance is placed on the increasing application of the available noninvasive diagnostic technology. It can be postulated that the hands and stethoscope of clinicians may gradually lose their importance in making accurate clinical diagnoses!

According to recent statistics, the number of diagnostic cardiac catheterizations and angiographic studies being performed has been significantly curtailed—up to 30–40%—due to the application of two-dimensional Doppler echocardiography. However, the total number of catheterization procedures remains about the same or has increased in some major centers, due to the introduction of therapeutic interventions including electrophysiologic studies and treatment using high-frequency ablation. I believe that this trend will continue as more experience with interventional procedures is acquired and more cardiac or vascular lesions can be safely and effectively treated using the "catheter" and devices delivered through it.

Concurrently, our surgical colleagues will concentrate on developing newer operative techniques to repair or palliate more complex malformations and improve survival. At the present time, more than 95% of infants born with significant congenital heart disease are potentially amenable to some form of medical or surgical treatment. This percentage includes patients with the most complex and otherwise inoperable or lethal malformations, in whom heart and/or lung transplantation can be offered as a means of surgical "palliation."

Advances in electrophysiology and pacemaker technology are contributing immensely to the welfare of infants and children with primary or secondary postoperative arrhythmias. Surgical and high-frequency ablations of aberrant pathways or automatic ectopic atrial arrhythmogenic foci are currently used as definitive treatment of certain patients with persistent supraventricular tachycardias unresponsive to drug therapy. These procedures are performed in certain medical centers where expertise, pediatric and/or medical, is available. Highly sophisticated miniaturized pacemaker devices with long life span are also available even for the smallest infants with congenital or acquired heart block.

Moreover, during the last decade or so, and with the advent of two-dimensional Doppler echocardiography and refinement of associated technology, a number of pediatric cardiologists and a few obstetricians have begun to focus their attention on prenatal diagnosis of fetal cardiovascular disease. Cardiac malformations can be detected as early as 16 weeks gestation. Sequential prenatal examinations of some fetuses are providing new insight into the pathogenesis of certain malformations. Progressive deterioration of certain lesions, such as pulmonic or aortic stenosis, has been observed and attributed to abnormal fetal blood flow patterns. Prenatal diagnosis and successful treatment of fetal supraventricular tachycardia is presently available. Based on animal experimentation, fetal surgical interventions (valvotomies) have been suggested as feasible by some and even attempted unsuccessfully by others. A new branch of pediatric cardiology, "fetal cardiology," is being developed and requires serious assessment of its impact and scope. The usefulness of prenatal diagnosis of congenital heart disease is somewhat controversial. Pregnancy termination is an option that is offered to the family only in cases of serious malformations. Application of fetal two-dimensional Doppler echocardiographic technology will illuminate hitherto unavailable physiologic and anatomic features of the normal human fetal circulation during fetal growth, and will provide important information regarding cardiovascular functional abnormalities induced by subacute or chronic hypoxia/asphyxia in complicated pregnancies. It is possible that such abnormalities may be detected well before heart rate disturbances appear, leading to earlier elective delivery and the avoidance of emergency delivery of a newborn who already has been seriously compromised by acidosis and hypoxemia.

The role of the pediatric cardiologist in the prevention of essential hypertension and coronary heart disease has been debated for many years. There is evidence that these diseases have a genetic predisposition and that their manifestations begin during childhood. Thus, in several major centers, interested pediatric cardiologists are concentrating their efforts in establishing special clinics for the offspring of parents with familial hypercholesterolemia. Dietary interventions, avoidance of smoking, and in rare cases pharmacologic cholesterol-reducing agents are used as a means of preventing development of atherosclerosis. In some instances, salt intake restriction and exercise are recommended for children and adolescents with pressure above the 95th percentile and a family history of hypertension. There are no hard data available as yet to confirm that such early interventions will prevent future development of these diseases and their complications.

In recent years, research in molecular biology and genetics has introduced powerful tools to study factors influencing the developing heart and to understand its orderly structural and functional development. It is possible that understanding these fundamentals of normal cardiac development may provide information regarding the pathogenesis of congenital malformations and may also reveal early control mechanisms in the development of acquired cardiovascular disease of adulthood.

The ultimate aim in medicine is to explore ways of preventing illness as well as treating it. Accordingly, the aim of pediatric cardiology must be the prevention of cardiac malformations. Talented young investigators are needed and must be supported in order to accomplish this goal. A serious commitment by the leaders of the subspecialty, and the discipline as a whole, is required in order to create the appropriate environment and resources necessary for such gifted and dedicated individuals to obtain competitive support and pursue their research interests. Unfortunately, the prevailing climate for the funding of medical care and the support of basic medical and biological research does not appear very promising. A long-range commitment by government, voluntary, and private sectors is urgently needed so that the progress that was started 50 years ago may continue with the same rate during the 21st century.

George C. Emmanouilides, MD

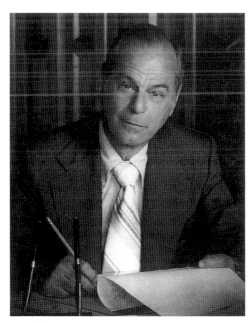

Arthur J. Moss, MD (1914–2004)
Pediatrician, Pediatric Cardiologist, Educator
Professor of Pediatrics, Emeritus
University of California, Los Angeles
Chairman, Department of Pediatrics (1967–1977)
Chairman, Executive Committee, Section on Cardiology,
American Academy of Pediatrics (1967–1968)

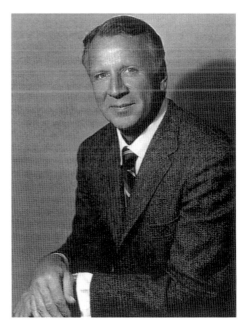

Forrest H. Adams, MD (1919...)
Pediatrician, Pediatric Cardiologist, Investigator, Educator
Professor of Pediatrics, Emeritus
University of California, Los Angeles
Director, Division of Cardiology
Department of Pediatrics (1952–1978)
Chair, Sub-board of Pediatric Cardiology (1967–1969)
President, American College of Cardiology (1971–1972)

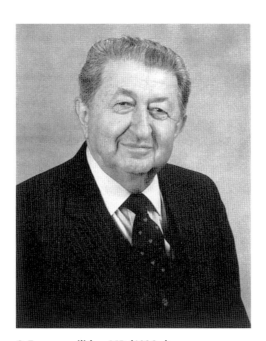

George C. Emmanouilides, MD (1926...)
Pediatrician, Pediatric Cardiologist, Educator, Advocate,
Neonatologist, Investigator
Professor of Pediatrics, Emeritus
University of California, Los Angeles
Chief, Division of Pediatric Cardiology
Department of Pediatrics
Harbor–UCLA Medical Center
Torrance, California (1963–1995)
Chair, Executive Committee of Section on Cardiology,
American Academy of Pediatrics (1978–1980)
Distinguished Physician Award—Hellenic Society of New York (1992)

PART I ■ STRUCTURE AND FUNCTION
OF THE CARDIOVASCULAR SYSTEM

CHAPTER 1 ■ CARDIAC ANATOMY AND EXAMINATION OF CARDIAC SPECIMENS

WILLIAM D. EDWARDS, MD

A fundamental understanding of cardiac anatomy forms the cornerstone of diagnostic pediatric cardiology and is a prerequisite for the proper interpretation of clinical cardiovascular imaging. In this chapter, cardiac anatomy is presented segmentally, with an emphasis on comparisons between analogous right-sided and left-sided structures. Although standard and commonly accepted anatomic terminology is used, anglicized forms are also provided in parentheses—for example, crista terminalis (terminal crest).

MEDIASTINUM

General Features

In keeping with their embryonic origins as midline structures, the heart and great vessels occupy the midthorax, within the mediastinum. The anatomic borders of the mediastinum are as follows:

1. Anteriorly, the sternum and its adjacent ribs
2. Posteriorly, the vertebral column and its adjacent ribs
3. Laterally, the medial aspects of the parietal pleuras (pleurae)
4. Superiorly, the plane of the first rib
5. Inferiorly, the diaphragm

The mediastinum, in turn, is divided into four regions (Fig. 1.1). The heart, aortic arch, and descending thoracic aorta are located in the middle, superior, and posterior regions, respectively. Also located within the mediastinum are the esophagus, trachea, right and left main bronchi, thymus, lymph nodes, autonomic nerves, thoracic duct, and small vessels (including bronchial, esophageal, azygos, and hemiazygos).

Cardiac Size

The size of the heart relative to the thoracic cage varies with age. Radiographically, the normal cardiothoracic ratio is 60% or less for newborns and 50% or less in children and adults (Fig. 1.2). However, these ratios are applicable only for full respiratory inspiration, a condition that may be difficult to attain in newborns and infants. Accurate assessment of the great vessels by chest radiography also may be hampered by the overlying thymus.

Cardiac size also is proportional to body size and correlates better with body surface area and weight than with height. In well-conditioned athletes, with physiologic cardiac hypertrophy, heart weights may approach or slightly exceed the upper limits of normal. Heart weight varies with gender as well and, for the same body size, is greater in girls than in boys during infancy and childhood. By the time a body weight of 25 kg is achieved, however, heart weights are similar between genders, and beyond 35 kg body weight, heart weights in boys exceed those in girls by about 10% (1). This trend continues throughout adult life and increases with body size, from 15% at 70 kg, to 20% at 100 kg, to 25% at 150 kg (2).

In general, the normal human heart is roughly the size of one's fist. In this regard, it is important to emphasize that a patient's heart size should be similar in size to the patient's fist, not the examiner's. This obvious fact can easily be forgotten when one is viewing cardiac images and not taking into account the size of the patient.

Cardiac Position

Within the mediastinum, the cardiac apex is normally directed leftward, anteriorly, and inferiorly, and this constitutes levocardia. In newborns, the apical direction is more horizontal than in children or adults.

However, once the heart is removed from the chest, whether literally at autopsy or technically by projecting an image onto a video monitor, the extracardiac reference points are lost, and orientation becomes a matter of convenience. Traditionally, photographs of cardiac specimens have been oriented with the apex down, and echocardiographic four-chamber images of the heart are often projected similarly. As a result, confusion has arisen concerning the true anatomic positions of the cardiac chambers and valves.

PERICARDIUM

General Features

The pericardium both covers the heart, as the epicardium, and surrounds it, as the parietal pericardium, much like a fluid-filled balloon covers a fist that is pressed into it. Between the two layers, within the pericardial sac, serous pericardial fluid (≤25 mL in adults) serves to lubricate the heart and allow its relatively friction-free movement within the chest. In addition, the parietal pericardium limits the diastolic dimensions of the heart.

Parietal Pericardium

The parietal pericardium represents a tough, flask-shaped sac that surrounds the heart and attaches along the great vessels, such that the ascending aorta and pulmonary trunk are primarily intrapericardial (Fig. 1.3A). Similarly, the terminal 2 to 4 cm of the superior vena cava (superior caval vein) are also

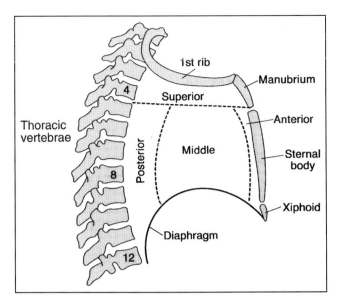

FIGURE 1.1 Mediastinum, shown schematically. Viewed from a right lateral perspective, the mediastinum has four divisions.

located within the pericardial sac, as are shorter lengths of the pulmonary veins and the inferior vena cava (inferior caval vein).

For patients with total anomalous pulmonary venous connection, the confluence of pulmonary veins is located within the pericardial sac behind the heart. In contrast, the right and left pulmonary arteries and the ductus arteriosus (ductal artery) are extrapericardial structures, and surgical procedures restricted to these vessels do not require a pericardial incision.

The parietal pericardium consists of an outer fibrous layer and an inner serous layer of mesothelial cells. The fibrous layer is densely collagenous and is ≤1 mm thick in adults. Its outer surface also normally contains variable amounts of adipose tissue, especially near the diaphragm, that can cause apparent thickening of the pericardium, as well as contributing to the cardiac silhouette radiographically.

Because the fibrous pericardium contains little elastic tissue, it cannot distend acutely. Consequently, the rapid accumulation of as little as 200 mL of pericardial fluid in adults generally produces hemodynamic features of cardiac tamponade. However, in the setting of chronic enlargement of the heart, as occurs with normal body growth or with cardiac dilation, stretching and growth of the parietal pericardium do take place to accommodate the increasing cardiac volume.

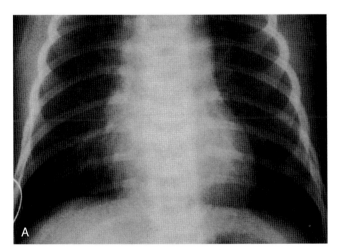

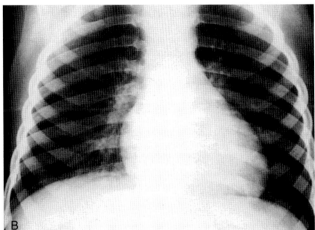

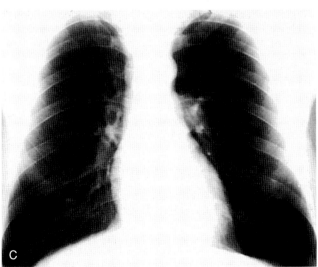

FIGURE 1.2 Cardiothoracic ratio. In posteroanterior chest radiograms, the relative size of the cardiac silhouette changes with age. **A:** Two-day-old newborn. **B:** Three-year-old child. **C:** Thirty-one-year-old man.

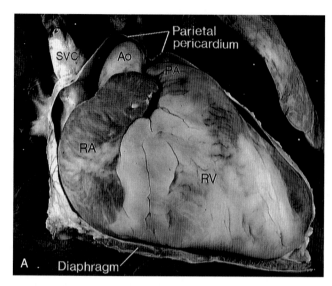
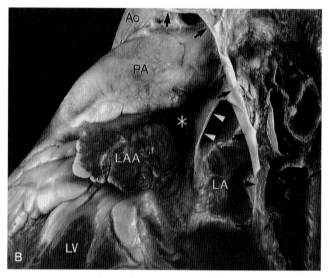

FIGURE 1.3 Parietal pericardium. **A:** With the anterior aspect of the parietal pericardium removed, the intrapericardial position of the great vessels is apparent. **B:** With most of the parietal pericardium excised, the pericardial reflection can be identified (*arrows*), as can the ligament of Marshall (*arrowheads*) and the transverse sinus (*asterisk*) (left lateral view). (See Appendix 1.1 for abbreviations.)

Visceral Pericardium (Epicardium)

The visceral pericardium, or epicardium, covers the heart and the intrapericardial portions of the great vessels. It consists of a delicate lining of mesothelial cells and the subjacent adipose tissue, coronary vessels, and nerves along the surface of the heart. Adipose tissue tends to accumulate within the atrioventricular, interventricular, and interatrial grooves (sulci) and along the acute margin of the right ventricle and the coronary branches. Prominent tags of fat cover the origins of the coronary arteries, between the aorta and the atrial appendages. With increasing age, epicardial fat increases in amount and may infiltrate into the atrial septum, particularly within the limbus of the fossa ovalis (limb of the oval fossa).

Because the heart must be compliant enough to enlarge during ventricular diastole and to contract during systole, the normal visceral pericardium has no dense fibrous component. Even so, it does have appreciable mechanical strength, as evidenced by the fact that, following coronary interventions complicated by arterial perforation, the overlying epicardium readily withstands coronary blood pressure and thereby deters rupture into the pericardial sac.

Pericardial Reflection

The line of junction between the parietal and visceral layers occurs along the great vessels and is known as the pericardial reflection. That portion involving the great veins forms the oblique sinus, a cul-de-sac (shaped like an inverted U) along the posterior aspect of the left atrium. Between the great arteries, anterosuperiorly, and the atrial walls, posteroinferiorly, is a tunnel-shaped structure, the transverse sinus (Fig. 1.3B). Nearby, the ligament of Marshall represents the embryonic remnant of a left superior vena cava.

Intraoperatively, in the setting of pulmonary atresia, if a remnant of the hypoplastic or atretic main pulmonary artery

exists, it will be found along the ascending aorta, anterosuperior to the transverse sinus. Conversely, a persistent left superior vena cava will abut the left pulmonary artery, posterior to the transverse sinus.

Following operative procedures that require an anterior pericardiotomy, the development of fibrinous pericarditis is the rule and may be accompanied by a friction rub. As healing takes place, fibrin is replaced by fibrovascular granulation tissue, from which oozing of blood may occur as small vessels are eroded by repeated contact between the parietal and visceral layers with each heartbeat. For this reason, the pericardium is generally left open postoperatively so that accumulations of blood or fluid can be drained into one of the pleural cavities and removed through a chest tube.

Within a few days, however, the raw and inflamed surfaces generally begin to adhere to the overlying sternum, effectively closing the pericardium. When this occurs, oozing of blood from the pericardial surfaces can result in the insidious development of postoperative cardiac tamponade. Furthermore, in supine patients, localized accumulations of blood within the oblique sinus can produce isolated left atrial tamponade.

Over time, organization of fibrinous exudates often results in the development of diffuse fibrous adhesions between the parietal pericardium and the epicardial surface, although progression to constriction is rare. However, fibrous adhesions may increase the risk of subsequent cardiac operations by obscuring the locations of epicardial coronary arteries or, when dissected free, by causing appreciable intraoperative bleeding while the patient is heparinized.

EXTERNAL TOPOGRAPHY

General Features

The atrioventricular groove (sulcus) defines the plane of the base of the heart, which contains the four cardiac valves. The anterior and inferior interventricular grooves indicate the plane of the ventricular septum. Normally, the two ventricles are similar in size and the atria are appreciably smaller than the ventricles. Along the surface of the heart, the right and circumflex coronary arteries travel in the right and left atrioventricular grooves, respectively, and the left anterior and posterior descending coronary arteries course along the anterior and inferior interventricular grooves, respectively. Thus, by external inspection alone, surgeons and pathologists can assess the location of the coronary arteries and the presence of hypoplastic or dilated chambers.

Base–Apex Characteristics

The ventricles, being roughly conical, have a base (at the base of the heart) and an apex. The base–apex direction (or axis) for both ventricles is leftward, anterior, and inferior, and the two directions are roughly parallel. However, in crisscross hearts, the ventricular apical directions cross and are often orthogonal.

Because the left base–apex length is normally greater than that of the right, the left ventricular apex generally forms the true apex of the heart. However, the right ventricle may form the cardiac apex when the left ventricle is hypoplastic or when the right ventricle is dilated. Rarely, the interventricular groove is quite deep apically and results in a heart with a bifid apex.

The cardiac apex is normally located along the left midclavicular line at the fourth or fifth intercostal space. Clinically, the point of maximal impulse usually corresponds to the anteroseptal region of the left ventricle rather than to the true cardiac apex.

External Landmarks

The junction between the anterior and inferior free walls of the right ventricle forms a sharp angle known as the acute margin, the basal aspect of which delineates the right shoulder of the heart. Analogously, the rounded lateral wall of the left ventricle forms an ill-defined obtuse margin, and its basal aspect represents the left shoulder of the heart. Thus, coronary vessels supplying this region are known as obtuse marginal branches of the circumflex artery. Along the inferior (diaphragmatic) aspect of the heart, the atrioventricular, interventricular, and interatrial grooves form a cross-shaped intersection called the crux cordis (crux of the heart).

Chambers and Great Vessels

To properly interpret the various cardiac imaging modalities, one must understand not only the normal size and shape of the cardiac chambers and great vessels but also their relative positions three-dimensionally (Fig. 1.4). In this regard, only the right atrium is anatomically named correctly. It is truly a right lateral chamber, whereas the left atrium lies in the midline posteriorly and is not a left-sided structure. The right ventricle is a right anterior chamber, and the left ventricle is a left posterior structure. Although not striking, the atria are located slightly superiorly relative to the ventricles. Positionally, the aorta arises posteriorly, inferiorly, and to the right of the main pulmonary artery. In patients with congenitally malformed hearts, the relative sizes and positions of the cardiac chambers and great vessels may vary considerably from normal.

GREAT VEINS

Superior Vena Cava

The internal jugular and subclavian veins merge to form brachiocephalic (or innominate) veins bilaterally (Fig. 1.5). Their junctions are usually guarded by venous valves (3). The brachiocephalic veins enter the mediastinum at the level of the first rib, posterior to the sternoclavicular joint. The left brachiocephalic or innominate vein is two to three times the length of its right-sided counterpart and lies along the anterosuperior aspect of the aortic arch and its brachiocephalic branches. Each innominate vein receives internal mammary (thoracic) and pericardiophrenic veins, and the left also receives the inferior thyroidal vein.

Both brachiocephalic veins merge to form the superior vena cava (superior caval vein), which lies just anteriorly to the right pulmonary artery and against the posterolateral aspect of the ascending aorta. The azygos vein arches over the right bronchus and empties into the superior vena cava posteriorly. The superior vena cava, as a right lateral structure, contributes to the right superior border of the radiographic frontal cardiac silhouette (Fig. 1.6). Approximately one third to one half of its length is intrapericardial as it approaches the right atrium.

The right internal jugular vein, right brachiocephalic vein, and superior vena cava provide a short and relatively straight intravascular route to the right atrium and tricuspid orifice that may be used for obtaining endomyocardial biopsy specimens from the right ventricle. Subclavian veins often are used for the placement of transvenous pacemaker leads, and both the subclavian and internal jugular veins are used for the insertion of pressure-monitoring catheters. Catheters and pacemaker leads quickly become coated with thrombus, particularly at sites of contact with vascular walls, which may become sites of embolization or infection.

Inferior Vena Cava

The inferior vena cava (inferior caval vein) receives systemic venous drainage from the legs, retroperitoneal viscera, and the portal circulation (Fig. 1.5). Because the veins from the abdominal digestive system drain through the liver, ingested substances are metabolized before they gain access to the remainder of the body. The suprahepatic portion of the inferior caval vein is only a few centimeters in length and, after traversing the diaphragm, joins the inferior surface of the right atrium.

The ostium of the inferior vena cava is guarded by a diminutive crescent-shaped flap of tissue, the eustachian valve. Although generally small, this structure can become so large that it produces a double-chambered right atrium (cor triatriatum dexter).

Interestingly, the vertebral venous plexus does not directly join the inferior vena cava. Rather, it drains into the intracranial, intercostal, lumbar, and lateral sacral veins, as well as into the portal system via the rectal venous plexus. Accordingly, infections or metastases may spread to the vertebral bodies or central nervous system through this vascular network.

Coronary Sinus

The coronary sinus travels in the left AV groove and receives not only the great cardiac vein but also the posterior, middle, and small cardiac veins. It empties into the right atrium near

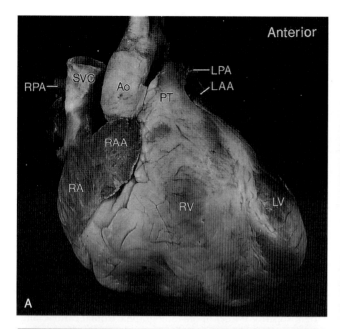

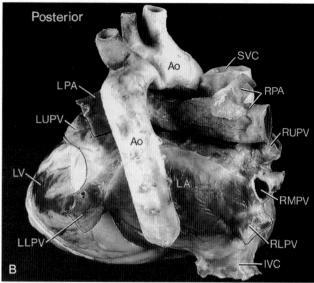

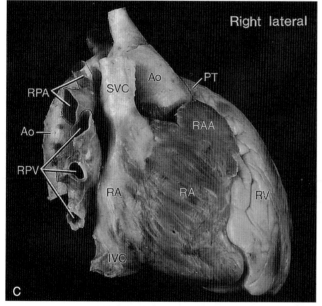

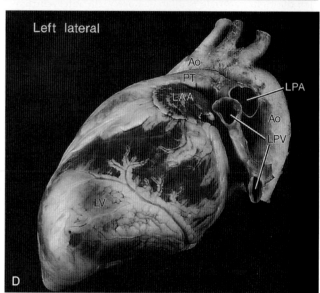

FIGURE 1.4 External cardiac anatomy. The heart and great vessels are shown from the anterior (**A**), posterior (**B**), right lateral (**C**), left lateral (**D**), superior (**E**), inferior (**F**), right anterior oblique (**G**), and left anterior oblique (**H**) anatomic perspectives, as indicated for each view. (See Appendix 1.1 for abbreviations.)

the atrial septum and the orifice of the inferior vena cava. During electrophysiologic studies in patients with the Wolff-Parkinson-White pre-excitation syndrome and left-sided bypass tracts, a multielectrode catheter can be positioned within the coronary sinus and great cardiac vein, adjacent to the mitral valve ring, to localize the aberrant conduction pathways. During cardiac operations, cardioplegic solution may be retrogradely administered into the coronary sinus.

The coronary sinus ostium is guarded by a crescent-shaped valvular remnant, the thebesian valve. When large and extensively fenestrated, this valve is known as a Chiari net. A commissure exists between the valves of the coronary sinus and

the inferior vena cava. From this commissure a small cord, the tendon of Todaro, travels just beneath the endocardium and inserts into the membranous septum. Rarely, an unroofed coronary sinus drains directly into the left atrium, or the coronary sinus ostium is atretic.

Pulmonary Veins

Superior (upper) and inferior (lower) pulmonary veins from each lung join the posterolateral aspects of the left atrium. Owing to the midline nature of the left atrium, the right-sided

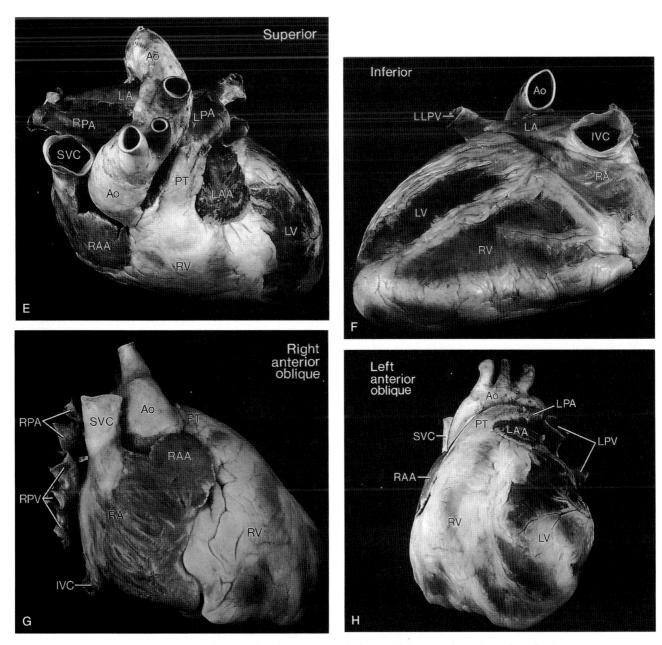

FIGURE 1.4 (*Continued*) External cardiac anatomy. The heart and great vessels are shown from the anterior (**A**), posterior (**B**), right lateral (**C**), left lateral (**D**), superior (**E**), inferior (**F**), right anterior oblique (**G**), and left anterior oblique (**H**) anatomic perspectives, as indicated for each view. (See Appendix 1.1 for abbreviations.)

veins are similar in length to their left-sided counterparts. As a variation of normal, a middle lobe vein from the right lung may enter the left atrium separately rather than first joining the upper lobe vein. In other cases, the upper and lower pulmonary veins, particularly from the left lung, can merge and join the left atrium as a single vein.

The right and left lower pulmonary veins each travel along the inferior aspect of the corresponding main bronchus. In contrast, the two upper veins each course anteriorly to their respective bronchus and, at the pulmonary hilum, lie anteriorly to the right intermediate and left main pulmonary arteries. Thus, because the upper pulmonary veins travel anteriorly and the pulmonary arteries travel posteriorly (moving from the

heart to the hilus), the veins are posterior to the arteries at the level of the left atrium but lie anteriorly to the arteries at the level of the pulmonary hilum.

Interestingly, the media of the pulmonary veins, within 1 to 3 cm of the left atrium, contain myocardial cells rather than smooth muscle cells. Consequently, these regions can function as sphincters during atrial systole and thereby minimize retrograde blood flow back into the lungs. Because the pulmonary veins are normally thin walled and distended under low pressure, they are prone to extrinsic compression either by a native structure, such as thrombus or neoplasm, or by synthetic materials, such as a conduit or surgical hemostatic packing material.

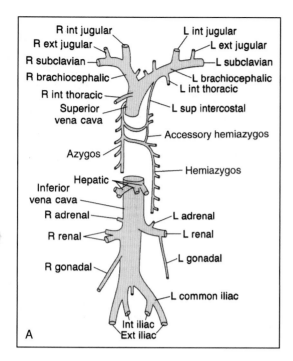

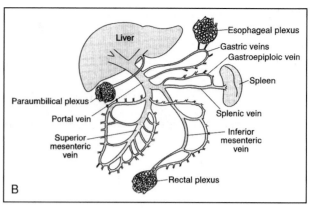

FIGURE 1.5 Systemic veins, shown schematically. **A:** The systemic veins include the superior and inferior venae cavae and their tributaries. **B:** The portal circulation drains the abdominal digestive system and the spleen. (See Appendix 1.1 for abbreviations.)

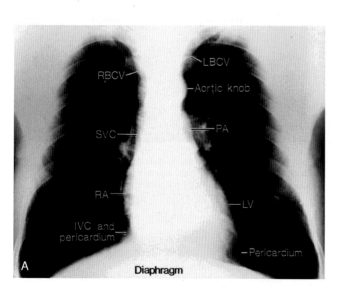

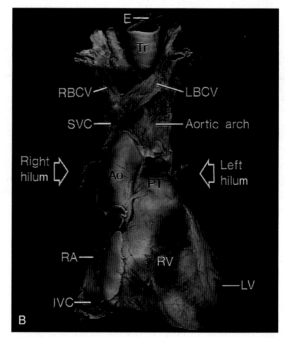

FIGURE 1.6 Heart and great vessels. **A:** The borders of the frontal cardiac silhouette are demonstrated on a chest radiogram. **B:** An anterior view of a cardiac specimen is shown, for comparison with **A.** (See Appendix 1.1 for abbreviations.)

ATRIA

General Features

The right and left atria serve as receiving chambers for blood returning from the systemic and pulmonary venous systems, respectively. They also have an endocrine function, particularly the right atrium. In the setting of right atrial dilation or congestive heart failure, atrial natriuretic peptide is released from secretory granules within myocytes, as part of the cardiorenal system for sodium and body fluid homeostasis.

Right Atrium

The right atrium is a right posterolateral chamber that, along with the venae cavae, forms the right lateral border of the radiographic frontal cardiac silhouette (Fig. 1.6). It receives blood from the two venae cavae, coronary sinus, and numerous small thebesian veins, and it expels blood across the tricus-

pid valve and into the right ventricle. Structurally, the right atrium consists of free-wall and septal components.

Right Atrial Free Wall

Internally, the free wall has a smooth posterior region and a more muscular anterior region (Fig. 1.7). The posterior aspect receives the two venae cavae and has a veinlike appearance, in keeping with its embryologic origin from the sinus venosus. In contrast, the anterior aspect exhibits a muscular wall and a large pyramidal appendage. A prominent C-shaped ridge of muscle, the crista terminalis (terminal crest), serves to separate the two regions and forms one of the tracts for internodal conduction.

Numerous pectinate muscles arise from the terminal crest and travel as parallel ridges along the anterior aspect of the free wall. *Pectinatus* is Latin for comb, and the crista terminalis and pectinate muscles may be likened to the backbone and teeth of a comb, respectively. An irregular arrangement of pectinate muscles is also found within the atrial appendage and, as a

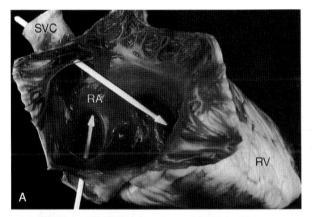
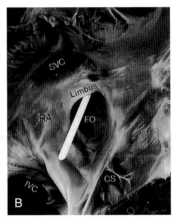
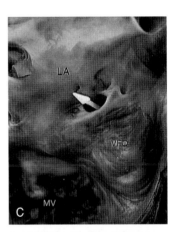
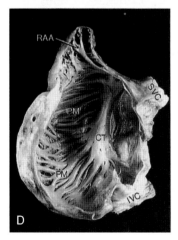
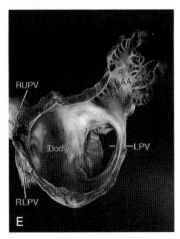
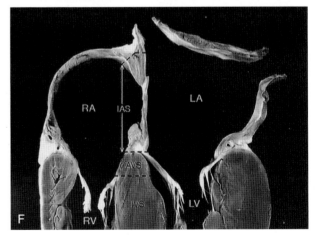

FIGURE 1.7 Comparison of right and left atria. **A:** Opened right atrium. Two arrow-shaped probes show that the superior vena cava is directed toward the tricuspid orifice and the inferior vena cava is directed toward the fossa ovalis. **B and C:** Atrial septum. A white probe in the patent foramen ovale passes between the limbus and valve of the fossa ovalis in the right atrium (**B**) and exits through the ostium secundum in the left atrium (**C**). **D and E:** Atrial free walls. The right atrial wall (**D**, viewed from a left lateral perspective) contains a crista terminalis and pectinate muscles, whereas the left atrial wall (**E**, viewed from an anterior perspective) contains neither of these structures. **F:** The interatrial and atrioventricular septa are demonstrated in a four-chamber slice of the heart. (See Appendix 1.1 for abbreviations.)

result, atrial pacemaker leads can readily be lodged in this area. The right atrial appendage rests against the ascending aorta and overlies the proximal right coronary artery.

When right atrial enlargement is associated with stasis to blood flow, thrombus may form between the pectinate muscles, particularly within the appendage. Transvenous pacemaker leads and intracardiac catheters often produce linear contact lesions at the cavoatrial junction, and these usually become lined by shallow mural thrombi.

It is important to note that the atrial wall between the ridges of pectinate muscles is generally <1 mm thick and can be perforated by catheters and pacemaker leads. Although the posterior half of the free wall (derived from the sinus venosus) is also only about 1 mm thick, it has a thicker endocardium is therefore less prone to perforation. In adolescents and adults, the pectinate muscles are 2 to 4 mm thick, and the crista terminalis may achieve a thickness of 3 to 6 mm.

Atrial Septum

When viewed from the right, the septum has an interatrial component (between the right and left atria) and an atrioventricular component (between the right atrium and left ventricle). The interatrial portion is relatively small, and its most prominent feature is the fossa ovalis (oval fossa) (4). This consists of a horseshoe-shaped muscular rim—the limbus (limb), which forms a pathway for internodal conduction—and a central sheet of thin fibrous tissue—the valve of the fossa ovalis (Fig. 1.7). In adolescents and adults, the limbus averages 4 to 8 mm in thickness, and the valve is about 1 mm thick. Embryologically, the valve of the fossa ovalis represents the first septum that develops (septum primum), and the limbus represents the second septum that forms (septum secundum).

During fetal and neonatal life, the valve of the fossa ovalis represents a paper-thin, delicate, translucent membrane. As such, it is readily torn (or stretched) during balloon atrial septostomy procedures. With increasing age, however, the progressive deposition of collagen and elastin produces a thicker, tougher, opaque valve (5). As a result, transseptal procedures may be more difficult in older children, adolescents, and adults.

In contrast to the fossa ovalis, the foramen ovale (oval foramen) represents a potential passageway between the two atria. It courses between the anterosuperior aspect of the limbus and the valve of the fossa ovalis and then through a natural valvular perforation, the ostium secundum, and into the left atrium (Fig. 1.7). Although the foramen ovale is patent throughout fetal life, it functionally closes soon after birth, as left atrial pressure begins to exceed that in the right atrium, and the valve of the fossa ovalis becomes pressed against the limbus, thereby effectively closing the foramen.

In approximately two thirds of individuals, the foramen ovale closes permanently during the first year of life, as fibrous tissue seals the valve to the limbus of the fossa ovalis. Thus, in about one third of infants, children, and adolescents, this flap valve closes only when the pressure in the left atrium exceeds that in the right atrium. During the Valsalva maneuver, for example, a small right-to-left shunt can be detected echocardiographically in persons with a patent foramen ovale. In adolescents and adults, the foramen ovale ranges from 2 to 10 mm in maximal potential diameter, with a mean size of 5 to 6 mm (6).

In the setting of pronounced atrial dilation, the atrial septum can be stretched to such an extent that the limbus no longer covers the ostium secundum, resulting in a valvular-incompetent patent foramen ovale—an acquired atrial septal defect. In contrast, fenestrations of the valve are the most common cause of congenital atrial septal defects. Excessive valve tissue may undulate during the cardiac cycle and form an aneurysm of the fossa ovalis.

Because the tricuspid valve annulus attaches to the septum lower (more apically) than the mitral annulus, septal myocardium is interposed between the right atrium and the left ventricle. This constitutes the atrioventricular septum (Fig. 1.7). Although this is primarily a muscular septum, averaging 10 mm thick in adults, it also contains a membranous portion that is only about 1 mm thick. The atrioventricular portion of the membranous septum is located at the anteroseptal tricuspid commissure (when viewed from the right side of the heart) and beneath the right posterior aortic commissure (as seen from the left side).

The atrioventricular septum corresponds to the triangle of Koch, an important anatomic surgical landmark because it contains the atrioventricular (AV) node and the proximal (penetrating) portion of the atrioventricular (His) bundle. Thus, during tricuspid annuloplasty procedures, care must be taken to avoid injury to the conduction system. When defects occur in the muscular atrioventricular septum, the mitral annulus usually drops to the same level as the tricuspid annulus, so that the defect becomes primarily interatrial, and the atrioventricular conduction tissues are displaced inferiorly.

Finally, a medial portion of the free wall lies against the right aortic sinus, which bulges somewhat into the atrial cavity as the torus aorticus (aortic bulge). This protuberance is bordered by the limbus of the fossa ovalis, the ostium of the appendage, the tricuspid annulus, and the atrioventricular septum. During transseptal procedures, care must be taken to stay within the confines of the valve of the fossa ovalis to avoid perforation along the aortic protuberance, which could result in trauma to the adjacent aortic root or coronary arteries.

Because of hemodynamic streaming within the right atrium during intrauterine life, poorly oxygenated blood from the superior vena cava is directed toward the tricuspid orifice, whereas well-oxygenated placental blood within the inferior vena cava is directed by the eustachian valve toward the foramen ovale and into the left atrium. Consequently, the most oxygenated blood in the fetal circulation travels, via the left side of the heart, to the coronary arteries, upper extremities, and the rapidly developing central nervous system. Throughout postnatal life, this orientation of the venae cavae is maintained (Fig. 1.7). As a result, transseptal procedures are more easily performed via the inferior vena cava, in contrast to right ventricular biopsies, which are more readily performed by a superior vena caval approach.

Left Atrium

The left atrium is a midline posterosuperior chamber that receives pulmonary venous blood and expels it across the mitral valve and into the left ventricle. By virtue of its posterior location, the body of the left atrium does not contribute to the borders of the radiographic frontal cardiac silhouette. However, the left atrial appendage, when enlarged, may produce a bulge along the left cardiac border, between the left ventricle and the left pulmonary artery.

Interposed between the left atrium and the vertebral bodies are the esophagus, to the right, and the descending thoracic aorta, to the left. Furthermore, the pulmonary artery bifurcation and left bronchus travel along the superior aspect of the left atrium, and the left and posterior aortic sinuses may indent the atrial wall as the aortic protuberance (torus aorticus). During transesophageal echocardiography, the transducer is placed close to the left atrium and provides excellent visualization of the atria, atrioventricular valves, and great vessels.

In the setting of left atrial dilation, the left bronchus is pushed upward, as can be seen radiographically, and the esophagus is displaced rightward. When a left superior vena cava persists, the coronary sinus into which it drains is generally quite dilated, in some cases indenting the left atrial wall, and should not be mistaken echocardiographically for the descending thoracic aorta. As on the right side, the left atrium consists of a free wall and a septum.

Left Atrial Free Wall

The free wall includes a dome-shaped body, which receives the pulmonary veins, and a fingerlike appendage. These two regions are separated externally by the left atrial coronary vein and ligament of Marshall and internally by the ostium of the appendage. The left atrial body, although 1 to 3 mm thick and infiltrated by cardiac myocytes, is derived embryologically from the common pulmonary vein and internally maintains a smooth veinlike appearance. The endocardium is opaque and gray-white, owing to the deposition of collagen and elastin, and is thicker and less compliant than that in the other three chambers.

The left atrial appendage rests along the left atrioventricular groove and covers the proximal circumflex coronary artery and, in some individuals, the left main coronary artery. The appendage contains numerous small pectinate muscles, has a variable number of lobes or blind-ended pouches, and is tortuous and may fold on itself. Outside the appendage, the body of the left atrium contains no pectinate muscles, and there is no crista terminalis.

As the left upper pulmonary vein joins the left atrium, an infolded ridge often forms where the ostium of the pulmonary vein is contiguous with that of the atrial appendage. This should not be mistaken as a partial form of cor triatriatum (triatrial heart).

Atrial Septum

When viewed from the left, the septum is entirely interatrial. Along its anterosuperior border, the valve of the fossa ovalis contains one or more fenestrations, representing the embryologic counterpart of the ostium secundum. If a probe passed through the fenestrations enters the right atrium, the foramen ovale is considered patent. Neither the limb of the fossa ovalis nor the atrioventricular septum is visible from within the left atrium. Several small thebesian veins drain directly into the left atrial cavity, particularly along the septum.

Comparison of the Atria

With regard to the atrial septum, the limbus of the fossa ovalis is a feature of the right atrium, and the ostium secundum is characteristic of the left atrium (Fig. 1.7). The free wall of the right atrium contains the crista terminalis and pectinate muscles, whereas that of the left atrium does not (Table 1.1). Moreover, the right atrial appendage is large and pyramidal, whereas the left atrial appendage is smaller and fingerlike.

TABLE 1.1

COMPARISON OF RIGHT-SIDED AND LEFT-SIDED ANATOMIC FRACTURES OF CARDIAC SEGMENTS

Right atrium	Left atrium
Limbus of fossa ovalis (limb of oval fossa)	Ostium secundum
Large pyramidal appendage	Small fingerlike appendage
Crista terminalis (terminal crest)	No crista terminalis
Pectinate muscles	No pectinate muscles
Receives venae cavae and coronary sinus[a]	Receives pulmonary veins[a]
Tricuspid valve	**Mitral valve**
Low septal annular attachment	High septal annular attachment
Septal cordal attachments	No septal cordal attachments
Triangular orifice (midleaflet level)	Elliptical orifice (midleaflet level)
Three leaflets and commissures	Two leaflets and commissures
Three papillary muscles	Two large papillary muscles
Empties into right ventricle	Empties into left ventricle
Right ventricle	**Left ventricle**
Tricuspid-pulmonary discontinuity	Mitral-aortic continuity
Muscular outflow tract	Muscular-valvular outflow tract
Septal and parietal bands	No septal or parietal band
Large apical trabeculations	Small apical trabeculations
Coarse septal surface	Smooth upper septal surface
Crescentic in cross sections[a]	Circular in cross section[a]
Thin free wall (3–5 mm)[a]	Thick free wall (12–15 mm)[a]
Receives tricuspid valve	Receives mitral valve
Pulmonary valve	**Aortic valve**
Empties into main pulmonary artery	Empties into ascending aorta

[a]Variable feature.

Although the superior vena cava and the pulmonary veins can anomalously join the contralateral atrium, the inferior vena cava almost invariably joins the morphologic right atrium.

Thus, the distinguishing features of a morphologic right atrium are the limbus of the fossa ovalis, connection of the inferior vena cava, and a large pyramidal appendage. The limbus can be detected with four-chamber imaging, and the course of the inferior vena cava and the morphology of the atrial appendage can be assessed by either invasive or noninvasive imaging. Identification of the crista terminalis and pectinate muscles is possible by direct inspection at operation or autopsy but not consistently by imaging procedures.

ATRIOVENTRICULAR VALVES

General Features

The atrioventricular valves serve to maintain unidirectional blood flow and to electrically separate the atria and ventricles. Each valve has five components. The annulus, leaflets, and commissures form the valvular apparatus, and the chordae tendineae (tendinous cords) and papillary muscles form the tensor apparatus.

The annulus of each valve is somewhat saddle shaped rather than being truly planar and represents an ill-defined ring of fibrous tissue from which the leaflets arise. Although the mitral annulus is a continuous ring of collagen, the tricuspid annulus is not and exhibits loose connective tissue at the points of annular discontinuity. Consequently, ventricular dilation leads more readily to annular dilation of the tricuspid valve than of the mitral valve. During the first two decades of life, valvular growth correlates better with age than with body height, weight, or surface area (1).

Leaflets represent delicate flaps of connective tissue. Owing to direct cordal insertions along their leading edges, the free edges have a serrated appearance. Tendinous cords also insert along the ventricular aspect of each leaflet (the valve pocket or undersurface) and thereby support the leaflet during ventricular systole. On the atrial aspect, the closing edge represents an ill-defined junction between the thinner body (or clear zone) and the thicker contact region (or rough zone) of the leaflet. During valve closure, apposing leaflets contact one another along the surfaces between the free and closing edges (Fig. 1.8). In about 50% of fetuses and infants, blood cysts occur as

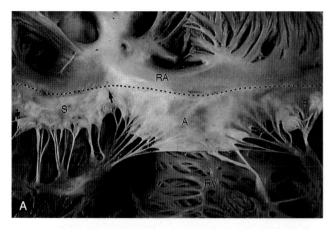
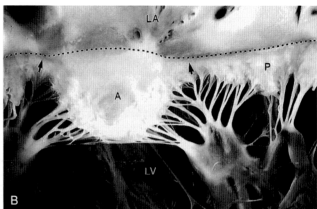
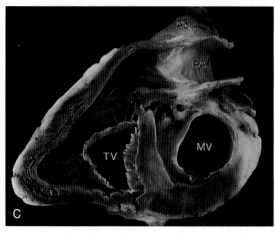
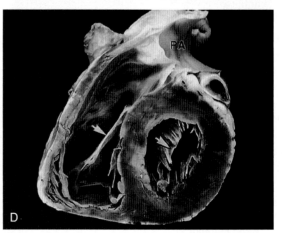

FIGURE 1.8 Comparison of right and left atrioventricular valves. **A:** The tricuspid valve normally has three leaflets. The membranous septum is located along its annulus (dashed line), at the anteroseptal commissure (*arrow*). **B:** The mitral valve has two leaflets, with papillary muscles beneath each commissure. **C and D:** In short-axis views, the tricuspid orifice is shaped like a reversed D at the annular level (**C**) and like a triangle at the midleaflet level (**D**). In contrast, the mitral orifice is elliptical at both levels. As shown in **D**, the anterior leaflet (*arrow*) of each valve is a midcavitary structure that divides its ventricle into inflow and outflow regions. (See Appendix 1.1 for abbreviations.)

small (<3 mm) purple nodules along the contact surfaces of the mitral and tricuspid valves and generally disappear within 1 year (7).

Microscopically, each leaflet exhibits two major layers. A fibrous layer (fibrosa) forms the strong structural backbone of the valve and is continuous from the annulus proximally to the sites of cordal insertion distally. In contrast, the spongy layer (spongiosa) acts as a shock absorber and becomes prominent along the contact regions of each leaflet. Because the leaflets are thin and compliant and are attached only at the annulus and papillary muscles, rapid opening and closure of the valve is possible.

A commissure represents the site along a valve annulus where two leaflets meet. Commissures always have an underlying papillary muscle and a fanlike array of tendinous cords that attach to both leaflets, in contrast to congenital clefts, which have neither. Although each leaflet has two major commissures, it also may be further divided into several regions, or scallops, by minor commissures, each of which has a small underlying papillary muscle.

The tendinous cords act as strong fibrous guy wires to anchor and support the leaflets. Accordingly, they restrict excessive valvular excursion during ventricular systole and prevent valvular prolapse into the atrium. Because a cord generally branches several times, more than 150 cords normally insert into the free edge or ventricular aspect of each valve, which tends to distribute the systolic force of ventricular blood evenly along the undersurface of each leaflet (8,9). If the tendinous cords are malformed, weakened, or insufficient in number, a portion of the leaflet can begin to bulge and prolapse, leading to valvular regurgitation. This commonly occurs not only with myxomatous valves, but with common atrioventricular valves and at least one of the two atrioventricular valves in a double-inlet left ventricle (10).

Papillary muscles can be single, multiheaded, or a fused group. By being positioned directly beneath a commissure and by receiving tendinous cords from two adjacent leaflets, a papillary muscle tends to pull its two leaflets toward each other during ventricular systole, thereby facilitating valve closure. Ventricular contraction also contributes to valve closure by decreasing the annular dimension and shortening the base–apex length of the chamber. Thus, papillary muscle ischemia or ventricular dilation may produce valvular regurgitation, as can be seen with the tricuspid valve after severe birth asphyxia or in the setting of persistent pulmonary hypertension of the newborn.

Tricuspid Valve

Because of the normal rightward bowing of the ventricular septum, the tricuspid annulus is shaped like a reversed D when viewed from its ventricular aspect (Fig. 1.8). However, at midleaflet level, the orifice becomes triangular. Annular dimensions vary with the cardiac cycle, decreasing by about 20% in circumference and 33% in area during systole, owing to contraction of the right ventricular myocardium (11). The plane of the tricuspid annulus faces toward the right ventricular apex.

Whereas the septal and posterior leaflets lie against the ventricular septum and inferior wall of the right ventricle, respectively, the anterior leaflet forms a prominent intracavitary curtain that partially separates the inflow and outflow tracts. The anterior leaflet is the most mobile of the three, and the septal leaflet, by virtue of its numerous direct cordal attachments along the ventricular septum, is the least mobile.

The relative sizes of the three leaflets vary appreciably from person to person (9).

Among the three papillary muscles, the anterior muscle is the largest and most well formed. It originates from the acute margin of the right ventricle, may be single or bifid, and provides cordal insertions to the anterior and posterior leaflets. The posterior papillary muscle arises from the inferior wall near the septum, and the posterior and septal leaflets receive cords not only from this small muscle but also from accessory papillary muscles and trabeculations. The medial papillary muscle (also called the papillary muscle of the conus or the muscle of Lancisi) emanates along the superior aspect of the septal band, at the level of the membranous septum, and has cordal attachments to the septal and anterior leaflets. Although prominent in infants and children, it commonly merges with the septal band and becomes small or absent by adulthood.

Of the three commissures, the anteroseptal is the most variable. It traverses the midportion of the membranous septum, dividing it into atrioventricular and interventricular regions. Leaflet tissue is deficient at this commissure in about 10% of hearts, and the membranous septum fills the 1- to 7-mm gap between the anterior and septal leaflets (12). This commissure is also characteristically deficient in partial atrioventricular septal defects.

Mitral Valve

The mitral annulus changes shape during the cardiac cycle, from circular in diastole to elliptical during systole. However, at the midleaflet level the diastolic orifice is elliptical or football shaped. The annular circumference and area also decrease by approximately 15% and 25%, respectively, during ventricular systole (13). Unlike the tricuspid annulus, the mitral annulus is directed more toward the midportion of the septum than toward the apex. Although the entire annular circumference connects to the overlying left atrium, only a C-shaped portion attaches to the underlying left ventricular free wall. The remaining 30% of the annulus is intracavitary, is attached to the anterior mitral leaflet, and is continuous with the aortic valve annulus.

Therefore, the anterior mitral leaflet, like the anterior tricuspid leaflet, forms an intracavitary curtain that partially separates the inflow and outflow tracts (Fig. 1.8). However, unlike its right-sided counterpart, it actually forms part of the outflow tract and may contribute to subaortic obstruction in such disorders as hypertrophic cardiomyopathy. Whereas the anterior leaflet is semicircular, the posterior leaflet is rectangular and is usually subdivided by minor commissures into three or more semicircular scallops. Only the mitral valve has just two leaflets; the other three valves each have three leaflets or cusps.

Interestingly, the surface areas of the anterior and posterior leaflets are almost identical and together provide nearly twice the area needed to close the systolic annular orifice (14). However, because some folding and puckering of leaflet tissue, as well as appreciable surface area for contact between leaflets, are needed to ensure a competent seal, the mitral leaflets are not as redundant as they might first appear.

The mitral valve has two major commissures, beneath which are located the two major papillary muscles, anterolateral and posteromedial. In addition to the usual tendinous cords, two thick and prominent strut cords, one from each papillary muscle, attach to the ventricular aspect of the anterior leaflet and offer additional support (15). In about 50% of subjects, cordal structures known as left ventricular pseudotendons arise from a papillary muscle and insert onto either the septum or the opposite papillary muscle. In contrast, attachment of cords from a mitral leaflet to the ventricular septum is distinctly abnormal and is usually associated with atrioventricular septal defects or straddling mitral valves.

Both papillary muscles originate from the left ventricular free wall and can have thicknesses similar to those of the ventricular wall. They occupy the middle third of the left ventricular base–apex length, not only in normal hearts but also in hypertrophied and dilated hearts. In the setting of hypertrophic cardiomyopathy, the mitral papillary muscles may be particularly prominent and occupy a substantial portion of the potential volume of the left ventricular chamber.

The anterolateral papillary muscle is commonly single with a midline groove and usually has a dual blood supply from the left anterior descending and circumflex coronary arteries. In contrast, the posteromedial papillary muscle is generally multiple or else bifid or trifid, and it most commonly is nourished solely by the right coronary artery. The anterolateral muscle is usually larger and extends closer to the mitral annulus than the posteromedial muscle.

Comparison of Atrioventricular Valves

The tricuspid valve has three leaflets, commissures, and papillary muscles, whereas the mitral valve has only two of each. Other differences also exist that may be of clinical use (Fig. 1.8 and Table 1.1).

From a practical standpoint, identification of the lower septal insertion of the tricuspid annulus, as distinct from the mitral, can be assessed with four-chamber images (Fig. 1.7F) in both normal and malformed hearts. Exceptions include partial atrioventricular septal defects and double-inlet ventricles, in which the two valves achieve the same annular level. Along the septum, the distance between the mitral and tricuspid insertions is <0.8 cm/m^2 body surface area in normal hearts and is greater than this in the Ebstein malformation (16).

The insertion of numerous cords directly onto the septum is a reliable distinguishing feature of the tricuspid valve. Finally, the tricuspid valve virtually always connects to a morphologic right ventricle, whereas the mitral valve connects to a morphologic left ventricle. Differences also exist between the two valves with regard to annular size and orifice shape.

VENTRICLES

General Features

Normally, a ventricle receives blood through an atrioventricular valve from an atrium and pumps it across a semilunar valve into a great artery. Because all four cardiac valves lie in the same plane, at the base of the heart, blood entering and exiting a ventricle follows a V-shaped course. During ventricular systole, both the base–apex length and the short-axis diameter decrease and not only expel blood from the chamber but also assist closure of the atrioventricular valve by decreasing its annular size.

Heart weight, which roughly corresponds to ventricular mass, is related to body surface area or weight for all age groups (1,2). During the first two decades of life, thicknesses of the right and left ventricular free walls and the ventricular septum correlate better with age than with body size. In normal hearts, the ratio between ventricular septal and left ventricular free-wall thicknesses is 1.1 (range 0.8 to 1.4), and the ratio between left and right ventricular thicknesses is 3 (range

2 to 5). Because of the effects of rigor mortis, autopsy measurements of wall thickness correspond to end-systolic rather than end-diastolic dimensions (17).

It is important to note that the right ventricle in fetuses and neonates differs from that in older persons. During fetal life, the presence of a patent ductus arteriosus is associated with equalization of aortic and pulmonary artery pressures and a state of physiologic pulmonary hypertension. Thus, during fetal and neonatal life, right ventricular hypertrophy is evident and the thickness of the right ventricle is similar to that of the left (Fig. 1.9).

Right Ventricle

As a right anterior chamber, the right ventricle normally does not contribute to the radiographic frontal cardiac silhouette. The anterior and inferior surfaces of its free wall merge along the acute margin of the heart and form an angle of 45 to 75 degrees. This, along with rightward bowing of the ventricular septum, results in a crescent-shaped chamber in the short-axis view. Conditions such as pulmonary hypertension that impose a pressure or volume overload on the right ventricle and cause its hypertrophy and dilation may be attended by straightening of the septum so that both ventricles become D-shaped on cross section. In extreme cases, such as an Ebstein anomaly or total anomalous pulmonary venous connection, leftward bowing of the septum can result not only in a reversal in ventricular short-axis shapes but also in possible obstruction of the left ventricular outflow tract.

Anatomically, the right ventricle can be divided into inlet, trabecular, and outlet regions. This concept of a tripartite chamber correlates well with the embryologic development of the right ventricle. The inlet portion is associated with the tricuspid valve, and its border is defined by the cordal insertions. Anteroapically, prominent muscle bundles traverse the chamber from septum to free wall and demarcate the trabecular region. It is in this region that biopsy tissue is obtained and transvenous pacemaker leads are lodged. The remainder of the ventricle is relatively smooth walled and forms the outlet region, which is a collar of myocardium known as the conus (meaning cone), infundibulum (meaning funnel), or right ventricular outflow tract.

Within the right ventricle, a nearly circular ring of muscle known as the crista supraventricularis (supraventricular crest) forms an unobstructed opening into the outlet region. It consists of a parietal band, outlet septum, septal band, and moderator band (Fig. 1.9). The parietal band is a free-wall structure that separates the tricuspid and pulmonary valves. Lying beneath the right-left commissure of both semilunar valves, the outlet septum separates the two ventricular outflow tracts and tilts approximately 45 degrees relative to the remainder of the ventricular septum. The septal band is a Y-shaped structure with a long, broad stem and smaller inferior and anterior limbs. The two limbs, in turn, cradle the outlet septum and give rise to the medial tricuspid papillary muscle. Apically, the septal band merges with the apical trabeculations and gives rise to the moderator band, which inserts at the base of the anterior tricuspid papillary muscle. The right bundle branch travels along the septal and moderator bands.

When viewed from a right anterior oblique perspective, the ventricular septum is shaped like a triangle, the vertexes of which correspond to the apex, pulmonary annulus, and the most inferior aspect of the tricuspid annulus. Normally, the distance from the apex to the pulmonary valve annulus is about 25% greater than that from the apex to the tricuspid annulus.

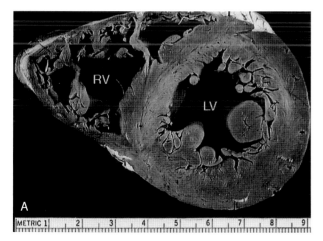

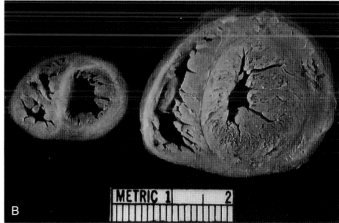

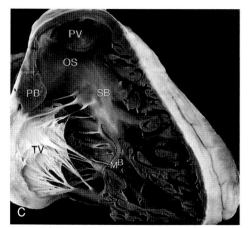

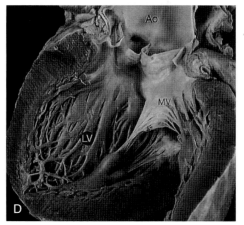

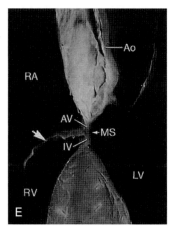

FIGURE 1.9 Comparison of right and left ventricles. **A:** In cross section, the right ventricle is crescent shaped, the left ventricle is circular, and the wall thickness of the left ventricle is three to four times that of the right ventricle. **B:** The fetal heart (to the left) exhibits prominent right ventricular hypertrophy, whereas by the age of 3 months, the infant's heart (to the right) shows regression of hypertrophy. **C:** The right ventricle receives a tricuspid valve, has prominent anteroapical trabeculations, and has a muscular outflow track that separates the tricuspid and pulmonary valves. The parietal and septal bands and the outlet septum form the crista supraventricularis (supraventricular crest). **D:** The left ventricle, in contrast, receives a mitral valve, has shallow apical trabeculations, and exhibits direct continuity between the mitral and aortic valves. **E:** The membranous septum is divided into atrioventricular and interventricular components by the septal tricuspid leaflet (*arrow*). (See Appendix 1.1 for abbreviations.)

The membranous septum lies midway between the pulmonary valve annulus and the inferior aspect of the tricuspid annulus.

Using these landmarks, the surface of the ventricular septum can be divided into six regions that are useful for localizing the position of septal defects (Fig. 1.10) (18). A line drawn from the membranous septum to the apex divides the septum into anterior and inferior halves. By dividing the base–apex length into thirds (basal, middle, and apical), the six regions are obtained. The basal and middle regions inferiorly correspond to the inlet portion of the right ventricle, and the two apical regions plus the anterior middle region match the anteroapical trabecular area. The remaining anterobasal region corresponds to the outlet septum.

Left Ventricle

The left ventricle is a left posterior chamber that forms the left border of the radiographic frontal cardiac silhouette (Fig. 1.6).

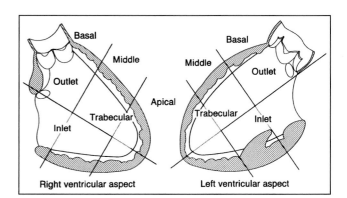

FIGURE 1.10 Ventricular septum, shown schematically. For each ventricle, the septum is roughly triangular-shaped. One side forms the anterior border, and one forms the inferior border. The third side is located at the cardiac base and is associated with atrioventricular and semilunar valves. (See text for further description.)

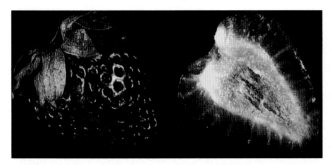

FIGURE 1.11 Three-dimensional shape of the left ventricle. The left ventricle in humans is shaped like a strawberry, here shown whole and in long-axis. Rather than being facetious, this analogy serves to emphasize the complex shape of the chamber. Thus, mathematical formulas used for the determination of chamber volume or myocardial mass are accurate only insofar as they also accurately reflect the actual shape of the left ventricle. In disease states that are commonly attended by appreciable alterations in ventricular shape, the use of standard formulas may result in determinations that are considerably inaccurate.

It consists of septal and free-wall components, and its entrance and exit are guarded by the mitral and aortic valves, respectively. The left ventricle is circular in short-axis cross section and is somewhat wedge shaped in the long-axis view. Three-dimensionally, it is shaped like a strawberry and is approximated mathematically as a truncated ellipsoid (Fig. 1.11). It is of interest that, whereas a conical chamber (as in aortic stenosis) uses the least energy for systolic contraction and a spherical chamber (as in dilated cardiomyopathy) requires the least expenditure of energy for diastolic filling, the normal elliptical left ventricular chamber expends the least total systolic and diastolic energy (19).

In the left ventricle, muscle bundles follow a spiral course from apex to base and also form several different layers that crisscross one another. As a result of this arrangement, systole is characterized by twisting or wrenching contractions that effectively wring blood out of the left ventricle, and diastole creates a vortex that literally sucks blood into the left ventricular chamber.

The free wall is thickest basally and then gradually tapers toward the apex. Interestingly, the tip of the apex, called the apical thin point, averages only 1 to 2 mm in thickness, even in hypertrophied hearts. In contrast, the muscular septum forms a rounded peak at its basal summit and becomes thickest at its midportion owing to the contribution of the right ventricular septal band. Then, after thinning a bit, the septum remains relatively constant in thickness and tapers only as it fuses with the apical portion of the free wall.

Direct fibrous continuity exists between the anterior mitral leaflet and the left and posterior aortic cusps, and this region is reinforced bilaterally by the right and left fibrous trigones (see Base of the Heart section later in this chapter). In some hearts, small bundles of myocytes are embedded in this fibrous tissue and afford a minor degree of muscular separation between the two valves. With persistence of the left parietal band (so-called double conus), this muscle bundle causes appreciable valvular separation as is often seen in a double-outlet right ventricle.

As in the right ventricle, the septal surface of the left ventricle is roughly triangular. However, in contrast, the distances from the apex to the mitral annulus and from the apex to the aortic annulus are similar. The inflow length is appreciably shorter than the outflow length only with atrioventricular septal defects. The membranous septum and the site of mitral-aortic valvular continuity lie at a level midway between the aortic valve annulus and the most inferior portion of the mitral annulus. Thus, in long-axis scans, a line drawn from the point of valvular continuity to the apex will divide the ventricle into an inferior inflow region and an anterosuperior outflow region and allow identification of the site of the membranous septum.

The ventricular apex is characterized by small, shallow trabeculations, and the apical one half to two thirds of the septal surface is also finely trabeculated. More basally, the septum is smooth walled, and subendocardially, the left bundle branch travels in this region. The membranous septum lies beneath the right posterior aortic commissure (Fig. 1.9). Because the septal tricuspid leaflet inserts along its midportion, the membranous septum consists of atrioventricular and interventricular components, and their relative sizes vary inversely, depending on the level of tricuspid insertion. Moreover, the entire membranous septum varies considerably in size among individuals and tends to be largest in patients with Down syndrome. Septal defects in this region are generally associated with focal elevation of the tricuspid annulus to the level of the mitral valve so that the communication is interventricular rather than atrioventricular.

The outflow tract of the left ventricle is formed by the upper septum, the anterobasal free wall, and the anterior mitral leaflet. Abnormalities in any of these structures may be associated with outflow tract obstruction. Examples include the discrete and tunnel forms of subaortic stenosis and hypertrophic cardiomyopathy. Along the anterior free wall, at the entrance to the outflow tract, is found the anterolateral muscle of the left ventricle, a prominent trabeculation that may cause outflow tract obstruction in association with certain anomalies (20,21). By cardiac imaging, such prominent trabeculations may be misinterpreted as mural thrombus.

Conditions such as aortic stenosis that impose a pressure overload on the left ventricle induce concentric hypertrophy without appreciable dilation (pressure hypertrophy). In contrast, disorders that produce a volume overload, such as chronic aortic regurgitation, are attended not only by concentric hypertrophy but also by chamber dilation (volume hypertrophy). Although pressure and volume hypertrophy each increase the ventricular mass, only pressure hypertrophy is consistently associated with an increased wall thickness. In volume hypertrophy, dilation masks the degree of hypertrophy and wall thicknesses are often normal (Fig. 1.12). Consequently, when the left ventricle is dilated, wall thickness cannot be used as a reliable indicator of hypertrophy.

As a general rule, only in myocarditis does the left ventricle become dilated without coexistent hypertrophy, owing to the acute nature of the disorder. It is also important to recognize that hypertrophy, with or without dilation, decreases myocardial compliance and may hinder diastolic filling. Many forms of congenital heart disease are associated with moderate to marked degrees of ventricular hypertrophy and, as a result, there may be difficulty in achieving adequate myocardial preservation during long operations. Moreover, marked hypertrophy does not always regress significantly following reparative procedures and may become a source for ischemic injury as the individual survives into adulthood.

Comparison of Ventricles

Because the atrioventricular valves travel with their corresponding ventricles, the identification of these valves (by noting their different annular insertion levels along the septum) provides an indirect but reliable clinical means of establishing

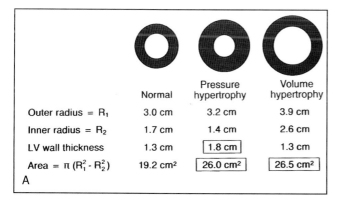

	Normal	Pressure hypertrophy	Volume hypertrophy
Outer radius = R_1	3.0 cm	3.2 cm	3.9 cm
Inner radius = R_2	1.7 cm	1.4 cm	2.6 cm
LV wall thickness	1.3 cm	1.8 cm	1.3 cm
Area = $\pi (R_1^2 - R_2^2)$	19.2 cm²	26.0 cm²	26.5 cm²

A

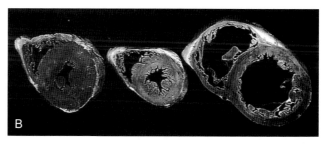

B

FIGURE 1.12 Geometry of left ventricular hypertrophy and dilation in short-axis views. **A:** As shown schematically, compared with the normal state, pressure hypertrophy produces an increase in both wall thickness and surface area, whereas volume hypertrophy (with chamber dilation) increases the surface area but not the wall thickness. **B:** Compared with a normal heart (center), the heart with pressure hypertrophy (left) has a thick left ventricular wall, but the one with volume hypertrophy (right) has a normal wall thickness.

ventricular morphology. The presence of continuity or discontinuity between the atrioventricular and semilunar valves is also useful and can be evaluated using various scanning techniques (Table 1.1). Coarse apical trabeculations, indicative of a right ventricle, are more readily identified by angiography than by echocardiography. Although differences in wall thickness and ventricular shapes are characteristic in normal hearts, they often do not apply in malformed hearts.

SEMILUNAR VALVES

General Features

The semilunar valves connect the ventricles to the great arteries and serve to maintain unidirectional blood flow. They consist of an annulus, cusps, and commissures. Because they have no tensor apparatus (tendinous cords and papillary muscles), the semilunar valves are simpler than the atrioventricular valves, and their opening and closure are primarily passive processes.

Behind each cusp is an outpouching of the great artery that imparts a tribulbous, or cloverleaf, shape to the arterial root. The junction between the sinus portion of a great artery and its distal tubular portion forms a prominent ridge, the sinotubular junction. From the right and left aortic sinuses, proximal to this junction, arise the right and left coronary arteries, respectively. These are often incorrectly called the right and left coronary sinuses; the coronary sinus, of course, is a venous structure that empties into the right atrium.

The annulus of each semilunar valve assumes the shape of a triradiate crown, the three points of which attain the level of the sinotubular junction and demarcate the commissures. A commissure, in turn, represents the site at which two cusps meet along the annulus. Because the valvular orifice approximates the level of the sinotubular junction, autopsy measurements of the arterial diameter and circumference at this level correlate well with clinical measurements of orifice size (1). During the first two decades of life, age is the best predictor of normal valve size.

As half-moon–shaped (semilunar) structures, the cusps represent pocketlike flaps of delicate fibrous tissue. The leading edge of each cusp is its free edge, beneath which lies a shallow biscalloped ridge, the closing edge, along the ventricular surface of the cusp (Fig. 1.13). At the center of each cusp, along the free edge, is a small fibrous mound, the nodule of Arantius. To either side of this nodule, between the free and closing edges, are two crescent-shaped areas called lunulae that represent the contact surfaces between adjacent cusps during valve closure. The arterial surface of each cusp, in conjunction with its arterial sinus, forms the valve pocket.

Like the atrioventricular valves, the semilunar valves histologically consist of fibrous (fibrosa) and spongy (spongiosa) layers. Cusps contain little elastic tissue and therefore have little elastic recoil. As passively mobile structures, they have no memory of shape and no tendency to assume either an opened or a closed position. During isovolumetric ventricular contraction, expansion of the arterial root may produce commissural separation and thereby initiate valvular opening. Each cusp moves in undulating fashion toward its arterial sinus during ventricular systole and then back toward the center of the arterial lumen during ventricular diastole as retrograde blood flow fills each valve pocket.

Pulmonary Valve

The pulmonary valve lies closest to the chest wall, near the upper left sternal border, and its orifice is directed toward the left shoulder. Because right ventricular myocardium extends onto the pulmonary sinuses, the valve appears partially submerged within a crater of infundibular muscle. The anterosuperior limb of the septal band extends onto the left pulmonary sinus, and trabeculations parallel to the parietal band insert onto the right pulmonary sinus. Trabecular extensions onto the anterior sinus are less prominent. In the setting of pulmonary atresia with an intact ventricular septum, failure to recognize these features has resulted in burrowing into the pericardial sac rather than into the pulmonary artery during closed operations (Brock procedure). Although this procedure is no longer performed, it is important to remember this potential complication during cardiac catheter manipulations.

Aortic Valve

The annulus of the aortic valve is a midline structure, and its orifice is directed toward the right shoulder. Consequently, its

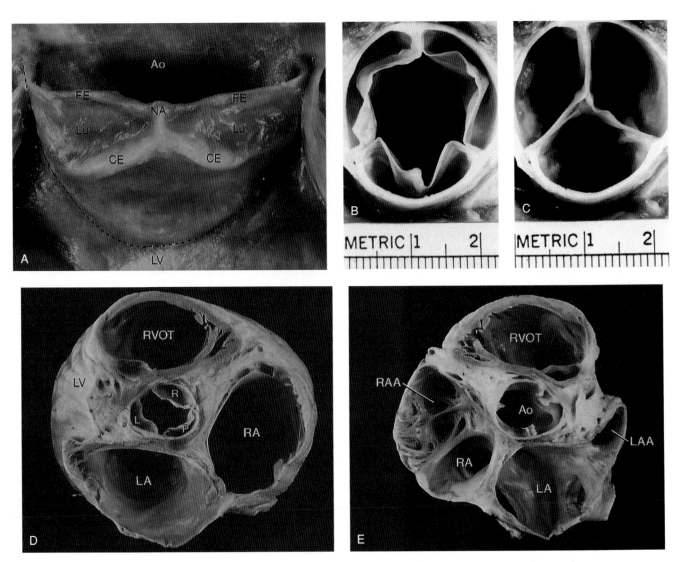

FIGURE 1.13 Semilunar valves. **A:** Each cusp is pocket shaped and has a free edge, a closing edge, a nodule of Arantius, and two contact regions (lunulae). The annulus (*dotted line*) for each cusp is U shaped. **B** and **C:** The aortic valve, viewed from above, is shown in simulated opened (**B**) and closed (**C**) positions. **D** and **E:** Tomographic sections at the level of the aortic valve show adjacent structures as viewed from above (**D**) and below (**E**). (See Appendix 1.1 for abbreviations.)

systolic murmurs are best heard along the upper right sternal border and radiate toward the neck. Although the valve cusps are similar in size, in only about 10% of hearts are they truly equal in size. Thus, a minor degree of inequality is the rule, and in two thirds of hearts, either the right or the posterior cusp is larger than the other two.

By virtue of its central position, the aortic valve and its sinuses contact all four cardiac chambers, an important consideration in evaluating aortic sinus aneurysms of congenital or infectious origin. The right aortic sinus abuts the ventricular septal summit and right ventricular parietal band and is covered in part by the right atrial appendage. In contrast, the left aortic sinus rests against the anterior left ventricular free wall and a portion of the anterior mitral leaflet, abuts the left atrial free wall, and is covered in part by the main pulmonary artery and left atrial appendage. Finally, the posterior aortic sinus overlies the ventricular septal summit and a part of the anterior mitral leaflet, forms part of the transverse sinus, abuts

the atrial septum, and indents both atrial free walls as the torus aorticus (aortic bulge).

Comparison of Semilunar Valves

The semilunar valves are named according to the great artery into which they empty, not the ventricle from which they arise. During fetal development and infancy, the aortic and pulmonary valves are virtually identical. However, during childhood, the aortic cusps begin to thicken and become more opaque than the pulmonary cusps as a result of higher left-sided pressures, and this process continues throughout life. The annular dimensions of the aortic and pulmonary valves are similar from birth through the first four decades of life, but beyond the age of 40 years, the rate of age-related annular dilation is greater for the aortic valve than for the pulmonary valve.

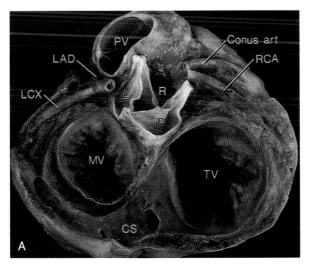

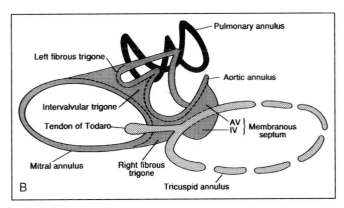

FIGURE 1.14 Base of the heart. **A:** The aortic valve is located centrally and abuts the other three cardiac valves. **B:** The cardiac skeleton, shown schematically, consists of four valvular annuli, three fibrous trigones, a membranous septum, and the tendon of Todaro. (See Appendix 1.1 for abbreviations.)

Base of the Heart

The cardiac base is defined by the plane of the atrioventricular groove (sulcus) and houses the four cardiac valves (Fig. 1.14). It also contains the fibrous cardiac skeleton, whose purpose is to weld together the valvular annuli (annuluses), to fuse together but also electrically separate the atria and the ventricles, and to provide a firm foundation against which the ventricles can contract. The cardiac skeleton contains not only the four valve annuli but also their intervalvular fibrous attachments (the right, left, and intervalvular fibrous trigones and the conus ligament).

The centrally located aortic valve forms the cornerstone of the cardiac skeleton, and its fibrous extensions anchor and support the other three valves. The intervalvular fibrous trigone is interposed between the left-posterior aortic commissure and the anterior mitral leaflet, and the left and right fibrous trigones project from each side and attach to the remainder of the anterior mitral leaflet. Thus, the left, intervalvular, and right fibrous trigones provide the anatomic substrate for direct mitral-aortic valvular continuity.

The membranous septum, in conjunction with the right fibrous trigone, fuses the right posterior aortic commissure to the anteroseptal tricuspid commissure. Therefore, the right fibrous trigone (also known as the central fibrous body) welds together the aortic, mitral, and tricuspid valves and forms the largest and strongest component of the cardiac skeleton. Even in the setting of a membranous ventricular septal defect, this connection is maintained, so that the region of mitral-tricuspid continuity forms the posterior wall of the defect. Near the right-left aortic commissure is a diminutive connection between the aortic and pulmonary valves, the conus ligament (or ligament of Krehl). Thus, each aortic valve commissure is fused to one of the other three valves: left-posterior commissure to mitral valve, right-posterior commissure to tricuspid valve, and right-left commissure to pulmonary valve.

Although schematic drawings of the cardiac base generally show the four valves in the same plane, they actually do not lie in the same plane or even in parallel planes. Because of the intertwining of the great arteries, the aortic and pulmonary valves are skewed 60 to 90 degrees as the valvular orifices are directed toward opposite shoulders. Moreover, the tricuspid and mitral valves are skewed 10 to 15 degrees, such that their annuluses approach one another at the membranous septum and diverge along the inferior wall as the coronary sinus is interposed between them. These angles may vary somewhat during the course of the cardiac cycle.

GREAT ARTERIES

General Features

The great arteries include the aorta, pulmonary arteries, and ductus arteriosus (ductal artery). Although the aorta and pulmonary artery represent elastic vessels, the ductus arteriosus has a unique microscopic appearance that changes during fetal and neonatal life.

In the fetus and neonate, the aorta and pulmonary arteries are similar in thickness and in the number of elastic laminae (laminas) within their medial layers. During the first several months of life, and consequent to the postnatal decrease in pulmonary artery pressure and resistance, the mediastinal pulmonary arteries attenuate and decrease in thickness and their elastic fibers become irregular and fragmented. Beyond the first year of life, the thickness of the main pulmonary artery is normally less than half that of the adjacent ascending aorta, although the diameters of the two great arteries remain similar.

Interestingly, for patients with persistent pulmonary artery hypertension after birth (as with ventricular septal defects not surgically treated), the medial thickness and elastic pattern in the pulmonary arteries remain similar to those in the aorta. In contrast, in patients who develop primary pulmonary hypertension later in life, their pulmonary arteries become thickened and the medial elastic layers retain the appearance of a pulmonary artery rather than that of an aorta.

Pulmonary Arteries

The main pulmonary artery emanates from the right ventricle and travels to the left of the ascending aorta in the general

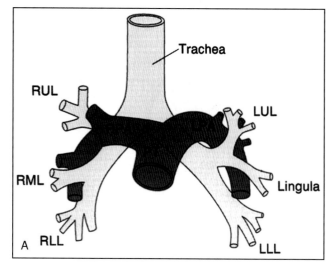

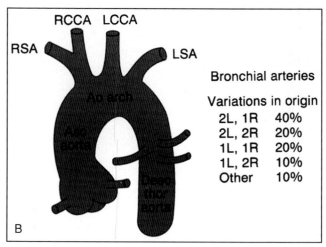

FIGURE 1.15 Pulmonary and bronchial arteries, shown schematically. **A:** The right and left pulmonary arteries are not mirror-image structures, and neither are the right and left bronchial trees. **B:** Bronchial arteries usually arise from the descending thoracic aorta at the level of the carina, but they vary in number. (See Appendix 1.1 for abbreviations.)

direction of the left shoulder. As it bifurcates, the left pulmonary artery continues as a smooth arch and courses over the left bronchus, whereas the right pulmonary artery arises at a right angle and travels beneath the aortic arch and behind the superior vena cava. Creation of a Glenn anastomosis between the superior vena cava and right pulmonary artery takes advantage of the close proximity of these two vessels. The main and left pulmonary arteries contribute to the left border of the radiographic frontal cardiac silhouette (Fig. 1.6). Because the pulmonary arteries do not exhibit bilateral mirror-image symmetry, the spatial relationship of the main and lobar arteries to their adjacent bronchi differs between the right and left lungs and can be used to determine pulmonary morphology and sidedness (Fig. 1.15; also see Figs. 2.5 and 2.6).

During childhood, the tracheobronchial cartilage is pliable and may be compressed by hypertensive pulmonary arteries. Chronic compression of the left main and right middle lobe bronchi may contribute to the development of recurrent bronchopneumonia or atelectasis in the corresponding lobes. Furthermore, rightward displacement of the aortic arch by a dilated and hypertensive pulmonary trunk can produce tracheal indentation, which may be detected radiographically, and hoarseness owing to compression of the left recurrent laryngeal nerve.

The pulmonary circulation is often referred to as the central or lesser circulation. Within the human lung, pulmonary arteries travel with their corresponding airways and pulmonary veins course within the interlobular septa (or septums, but *not* septae) (22). Because the pulmonary circulation represents a low-pressure and low-resistance system, its arteries and veins are normally thin walled. In general, pulmonary arteries >1 mm in diameter are elastic vessels, and those <1 mm represent muscular resistance arteries. Because pulmonary arterioles normally contain little medial muscle, the term arteriolar resistance is inaccurate.

During fetal life, a state of physiologic pulmonary hypertension exists owing to patency of the ductus arteriosus and equalization of aortic and pulmonary arterial pressures. As a result, the medial thickness of muscular pulmonary arteries resembles that of systemic arteries. After birth, as the ductus

arteriosus closes and pulmonary arterial pressure decreases, attenuation of medial smooth muscle occurs, such that the ratio of medial thickness to external diameter decreases from 20% to 25% in fetuses to <10% in infants 3 to 6 months of age (Fig. 1.16).

The pulmonary arteries serve to transport systemic venous blood to the lungs for oxygenation and for the release of carbon dioxide. In contrast, nutrition of the bronchial and pulmonary vascular walls is provided by bronchial arteries that arise from the descending thoracic aorta (Fig. 1.15).

Aorta

The aorta is the major elastic artery of the systemic circulation. It arises at the level of the aortic valve annulus and terminates at its bifurcation into the common iliac arteries, at the level of the umbilicus and the fourth lumbar vertebra. The aorta may be divided into four regions: ascending aorta, aortic arch, descending thoracic aorta, and abdominal aorta (Fig. 1.17).

The ascending aorta lies to the right of the main pulmonary artery and is located almost entirely within the pericardial sac. It consists of sinus and tubular portions, which are demarcated by the sinotubular junction, the site at which the discrete form of supravalvular aortic stenosis occurs. The right and left coronary arteries, as the only major branches from the ascending aorta, arise from the right and left aortic sinuses, respectively. During childhood and adolescence, the dimensions of the ascending aorta are related to age and body size.

The aortic arch normally travels over the left bronchus, defining a left aortic arch, and over the right pulmonary artery. From the top of the arch, the brachiocephalic (or innominate), left common carotid, and left subclavian arteries arise, in that order. In about 10% of individuals, the left common carotid artery originates from the brachiocephalic artery, and in 5%, the left vertebral artery arises from the aorta, between the left common carotid and left subclavian arteries. The aortic arch contributes to the left superior border of the radiographic frontal cardiac silhouette and forms the aortic knob.

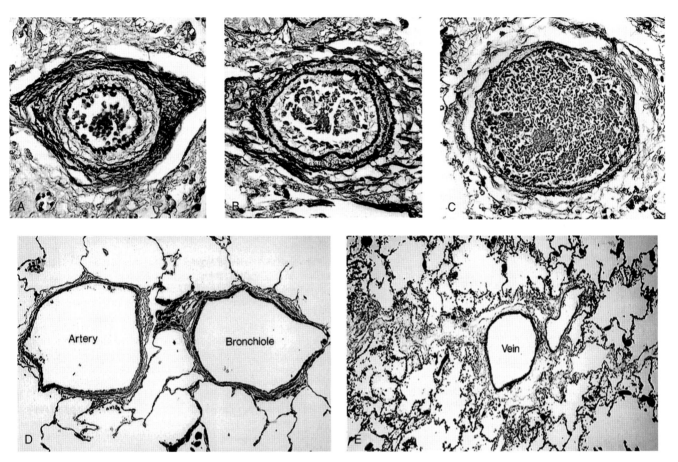

FIGURE 1.16 Microscopic appearance of the pulmonary circulation. **A–C:** The medial thickness of muscular pulmonary arteries changes after birth, as shown at birth (**A**), in a 5-month-old (**B**), and in a 7-month-old (**C**). **D** and **E:** Pulmonary arteries (**D**) travel with their airways, and pulmonary veins (**E**) travel within the interlobular septa. (Elastic van Gieson stain; **A–C**, high power; **D** and **E**, medium power.)

When the aorta courses over the right bronchus, a right aortic arch exists, and the arch vessels show mirror-image branching. Aberrant retroesophageal subclavian arteries arise from the side of the arch rather than from its top. Most aortic coarctations occur opposite the ductus arteriosus, just distal to the left subclavian artery.

The descending thoracic aorta lies adjacent to the left atrium, esophagus, and vertebral column. Its posterolateral branches are the paired intercostal arteries, and its anterior branches include the bronchial, esophageal, mediastinal, pericardial, and superior phrenic arteries. The bronchial arteries also may arise from the intercostal or subclavian arteries or, rarely, from a coronary artery. Bronchial veins drain not only into the azygos and hemiazygos veins but also into the pulmonary veins (23).

The abdominal aorta lies to the left of midline, adjacent to the vertebral column. Its major lateral branches are retroperitoneal and include the renal, adrenal, lumbar, and inferior phrenic arteries. Although the gonadal arteries originate more anteriorly, they too are retroperitoneal. In contrast, all other branches that arise anteriorly represent intraperitoneal arteries that supply the digestive system, including the celiac artery (with its left gastric, splenic, and hepatic branches) and the superior and inferior mesenteric arteries. Distally, the aorta bifurcates into the common iliac arteries and also gives rise to the middle sacral artery.

Ductus Arteriosus (Ductal Artery)

During fetal life, the ductus arteriosus provides an avenue for communication between the pulmonary and systemic circulations. It is interposed between the proximal portion of the left pulmonary artery and the undersurface of the aortic arch; during intrauterine life, its diameter is similar to that of the descending thoracic aorta and is larger than that of the right or left pulmonary artery. Most of the right ventricular output bypasses the lungs and enters the aorta via the ductus arteriosus. However, within 24 hours after birth and with expansion of the lungs, the ductus functionally closes, pulmonary vasodilation occurs, and the entire right cardiac output passes through the lungs (see Chapters 29 and 33).

Throughout gestation, structural changes take place that prepare the ductus arteriosus for rapid functional closure soon after birth (24). Initially, this vessel has the appearance of a muscular artery, in contrast to the elastic arteries to which it connects. During the third trimester, proliferative fibroelastic intimal cushions become prominent and medial thickening results from smooth muscle proliferation and the deposition of collagen, elastin, and glycoproteins. Ultrastructurally, medial smooth muscle cells change from the secretory to the contractile type. Blurring of intimal-medial junctions, coupled with haphazard arrangement of muscle bundles, produces an

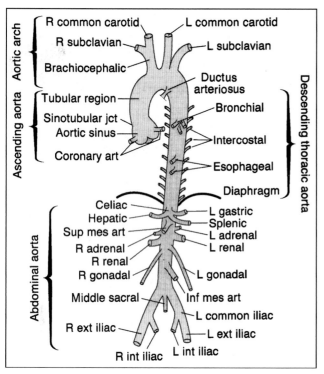

FIGURE 1.17 Systemic arteries, shown schematically. The aorta consists of ascending, arch, descending thoracic, and abdominal regions. (See Appendix 1.1 for abbreviations.)

appearance similar to that of fibromuscular dysplasia. Adventitial elastic fibers become prominent, particularly at each end of the artery.

During the latter part of the third trimester, the number of receptors on medial and intimal smooth muscle cells increases. As a result, the ductus arteriosus responds to a postnatal increase in oxygen tension by vasoconstriction. Not surprisingly, ductal closure is hampered in premature infants and infants born at high altitude. Other factors that contribute to ductal closure, in addition to vasoconstriction, include focal medial necrosis, medial edema, disruption of the internal elastic lamina, and mural thrombosis. With time, the deposition of elastin within the arterial wall becomes marked and focal areas of calcification are the rule.

In general, closure of the ductus arteriosus begins near the pulmonary artery and progresses toward the aorta. If this process is incomplete, a small ductal diverticulum remains that characteristically emanates from the undersurface of the aortic arch. Rarely, ductal aneurysms, dissections, or ruptures occur and may be linked to neonatal treatment with prostaglandin E1.

CORONARY CIRCULATION

Coronary Arteries

The right and left coronary arteries arise from their corresponding aortic sinuses. Their ostia (ostiums) are circular to elliptical and originate midway between the aortic valve commissures and about two thirds of the distance between the annulus and the sinotubular junction. The right coronary artery originates nearly perpendicularly from the right aortic sinus. In contrast, the left main coronary artery arises at an acute downward angle and travels parallel to its aortic sinus wall.

The major epicardial arteries include the left main, left anterior descending, circumflex, and right coronary arteries. Branches of the left anterior descending artery are called diagonals, whereas branches of the right and circumflex arteries are called marginals (Fig. 1.18). Septal perforators represent long intramural branches of the anterior and posterior descending arteries that supply the ventricular septum and, hence, are not epicardial branches.

Proximally, the right coronary artery travels between the main pulmonary artery and the right atrium and is covered by the right atrial appendage. Throughout its course within the right atrioventricular groove, the right coronary artery is embedded in epicardial adipose tissue. In about 60% of subjects, the first branch is the conus coronary artery, which supplies the right ventricular outflow tract; in the other 40%, this artery arises independently from the right aortic sinus (25). The descending septal artery nourishes the infundibular septum. Marginal branches include several small vessels and a prominent acute marginal artery.

Beyond the acute margin, along the inferior surface of the heart, the length of the right coronary artery varies inversely with that of the circumflex artery. In about 70% of human hearts, the right coronary artery gives rise not only to the posterior descending branch, as the dominant coronary artery, but also to posterolateral branches, thereby nourishing the right ventricular free wall, the inferoseptal wall of the left ventricle, and the posteromedial mitral papillary muscle.

The left main coronary artery lies between the main pulmonary artery and the left atrium and is covered by the left atrial appendage. It bifurcates into left anterior descending and circumflex branches in most individuals but trifurcates in some, with an intermediate artery emanating between the other two vessels. A short (<8 mm) left main artery is often associated with left coronary dominance.

Traveling within the anterior interventricular groove, the left anterior descending artery wraps around the apex and extends for a variable distance in the posterior interventricular groove. Including its diagonal and septal perforating branches, this vessel supplies the anteroseptal and anterolateral walls, part of the anterolateral mitral papillary muscle, and the entire apex of the left ventricle. Bridges of myocardium cover small lengths of the left anterior descending artery in about 10% of human hearts, produce critical systolic narrowing in <2%, and have a benign prognosis in most cases (26).

The circumflex coronary artery travels within adipose tissue in the left atrioventricular groove. It generally terminates just beyond its obtuse marginal branches and nourishes the lateral wall of the left ventricle and part of the anterolateral mitral papillary muscle. In about 10% of subjects, the circumflex artery also supplies the posterior descending branch, constituting left coronary dominance, and the inferoseptal wall of the left ventricle and the posteromedial mitral papillary muscle. About 20% of human hearts exhibit shared coronary dominance, such that both the right and circumflex arteries provide posterior descending branches.

The sinus nodal artery arises from the right coronary artery in about 60% of hearts and from the circumflex artery in 40%, but its artery of origin does not depend on patterns of coronary dominance. In contrast, the AV nodal artery arises from the dominant coronary artery and, therefore, originates from the right coronary artery in 90% of human hearts. The AV (His) bundle receives a dual blood supply from the AV nodal artery and the first septal perforator of the left anterior descending artery. Nourishment for the right and left bundle

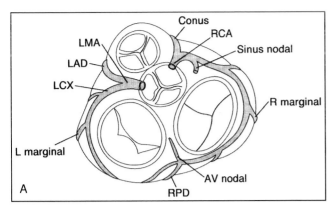

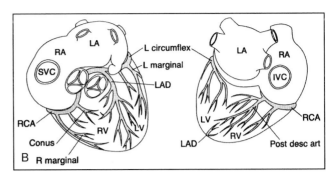

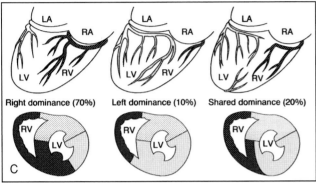

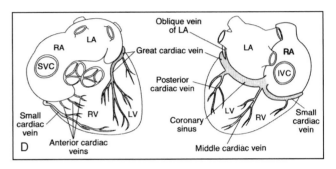

FIGURE 1.18 Coronary circulation, shown schematically. **A:** The right and circumflex arteries travel in the atrioventricular groove, near the tricuspid and mitral valves, respectively (cardiac base). **B:** The anterior and posterior descending arteries travel in the interventricular groove and demarcate the plane of the ventricular septum (superior and inferior views). **C:** Coronary dominance is determined by the origin of the posterior descending branch. **D:** The anterior cardiac veins empty directly into the right atrium, whereas the other major epicardial veins drain into the coronary sinus. (See Appendix 1.1 for abbreviations.)

branches is provided by other septal perforator branches of the anterior and posterior descending arteries.

The right and circumflex coronary arteries travel in the atrioventricular groove and thereby define the plane of the cardiac base. Similarly, the anterior and posterior descending coronary arteries course within the interventricular grooves and indicate the plane of the ventricular septum. Consequently, for surgeons and pathologists, the epicardial coronary arteries are reliable external landmarks for determining relative chamber sizes and valve locations.

Coronary Veins

The coronary veins and cardiac lymphatics work in concert to remove excess fluid from the myocardial interstitium and the pericardial sac. The venous circulation of the heart consists of a coronary sinus system, an anterior cardiac venous system, and a thebesian venous system (Fig. 1.18). The great cardiac vein travels beside the left anterior descending and circumflex coronary arteries to merge with the coronary sinus. The coronary sinus, in turn, receives the left-posterior, middle, and small cardiac veins, as well as several smaller tributaries, before joining the right atrium. Along the anterobasal aspect of the right ventricular free wall, three or four anterior cardiac veins either empty directly into the right atrium or first join a common collecting vein. Finally, numerous small thebesian veins drain directly into a cardiac chamber, particularly the right atrium or right ventricle.

Cardiac Lymphatics

Within the ventricular myocardium is an interconnecting network of delicate lymphatic channels that drain toward the epicardial surface. Along the epicardial surface, the right and left lymphatic channels form and accompany their respective coronary arteries in retrograde fashion toward the aortic root. These are joined by lymphatic channels from the conduction system and a few sparse lymphatic vessels from the atria and the valves (27). As the right and left lymphatic channels coalesce, they travel along the ascending aorta to the undersurface of the aortic arch and drain into a pretracheal lymph node. Next, they course between the superior vena cava and the brachiocephalic artery to join a cardiac lymph node before emptying into the right lymphatic duct. Lymphatics from the parietal pericardium drain into either the right lymphatic duct or the thoracic duct.

CARDIAC CONDUCTION SYSTEM

General Features

The cardiac conduction system consists of the sinus node, internodal tracts, and atrioventricular (AV) conduction tissues (Fig. 1.19). Its function is influenced by sympathetic and parasympathetic innervation, circulating catecholamines, patency of its nutrient blood supply, regional acid-base or

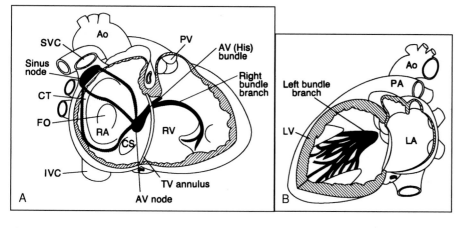

FIGURE 1.19 Cardiac conduction, shown schematically. **A:** Right heart. The sinus node and atrioventricular (AV) node are both right atrial structures, whereas the AV (His) bundle travels through the right fibrous trigone to reach the summit of the ventricular septum. The right bundle branch travels along the septal and moderator bands. **B:** Left heart. The left bundle branch forms a broad sheet of fibers along the septal surface. (See Appendix 1.1 for abbreviations.)

electrolyte disturbances, and mechanical trauma (such as sutures, synthetic patches, or ablation procedures).

The sinus and AV nodes are both right atrial structures with similar microscopic features, conduction velocities, and action potentials (Table 1.2). Similarities also exist in the structure, conduction velocities, and action potentials of the AV (His) bundle, right and left bundle branches, and working cardiac myocytes.

Sinus Node

As the primary pacemaker of the heart, the sinus node represents a right atrial structure that is located subepicardially, along the terminal groove near the superior cavoatrial junction (Fig. 1.20 and Table 1.2). Because it is found at the border between areas derived from the sinus venosus and the embryonic atrium, the pacemaker is often referred to as the sinoatrial node. It is shaped like a flattened ellipse, through which a prominent sinus nodal artery passes. Numerous autonomic nerves approach the sinus node at both its poles.

Microscopically, the node is characterized by a complex interwoven pattern of P cells and transitional cells, within a fibrous stroma, and an outer coat of working atrial myocytes (28). Because these specialized cells are primarily concerned with conduction rather than contraction, they have fewer contractile elements and expend less energy than working myocytes. Although P cells are thought to be the source of impulse formation, changes in autonomic input may alter the actual pacing site within the node.

Among patients with the asplenia syndrome and right isomerism, bilateral sinus nodes may be encountered. In contrast, in the setting of polysplenia and left isomerism, the sinus node can be congenitally absent or malpositioned. During surgical operations such as the Mustard and Fontan procedures, the sinus node and its artery are susceptible to injury.

Internodal Tracts

Whether specialized conduction pathways exist between the sinus and AV nodes has been the subject of much controversy. Electrophysiologic studies support the concept of preferential pathways, but morphologic studies do not. Recent investigations

TABLE 1.2

COMPARISON OF COMPONENTS OF THE CARDIAC CONDUCTION SYSTEM

Site	Location	Cell types	Cell diameter (mm)	Conduction velocity (m/s)	Action potential
Sinus node	Right atrial subepicardium	P cells Transitional cells	5–10 5–10	<0.05	
Internodal tracts	Atrial septum and free walls	Atrial myocytes	10–15	0.3–0.4	
AV node	Right atrial subendocardium	P cells Transitional cells Purkinje cells	5–10 5–10 30–60	0.1	
AV (His) bundle	Tricuspid valve annulus and ventricular septal summit	Purkinje cells Ventricular myocytes	30–60 10–20	2–3	
Bundle branches	Ventricular subendocardium	Purkinje cells Ventricular myocytes	30–60 10–20	2–3	
Ventricular myocardium	Ventricular septum and walls	Ventricular myocytes	10–20	0.3–0.4	

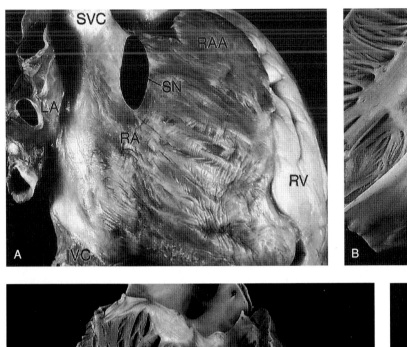

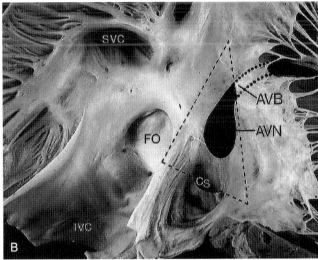

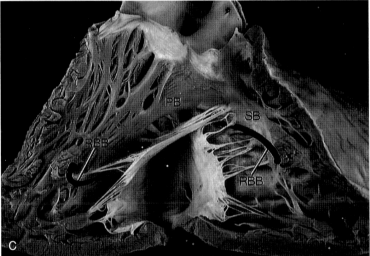

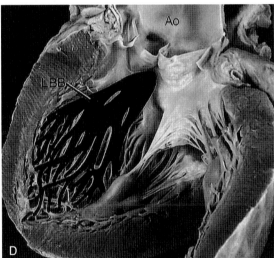

FIGURE 1.20 Location of the cardiac conduction system (indicated in *black ink*). **A:** The sinus node lies subepicardially in the terminal groove of the right atrium (right lateral view). **B:** The atrioventricular (AV) node represents a subendocardial right atrial structure that lies within the triangle of Koch (*dashed lines*), and the AV (His) bundle travels through the tricuspid annulus to rest along the summit of the ventricular septum. **C:** The right bundle branch is a small cordlike structure that courses along the septal and moderator bands (opened right ventricle). **D:** In contrast, the left bundle branch represents a broad sheet of fibers that travels subendocardially along the left side of the ventricular septum. (See Appendix 1.1 for abbreviations.)

suggest that both views may be correct. The three internodal tracts identified electrophysiologically correspond to those regions of the atrial septum and right atrial free wall, such as the crista terminalis, that contain the greatest concentration of myocytes. Thus, microscopically, these regions consist of working atrial myocytes rather than specialized P, transitional, or Purkinje cells.

Because the septal preferential pathways near the fossa ovalis travel anterosuperiorly in its limbus, internodal conduction disturbances would not be expected following a Rashkind balloon atrial septostomy, in which the valve of the oval fossa is torn, or a Blalock–Hanlon posterior atrial septectomy. However, for operations in which the atrial septum is resected, as in the Mustard and Fontan procedures, such disturbances can occur. Similarly, disruption of the crista terminalis may interfere with normal internodal conduction.

Atrioventricular Node

Like the sinus node, the AV node is a right atrial structure that is richly innervated by parasympathetic and sympathetic fibers. In contrast, it is located sub*endo*cardially, rather than sub*epi*cardially, within the triangle of Koch and adjacent to the right fibrous trigone (or central fibrous body). The triangle of Koch, in turn, corresponds to the atrioventricular septum and is bordered by the septal tricuspid annulus, coronary sinus ostium, and tendon of Todaro, a subendocardial fibrous cord that travels from the thebesian-eustachian valvular commissure to the membranous septum (Fig. 1.20). The AV nodal artery, or several of its branches, travels near the node but not necessarily through it, and venous and lymphatic channels are abundant in and around the node.

Microscopically, the AV node consists of a complex interwoven pattern of specialized cardiac muscle cells within a fibrous matrix, similar to the sinus node (28). Proximally, at its junction with the internodal tracts, the AV nodal tissues are loosely arranged and consist primarily of transitional cells and a few working atrial myocytes. Centrally, the node is more compact and is characterized by an interlacing arrangement of P cells. Distally, Purkinje cells begin to form parallel bundles as the node merges with the His bundle. Around its periphery, the AV node contains transitional cells and an outer insulating coat of collagen.

Because of its right atrial location near the tricuspid annulus, the AV node is susceptible to injury during annuloplasty procedures for tricuspid regurgitation and during plication procedures for the Ebstein malformation. In the setting of atrioventricular septal defects, involving the expected site of the AV node, the node and His bundle are displaced posteroinferiorly and are associated with relatively specific electrocardiographic alterations. Interestingly, in hearts affected by corrected transposition of the great arteries, both anterior and posterior AV nodes are observed, usually with a sling of His bundle tissue between the two.

Atrioventricular (His) Bundle

The AV (His) bundle arises from the distal portion of the AV node and travels through the central fibrous body (right fibrous trigone) to reside along the summit of the ventricular septum, adjacent to the membranous septum. It thereby represents the only normal avenue for electrical conduction between the atrial and ventricular myocardium. Within the central fibrous body, the AV bundle is closely related to the annuli of the aortic, mitral, and tricuspid valves, and its location is somewhat variable along the septal summit. Thus, during operative procedures involving these valves or a membranous ventricular septal defect, care must be taken to avoid injury to the His bundle. In some cases of congenital heart block, discontinuity exists between the AV node and the AV bundle.

Microscopically, the AV bundle can be divided into two regions: the penetrating portion, which courses through the central fibrous body, and the branching portion, which gives rise to the right and left bundle branches. Both regions are characterized by numerous parallel bundles of Purkinje cells and working ventricular myocytes, separated by delicate fibrous tissue (28). During fetal and neonatal life, these conduction bundles are often dispersed or separated within the central fibrous body. The final destination of each bundle within the right or left ventricle is probably determined by its position proximally within the penetrating portion of the His bundle. Like an electrical wire, the entire AV bundle is insulated by a dense fibrous sheath.

In many individuals, additional connections exist between the AV conduction system and the atrial and ventricular myocardium. In some, atrial myocardium either joins the distal AV node via the atrionodal bypass tracts of James or connects to the AV bundle through the atriofascicular tracts of Brechenmacher. In others, nodoventricular and fasciculoventricular bypass fibers of Mahaim link the AV node and AV bundle, respectively, to the underlying ventricular septal myocardium. These accessory pathways are apparently nonfunctional in most individuals, although they may produce ventricular pre-excitation in some.

However, ventricular pre-excitation is more often associated with aberrant bypass tracts that span the annulus of the tricuspid or mitral valve, traveling either through the fibrous ring or within the adipose tissue in the atrioventricular groove. Such bypass tracts can be single or multiple and may be identified by electrophysiologic mapping. In contrast, nodules of specialized conduction tissue, representing the bundles of Kent, are located in the right lateral atrioventricular groove but usually do not provide a connection between atria and ventricles.

Bundle Branches

The right bundle branch emanates from the distal portion of the AV (His) bundle and forms a cordlike structure that travels along the septal and moderator bands toward the anterior tricuspid papillary muscle. In contrast, the left bundle branch represents a broad fenestrated sheet of subendocardial conduction fibers that spreads along the septal surface of the left ventricle. As it courses toward the ventricular apex and both mitral papillary muscles, the left bundle branch may separate into two or three indistinct fascicles. Left ventricular pseudotendons also may contain conduction tissue from the left bundle branch (29). Microscopically, the bundle branches consist of Purkinje cells and ventricular myocytes (28).

In the setting of a membranous ventricular septal defect, the AV conduction tissues travel along the posteroinferior rim of the defect. However, if atrioventricular discordance coexists, the conduction fibers course along the anterosuperior aspect of the defect. For the outlet, inlet, and muscular forms of ventricular septal defect, the AV conduction tissues are generally remote from the defect. Interestingly, following a right ventriculotomy for reconstruction of the right ventricular outflow tract, the electrocardiogram characteristically exhibits a pattern of right bundle branch block, even though the right bundle has not been disrupted.

Cardiac Innervation

Because the embryonic heart tube first forms in the future neck region, its autonomic innervation also originates from this level. From the cervical ganglia arise three pairs of cervical sympathetic cardiac nerves, which intertwine as they join the cardiac plexus between the great arteries and the tracheal bifurcation. Several thoracic sympathetic cardiac nerves arise from the upper thoracic ganglia and also join the cardiac plexus. From the parasympathetic vagus nerves emanate the superior and inferior cervical vagal cardiac nerves and the thoracic vagal cardiac nerves, which also enter the cardiac plexus. These nerves then descend from the cardiac plexus onto the heart and innervate the coronary arteries, conduction system, and myocardium. In addition, afferent nerves concerned with pain and various reflexes ascend from the heart toward the cardiac plexus.

Transplanted hearts are completely denervated early after transplantation and can respond only to circulating substances, such as catecholamines, but not to autonomic impulses. Moreover, because afferent pathways are also lost, coronary obstruction owing to chronic transplant vasculopathy may be associated with undetected myocardial infarctions, because chest pain cannot develop.

EXAMINATION OF CARDIAC SPECIMENS

General Features

Evaluation of cardiopulmonary specimens from patients with congenital heart disease entails more than documentation of the underlying anomalies, although this is certainly important.

The recognition of malformations in other organ systems is necessary for the identification of various syndromes, which can have implications for genetic counseling. In addition, the presence of secondary obstructive lesions in the pulmonary vasculature may be more significant in explaining the demise of a patient than the underlying cardiac anomalies. Other processes, such as infections or protein-losing enteropathy, also may be important.

In the 21st century, it is distinctly uncommon for subjects with congenital heart disease to have received no interventional therapy, either in the operating room or in the cardiac catheterization laboratory. Hence, the investigation of cardiopulmonary specimens also entails an evaluation of old and recent procedures, addressing not only their effectiveness but also their secondary effects on the heart and the pulmonary circulation. This includes recognition not only of the complications of therapy but also of the beneficial effects, such as the regression of obstructive pulmonary vascular disease.

Pathologists who evaluate treated forms of congenital heart disease often act in the capacity of a medical archeologist, searching for the telltale results of procedures performed at various times in the past. In complex cases, accurate conclusions can be reached only if accurate and complete historical information is available concerning clinical diagnoses and previous procedures. For example, in patients with multiple interventions, the results of reconstruction and takedown procedures may so alter the underlying morphology that identification of the original anomalies or even previous procedures becomes difficult or impossible.

To relay this information to one's clinical colleagues, a pathologist should not only provide a written report, often with schematic diagrams, but also be prepared to review the actual specimen with others. Such reviews may represent informal sessions, formal conferences, or publications, and therefore can involve the specimen itself or its photographs. In this regard, methods of dissection and photography should be chosen that display the lesions most clearly and accurately. Details of these various methods are discussed below. If one does not have the time, training, or interest to dissect operated hearts with congenital anomalies, referral to a pathologist who does represents a reasonable option.

In the past, for the dissection of congenitally malformed hearts, it was recommended that the heart and lungs be maintained as one intact specimen. Based on personal experience, however, if the pulmonary arterial and venous connections are normal, then the lungs can be removed from the heart without compromising the accuracy of the evaluation. In fact, both the inspection and photography of the heart are generally easier if the lungs and tracheobronchial tree are removed (but not discarded). In contrast, the entire thoracic aorta with appreciable lengths of its brachiocephalic branches should remain attached to the cardiac specimen.

Inflow–Outflow Method

In the inflow–outflow method, the heart is opened according to the direction of blood flow (30). First, scissors are used to make an incision from the inferior vena cava to the right atrial appendage. The superior vena cava is left unopened so as not to disturb the region of the sinus node. Both the inflow and outflow cuts for the right ventricle are made about 0.5 cm from the ventricular septum, with either scissors or a knife, from the right atrium to the ventricular apex and then from the apex to the pulmonary artery. Contrary to older recommendations, there is no reason to avoid cutting through an abnormal valve when using this method of dissection.

The left atrium is best opened from a point between the right upper and lower pulmonary veins to the tip of the left atrial appendage. In contrast to the right ventricle, the left ventricular inflow tract is opened not along the septum but rather along the lateral wall, between the mitral papillary muscles, from the left atrium to the left ventricular apex. From the apex to the aortic valve, the outflow cut follows the junction with the ventricular septum, generally forming a gentle inverted S-shaped curve. Whereas the inflow cut is best made with a long knife, the outflow cut is best accomplished using a scalpel.

Once the aortic annulus is crossed, scissors can be used to continue cutting through the left aortic cusp. Because of the normal intertwining of the great arteries, further dissection into the ascending aorta requires transection of the main pulmonary artery. The aortic arch is then opened along its left lateral border and, as a continuous dissection, the descending thoracic aorta is opened posteriorly, between the paired intercostal arteries. Once the great arteries are opened, the origins of the coronary arteries and the patency of the ductus arteriosus can be evaluated.

The inflow–outflow method of cardiac dissection is easy to learn and quick to perform. Although it has withstood the test of time and is currently the most popular dissection method among pathologists, it is recommended primarily for normal hearts and perhaps for simple or unoperated forms of congenital heart disease (Fig. 1.21A, B).

Base-of-Heart Method

Removal of the atria and the great arteries just above their corresponding valves allows visualization and inspection of the cardiac base (Fig. 1.14). This method is useful for the evaluation of valvular anomalies or the effects of valvular surgery on nearby structures (Fig. 1.21C). For example, following tricuspid annular plication for an Ebstein anomaly, possible kinking of the right coronary artery may be investigated by this method.

Window Method

In selected cases, hearts prepared by perfusion fixation, paraffin infiltration, or plastination may be examined by cutting windows from the cardiac chambers or great vessels (Fig. 1.21D). In this manner, the interior of the heart or vessels can be viewed without greatly disturbing the internal structures. Although such specimens can be visually stunning, their preparation and photography can be difficult.

Tomographic Method

In the tomographic method, the heart is bisected (divided into two pieces) by one plane of section. With the bread-slice technique, multiple sections are made parallel to the atrioventricular groove, producing numerous ventricular slices. For the past several decades, this popular method has been used by pathologists for the evaluation of ischemic heart disease. It is identical to the short-axis method used in clinical imaging and represents the most common method of cardiac dissection used at our institution for the evaluation of acquired heart disease. It also may be performed concomitantly with the base-of-heart method.

In addition to the short-axis method, the long-axis and four-chamber planes represent other tomographic sections commonly obtained clinically and may be correlated with

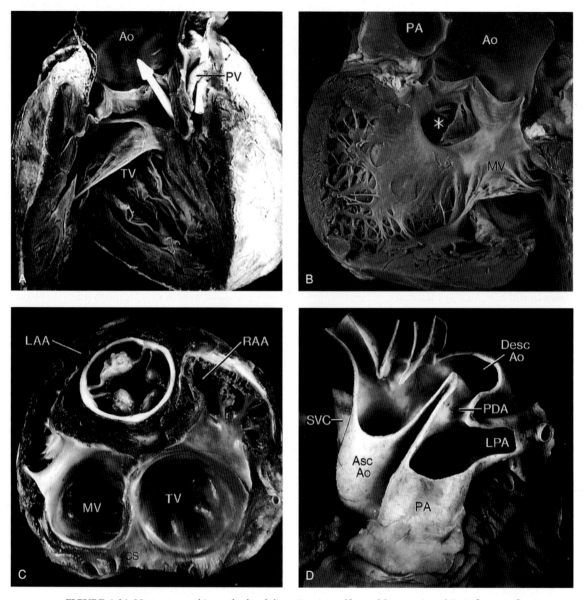

FIGURE 1.21 Nontomographic methods of dissection in malformed hearts. **A** and **B:** Inflow–outflow method. In **A**, the right ventricle in a specimen with tetralogy of Fallot is opened to display the ventricular septal defect (with an arrow-shaped probe coming from the left ventricle), overriding aorta, and pulmonary stenosis (probe). In **B**, an opened left ventricle demonstrates the position of a membranous ventricular septal defect (*). **C:** Base-of-heart method. The atria and great arteries have been removed to show the cardiac valves in a case of truncus arteriosus. **D:** Window method. The great arteries have been unroofed to demonstrate a patent ductus arteriosus. (See Appendix 1.1 for abbreviations.)

anatomic features in normal hearts. Other planes, parallel to the standard anatomic directions, also have been used clinically, not only for transesophageal echocardiography but also for magnetic resonance imaging (31). These include frontal (coronal), parasagittal (lateral), and horizontal (transverse) planes of section. In cardiac specimens, any of the aforementioned tomographic planes can be applied not only to normal hearts but also to acquired and congenital forms of heart disease (Figs. 1.22 to 1.25) (32).

Although the tomographic method of cardiac dissection has been used by anatomists and pathologists for more than a century, it has not been widely accepted, probably because it is time

consuming and requires prior fixation (preferably perfusion fixation). Nonetheless, perhaps no other technique allows the assessment of intracardiac relationships as well as the cross-sectional method. For congenitally malformed hearts, tomographic sections are particularly well suited for demonstrating not only the primary anomalies and various interventions but also their secondary effects on the heart. Thus, photographs of specimens dissected tomographically provide clarity as teaching tools and correlate well with current clinical imaging modalities.

Technically, the best cardiac cross sections are generally achieved when a perfusion-fixed specimen is cut in one continuous cut with a very sharp knife. Sawing motions are to be

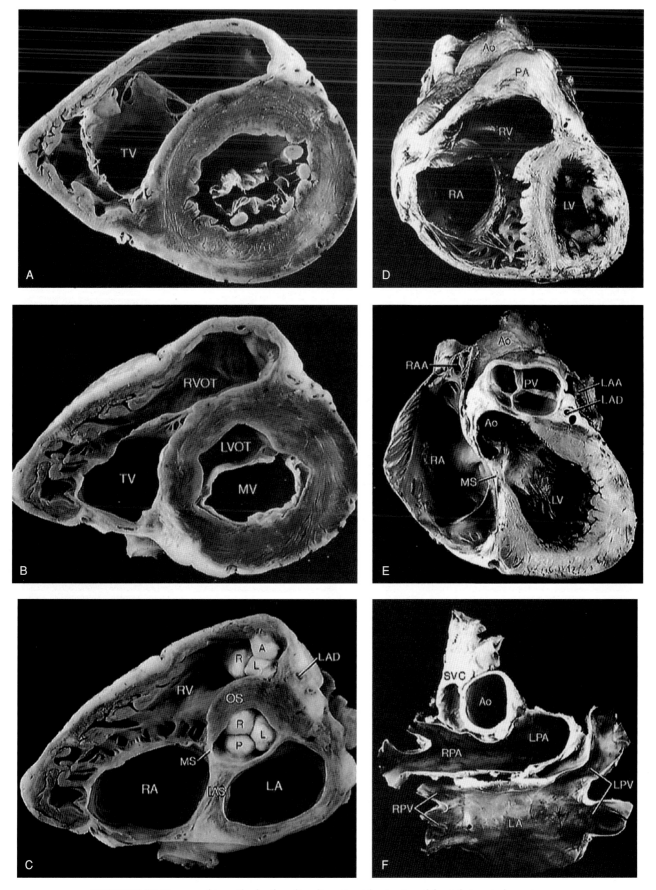

FIGURE 1.22 Tomographic methods of cardiac dissection (short-axis and frontal views), shown in normal hearts. **A–C:** Short-axis views, at the levels of the mitral valve orifice (**A**), left ventricular outflow tract (**B**), and aortic valve (**C**). **D–F:** Frontal (coronal) views, at the levels of the ventricular septum (**D**), membranous septum (**E**), and left atrium (**F**). (See Appendix 1.1 for abbreviations.)

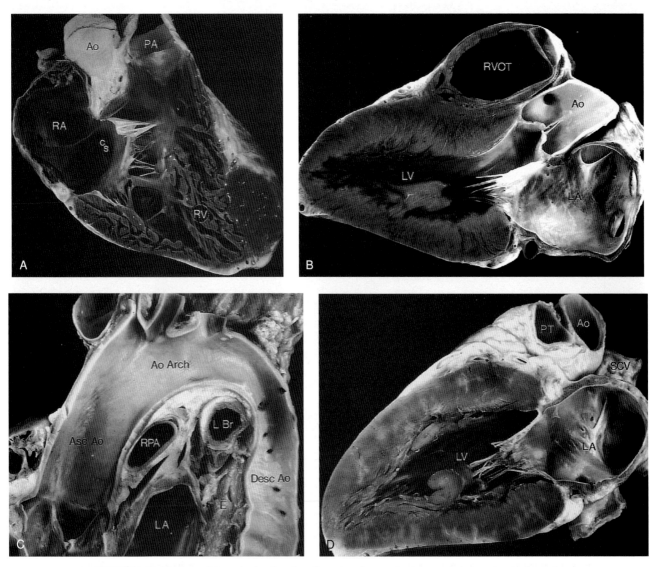

FIGURE 1.23 Tomographic methods of cardiac dissection (long-axis and two-chamber views), shown in normal hearts. **A** and **B:** Long-axis views show inflow and outflow tracts of right ventricle (**A**) and left ventricle (**B**). **C:** Long-axis view of thoracic aorta shows left bronchus and right pulmonary artery traveling beneath aortic arch. **D:** Two-chamber view demonstrates inflow tract of left ventricle. (See Appendix 1.1 for abbreviations.)

avoided. Moreover, after one section has been made and documented photographically, the specimens can be glued back together and resectioned along another tomographic plane. For this purpose, any of the readily available cyanoacrylate glues (such as Krazy Glue or Super Glue) will suffice. The best results are attained with smooth dry surfaces; roughened surfaces (such as those produced by using scissors) may adhere poorly.

Photography of Cardiac Specimens

It is difficult to overestimate the role of photography in the teaching of congenital heart disease. Although schematic diagrams are helpful, the visualization of actual specimens is often necessary for an appreciation of three-dimensional features. In this regard, the well-planned dissection and photography of a classic lesion may be remembered far longer than written words (33). Having access to the most expensive photographic equipment, however, does not guarantee good results. Careful planning and attention to detail are more important.

The use of a high-resolution digital camera has essentially replaced film-based cameras in the field of specimen photography. However, certain basic rules of photography still apply. For example, to increase the depth of field of focus, the aperture should be as small as possible (achieved by setting the f-stop as large as possible, preferably 16 or greater). One of the simplest yet most important factors for attaining high-quality photographs is the initial focusing of the camera. Few things can ruin a photograph as quickly and irreversibly as failure to attend to sharp focusing.

The use of black or white backgrounds is favored over backlighting through translucent sheets of colored plastic. In this regard, it is important to note that standard black poster

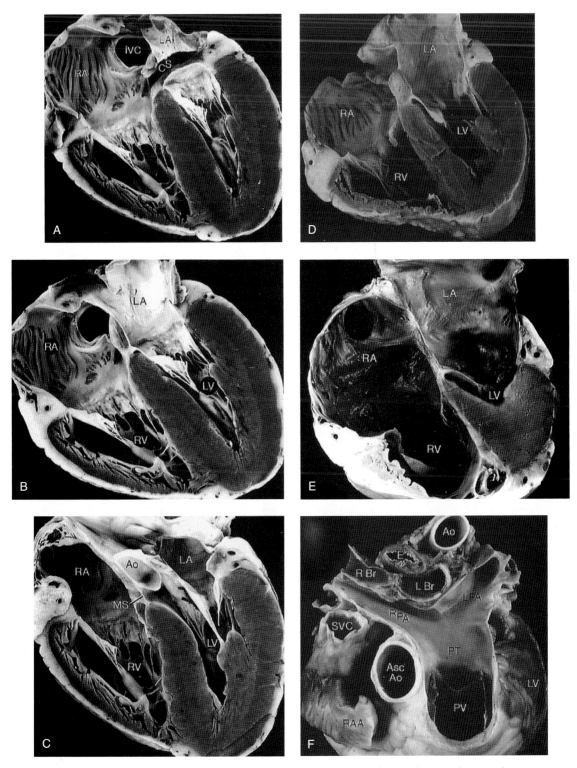

FIGURE 1.24 Tomographic methods of cardiac dissection (four-chamber and horizontal views) shown in normal hearts. **A–C:** Four-chamber views, at levels of coronary sinus (**A**), fossa ovalis (**B**), and aortic valve (**C**). **D–F:** Horizontal (transverse) views at levels of ventricular inflow (**D**) and outflow (**E**) tracts and pulmonary artery (**F**). (See Appendix 1.1 for abbreviations.)

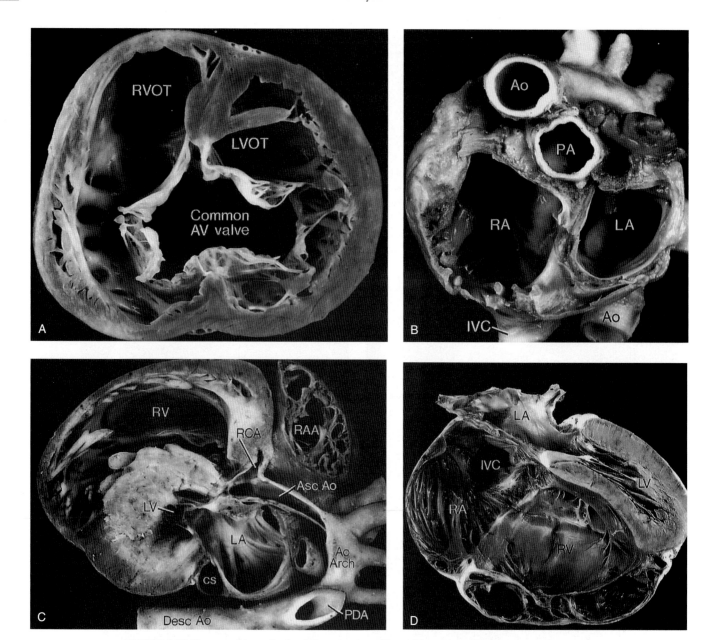

FIGURE 1.25 Tomographic methods of dissection in malformed hearts. **A:** Short-axis view of common atrioventricular valve in complete atrioventricular septal defect. **B:** Short-axis view of right anterosuperior aorta in complete transposition of the great arteries. **C:** Long-axis view of hypoplastic left ventricle in aortic atresia. **D:** Four-chamber view of right-sided dilation in an Ebstein malformation. (See Appendix 1.1 for abbreviations.)

board, available from art supply stores, is generally made with water-soluble ink and will stain the specimens.

Because fresh specimens have shiny surfaces that produce extensive glare, tissues should be fixed before being photographed. Maintenance of lifelike colors can be achieved by fixation in formalin for only brief periods (5 to 15 minutes) or in nonformalin fixatives such as Kaiserling or Jores (32). For perfusion-fixed specimens that have been in formalin less than a week, colors may be partially restored by soaking the tissues in 80% ethanol for 15 to 30 minutes. Specimens are then thoroughly dried with paper towels to eliminate reflective glare.

In some cases, pins are necessary to hold thin or collapsible structures in position. From a technical perspective, a piece of black cardboard is placed on a piece of similarly sized corkboard, and the specimen is placed on the cardboard. Pins of various sizes are then used to stabilize the specimen, and the heads of the pins are removed with cutting pliers so they will not be visible in the photograph (32). For example, 46 pins were used in Fig. 1.7E to hold the atrial walls and valve leaflets upright. Probes, arrows, transillumination, and normal specimens (for comparison) also may be used to highlight specific morphologic features.

APPENDIX 1.1 ■ ABBREVIATIONS USED IN FIGURES IN CHAPTERS 1 AND 2

A, anterior
A, atrium (Fig. 2.1 only)
AML, anterior mitral leaflet
Ao, aorta
Art, artery
AS, atrial septum
Asc, ascending
ATL, anterior tricuspid leaflet
AV, atrioventricular
AVB, atrioventricular (His) bundle
AVN, atrioventricular node
AVS, atrioventricular septum
Br, bronchus
C, cecum
CE, closing edge
CS, coronary sinus
CT, crista terminalis
Desc, descending
E, esophagus
Ext, external
FE, free edge
FO, fossa ovalis
IAS, interatrial septum
Inf, inferior
Int, internal
IV, interventricular
IVC, inferior vena cava
IVS, interventricular septum
Jct, junction
L, left
LA, left atrium
LAA, left atrial appendage
LAD, left anterior descending coronary artery
LAO, left anterior oblique
LBB, left bundle branch
LBCV, left brachiocephalic vein
LCCA, left common carotid artery
LCX, left circumflex coronary artery
LDA, left ductus arteriosus
LPA, left pulmonary artery
LLL, left lower lobe of lung
LLPV, left lower pulmonary vein
LMA, left main coronary artery
LPA, left pulmonary artery
LPV, left pulmonary veins
LSA, left subclavian artery
LSVC, left superior vena cava
Lu, lunula
LUL, left upper lobe of lung
LUPV, left upper pulmonary vein
LV, left ventricle
LVOT, left ventricular outflow tract
MB, moderator band

Mes, mesenteric
MLB, morphologic left bronchus
MO, mitral orifice
MRB, morphologic right bronchus
MS, membranous septum
MV, mitral valve
NA, nodule of Arantius
OS, outlet (infundibular) septum
OS, ostium secundum (Fig. 2.9 only)
P, posterior
PA, main pulmonary artery
PB, parietal band
PDA, patent ductus arteriosus
PM, pectinate muscles
Post, posterior
PT, pulmonary trunk
PV, pulmonary valve
R, right
RA, right atrium
RAA, right atrial appendage
RBB, right bundle branch
RBCV, right brachiocephalic vein
RCA, right coronary artery
RCCA, right common carotid artery
RDA, right ductus arteriosus
RLL, right lower lobe of lung
RLPV, right lower pulmonary vein
RML, right middle lobe of lung
RMPV, right middle pulmonary vein
RPA, right pulmonary artery
RPD, right posterior descending coronary artery
RPV, right pulmonary veins
RSA, right subclavian artery
RSVC, right superior vena cava
RUL, right upper lobe of lung
RUPV, right upper pulmonary vein
RV, right ventricle
RVOT, right ventricular outflow tract
S, septal
S, spleen (Fig. 2.7 only)
SB, septal band
SN, sinus node
St, stomach
STL, septal tricuspid leaflet
Sup, superior
SVC, superior vena cava
TA, truncal artery
TO, tricuspid orifice
Tr, trachea
TV, tricuspid valve
V, ventricle
VS, ventricular septum
VFO, valve of fossa ovalis

References

1. Scholz DG, Kitzman DW, Hagen PT, et al. Age-related changes in normal human hearts during the first 10 decades of life. Part I (Growth): A quantitative anatomic study of 200 specimens from subjects from birth to 19 years old. *Mayo Clin Proc* 1988;63:126–136.

2. Kitzman DW, Scholz DG, Hagen PT, et al. Age-related changes in normal human hearts during the first 10 decades of life. Part II (Maturity): A quantitative anatomic study of 765 specimens from subjects 20 to 99 years old. *Mayo Clin Proc* 1988;63:137–146.

3. Harmon JV Jr, Edwards WD. Venous valves in subclavian and internal jugular veins: Frequency, position, and structure in 100 autopsy cases. *Am J Cardiovasc Pathol* 1987;1:51–54.

4. Sweeney LJ, Rosenquist GC. The normal anatomy of the atrial septum in the human heart. *Am Heart J* 1979;98:194–199.

5. Hutchins GM, Moore GW, Jones JF, et al. Postnatal endocardial fibroelastosis of the valve of the foramen ovale. *Am J Cardiol* 1981;47:90–94.

6. Hagen PT, Scholz DG, Edwards WD. Incidence and size of patent foramen ovale during the first 10 decades of life: An autopsy study of 965 normal hearts. *Mayo Clin Proc* 1984;59:17–20.

7. Zimmerman KG, Paplanus SH, Dong S, et al. Congenital blood cysts of the heart valves. *Hum Pathol* 1983;14:699–703.

8. Seccombe JF, Cahill DR, Edwards WD. Quantitative morphology of normal human tricuspid valve: Autopsy study of 24 cases. *Clin Anat* 1993;6:203–212.

9. Roberts WC. Morphologic features of the normal and abnormal mitral valve. *Am J Cardiol* 1983;51:1005–1028.

10. Becker AE, de Wit APM. Mitral valve apparatus: A spectrum of normality relevant to mitral valve prolapse. *Br Heart J* 1979;42:680–689.

11. Tei C, Pilgrim JP, Shah PM, et al. The tricuspid valve annulus: Study of size and motion in normal subjects and in patients with tricuspid regurgitation. *Circulation* 1982;66:665–671.

12. Restivo A, Smith A, Wilkinson JL, et al. Normal variations in the relationship of the tricuspid valve to the membranous septum in the human heart. *Anat Rec* 1990;226:258–263.

13. Ormiston JA, Shah PM, Tei C, et al. Size and motion of the mitral valve annulus in man. I: A two-dimensional echocardiographic method and findings in normal subjects. *Circulation* 1981;64:113–120.

14. Ranganathan N, Lam JHC, Wigle ED, et al. Morphology of the human mitral valve. II: The valve leaflets. *Circulation* 1970;41:459–467.

15. Lam JHC, Ranganathan N, Wigle ED, et al. Morphology of the human mitral valve. I: Chordae tendineae: A new classification. *Circulation* 1970;41:449–458.

16. Shiina A, Seward JB, Tajik AJ, et al. Two-dimensional echocardiographic–surgical correlation in Ebstein's anomaly: Preoperative determination of patients requiring tricuspid valve plication vs replacement. *Circulation* 1983;68:534–544.

17. Prakash R, Umali SA. Comparison of echocardiographic and necropsy measurements of left ventricular wall thickness in patients with coronary artery disease. *Am J Cardiol* 1984;53:838–841.

18. Hagler DJ, Edwards WD, Seward JB, et al. Standardized nomenclature of the ventricular septum and ventricular septal defects, with applications for two-dimensional echocardiography. *Mayo Clin Proc* 1985;60:741–752.

19. Hutchins GM, Bulkley BH, Moore GW, et al. Shape of the human cardiac ventricles. *Am J Cardiol* 1978;41:646–654.

20. Wafae N, Warde M, Vieira MC. Morphologic study of one septal trabecula carnea of the left ventricle. *Bull Assoc Anat (Nancy)* 1990;74:33–36.

21. Draulens-Noe HA, Wenink AC. Anterolateral muscle bundle of the left ventricle in atrioventricular septal defect: Left ventricular outflow tract and subaortic stenosis. *Pediatr Cardiol* 1991;12:183–188.

22. Edwards WD. Pathology of pulmonary hypertension. *Cardiovasc Clin* 1988;18:321–359.

23. Cudkowicz L. Bronchial arterial circulation in man: Normal anatomy and responses to disease. *Lung Biol Health Dis* 1979;14:111–232.

24. Silver MM, Freedom RM, Silver MD, et al. The morphology of the human newborn ductus arteriosus: A reappraisal of its structure and closure with special reference to prostaglandin E1 therapy. *Hum Pathol* 1981;12:1123–1136.

25. Edwards BS, Edwards WD, Edwards JE. Aortic origin of conus coronary artery: Evidence of postnatal coronary development. *Br Heart J* 1981;45:555–558.

26. Kramer JR, Kitazume H, Proudfit WL, et al. Clinical significance of isolated coronary bridges: Benign and frequent condition involving the left anterior descending artery. *Am Heart J* 1982;103:283–288.

27. Miller AJ. *Lymphatics of the Heart*. New York: Raven Press, 1982:107–180, 318–325.

28. Ferrans VJ, Rodriguez ER. Ultrastructure of the normal heart. In: Silver MD, ed. *Cardiovascular Pathology*. New York: Churchill Livingstone, 1991:43–101.

29. Abdulla AK, Frustaci A, Martinez JE, et al. Echocardiography and pathology of left ventricular "false tendons." *Chest* 1990;98:129–132.

30. Layman TE, Edwards JE. A method for dissection of the heart and major pulmonary vessels. *Arch Pathol* 1966;82:314–320.

31. Seward JB, Khandheria BK, Freeman WK, et al. Multiplane transesophageal echocardiography: Image orientation, examination technique, anatomic correlations, and clinical applications. *Mayo Clin Proc* 1993;68:523–551.

32. Ackermann DM, Edwards WD. Anatomic basis for tomographic analysis of the pediatric heart at autopsy. *Perspect Pediatr Pathol* 1988;12:44–68.

33. Edwards WD. Photography of medical specimens: Experiences from teaching cardiovascular pathology. *Mayo Clin Proc* 1988;63:42–57.

CHAPTER 2 ■ CLASSIFICATION AND TERMINOLOGY OF CARDIOVASCULAR ANOMALIES

WILLIAM D. EDWARDS, MD

PERSPECTIVES ON NOMENCLATURE

Through 5,000 years of recorded human history, only during the past 50 have treatments become available to substantially improve the quality of life and increase the longevity of children with cardiac anomalies. Within these 50 years, diagnostic and interventional procedures have been developed that have defined the frontiers of medical technology and creativity. During these exciting and innovative times, however, seeds were also sown, in the form of redundant and overlapping terminology, that have inadvertently led to difficulty and confusion for those interested in the subject of congenital heart disease.

Diversity of Terminology

Drawings and descriptions of malformed hearts date back to the eighteenth century, and in the mid-nineteenth century Peacock published 18 cases in his classic series (1). However, it is the categorization of 1,000 malformed hearts by Dr. Maude E. Abbott at McGill University, published by the American Heart Association in 1936, that stands as a landmark in the classification of congenital heart disease (2). Since that time, others have examined large numbers of cases, both from autopsies and from living patients, and have proposed different systems of classification and nomenclature (3–13). Furthermore, numerous classifications have been adopted for individual anomalies, such as ventricular septal defects, and for groups of anomalies, such as hearts with univentricular atrioventricular connections.

Each new system, however, has reflected not only the state of knowledge at the time of its formulation, but also the particular interests or biases of its creators. Thus, among the various classifications, some researchers have emphasized surgical anatomy, some embryogenesis, others spatial relationships such as atrial sidedness and the positions of ventricles and great arteries, and still others clinical features such as cyanosis and altered pulmonary blood flow. Not surprisingly, the introduction of new systems of classification has been attended by changes in terminology, primarily to clarify or simplify certain concepts. But as newer terms have been introduced, older terms have rarely been abandoned. As a result, the nomenclature for congenital heart disease has become a sea of synonyms, adding confusion rather than clarity to an already complex subject (Appendix 2.1).

Unity from Diversity

Is the development of a unified system of nomenclature a realistic and worthwhile goal? If so, who should decide on the acceptable terminology? And what price will be paid to gain unity at the expense of diversity? Although such a system would limit the confusing number of synonyms that now exist, it also could limit our perspective as certain terms (such as those with an embryologic basis) are purged from our rich and diverse heritage.

Nevertheless, a movement is already well underway to establish such a unified system. Uniform acceptance, however, will probably be achieved only following the publication of a consensus report from an international group that represents all disciplines dealing with congenital heart disease. To date, such attempts have met with only limited success (14). The system that is eventually chosen should be accurately descriptive, internally consistent, clinically usable, readily codable in a database, and applicable to all forms of congenital heart disease. New terms should be accepted only if they are necessary, brief, and specific (3).

Until such a consensus report is available, it is premature to endorse a specific system of nomenclature. However, at least at an institutional level, those dealing with patients having congenital heart disease should agree to speak the same clinical language and to prescribe to a single system of terminology. For this chapter, the approach and terminology suggested by Anderson et al. (4) are emphasized, with some modifications. For commonly used Latin terms, their anglicized counterparts are also provided in parentheses—for example, ductus arteriosus (ductal artery), and these are also listed in Appendix 2.2.

Although the notation system proposed by Van Praagh (3) is not emphasized in this chapter, it is favored at some institutions and warrants summarization. The situs (sidedness) is determined separately for the atria, ventricles, and great arteries. Atrial situs may be solitus (S), inversus (I), or ambiguous (A). Ventricular situs is solitus or D-loop (D), inversus or L-loop (L), or ambiguous (X). Great arterial situs is designated as solitus (S), inversus (I), D-transposition/malposition (D), L-transposition/malposition (L), or ambiguous or anterior transposition/malposition (A). Abbreviations are listed within the parentheses, with the ventriculoarterial arrangement included before the parentheses and any atrioventricular malalignments or other anomalies stated after the parentheses. Thus, TGA {S,D,D} would correspond to complete transposition of the great arteries.

SEQUENTIAL SEGMENTAL ANALYSIS

For evaluating patients with suspected congenital heart disease, it is helpful to consider the heart as a segmented structure represented by three regions—atria, ventricles, and great arteries (3–6). Each region, in turn, is partitioned into two components, usually right-sided and left-sided. Atrioventricular valves serve as connectors between atria and ventricles, and semilunar valves join the ventricles to the great arteries. There are only a limited number of possible connections between the three major regions, regardless of their spatial orientations. In practice, each region is evaluated independently, following the direction of blood flow: (a) systemic and pulmonary veins, (b) atria, (c) atrioventricular valves, (d) ventricles and right ventricular outflow tract (infundibulum or conus), (e) semilunar valves, and (f) great arteries.

In a systematic manner, right-sided and left-sided structures at each level are evaluated according to their morphology, their relative positions, their connections to proximal and distal segments, and the presence and location of shunts, obstructions, and valvular regurgitation (7). This constitutes the sequential segmental method for the investigation of congenital heart disease, and it represents a diagnostic cornerstone both for clinicians and for pathologists. Before applying this method, however, it is important to determine the cardiac position and the visceral situs (sidedness).

CARDIAC POSITION

With regard to the position of the heart in the chest, two questions arise that can be answered independently: Where is the heart located, and what is the direction of the cardiac apex? Unfortunately, the terms levocardia, dextrocardia, and mesocardia are commonly used to answer both questions, thus imparting an element of ambiguity (3,4). Although the approach described below is not universally accepted, it does provide clarity by defining the cardiac location and apical direction separately and by avoiding the ambiguous Latin terms.

Location in the Chest

Within the thorax, the heart can be described positionally as left-sided (normal), right-sided, or midline. This designation is particularly useful radiographically, before a patient has been evaluated by other imaging techniques.

The position of the heart in the mediastinum is affected not only by underlying cardiac malformations but also by abnormalities in adjacent structures. It can be displaced by conditions that distort the shape of the thorax, such as severe scoliosis or an elevated diaphragm, or that alter the size of thoracic structures, such as a hypoplastic lung or diaphragmatic hernia. Rightward displacement of the heart constitutes dextroposition, a leftward shift represents levoposition, and shifts toward the midline are called mesoposition.

In rare instances, sternal or diaphragmatic defects exist and are associated with an extrathoracic heart, or ectopia cordis (ectopic heart). This condition may be partial or complete and can be further categorized as cervical, thoracocervical, thoracic, thoracoabdominal, or abdominal.

Orientation in the Chest

The direction in which the ventricles are aligned defines the base–apex axis of the heart and may be leftward, rightward, or midline (Figs. 2.1 and 2.2). Leftward ventricles represent the normal state and are characterized by an apex that is directed leftward, anteriorly, and somewhat inferiorly. The extent of these three directions is variable and is influenced by age, body build, and the level and functional state of the diaphragm. Ventricles with a rightward apex are directed to the right of midline. In contrast, midline ventricles are often box shaped and exhibit two apexes that are directed anteriorly and inferiorly (7).

The base–apex axis is independent of cardiac location and displacements. For example, a patient with a hypoplastic right lung could have a right-sided heart, owing to dextroposition, and still exhibit a leftward apex (Fig. 2.1B).

The base–apex axis is also independent of cardiac sidedness. Thus, the presence of a leftward apex does not necessarily imply situs solitus (normal sidedness), and a right-sided apex does not always coincide with situs inversus (mirror-image sidedness). A midline apex, on the other hand, usually is associated with situs ambiguus (cardiac isomerism).

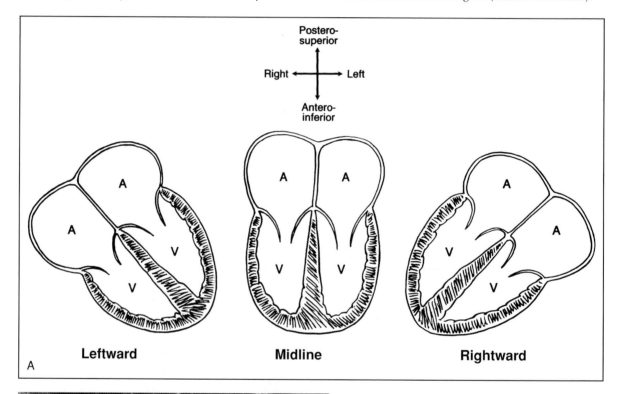

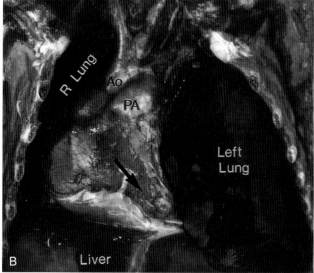

FIGURE 2.1 Cardiac base–apex axis. **A:** The three types are shown schematically and are independent of cardiac position or situs. **B:** The ventricular apex is leftward (*arrow*), even though a hypoplastic right lung has caused dextroposition of the entire heart. (See Appendix 1.1 for abbreviations.)

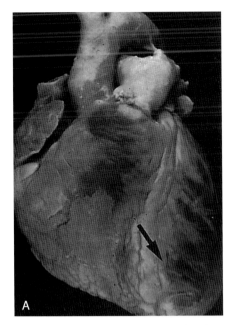 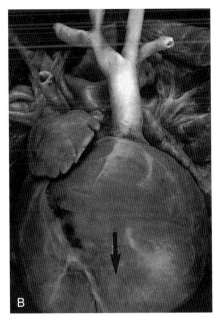 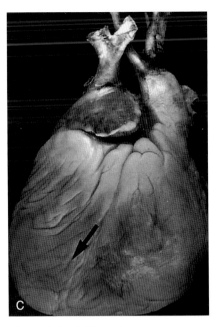

FIGURE 2.2 Cardiac base–apex axis (*arrows*) shown in three specimens, viewed anteriorly. **A:** Normal heart, with a leftward apex. **B** and **C:** Congenitally corrected transposition of the great arteries, showing a box-shaped midline apex (**B**) and a rightward apex (**C**).

VISCERAL SITUS (SIDEDNESS)

All major organ systems begin their embryologic development as midline structures with bilateral mirror-image symmetry. However, three organ systems (cardiovascular, respiratory, and digestive) later acquire asymmetry and are thereby characterized by situs (sidedness or handedness), which appears to be genetically determined. Situs may be solitus (normal), inversus (mirror-image), or ambiguus (isomeric or indeterminate). Right isomerism indicates bilateral right-sidedness, whereas left isomerism denotes bilateral left-sidedness.

Isomerism and Splenic Anomalies

The relationship between isomerism and splenic anomalies is intriguing (8). The splenic anlage, rather than originating as a midline structure, appears to be left-sided from its inception. Thus, when right isomerism exists, the spleen is usually absent (asplenia). Left isomerism, in contrast, is generally associated with multiple spleens (polysplenia) that are confined to only one side of the vertebral column. Occasionally, subjects with asplenia or polysplenia have normal hearts, and, rarely, those with atrial isomerism have normal spleens.

Abnormalities may affect the entire body, as in situs inversus totalis (total mirror-image sidedness), or can involve individual organ systems. Moreover, situs may vary between systems, particularly in conditions associated with isomerism. Although the term atriovisceral situs enjoys common usage, it does not always allow an accurate description of sidedness in the asplenia and polysplenia syndromes. Consequently, it is recommended that the situs of cardiovascular, respiratory, and digestive systems be designated separately (7).

Cardiac Situs (Sidedness)

Cardiac situs is determined by the position of the morphologic right atrium (Fig. 2.3). It is not determined by the direction of the cardiac apex, the positions of the ventricles or great arteries, or the sidedness of noncardiac viscera. The morphologic right atrium is normally right-sided but is left-sided in situs inversus. Bilateral right atria define right cardiac isomerism, and bilateral left atria constitute left cardiac isomerism (Fig. 2.4) (14). In some cases of polysplenia, one chamber represents a left atrium, but the other has a hybrid appearance that is morphologically neither left nor right; this constitutes indeterminate cardiac sidedness. In practice, an accurate determination of cardiac situs depends on an accurate distinction between right and left atrial morphology, as discussed in this chapter and in Chapter 1. Although all investigators agree on the concept of normal and mirror-image cardiac sidedness, some have questioned the existence of atrial isomerism (9).

Pulmonary Situs (Sidedness)

Pulmonary situs is determined by the positions of the morphologic right and left lungs (Fig. 2.5). Pulmonary morphology, in turn, is defined by the relationship of the pulmonary arteries to their adjacent bronchi, and not by the number of lobes. The pulmonary artery of a morphologic right lung travels anterior to its upper and intermediate bronchi, whereas that of a morphologic left lung travels over its main bronchus and posterior to the upper lobe bronchus.

Clinically, pulmonary situs may be inferred by comparing the relative lengths of the two main bronchi, as measured on a chest radiograph that shows an air bronchogram. Normally, the distance from the carina to the origin of the upper lobe bronchus is 1.5 to 2.5 times greater for the morphologic

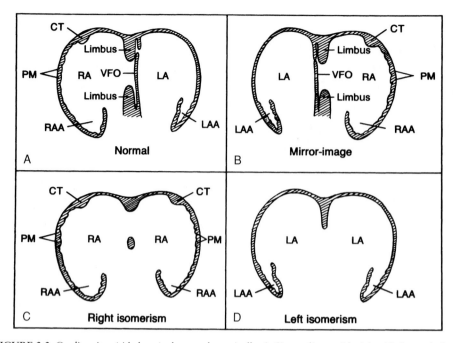

FIGURE 2.3 Cardiac situs (sidedness), shown schematically. **A:** Situs solitus, with right-sided morphologic right atrium. **B:** Situs inversus, with left-sided morphologic right atrium. **C** and **D:** Situs ambiguus, with bilateral morphologic right atria (**C**) and bilateral morphologic left atria (**D**). (See Appendix 1.1 for abbreviations.)

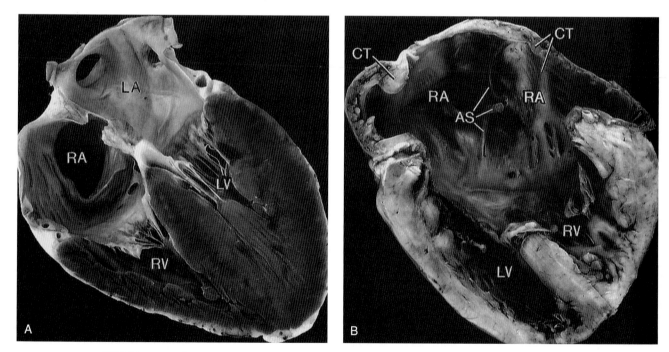

FIGURE 2.4 Cardiac situs in two specimens, displayed in the four-chamber format. **A:** Situs solitus (normal cardiac sidedness). **B:** Situs ambiguus, with right isomerism. A crista terminalis is present bilaterally. Ventricular inversion is also present but plays no role in determining cardiac sidedness. (See Appendix 1.1 for abbreviations.)

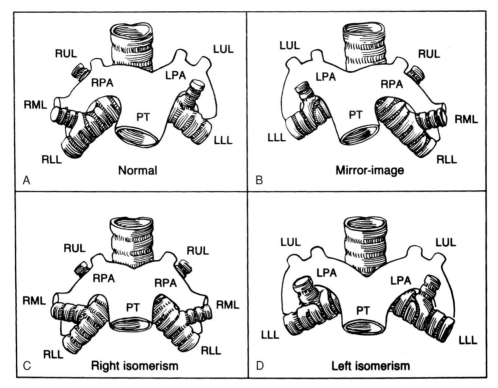

FIGURE 2.5 Pulmonary situs (sidedness), shown schematically. **A:** Situs solitus, with right pulmonary anterior to its upper lobe bronchus and with left pulmonary artery posterior to its upper lobe bronchus. **B:** Situs inversus, with mirror-image morphology. **C** and **D:** Situs ambiguus, with bilateral morphologic right lungs (**C**) and bilateral morphologic left lungs (**D**). (See Appendix 1.1 for abbreviations.)

left lung than for the right lung, and this ratio holds true regardless of the sidedness of the aortic arch (which is determined by the bronchus over which the aorta travels) (10). With pulmonary isomerism, this ratio approaches unity because the lengths of the two mirror-image bronchi are similar (Fig. 2.6).

Although most examples of bilateral trilobed lungs do correspond to cases of right isomerism or asplenia, bilateral bilobed lungs more often occur as a variation of normal morphology than as a manifestation of left isomerism or polysplenia.

Abdominal Situs (Sidedness)

Abdominal situs is determined by the location of the liver and stomach, with the spleen and pancreas generally on the same side of the vertebral column as the stomach (Fig. 2.7). The state of the spleen can be evaluated by clinical imaging, thus supplanting the less reliable method of identifying Howell-Jolly bodies in peripheral blood smears. At autopsy, splenic morphology should always be designated in patients with congenital heart disease.

In the asplenia syndrome, the liver is commonly midline with two mirror-image right lobes (right hepatic isomerism), and the biliary tree is patent and is usually associated with a single gallbladder (Fig. 2.8). The position of the stomach and pancreas can be left-sided, right-sided, or midline. Malrotation of the bowel is the rule, such that the cecum and appendix

may be located in any of the abdominal quadrants. Finally, the aorta and inferior vena cava travel together on the same side of the vertebral column, a unique feature that can be demonstrated by abdominal imaging.

Interestingly, with the polysplenia syndrome, the situs of the abdominal viscera may be ambiguus (indeterminate), inversus (mirror-image), or even solitus (normal). Although the spleens are multiple, they are all located on the same side of the vertebral column as the stomach. The gallbladder is single, but biliary atresia may occur. As a rule, the inferior vena cava fails to join the heart directly and exhibits azygos continuation, with connection to the superior vena cava.

MORPHOLOGY OF CARDIAC SEGMENTS

Accurate identification of right-sided and left-sided structures is an essential feature of the sequential segmental approach to the diagnosis of congenital heart disease. For consistency and reproducibility of diagnoses, definitions of even the most commonly used terms are helpful.

In this regard, a distinction between the terms connection and drainage is necessary because the two are not synonymous. *Connection* is an anatomic term that implies a direct link between two structures. In contrast, *drainage* is a hemodynamic term that refers to the direction of blood flow.

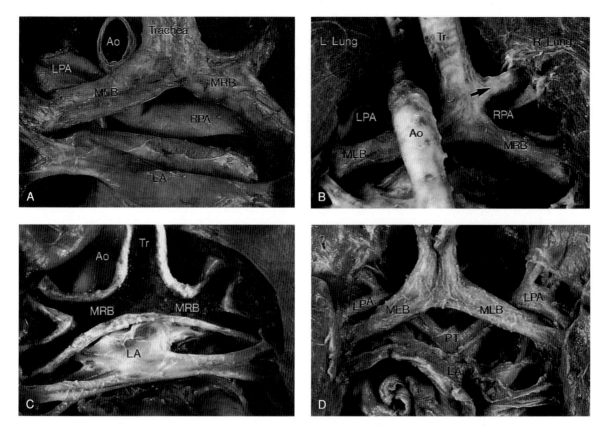

FIGURE 2.6 Pulmonary situs in four specimens, viewed posteriorly. **A:** Normal situs, with long left bronchus and short right bronchus. **B:** Normal situs, with tracheal origin of the right upper lobe bronchus (bronchus suis) (*arrow*). **C:** Right pulmonary isomerism, with short bronchi of similar length (the posterior wall of the airways has been removed). **D:** Left pulmonary isomerism, with long bronchi of similar length. (See Appendix 1.1 for abbreviations.)

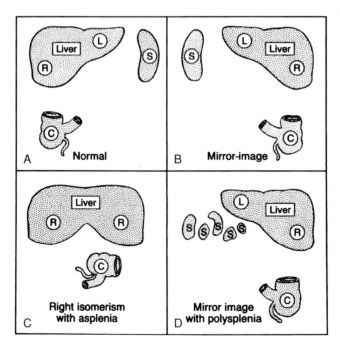

FIGURE 2.7 Abdominal situs (sidedness), drawn schematically. **A:** Situs solitus, with right-sided liver, left-sided spleen (also stomach and pancreas, not shown), and cecum in right lower quadrant. **B:** Situs inversus, with mirror-image morphology. **C:** Situs ambiguus with right isomerism shows liver with two right lobes, malrotation of the bowel (indicated by the abnormal position of the cecum), and asplenia. **D:** Situs ambiguus with left isomerism shows polysplenia; other features are variable. (See Appendix 1.1 for abbreviations.)

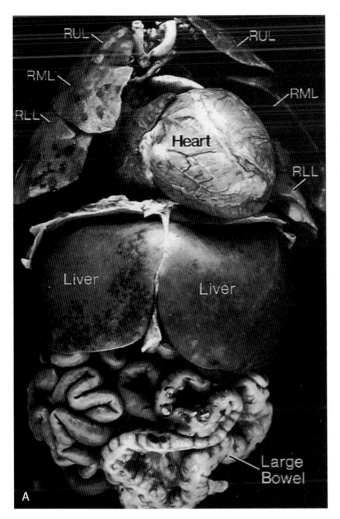
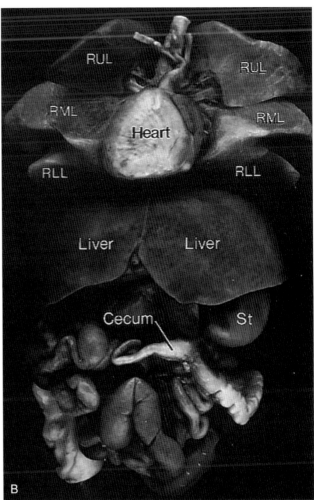

FIGURE 2.8 Abdominal situs in two patients, with thoracoabdominal organs viewed anteriorly. **A** and **B:** Both patients had the asplenia syndrome, with right isomerism of the heart, lungs, and abdominal organs. Both exhibit a midline symmetric liver and malrotation of the bowel (with the small bowel to the right and the large bowel to the left). (As an aside, cardiac situs is not affected by the cardiac base–apex axis, which is leftward in **A** and rightward in **B**.) (See Appendix 1.1 for abbreviations.)

A distinction also should be drawn between single and common, as applied to cardiac chambers and valves. *Single* implies that the corresponding contralateral structure is entirely absent. Tricuspid atresia with a single-inlet ventricle is one example. In contrast, the term *common* indicates bilateral components with absent septation. Examples are a common atrium, a common atrioventricular valve, and a common truncal artery (truncus arteriosus).

Superior Vena Cava (Superior Caval Vein)

When the superior vena cava is single and right-sided, as normally occurs, no further designation is necessary. The term left superior vena cava is recommended for its left-sided counterpart, and distinction should be made between right-sided and left-sided structures in the setting of bilateral venae cavae. With bilateral veins, the presence or absence of a brachiocephalic, or innominate, venous bridge between the two should also be described.

Inferior Vena Cava (Inferior Caval Vein)

The inferior vena cava, or at least its suprahepatic segment, almost invariably connects to the inferior aspect of the morphologic right atrium. Rarely, and usually in patients with polysplenia, this connection is interrupted, and the vein empties into the superior vena cava through a direct connection with the azygos or hemiazygos vein, representing azygos continuation of the inferior vena cava. In such cases, the hepatic veins generally connect directly to one or both atria via the suprahepatic segment of the inferior vena cava (9).

Coronary Sinus

The coronary sinus normally joins the right atrium. Rarely, its ostium is atretic. Moreover, variable portions of the vein may be unroofed and produce a left atrial fistula. Complete unroofing is commonly referred to as absence of the coronary sinus and is often associated with asplenia and direct left atrial connection of a left superior vena cava.

Pulmonary Veins

Normally, the four pulmonary veins join the body of the left atrium separately. As a variant of normal, the upper and lower veins, most commonly from the left lung, merge and connect to the left atrium as a single vein. Another variant is independent connection of the right middle lobar vein directly to the left atrium.

In the setting of anomalous pulmonary venous connection or severe left-sided obstructive lesions, a vessel connecting the pulmonary veins to the left brachiocephalic, or innominate, vein has been referred to as a persistent superior vena cava, vertical vein, or a levo-atrial cardinal vein. For these anomalies, perhaps the term collateral vein would suffice (analogous to collateral arteries in cases of pulmonary atresia with ventricular septal defect).

Atria

Definition

By definition, an atrium is a cardiac receiving chamber that usually is interposed between the great veins and an atrioventricular valve. Occasionally, it may exist either between the great veins and an adjacent atrium, as in tricuspid atresia or cor triatriatum (triatrial heart), or between an atrium and an atrioventricular valve, as in total anomalous pulmonary venous connection. Triatrial hearts can be described as having a subdivided left atrium, a double-chamber left atrium, or an accessory left atrial chamber. Rarely, the right atrium is subdivided by an enlarged valve of the inferior vena cava.

Right Atrium

The morphologic right atrium is characterized by connections from the venae cavae and coronary sinus and by connections to one or both atrioventricular valves, with drainage into one or both ventricles. Its septal surface is defined by an interatrial portion, with the limbus and valve of the fossa ovalis (oval fossa), and by an atrioventricular portion. The free wall harbors not only a large pyramidal appendage, but also a crista terminalis (terminal crest) and numerous pectinate muscles outside the appendage (11). The terminal crest forms a boundary between the smooth-walled posterior aspect of the free wall, derived from the sinus venosus, and the muscular anterior aspect, derived from the embryologic right atrium.

Left Atrium

In contrast, the morphologic left atrium has neither a crista terminalis nor pectinate muscles. Its appendage is more finger-shaped than pyramidal, with several small outpouchings or lobes. The main body of the left atrium is smooth walled, like the common pulmonary vein from which it is derived, and only the appendage remains as a remnant of the embryologic atrium. The left side of the atrial septum is entirely interatrial. Its smooth surface is interrupted only by a crescentic rim that forms the residual border of the ostium secundum.

Common Atrium

A common atrium is the result of absence, or near absence, of the atrial septum. It almost always is associated with an atrioventricular septal defect, with or without asplenia. In most cases, a characteristic band or bar of myocardium spans the midportion of the atrium as the only septal remnant. The two atrial free walls can be morphologically right and left, or they may be bilaterally right or bilaterally left.

Indeterminate Atrial Morphology

Occasionally, atrial morphology may be impossible to determine with certainty. This most often occurs in patients with asplenia or polysplenia syndromes. With polysplenia in particular, one atrium often has a hybrid structure with some anatomic features of each atrium. In addition, previous surgical procedures with ligation of the atrial appendages or excision of the atrial septum may so distort the chambers that determination of atrial morphology is impossible.

Diagnostic Criteria

From a practical standpoint, the most reliable anatomic criteria for distinguishing morphologic right and left atria are the connection of the inferior vena cava, the presence of a large pyramidal appendage, and identification of the limbus of the fossa ovalis, all of which are indicative of a morphologic right atrium (10) (Fig. 2.9). In complex cases, particularly if the atrial septum is absent, it is recommended that a combination of anatomic structures be examined rather than relying on only one of the above criteria. Morphologic features of the atrial appendages can be assessed angiographically, and those of the atrial septum can be evaluated echocardiographically. The atrial connection of the inferior vena cava can be determined by either method. In addition, all three structures are accessible to direct inspection by surgeons and pathologists.

Atrioventricular Valves

Definition

Atrioventricular valves are fibrous tissue flaps that not only connect the atria to the ventricles but also serve to separate them electrically. Because the valves tend to travel with their respective ventricles, a morphologic tricuspid valve almost invariably connects to a morphologic right ventricle, and a morphologic mitral valve connects to a morphologic left ventricle. In normal hearts, viewed in a four-chamber format, the tricuspid valve ring attaches to the septum more apically than does the mitral annulus (Fig. 2.9). Identification of this arrangement by clinical imaging allows determination not only of atrioventricular valve morphology, but also of ventricular morphology.

Tricuspid Valve

The normal tricuspid valve consists of three leaflets, three major commissures, and three papillary muscles. Although its annulus is elliptical, the shape of its orifice at the midleaflet (or midventricular) level is more triangular. The septal tricuspid leaflet has numerous direct cordal insertions along the ventricular septum, and the anterior leaflet forms an intracavitary curtain that separates the inflow and outflow tracts. Additionally, the tricuspid and pulmonary valves are separated by the muscular right ventricular outflow tract (infundibulum or conus).

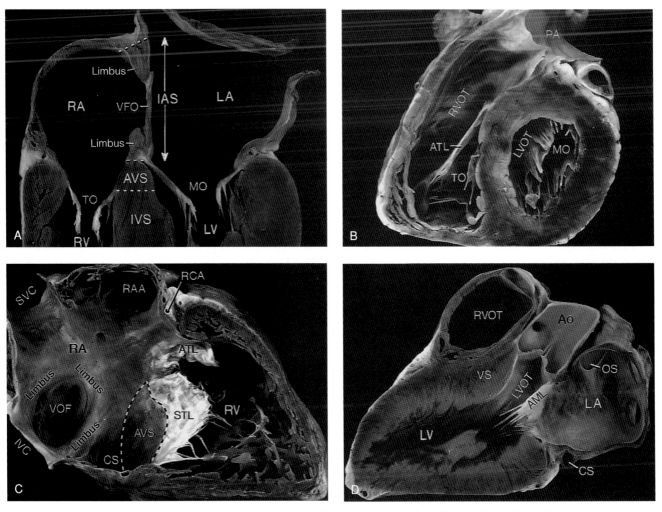

FIGURE 2.9 Characteristic anatomic features of atria, atrioventricular valves, and ventricles in four specimens of normal hearts. **A:** The atrioventricular septum and the more apical attachment of the tricuspid valve ring, compared with the mitral valve, are best evaluated in a four-chamber view. **B:** The triangular tricuspid orifice and elliptical mitral orifice, at midleaflet level, are shown in a short-axis view, as are the septal insertions of tendinous cords from the septal tricuspid leaflet. **C** and **D:** Right-sided and left-sided features can readily be compared between a two-chamber view of the right heart (**C**) and a long-axis view of the left heart (**D**). (See Appendix 1.1 for abbreviations.)

Mitral Valve

Like the tricuspid valve, the mitral valve has an elliptical annulus and an intracavitary anterior leaflet that separates the inflow and outflow tracts. However, the mitral valve has only two leaflets, two major commissures, and two papillary muscle groups rather than three, and because the papillary muscles attach to the left ventricular free wall, there are normally no septal insertions of tendinous cords. Moreover, in contrast to the muscular separation that exists between the tricuspid and pulmonary valves, the mitral annulus is in direct continuity with the aortic valve ring, such that the anterior mitral leaflet forms a part of the left ventricular outflow tract.

Common Atrioventricular Valve

With complete atrioventricular septal defects, the presence of a common valve, rather than distinct tricuspid and mitral

valves, renders four-chamber imaging unsuitable for determining ventricular morphology. Similarly, in partial atrioventricular septal defects, the mitral valve ring generally attaches to the septum at the same level as the tricuspid annulus, producing an interatrial septal defect and interfering with the identification of ventricular morphology.

Right and Left Atrioventricular Valves

A double-inlet left ventricle is characterized by papillary muscle insertions from both atrioventricular valves into the morphologic left ventricle. In many cases, the valves have mirror-image mitral morphology or one of the valves has indeterminate, or hybrid, morphology with mitral and tricuspid features. Designation simply as right-sided or left-sided atrioventricular valves rather than as mitral, tricuspid, or hybrid minimizes the likelihood of confusion.

Diagnostic Criteria

The most reliable feature that allows distinction between tricuspid and mitral valves is the more apical septal attachment of the tricuspid valve when viewed in a four-chamber format. For conditions in which this cannot be assessed, other features should be assessed, including septal cordal attachments, indicative of a tricuspid valve, and direct continuity with a semilunar valve, indicative of a mitral valve.

Ventricles

Definition

A ventricle represents an endocardial-lined chamber within the ventricular muscle mass. Other proposed definitions have been a source of disagreement and controversy (12,13). Although normal ventricles are characterized by inlet, trabecular, and outlet regions, they are not defined by the presence of all three or by the presence of any one in particular. Hypoplastic ventricles, as described below, frequently consist of only one or two components. It is important to emphasize that, with only rare exceptions, virtually all human hearts contain two ventricular chambers. Hence, the terms single ventricle and univentricular heart are inaccurate.

Right Ventricle

A morphologic right ventricle is characterized by a heavily trabeculated anteroapical region (4). Other definitive features relate to the inlet region and the anatomic details of the tricuspid valve, as discussed earlier. The normal right ventricular outflow tract (infundibulum or conus) represents a collar of muscle that separates the tricuspid and pulmonary valves. Rarely, in the case of a double-outlet left ventricle, the infundibular region may originate entirely from the contralateral ventricle. To conceptualize this and other conotruncal anomalies, the heart may be considered as consisting of five chambers (two atria, two ventricles, and an infundibulum) in which the infundibulum can attach to one or both ventricles, in various orientations (15).

Left Ventricle

A morphologic left ventricle has fine apical trabeculations. However, in patients with a double-inlet left ventricle, the presence of four sets of papillary muscles produces a muscular apex that can be misinterpreted as a morphologic right ventricle, particularly by echocardiography.

Common Ventricle

A common ventricle is characterized by virtual absence of the ventricular septum and by a free wall that morphologically is part right ventricle and part left ventricle. This represents an exceedingly rare condition. Accordingly, other anomalies that resemble a common ventricle should be considered before rendering a diagnosis. Among patients with a common-inlet right ventricle, the hypoplastic left ventricle may be so diminutive that it is difficult to identify even at autopsy and may lead to a misdiagnosis of common ventricle.

Ventricular Morphology

If ventricular morphology cannot be determined with confidence, the term indeterminate may be applied. This designation is usually reserved for the rare condition in which only one ventricular chamber can be identified. Such a chamber has either ambiguous morphologic features (a true single ventricle) or right and left ventricular free walls with an absent ventricular septum (a true common ventricle).

Hypoplastic Ventricle

Underdeveloped ventricles have an appreciably smaller chamber size than expected, although their muscular walls may either be normal in thickness or hypertrophied, depending on the pressures generated within the chamber. Structurally, either they exhibit inlet, trabecular, and outlet components or they are deficient and consist of only one or two of these regions.

In the setting of tricuspid or mitral atresia, for example, the inlet portion of the affected ventricle is either absent or very diminutive. Similarly, with pulmonary or aortic atresia, the outlet region is usually incompletely formed. For combined tricuspid and pulmonary atresia or combined mitral and aortic atresia, the interposed ventricle is severely hypoplastic and generally consists primarily of a trabecular component.

A hypoplastic ventricle that is positioned along the anterosuperior surface of the heart and gives rise to a great artery is virtually always a morphologic right ventricle. Conversely, a small chamber that occupies the posteroinferior aspect of the heart and does not connect to a great artery is almost invariably a morphologic left ventricle. Thus, the use of terms such as outlet chamber, trabecular pouch, and rudimentary chamber is probably unnecessary.

Criteria

In practice, the most reliable features that allow distinction between morphologic right and left ventricles are the nature of the apical trabeculations, the morphology of the associated atrioventricular valve, and the state of continuity between the atrioventricular and semilunar valves (Fig. 2.9). Even in the setting of a hypoplastic ventricle, the other ventricle should be assessable at all three levels. Trabeculations and valvular discontinuity can be determined angiographically, and valvular morphology and discontinuity are readily evaluated echocardiographically.

In normal hearts, the short-axis shapes and wall thicknesses of the ventricles differ appreciably. The left ventricle has a thick wall and a circular chamber, whereas the right ventricle is thin walled and more crescent shaped. Neither of these features, though, is reliable for distinguishing ventricular morphology. Right ventricular hypertrophy or left ventricular atrophy is encountered relatively frequently and produces either ventricles of similar thickness or a thick right ventricle and thin left ventricle, respectively. Likewise, straightening or leftward bowing of the ventricular septum may occur and result in mirror-image D-shaped chambers or a crescentic left ventricle, respectively.

Semilunar Valves

A semilunar valve serves to connect a ventricle to a great artery and is named according to the artery into which it empties. It is not named according to the ventricle from which it emanates or according to its relative position in the chest. Semilunar valves include aortic, pulmonary, and truncal valves. Normal semilunar valves consist of three pocketlike cusps, three commissures, and a fibrous annulus shaped like a triradiate crown. When malformed, they can have an abnormal number of

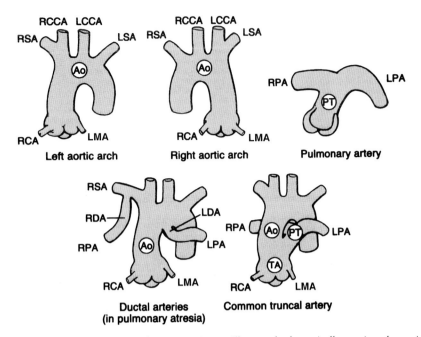

FIGURE 2.10 The different types of great arteries are illustrated schematically, as viewed anteriorly. A right aortic arch travels over the right main bronchus, and its brachiocephalic branching is the mirror-image of normal. (See Appendix 1.1 for abbreviations.)

cusps, be hypoplastic or dysplastic, or exhibit a combination of these features.

Great Arteries

Definition

The great arteries include the aorta, main pulmonary artery, truncus arteriosus (truncal artery), and ductus arteriosus (ductal artery). Distinction between the aorta, pulmonary artery, and truncal artery is based solely on their branching patterns (Fig. 2.10); there are no other distinguishing features. In contrast, the identification of a ductus arteriosus is based on its position and its lack of tortuosity or branching.

Aorta

The aortic arch is normally left-sided, traveling over the left bronchus. In contrast, a right aortic arch travels over the right bronchus and is almost always associated with mirror-image brachiocephalic arterial branching. A double aortic arch, although rare, travels over both bronchi. The sidedness of the aortic arch is not associated with appreciable lengthening of the subjacent bronchus and therefore does not interfere with the radiographic determination of pulmonary situs (10). Consequently, even with a right aortic arch, the length of the right bronchus will be substantially less than that of the left bronchus.

Pulmonary Artery

The mediastinal pulmonary arteries maintain their characteristic Y shape when severely hypoplastic and occasionally even when atretic. They do not branch further before entering the lungs. Rarely, the right or left pulmonary artery anomalously arises from the ascending aorta. In contrast, the smaller bronchial arteries originate from the descending thoracic aorta, often form several branches, and course along the major bronchi to enter the lungs. Systemic collateral arteries usually have a similar origin and distribution.

Truncus Arteriosus (Common Truncal Artery)

The truncus arteriosus represents a common vessel that has not divided into the ascending aorta and main pulmonary artery. Accordingly, it gives rise to the coronary, systemic, and pulmonary circulations. In patients with pulmonary atresia and a ventricular septal defect, in whom no remnant of the main pulmonary artery can be identified, the single artery that emanates from the heart is an aorta and not a common truncus arteriosus, because the right and left pulmonary arteries do not originate from it.

Ductus Arteriosus (Ductal Artery)

The left ductus arteriosus travels between the most proximal portion of the left pulmonary artery and the undersurface of the aortic arch. In the setting of a left aortic arch, a right ductal artery, if present, will connect the proximal portion of the right subclavian artery to the right pulmonary artery. For a right aortic arch with mirror-image brachiocephalic branching, the opposite applies. Ductal arteries are not tortuous and do not form branches.

POSITIONS OF CARDIAC SEGMENTS

Once the cardiac segments are defined morphologically, their spatial orientations are next recorded. Three segments are evaluated: atria, ventricles, and great arteries. The positions of the atrioventricular and semilunar valves are addressed later when segmental connections are evaluated.

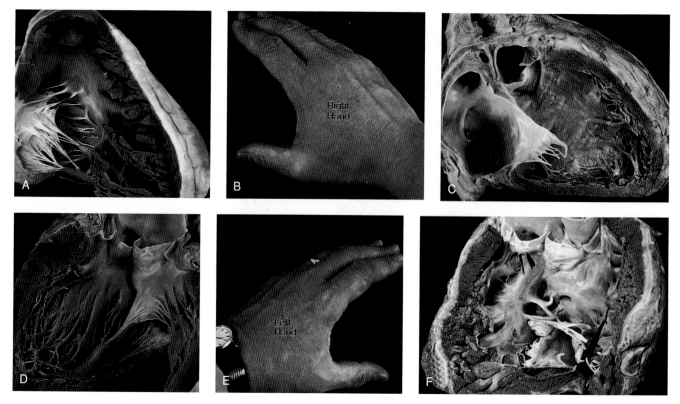

FIGURE 2.11 Ventricular sidedness (handedness). **A–C:** Right-handed ventricles. A normal right-handed morphologic right ventricle has been dissected by removal of its free wall (**A**). By analogy with a right hand, the thumb and fingers correspond to the inlet and outlet regions, respectively, and the palm of the hand represents the trabecular zone (**B**). A mirror-image right-sided (and right-handed) morphologic left ventricle is shown from a patient with atrioventricular discordance (**C**). **D–F:** Similar views are provided of a normal morphologic left ventricle (**D**), a left hand (**E**), and a mirror-image left-sided (and left-handed) morphologic right ventricle from a patient with atrioventricular discordance (**F**).

Atria

The spatial relationship between the atria is important because the position of the morphologic right atrium determines cardiac situs (Figs. 2.3 and 2.4). If the right atrium is right-sided, then the cardiac situs is solitus, or normal. On the other hand, if it is left-sided, then the situs is inversus, or mirror-image.

Ventricles

The location of the ventricles is determined by the position of the cardiac apex and the plane of the ventricular septum. In hearts with a leftward apex, the two ventricles occupy right-anterior and left-posterior positions. Conversely, with a rightward apex, they are usually right-posterior and left-anterior. A midline apex is generally characterized by a vertical midline septum with side-by-side ventricles.

For hearts with univentricular atrioventricular connections and a hypoplastic right ventricle, the ventricular septum is often tilted midway between vertical and horizontal. Rarely, the septum is horizontal, resulting in superoinferior ventricles, with the morphologic right ventricle on top. Finally, in crisscross hearts with twisted atrioventricular connections, the ventricular septum may also acquire a partial

spiral twist, such that the relative positions of the ventricular chambers change as one travels from the cardiac base toward the apex.

In each of the aforementioned positions, the ventricles may be normal or mirror image in morphology. Mirror-image ventricles have also been referred to by various researchers as l-loop ventricles, ventricular situs inversus, or ventricular inversion (3). More recently, the normal and mirror-image states have been likened to right and left hands (16) (Fig. 2.11).

Great Arteries

The position of the ascending aorta is generally described in relation to the main pulmonary artery (Fig. 2.12). Normal hearts are characterized by a right-posterior aorta. Abnormalities in aortic position are important to assess because each generally occurs in only a limited number of conditions. For the vast majority of malformed hearts, the aortic position is either normal or occupies a position that is dextroposed, right lateral, right anterior, or left anterior (Fig. 2.13). Only rarely are other positions encountered.

A slightly anterior shift of the aorta, to a position midway between right posterior and right lateral, is termed dextroposition of the aorta (in contrast to dextroposition of the entire

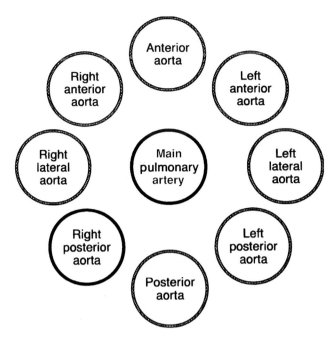

FIGURE 2.12 The possible positions of the ascending aorta relative to the main pulmonary artery are shown schematically, as viewed from below (from apex toward base).

heart) and is commonly encountered in tetralogy of Fallot, double-outlet right ventricle, and atrioventricular septal defects. A right-anterior aorta is most frequently associated with complete transposition of the great arteries, and a left-anterior aorta most often occurs in patients with either congenitally corrected transposition of the great arteries or a double-inlet left ventricle.

CONNECTIONS OF CARDIAC SEGMENTS

Once the morphology and positions of the cardiac segments are determined, the manner in which they join to one another can be evaluated. Connections exist at three levels: venoatrial, atrioventricular, and ventriculoarterial. Abnormal venoatrial connections are related to malformations involving the sinus venosus, common pulmonary vein, and their derivatives.

In contrast, cardiac valves form the mortar that connects atria to ventricles and ventricles to great arteries. These connections, however, do not necessarily imply patency for blood flow. For example, in aortic atresia, identification of an imperforate valve between the left ventricle and the ascending aorta is indicative of a concordant connection, despite the fact that blood does not flow between the two. The presence of overriding valves can interfere with the determination of atrioventricular and ventriculoarterial connections, as discussed below.

Venoatrial Connections

Normally, the superior and inferior venae cavae and the coronary sinus connect to the morphologic right atrium and the pulmonary veins join the morphologic left atrium. Anomalies may involve the systemic veins, pulmonary veins, or both, and they can involve all or only some of the veins. Consequently, the connection of each venous structure should be evaluated separately.

Atrioventricular Connections

Only four possible modes of atrioventricular connection exist: concordance, discordance, univentricular, and ambiguous (Figs. 2.4B, 2.14, and 2.15). The univentricular connections, in turn, include three subtypes: double inlet, single inlet, and common inlet.

If an atrioventricular valve is atretic, it is important to distinguish between the presence of an imperforate fibrous membrane, in which the connection can be determined, and absence of the atrioventricular connection on that side of the heart. Most cases of tricuspid atresia, for example, are characterized by an absent right atrioventricular connection rather than by an identifiable valvular plug. By clinical imaging, the membranous septum should not be misinterpreted as an imperforate tricuspid valve.

Concordance and Discordance

Concordance denotes the normal state and indicates that the morphologic right atrium is connected to the morphologic right ventricle, and that the left atrium is connected to the left ventricle. In contrast, connection of the right atrium to the left ventricle and of the left atrium to the right ventricle constitutes atrioventricular discordance, which corresponds to ventricular inversion or l-loop ventricles.

Univentricular Atrioventricular Connections

When both atria are joined to only one ventricle, the connection is univentricular, and three variants are recognized: Double-inlet ventricle, in which two atrioventricular valves are present; single-inlet ventricle, in which only one valve is present and there is no grossly identifiable remnant of the other valve; and common-inlet ventricle, in which a common atrioventricular valve connects both atria to only one ventricle. Thus, it is the connection, and not the heart, that is univentricular.

Ambiguous Atrioventricular Connection

With either right or left cardiac isomerism, the atrioventricular connection, by definition, is ambiguous or mixed. In the setting of right isomerism, for example, the right-sided morphologic right atrium might be connected to a morphologic right ventricle (concordance), and the left-sided morphologic right atrium would then join a morphologic left ventricle (discordance). For complex cases such as this, a description of the atrioventricular connection is recommended.

Ventriculoarterial Connections

Like connections at the atrioventricular level, those at the ventriculoarterial level are limited in number. Possibilities include concordance, discordance, and double, single, and common outlets (Figs. 2.16 and 2.17). Occasionally, with an atretic pulmonary or aortic valve, the ventricle to which the corresponding great artery is connected cannot be distinguished with certainty, and the ventriculoarterial connection is considered indeterminate.

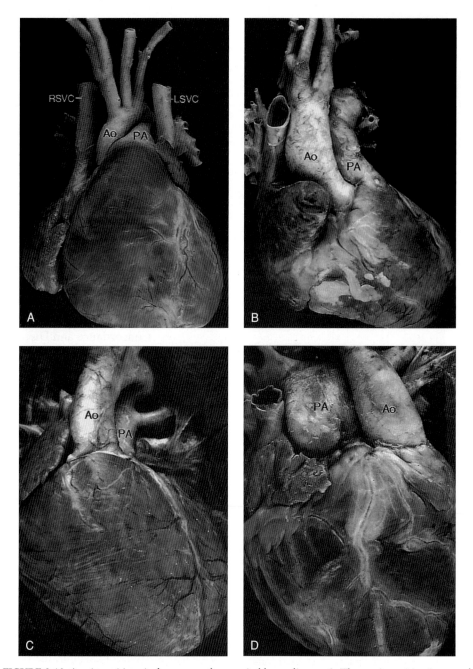

FIGURE 2.13 Aortic positions in four types of congenital heart disease. **A:** The aortic position is normal in this example of supravalvular aortic stenosis with bilateral superior venae cavae. **B:** A right lateral aorta is associated with tetralogy of Fallot and a right aortic arch with mirror-image brachiocephalic branching. **C:** The aorta is right-anterior in this case of complete transposition of the great arteries. **D:** The aortic position in this patient is left-anterior and is associated with a double-inlet left ventricle. (See Appendix 1.1 for abbreviations.)

Concordance and Discordance

Concordance refers to the normal state, in which the morphologic right ventricle is connected to the pulmonary artery and the morphologic left ventricle is linked to the aorta. By comparison, discordance corresponds to right ventricular origin of the aorta and left ventricular origin of the pulmonary artery and is synonymous with transposition of the great arteries.

When the atrioventricular connection is concordant and the ventriculoarterial connection is discordant, the malformation is called complete transposition, which results in complete separation of the systemic and pulmonary circulations, except at the sites of shunts. In contrast, congenitally corrected transposition is characterized by ventriculoarterial discordance and atrioventricular discordance, which results in normal blood flow but a systemic workload on the morphologic right

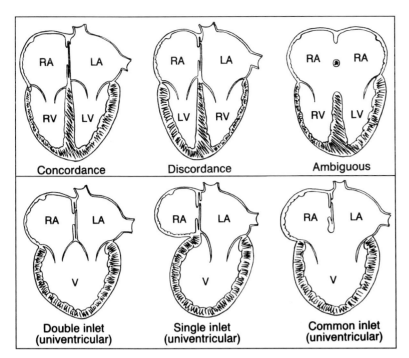

FIGURE 2.14 The six possible atrioventricular connections are shown schematically. **Upper panel:** Concordance is synonymous with the normal state, and discordance is synonymous with ventricular inversion. For either right or left cardiac isomerism, the atrioventricular connection is always ambiguous. **Lower panel:** There are three possible univentricular atrioventricular connections: double inlet, single inlet, and common inlet. (See Appendix 1.1 for abbreviations.)

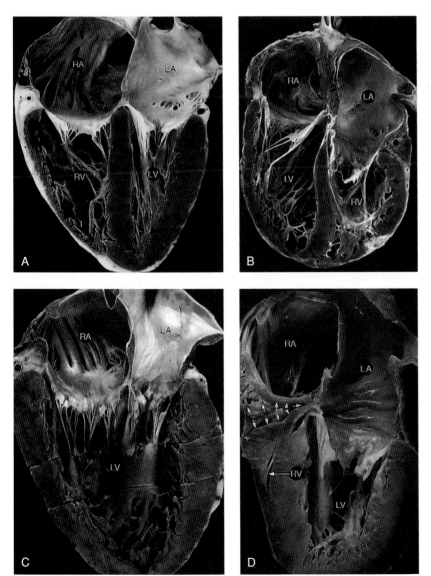

FIGURE 2.15 Four types of atrioventricular connection, shown in a four-chamber (or three-chamber) format. **A:** Concordance. **B:** Discordance. **C:** Double-inlet left ventricle. **D:** Tricuspid atresia with single-inlet left ventricle and absent right atrioventricular connection (*arrows*). (See Appendix 1.1 for abbreviations.)

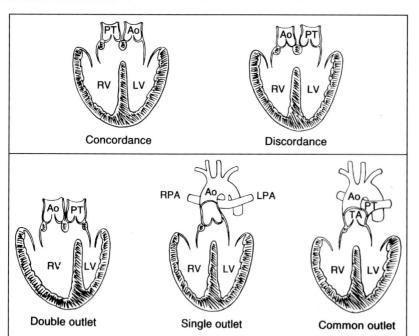

FIGURE 2.16 The five possible ventriculoarterial connections are shown schematically. **Upper panel:** Concordance indicates the normal state, and discordance is synonymous with transposition of the great arteries. **Lower panel:** There are three other possible connections: double outlet, which usually involves a right ventricle; single outlet, which includes pulmonary atresia with ventricular septal defect; and common outlet, which represents truncus arteriosus (TA). (See Appendix 1.1 for abbreviations.)

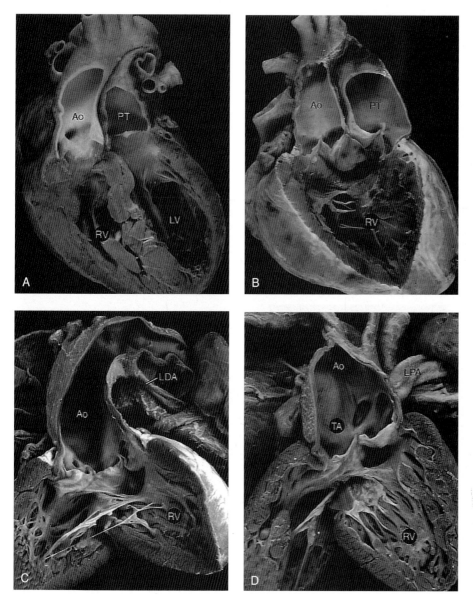

FIGURE 2.17 Four types of ventriculoarterial connection, viewed anteriorly. **A:** Discordance, in complete transposition of the great arteries. **B:** Double-outlet connection, in double-outlet right ventricle. **C:** Single-outlet connection, in pulmonary atresia with a ventricular septal defect and ductal origin of the pulmonary arteries. **D:** Common-outlet connection, in truncus arteriosus (TA). (See Appendix 1.1 for abbreviations.)

ventricle. Because the term great vessels refers to either the great arteries or the great veins, use of the term great arteries is favored for the transposition complexes.

Double, Single, and Common

When both great arteries emanate from only one ventricular chamber, the ventriculoarterial connection is considered double outlet. It is important to recognize that a double-outlet connection is not synonymous with the diagnostic entity known as double-outlet right ventricle. This form of connection includes not only double-outlet right ventricle but also double-outlet left ventricle and most cases of tetralogy of Fallot.

Morphologic criteria exist to distinguish tetralogy of Fallot from cases of double-outlet right ventricle with subpulmonary stenosis and a subaortic ventricular septal defect. Interestingly, patients with tetralogy of Fallot and a complete atrioventricular septal defect usually have Down's syndrome and a low surgical mortality rate, whereas those with double-outlet right ventricle and a complete atrioventricular septal defect characteristically have atrial isomerism and a high surgical mortality rate.

Among patients with pulmonary atresia and a ventricular septal defect, there exists a group in whom no remnant of the pulmonary valve or proximal portion of the pulmonary artery can be identified. As a result, only the aorta arises from the ventricles, constituting a single-outlet ventriculoarterial connection. In general, this situation does not pertain to aortic valve atresia because the ascending aorta, although hypoplastic, must remain patent to provide coronary blood flow, thus allowing its ventricular connection to be readily determined.

A common-outlet connection is characteristic of truncus arteriosus (truncal artery), in which this vessel represents the undivided aortic and pulmonary roots. Although hearts with single-outlet and common-outlet connections are quite similar, only in the setting of truncus arteriosus do the pulmonary arteries arise proximally from this vessel rather than from the ductus arteriosus or systemic collateral arteries.

Overriding and Straddling Valves

Definition of Overriding Valves

Overriding may be defined as biventricular emptying of an atrioventricular valve or biventricular origin of a semilunar valve. It is a property of the valve annulus and is always associated with a malalignment ventricular septal defect. The presence of annular overriding may interfere with accurate determination of cardiac connections. As a further complication in living patients, the extent of overriding may vary throughout the cardiac cycle and may appear to vary with different angles of view.

Malalignment

For overriding atrioventricular valves, the atrial and ventricular septa are malaligned. This may represent a lateral shift, a rotational shift, or a combination of the two (Fig. 2.18). The ventricular septal defect tends to involve the basal portion of the inlet septum. For the assessment of atrioventricular connections, an atrium is considered to join the ventricle into which >50% of the valve orifice empties (Fig. 2.19). A common atrioventricular valve is usually associated with concordant or discordant connections, although a common-inlet arrangement applies if >75% of the valve orifice empties into only one of the two ventricles.

Overriding of the semilunar valves is associated with malalignment of the outlet septum relative to the remainder of the ventricular septum. Malalignment can be lateral, rotational, or a combination of these (Figs. 2.18 and 2.20). The ventricular septal defect is located beneath the overriding

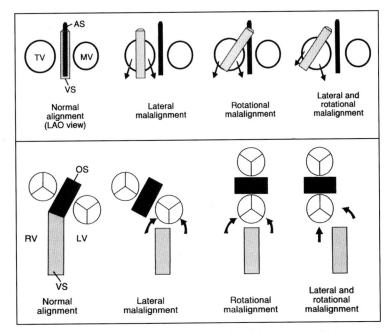

FIGURE 2.18 The types of annular overriding and septal malalignment are illustrated schematically. **Upper panel:** Atrioventricular valves are shown, with lateral and rotational malalignments between the atrial and ventricular septa. **Lower panel:** Semilunar valves are shown, with lateral and rotational malalignments between the ventricular and outlet septa. (See Appendix 1.1 for abbreviations.)

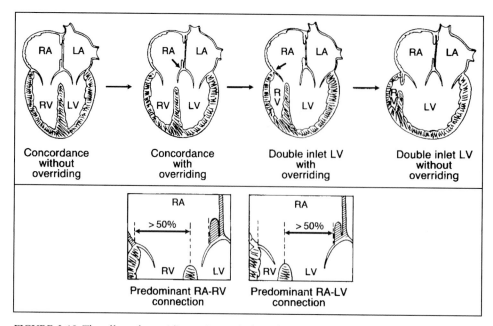

FIGURE 2.19 The effect of overriding atrioventricular valves on the determination of atrioventricular connections. **Upper panel:** With progressive leftward shifting of the atrial septum, the connections change from concordant to double-inlet left ventricle. **Lower panel:** The two insets illustrate the 50% rule. (See Appendix 1.1 for abbreviations.)

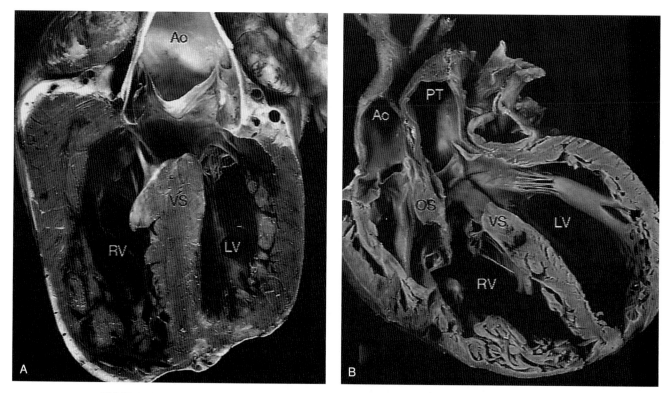

FIGURE 2.20 Overriding semilunar valves, in two cardiac specimens. **A:** An overriding aortic valve in tetralogy of Fallot. **B:** An overriding pulmonary valve in complete transposition of the great arteries. (See Appendix 1.1 for abbreviations.)

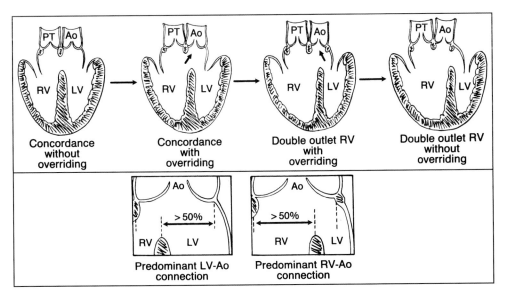

FIGURE 2.21 The effect of overriding semilunar valves on the determination of ventriculoarterial connections. **Upper panel:** With progressive rightward shifting of the outlet septum, the connection changes from concordant to double-outlet right ventricle. **Lower panel:** The two insets illustrate the 50% rule. (See Appendix 1.1 for abbreviations.)

artery and is either membranous or outlet in location, or a combination of the two. As with the atrioventricular valves, the 50% rule also applies to the semilunar valves (Fig. 2.21).

Definition of Straddling Valves

In contrast to annular overriding, *straddling* involves the anomalous insertions of chordae tendineae (tendinous cords) or papillary muscles into the contralateral ventricle (Figs. 2.22 and 2.23). Thus, straddling involves only the atrioventricular valves and requires the presence of a ventricular septal defect. Although straddling does not affect the evaluation of atrioventricular connections, it is important that it be identified preoperatively because its presence may preclude certain types of surgical repair or may necessitate valve replacement. Cordal straddling may occur alone or in conjunction with annular overriding.

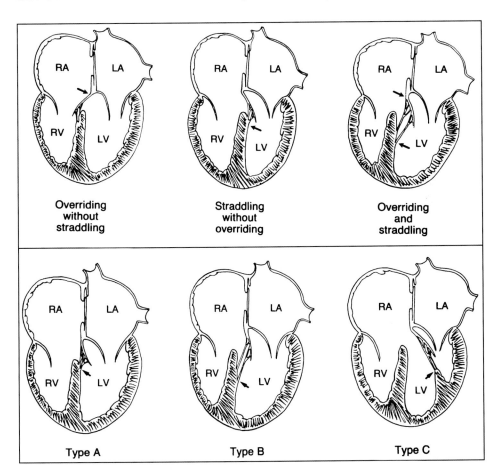

FIGURE 2.22 Overriding and straddling atrioventricular valves are shown schematically. **Upper panel:** Overriding and straddling are compared (see text for definitions). **Lower panel:** The three types of straddling are determined by the sites or cordal insertion into the contralateral ventricle along the crest (type A) or body (type B) of the ventricular septum, or onto the ventricular free wall (type C). (See Appendix 1.1 for abbreviations.)

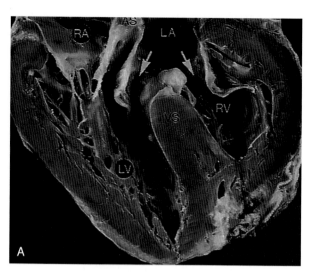
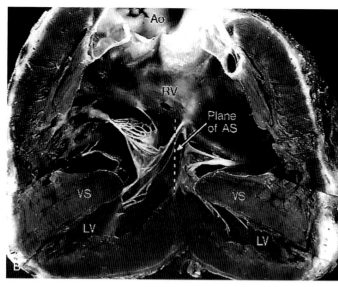

FIGURE 2.23 Overriding and straddling atrioventricular valves in two specimens. **A:** Straddling without overriding of the left-sided tricuspid valve (*arrows*) in a heart with atrioventricular discordance. **B:** Overriding and straddling of both atrioventricular valves is associated with rotational malalignment of the atrial and ventriculare septa in a case of superoinferior ventricles with a horizontal ventricular septum. (See Appendix 1.1 for abbreviations.)

APPENDIX 2.1 ■ SYNONYMS FOR COMMONLY USED DIAGNOSTIC TERMS

Preferred Term	Synonyms
AP septal defect	AP window or fenestration
AV discordance	Ventricular inversion; l-loop ventricles
AV septal defect	AV canal defect; endocardial cushion defect; AV commune; common AV orifice
Common-inlet RV	Cor biloculare
Complete TGA	d-TGA; complete transposition of the great vessels
Congenitally corrected TGA	Corrected TGA; 1-TGA
Dilated cardiomyopathy with EFE	Primary EFE
DORV with subpulmonary VSD	Taussig–Bing heart
Double-inlet LV	Single LV; univentricular heart of LV type; common ventricle; cor triloculare biatriatum
Extrathoracic heart	Ectopic heart; ectopia cordis
Inlet VSD	Subtricuspid or AV canal VSD
Left isomerism	Polysplenia syndrome; bilateral left-sidedness
Leftward base–apex axis	Levocardia; left-sided heart
Membranous VSD	Paramembranous, perimembranous, or infracristal VSD
Midline base–apex axis	Mesocardia; midline heart
Muscular VSD	Persistent bulboventricular foramen
Outlet or infundibular VSD	Subarterial, subaortic, subpulmonary, supracristal, conal, or doubly committed juxta-arterial VSD
Right isomerism	Asplenia syndrome; bilateral right-sidedness
Rightward base–apex axis	Dextrocardia; right-sided heart
RPA or LPA from aorta	Hemitruncus
Arrhythmogenic RV cardiomyopathy	Arrhythmogenic RV dysplasia; Uhl's parchment heart
Primum ASD	Ostium primum ASD; partial AV septal defect
Pulmonary atresia with VSD	Tetralogy with pulmonary atresia; truncus arteriosus (type IV); pseudotruncus
Secundum ASD	Ostium secundum ASD; ASD at fossa ovalis
Sinus venosus defect	Sinus venosus ASD
Superoinferior ventricles	Upstairs-downstairs or over-and-under heart
Tricuspid atresia	Single-inlet LV; absent right AV connection
Twisted AV connection	Criss-cross heart
VA discordance	Transposed great arteries (as a type of connection)

AP, aortopulmonary; ASD, atrial septal defect; DORV, double-outlet right ventricle; EFE, endocardial fibroelastosis; TGA, transposition of the great arteries; VA, ventriculoarterial; VSD, ventricular septal defect. (See Appendix 1.1 for other abbreviations.)

APPENDIX 2.2 ■ LATIN TERMS AND THEIR CORRESPONDING ANGLICIZED TERMS

Latin Term (Plural)	Anglicized Equivalent (Plural)
Annulus (annuli)	Annulus (annuluses), or valve ring
Aorta (aortae)	Aorta (aortas)
Apex (apices)	Apex (apexes)
Apex cordis	Cardiac apex
Atrium (atria)	Atrium (atriums)
Atrium dextrum	Right atrium
Atrium sinistrum	Left atrium
Auricula dextra	Right atrial appendage
Auricula sinistra	Left atrial appendage
Chorda tendinea (chordae tendineae)	Tendinous cord (cords)
Crista supraventricularis	Supraventricular crest or ridge
Crista terminalis	Terminal crest or ridge
Conus arteriosus	Right ventricular outflow tract, or infundibulum
Cor biloculare	Common atrium with common-inlet ventricle
Cor triatriatum	Triatrial heart, or double-chamber left atrium
Cor triatriatum dexter	Double-chamber right atrium
Cor triloculare biatriatum	Double-inlet left ventricle
Dextrocardia	Right-sided heart or apex
Ductus arteriosus (ductus arteriosi)	Ductal artery, or arterial duct
Ductus venosus	Ductal vein, or venous duct
Ectopia cordis	Ectopic heart, or extrathoracic heart
Foramen ovale	Oval foramen
Fossa ovalis	Oval fossa
Inferior vena cava	Inferior caval vein
Infundibulum (infundibuli)	Infundibulum (infundibulums)
Levocardia	Left-sided heart or apex
Ligamentum arteriosum	Arterial ligament
Ligamentum teres hepatis	Round ligament of liver
Ligamentum venosum	Venous ligament
Limbus fossae ovalis, or anulus ovalis	Limb or rim of the oval fossa
Mesocardia	Midline heart or apex
Musculus papillaris	Papillary muscle
Musculi pectinati	Pectinate muscles
Ostium (ostia)	Ostium (ostiums), or orifice
Ostium primum	First ostium or orifice
Ostium secundum	Second ostium or orifice
Pars membranacea septi	Membranous septum
Patent ductus arteriosus	Patent ductal artery
Patent foramen ovale	Patent oval foramen
Septum (septa, not septae)	Septum (septums)
Septum atriorum	Atrial septum
Septum interatriale	Interatrial septum
Septum interventriculare	Interventricular septum
Septum primum	First septum
Septum secundum	Second septum
Septum ventriculorum	Ventricular septum
Sinus coronarius	Coronary sinus
Sinus venosus	Venous sinus, or sinus vein
Situs ambiguus	Isomerism, or indeterminate sidedness
Situs inversus	Mirror-image sidedness
Situs solitus	Normal sidedness
Sulcus coronarius	Coronary or atrioventricular groove
Sulcus interventricularis anterior	Anterior interventricular groove
Sulcus interventricular posterior	Posterior interventricular groove
Sulcus terminalis	Terminal groove
Superior vena cava	Superior caval vein
Trabecula carnea (trabeculae carneae)	Trabeculation(s)
Trabecula septomarginalis	Septal band, or moderator band
Trigonum fibrosum dextrum	Right fibrous trigone
Trigonum fibrosum sinistrum	Left fibrous trigone
Truncus arteriosus	Truncal artery, or arterial trunk
Vena cava (venae cavae)	Caval vein(s)
Ventricularis dexter	Right ventricle
Ventricularis sinister	Left ventricle

References

1. Peacock TB. *On Malformations of the Human Heart.* London: John Churchill, 1858.
2. Abbott ME. *Atlas of Congenital Cardiac Disease.* New York: American Heart Association, 1936.
3. Van Praagh R. Diagnosis of complex congenital heart disease: Morphologic-anatomic method and terminology. *Cardiovasc Intervent Radiol* 1984;7:115–120.
4. Anderson RH, Becker AE, Freedom RM, et al. Sequential segmental analysis of congenital heart disease. *Pediatr Cardiol* 1984;5:281–288.
5. Van Praagh R. The segmental approach to diagnosis in congenital heart disease. *Birth Defects* 1972;8:4–23.
6. de la Cruz MV, Nadal-Ginard B. Rules for the diagnosis of visceral situs, truncoconal morphologies and ventricular inversions. *Am Heart J* 1972;84:19–32.
7. Edwards WD. Congenital heart disease. In: Schoen FJ, ed. *Interventional and Surgical Cardiovascular Pathology: Clinical Correlations and Basic Principles.* Philadelphia: WB Saunders, 1989:281–367.
8. Anderson C, Devine WA, Anderson RH, et al. Abnormalities of the spleen in relation to congenital malformations of the heart: A survey of necropsy findings in children. *Br Heart J* 1990;63:122–128.
9. Van Praagh R, Van Praagh S. Atrial isomerism in the heterotaxy syndromes with asplenia, or polysplenia, or normally formed spleen: An erroneous concept. *Am J Cardiol* 1991;66:1504–1506.
10. Macartney FJ, Partridge JB, Shinebourne EA, et al. Identification of atrial situs. In: Anderson RH, Shinebourne EA, eds. *Paediatric Cardiology 1977.* Edinburgh: Churchill Livingstone, 1978:16–26.
11. Sharma S, Devine W, Anderson RH, et al. The determination of atrial arrangement by examination of appendage morphology in 1842 autopsied specimens. *Br Heart J* 1988;60:227–231.
12. Van Praagh R, David I, Van Praagh S. What is a ventricle? The single ventricle trap. *Pediatr Cardiol* 1982;2:79–84.
13. Anderson RH, Macartney FJ, Tynan M, et al. Univentricular atrioventricular connection: The single ventricle trap unsprung. *Pediatr Cardiol* 1983;4:273–280.
14. Van Mierop LHS. Diagnostic code for congenital heart disease. *Pediatr Cardiol* 1984;5:331–362.
15. Van Praagh R, Van Praagh S. Embryology and anatomy: Keys to the understanding of complex and congenital heart disease. *Coeur* 1982;13: 315–336.
16. Van Praagh S, LaCorte M, Fellows KE, et al. Supero-inferior ventricles: Anatomic and angiocardiographic findings in 10 postmortem cases. In: Van Praagh R, Takao A, eds. *Etiology and Morphogenesis of Congenital Heart Disease.* Mount Kisco, NY: Futura, 1980:317–378.

PART II ■ DIAGNOSTIC METHODS

CHAPTER 3 ■ HISTORY AND PHYSICAL EXAMINATION

HUGH D. ALLEN, MD, ScD (Hon), JOHN R. PHILLIPS, MD, AND DAVID P. CHAN, MD

Despite the availability of advanced imaging technologies, a thorough history and physical examination are the core of evaluating children with suspected heart disease. Although the basics of obtaining a history and physical examination are similar in all patients, this chapter emphasizes specific issues when evaluating a child with possible cardiac pathology.

HISTORY

To obtain an accurate history, it is important to establish a relationship with the patient and parents. Meetings are often short and first impressions are lasting, so the first encounter is critical. The history is the predominant vehicle that defines the first encounter.

Parents often research their child's illness on the Internet or through the media and may come to a visit with preconceived notions and, perhaps, opinionated or anecdotal information. The examiner must be prepared for this and discuss the patient's condition in a nonconfrontational and open manner. In that way, an honest and positive patient–physician relationship will be established.

Many aspects of the history are age specific. Therefore, historical information should be elicited from both the patient and the parents.

Newborns and Infants

When evaluating a newborn for the first time, it is important to obtain details about the pregnancy. The infant of a mother with gestational diabetes, for example, has an increased risk of cardiac defects. Similarly, the relationship between maternal lupus and congenital heart block is well recognized. Maternal exposure to teratogens associated with cardiac defects (Table 3.1) should be part of the prenatal history (see Chapters 25 and 28). Smoking during pregnancy has been linked to small-for-gestational-age newborns but not specific cardiac defects. Congenital infections may lead to specific types of cardiac diseases. One example is rubella, which has been associated with patent ductus arteriosus (PDA) and pathologic peripheral pulmonary stenosis. The use of illicit drugs may indicate an increased risk for human immunodeficiency virus infection, which has been associated with infantile cardiomyopathy. The age of the mother is important to determine her risk for offspring with chromosomal abnormalities such as trisomy 21.

A family history of relatives, especially siblings, born with heart defects indicates a higher than normal risk of congenital heart defects. For a couple who have already had a child with a left-sided obstructive lesion (i.e., hypoplastic left heart syndrome) the risk of congenital heart defects in subsequent children is increased. In most centers, a history of siblings with significant congenital heart lesions would prompt a referral to a pediatric echocardiographer for detailed fetal echocardiography. A complete family history also should include the presence or absence of syndromes associated with congenital heart disease such as Marfan syndrome, Holt–Oram syndrome, long-QT syndrome, and idiopathic sudden death. A positive family history for these diseases may warrant screening of other family members.

The perinatal history of the child can be helpful in suggesting the type of cardiac defect. Complications such as toxemia, birth asphyxia, fetal distress, and low birth weight may result in perinatal insult to the myocardium, leading to a generalized cardiomyopathy. The infant's Apgar scores should be noted, and cyanosis, color, and perfusion status should be assessed.

The time at which signs and symptoms of heart disease begin may be a clue to the type of cardiac lesion. Commonly, murmurs detected early in the neonatal period originate from atrioventricular (AV) valve regurgitation or semilunar valve stenosis. Most newborns with congenital heart disease are asymptomatic at birth. As perinatal changes are completed, symptoms specific to the physiology of the defect become evident. For example, ductal-dependent left-sided obstructive lesions usually present in the first 2 weeks of life as the ductus arteriosus closes. This results in a marked decrease in cardiac output and signs of shock. On the other hand, children with significant left-to-right shunt lesions typically are asymptomatic until 4 weeks of age when pulmonary vascular resistance decreases to near normal levels and heart failure ensues.

Because an infant's primary physical exertion is eating, a thorough feeding history should be obtained. If the mother has had previous children, she may offer insight into differences in feeding habits between the patient and her other children. Frequency of feeding, amount consumed, and the length of time to finish a feeding should be obtained. Most infants feed every 2 to 3 hours. It is common for children with congestive heart failure to fall asleep during feeding only to awaken after a few minutes and feed a small amount again. Infants should be able to complete their feeding in less than 30 minutes. A longer time to finish each feeding, low volume consumed, excessive diaphoresis, and dyspnea with feeding are signs of heart failure or poor cardiac output. As pulmonary vascular resistance declines, irritability and fussiness with feeding may indicate angina and ischemia in a child with an anomalous left coronary artery from the pulmonary artery.

The presence of cyanosis should be determined, recognizing that acrocyanosis is normal. Central cyanosis is characterized by blueness of the tongue and oral mucosa. Central cyanosis most likely is related to cardiac or respiratory disease. If the source of cyanosis is cardiac, it is constant. Children in shock also may appear cyanotic owing to venous

TABLE 3.1

COMMON TERATOGENS AND THEIR ASSOCIATED CARDIAC DEFECTS

Teratogen	Cardiac Defect
Alcohol	ASD, VSD
Lithium	Ebstein's anomaly
Retinoic acid	Conotruncal abnormalities
Valproic acid	ASD, VSD, AS, PA/IVS, CoA

AS, aortic valve stenosis; ASD, atrial septal defect; CoA, coarctation of the aorta; PA/IVS, pulmonary atresia with intact ventricular septum; VSD, ventricular septal defect.

stasis, right-to-left intrapulmonary shunting, and increased peripheral oxygen extraction.

The infant's breathing patterns should be documented. Unlabored tachypnea often accompanies cyanotic heart disease, whereas grunting and dyspnea are associated with left-sided obstructive lesions or respiratory illness.

Even in a patient beyond infancy, the child's history regarding pregnancy, labor and delivery, and neonatal course are important. Growth and development now are important areas to document. Poor growth and development may be related to cardiac disease. Activity level, especially in comparison with siblings, should be assessed. Does the child fatigue easily? Does the child experience cyanosis and dyspnea with exercise? A child with tetralogy of Fallot may squat after exercise to increase pulmonary blood flow. Syncope with exercise is an ominous sign and suggests an arrhythmia, coronary abnormalities, or severe aortic obstruction.

Children and Adolescents

When evaluating children and adolescents, the primary historian should be the patient. The parents should be asked additional pertinent historical information. Adolescents should have the right to speak privately, especially about sexual and personal matters. A clinician should not betray their confidentiality and should not divulge to others the information revealed in confidence.

The patient's reasons for consultation should be ascertained. Chest pain is a common reason for referral and anxiety. The patient should describe the location, quality, and timing of the pain. The clinician should ask what relieves the pain. Is it associated with exercise? Pain associated with chest "pounding" may indicate an arrhythmia. This information will help the examiner to differentiate between noncardiac chest pain and abnormalities of the coronary arteries or left-sided obstructive lesions.

The past medical history should include documentation of significant illnesses, previous hospitalization, previous operations, immunization status, and symptoms of poor growth as an infant.

A review of systems and social history should include specific information regarding the patient's eating and exercise habits. School performance and participation should be assessed. Is the patient capable of keeping up with peers? The clinician should make a private interview available to the adolescent. A history of tobacco and illicit drug use can then be determined. A discussion of personal habits gives the examiner

an opportunity to advise about risk factors for coronary artery disease. This information is pertinent to the cardiac evaluation and aids in building the patient–physician relationship.

In the family history, one should identify the presence of premature myocardial infarction and hypercholesterolemia that may prompt cholesterol screening. As in the infant, a family history of idiopathic sudden death in a close relative should prompt careful evaluation of the patient's QTc interval on a surface electrocardiogram.

PHYSICAL EXAMINATION

The cardiac physical examination consists of five parts: Vital signs assessment, inspection, palpation, percussion, and auscultation. For the physician to perform a successful examination, the patient must be cooperative. This requires tact, patience, and innovation on the part of the examiner. If the infant is happiest in the mother's lap, then he or she should be allowed to stay there. The mother should feed or play with the child during inspection or palpation. The order of the examination can be adjusted to obtain the most information. For example, if the child is asleep, auscultation should be performed before palpation. The privacy and modesty of older children and adolescents must be respected. A staff member chaperone should be present during the examination of a patient of the opposite sex. Every child is different, so each examination must be individualized to be successful.

VITAL SIGN ASSESSMENT

Heart rate, respiratory rate, and blood pressure are vital to a complete cardiac examination. They should be assessed at each visit.

Heart Rate and Respiratory Rate

The importance of changes in heart rate and respiratory rate are noted throughout this chapter. Often, changes in heart rate and respiratory rate are the first harbingers of myocardial dysfunction, pulmonary congestion, or arrhythmia, even before changes in blood pressure occur.

Blood Pressure Measurement

On the initial visit, blood pressures should be measured in both upper extremities and one lower extremity. Although many hospitals are phasing out mercury manometers, they are the most accurate tools for blood pressure measurement. Aneroid instruments are the next most reliable, and although Dinamap pressures are easy to obtain, diastolic pressures are often questionable. The standard technique for measuring blood pressure should be used. First, the length of the bladder of the cuff should be 80% of the circumference of the limb and the width of the cuff should cover at least two thirds of the length of the extremity. Second, the patient should be sitting. Finally, to obtain an accurate measurement, the cuff should be deflated slowly. Listening to the brachial or popliteal arteries yields the Korotkoff sounds that are used; first and fifth are now the standard. If the sounds cannot be heard, systolic pressure can be obtained by palpating the first pulsation of an artery distal to the cuff or by using a handheld

Doppler probe over the distal artery. Another alternative, especially in infants, is using the flush technique, done by squeezing the hand or foot, inflating the blood pressure cuff, releasing the hand or foot, and slowly deflating the cuff until intense redness is seen in the previously pale extremity; this technique will estimate mean arterial pressure.

INSPECTION

The examiner should take advantage of the time while interviewing the parent to inspect the child. The physical examination actually starts here. Each patient should be inspected for general appearance, nutritional status, dysmorphic features, color, and comfort. A thorough inspection often will clue the examiner to the cause and severity of an illness.

General Appearance

The child's general appearance and comfort should be noted. Is he or she fussy or playful? Is the child well nourished? Are dysmorphic features or chromosomal abnormalities present? As discussed elsewhere in the text, specific cardiac lesions will accompany specific syndromes. The child's breathing pattern should be observed. Patients with severe heart failure, pulmonary edema, or pericardial restriction (tamponade, constrictive pericarditis) prefer sitting up. Forcing such a patient into the supine position may result in respiratory failure. Patients should be allowed to determine the position in which they are most comfortable.

Chest wall surgical scars suggest particular lesions. A right thoracotomy is used for placement of a right Blalock–Thomas–Taussig shunt, atrial septal defect repair, or mitral valve surgery. A midline sternotomy is used for most heart operations, especially if cardiopulmonary bypass is used. A left thoracotomy is used for patent ductus ligation, coarctation repair, and placement of a left Blalock–Thomas–Taussig shunt.

The clinician should inspect the chest. The transverse aorta sits under the suprasternal notch. Pulsations of the suprasternal notch may be visible in the presence of significant aortic runoff lesions such as aortic regurgitation. A left parasternal precordial bulge often is noted in patients with right ventricular volume overload (i.e., atrial septal defect). Because the dilated right ventricle is below the left precordium, the developing cartilaginous rib cage will expand to accommodate the structure. As the ribs ossify, the left precordial bulge remains. With the patient supine and the examiner at the feet of the patient, the point of maximal impulse (PMI) can be observed. It is usually located in the left fourth intercostal space in the midclavicular line. In dextrocardia, it is on the right. It is displaced downward and laterally with left ventricular volume overload. Left ventricular hypertrophy does not usually alter the PMI's location.

Color

The child's color (i.e., pink, cyanotic, pale) should be noted. True cyanosis requires desaturation of 5 g% of hemoglobin and is difficult to detect unless the arterial saturation is ≤85% in a child with normal hemoglobin levels. The best indicator of cyanosis is the tongue. It has a rich vascular supply and is free of pigmentation. Acrocyanosis that occurs in a cold environment or after bathing nearly always is a normal finding and is not true cyanosis. In the older child, long-standing cyanosis is usually accompanied by digital clubbing. The loss of the angle between the nail and the cuticle area is a consistent finding of clubbing. Cyanosis also results from respiratory disease or central nervous system disorders. If cyanosis is suspected, pulse oximetry should be obtained. Pulse oximetry is not necessary as a serial test in acyanotic patients.

Comfort

The child's activity level should be observed. In the infant, feeding constitutes exercise, which may elicit dyspnea, tachypnea, or diaphoresis. While the toddler or young child is playing, the clinician should ask about early cessation of activity, especially if accompanied by dyspnea. Exercise intolerance may indicate inadequate cardiac output.

Breathing Pattern

Resting breathing patterns can offer information regarding the patient's hemodynamic state. If the infant has central cyanosis, it is usually accompanied by a nonlabored tachypnea that results from hypoxic respiratory drive. Grunting is a physiologic means of producing positive end-expiratory pressure and often accompanies pulmonary edema. Nasal flaring and intercostal and subcostal retractions may be present. If the infant is severely distressed, the head will bob with respiratory effort.

Neck Veins

Neck vein distention suggests impaired right ventricular filling. It is best observed with the patient positioned 30 degrees upright. Cannon A waves may be seen in patients with atrial flutter and a closed tricuspid valve. Bobbing of the head may be seen in patients with significant aortic regurgitation. This is caused by increased carotid arterial pulsations striking the angles of the mandibles. The patient appears to be nodding "yes." Patients with significant tricuspid regurgitation will exhibit lateral head movement. This occurs when regurgitant blood in the superior vena cava strikes the right mandibular angle. The patient appears to be nodding "no."

PALPATION

The clinician should first wash his or her hands. Before the clinician proceeds with the examination, the patient should undress. The child may be covered with a blanket or wear a medical examination gown. Palpation of peripheral pulses, the chest, the abdomen, and the back should be included in each cardiac examination.

Pulses

Pulse rate should be assessed, noting regularity and quality of the pulsations. Pulse rate changes with the age of the patient. A fast pulse rate for age may indicate arrhythmia or congestive heart failure. A slow pulse rate usually reflects athletic conditioning; however, atrioventricular block or drug effect should be considered. Irregularity of pulse rate may indicate an arrhythmia. However, a change in pulse rate with respiration is normal (sinus arrhythmia).

Palpate pulses simultaneously in the upper and lower extremities. Brachial pulses should be palpated simultaneously as well. If there is a delay between the upper and lower extremity pulses or absence of femoral pulsations, coarctation of the aorta should be considered. Diminished pulses are ominous in children and may suggest cardiac failure or shock. Absent or weak pulses in the arm may result from previous subclavian flap repair of a coarctation of the aorta or systemic-to-pulmonary artery shunts (i.e., classic Blalock–Thomas–Taussig shunt). Bounding pulses reflect aortic runoff as in aortic regurgitation, PDA, or arteriovenous malformations.

Capillary refill time is the time required for blanching to disappear after manually pressing on an extremity. While testing capillary refill, the clinician should examine the extremities for abnormalities associated with congenital heart disease, such as clubbing, fingerlike thumbs (Holt–Oram syndrome), webbing of the digits, or polydactyly.

Chest

The chest should be palpated for the PMI, precordial activity, and thrills. The location of the PMI suggests the ventricular dominance. The chest should be palpated with a fingertip to confirm its location. With left ventricular dominance, the PMI is palpated at the left midclavicular line or apex. A PMI located at the lower left sternal border or xiphoid process suggests right ventricular dominance. Patients with dextrocardia will have a PMI on the right side of the chest. Occasionally, an impulse will have a double contour or heave in the presence of volume overload (i.e., mitral regurgitation). In the face of pressure overload, a well-localized, sharp rising impulse or tap may be detected.

Precordial activity should be assessed. A hyperactive precordium suggests heart disease with volume overload. Volume overload may result from a large left-to-right shunt (i.e., a large ventricular septal defect [VSD] or PDA) or severe valvular regurgitation (i.e., aortic and mitral insufficiency). In addition, left precordial bulging often is noted in patients with significant right ventricular volume overload.

Thrills are vibrations detected distal to jet lesions. Left precordial thrills are best felt with the metacarpal heads of the right hand while the examiner is positioned to the right of the supine patient. Gently placing a fingertip in the suprasternal notch will allow detection of aortic pulsations and thrills in patients with aortic valve stenosis (AS), pulmonary valve stenosis (PS), aortic insufficiency (AI), PDA, or coarctation of the aorta. In these lesions, a thrill also may be palpable over the carotid arteries.

Thrills located over the right upper sternal border are aortic in origin and are felt in patients with AS. Left upper sternal border thrills are pulmonic in origin and indicate PI, PS, or, occasionally, PDA. A thrill may be felt over the jet of a restrictive VSD as it strikes the endocardial surface of the right ventricle and transmits to the chest wall. Stenotic right ventricle-to-pulmonary artery conduits may produce a thrill. These are usually felt along the left sternal border.

In patients with pulmonary hypertension and elevated pulmonary arterial diastolic pressure, the pulmonic valve closure is often palpable at the left upper sternal border.

Abdomen

The abdominal examination is important and often fraught with difficulty, especially in the infant. To conduct a thorough examination, it may be best to palpate the abdomen last. The clinician should remember to warm his or her hands before starting. A child who is tense or ticklish may be distracted by bending his or her knees so that the abdominal muscles relax. The patient's expiration should be the examiner's cue to palpate the deeper aspects of the abdomen and maintain pressure during inspiration. The size and texture of the liver and spleen should be assessed, palpating above the pelvic brim and working slowly upward until the liver edge or spleen tip is felt. With increased venous pressure, the liver will be enlarged and its capsule may be tender.

Back

Patients with congenital heart disease, especially those with chronically enlarged hearts and connective tissue disorders, have a high incidence of scoliosis. Therefore, examination of the spine for the presence of scoliosis should be part of the cardiac physical.

PERCUSSION

The primary role of percussion is to evaluate the total span of the liver. This is particularly useful if the lungs are hyperinflated. Hyperinflation pushes the liver below the costal margin, giving a false impression of liver enlargement. In this case, percussion is a more accurate method for assessing liver size.

Percussion of the chest will help detect pulmonary consolidation or effusion. Occasionally, a "heart border" is percussed well beyond the PMI and may indicate a pericardial effusion.

AUSCULTATION

"Sound is the organized movement of molecules caused by a vibrating body in some medium" (1). In the case of heart sounds and murmurs, the medium is blood. Vibrations are produced by the cessation or propulsion of blood within the heart that, in turn, create sound that then radiates through the thorax, across the skin, and ultimately to the examiner through a stethoscope. The ability to identify heart sounds and murmurs and relate them to other clinical findings is a paramount step in the evaluation of heart disease.

Heart Sounds

Vibration of the valve apparatus, myocardium, pericardium, and chest wall have all been implicated in the production of heart sounds (2–5). The timing of the first heart sound corresponds to the closure of the AV valves. The second heart sound corresponds to the closure of the semilunar valves. It has been shown that these sounds are not produced by coaptation of the valve leaflets, but rather the sudden deceleration of blood flow following closure of the valves. In turn, deceleration and cessation of blood flow cause surrounding cardiac structures and tissue to vibrate, producing audible sound (6,7).

During systole, atrial pressure increases and eventually exceeds that of the ventricles. The AV valves are forced open and blood flows down the pressure gradient into the ventricles. Early in diastole, rapid ventricular filling causes vibration of the cardiac structures, thus producing the third heart sound. Most children will have a normal soft S3. Later in diastole, atrial contraction augments ventricular filling. If the ventricle is resistant to further distention, as in cardiomyopathy, the poorly compliant myocardium will vibrate, producing a fourth heart sound.

Heart Murmurs

Turbulence is described as highly disturbed flow that produces random fluctuations of velocity and pressure within the blood and vibration of the surrounding tissue. Audible vibrations from turbulence are thought to be the cause of murmurs.

"The Reynolds number is a dimensionless quantity often used to describe the characteristics of steady flow through straight tubes at which transition from laminar to turbulent flow would occur" (8). The Reynolds number is defined as:

$$Re = [(\text{density of fluid})(\text{velocity})(\text{tube diameter})]/\text{viscosity of fluid}$$

Although the cardiovascular system varies from the steady state conditions noted above, the transition to turbulent blood flow is thought to typically occur at a Reynolds number >2,000. There is debate whether murmurs are a direct result of turbulence or a consequence of turbulence.

Turbulent blood flow produces vibrations of the surrounding vessel in several ways. Direct impact of a jet against cardiac structures is the easiest to comprehend. However, several other mechanisms of creating vibration have been suggested (8). Eddy currents, for example, are produced adjacent to high-velocity jets. Like ripples in a pond, they produce vibrations as they strike the vessel wall. Second, pressure is lower in a moving fluid compared with stationary fluid. Therefore, the higher pressure outside of the moving fluid pushes the vessel wall toward the lower pressure fluid. This is called the Bernoulli effect. Fluctuations in the intensity of the Bernoulli effect may cause vibration of the vessel wall. Last, high turbulent flow can cause cavitation or the forming of bubbles of vapor in a liquid. Theoretically, these bubbles cause vibrations as they strike the vessel wall.

Equipment

The choice of the best stethoscope is personal. Some advocate single tubing, whereas others prefer double-tubed devices. Some of the newer digital stethoscopes are quite useful. Whichever the instrument, the tubing must be intact and the earpieces must fit comfortably into the examiner's ears. Chest pieces vary in size. Chest pieces with a diaphragm and bell are essential to evaluate both high- and low-frequency sounds, respectively. In infants and small children, it is possible to hear high-frequency sounds by pressing on the bell, thereby creating a diaphragm with the skin.

Examination

In anxious toddlers and infants, often it is useful to auscultate before palpating. Distracting a toddler or feeding an infant may help to keep them quiet while the clinician listens. On rare occasions, sedation is necessary to perform a proper examination.

The clinician should develop a routine (and stay with it) for listening to heart sounds so that each portion of the cardiac cycle is examined at several locations. Most examiners start at the apex and work to the left lower (LLSB) and left upper (LUSB) sternal borders, then right upper sternal border (RUSB). The clinician should be sure to auscultate the left subclavicular area, both axillae, the liver, the head, and the back. At each location, one must listen to the first heart sound, throughout systole, the second heart sound, and throughout diastole. The process should be repeated with the patient in a different position. Adolescents and patients with collagen vascular disorders should be examined supine and upright, including squatting to standing (dynamic auscultation) to detect the click and murmur of mitral valve prolapse or the ejection murmur of hypertrophic cardiomyopathy. This maneuver first places increased afterload on the heart, enlarging the left ventricle. Then, with standing, the ventricle is relatively unloaded, allowing mitral valve prolapse or dynamic outflow obstruction to be more manifest to the examiner.

Arteriovenous malformations may be responsible for unexplained cardiomegaly. In those instances, the clinician should listen for a bruit over the fontanel or liver. In severe aortic regurgitation, one should listen over the femoral arteries for "pistol shot" sounds. The lungs should be examined for wheezing, rales, or abnormal breath sounds.

HEART SOUNDS

First Heart Sound (S1)

The first heart sound occurs with closure of the mitral and tricuspid valves. There are four components to the first heart sound, but only the second and third are audible to the human ear. The first heart sound is usually single in infancy. As the patient grows older, the heart rate slows, allowing detection of both audible components. The first audible component correlates with the effects of mitral valve closure and is best heard at the apex. The second audible component correlates with the effects of tricuspid valve closure and is best appreciated at the LLSB.

Second Heart Sound (S2)

The second heart sound has two components that coincide with aortic and pulmonary valve closure. The aortic component (A2) precedes the pulmonary component (P2) because left ventricular contraction ends slightly before right ventricular contraction. With the exception of some newborns, a split in the second heart sound can be detected in normal patients. S2 normally splits with respiration. The split is accentuated with inspiration because of increased right ventricular filling and subsequently longer ejection time. It is single with expiration because of shortened right ventricular ejection time.

Abnormal splitting of S2 is an important finding when diagnosing heart disease. Wide and sometimes fixed splitting will be heard in conditions that prolong right ventricular ejection time, such as atrial septal defects, total anomalous pulmonary venous drainage, pulmonary stenosis, some VSDs, and right bundle branch block. Narrow splitting of S2 occurs with early closure of the pulmonary valve (i.e., pulmonary hypertension) or delayed aortic valve closure (i.e., severe AS). A single S2 occurs when there is a single semilunar valve (i.e., pulmonary or aortic valve atresia), an inaudible P2 (i.e., transposition of the great arteries), delayed aortic valve closure (i.e., severe AS), and early pulmonary valve closure (i.e., pulmonary vascular obstructive disease). Paradoxical splitting occurs when the aortic valve closes later than the pulmonary valve (i.e., severe AS, left bundle branch block).

Ordinarily, P2 is softer than A2. Elevated pulmonary arterial diastolic pressure, as seen with pulmonary vascular obstructive disease, will cause the pulmonic valve to close crisply and accentuate P2.

Third Heart Sound (S3)

The third heart sound is heard early in diastole with the rapid filling phase. It is a low-frequency sound, best appreciated with the bell of the stethoscope at the apex or LLSB. An apical S3 is frequently heard in normal children and competitive athletes.

Fourth Heart Sound (S4)

A fourth heart sound is always abnormal. It is a low-frequency sound heard at the end of diastole just before S1. It is associated with rapid filling of the ventricle during atrial contraction and is heard in congestive heart failure and conditions of decreased ventricular compliance (i.e., cardiomyopathy). When ventricular compliance is abnormal, there is often a louder-than-normal third sound as well.

Clicks

Ejection clicks occur soon after S1 and are associated with semilunar valve stenosis (i.e., AS, PS) and dilated great arteries. Aortic valve clicks are heard at the apex or RUSB and do not vary with respiration. Pulmonary valve clicks are heard along the left sternal border and are louder with expiration. Clicks associated with dilation of the aorta or pulmonary arteries are best heard over the vessel, at the right and left upper sternal borders, respectively.

A midsystolic, apical click is heard with mitral valve prolapse and may be accompanied by a late systolic murmur. Evaluation of the mitral valve when the patient stands after squatting may accentuate a mitral valve click or regurgitant murmur.

HEART MURMURS

Heart murmurs should be evaluated in terms of intensity (i.e., loudness; grades 1–6), timing, location, transmission, and quality (i.e., harsh, vibratory, etc.).

Intensity

The intensity of a murmur is graded from I to VI:

Grade I. Barely audible and may require several cycles to detect
Grade II. Soft, but easily audible
Grade III. Moderately loud murmur without a thrill
Grade IV. Loud murmur with a thrill
Grade V. Loud murmur heard with the stethoscope barely off the chest
Grade VI. Loud murmur heard without the stethoscope touching the chest

Timing

Classification of heart murmurs is based on their timing during the cardiac cycle (Fig. 3.1). The three types of heart murmurs are the following:

Systolic murmurs: ejection and S1 coincident (often holosystolic)
Diastolic murmurs: early diastolic, middiastolic, and late diastolic/presystolic
Continuous murmurs

Systolic Murmurs

Systolic murmurs can be classified further as ejection or S1 coincident, based on the onset of the murmur relative to S1.

Ejection Murmurs

The onset of ejection murmurs occurs a short time after S1. They may be long or short and usually have a crescendo-decrescendo quality. They may end prior to S2. Ejection murmurs are the result of obstructed blood flow through a stenotic semilunar valve or excessive volume through a normal semilunar valve. They are heard best over the site of altered flow (i.e., aortic, RUSB; pulmonary, LUSB) and radiate in the direction of flow.

Ejection murmurs associated with obstructed blood flow are heard with semilunar valve stenosis, subvalvular or supravalvular aortic or pulmonary stenosis, branch pulmonary artery stenosis, and hypertrophic cardiomyopathy. Ejection murmurs caused by excessive volume across the pulmonary valve are heard in atrial septal defects, pulmonary valve regurgitation, and anomalous pulmonary venous drainage. Commonly, an ejection murmur across the pulmonary valve is detected during pregnancy because of increased intravascular volume. Ejection murmurs caused by excessive volume across the aortic valve are heard with aortic regurgitation, PDA, and systemic arteriovenous malformations. Ejection murmurs are also heard when blood volume is low or viscosity is altered, such as with anemia.

S1-Coincident Murmurs

S1-coincident murmurs start with S1. They usually last throughout systole and are thus referred to as holosystolic or pansystolic murmurs (Fig. 3.2). S1-coincident murmurs occur when blood flows from a high-pressure chamber to a low-pressure chamber. They are associated with VSD and mitral or tricuspid valve regurgitation. Their location, therefore, corresponds with the tricuspid (LLSB) and mitral (apex) valves. In the case of a VSD, an S1-coincident murmur is heard along the left sternal border and may radiate to the right. The frequency or pitch of a VSD murmur is directly proportional to the pressure drop through the defect; the higher the frequency, the smaller the VSD (9).

Diastolic Murmurs

Diastolic murmurs are differentiated based on the timing of their onset during diastole: early diastolic, middiastolic, and late systolic/presystolic.

Early Diastolic Murmurs

Early diastolic murmurs begin immediately after S2 and are decrescendo as the ventricle fills. They are the result of early

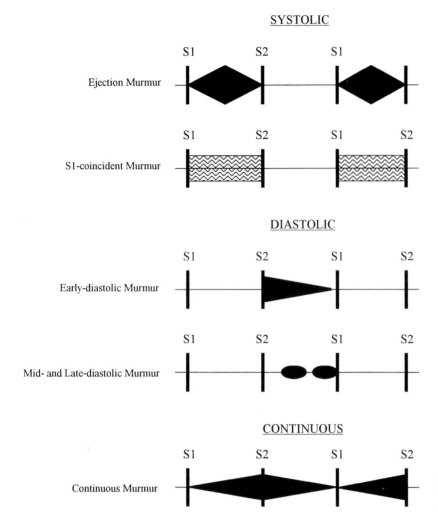

SYSTOLIC

Ejection Murmur

S1-coincident Murmur

DIASTOLIC

Early-diastolic Murmur

Mid- and Late-diastolic Murmur

CONTINUOUS

Continuous Murmur

FIGURE 3.1 Classification of heart murmurs. This figure demonstrates the classification of heart murmurs based on their timing during the cardiac cycle.

diastolic backflow from the great vessel into the heart through an incompetent semilunar valve.

Aortic regurgitant murmurs arise from the higher diastolic pressure in the aorta and are therefore high pitched. They are heard best with the diaphragm of the stethoscope at the left midsternal border and radiate toward the apex. As the dia-

stolic pressure gradient equalizes, the murmur decreases in intensity. Listening while the patient leans forward and exhales accentuates the aortic regurgitant murmur.

Pulmonary regurgitant murmurs are also heard in early diastole. They are medium-pitched murmurs unless there is diastolic pulmonary hypertension, in which case they are high

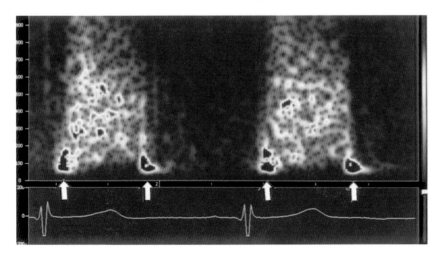

FIGURE 3.2 Digital phonocardiographic image demonstrating the S1-coincident murmur of a ventricular septal defect. The scale on the left denotes frequency of sound. The color scale on the right depicts intensity of sound. The corresponding electrocardiogram is plotted below. Arrows correspond to S1 and S2. The color display between S1 and S2 represents the various frequencies and intensities of the murmur. (From Balster DA, Chan DP, Rowland DG, et al. Digital acoustic analysis of precordial innocent versus ventricular septal defect murmurs in children. *Am J Cardiol* 1997;79:1552–1555, with permission.)

pitched. They are heard from the left upper to midsternal border and radiate down the left sternal border. In the infant, they sound like a saw cutting wood with the to and fro diastolic backflow and forward volume load during ejection across the pulmonary valve.

Middiastolic Murmurs

Middiastolic murmurs occur during the rapid filling phase of diastole when blood crosses the AV valves. They are low pitched and best heard with the bell of the stethoscope. Pathologic narrowing or thickening of the mitral or tricuspid valves (i.e., mitral and tricuspid stenosis) causes middiastolic murmurs. Excessive volume across a normal-sized AV valve is heard as a middiastolic rumble and is erroneously referred to as "relative stenosis." If the valve is held partially closed by an aortic regurgitant jet, a middiastolic murmur results, called the Austin-Flint murmur.

Mitral valve stenosis (obstruction), VSD, PDA, and mitral regurgitation (volume) cause mitral valve middiastolic murmurs that are heard at the apex. Tricuspid valve stenosis (obstruction), ASD, and anomalous pulmonary venous return (both volume) cause tricuspid valve middiastolic murmurs that are heard along the LLSB.

Late Diastolic Murmurs

Presystolic murmurs also are caused by flow across narrowed AV valves. They occur late in diastole as a result of atrial contraction pushing blood through the narrowed valve into the ventricle. The murmur will accentuate with atrial contraction and will be absent if the patient is in atrial fibrillation. They are low-frequency murmurs heard in true mitral and tricuspid valve stenosis. They are rare in children, paralleling the low numbers of children with true AV-valve stenosis.

Continuous Murmurs

Continuous murmurs begin in systole and are heard into, and often, through diastole. These murmurs almost always are vascular in origin. They are caused by aortopulmonary (dependent) (i.e., PDA, surgical aorticopulmonary shunts) or arteriovenous (obligate) connections (AV fistula, coronary-cameral fistula), turbulent flow in arteries (coarctation, severe branch pulmonary artery stenosis), or turbulent flow through veins (venous hum).

The most common aortopulmonary continuous murmur is heard in PDA. It is loudest in systole and softest during diastole, giving it a "machinery" characteristic. It is continuous because of the constant pressure gradient between the aorta and pulmonary arteries and increases during systole because of a larger pressure gradient. In patients with levocardia, it is best heard at the left infraclavicular area. A surgically placed aorticopulmonary shunt murmur sounds similar to that of the PDA.

Other continuous murmurs arising from arterial malformations include coronary artery fistulas, pulmonary arteriovenous fistulas, bronchial collateral vessels, and pulmonary vessels arising from a truncus arteriosus. Coronary artery fistulas may empty into the right atrium, right ventricle, left ventricle, or pulmonary artery. These continuous murmurs may be louder in diastole. The location of the murmur will differ with each abnormality; however, it will usually be located on the lower pressure side of the abnormal connection.

Continuous murmurs occasionally are heard in patients with peripheral pulmonary arterial stenosis in whom flow into distal vessels varies and in patients with coarctation of the aorta who have large collateral vessels. These murmurs will be heard in the axillae and over the back, respectively.

Venous murmurs are often benign, as in the venous hum. They usually are heard over the left or right upper chest and disappear with changes in head position or compression of the jugular vein. They vary with respiration and are best heard with the patient upright.

In obstructed forms of total anomalous pulmonary venous return, a soft, high-pitched continuous murmur may be heard over the site of obstruction. The site of the murmur is determined by the locus of drainage, for example, over the liver.

The so-called to-and-fro murmur is the combination of a systolic and diastolic murmur, as in aortic stenosis and regurgitation. The systolic component of such a murmur ends prior to the start of the diastolic component, thus differentiating it from a continuous murmur. The characteristic murmur in absence of the pulmonary valve has a distinctive "sawing" quality.

INNOCENT MURMURS

Innocent murmurs are the sound of noisy blood flow coursing through a normally structured heart. They are heard in ≤80% of children at some time or another, particularly at around 3 or 4 years of age. They are accentuated by increased cardiac output, as when a child is excited, anemic, or febrile. Auscultation with the ability to differentiate pathologic murmurs from benign murmurs is the method of choice for diagnosing innocent murmurs.

The exact cause of the innocent murmur has yet to be defined. Suggestions include relatively smaller aortic size resulting in increased velocity of blood across the aorta during ejection, left ventricular false tendons, exaggerated vibrations with ventricular contraction, and increased cardiac output (10–12). Whatever the cause, the heart is normal and a detailed imaging evaluation is unnecessary for diagnosis.

Still's Murmur

The most common innocent systolic murmur of childhood is Still's murmur. It has many names, including innocent, vibratory, functional, normal, and physiologic murmur. It is a midsystolic murmur heard loudest at the midpoint between the left midsternal border and the apex. Described as having a vibratory, musical, or twanging string quality, its usual intensity is 2 to 3/6. It is a low-frequency murmur in the range of 150 Hz (13). The murmur is heard best with the patient supine. As with all innocent murmurs, the ECG and chest radiograph are normal.

Pulmonary Flow Murmur of Childhood

A second innocent ejection murmur is the pulmonary flow murmur. Commonly detected in thin-chested adolescents between 8 and 14 years of age, it is heard maximally over the pulmonary outflow area. Although it resembles the ejection murmur of PS, it is not accompanied by a click or thrill. Its intensity is 1 to 3/6, and the P2 component of the second heart sound is normal.

Pulmonary Flow Murmur of Infancy

Also referred to as a peripheral pulmonary stenosis (PPS) murmur, this murmur is commonly heard during the newborn period, particularly in premature infants. It is an ejection murmur that radiates from the LUSB to both axillae and the back. Theories of its origin include the relatively small size of the branch pulmonary arteries immediately after birth, as well as their angle of the takeoff from the main pulmonary artery during the newborn period (14,15). Whatever the cause, it usually disappears by 6 months of age. If the murmur persists past

6 months of age, structural abnormalities of the pulmonary artery tree should be considered.

Venous Hum

The venous hum murmur is discussed above.

References

1. Stevens SS, Warshofsky F. *Sound and Hearing.* Alexandria, VA: Time-Life Science Library, 1980.
2. Dock W, Grandell F, Taubman F. The physiologic third sound, its mechanism and relation to protodiastolic gallop. *Am Heart J* 1955;50:449–464.
3. Ozawa Y, Smith D. Origin of the third heart sound: 1. Studies in dogs. *Circulation* 1983;67:393–398.
4. Dunn FL, Dickerson WJ. Third heart sound: Possible role of pericardium in its production. *Circ Res* 1955;3:51–55.
5. Reddy PS, Meno F, Cutiss EI, et al. The genesis of gallop sounds: Investigation by quantitative phono- and apex cardiography. *Circulation* 1981;63:922–933.
6. Leatham A. *Auscultation of the Heart and Phonocardiography.* London: J & A Churchill, 1970.
7. Shaver JA, Leonard JJ, Leon DF. *Examination of the Heart. Part 4: Auscultation of the Heart.* Dallas: American Heart Association, 1990.
8. Nichols WW, O'Rourke MF. *McDonald's Blood Flow in Arteries.* Philadelphia: Lea & Febiger, 1990.
9. Balster DA, O'Connell D, McCreary M, et al. Frequency analysis of heart murmurs correlates to severity of ventricular septal defect. Paper

presented at the American Academy of Pediatrics; October, 2004; San Francisco, CA.
10. Klewer SE, Donnerstein RL, Goldberg SJ. Still's-like innocent murmur can be produced by increasing aortic velocity to a threshold value. *Am J Cardiol* 1991;68:810–812.
11. Stein P, Sabbah H. Aortic origin of innocent murmurs. *Am J Cardiol* 1977;39:665–671.
12. Stein P, Sabbah H, Lakier J. Origin and clinical relevance of musical murmurs. *Int J Cardiol* 1983;4:103–112.
13. Balster DA, Chan DP, Rowland DG, et al. Digital acoustic analysis of precordial innocent versus ventricular septal defect murmurs in children. *Am J Cardiol* 1997;79:1552–1555.
14. Danilowicz DA, Rudolph AM, Hoffman JIE, et al. Physiologic pressure differences between main and branch pulmonary arteries in infants. *Circulation* 1972;45:410–419.
15. Miyake T, Yokoyama T. Evaluation of transient heart murmur resembling pulmonary artery stenosis in term infants by Doppler and M-mode echocardiography. *Jpn Circ J* 1993;57:77–83.

CHAPTER 4 ■ SPORTS SCREENING AND PARTICIPATION

ALBERT P. ROCCHINI, MD

Participation in competitive athletics is a rewarding experience both physically and emotionally. However, for some children with congenital cardiovascular disease this activity has the potential to end tragically with severe disability or even death. While the absolute number of children dying during sports participation is extremely small, especially compared with children of the same age who die each year from trauma, some of the sports-related deaths in children with congenital heart disease are at least theoretically preventable (1). Additionally, sports related deaths get wider publicity and therefore have increased visibility. Common sense dictates that children with severe heart disease should be restricted form strenuous competitive physical activity. Yet there are little available data that we can use to make evidence-based recommendations (2–7). Much of the data are empiric; therefore many children are restricted on the basis of personal prejudices rather than on objective data.

Remarkable progress has been made in the treatment of children with congenital heart disease during the past five decades. Children with defects that were once considered fatal are now living relatively normal lives. Thus, physicians are faced with a new patient population: Adolescents and young adults with corrected congenital heart disease who want to be able to live normal lifestyles that include competitive sports. To empirically restrict some of these individuals from participating in competitive sports may be tragic, since being a member of a sports team can be a critical part of normal adolescent maturation. To label a child a "cardiac cripple" and deprive him or her of the benefits of participation on the basis of whim rather than data does a disservice.

This chapter will describe what screening should be done before permitting patients to participate in competitive physical activity, review the normal cardiovascular response to exercise, and review the hemodynamic responses to exercise in patients with repaired or unrepaired congenital heart disease. Recommendations regarding appropriate activity restrictions will be offered.

PRE–ATHLETIC PARTICIPATION SCREENING

Pre–athletic participation screening for the early identification of "silent" cardiovascular disease that might cause sudden death is a strategy that is used to prevent sudden death during athletic competition (8–11). Suspicion of heart disease during preparticipation screening is raised by the presence of cardiac symptoms including dyspnea, chest pain, syncope, or near syncope; a family history of heart disease or sudden unexpected death; and/or by the presence of a pathologic heart murmur. In 2003, Corrado et al. (12) reported the incidence of sudden death in the athletic and nonathletic young population (12 to 35 years) in the Veneto region of Italy. These authors demonstrated that participating in competitive sports increased the risk of sudden death in adolescents and young adults by 250%. They reported an incidence of sudden death of 2.3 (2.62 in the males and 1.07 in females) per 100,000 athletes per year from all causes and of 2.1 per 100,000 athletes per year from cardiovascular disease. Maron (13) estimated the prevalence of sudden death in young athletes in the United States to be ≤0.3%. In Corrado's study (12), young athletes who died suddenly had silent cardiovascular diseases, predominately hypertrophic cardiomyopathy, premature coronary artery disease, congenital coronary anomalies (origin of the left main coronary artery arising from the right sinus of Valsalva, acute angle of the origin of a coronary artery, stenosis of the ostia, and anomalous origin of the left coronary artery from the pulmonary artery) and dysrhythmias (prolonged QT syndrome, arrhythmogenic right ventricular cardiomyopathy and Brugada's syndrome). Other cardiac conditions associated with sudden death include valvar aortic stenosis and Marfan syndrome (11,13).

In the United States, it is customary to screen high school and college athletes for silent cardiovascular disease by taking a history and performing a physical examination. Performing a 12-lead ECG is not routine. This screening method has been recommended by the American Heart Association Sudden Death and Congenital Defects Committee (14). However, the quality of the cardiovascular screening for United States athletes has come under scrutiny because of inadequacies of questionnaires used for history taking and the level of training and expertise of individuals performing the examinations (15,16). One retrospective analysis of 134 high school and collegiate athletes who died suddenly demonstrated that cardiovascular abnormalities were suspected by standard history and physical examination screening in only 3% of the examined athletes and eventually, <1% received an accurate diagnosis (17).

In contrast to the United States, Italian law mandates that every subject engaged in competitive sports activity must undergo a clinical evaluation and a 12-lead electrocardiogram before obtaining eligibility for participation in sports (18). This has been the practice in Italy for >25 years (15,19). Corrado et al. (19) reported on a 17-year experience from this type of preparticipation screening. During 1979 to 1996, a consecutive series of 33,735 young athletes was evaluated. Of these, 1,058 were disqualified for medical reasons, 621 (1.8%) of them because of the recognition of clinically relevant cardiovascular abnormalities. The most frequent conditions were rhythm and conduction abnormalities (38.3%), hypertension (27%), valvular disease (21.4%), and hypertrophic cardiomyopathy (3.6%). Among the 33,735 athletes screened, 22 (0.07%) showed both clinical and echocardiographic evidence of hypertrophic cardiomyopathy, a prevalence rate similar to the 0.1% reported in young white individuals in the United States (20).

ECG screening is associated with a substantial proportion of false-positive results. Of the 33,735 athletes screened, 3,019 (8.9%) were referred for echocardiographic evaluation and only 22 ultimately showed definitive evidence of hypertrophic cardiomyopathy. Despite this high incidence of false-positive ECGs, the European Society of Cardiology has recommended that preparticipation cardiovascular evaluation of young competitive athletes should include a 12-lead ECG in addition to a complete history and physical examination (10).

In the United States, obstacles exist to implementation of an obligatory national screening of competitive athletes with an ECG. These include the large population of athletes to be screened (about 10 to 12 million), major cost–benefit considerations, and the recognition that it is impossible to absolutely eliminate the risks associated with competitive sports (12). For example, since there are >10 million athletes in the United States, if an electrocardiogram costs $50, it would cost $500 million for electrocardiographic screening of all athletes. Additionally, based on the Italian experience, 890,000 electrocardiograms will be positive. This will result in ordering an echocardiogram at an approximate cost of $1,500 per test. Thus, the total cost of an Italian/European-based screening program in the United States would be $1.835 billion. A potential alternative strategy for athletic screening in the United States could be a structured history and physical examination for *all* individuals participating in competitive athletics; however, for elite athletes (college and Olympic-caliber athletes) pre–athletic participation screening should also include a 12-lead electrocardiogram. If the 12-lead electrocardiogram is abnormal, an echocardiogram or other appropriate diagnostic studies would result. If this type of strategy were used at the University of Michigan, which has 750 varsity athletes, the cost would be $137,500 ($37,500 for electrocardiograms and $100,000 for echocardiograms performed because of a false-positive "abnormal" electrocardiogram).

Diagnostic Testing Strategies

When a cardiovascular abnormality is initially suspected by formal screening diagnostic testing, strategies should focus on the systematic exclusion of those conditions that are known to cause sudden death. The most common noninvasive diagnostic tests are the ECG, echocardiography, Holter ECG, and exercise test.

Electrocardiography

The 12-lead ECG should be used as the first diagnostic test for identifying cardiovascular disease in young athletes. It has been shown to be a practical and cost-effective alternative to the routine use of echocardiography for population-based screening. For example, the ECG is abnormal in ≤75% to 95% of individuals with hypertrophic cardiomyopathy (11,21). The ECG will also identify many individuals with long QT syndrome, Brugada's syndrome, and other

TABLE 4.1

CRITERIA FOR A POSITIVE 12-LEAD ECG

- Abnormal P wave:
  - LA enlargement: negative P in V1 ≥0.1 mV in depth and ≥0.04 s in duration
  - RA enlargement: peaked P wave in leads II, III, or V1 ≥0.25 mV in amplitude
- QRS complex:
  - QRS axis right of ≥+120 or left of −30 to −90 degrees
  - Inc. voltage R or S standard leads ≥2 mV, S wave in V1 or V2 ≥3 mV or R in V5 or V6 ≥3 mV
  - R or R' in V1 ≥0.5 mV and R/S ≥1
  - Abnormal Q waves ≥0.04 s in duration or ≥25% of the height of the ensuing R wave or a QS pattern in two or more leads
- ST segment, T wave, and QT interval:
  - ST depression or T-wave flattening or inversion in two or more leads
  - QT prolongation if corrected interval is ≥0.44 s males and ≥0.46 s females
- Rhythm and conduction abnormalities:
  - Right of left bundle branch block QRS ≥0.12 s
  - Premature beats or more severe ventricular arrhythmias
  - Supraventricular tachycardia, atrial flutter or fibrillation
  - Short PR interval <0.12 s with or without delta wave
  - Sinus bradycardia with a resting heart rate <40 and increasing <100 beats/min during light exercise
  - Any degree of AV block

Modified from Corrado D, Basso C, Schiavon M, et al. Screening for hypertrophic cardiomyopathy in young athletes. *N Engl J Med* 1998;339:364–369, with permission.

inherited syndromes associated with ventricular arrhythmias. Table 4.1 outlines the criteria for a positive 12-lead ECG. It is important to remember that an abnormal 12-lead ECG pattern may exist in about 40% of elite athletes, for example, increased R- or S-wave voltages, Q waves, and repolarization "abnormalities" (22). Athletes with truly abnormal electrocardiograms should be referred for additional testing such as echocardiography, 24-hour ambulatory Holter monitoring, and exercise testing.

Echocardiography

A two-dimensional echocardiogram with Doppler is an excellent tool for evaluating structural heart disease. It can also assess overall cardiac function. However, function may appear normal at rest and be significantly abnormal with exercise, for example, in patients with congenital abnormalities of the coronary arteries. In individuals with a negative history, physical examination, and electrocardiogram, echocardiographic screening is of low yield and high cost. The two-dimensional echocardiogram is the major diagnostic test for the clinical identification of hypertrophic cardiomyopathy. However, it may be difficult to differentiate between a normal variant, athlete's heart (22–25), and pathologic hypertrophy. Conditioned athletes often develop adaptive cardiac changes to increase stroke volume. These include thickening of the left ventricular walls and enlargement of chambers. These changes are normal adaptations to chronic exercise. In general, a maximal left ventricular end-diastolic wall thickness in the adult of ≤15 mm or in the child greater than two standard deviations above the mean relative to body surface area are the absolute dimensions generally accepted for clinical diagnosis of hypertrophic cardiomyopathy (20,21,26). However, it is important to remember that, theoretically, any specific left ventricular wall thickness (including normal) is compatible with the presence of a mutant hypertrophic cardiomyopathy gene (26).

Ambulatory Holter Monitoring

Ambulatory Holter monitoring is a good screening tool for individuals who are suspected of having paroxysmal arrhythmias. The monitor allows evaluation of the cardiac rhythm during the individual's daily activities for 24 to 48 hours.

Exercise Testing

Exercise testing is used to determine physical working capacity. It is a provocative test for detecting either ischemia or arrhythmias. In most cases, it is best used to determine if exercise can be performed safely without risk of compromise or adverse events. Exercise studies can be performed using either a bicycle ergometer or treadmill. It is important to test exercise tolerance to the level of activity the athlete is likely to achieve in competition. A comprehensive exercise evaluation should include pre-exercise and postexercise assessment of pulmonary function; measurements of heart rate, blood pressure, and oxygen saturation; and ventilatory measures including maximal oxygen consumption, minute ventilation, carbon dioxide production, and anaerobic threshold.

NORMAL CARDIOVASCULAR RESPONSES TO EXERCISE

Most exercise can be classified as either isometric (static) or isotonic (dynamic). Isometric exercise involves the development of high muscle tension without active shortening. A good example of isometric exercise is weight lifting or performing a handstand. Isotonic (dynamic) exercise involves active changes in muscle length, usually with frequent rhythmic contraction, such as in running and swimming. However, most sports cannot be simply classified as either solely isometric or isotonic since they include both isotonic and isometric exercise. A football player performs isotonic exercise

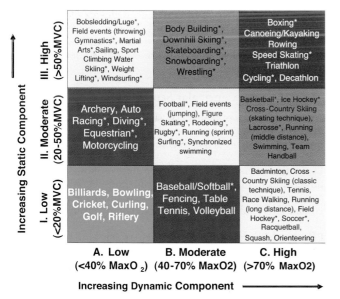

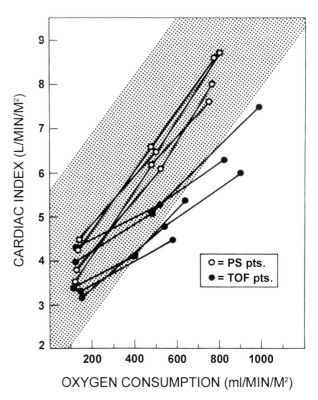

FIGURE 4.1 Classification of sports. This classification is based on peak static and dynamic components achieved during competition. It should be noted that higher values may be reached in training. The increasing dynamic component is defined in terms of the estimated percent of maximal oxygen consumption (Max O_2) achieved and results in an increasing cardiac output. The increasing static component is related to the estimated percent of maximal voluntary contraction (MVC) reached and results in an increasing blood pressure load. The lowest total cardiovascular demands (cardiac output and blood pressure) are shown in green and the highest in red. Blue, yellow, and orange depict low moderate, moderate, and high moderate total cardiovascular demands, respectively. (From Mitchell JH, Haskell W, Snell P. Task Force 8: classification of Sports. *J Am Coll Cardiol* 2005;45:1364-1367, with permission.)

FIGURE 4.2 Relation between cardiac index and indexed oxygen consumption at rest and during supine bicycle exercise in four patients with mild pulmonary stenosis (PS) and five with repaired tetralogy of Fallot (TOF). The hatched area represents the normal range. The tetralogy patients are below the normal range whereas the pulmonary stenosis patients have a normal relationship between oxygen consumption and cardiac output. (From Rocchini AP. Hemodynamic abnormalities in response to supine exercise in patients after operative correction of tetrad of Fallot after early childhood. *Am J Cardiol* 1981;48:325–330, with permission.)

when he runs but performs isometric exercise when blocking and tackling.

Sports have been classified into nine categories based on intensity of both the dynamic and static component of the exercise (27) (Fig. 4.1). Weight lifting and gymnastics are classified as high static and low dynamic, whereas running and soccer are classified as high dynamic and low static.

With isotonic exercise, there is an increase in oxygen demand resulting in increased oxygen consumption (28,29,30) (Table 4.2). Cardiac output increases almost linearly with the increase in oxygen consumption and may increase by as much as 400% to 500% with peak exercise (Fig. 4.2). Increased cardiac output is caused by both greater stroke volume (25% to

50% increase) and accelerated heart rate (300% to 400% increase). The increase in cardiac output is directed toward the involved working skeletal muscles and heart whereas blood flow to the nonexercising tissues (kidney, brain, splanchnic bed) remains unchanged or is reduced. Because of systemic vasodilation and the increased cardiac output associated with exercise, systolic blood pressure increases, diastolic blood pressure decreases, and mean blood pressure remains unchanged.

TABLE 4.2

HEMODYNAMIC RESPONSES TO DYNAMIC AND STATIC EXERCISE

	Dynamic	Static
Heart rate	↑↑↑	↑
Systemic systolic pressure	↑	↑↑↑
Systemic diastolic pressure	↓	↑↑
Systemic mean pressure	No change	↑↑
Systemic vascular resistance	↓↓	↑↑
Cardiac output	↑↑↑	↑
Left ventricular stroke volume	↑	No change

Pulmonary vasodilation is more limited, and pulmonary artery pressures typically increase by as much as 50%. Thus, dynamic exercise primarily imposes a volume load on the heart. The normal heart performs the increased volume work associated with dynamic exercise with assistance from the Frank-Starling mechanism (increased venous return), enhanced contractility (increased catecholamines), increased heart rate (increased sympathetic and reduce parasympathetic tone), and reduced afterload (decreased peripheral resistance).

Isometric exercise, such as weight lifting, involves sustained muscular contraction against a large resistance (Table 4.2). There is usually a marked increase in systemic arterial systolic, diastolic, and mean blood pressure, a slight increase in cardiac output, and a significant increase in peripheral vascular resistance (30,31). Intra-arterial pressure can reach 320/250 mm Hg in response to weight lifting (31). This increased afterload is usually associated with a constant or slightly decreased stroke volume and a small to moderate increase in end-diastolic pressure. Thus isometric exercise primarily imposes a pressure load on the heart.

RECOMMENDATIONS REGARDING ACTIVITY RESTRICTION IN PATIENTS WITH CONGENITAL HEART DISEASE

Most recommendations that will be made in this section come from the consensus panel recommendations of the 36th Bethesda Conference for eligibility and disqualification of competitive athletes (7,9,27). These recommendations are intended to provide broad guidelines for the participation of patients with congenital heart disease in competitive athletics.

Left-to-Right Shunt Lesions

Atrial Septal Defects

Most patients with atrial septal defect are asymptomatic. There is minimal right ventricular volume overload with a small atrial septal defect. There can be marked right ventricular volume overload with moderate to large defects. Pulmonary hypertension is unusual in individuals with atrial septal defect.

Evaluation. Atrial septal defects often can be diagnosed by physical examination. The chest radiograph and echocardiogram are useful in determining the degree of right ventricular volume overload and defect size.

Effects of Exercise. Dynamic exercise is well tolerated in most patients with atrial septal defects. In patients with marked right ventricular volume overload, exercise endurance may be limited by the ability of the right ventricle to maintain the high cardiac output necessary at peak exercise.

Recommendations

1. Since most children have atrial septal defects closed before they are active in competitive sports, exercise usually is not restricted. The only patients in whom exercise should be restricted are those with a large atrial septal defect and mild pulmonary artery hypertension. Low-intensity competitive sports (IA) are recommended until the defect is closed (7).

2. For those athletes with surgical or device closure of an atrial septal defect, if the patient has no evidence of pulmonary hypertension or ventricular or atrial ectopy, they can participate in all sports 3 to 6 months after the operation or device closure (7).

Ventricular Septal Defects

As with atrial septal defects, significant ventricular septal defects are usually closed in early childhood well before the individual becomes active in competitive sports.

Evaluation. Ventricular septal defects are usually diagnosed by physical examination. The echocardiogram, chest radiograph, and electrocardiogram are useful in determining left ventricular volume overload and elevation of pulmonary artery pressure.

Effects of Exercise. Small ventricular septal defects with a pulmonary-to-systemic flow ratio (Qp/Qs) of <1.5/1 do not effect the cardiovascular response to exercise. Moderate-size defects (Qp/Qs 1.5 to 2/1) with low pulmonary artery pressure and resistance usually have only mild left ventricular volume overload. As a result, dynamic exercise is well tolerated; however, isometric exercise may be less well tolerated. Since isometric exercise increases systemic afterload much more than pulmonary afterload, isometric exercise can result in an increase in both pulmonary flow and Qp/Qs.

Large ventricular septal defects (Qp/Qs >2) with normal pulmonary pressures and resistances have similar exercise hemodynamics to the moderate-size defects; however, if pulmonary hypertension is present, either dynamic or isometric exercise is usually not well tolerated. With both types of exercise, the pulmonary vascular bed is unable to handle the increased blood flow associated with the exercise; right-to-left shunting may occur.

Recommendations

1. Athletes with small to moderate ventricular septal defects and normal pulmonary artery pressure can participate in all sports (7).
2. Athletes with large defects and normal pulmonary artery pressure can participate after defect closure (7).
3. Athletes with large defects and elevated pulmonary vascular resistance cannot participate in any competitive sports (7).
4. For those athletes with surgical or device closure of a ventricular septal defect, if the patient does not have evidence of pulmonary hypertension or ventricular or atrial ectopy, he or she can participate in all sports 3 to 6 months after successful intervention (7).

Patent Ductus Arteriosus (PDA)

Moderate to large PDAs are usually closed in infancy well before the patients would participate in competitive sports. Those with a small PDA should have no restrictions from competitive sports since the defect should not adversely affect the cardiovascular response to either isometric or isotonic exercise. Competitive sports should be restricted in the rare patient with a moderate to large PDA until the defect has either been surgically or device closed. Although the 36th Bethesda Conference report (7) suggests that patients with normal pulmonary pressures and left ventricular chamber sizes after PDA closure should wait for 3 months before participating in competitive sports, most pediatric cardiologists let these patients start athletic participation within 1 to 2 weeks after device closure and within 6 weeks after surgical closure.

Atrioventricular Septal Defects

Patients with an atrioventricular septal defect should follow the same recommendations as for a ventricular septal defect. The only exception is those individuals who have significant mitral regurgitation. Those with moderate to severe mitral regurgitation should be restricted from exercise if they have either severe volume overload of the left atrium and/or left ventricle or evidence of pulmonary hypertension.

Valvular Lesions

Pulmonary Valve Stenosis

Pulmonary stenosis is quantified, depending on the peak systolic right ventricular outflow tract gradient, as being mild (gradients of <40 mm Hg), moderate (gradients of between 40 and 60 mm Hg), or severe (gradients of >60 mm Hg).

Evaluations. The degree of pulmonary stenosis can be accurately diagnosed by physical examination, electrocardiogram, and Doppler echocardiogram. The echocardiogram is especially useful in quantitating the degree of pulmonary regurgitation that may be present following valvuloplasty.

Response to Exercise. During dynamic isotonic exercise, the associated increase in cardiac output and right ventricular outflow stroke volume causes the right ventricular outflow tract gradient to increase. With severe stenosis, the stroke volume can remain unchanged or even decrease during exercise (32–34). In patients with mild to at most moderate pulmonary stenosis, increased stroke volume is associated with decreased right ventricular end-diastolic pressure, whereas with severe stenosis, right ventricular end-diastolic pressure can increase (34,35). Increased right ventricular end-diastolic pressure with exercise may represent a ventricular compliance abnormality. Isometric exercise usually has little effect on patients with pulmonary stenosis because pulmonary pressure and resistance only mildly increase.

Recommendations

1. Athletes with mild pulmonary stenosis and normal right ventricular function can participate in all forms of exercise (7).
2. Athletes with right ventricular outflow tract gradients of >40 mm Hg should participate in only low-intensity competitive sports (IA and IB) until after pulmonary valvuloplasty has been performed (7).
3. Exercise hemodynamics improve rapidly following valvuloplasty, with marked decrease in exercise-augmented outflow obstruction and improved right ventricular end-diastolic pressure with exercise (33) (Fig. 4.3). However, since most patients with severe valvar pulmonary stenosis also have some degree of dynamic subpulmonary stenosis, it may take ≤6 months before maximal gradient relief is achieved. After valvuloplasty, athletes with no or only mild residual pulmonary stenosis and normal ventricular function can participate in all types of competitive exercise. Participation can begin 2 to 4 weeks after balloon valvuloplasty or 3 months after surgical valvuloplasty (7).
4. Athletes with severe pulmonary regurgitation after valvuloplasty characterized by marked right ventricular enlargement can participate in only class IA and IB types of exercise (7).

Pulmonary Valve Regurgitation

Isolated pulmonary regurgitation is uncommon. The most common cause of severe pulmonary regurgitation occurs after repair of tetralogy of Fallot.

Aortic Stenosis

Aortic stenosis (either valvar, subvalvar, or supravalvar) is one of the very few types of congenital heart disease associated with sudden death during sports participation (11,13,36). Aortic stenosis is quantified, depending on the peak systolic left ventricular outflow tract gradient, as being mild (gradients <30 mm Hg), moderate (gradients between 30 and 50 mm Hg), or severe (gradients >50 mm Hg) (7).

Evaluation. Differentiation between mild, moderate, and severe stenosis can be made by physical examination, electrocardiogram, and Doppler echocardiogram. Patients with aortic stenosis can develop symptoms with exercise including fatigue, light-headedness, dizziness, syncope, chest pain, and sudden death. Sudden death is more likely to occur in patients with severe left ventricular hypertrophy, resting ST-segment depression, exertional syncope, and chest pain (37). Symptomatic patients deserve complete evaluation including cardiac catheterization. Graded treadmill exercise testing should be performed in all athletes who are suspected to have moderate aortic stenosis.

Response to Exercise. Several abnormal responses to dynamic exercise have been described in children with aortic stenosis. These include ischemic ST segments (Fig. 4.4), angina, ventricular arrhythmias, and suboptimal systolic systemic arterial pressure response (38–42). Most of these abnormalities are the consequence of exercise-induced pressure overload. During dynamic exercise, since the valve area remains constant, increased cardiac output and left ventricular stroke volume cause the left ventricular outflow tract gradient to increase (39). In severe stenosis, if the left ventricle cannot increase stroke volume to compensate for the decreased systemic vascular resistance associated with vasodilation of the working muscle, systolic aortic pressure will either only minimally increase or even decrease with exercise (43). Decreased arterial pressure with exercise can explain the light-headedness, dizziness, and syncope associated with exercise in certain patients with aortic stenosis. In patients with aortic stenosis, Kveselis et al. (38) found that during supine bicycle exercise aortic gradients increased from a mean of 48 to 94 mm Hg and left ventricular systolic pressures increased from 166 to 231 mm Hg. In those children who developed ST-segment depression with exercise, they found that the ST-segment depression was related to increased left ventricular end-diastolic pressure (17 to 25 mm Hg) and decreased left ventricular supply/demand ratio (13.9 to 6.4). Isometric exercise is not well tolerated in individuals with aortic stenosis since increased systemic vascular resistance can result in depressed myocardial oxygen supply/demand ratio (39).

Recommendations

1. Because of the abnormal hemodynamic responses to exercise associated with aortic stenosis only athletes with mild aortic stenosis, a normal resting electrocardiogram, and no history of exercise-related symptoms can participate in all forms of competitive sports. However, since aortic stenosis is a progressive disease, patients with mild stenosis should be re-evaluated periodically to continue with their competitive sport (7).

PRE PULMONARY VALVULOPLASTY

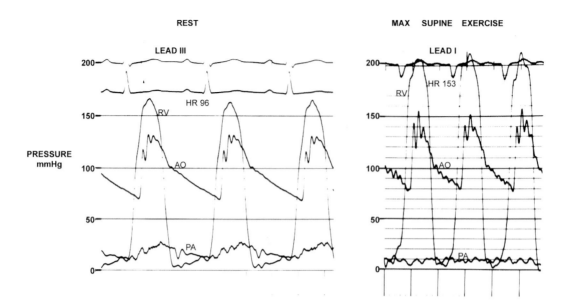

POST PULMONARY VALVULOPLASTY

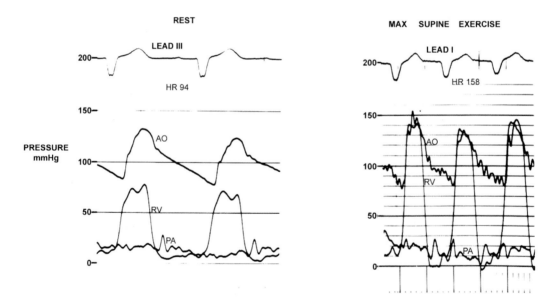

FIGURE 4.3 Simultaneous right ventricular (RV), aortic (AO), and pulmonary artery (PA) pressures and heart rate (HR) at rest and during maximal (MAX) supine bicycle exercise before (pre) and immediately after (post) balloon valvuloplasty. Before the valvuloplasty, right ventricular pressure was mildly suprasystemic and increased well above systemic pressure at peak exercise, whereas after valvuloplasty with incomplete relief of stenosis, right ventricular pressure decreased to less than half systemic pressure. With maximal supine exercise, right ventricular pressure still reached systemic level. (From Rocchini AP, Kveselis DA, Crowley D, et al. Percutaneous balloon valvuloplasty for treatment of congenital pulmonary valvular stenosis in children. *J Am Coll Cardiol* 1984;3:1005–1012, with permission.)

2. Athletes with moderate aortic stenosis who have mild or no left ventricular hypertrophy, normal response to treadmill exercise testing, and no exercise-induced symptoms can participate in low static/low to moderate dynamic, and moderate static/low to moderate dynamic exercise (classes IA, IB, and IIA) (7).

3. Athletes with severe aortic stenosis cannot participate in any form of competitive sports (7).

4. Surgical or balloon valvuloplasty can reduce the degree of aortic stenosis but frequently is associated with some degree of aortic regurgitation. Patients with residual mild, moderate, or severe stenosis after either balloon or surgical

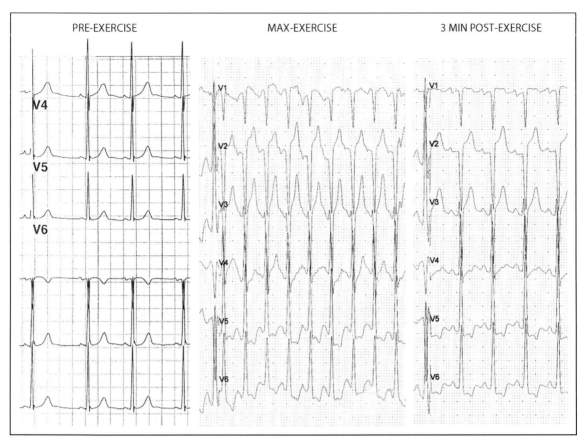

PRE-EXERCISE   MAX-EXERCISE   3 MIN POST-EXERCISE

FIGURE 4.4 An exercise test on a 12-year-old boy with aortic stenosis. The resting chest leads for the electrocardiogram demonstrate normal ST segments and T waves; however, at maximal exercise (stage 4 of the Bruce protocol) he developed 0.25 mV ST-segment depression in leads V5 and V6 and negative T waves. ST-segment depression (0.2 mV) was present in these same leads 3 minutes after recovery.

intervention should follow the same recommendations as previously stated for untreated individuals, provided moderate or severe aortic regurgitation is not present (7).

Aortic Regurgitation

Aortic regurgitation in childhood is usually seen in association with a congenital bicuspid aortic valve, following surgical or balloon valvuloplasty, as a result of endocarditis, associated with rheumatic heart disease, and/or owing to aortic root disease such as seen in Marfan syndrome. Individuals with severe aortic regurgitation can remain asymptomatic and athletic for many years. Sudden death is rare in asymptomatic patients with aortic regurgitation (>0.2% per year) (44).

Evaluation. Aortic regurgitation can be adequately assessed by physical examination, chest radiograph, and echocardiography. Doppler echocardiography is a sensitive method for detecting aortic regurgitation; however, it can be difficult to quantitatively differentiate between moderate and severe aortic regurgitation. Exercise testing and Holter monitoring can be useful for assessing exercise capacity and detecting ventricular arrhythmias, especially in those patients who wish to be involved in competitive sports. Aortic regurgitation is classified as mild (absent or slight peripheral signs such as wide pulse pressure, bounding pulses, and normal LV size); moderate (peripheral signs of aortic regurgitation, increased left ventricular size but normal left ventricular function); and severe (peripheral signs of

aortic regurgitation and significant left ventricular enlargement with or without left ventricular dysfunction) (45).

Effects of Exercise. Aortic regurgitation increases left ventricular diastolic volume and stroke volume. With dynamic exercise, the regurgitant volume decreases because of the decreased peripheral vascular resistance and decreased diastolic filling period that accompanies an increased heart rate (46). Isometric exercise has the opposite effect since regurgitant volume can be increased owing to markedly increased peripheral vascular resistance and aortic pressure with little to no decrease in the diastolic filling period.

Recommendations

1. Athletes with mild or moderate aortic regurgitation who have a left ventricular end-diastolic size that is similar to that seen with athletic training can participate in all competitive sports (7,45).
2. According to the 36th Bethesda conference report (7,45), in selected instances, athletes with aortic regurgitation and moderate left ventricular enlargement (>95th percentile for body surface area in children or 60 to 65 mm for an adult) can engage in low and moderate static and low, moderate, and high dynamic competitive sports (classes IA, IB, IC, IIA, IIB, and IIC), if exercise testing to at least the level of activity achieved in competition demonstrates no symptoms or ventricular arrhythmias (7,45).

3. Athletes with severe aortic regurgitation and left ventricular diastolic diameters >65 mm as well as those with mild or moderate aortic regurgitation and symptoms should not participate in competitive sports (7,45).
4. Those patients with aortic regurgitation and some dilation of the proximal aorta (<45 mm) can engage in low-intensity competitive sports (class IA), providing they do not have Marfan syndrome. Patients with Marfan syndrome and aortic regurgitation should not participate in any form of competitive sports (7,45).

Mitral Stenosis

As an isolated lesion, mitral stenosis is extremely uncommon in children. Competitive exercise is possible in patients with only mild to moderate stenosis.

Evaluation. Severity of mitral stenosis can usually be determined from history, physical examination, electrocardiogram, and echocardiogram. In patients with mild to moderate mitral stenosis, an exercise test should be performed before the patient is permitted to participate in competitive activity. The severity of mitral stenosis is categorized as mild (mitral valve area >1.5 cm², resting pulmonary artery systolic pressure <35 mm Hg), moderate (mitral valve area between 1 and 1.5 cm², or resting pulmonary systolic pressure <50 mm Hg), and severe (mitral valve area <1 cm² and resting pulmonary systolic pressures >50 mm Hg) (45).

Effects of Exercise. In patients with significant mitral stenosis, increased cardiac output and heart rate during dynamic exercise can cause sudden and marked increases in pulmonary artery and capillary pressures and at times can result in sudden acute pulmonary edema. As heart rate increases, diastolic filling time decreases and the pressure gradient across the mitral valve will increase (47).

Recommendations

1. Patients with mild mitral stenosis and sinus rhythm can participate in all competitive sports. Chronic atrial fibrillation or a history of atrial flutter/fibrillation resulting in systemic anticoagulation disallows participation in any competitive sport that involves risk for bodily contact or possible trauma (7,45).
2. Patients with moderate mitral stenosis and sinus rhythm can participate in low to moderate static and low to moderate dynamic competitive sports (classes IA, IB, IIA, and IIB) (7,45).
3. Patients with severe mitral stenosis should not compete in any form of competitive sports (7,45).

Mitral Regurgitation

As an isolated lesion, mitral regurgitation is uncommon in childhood. However, mitral regurgitation is quite common in association with a repaired atrioventricular septal defect. Other causes of mitral regurgitation include mitral valve prolapse, either idiopathic or in association with other connective tissue disease (i.e., Marfan syndrome), rheumatic heart disease, and endocarditis.

Evaluation. Mitral regurgitation can be diagnosed by physical examination. The echocardiogram is useful for assessing severity of mitral regurgitation. In general, the left ventricular end-diastolic dimension reflects the severity of the regurgitation.

However, the upper limit of left ventricular size is increased in the highly trained athlete. In elite athletes, echocardiographic left ventricular end-diastolic dimensions have been recorded as high as 66 mm in women (mean 48 mm) and ≤70 mm in men (mean 55 mm) (9,23,25). Mild to moderate regurgitation is usually present with left ventricular end-diastolic dimensions that are <95th percentile for body surface area or, in the adult, <60 mm. Regurgitation is considered severe if dimensions are >95th percentile or >60 mm with increasing left ventricular end-systolic dimensions.

Effects of Exercise. Isometric exercise markedly increases the left ventricular afterload, which will significantly increase the amount of mitral regurgitation and as a result will also significantly increase both pulmonary venous and arterial pressures. Isotonic exercise is usually much better tolerated than isometric exercise, since although isotonic exercise increases the volume load of an already volume stressed left ventricle, decreased ventricular afterload associated with vasodilation in the exercising muscles helps, in part, to compensate for the deleterious affects of the increased volume stress. The failure of exercise to increase the left ventricular ejection fraction is used as an indication for surgery in patients with severe mitral and aortic regurgitation.

Recommendations

1. Patients with mild to moderate mitral regurgitation and sinus rhythm can participate in all competitive sports (7,45).
2. Patients with moderate mitral regurgitation with normal left ventricular systolic function and mild to moderate left ventricular enlargement (≤95th percentile for body surface area or ≤60 mm) can participate in some low and moderate static and low, moderate, and high dynamic competitive sports (classes IA, IB, IC, IIA, IIB, IIC) (7,45).
3. Patients with severe mitral regurgitation should not participate in any competitive sports (7,45).
4. Patients who have had surgical mitral valve repair should not engage in sports involving the risk of bodily contact or the danger of trauma that might disrupt the repair. They can participate in low-intensity competitive sports (class IA) and in selected athletes, in low and moderate static and low and moderate dynamic competitive sports (classes IA, IB, and IIA) (7,45).

Prosthetic Heart Valves

This section will deal with exercise recommendations for individuals with prosthetic (mechanical or bioprosthetic) mitral and aortic heart valves. Exercise recommendations for patients with right ventricular to pulmonary artery valved conduits should follow recommendations the same as with repaired tetralogy of Fallot. Although most who have a prosthetic heart valve will be asymptomatic, long-term mortality after valve replacement is significantly greater than that for the general population. Additionally, although resting cardiovascular hemodynamics may be near normal, many patients will have an abnormal exercise response.

Effects of Exercise. There are few to no data showing whether vigorous competitive exercise has any effect on long-term valve function. Mechanical and most bioprosthetic valves have a reduced effective valve area and many have small transvalvar gradients at rest. With dynamic exercise, some can develop large gradients.

Recommendations

1. Athletes with a bioprosthetic mitral or aortic valve who are not taking anticoagulants and who have normal valve function and near normal left ventricular function can participate in low and moderate static and low and moderate dynamic competitive sports (class IA, IB, IIA, IIB). Athletes should undergo yearly exercise testing to at least the level of activity achieved in competition to evaluate exercise tolerance, symptoms, and hemodynamic responses (7,45).
2. There is little information in the literature to make recommendations for patients who have had a Ross operation, but it seems reasonable to follow the recommendations for a bioprosthetic aortic valve (7,45). Coronary adequacy must be considered as well.
3. Patients who have a mechanical valve and are taking anticoagulation therapy should not engage in sports involving the risk of bodily contact or the danger of trauma (7,45).

Coarctation of the Aorta

Virtually all patients with coarctation of the aorta have had either surgical repair or balloon dilation/stenting. The only exception is patients with mild coarctation with aortic arch systolic gradients of ≤ 15 mm Hg and normal upper extremity blood pressures. Several abnormalities may persist following coarctation repair. A residual resting systolic gradient is frequently found, especially if the patient was operated on in infancy. Upper extremity hypertension occurs in $\leq 40\%$ of patients after coarctation repair (48–51). Patients are at risk for aneurysm formation or dissection either at the site of the repair or in the ascending aorta (48–51). Associated cardiovascular abnormalities are common, including valvar or subvalvar aortic stenosis, aortic regurgitation, mitral valve stenosis or regurgitation, and intracerebral berry aneurysms (48–51).

Evaluation

Patients with coarctation should be evaluated by physical examination, echocardiogram, exercise testing, and magnetic resonance imaging. Magnetic resonance imaging or CT scanning is useful to determine the status of the repair site and the presence of aortic aneurysms (both at the repair site and in the ascending aorta). Exercise testing is critical for those who plan to participate in competitive sports since exercise-induced hypertension is extremely common following coarctation repair.

Effects of Exercise

With dynamic exercise, increased cardiac output directed to the lower extremity working muscles can cause a flow-mediated gradient across the repair site. This flow-mediated gradient can result in significant upper extremity hypertension (52–56). Exercise-induced changes in systolic coarctation gradient were evaluated in 126 postoperative coarctation patients aged 7 to 28 years who had treadmill exercise testing at the University of Michigan from 1986 to 2005. The arm/leg systolic gradient increased from 5 ± 8 to 39 ± 12 mm Hg with exercise and was associated with increased upper extremity systolic pressure from 109 ± 10 to 185 ± 12 mm Hg. In addition to a residual gradient across the coarctation site being responsible for the marked systolic hypertension associated with dynamic exercise, other factors such as altered baroreceptor function and peripheral vascular reactivity may also play a role (52–58). Isometric exercise also results in a marked increase in both systolic and diastolic pressures. The increased systemic afterload

associated with exercise with coarctation can also result in ischemic ST-segment changes.

Recommendations

1. Patients with unrepaired mild coarctation can participate in all competitive sports provided they do not have significant aortic root dilation (Z-score +2 or less), have a normal exercise test with only a small pressure gradient at rest (<20 mm Hg), normal resting upper extremity blood pressures, and a peak systolic blood pressure of ≤ 230 mm Hg with exercise (7).
2. Patients with a systolic arm/leg gradient of >20 mm Hg, exercise-induced hypertension, and peak exercise systolic blood pressure of >230 mm Hg can engage in only low-intensity competitive sports (classes IA and IB) (7).
3. If the patient had surgical repair or a catheter intervention, participation in sports is permitted ≥ 3 months after the procedure provided he or she has findings similar to those described for mild unrepaired coarctation. Although the Bethesda Conference recommendations (7) suggest that patients with repaired coarctation should refrain from high-intensity static exercise (class IIIA, IIIB, IIIC), if no aortic dilation is present, there are few objective data to support this recommendation.
4. Athletes with evidence of significant aortic dilation, wall thinning, or aneurysm formation should be restricted to low-intensity competitive sports (classes IA and IB) (7).

Cyanotic Heart Disease

Tetralogy of Fallot

Virtually all patients with tetralogy of Fallot will have had complete repair prior to starting school. Their ability to participate in completive sports depends on the extent of the residua and/or sequelae of their surgical repair including pulmonary stenosis, pulmonary regurgitation, ventricular septal defects, and conduction abnormalities (57).

Evaluation. Prior to permitting a patient with repaired tetralogy of Fallot to participate in competitive sports, he or she should have a diagnostic evaluation that includes a complete physical examination, echocardiogram, chest radiograph, Holter monitoring, exercise testing, and magnetic resonance imaging. Magnetic resonance is especially useful in evaluating right ventricular function and the degree of pulmonary regurgitation (58,59). Patients with important residual abnormalities such as a significant left-to-right shunt, right ventricular hypertension, moderate to severe pulmonary regurgitation or right ventricular dysfunction, or a history of syncope and/or arrhythmia may be at risk of sudden death (60).

Effect of Exercise. Responses to dynamic exercise after tetralogy of Fallot repair are often abnormal including diminished total work capacity, decreased maximal oxygen consumption, suboptimal heart rate response, and ventricular and atrial arrhythmias (60–67). Garson et al. (60) observed exercise-induced ventricular arrhythmias in 31 of 104 patients with repaired tetralogy of Fallot. Only 10 of 31 had an arrhythmia detected on resting electrocardiogram. With supine bicycle exercise during cardiac catheterization (64–66), all patients with residual pulmonary stenosis increased their gradients with exercise. In some patients, exercise uncovered evidence of

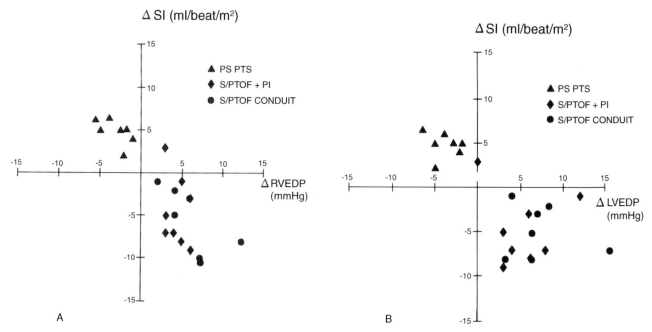

FIGURE 4.5 A: Exercise-induced changes in stroke index (ΔSI) and right ventricular end-diastolic pressure (ΔRVEDP) in seven patients without pulmonary insufficiency (PI) after repair of tetralogy of Fallot (TOF) (*circles*), eight patients with moderate PI after repair of tetralogy of Fallot (*diamonds*), and seven nonsurgically treated patients with mild pulmonary stenosis (PS) (*triangles*). Responses were abnormal in both groups of surgically treated patients. **B:** Exercise-induced changes in stroke index (ΔSI) and left ventricular end-diastolic pressure (ΔLVEDP) in seven patients without PI after repair of S/PTOF (*circles*); eight patients with moderate PI after repair of S/PTOF (*diamonds*) and seven nonsurgically treated patients with mild PS (*triangles*). Responses were abnormal in both groups of surgically treated patients. (From Rocchini AP. Hemodynamic abnormalities in response to supine exercise in patients after operative correction of tetrad of Fallot after early childhood. *Am J Cardiol* 1981;48:325–330, with permission.)

biventricular dysfunction with suboptimal increases in cardiac output and stroke volume together with elevation in right ventricular end-diastolic pressures (Fig. 4.5A, B). Borow et al. (67) found evidence of left ventricular dysfunction in response to afterload stress (methoxamine infusion) in teenagers who were repaired after 2 years of age.

Recommendations

1. After tetralogy repair, athletes with normal or near-normal right ventricular pressure, no or only mild right ventricular volume overload, no evidence of significant residual shunt, and no atrial or ventricular arrhythmias on ambulatory electrocardiographic monitoring and/or exercise testing should be allowed to participate in all sports (7).
2. Athletes with marked pulmonary regurgitation and right ventricular volume overload, residual right ventricular hypertension (peak systolic right ventricular pressure >50% of systemic pressure), or atrial or ventricular tachyarrhythmias should participate in only low-intensity competitive sports activities (class IA) (7).

Transposition of the Great Arteries

Postoperative Mustard or Senning. Senning and Mustard operations for d-transposition of the great arteries involve an intra-atrial baffle that reroutes systemic venous return to the

left ventricle and pulmonary arteries and pulmonary venous return to the right ventricle and aorta. The major limitation following a Mustard or Senning operation is the capacity of the right ventricle to perform systemic work effectively over a lifespan (68,69). Other hemodynamic abnormalities following intra-atrial repair of transposition can include obstruction of systemic and/or pulmonary venous return, pulmonary stenosis, pulmonary hypertension, tricuspid regurgitation, and significant atrial or ventricular arrhythmias (70,71).

Evaluation. Prior to permitting a patient with Mustard or Senning repair of transposition to participate in competitive sports, he or she should have a diagnostic evaluation including a complete physical examination, echocardiogram, chest radiograph, Holter monitoring, exercise testing, and magnetic resonance imaging. Magnetic resonance imaging is especially useful for evaluation of right ventricular function and the presence of systemic venous baffle obstruction and/or pulmonary venous baffle obstruction (72,73).

Effects of exercise. Response to dynamic exercise following intra-atrial repair of d-transposition is often abnormal. Mathews et al. (74) reported results of graded treadmill exercise testing in 21 children an average of 9 years following the Mustard operation. Compared with normal children, patients had diminished exercise endurance, lower maximal oxygen consumption, and lower maximal exercise systolic blood pressure.

Radionucleotide studies have also shown an abnormal right ventricular ejection fraction response to dynamic exercise following intra-atrial repair of transposition (75,76). Right ventricular dysfunction can be unmasked by afterload stress (methoxamine infusion), suggesting that the increase in systemic resistance that occurs with isometric exercise may have a deleterious effect (77). Heart rate response to exercise is often suboptimal, a manifestation of sick sinus syndrome.

Recommendations

1. If the athlete has mild or no cardiac chamber enlargement; no history of atrial flutter, supraventricular tachycardia, or ventricular tachycardia; no history of syncope or other cardiac symptoms; and a normal exercise test defined as normal duration, normal workload, heart rate, electrocardiogram, and blood pressure response, he or she can engage in low to moderate static/low dynamic sports (classes IA and IIA) (7).

Postoperative Arterial Switch Repair. Since the mid-1980s, the arterial switch operation has become the surgical treatment of choice for children with d-transposition of the great arteries. Short-term to midterm follow-up of these patients has been excellent (78–81). Potential residua and sequelae of the arterial switch operation include supravalvar and branch pulmonary stenosis, coronary artery occlusion, aortic root dilation, and aortic regurgitation.

Evaluation. Prior to participation in competitive sports, a diagnostic evaluation should include a complete physical examination, echocardiogram, chest radiograph, Holter monitoring, and exercise testing. Magnetic resonance imaging allows evaluation of aortic root dilation and branch pulmonary artery obstruction (82).

Effects of exercise. Heart rate and blood pressure response to exercise, endurance times, peak oxygen consumption, and aerobic capacity, assessed by determination of the ventilatory anaerobic threshold, are normal in most children who have had an arterial switch operation (79–81). However, a few patients have been reported to have chronotropic impairments and/or ST-segment depression with strenuous exercise (80). Many of the patients with chronotropic impairments and ST-segment depression have coronary occlusion or stenosis. Sachweh et al. (83) reported that three of five patients with an intramural coronary artery developed angiographic evidence of coronary occlusion. Hui et al. (78) demonstrated that despite being asymptomatic, a significant number of children (23 of 31) had impaired baseline left ventricular contractility, reversible myocardial perfusion defects, and mild wall motion abnormalities during dobutamine stress. Hauser et al. (84) demonstrated that, after the arterial switch operation, asymptomatic children who have no signs of coronary dysfunction can have stress-induced perfusion defect and attenuated coronary flow reserve on positron emission tomography. Thus, careful and serial evaluations of arterial switch patients are necessary before permitting them to participate or continue in competitive sports.

Recommendations

1. Athletes with normal ventricular function, a normal exercise test, and no atrial or ventricular tachyarrhythmias can participate in all sports (7).
2. Athletes with more than mild hemodynamic abnormalities or ventricular dysfunction can participate in low and moderate static/low dynamic competitive sports (classes IA, IB, IC, IIA), provided that exercise testing is normal (7).

Congenitally Corrected Transposition of the Great Arteries

Isolated congenitally corrected transposition of the great arteries is rare. Most individuals with congenitally corrected transposition have other associated cardiovascular anomalies such as ventricular septal defect, pulmonary stenosis or atresia, and tricuspid valve regurgitation. The extent of these other anomalies usually dictates the level of competitive exercise. Heart block is common as well. Participation in competitive sports should be restricted in the small subset of patients with isolated congenitally corrected transposition.

Evaluation. Prior to permitting a patient with congenitally corrected transposition to participate in competitive sports, he or she should have a diagnostic evaluation including a complete physical examination, echocardiogram, chest radiograph, Holter monitoring, and exercise testing.

Response to Exercise. With exercise, children with isolated congenitally corrected transposition have lower peak exercise VO_2, chronotropic incompetence, impaired stroke volume response of the morphologic right ventricle, and reduced exercise capacity when compared with control subjects (85). These abnormalities in exercise capacity worsen with time. Fredriksen et al. (86) demonstrated that aerobic capacity in adult patients with isolated congenitally corrected transposition was severely diminished, varying from 30% to 50% of results achieved in healthy subjects.

Recommendations

1. Because of the abnormal responses to exercise in patients with isolated congenitally corrected transposition, eligibility for participation in completive sports should be limited to classes IA and IIA. Patients may participate in these types of sports if they have no systemic ventricular enlargement, no evidence of atrial or ventricular tachyarrhythmias, and a normal or near-normal exercise test. Periodic re-evaluation is important to detect deterioration of ventricular function, development of systemic atrioventricular valve regurgitation, and/or the development of arrhythmias (7).

Ebstein's Anomaly

The severity of Ebstein's anomaly depends on the degree of tricuspid regurgitation, the magnitude of right heart enlargement, and atrial level right-to-left shunting. symptomatic patients with severe Ebstein's anomaly are at increased risk of sudden death associated with exercise (87). Some with even mild Ebstein's anomaly may have significant and potentially life-threatening arrhythmias.

Evaluation. Prior to permitting a patient with Ebstein's anomaly of the tricuspid valve to participate in competitive sports, he or she should have a diagnostic evaluation that includes a complete physical examination, echocardiogram, chest radiograph, Holter monitoring, and exercise testing.

Effects of Exercise. The major predictor of exercise tolerance in asymptomatic patients with Ebstein's anomaly is oxygen saturation at peak exercise (88,89). After surgery, if the atrial septal defect is closed, exercise tolerance is predominantly influenced by heart size. Those with the largest hearts on chest x-ray views have the worse exercise tolerance (89). Other abnormalities associated with exercise include reduced maximal oxygen consumption and a blunted heart rate responses to exercise. Many patients with Ebstein's anomaly will develop significant tachyarrhythmias with exercise.

Recommendations

1. Athletes with Ebstein's anomaly who have normal right ventricular size, no right-to-left shunting at rest or with exercise, and no evidence of atrial or ventricular arrhythmias can participate in all competitive sports (7).
2. Athletes with Ebstein's anomaly and moderate tricuspid insufficiency and mild to moderate increase in right ventricular size and no atrial or ventricular arrhythmias should participate in only low-intensity competitive sports (Class IA) (7).
3. Athletes with severe Ebstein's should be prohibited from participating in any competitive sports. If they have surgical correction, the exercise level should be dictated by the degree of tricuspid regurgitation, heart size, and degree of atrial and ventricular dysrhythmias (7).

Postoperative Fontan Operation

Patients with a functionally single ventricle who have the Fontan procedure continue to have exercise tolerance limitations (90–97). Postoperative arrhythmias have been associated with significant morbidity and mortality.

Evaluation. Prior to permitting a Fontan patient to participate in competitive sports, he or she should have a diagnostic evaluation that includes a complete physical examination, echocardiogram, chest radiograph, Holter monitoring, and exercise testing.

Effects of Exercise. Fontan patients have lower peak VO_2 (92–97), lower maximal heart rate (92–95), lower maximal arterial blood oxygen saturation (92–97), lower pulmonary function parameters (95,96), and higher ventilatory equivalents (92,93) compared with healthy subjects. Brassard et al. (97) demonstrated that skeletal muscle function is abnormal in Fontan patients, which contributes to their reduced exercise tolerance.

Recommendation. After a Fontan procedure, patients can participate in low-intensity competitive sports (class IA) (7).

Coronary Artery Anomalies

Congenital Coronary Anomalies

Congenital coronary anomalies are the second most common cardiovascular cause of sudden death in young athletes (13). Their identification can be difficult and sometimes impossible to make before the athlete experiences sudden death, since many do not experience warning symptoms. Even if they have electrocardiograms at rest and exercise, the results are usually normal. Coronary artery anomalies should be considered in athletes who develop exertional syncope or symptomatic ventricular arrhythmias. Appropriate diagnostic tests include echocardiography, cardiac magnetic resonance imaging, ultrafast computer tomography, and coronary angiography. Surgery is indicated in almost all of these patients.

Recommendations

1. Detection of a coronary anomaly associated with sudden death should result in exclusion from all competitive sports (7).

2. Participation in all sports 3 months after a successful operation should be permitted for athletes without ischemia, ventricular tachyarrhythmia, or ventricular dysfunction during maximal exercise testing (7).

Kawasaki's Disease

Kawasaki's disease is the most common cause of acquired heart disease in children (98). Coronary aneurysms, together with progressive coronary artery stenosis, can lead to ischemic heart disease, myocardial infarction, or even sudden death (99). The extent of coronary artery disease can change over time. For the first 20 years after the onset of Kawasaki's disease, patients without evidence of coronary artery disease on echocardiography at any stage of the illness appear to have a risk for ventricular tachyarrhythmias and sudden death no greater than that of the normal population (99). Patients with aneurysms that regress to normal lumen diameter may have persisting structural and functional coronary abnormalities (100). Patients with persistent aneurysms may develop stenoses or occlusion, increasing the risk of myocardial ischemia. Risk associated with competitive sports in patients who have had Kawasaki's disease depends on the degree of coronary involvement.

Evaluation. The evaluation of a patient who has had Kawasaki's disease should include echocardiography, exercise testing, and exercise testing with myocardial perfusion imaging.

Recommendations

1. Patients with no coronary artery abnormalities or transient coronary artery ectasia resolving during the convalescent phase of the disease are encouraged to participate in all sports after 6 or 8 weeks (7).
2. Patients with regressed aneurysms can participate in all competitive sports if they have no evidence of exercise-induced ischemia by stress testing with myocardial perfusion imaging (7).
3. Patients with isolated small to medium-sized aneurysms in one or more coronary arteries and normal left ventricular function, and absence of exercise-induced ischemia or arrhythmia, are judged to be at low risk for ischemic complications. They may participate in low to moderate static and dynamic competitive sports (class IA, IB, IIA, IIB). Stress testing with evaluation of myocardial perfusion should be repeated at 1- to 2-year intervals to monitor development of ischemia (7).
4. Patients with one or more large coronary aneurysms or multiple (segmented) or complex aneurysms with or without obstruction to coronary flow may participate in class IA and IIA sports if they have no evidence of reversible ischemia on stress testing, normal left ventricular function, and absence of exercise-induced arrhythmias. Stress testing with evaluation myocardial perfusion should be repeated at 1-year intervals to monitor development of ischemia (7).
5. Patients with recent myocardial infarction or revascularization should avoid competitive sports until their recovery is complete; usually 6 to 8 weeks. Those with normal left ventricular ejection fraction, exercise tolerance, absence of reversible ischemia on myocardial perfusion testing, and absence of exercise-induced arrhythmias can participate in class IA and IB sports. Those with a left ventricular ejection fraction <40%, exercise intolerance, or exercise-induced ventricular tachyarrhythmias should not participate in competitive sports (7).

6. Patients with coronary lesions who are taking anticoagulants and/or antiplatelet drugs (aspirin, clopidogrel) should not participate in sports that pose a danger of high-speed collision (7).

Summary

Although the presence of congenital heart disease may limit a patient from participating in competitive athletics, as discussed in this chapter, many who have had correction of these defects can participate in all type of competitive athletics. Screening an athlete for the early identification of "silent" cardiovascular disease that might cause sudden death is important. Residual hemodynamic abnormalities that can occur after correction of congenital heart disease and the effect of these abnormalities on the patient's response to exercise influence exercise recommendations. Even though a given patient with corrected congenital heart disease can be cleared to participate in competitive sports, it is important to perform periodic re-evaluation, since hemodynamics and residual abnormalities can change as the child grows and matures into adulthood.

References

1. Rose KD. The potential for cardiovascular accidents in athletes with a heart problem. *Med Sci Sports* 1969;1:144–151.
2. Freed MD. Recreational and sports recommendations for the child with heart disease. *Ped Clin N Am* 1984;31:1307–1319.
3. Engle MA, Chairman, Congenital Heart Disease Study Group. Resources for optimal long-term care of congenital heart disease. *Circulation* 1971; 44:A205–219.
4. Strauzenberg SE. Recommendations for physical activity and sports in children with heart disease. *J Sports Med* 1982;22:401–406.
5. Beekman RH. Exercise recommendations for adolescents after surgery for congenital heart disease. *Pediatrician* 1986;13:210–219.
6. Mitchell JH, Maron BJ, Epstein SE. 16th Bethesda Conference: Cardiovascular abnormalities in the athlete: Recommendations regarding eligibility for competition: October 3–5, 1984. *J Am Coll Cardiol* 1985;6:1186–1232.
7. Graham TP Jr, Driscoll DJ, Gersony WM, et al. Task Force 2: Congenital heart disease. *J Am Coll Cardiol* 2005;45:1326–1333.
8. Maron BJ, Bodison SA, Wesley YE, et al. Results of screening a large group of intercollegiate competitive athletes for cardiovascular disease. *J Am Coll Cardiol* 1987;10:1214–1221.
9. Maron BJ, Douglas PS, Graham TP, et al. Task Force 1: Pre-participation screening and diagnosis of cardiovascular disease in athletes. *J Am Coll Cardiol* 2005;45:1322–1326.
10. Corrado D, Pelliccia A, Bjornstad HH, et al. Cardiovascular pre-participation screening of young competitive athletes for prevention of sudden death: Proposal for a common European protocol. *Eur Heart J* 2005;26:516–524.
11. Cava JR, Danduran MJ, Fedderly RT, et al. Exercise recommendations and risk factors for sudden cardiac death. *Pediatr Clin N Am* 2004;51:1401–1420.
12. Corrado D, Basso C, Rizzoli G, et al. Does sports activity enhance the risk of sudden death in adolescents and young adults? *J Am Coll Cardiol* 2003;42:1959–1963.
13. Maron BJ. Sudden death in young athletes. *N Engl J Med* 2003;349:1064–1075.
14. Maron BJ, Thompson PD, Puffer JC, et al. Cardiovascular pre-participation screening of competitive athletes. A statement for health professionals from the Sudden Death Committee (clinical cardiology) and Congenital Cardiac Defects Committee (cardiovascular disease in the young), American Heart Association. *Circulation* 1996;94:850–856.
15. Pelliccia A, Maron BJ. Pre-participation cardiovascular evaluation of the competitive athlete: Perspectives from the 30-year Italian experience. *Am J Cardiol* 1995;75:827–829.
16. Grafe MW, Paul GR, Foster TE. The pre-participation sport examination for high school and college athletes. *Clin Sports Med* 1997;16:570–591.
17. Maron BJ, Shirani J, Poliac LC, et al. Sudden death in young competitive athletes. Clinical, demographics and pathological profiles. *JAMA* 1996;276:199–204.
18. Decree of the Italian Ministry of Health, February 18, 1982. Norme per la tutela sanitaria dell'attivita sportiva agonistica (rules concerning the medical protection of athletic activity). *Gazzetta Ufficiale* March 5, 1982:63.
19. Corrado D, Basso C, Schiavon M, et al. Screening for hypertrophic cardiomyopathy in young athletes. *N Engl J Med* 1998;339:364–369.
20. Maron BJ, Gardin JM, Flack JM, et al. Prevalence of hypertrophic cardiomyopathy in a general population of young adults: Echocardiographic analysis of 4111 subjects in CARDIA study. *Circulation* 1995;92:785–789.
21. Maron BJ, McKenna WJ, Danielson GK. American College of Cardiology/ European Society of Cardiology clinical expert consensus document on hypertrophic cardiomyopathy: A report of the American College of Cardiology Foundation Task Force on Clinical Expert Consensus Documents and the European Society of Cardiology Committee for Practice Guidelines. *J Am Coll Cardiol* 2003;42:1687–1713.
22. Pelliccia A, Maron BJ, Culasso F. Clinical significance of abnormal electrocardiographic patterns in trained athletes. *Circulation* 2000;102:278–284.
23. Pluim BM, Zwinderman AH, van der Laarse A, et al. Athlete's heart: A meta-analysis of cardiac structure and function. *Circulation* 2000;101:336–344.
24. Biffi A, Pelliccia A, Verdile L. Long-term clinical significance of frequent and complex ventricular tachyarrhythmias in trained athletes. *J Am Coll Cardiol* 2002;40:446–452.
25. Pelliccia A, Culasso F, Di Paola FM, et al. Physiologic left ventricular cavity dilatation in elite athletes. *Ann Intern Med* 1999;130:23–31.
26. Klues HG, Schiffers A, Maron BJ. Phenotypic spectrum and patterns of left ventricular hypertrophy in hypertrophic cardiomyopathy: Morphologic observations and significance as assessed by two-dimensional echocardiography in 600 patients. *J Am Coll Cardiol* 1995;26:1699–1708.
27. Mitchell JH, Haskell W, Snell P, et al. Task Force 8: Classification of Sports. *J Am Coll Cardiol* 2005;45:1364–1367.
28. Ellestad MH. Cardiovascular responses to exercise. In: *Stress Testing: Principles and Practice*. 2nd ed. Philadelphia: Davis, 1980:9–38.
29. Lock JE, Einzig S, Moller JH. Hemodynamic responses to exercise in normal children. *Am J Cardiol* 1978;41:1278–1284.
30. Asmussen E. Similarities and dissimilarities between static and dynamic exercise. *Circulation Res* 1981;48(suppl 1):3–10.
31. MacDougall JD, Tuxen D, Sale DG, et al. Arterial blood pressure response to heavy resistance exercise. *J Appl Physiol* 1985;85:785–790.
32. Graham TP Jr, Jarmakani JM, Atwood GF, et al. Right ventricular volume determinations in children. Normal values and observations with volume or pressure overload. *Circulation* 1973;47:144–153.
33. Rocchini AP, Kveselis DA, Crowley D, et al. Percutaneous balloon valvuloplasty for treatment of congenital pulmonary valvular stenosis in children. *J Am Coll Cardiol* 1984;3:1005–1012.
34. Moller JH, Roa BNS, Lucus RF Jr. Exercise hemodynamics of pulmonary valvar stenosis. *Circulation* 1972;40:1018–1026.
35. Rocchini AP. Hemodynamic abnormalities in response to supine exercise in patients after operative correction of tetrad of Fallot after early childhood. *Am J Card* 1981;48:325–330.
36. Driscoll DJ, Edwards WD. Sudden unexpected death in children and adolescents. *J Am Coll Cardiol* 1985;5:118B–121B.
37. Doyle EF, Arumugham P, Lara E, et al. Sudden death in young patients with congenital aortic stenosis. *Pediatrics* 1974;53:481–489.
38. Kveselis DA, Rocchini AP, Rosenthal A, et al. Hemodynamic determents of exercise-induced ST-segment depression in children with valvar aortic stenosis. *Am J Cardiol* 1985;55:1133–1139.
39. Rosenthal A, Freed M, Keane JF. Isometric exercise in adolescents with congenital aortic stenosis [abstract]. *Circulation* 1976;54(suppl 2):48.
40. Chandramouli B, Ehmke DA, Lauer RM. Exercise-induced electrocardiographic changes in children with congenital aortic stenosis. *J Pediatr* 1975;87:725–730.
41. Barton CW, Katz B, Schork MA, et al. Value of treadmill exercise test in pre- and postoperative children with valvular aortic stenosis. *Clin Cardiol* 1983;6:473–477.
42. Whitmer JT, James FW, Kaplan S, et al. Exercise test in children before and after surgical treatment of aortic stenosis. *Circulation* 1981;63:245–262.
43. Battle RW, Crumb S, Tischler MD. Hemodynamic characteristics of congenital aortic stenosis. A quantitative stress echocardiography study. *Am Heart J* 2000;139:346–351.
44. Bonow RO, Carabello B, De Leon AC, et al. ACC/AHA guidelines for the management of patients with valvular heart disease: A report of the American College of Cardiology/American Heart Association Task Force on Practice Guidelines (Committee on Management of Patients with Valvular Heart Disease). *J Am Coll Cardiol* 1998;32:1486–1582.

45. Bonow RO, Cheitlin MD, Crawford MH, et al. Task Force 3, Valvular Heart Disease. *J Am Coll Cardiol* 2005;45:1334–1340.
46. Dehmer GJ, Firth BG, Hillis LD, et al. Alterations in left ventricular volumes and ejection fraction at rest and during exercise in patients with aortic regurgitation. *Am J Cardiol* 1981;48:17–27.
47. Rahimtoola SH, Durairaj A, Mehra A, et al. Current evaluation and management of patients with mitral stenosis. *Circulation* 2002;106:1183–1188.
48. Toto-Salazar OH, Steinberger J, Thomas W, et al. Long-term follow-up of patients after coarctation of the aorta repair. *Am J Cardiol* 2002;89:541–547.
49. Presbitero P, Demarie D, Villani M, et al. Long-term results (15–30 years) of surgical repair of aortic coarctation. *Br Heart J* 1987;57:462–467.
50. Cohen M, Fuster V, Steele PM, et al. Coarctation of the aorta. Long-term follow-up and prediction of outcome after surgical correction. *Circulation* 1989;80:840–845.
51. Stewart AB, Ahmed R, Travill CM, et al. Coarctation of the aorta life and health 20–44 years after surgical repair. *Br Heart J* 1993;69:65–70.
52. Markel H, Rocchini AP, Beekman RH, et al. Exercise-induced hypertension after repair of coarctation of the aorta: arm versus leg exercise. *J Am Coll Cardiol* 1986;8:165–171.
53. Beekman RH, Katz BP, Moorehead-Steffens C, et al. Altered baroreceptor function in children with systolic hypertension after coarctation repair. *Am J Cardiol* 1983;52:112–117.
54. Gidding S, Rocchini AP, Moorehead C, et al. Increased forearm vascular reactivity in patients with hypertension after repair of coarctation. *Circulation* 1985;71:495–499.
55. James FW, Kaplan S. Systolic hypertension during submaximal exercise after correction of coarctation of the aorta. *Circulation* 1974;50(suppl 2):27–33.
56. Freed MD, Rocchini AP, Rosenthal A, et al. Exercise-induced hypertension after surgical repair of coarctation of the aorta. *Am J Cardiol* 1979;43:253–258.
57. Morriss JH, McNamara DG. Residua, sequelae and complications of surgery for congenital heart disease. In: Rosenthal A, Sonnenblick EH, Lesch M, eds. *Postoperative Congenital Heart Disease*. New York: Grune & Stratton, 1975:3–28.
58. Geva T, Sandweiss BM, Gauvreau K, et al. Factors associated with impaired clinical status in long-term survivors of tetralogy of Fallot evaluated by magnetic resonance imaging. *J Am Coll Cardiol* 2004;43:1068–1074.
59. van Straten A, Vliegen HW, Hazekamp MG, et al. Right ventricular function late after total repair of tetralogy of Fallot. *Eur Radiol* 2005;15:702–707.
60. Garson AJ, Gillette PC, Gutgesell HP, et al. Stress-induced ventricular arrhythmia after repair of tetralogy of Fallot. *Am J Cardiol* 1980;46:1006–1012.
61. Kavey REW, Thomas FD, Byrum CJ, et al. Ventricular arrhythmias and biventricular dysfunction after repair of tetralogy of Fallot. *J Am Coll Cardiol* 1984;4:126–131.
62. Wesel HU, Cunningham WJ, Paul MH, et al. Exercise performance in teratology of Fallot after intracardiac repair. *J Thorac Cardiovasc Surg* 1980;80:582–593.
63. James FW, Kaplan S, Swarrtz DC, et al. Response to exercise in patients after total surgical correction of tetralogy of Fallot. *Circulation* 1976;54:671–679.
64. Rocchini AP. Hemodynamic abnormalities in response to supine exercise in patients after operative correction of tetrad of Fallot after early childhood. *Am J Cardiol* 1981;48:325–330.
65. Hirschfeld S, Tuboku-Metzger AJ, Borkat G, et al. Comparison of exercise and catheterization results following total surgical correction of tetralogy of Fallot. *J Thorac Cardiovasc Surg* 1978;75:446–451.
66. Cumming GR. Maximal supine exercise haemodynamics after open heart surgery for Fallot's tetralogy. *Br Heart J* 1979;41:683–691.
67. Borow KM, Green LH, Castenada AR, et al. Left ventricular function after repair of tetralogy of Fallot and its relationship to age at surgery. *Circulation* 1980;61:1150–1158.
68. Graham TP. Ventricular performance in adults after operation for congenital heart diseases. *Am J Cardiol* 1982;50:612–619.
69. Ninomiya K, Duncan WJ, Cook DH, et al. Right ventricular ejection fraction and volumes after Mustard repair: Correlation of two-dimensional echocardiograms and cineangiograms. *Am J Cardiol* 1981;48:317–324.
70. Flinn CJ, Wolff GS, Dick M, et al. Cardiac rhythm after the Mustard operation for complete transposition of the great arteries. *N Engl J Med* 1984;310:1635–1638.
71. Graham TP Jr. Hemodynamic residua and sequelae following intra-atrial repair of transposition of the great arteries: A review. *Pediatr Cardiol* 1982;2:203–213.
72. Theissen P, Kaimmierer H, Sechtem U, et al. Magnetic resonance imaging of cardiac function and morphology in patients with transposition of the great arteries following Mustard procedure. *Thorac Cardiovasc Surg* 1991;39(suppl 3):221–224.
73. Chung KJ, Simpson IA, Glass RF, et al. Cine magnetic resonance imaging after surgical repair in patients with transposition of the great arteries. *Circulation* 1988;77:104–109.
74. Mathews RA, Fricker FJ, Beerman LB, et al. Exercise studies after the Mustard operation in transposition of the great arteries. *Am J Cardiol* 1983;51:1526–1529.
75. Parrish MD, Graham TP, Bender HW, et al. Radionuclide angiographic evaluation of right and left ventricular function during exercise after repair of transposition of the great arteries. *Circulation* 1983;67:178–183.
76. Benson LN, Vonet J, McLauglin P, et al. Assessment of right ventricular function during supine bicycle exercise after Mustard's operation. *Circulation* 1982;65:1052–1059.
77. Borow KM, Keane JF, Casteñeda AR, et al. Systemic ventricular function in patients with tetralogy of Fallot, ventricular septal defect and transposition of the great arteries repaired during infancy. *Circulation* 1981;64:878–885.
78. Hui L, Chau AK, Leung MP, et al. Assessment of left ventricular function long term after arterial switch operation for transposition of the great arteries by dobutamine stress echocardiography. *Heart* 2005;91:68–72.
79. Hovels-Gurich HH, Kunz D, Seghaye M, et al. Results of exercise testing at a mean age of 10 years after neonatal arterial switch operation. *Acta Paediatr* 2003;92:190–196.
80. Mahle WT, McBride MG, Paridon SM. Exercise performance after the arterial switch operation for D-transposition of the great arteries. *Am J Cardiol* 2001;87:753–758.
81. Reybrouck T, Eyskens B, Mertens L, et al. Cardiorespiratory exercise function after the arterial switch operation for transposition of the great arteries. *Eur Heart J* 2001;22:1052–1059.
82. Mussatto K, Wernovsky G. Challenges facing the child, adolescent, and young adult after the arterial switch operation. *Cardiol Young* 2005;15 (suppl 1):111–121.
83. Sachweh JS, Tiete AR, Jockenhoevel S, et al. Fate of intramural coronary arteries after arterial switch operation. *Thorac Cardiovasc Surg* 2002;50:40–44.
84. Hauser M, Bengel FM, Kuhn A, et al. Myocardial blood flow and flow reserve after coronary reimplantation in patients after arterial switch and Ross operation. *Circulation* 2001;103:1875–1880.
85. Ohuchi H, Hiraumi Y, Tasato H, et al. Comparison of the right and left ventricle as a systemic ventricle during exercise in patients with congenital heart disease. *Am Heart J* 1999;137:1185–1194.
86. Fredriksen PM, Chen A, Veldtman G, et al. Exercise capacity in adult patients with congenitally corrected transposition of the great arteries. *Heart* 2001;85:191–195.
87. Pelech AN, Neish SR. Sudden death in congenital heart disease. *Pediatr Clin North Am* 2004;51:1257–1271.
88. Lupoglazoff JM, Denjoy I, Kabaker M, et al. Cardiorespiratory exercise tolerance in asymptomatic children with Ebstein's anomaly. *Pediatr Cardiol* 1999;20:189–194.
89. Maclellan-Tobert SG, Driscoll DJ, Mottram CD, et al. Exercise tolerance in patients with Ebstein's anomaly. *J Am Coll Cardiol* 1997;29:1615–1622.
90. Driscoll DJ, Durongpisitkul K. Exercise testing after the Fontan operation. *Pediatr Cardiol* 1999;20:57–59.
91. Driscoll DJ, Danielson GK, Puga FJ, et al. Exercise tolerance and cardiorespiratory response to exercise for tricuspid atresia or functional single ventricle. *J Am Coll Cardiol* 1986;7:1087–1094.
92. Toutman WB, Barastow TJ, Galindo AJ, et al. Abnormal dynamic cardiorespiratory responses to exercise in pediatric patients after Fontan procedure. *J Am Coll Cardiol* 1998;31:668–673.
93. Grant GP, Mansell AL, Garofano RP, et al. Cardiorespiratory response to exercise after the Fontan procedure for tricuspid atresia. *Pediatr Res* 1988;24:1–5.
94. Rosenthal M, Bush A, Deanfield J, et al. Comparison of cardiopulmonary adaptation during exercise in children after the atriopulmonary and total cavopulmonary connection Fontan procedures. *Circulation* 1995;91:372–378.
95. Fredriksen PM, Therrien J, Veldtman G, et al. Lung function and aerobic capacity in adult patients following modified Fontan procedure. *Heart* 2001;85:295–299.
96. Larsson ES, Eriksson Bo, Sixt R. Decreased lung function and exercise capacity in Fontan patients. A long-term follow-up. *Scand Cardiovasc J* 2003;37:58–63.
97. Brassard P, Poirier P, Martin J, et al. Impact of exercise training on muscle function and ergoreflex in Fontan patients: A pilot study. *Int J Cardiol* 2005;23:1–10.
98. Newberger JW, Takahashi M, Gerber MA. Diagnosis, treatment, and long-term management of Kawasaki disease: A statement for health professionals from the Committee on Rheumatic Fever, Endocarditis and Kawasaki Disease, Council on Cardiovascular Disease in the Young. *Circulation* 2004;110:2747–2771.
99. Kato H, Sugimura T, Akagi T. Long-term consequences of Kawasaki disease: A 10 to 21 year follow-up study of 594 patients. *Circulation* 1996;94:1379–1385.
100. Tsuda E, Kamiya T, Kimura K, et al. Coronary artery dilatation exceeding 4.0 mm during acute Kawasaki disease predicts a high probability of subsequent late intima-medial thickening. *Pediatr Cardiol* 2002;23:9–14.

CHAPTER 5 ■ EXERCISE TESTING

PAOLO T. PIANOSI, MD, AND DAVID J. DRISCOLL, MD

The ability to perform work or to exercise is a basic function of life, and many disease states affect this ability. Accurate and reproducible measurement of work performance or exercise capacity provides a means to quantify a dimension of disease severity and assess one aspect of quality of life; to assess the effects of treatment and training; and, in some instances, to identify previously unrecognized disease. Much of our knowledge of exercise physiology comes from studies in adults, and the field of pediatric work physiology has had to draw many parallels and extrapolations from these studies. There are obvious inherent flaws in this approach, which readers must bear in mind while reading this chapter.

BASIC EXERCISE PHYSIOLOGY

Work, Energy, and Power

Exercise involves the conversion of energy and its consumption by the performance of work. Because work equals force multiplied by distance, the unit for work is the Newton-meter, or joule (J). There is a constant relationship between energy and work as described by the relationship of one kilocalorie (Kcal) being equal to 4.1868 joules (J). Power is work performed per unit of time and can be expressed as joules per second (J/sec). A common expression of power is the watt (W): 1 W = 1 J/sec [SI units] = 6.12 KPM/min. Older nomenclature used the kilopond-meter (KPM), derived from the relationship: one kilopond is the force acting on a mass of l kg at the normal acceleration owing to gravity (9.8 m/sec^2), or 9.8 Newtons (N); and 1 joule = 1 newton-meter.

There are two types of exercise: isotonic (dynamic) and isometric (static). Isotonic exercise implies alternate rhythmic contraction (shortening) and relaxation (lengthening) of muscles against a nonfixed resistance. Isometric exercise involves muscular contraction against a fixed resistance with little (if any) muscle shortening. Clinical exercise testing can be done using either isotonic or isometric exercise. Usually, however, clinical exercise testing is done using isotonic forms of exercise, such as cycling, walking, and running.

The amount of work a person can perform could be used to define exercise capacity, but it is difficult to measure work accurately. Although many different indices can be used to describe fitness or maximal exercise capacity, the maximum aerobic power or maximum oxygen uptake ($\dot{V}O_2 max$) that can be achieved during exercise is probably the best. The term *maximum aerobic power* has been used to indicate the highest achievable level of $\dot{V}O_2$ during exercise and will be used throughout this chapter. Because energy is necessary to perform work and requires combustion of oxygen, there is a predictable relationship between aerobic work and $\dot{V}O_2$, and in normal adults this approximates 10 mL O_2 per minute per watt. However, the oxygen cost of work (mechanical efficiency) tends to

be higher in children (Fig 5.1), and this phenomenon is age dependent (reviewed in reference 1). Technically, $\dot{V}O_2 max$ is defined by the plateau of $\dot{V}O_2$ that occurs despite continued work. The plateau of $\dot{V}O_2$ that occurs with additional work illustrates the fact that work can be performed using anaerobic mechanisms of energy production, but the amount of work that can be performed using anaerobic means is limited. Thus a plot of $\dot{V}O_2$ versus work will reach an asymptotic $\dot{V}O_2 max$ if and only if the subject is able and willing to continue to exercise until this zenith is reached. In assessing the cardiorespiratory responses to exercise, it is important to know the subject's degree of effort, as maximum effort is necessary to accurately measure $\dot{V}O_2 max$. Unfortunately, it is difficult to motivate many untrained subjects and most children to exercise to that asymptote, as continued exercise becomes uncomfortable. Because of this, the terms *peak* $\dot{V}O_2$, peak exercise, or peak work capacity have been coined to refer to a symptom- or discomfort-limited clinical exercise test—so-called voluntary exhaustion. In such tests, a true $\dot{V}O_2 max$ may not have been attained.

Determinants of Exercise Performance and Maximal Aerobic Power

Exercise requires a complex and intricate interaction of multiple organ systems, and abnormalities in any of these organ systems will affect and potentially limit work performance. When any one of these organ systems reaches maximal functional capacity, the performance of additional work will be limited. A more simplistic but fundamental approach is to ask whether oxygen supply or oxygen use (substrate or enzyme availability) imposes the limiting factor in determination of maximum work done. In general, the scale tips toward oxygen supply as the limiting step, and thus the pulmonary, cardiovascular, blood, and skeletal muscle are the most important organ systems in facilitating and regulating work performance. Rather than provide a specific diagnosis in a patient presenting with exercise intolerance, an exercise test has the potential to reveal the limiting organ system by applying the engineering principle of stress testing. The four principal systems involved in transferring oxygen from the atmosphere to the myocytes and mitochondria—lungs, heart, blood, and muscle—are intimately linked in series, and overall transport and use of oxygen depends on all components functioning optimally and in concert. In a maximal exercise test to voluntary exhaustion, most healthy subjects cease exercise because of leg discomfort or exhaustion, although some will complain of dyspnea as the reason for being unable to continue. In terms of organ systems, the cardiovascular system and specifically total oxygen transport capacity ($\dot{Q}O_2$ = product of cardiac output and O_2 carrying capacity) appear to be the limiting factor in maximum work achievable. Maximum cardiac

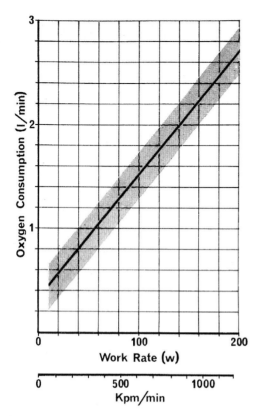

FIGURE 5.1 Diagrammatic illustration of the relationship between oxygen consumption and workload. (From Godfrey S. *Exercise Testing in Children*. London: WB Saunders, 1974, with permission.)

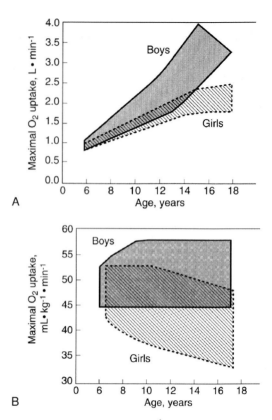

FIGURE 5.2 A: A composite graph of $\dot{V}O_2$ max in absolute terms versus age in children. **B:** The relationship with $\dot{V}O_2$ max normalized for body mass. (From Bar-Or O, Rowland TW. Pediatric exercise medicine. In: *Physiologic Principles to Health Care Application*. Champaign IL: Human Kinetics, 2004, with permission.)

output is closely correlated with maximum oxygen uptake: Reductions in cardiac output (and in certain situations, hemoglobin level) will reduce $\dot{V}O_2$ *max*, and experimentally increasing $\dot{Q}O_2$ will raise $\dot{V}O_2$ *max* (2,3).

The maximum $\dot{V}O_2$ achieved during work will depend on the type of work performed. For example, one could repetitively flex one's index finger until the finger was exhausted and could no longer be flexed despite continued volitional command to do so. This is the essence of true muscle fatigue, a state of neuromechanical dissociation. Maximum oxygen uptake during this maximal activity would not be high, however, because only a small muscle group was at work. In contrast, $\dot{V}O_2$ *max* would be considerably higher if one repetitively flexed a hip or knee because larger muscle masses are working and more work is being performed. Similarly, higher $\dot{V}O_2$ *max* can be achieved during treadmill than during cycle exercise because more muscle groups are working during exercise on a treadmill. The larger exercising muscle mass is an important determinant of many exercise parameters, and some measure of leg volume or muscle cross-sectional area is perhaps the single best predictor of $\dot{V}O_2$ *max*. There is some evidence that as children grow into adults, their leg volume increases in greater proportion to their body mass. Indeed, from the physiologic perspective, the proximal leg mass among mammals ranging from the shrew to the elephant constitutes a greater proportion of muscle mass to body mass in the larger animal. The greater muscle mass involved in exercise also dictates the relative contribution of stroke volume and heart rate in determining cardiac output in exercising humans.

Because body mass—or better still, lean leg mass—increases considerably during the period of growth and maturation, $\dot{V}O_2$

max rises considerably when expressed in absolute terms (L/min), particularly after puberty (Fig. 5.2A). If $\dot{V}O_2$ *max* is related to lean body mass, there ought to be no difference between boys and girls in achievable values of $\dot{V}O_2$ *max*, at least not before puberty. On the other hand, if $\dot{V}O_2$ *max* is normalized for weight (mL/kg/min) it remains *relatively* constant for boys between ages 6 and 18 years, whereas in girls $\dot{V}O_2$ *max* also remains relatively constant between the ages of 6 and 13 years but levels off after puberty and even declines slightly over that age range (Fig. 5.2B). This decline in girls probably represents the effect of increased body fat (or decreased lean body mass) coupled with the recently demonstrated trend in decreasing levels of daily physical activity in adolescent girls. Thus, in adolescence it is fair to say that boys have a higher $\dot{V}O_2$ *max* than girls, whether expressed in absolute or relative terms, but apart from this generalization the waters are murky. Prior to adolescence, boys and girls differ little in terms of $\dot{V}O_2$ *max*, although even this conclusion depends on the study and methods.

There are two important caveats to any conclusion or statement about $\dot{V}O_2$ *max* in pediatrics: one concerns longitudinal versus cross-sectional study data; and the other concerns the method of scaling or normalization of the data (as noted above). Investigators have searched for the best method of indexing $\dot{V}O_2$, and considerable controversy persists as to the best method, if one indeed exists. Based on the dimensionality theory, an exponent of body length was proposed using an exponent from 1.5 to 3.21, and Astrand and Rodahl (4) suggested using length to the 2.9 power. Body weight (mass) expressed simply in kilograms has been criticized as a method for explaining growth-related changes because it led to spurious correlations, misinterpretation of data, and erroneous conclusions. Alternatively, mass raised to an exponent seems more robust although the reported exponents ranged from 0.7 to 1.0 (5,6). In the final analysis, the most commonly accepted and simplest method of indexing $\dot{V}O_2$ in clinical exercise testing is to use body weight (kilograms) but with recognition of the limitations of this approach. Said limitations become particularly relevant to compilation of normal reference standards, which are inevitably derived from large cross-sectional sampling of a pediatric population, usually without regard to stage of physical development and pubertal maturation. Longitudinal studies have clearly shown that there are differences in the change of $\dot{V}O_2\,max$ over the age span 8 to 16 years. There are different individual trajectories for $\dot{V}O_2\,max$ during these growth years, which depend not only on age, sex, height, and weight, but also on training (physical activity). In essence, the so-called normal range is merely a composite of individual single time-point data. Thus, if one studies the same individual repeatedly over his or her growth years, which is probably more meaningful in the clinical arena, one must bear in mind the pitfalls of applying normal population reference standards to an individual patient.

There appear to be minor racial differences in $\dot{V}O_2\,max$, at least in North American studies. Several small studies have shown lower $\dot{V}O_2\,max$ in African American children compared with white children. African American children have slightly smaller lung volumes than white children of similar standing height, and this alters ventilatory strategy during exercise slightly, but ventilation is not thought to limit exercise in health. One study concluded that slightly lower hemoglobin values and levels of habitual activity in African American children accounted for part of the lower $\dot{V}O_2\,max$ observed (7).

Considerable attention has focused on the so-called anaerobic threshold as a surrogate measure of maximal aerobic power. Theoretically, it might allow assessment of exercise capacity using a submaximal exercise study, a potential advantage in children who have difficulty achieving a true $\dot{V}O_2\,max$. The term *anaerobic threshold* has given way to the term *ventilatory threshold* in recent years, in recognition of the fact that this time point during incremental exercise does not reflect the onset of anaerobic metabolism as was once hypothesized (8). The ventilatory (anaerobic) threshold (VAT or VT) is defined as the $\dot{V}O_2$ at which there is a disproportionate increase in minute ventilation ($\dot{V}_E$) relative to oxygen uptake. A rise in mixed expired O_2 concentration is observed at this point. There frequently is a disproportionate rise in lactate production at this point as well; hence the term anaerobic threshold (Fig. 5.3), but an increased lactate is not necessary for the disproportionate rise in $\dot{V}_E$ to occur. Therefore, this

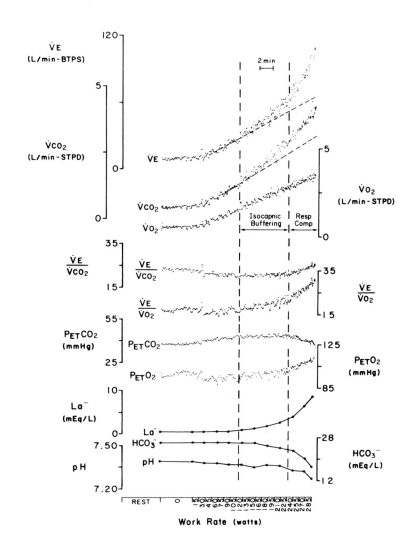

FIGURE 5.3 Changes in ventilatory indices, serum lactate, bicarbonate, and pH with increasing work. The vertical lines represent the onset of the ventilatory anaerobic threshold (left) and the threshold for decompensated acidosis (right). (From Wasserman K, Hansen J, Sue D, et al. *Principles of Exercise Testing and Interpretation*. Philadelphia: Lea & Febiger, 1987, with permission.)

term is a misnomer. Breath-by-breath measurements of ventilatory indices and brief incremental workloads are preferable for determining the anaerobic threshold. There are several methods of identifying this point, but the V-slope method is the most common and likely the most reliable in pediatrics (9). This point must also be distinguished from the second ventilatory threshold or respiratory compensation point. At this juncture during incremental exercise, $\dot{V}_E$ increases out of proportion to $\dot{V}CO_2$, such that $\dot{V}_E / \dot{V}CO_2$ also begins to rise and end-tidal $P_{ET}CO_2$ partial pressure begins to fall. This change is attributed to the H^+-mediated drive to breathe created by blood lactic acid accumulation that has outstripped buffering capacity. Reybrouck et al. (10) reported an inability to detect a VAT in 10% of children. In normal boys, they found a gradual decrease in VAT between ages 8 and 16 years. VAT was lower for girls than for boys. When expressed as a percentage of $\dot{V}O_2\,max$, VAT declined from approximately 65% in 8-year-old boys to approximately 55% in 16-year-old boys. It decreased from 62% in 8-year-old girls to approximately 55% in 16-year-old girls, similar to adult values.

CARDIAC RESPONSES TO EXERCISE

The essential function of the cardiovascular system is to propel blood to and from tissues, and the basic measurement of that function is cardiac output. Cardiac output ($\dot{Q}$) rises linearly with increasing $\dot{V}O_2$ (Fig. 5.4), the relationship described by

$$\dot{Q} = k\dot{V}O_2 + 4$$

where k averages somewhere between 5 and 6 (11). The intercept, 4, is obviously somewhat dependent on the size of the subject, but is a good approximation for children within the testable age range. Cardiac output is the product of heart rate × stroke volume, and stroke volume (SV) is dependent on preload, afterload, and contractility. Clinically useful proxy measures for these could be end-diastolic volume (EDV), blood pressure, and shortening fraction or preferably ejection fraction, respectively. Since ejection fraction (EF) = 100(SV/EDV), the basic determinants of cardiac output are heart rate, end-diastolic volume, and ejection fraction.

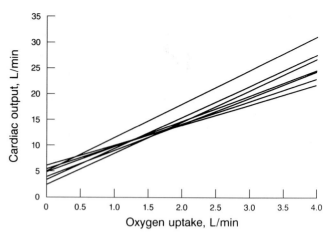

FIGURE 5.4 The relationship of cardiac output to oxygen uptake for normal persons. The various lines represent measurements from different laboratories using various techniques for measuring cardiac output.

Heart Rate

For normal persons, increased heart rate (HR) during exercise is the major determinant of increased cardiac output. There is a more or less linear relationship between heart rate and work (Fig. 5.5). The more or less qualification is warranted because some children will show a lesser increment in HR with step changes in work at near-maximal exercise. Indeed, Godfrey et al. (12) have shown that a plot of HR versus logarithm $\dot{V}O_2$ yields a linear plot. It can be seen from Figure 5.5 that, in general, smaller children will have higher HRs than larger children at any given work, and girls will have slightly higher HRs than boys, particularly after puberty. The maximum heart rate (HRmax) that can be achieved is an important determinant of $\dot{V}O_2\,max$. For subjects between 5 and 20 years of age, HRmax is about 195 to 215 beats per minute (bpm). The HRmax for children younger than 5 years of age probably is similar, but it is difficult to motivate these young children to perform a truly maximal test. For subjects older than 20 years, HRmax is

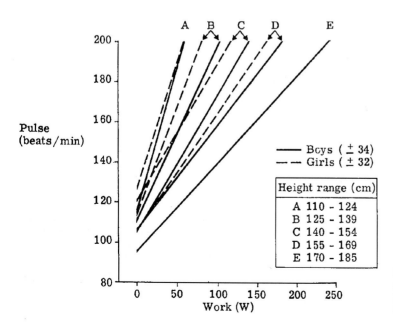

FIGURE 5.5 Heart rate versus work in children, illustrating sex and size (height) differences. (From Godfrey S. *Exercise Testing in Children*. London: WB Saunders, 1974, with permission.)

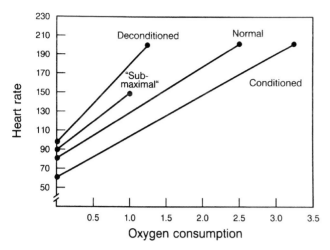

FIGURE 5.6. Diagrammatic representation of the relationship between heart rate response to exercise and oxygen consumption. Four conditions are depicted.

equal to $210 - 0.65 \times$ age. The reasons for the decline of HRmax with age are unclear but may be related to fibrosis and scarring of the sinoatrial node. The maximum heart rate will vary slightly depending on the exercise protocol used and the type of exercise performed. For example, a slightly higher HRmax is obtained for treadmill than for cycle exercise.

Four typical heart rate responses to exercise are illustrated in Figure 5.6. The "normal" graph represents the heart rate response of a normal subject with an HRmax of 200 bpm and $\dot{V}O_2\,max$ of 2.5 L/min. Although achieving predicted HRmax could be considered indicative of a maximum effort, very fit

individuals can continue exercising while the heart rate remains at its maximum value for 1 to 2 minutes. Obviously, this can occur only at the expense of extreme anaerobiosis. The curve labeled *Conditioned* illustrates the heart rate response if the subject improves his or her physical fitness. With improved fitness, the resting heart rate declines, the so-called training bradycardia. The maximum heart rate does not increase, but it occurs at a higher $\dot{V}O_2\,max$. The curve labeled *Deconditioned* illustrates the effect on heart rate response of deconditioning. The resting heart rate is higher than the control, and HRmax occurs at a lower $\dot{V}O_2\,max$. The curve labeled *Submaximal* could represent simply inadequate effort, but this curve also is typical of patients with chronotropic insufficiency, i.e., HRmax is low. This occurs in many patients with heart disease with or without prior cardiac operation.

Stroke Volume

In contrast to the relative ease with which HR is measured, stroke volume (SV) measurement has been a daunting challenge because of the invasive nature of methods available in the past. Therefore, our understanding of the behavior of stroke volume during exercise in children has largely been by extrapolation of work done in adults, or based on a limited number of small studies. The past decade has witnessed a minor explosion of pediatric studies reporting stroke volume during exercise, largely by Rowland et al. (13). Changes in stroke volume during exercise depend to some extent on the position in which exercise is performed. Stroke volume increases in humans in the supine position, such that when supine exercise is performed there is a limited rise in SV. The change in SV that occurs with exercise in the upright position is illustrated in Figure 5.7. Stroke

Stroke Index vs Oxygen Uptake

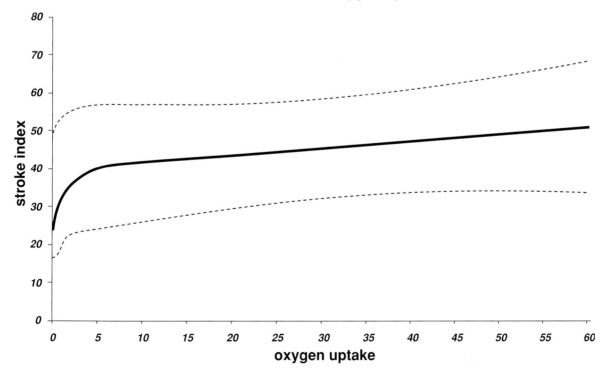

FIGURE 5.7 Normal range of stroke volume in healthy children plotted against oxygen uptake, with 95% confidence interval. (From Pianosi P, unpublished data).

volume increases primarily early in exercise and increases little thereafter. Thus, the change in cardiac output effected by change in SV occurs early in exercise, and additional changes of cardiac output depend predominantly on the heart rate.

It is important to appreciate the dynamics of this process, i.e., the mechanisms leading to the rise in stroke volume with exercise, as this provides insights into the regulation of circulation. Many physiologic systems involving bulk flow (blood, air) have models in basic physics such as electrical analogues, e.g., voltage = current × resistance. A circuit is characterized by a capacitance or an inductance, and inductance can be in phase or out of phase. Inductance is defined as the property of a circuit to oppose any change in current, and when a circuit has an inductive component, current lags voltage. Capacitance is the property of a circuit to oppose any change in voltage, and current leads voltage in a capacitance circuit. The circulatory equivalents are obviously pressure (voltage) and flow (current). Conceptualizing the cardiovascular system as a capacitance circuit is a useful paradigm. During exercise, the heart must pump more per beat into a systemic circulation under higher pressure, and in turn receives more blood return from the exercising limbs via the muscle pump phenomenon. Blood pressure rises in response to this increased flow through the circuit, but there are concomitant changes in other vascular beds to maintain central

blood volume and perfusion through exercising muscles. For this process to accommodate the requirements of dynamic exercise of increasing intensity, total peripheral vascular resistance must fall significantly. Whether pressure leads flow or lags flow in the cardiovascular system is a subject of intense interest to physiologists because of the importance of control of circulation during exercise.

With exercise, EDV must increase and EF usually increases as well, accounting for the rise in stroke volume and fall in end-systolic volume (ESV). The limits of SV augmentation will be reached when the rapidly increasing HR limits ventricular filling during diastole. Since most ventricular filling occurs in early diastole, left ventricular relaxation and compliance become important variables in the EDV response to exercise. In adults, conventional wisdom states that *on average*, SV levels off beyond 30% to 40% $\dot{V}O_2$ *max*, and most studies in children are in agreement. However, there is evidence that stroke volume falls slightly in adults during exercise above the ventilatory anaerobic threshold, perhaps because of reduced diastolic filling time. In contrast, Eriksson et al. (14), in one of the few invasive studies of upright cardiac output in children, noted that six of eight subjects achieved their largest stroke volume at maximal exercise. Healthy children should be able to continuously increase SV during progressive exercise, presumably because the younger myocardium has better relaxation kinetics and compliance. Although this supposition

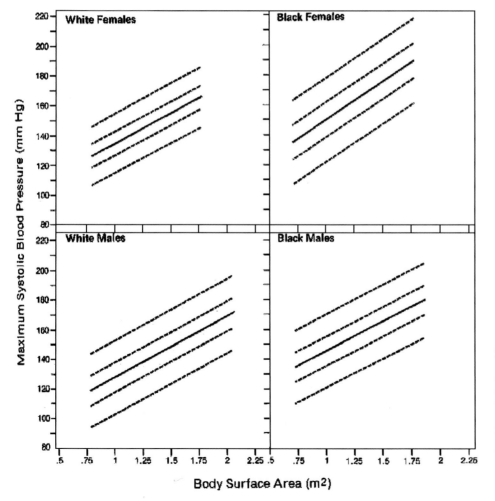

FIGURE 5.8 Nomograms for systolic blood pressure at peak exercise in children according to race and sex. Solid lines represent 50th percentiles, and dashed lines represent (top to bottom) 95th, 75th, 25th, and 5th, percentiles respectively. (From Alpert BS, Flood NL, Strong WB, et al. Responses to ergometer exercise in a healthy biracial population of children. *J Pediatr* 1982; 101:538–545. Copyright Mosby–Year Book. Reprinted with permission.)

TABLE 5.1

PHYSIOLOGIC CHANGES ASSOCIATED WITH TRAINED OR CONDITIONED STATE

Cardiovascular		Ventilatory		Cellular (muscle)	
Heart volume	↑	Maximal minute volume	↑	Glycogen stores	↑
LV dimension	↑	Ventilatory equivalents Submaximal or maximal	N or ↓	Oxidative enzymes succinyl dehydrogenase, cytochrome C oxidase, acyl CoA synthetase	↑
LV thickness	↑			Mitochondria—number[a]	↑
Ventricular filling	↑			Mitochondria—volume[a]	↑
Stroke volume	↑			Myoglobin content[a]	↑
Submaximal HR	↓				
Maximal HR	N				

N, no change.
[a]Demonstrated only in adults, not in children.
Adapted from Bar-Or O Rowland TW. *Pediatric Exercise Medicine*. Champaign, IL: Human Kinetics, 2004, with permission.

remains to be proven, recent work suggests a steady rise in SV in children during progressive exercise (15).

Blood Pressure

During isotonic exercise, systolic blood pressure increases whereas diastolic blood pressure changes little during exercise, although (on average) it may vary within 10 mm Hg from resting level. Larger children have higher blood pressures at submaximal and maximal exercise than smaller children (Fig. 5.8). Among similar-sized children, boys have higher peak systolic blood pressure than girls. African American children have a greater blood pressure response to exercise than white children (16). Blood pressure increases during isotonic exercise are owing to increased cardiac output, despite a rather marked reduction in total systemic resistance (P = R × $\dot{Q}$, where P is mean arterial pressure). In contradistinction to this pattern, blood pressure response to isometric exercise is quite different from that during isotonic exercise. With isometric exercise, both systolic and diastolic pressure will increase. Indeed, with power weight lifting, systolic blood pressure may reach 400 mm Hg.

Fitness

Improved fitness occurs with repetitive exercise. From a strict physiologic standpoint, improved fitness implies an increase in aerobic power ($\dot{V}O_2\ max$). Many studies in adults have demonstrated increases in $\dot{V}O_2\ max$ as a result of a conditioning or fitness program. In children, it has been more difficult to demonstrate this effect, probably because "normal" children simply are more fit than "normal" adults to begin with; hence, it is more difficult to demonstrate a change in fitness in normal children. However, a recent longitudinal study in athletic children demonstrated that the type of physical activity did indeed affect the change in $\dot{V}O_2\ max$ during childhood (17). The importance of this observation may become more

relevant in this era of increasing childhood obesity and decreasing fitness levels in today's youth.

As demonstrated in Figure 5.6, the resting heart rate decreases with improved fitness, and HRmax is achieved at a greater $\dot{V}O_2\ max$. It is apparent from this figure that submaximal heart rate is lower at any $\dot{V}O_2$ in the fit person compared with that in the unfit person. These adjustments of heart rate occur because of the increase in stroke volume that occurs with conditioning. Also, changes in the parasympathetic and sympathetic regulation of heart rate probably play an important role, with a relatively greater parasympathetic (vagal) influence on heart rate in the fit person. Changes in fitness or conditioning are not limited to changes in function of the cardiovascular system. The ventilatory changes listed are not the result of changes in resting lung function, but owing to improved oxygen delivery and use, which thereby reduce ventilatory requirements in heavy exercise. Important changes also occur in subcellular changes in muscle, and indeed, it is these changes that can contribute more to improved fitness with training. These are listed in Table 5.1. Fitness can be improved with regular episodes of sustained exercise. Conversely, deconditioning occurs if regular exercise is not done. Because children with heart disease may be sedentary, some component of reduced aerobic capacity in these patients may result from deconditioning.

VENTILATORY RESPONSE TO EXERCISE

Ventilation increases because of increases in both tidal volume and breathing frequency (Fig. 5.9). Similar to heart rate, submaximal respiratory rates (RRs) are higher in younger children at any given work rate. As children grow, the respiratory rate at peak exercise declines particularly above age 12 to 13 years. Younger children will typically achieve a peak RR of 60 breaths per minute; whereas older children will generally achieve a RR of 50 breaths per minute in early adolescence to 40 breaths per minute in late adolescence, at maximal exercise. In part this is because of the obligate dead space ventilation,

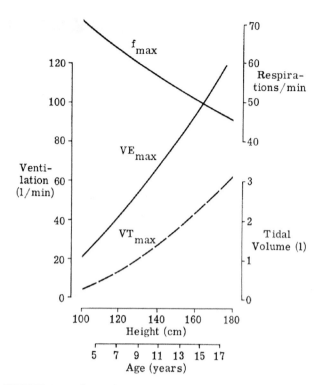

FIGURE 5.9 Relationships between ventilatory variables at maximum exercise in healthy children of varying age and height. (From Godfrey S. *Exercise Testing in Children*. London: WB Saunders, 1974, with permission.)

exercise when $\dot{V}_E/\dot{V}O_2$ begins to increase describes the ventilatory anaerobic threshold (VAT). $\dot{V}CO_2$ also creeps up during exercise, but at a slightly faster rate than $\dot{V}O_2$ with increasing work rate. This gradual rise in $\dot{V}CO_2$ relative to $\dot{V}O_2$ means that the gas exchange ratio ($\dot{V}O_2/\dot{V}CO_2$) goes from its resting value (usually approximately 0.8) toward unity. Beyond this point $\dot{V}CO_2$ continues to rise disproportionately to $\dot{V}O_2$ as exercise continues above the VAT. Minute volume ($\dot{V}_E$), which was also linearly related to $\dot{V}CO_2$ from the onset of exercise, maintains this tight coupling for a variable period even after the point when $\dot{V}_E/\dot{V}O_2$ begins to increase (VAT). However, as the work rate inches further toward maximum, $\dot{V}_E$ begins to increase disproportionately even to $\dot{V}CO_2$. This constitutes the so-called respiratory compensation point. In other words, at VAT the slope of $\dot{V}_E/\dot{V}O_2$ increases, but the slope of $\dot{V}_E/\dot{V}CO_2$ does not, until increasing work rate results in acidosis. At this point $\dot{V}_E$ increases disproportionately to $\dot{V}CO_2$ resulting in a rise in $\dot{V}_E/\dot{V}CO_2$. This point has been termed the *respiratory compensation point* and is characterized by hyperventilation with a reduction of $PaCO_2$ and end-tidal pCO_2, generally into the low thirties (mm Hg)—lower in younger compared with older children (19).

Normal subjects terminate exercise because cardiac output can increase no further. When exercise ceases at the point of voluntary exhaustion, $\dot{V}_E$ is 60% to 70% of maximum ventilation volume (MVV), leaving a ventilatory reserve of roughly 30% to 40%. Persons with pulmonary disease who encroach on this breathing reserve typically achieve maximal $\dot{V}_E$ >70% of MVV. Caution must be used, however, in assessing the relationship between $\dot{V}_E$ during exercise and resting MVV because obtaining a true measure of resting MVV depends greatly on subject effort. If the subject does not make a good effort, a factitiously low MVV will be recorded and the relationship with $\dot{V}_E$ during exercise will be misleading. A true MVV should approximate 1-second forced expiratory volume (FEV_1) × 35 or 40. This long-held index has other limitations, principally because the operating lung volume of the resting MVV maneuver differs from the actual operating lung volume during exercise. A better way to determine whether exercise is limited by ventilation is by measurement of tidal flow-volume loops during exercise (20), which has the added advantage of detecting vocal cord dysfunction, an increasingly recognized cause of exertional dyspnea. This is depicted in Figure 5.10, and has recently been studied in normal children (21). In a manner analogous to stroke volume, tidal volume normally is increased both by breathing at a lower end-expiratory lung volume (equivalent to LVESV) and attaining a higher end-inspiratory lung volume (higher LVEDV).

Diffusion limitation is seldom, if ever, a problem during routine clinical exercise testing. It may become a factor at extremes of exercise in high-performance athletes, as transit time through the pulmonary capillaries may be short enough (very high levels of cardiac output) to preclude equilibration of alveolar and end-capillary pO_2. Such an individual might even experience arterial desaturation if the person had an intrinsically low hypoxic ventilatory response (22). Normal healthy children should not exhibit desaturation even at maximal exercise, but this area has not been studied specifically in children with the exception of one report (23). These authors concluded (with a few caveats) that exertional desaturation can occur in 25% to 33% of physically active children with normal (versus supranormal) *peak* $\dot{V}O_2$ values. Given the technical difficulties in precise determination of oxygen saturation by pulse oximetry during exercise, healthy skepticism seems warranted.

but is largely owing to the relatively larger increase in vital capacity with growth, allowing more room for tidal volume recruitment. Unlike the stroke volume response, tidal volume in general does not level off with increasing exercise intensity, although some individuals with marked hyperventilation at maximal exercise will actually sacrifice tidal volume for faster breathing frequency. Tidal volume increases commensurate with growth in vital capacity during childhood and adolescence, but at maximal exercise tidal volume reaches a level at least 40% and as much as 60% of vital capacity regardless of age. This is accomplished by encroaching somewhat on the expiratory reserve volume but predominantly by tapping into the larger inspiratory reserve volume. This strategy has important implications in determining the cause(s) of exertional dyspnea.

The relationship between $\dot{V}_E$ or $\dot{V}_I$ (depending on whether one measures inspired or expired ventilation) and work is linear until the ventilatory anaerobic threshold is attained. Ventilation most closely tracks carbon dioxide output ($\dot{V}CO_2$) during exercise, and the ventilatory response to progressive exercise can be characterized as $\Delta\dot{V}_E/\Delta\dot{V}CO_2$. This slope falls slightly with age and growth during childhood (18). The ventilatory equivalent for CO_2 ($\dot{V}_E/\dot{V}CO_2$) dictates the volume of air breathed relative to the volume of CO_2 produced. By analogy, the ventilatory equivalent for O_2 ($\dot{V}_E/\dot{V}O_2$) describes the volume of air breathed relative to the volume of O_2 consumed. Figure 5.3 illustrates the time course of $\dot{V}_E/\dot{V}O_2$ and $\dot{V}_E/\dot{V}CO_2$ during an incremental exercise test. $\dot{V}_E/\dot{V}O_2$ declines early in exercise as a result of better ventilation and blood flow matching in the lungs as pulmonary blood flow increases and flow redistributes to the apices of the lungs. The point during

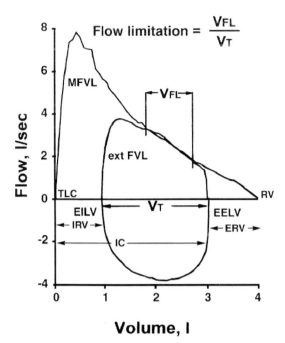

$$\text{Flow limitation} = \frac{V_{FL}}{V_T}$$

FIGURE 5.10 New method to assess ventilatory limitation to exercise. Exercise tidal flow volume loops (ext FVL) are superimposed within the maximal flow volume loop (MFVL) determined at rest, and any overlap is considered evidence of flow limitation (VFL). EELV and EILV are end-expiratory and end-inspiratory lung volumes, respectively; whereas IRV and ERV are inspiratory and expiratory reserve volumes, respectively. Lung volume is plotted on the abscissa with total lung capacity (TLC) at the origin; flow is on the ordinate, with expiration above the volume axis and inspiration below. (From Johnson BD, Weisman IM, Zeballos RJ, et al. Emerging concepts in the evaluation of ventilatory limitation during exercise: the exercise tidal flow-volume loop. *Chest* 1999;116:488–503, with permission.)

METHODOLOGY OF EXERCISE TESTING

Types of Exercise and Ergometers

Treadmill and stationary cycles are the two most frequently used ergometers for clinical exercise testing. Neither is inherently superior to the other; each has advantages and disadvantages. Most people can walk reasonably efficiently, but not everyone can cycle efficiently. Children younger than 4 or 5 years of age may have more difficulty using a cycle ergometer than a treadmill. On the other hand, a treadmill may be more dangerous than a cycle because the subject can fall from the treadmill. Also, it is more difficult to hear the Korotkoff sounds when the subject is running or jogging on a treadmill than when he or she is cycling. If the subject is connected to numerous monitoring devices, cycling may be preferable because it involves less movement of the trunk and extremities. In general, it is easier to calibrate a treadmill than a cycle ergometer.

The two general types of cycle ergometers are the mechanically braked and electronically braked. With a mechanically braked cycle ergometer, power changes with changes of pedaling frequency. With an electronically braked cycle ergometer, moderate changes in pedaling frequency do not affect power substantially. Thus, for untrained subjects, who may have difficulty maintaining a steady pedaling frequency, electronically braked cycles are preferable. Other less frequently used ergometers are handgrip ergometers and arm-crank ergometers. The arm-crank ergometer is useful for subjects who are unable to walk or cycle or for whom physiologic measurement of upper extremity function is of interest.

Exercise Protocols

There is no best exercise protocol. Examiners should select or create a protocol that best allows measurement of the responses to exercise that are of particular interest. One may use a protocol that has been standardized in another laboratory. Ideally, protocols should be standardized and data obtained for a "normal" population in the laboratory in which the clinical exercise testing is done.

In general, exercise protocols should be designed such that the duration of the exercise test is 8 to 12 minutes. Subjects become bored with longer tests. Also, it is important that the increments of workload not be excessive. Otherwise, some subjects may stop exercise before a maximum cardiorespiratory effort has been achieved. Three well-standardized protocols for treadmill exercise are detailed in Tables 5.2 through 5.4. The Bruce protocol is quite popular. For children and subjects incapable of much exercise, a modified Bruce protocol can be used in which the initial two steps use a belt speed of 1.7 mph and an incline of 0% and 5%, respectively.

For cycle testing, the James protocol (24) (Table 5.4) is popular. A disadvantage of this protocol is the relatively large work increments. The so-called ramp protocol may come to be used more and more frequently as investigators acquire the equipment to perform this type of study. The ramp protocol uses a constantly increasing workload for which the increment, regardless of magnitude, occurs as a gradual and continuous procedure instead of a step each minute. Obviously, this protocol is not suited for assessing physiologic functions that require steady-state exercise. A good compromise is the standard incremental cycle ergometer protocol with increments in work every minute, with the size of the increments tailored to the anticipated maximum capacity for each subject, such that test duration is 8 to 12 minutes.

TECHNIQUES OF SPECIFIC MEASUREMENTS

Heart Rate and Electrocardiogram

Heart rate, one of the basic indices of cardiac response to exercise, is measured from the electrocardiogram (ECG), which can be done manually by averaging several R-R intervals. Alternatively, the ECG signal can be processed through a tachometer, and a direct recording of heart rate based on one or more R-R intervals can be obtained. At least three leads of the standard surface ECG should be displayed or recorded continuously during, and for 5 to 10 minutes after completion of, an exercise test. The examiner should have the option of viewing various combinations of leads so that inferior (leads 2, 3, and AVF), anterior right (V1 or V2), and anterior left (V5 or V6) cardiac events can be assessed. A complete ECG should be recorded at rest at least once during each workload and for several intervals after exercise. Ideally, the ECG should have several recording speeds. Obtaining an ECG at a speed of 50 mm/sec facilitates assessment of ST segment changes. Continuous recording of the

TABLE 5.2

BRUCE TREADMILL PROTOCOL

Stage[a]	Belt speed (mph)	Incline (% grade)	METs[b]
(Modified Bruce)	1.7	0	2.3
(Modified Bruce)	1.7	5	3.5
1	1.7	10	4.5
2	2.5	12	7.0
3	3.4	14	10.0
4	4.2	16	12.9
5	5.0	18	15.0
6	5.5	20	16.9
7	6.0	22	19.1

[a]Three-minute stages.
[b]METs are multiples of resting O_2 uptake. One MET equals an O_2 uptake of 3.5 ml/kg/min.
From Bruce R. Exercise testing in coronary artery disease. *Ann Clin Res* 1971;3:323–332, with permission.

ECG at 5 mm per second paper speed facilitates detection of arrhythmias.

Appropriate application of the ECG electrodes and leads and electric shielding of the cable connecting the leads to the electrocardiograph are important for obtaining high-quality, artifact-free recordings. The subject's skin should be cleansed with alcohol and abraded lightly with no. 240 emery paper to reduce electric skin resistance. Most commercially available electrodes are prepackaged with electrode paste; occasionally, however, no paste is present, and these electrodes must be discarded or paste applied before using them. Note that pregelled electrodes have a limited shelf life owing to chemical changes in the conducting paste; they should be discarded if they are old and signal quality visibly deteriorates. The wire leads connecting the individual electrodes to the ECG cable should be secured to the subject's torso to minimize artifact from movement of these electrodes during exercise. This can be accomplished by loosely wrapping the torso with an elastic bandage or by using a commercially available knit shirt. The presence of artifact on the ECG usually indicates a loose lead–electrode interface, a poorly applied electrode, or inadequate electrode paste.

Blood Pressure

Blood pressure is an essential measurement in evaluating the cardiovascular response to exercise. Blood pressure can be measured directly with an indwelling arterial catheter or, more commonly, indirectly with a cuff, a sphygmomanometer, and a stethoscope. Numerous commercially available electronic units are available to measure blood pressure indirectly during exercise. The accuracy and precision of these "black boxes," however, must be a concern. Devices designed to inflate and deflate the cuff automatically and a microphone that can be secured over the brachial artery are useful. It is critical to use an appropriate-size cuff. The bladder of the cuff should encircle the arm completely, and the width of the cuff should be at least two-thirds the length of the upper arm. An oversized cuff should be available to measure leg blood pressure when indicated. It should be remembered that accurate measurement of diastolic blood pressure during exercise is extremely difficult, particularly during treadmill exercise, because the pounding

TABLE 5.3

BALKE TREADMILL PROTOCOL

Stage[a]	Belt speed (mph)	Incline (% grade)
1	3.3	0
2	3.3	2
3	3.3	3
4	3.3	4
5	3.3	5
6	3.3	6
7	3.3	7
Etc.	Etc.	Etc.

[a]One-minute stages.
From Balke J, Ware R. An experimental study of physical fitness of Air Force personnel. *US Armed Forces Med J* 1959; 10:675–688, with permission.

TABLE 5.4

JAMES CYCLE PROTOCOL

Stage[a]	KPM/min		
	<1 m² BSA	1–1.19 m² BSA	>1.2 m² BSA
1	200	200	200
2	300	400	500
3	500	600	800
4	600	700	1,000
5	700	800	1,200
6	800	900	1,400
7	900	1,000	1,600
8	1,000	1,100	1,800

BSA, body surface area.
[a]Three-minute stages.
From James FW, Kaplan S, Glueck CJ, et al. Responses of normal children and young adults to controlled bicycle exercise. *Circulation* 1980;61:902–912, with permission.

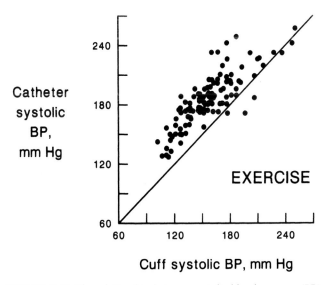

FIGURE 5.11 The relationship between systolic blood pressure (BP) measured using an indwelling radial artery cannula and arm blood pressure measured with a sphygmomanometer. Note that the blood pressures measured using a radial artery catheter are greater than those using a sphygmomanometer. (Reproduced from Rassmussen P, Staats B, Driscoll D, et al. Comparison of direct and indirect blood pressure during exercise. *Chest* 1985;87:743–748, with permission.)

feet and the noise of the treadmill make it difficult to hear Korotkoff sounds. Direct blood pressure measurement allows nearly instantaneous beat-to-beat monitoring of blood pressure with a high level of precision. Because of peripheral amplification, however, measurement of blood pressure in the distal vascular system (radial or brachial artery) overestimates central aortic blood pressure (Fig. 5.11). In addition,

this technique is invasive and potentially painful, which limits its usefulness in children.

Cardiac Output and Stroke Volume

The two techniques used most frequently to measure cardiac output ($\dot{Q}$) relatively noninvasively and without the need for radioactive material are the CO_2 and the acetylene helium rebreathing techniques (25). The CO_2 rebreathing technique (Fig. 5.12) is based on the Fick principle for CO_2:

$$\dot{Q} = \frac{\dot{V}CO_2}{C\bar{v}CO_2 - CaCO_2}$$

where $\dot{V}CO_2$ is the volume of carbon dioxide produced, $C\bar{v}CO_2$ is mixed venous blood CO_2 content, and $CaCO_2$ is the systemic arterial blood CO_2 content. $\dot{V}CO_2$ is directly measured; arterial CO_2 content is calculated from the measurement of systemic arterial blood pCO_2; mixed venous CO_2 content is calculated from the measurement of end-tidal (alveolar) pCO_2, assuming equilibrium with mixed venous pCO_2 and alveolar pCO_2 during the rebreathing maneuver. The latter maneuver can be done by the classic equilibrium (26) or the exponential technique (27). The latter is simpler during incremental exercise and better tolerated because it uses lower CO_2 concentration in the rebreathing mixture—inhaled CO_2 can create an unpleasant taste and transient headache in high concentrations. The need to measure systemic arterial pCO_2 is a disadvantage of this technique because it is invasive. Systemic arterial pCO_2 can be estimated from end-tidal pCO_2, or by assuming a normal anatomic dead space *in a subject with normal pulmonary function* and solving for $PaCO_2$ using the Bohr equation,

$$\frac{V_D}{V_T} = \frac{PaCO_2 - PeCO_2}{PaCO_2}$$

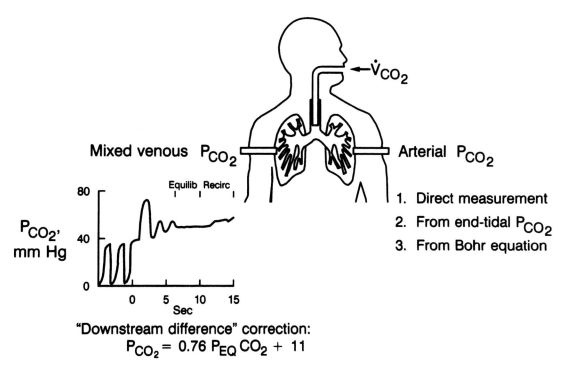

FIGURE 5.12 Diagrammatic representation of the CO_2 rebreathing method of assessing cardiac output. See text for determination of $PaCO_2$.

since all parameters in this equation are directly measured except for $PaCO_2$. Note that one must account for instrument dead space (mouthpiece, rebreathing technique). Ultimately however, such approximations introduce additional potential error into the technique. In addition, the concentration of CO_2 in the rebreathing mixture as well as the volume of the rebreathing mixture must be adjusted to the patient's size and exercise intensity. The future of this method is uncertain because of two recently described methodologic issues: the accuracy of measuring pCO_2 in a high O_2 mixture (28), and the solution to the equation relating CO_2 partial pressures to contents (29). The former problem, known as the collision-broadening effect, effectively limits the CO_2 rebreathing technique to laboratories using a mass spectrometer to measure exhaled gas concentrations; whereas the latter underscores the need to know (rather than assume) blood pH and pCO_2. Until these issues are clarified, healthy critical evaluation of papers using the indirect Fick (CO_2) technique would seem justified.

The acetylene-helium (C_2H_2-He) rebreathing technique to measure cardiac output is based on the principle that acetylene diffuses from the alveolus to the pulmonary capillary (30). The concentration of the acetylene in the rebreathing system declines relative to the volume of effective pulmonary blood flow (Fig. 5.13). This technique actually measures effective pulmonary blood flow rather than systemic blood flow, but in the absence of significant right-to-left or left-to-right intracardiac or intrapulmonary shunt, it is a reliable approximation of cardiac output. The other caveat is that the technique is dependent on even distribution of the inspired gas and will thus be less accurate in patients with lung disease characterized by mismatching of ventilation and perfusion. It is necessary to include a gas that does not diffuse out of the alveolus (e.g., helium) to determine the volume of the entire respiratory system and rebreathing apparatus. This technique is completely noninvasive and tolerated well by children. Technically, it is simpler to perform the C_2H_2-He than the CO_2 rebreathe maneuver because the concentration of acetylene, helium, oxygen, and nitrogen used as the rebreathe mixture is constant; only the volume of the mixture needs to be altered, depending on the subject's size and exercise intensity. Subjects

find the C_2H_2-He rebreathing technique more comfortable (with less feeling of dyspnea during the procedure) than with CO_2 rebreathing.

There are several publications on echocardiographic measurement of cardiac output during exercise. With this method, stroke volume is estimated by standard Doppler echocardiographic techniques (31). The cross-sectional area of the ascending aorta is first calculated at rest with subjects in the sitting position from the maximal diameter of the aorta measured by two-dimensional echocardiography (long-axis view) at the sinotubular junction (inner edge to inner edge) assuming the aorta to be circular. The velocity of ascending aorta blood flow is determined with a continuous-wave transducer positioned in the suprasternal notch. The velocity-time integral (VTI) for each beat is calculated off-line by tracing the velocity curve contour over time. The termination of each contour is marked by aortic valve closure. Five to eight curves with the highest values and most distinct spectral envelopes should be averaged for each workload. Stroke volume is estimated as the product of the mean VTI and the cross-sectional area of the ascending aorta. The method is reasonably accurate, provided enough beats are averaged to compute stroke volume, since SV is affected by phase of breathing (32); however, one risks overestimation of SV and hence cardiac output if one chooses the best-looking VTI. The technique is also critically dependent on accurate measurement of aortic valve area. Moreover, obtaining a satisfactory window at the suprasternal notch during heavy exercise can be a challenge both to the person holding the transducer and to the hyperpneic subject. Thus, echocardiographic measurement of cardiac output is very operator dependent, but despite these limitations the method is a choice among the noninvasive options.

There is potential usefulness for impedance cardiography as a clinical and research tool in the pediatric exercise laboratory. It has never gained widespread acceptance because of uncertainty over its theoretical foundations, and because of equivocal findings of previous reports comparing this method with more accepted methods of measuring cardiac output. Very recent work may change this thinking (15,33), so a brief description would seem worthwhile. The theory behind the

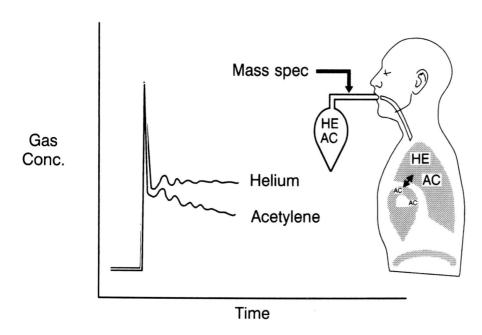

FIGURE 5.13 Diagram of the acetylene-helium rebreathing technique for measuring effective pulmonary blood flow. Note that with rebreathing there is a constant decay in the concentration of acetylene in the rebreathing system. This occurs because acetylene passes across the alveolar membrane and is taken up by the pulmonary blood flow.

method models the thorax as a cylinder or truncated cone whose electrical impedance changes in proportion to the electrical conductivity of the blood within, simultaneously with mechanical systole. A tiny, biologically inactive AC current is discharged by one set of electrodes, while another set measures the impedance of the thoracic contents to this current. Stroke volume is computed from thoracic impedance as follows:

$$SV = r(L^2/Z_0^2)(VET)(dZ/dt_{min})$$

where r = blood resistivity, a function of packed cell volume, L = distance between electrodes (measured), Z = baseline thoracic impedance, VET = ventricular ejection time (sec), dZ/dt_{min} = maximum rate of fall in impedance. Future studies will determine its role, but it offers a simple, unobtrusive method that yields results comparable to other methods for measuring cardiac output during exercise.

Ventilation Measurements

In the past 20 years, tremendous technical advances have been made in the measurement of ventilatory function at rest and during exercise. No longer is it necessary to use cumbersome Douglas bags and Tissot spirometers. Reliable respiratory mass flow sensors and high-speed gas analyzers are readily available. In addition, hardware and software are available to measure indices of ventilation in a breath-by-breath fashion. In general, these systems cost approximately $100,000. One must remember to use appropriate quality control measures even for prepackaged commercially available equipment.

The following indices of ventilation are measured: respiratory rate (RR), tidal volume (V_T), minute ventilation (typically $\dot{V}_E$), oxygen uptake ($\dot{V}O_2$), CO_2 production ($\dot{V}CO_2$), end-tidal CO_2 and O_2, and mixed expired CO_2 and O_2. From these measurements, the ventilatory equivalents for O_2 ($\dot{V}_E/\dot{V}O_2$) and CO_2 ($\dot{V}_E/\dot{V}CO_2$) and the respiratory gas-exchange ratio (R) can be measured. Noninvasive (ear or finger oximetry) measurement of blood oxygen saturation is useful for documenting the presence or absence, and degree, of hypoxemia. There is excellent correlation between blood oxygen saturation measured by oximetry and that measured by direct blood gas analysis (Fig. 5.14) at least for saturation levels >75%.

Measurement of ventilatory indices requires the use of a mouthpiece and a nose clip or a tightly fitting mask, and the latter can be oronasal or partition oral and nasal flow. Most children will tolerate a mouthpiece and nose clip. It is important, however, to have different-sized mouthpieces and three-way respiratory valves available so that the dead space of the system can be minimized for small children. We use a valve with 35 cm^3 dead space for children <1 m^2 BSA (body surface area) and a valve with 59 cm^3 dead space for patients of >1 m^2 BSA.

Safety Issues and Contraindications to Exercise

A properly supervised exercise study is safe. It is important that the examiner pay close attention to the subject during the study, especially during treadmill exercise. The major safety concern during treadmill exercise is the subject falling, which can occur as the treadmill is started because the subject may not be ready to walk. In general, the subject should stand with his or her feet astride the treadmill belt until the belt has achieved a steady speed. With one foot, the subject can test the speed of the belt before walking with both feet. A fall may occur as the subject becomes fatigued and either collapses or is swept off the device by the motion of the belt. Fatigue or dizziness leading to collapse is also a risk on the cycle ergometer. Thus, one must be alert to stopping the treadmill, or physically supporting the patient on the bike, when the patient can no longer exercise or appears to be in jeopardy. At these times, an observer should be positioned to assist the subject. Small children must be kept clear of the rollers of the moving treadmill so that they will not insert a digit or extremity into the moving machinery.

CARDIAC REHABILITATION

Some investigators advocate formal cardiac rehabilitation programs for children with congenital heart defects. Most children will resume reasonably normal physical activity after cardiac operation; hence, it is unclear, from a cost–benefit standpoint, which children should be enrolled in a formal exercise rehabilitation program. The following summarizes the state of the art of cardiac rehabilitation:

1. With a supervised exercise rehabilitation program, exercise efficiency and perhaps aerobic capacity can be improved in children who have had an operation for congenital heart disease. It is unclear, however, whether these changes

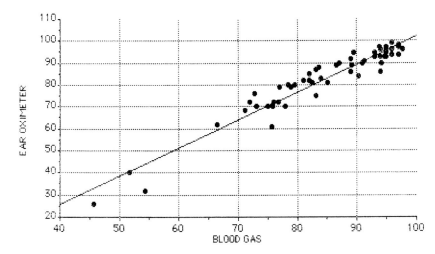

FIGURE 5.14 The relationship between arterial blood oxygen saturation estimated using ear oximetry and measured from blood. (From Driscoll D. Diagnostic use of exercise testing in pediatric cardiology: Noninvasive approach. In: Bar-Or O, ed. *Advances in Pediatric Sport Sciences.* Vol 3. Champaign, IL: Human Kinetics, 1989:223–251, with permission.)

would have occurred in the absence of a supervised exercise rehabilitation program.

2. Most children return to a reasonably normal lifestyle and level of physical fitness after repair of congenital heart defects.

3. Supervised exercise rehabilitation programs may be useful in returning selected children to an improved level of aerobic capacity and exercise efficiency.

4. There is insufficient information available at present to justify the cost of supervised exercise rehabilitation programs for all children after cardiac surgery.

5. Further studies are necessary to define clearly the medical efficacy, ideal population to target, and cost effectiveness of supervised exercise rehabilitation programs for children with congenital heart defects.

References

1. Bar-Or O, Rowland TW. *Pediatric Exercise Medicine—From Physiologic Principles to Health Care Application.* Champaign IL: Human Kinetics, 2004.

2. Wagner PD. Determinants of maximal transport and utilization. *Annual Rev Physiol* 1996;58:21–50.

3. di Prampero PE. Factors limiting maximal performance in humans. *Eur J Appl Physiol* 2003;90:420–429.

4. Astrand P-O, Rodahl K. *Textbook of Work Physiology: Physiological Basis of Exercise.* New York: McGraw-Hill, 1977:450.

5. Welsman JR, Armstrong N, Nevill AM, et al. Scaling VO_{2max} for differences in body size. *Med Sci Sports Exerc* 1996;28:259–265.

6. Cooper DM, Weiler-Ravell D, Whipp BJ, et al. Aerobic parameters of exercise as a function of body size during growth in children. *J Appl Physiol* 1984;56:628–634.

7. Andreacci JL, Robertson RJ, Dube JJ, et al. Comparison of maximal oxygen consumption between black and white prepubertal and pubertal children. *Pediatr Res* 2004;56:706–713.

8. Washington RL. Cardiorespiratory testing: Anaerobic threshold/respiratory threshold. *Pediatr Cardiol* 1999;20:12–15.

9. Hebestreit H, Staschen B, Hebestreit A. Ventilatory threshold: A useful method to determine aerobic fitness in children? *Med Sci Sports Exerc* 2000;32:1964–1969.

10. Reybrouck T, Weymans M, Stijns H, et al. Ventilatory anaerobic threshold in healthy children: Age and sex differences. *Eur J Appl Physiol* 1985;54:278–284.

11. Rowell LB. Circulatory adjustments to dynamic exercise. In: Rowell LB, ed. *Human Circulation Regulation during Physical Stress.* New York: Oxford University Press, 1986:213–256.

12. Godfrey S, Davies CTM, Wozniak E, et al. Cardio-respiratory response to exercise in normal children. *Clin Sci* 1971;40:419–431.

13. Rowland T, Potts J, Potts T, et al. Cardiac responses to progressive exercise in normal children: A synthesis. *Med Sci Sports Exerc* 2000;32:253–259.

14. Eriksson BO, Grimby G, Saltin B. Cardiac output and arterial blood gases during exercise in pubertal boys. *J Appl Physiol* 1971;31:348–352.

15. Pianosi P. Measurement of exercise cardiac output by thoracic impedance in healthy children. *Eur J Appl Physiol* 2004;92:425–430.

16. Strong W, Miller M, Striplin M, et al. Blood pressure response to isometric and dynamic exercise in healthy black children. *Am J Dis Child* 1978;132:587–591.

17. Baxter-Jones A, Goldstein H, Helms P. The development of aerobic power in young athletes. *J Appl Physiol* 1993;75:1160–1167.

18. Cooper DM, Kaplan MR, Baumgarten L, et al. Coupling of ventilation and CO_2 production during exercise in children. *Pediatr Res* 1987;21:568–572.

19. Ohuchi H, Kato Y, Tasato H, et al. Ventilatory response and arterial blood gases during exercise in children. *Pediatr Res* 1999;45:389–396.

20. Johnson BD, Weisman IM, Zeballos RJ, et al. Emerging concepts in the evaluation of ventilatory limitation during exercise: The exercise tidal flow-volume loop. *Chest* 1999;116:488–503.

21. Nourry C, Deruelle F, Fabre C, et al. Exercise flow-volume loops in prepubescent aerobically trained children. *J Appl Physiol* 2005;99:1912–1921.

22. Dempsey JA, Wagner PD. Exercise-induced arterial hypoxemia. *J Appl Physiol* 1999;87:1997–2006.

23. Nourry C, Fabre C, Bart F, et al. Evidence of exercise-induced arterial hypoxemia in prepubescent trained children. *Pediatr Res* 2004;55:674–681.

24. James F, Kaplan S, Glueck C, et al. Responses of normal children and young adults to controlled bicycle exercise. *Circulation* 1980;61:902–912.

25. Driscoll D. Diagnostic use of exercise testing in pediatric cardiology: The noninvasive approach. In: Bar-Or O, ed. *Advances in Pediatric Sport Sciences.* Champaign, IL: Human Kinetics, 1989:223–251.

26. Godfrey S. *Exercise Testing in Children.* London: WB Saunders, 1974.

27. Jacob SV, Hornby L, Lands LC. Estimation of mixed venous PCO_2 for determination of cardiac output in children. *Chest* 1997;111:474–480.

28. Hornby L, Coates AL, Lands LC. Effect of analyzer on determination of mixed venous PCO_2 and cardiac output during exercise. *J Appl Physiol* 1995;79:1032–1038.

29. Sun XG, Hansen JE, Stringer WW, et al. Carbon dioxide pressure-concentration relationship in arterial and mixed venous blood during exercise. *J Appl Physiol* 2001;90:1798–1810.

30. Triebwasser J, Johnson R, Burpo R, et al. Noninvasive determination of cardiac output by a modified acetylene rebreathing procedure utilizing mass spectrometer measurements. *Aviat Space Environ Med* 1977;48:203–209.

31. Calafiore P, Stewart WJ. Doppler echocardiographic quantitation of volumetric flow rate. *Cardiol Clin* 1990;8:191–202.

32. Du Quesnay MC, Stoute GJ, Hughson RL. Cardiac output in exercise by impedance cardiography during breath holding and normal breathing. *J Appl Physiol* 1987;62:101–107.

33. Tordi N, Mourot L, Matusheski B, et al. Measurements of cardiac output during constant exercise: Comparison of two non-invasive techniques. *Int J Sports Med* 2004;25:145–149.

CHAPTER 6 ■ ECHOCARDIOGRAPHY

THOMAS R. KIMBALL, MD, AND ERIK C. MICHELFELDER, MD

Improvement in transducer resolution and the development of color Doppler technology have positioned echocardiography as the principal diagnostic modality in the field of pediatric cardiology (1). The echocardiography laboratory is often the patient's last diagnostic stop before surgical or catheter intervention, which necessitates the most complete anatomic and physiologic description of the cardiovascular system possible and requires unprecedented detail in the echocardiographic evaluation.

HISTORY

In 1877, Pierre Curie, then only 18 years old, and his older brother, Jacques, launched the field of ultrasound by discovering the piezoelectric effect in which mechanical distortion of crystals produces an electric potential and vice versa. Although the piezoelectric effect forms the basis for ultrasound, it was not until many years later, in fact not until after the 1912 sinking of the Titanic (which catalyzed efforts to create systems aiding ships in earlier detection of icebergs), that the field of ultrasound began to develop (2). Finally, in World War II, ultrasound waves formed the basis of sonar (*sound navigation ranging*) (3).

The successful use of ultrasound as a diagnostic medical technique was simultaneously pioneered in the 1940s and 1950s by four groups: (a) the Massachusetts Institute of Technology (MIT; Bolt, Ballatine, Ludwig, and Heuter), (b) the University of Illinois (Fry, Fry, and Kelly), (c) the University of Colorado (Howry and Holmes), and (d) the University of Minnesota (Wild and Reid). The MIT group developed A (amplitude)-mode ultrasound, a method of displaying reflected waves as spikes of various heights on an oscilloscope. The Illinois group is renowned for using ultrasound to detect breast cancer. The Colorado group developed B (brightness)-mode imaging, a method of displaying the intensity of the reflected ultrasound waves as dots of various brightness along a single scan line, the progenitor to two-dimensional (2-D) ultrasound. They expanded this concept by creating the B-29 gun turret water-bath scanner in which both patient and transducer were immersed. The Minnesota group perfected pulsed ultrasound techniques that permit a single transducer to act as both a transmitter and a receiver in real time and, by incorporating a water interface in the transducer head, creating the first handheld scanner, thus eliminating the need for patient immersion (2,3).

Applying ultrasound for cardiac diagnosis was first performed at the University of Lund, Sweden (Edler and Hertz), in 1953. A B-mode detector with continuous moving film to obtain real-time images of the heart in waveform provided the first M (motion)-mode echocardiogram (2,3). Twenty years later, M-mode echocardiography was applied to congenital heart disease by Goldberg, Allen, Sahn, Meyer, and others (4,5). In the late 1970s and early 1980s, the application of 2-D echocardiography to congenital heart disease allowing complete, accurate, and detailed diagnoses was successfully completed by pioneers such as Snider, Silverman, Williams, Stevenson, and others (6–15). Each stressed a thoughtful, considered approach that coupled the evolving field of echocardiography to the established fields of cardiac morphology, pathology, and embryology, eventually forging the way for children, infants, and neonates to receive medical and surgical treatment after an assessment that was completely noninvasive. In the 1990s and early 2000s, ultrasound technology became increasingly miniaturized so echocardiography is poised for broader use including as a bedside adjunct to the physical examination in more unique settings such as the emergency room and the intensive care unit. Such applications create special challenges for the pediatric echocardiography community, which must respond to the training and quality assurance issues associated with a wider user base without being exclusionary.

PHYSICS OF TWO-DIMENSIONAL ECHOCARDIOGRAPHY

The piezoelectric effect occurs when an electric potential applied to a crystal results in mechanical distortion because of alignment of the crystal's molecular dipoles. This, in turn, causes the crystal to resonate, producing ultrasonic waves. A sound wave requires a deformable medium for its propagation because it is mechanical in nature, consisting of a series of compressions and expansions (rarefaction) of the molecules in the medium. The velocity of sound depends on the type of tissue through which it is traveling (1,540 m/s in soft tissue, 330 m/s in air). The wave has characteristics that define its existence (Fig. 6.1).

The echocardiographic transducer does not emit ultrasound continuously, but rather, emits pulses rapidly (approximately 1,000 pulses per second) and quickly (approximately 1 microsecond for every pulse). Therefore, the transducer is operating as a transmitter for an extremely short time (0.1% of the time). During a 30-minute examination, the transducer has transmitted pulses for <2 seconds. When the transducer is not emitting sound waves, it is in its receiver mode awaiting the return of reflected ultrasound.

Eight Equations That Form the Basis of Two-Dimensional and Doppler Echocardiography

Equation 1: The Basis of Image Generation

$$\%R = \{(Z_2 - Z_1) / (Z_2 + Z_1)\}^2 \times 100 \qquad [1]$$

where

$\%R$ = percent reflection of ultrasound signal
Z_n = impedance in medium$_n$ = $\rho_n c_n$
ρ_n = density of medium$_n$
c_n = speed of sound in medium$_n$

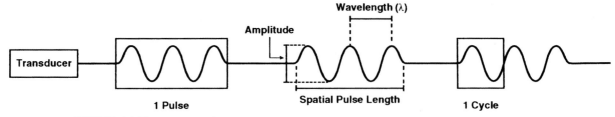

FIGURE 6.1 The anatomy of a wave. The wavelength is the distance between two consecutive and equivalent parts. The frequency is the number of compressions per unit of time expressed in Hertz. The amplitude is the pressure difference between nadir and peak. In echocardiography, waves are emitted as pulses consisting of wave cycles. Therefore, the spatial pulse length is the distance from the beginning of a single pulse train to its end.

As an ultrasound beam travels through the body, some of its energy will be reflected back to the transducer and some of its energy will continue to be transmitted forward. In considering the amount of reflected energy, it is helpful to consider the concept of momentum, which is the product of mass (m) of an object and its velocity (v) (momentum = mv). A speeding semi-tractor trailer (high velocity, huge mass) has much greater momentum than a pedaling bicyclist (slow velocity, small mass). Consider the well-known novelty of a set of metallic balls suspended adjacent to each other as a pendulum (Fig. 6.2). An outside ball is drawn away from the stationary balls and is released, striking the stationary balls, resulting in the outside ball on the opposite side moving away from the stationary balls. If the first outside ball were the size of a pea, it would strike the stationary balls and merely bounce away from them. It does not have sufficient momentum (because of relatively small mass) to cause any perturbation in the stationary balls. It is therefore merely reflected backwards.

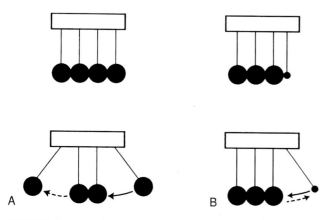

FIGURE 6.2 In mechanics, energy transfer is dependent on momentum. **A:** After an outside ball of equivalent size to the stationary balls is released, it strikes the stationary balls, resulting in movement of the outside ball on the opposite side. The ball has sufficient momentum to cause effective energy transfer to the stationary balls. **B:** After an outside ball of smaller size is released, it strikes the stationary balls and is reflected off of them. This ball has insufficient momentum to result in energy transfer. Acoustic impedance is the ultrasound equivalent to momentum. In ultrasound, energy transfer is dependent on impedance. If the impedances between two media are similar, ultrasound will be readily transmitted. If there is a mismatch in impedance, ultrasound will be reflected.

Acoustic impedance is the ultrasound equivalent to momentum; density replaces mass, and speed of sound replaces velocity in the equation (16). If the acoustic impedance is the same in two media, ultrasound will be readily transmitted through the media interface; however, a mismatch in the impedance of the two media will result in reflection of ultrasound.

Equation 2: The Basis of Image Resolution (Part I)

$$SPL = n(\lambda) = n(c/v) \qquad [2]$$

where

SPL = spatial pulse length
λ = wavelength
n = number of cycles in a pulse of ultrasound
c = speed of sound
v = transmission frequency

Axial resolution (resolution along the axis of the ultrasound beam) of a nonpulsed wave is approximately equivalent to its wavelength. A bat feeding at twilight emits ultrasound waves at a frequency of 100 kHz, which provides excellent resolution for catching insects in air ($\lambda = c/v = 330$ m/s ÷ 100,000 cycles/s = 3.3 mm) but provides an unacceptable resolution if an eccentric bat were to try fatuously to echo-locate cardiac anatomy through soft tissue (1,540 m/s ÷ 100,000 cycles/s = 15.4 mm). With pulsed ultrasound, the axial resolution is dependent on having a short spatial-pulse length. This can be achieved by either decreasing the number of wave cycles in an ultrasound pulse or decreasing the wavelength (i.e., increasing the transmission frequency). The best possible axial-point separation resolution is equal to ½ of the spatial-pulse length (Fig. 6.3). Using Equation 2, a 10-MHz transducer emitting a train of three pulsed ultrasonic waves will yield a point separation resolution of approximately 0.46 mm (3 × 154,000 cm/s ÷ 10,000,000 cycles/s). A 2.5-MHz transducer will have an approximate resolution of 1.8 mm. The poorer axial resolution of a transducer of this frequency therefore limits its usefulness in evaluating anatomy of smaller magnitude, for example, the luminal diameter of a coronary artery or the diameter of a small septal defect.

Equation 3: The Basis of Image Resolution (Part II)

$$D = (d^2v)/(4c) \qquad [3]$$

where

D = depth of near field
d = diameter of transducer
v = transmission frequency of transducer
c = speed of sound

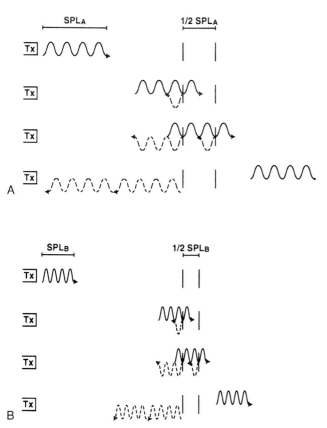

FIGURE 6.3 The axial resolution (resolution along the axis of the ultrasound beam) is dependent on the spatial pulse length (SPL). The shorter the SPL, the better the resolution. Resolution can be no better than $\frac{1}{2}$ of the SPL. **A:** The transducer emits pulses of sound waves (*solid line*) with a relatively long SPL of SPL_A. This train of pulses can distinguish two objects that are separated by a distance of $\frac{1}{2}$ SPL_A but no closer because the transducer would not be finished receiving the reflected wave from the proximal object before arrival of the reflected wave from the distal object. **B:** The transducer emits pulses of sound with a shorter SPL of SPL_B. These train of pulses can distinguish two objects that are closer together but still no closer than $\frac{1}{2}$ SPL_B (reflected waves shown as *dashed lines*).

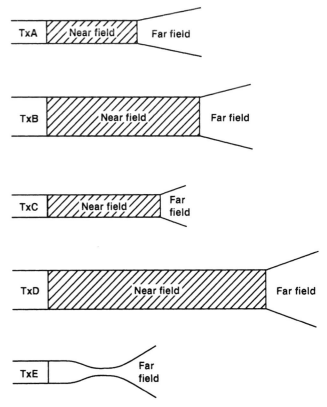

FIGURE 6.4 The lateral resolution (resolution perpendicular to the axis of the ultrasound beam) is dependent on the beam width of the transducer. The beam is relatively narrow in the near field of the transducer. In the far field, the ultrasound beam begins to diverge and lateral resolution deteriorates. Transducer A has a relatively small diameter and, therefore, a relatively shallow near field. The diameter of transducer B is larger, thereby extending the near field. Near-field depth can be increased even when using a smaller-diameter transducer if transducer frequency is increased (transducer C). Near-field depth is optimized with transducers having relatively large diameters and emitting ultrasound of high frequency (transducer D). Lateral resolution can be improved by focusing the transducer crystal; however, focusing has the disadvantage of the beam diverging rapidly beyond the focal zone (transducer E).

Lateral resolution is the ability to resolve objects that are perpendicular to the beam axis and, in general, is dependent on the beam width. For a nonfocused transducer, the ultrasonic beam consists of a near field with narrow beam width and good lateral resolution (the Fresnel zone) and a far field where the beam width diverges rapidly limiting resolution (the Fraunhofer zone) (16). The depth of the near field is extended by increasing the frequency or the footprint diameter of the transducer (Equation 3 and Fig. 6.4).

An example is afforded by imaging a newborn. For the parasternal and apical views, a small-diameter, high-frequency probe is advantageous because the cardiac structures are not at a deep depth and the small footprint can be placed between the acoustically unfriendly ribs. For subcostal imaging, a larger-diameter transducer provides great advantage by extending the near field to the level of the cardiac structures, improving their resolution.

Lateral resolution can be improved by focusing, which causes the beam width to narrow. Focusing can be accomplished by external devices (such as mirrors or lenses) or by electronic means; however, focusing results in two important disadvantages: first, the focal zone is closer to the transducer face than the nonfocused near-field zone, and second, the far-field divergence of a focused beam is greater than the divergence of a nonfocused beam.

Equation 4: The Ying-Yang Relationship between Resolution and Penetration

$$L = \mu v z \qquad [4]$$

where

L = intensity attenuation loss (in decibels)
μ = intensity attenuation coefficient (~0.8 dB/cm/MHz for soft tissue)
v = transducer frequency (in MHz)
z = distance traveled in the medium by ultrasound wave (in cm)

The energy of the ultrasound wave is decreased by tissue interactions. Attenuation describes the loss of intensity resulting from scattering (reflection at small interfaces) and absorption (energy transformation) (16). Equation 4 makes it clear that intensity loss is greatest (or penetration is poorest) when using a transducer with a higher frequency, precisely the frequency needed to enhance resolution (Equations 2 and 3). Thus, echocardiography requires a constant balancing act between optimizing resolution without sacrificing penetration and vice versa.

Equation 5: The Basis of Temporal Resolution

$$F = (c)/(2DNn) \qquad [5]$$

where

F = frame rate
c = speed of sound
D = sampling depth
N = number of sampling lines per frame
n = number of focal zones used to produce one image

Motion during 2-D echocardiography is portrayed by rapid presentation of successive single image frames, similar to viewing a motion picture film. A single image frame is generated by successive electronic stimulation of each element in the transducer to initiate an ultrasound pulse, which propagates down (and is received up) successive scan lines (one scan line typically extends through 1 to 3 degrees of the sector). In addition, the superimposition of a color Doppler sector on the image increases the time for a pulse to propagate down and up a scan line. The time required for the pulse to travel down one scan line to the depth of interest and back to the transducer imposes a restriction on how quickly the next element is stimulated, how rapidly a frame is acquired, and how soon the next frame can be produced. The frame rate (expressed in Hz) quantitates the speed of this process (16).

Temporal resolution can be optimized by narrowing the sector size (of both the image and the color Doppler region), thereby decreasing the number of scan lines, or by decreasing the depth range (Equation 5 and Fig. 6.5). A practical, easy-to-remember rule of thumb to optimize frame rate is to ensure

that the subject of interest fills the sector wedge completely, eliminating imaging of superfluous tissue at the lateral and inferior aspects of the sector. Since M-mode and Doppler echocardiography have better temporal resolution, these modalities may be more useful when measuring events that are occurring quickly.

Equation 6: The Doppler Equation

$$f_d = [2f_0(V)(\cos \theta)] \div c \qquad [6]$$

where

f_d = the observed Doppler frequency shift
f_0 = the transmitted frequency of sound
V = blood flow velocity
θ = the intercept angle between the ultrasound beam and the direction of blood flow
c = the velocity of sound in human tissue

The Doppler principle states that the frequency of a transmitted wave is altered when the source of the wave is in motion. The principle is also applicable when the source of the wave is stationary and the receiver of the wave is in motion. The observed change in frequency under these circumstances is termed the Doppler shift, after Christian Johann Doppler, who described this phenomenon in 1843. The phenomenon is apparent in daily life when an ambulance approaching with its siren wailing is perceived as having an increased pitch and when it moves past appears to have decreased pitch, or when a highway patrol person aims a microwave-emitting radar gun to measure a car's speed.

In medical ultrasound and echocardiography, the Doppler principle is applied using transmitted sound waves to strike moving red blood cells. Sound waves are transmitted by a stationary transducer, strike red blood cells in motion, and the returning backscattered sound pulses are Doppler shifted in frequency in relation to the velocity and direction in which the blood cells are moving. Doppler principles can also be applied—using modern ultrasound systems—to evaluate tissue motion by Doppler tissue imaging.

Doppler ultrasound is used primarily to assess velocity of moving structures, whether it be the velocity of blood flow

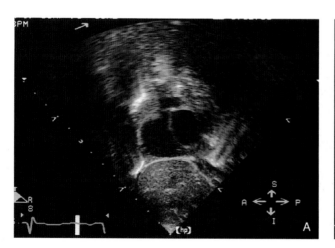
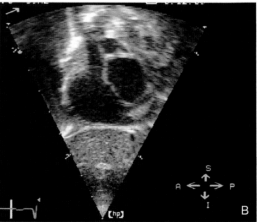

FIGURE 6.5 Two subcostal sagittal images demonstrate the factors that impact temporal resolution (*arrows*). **A:** The sampling depth is 13 cm, and the sector size is wide, yielding a frame rate of 38 Hz. **B:** The sampling depth has been decreased to 9 cm and the sector scan narrowed so that the image fills the entire sector and the frame rate has increased to 69 Hz.

through the heart and vasculature or the velocity of the ventricular myocardium. It is therefore appropriate to rearrange the Doppler equation to solve for velocity:

$$V = [c(f_d)] \div [2f_o \cos \theta]$$

As the speed of sound (c) and the transmitted frequency (f_o) are constant, and the frequency shift (f_d) can be very accurately measured, it becomes apparent that the main source of potential error in Doppler estimation of velocity arises from the intercept angle, θ, between the sound beam and the direction of blood/tissue motion. For intercept angles <20 degrees, $\cos \theta$ is small and is not felt to result is significant underestimation of the flow velocity. At greater intercept angles, correction for $\cos \theta$ is needed (Fig. 6.6). In clinical application, Doppler evaluation is generally avoided at higher intercept angles to avoid inaccuracy and the need for angle correction.

Equation 7: The Basis of Aliasing

$$V_{max} = (c^2) \div [8f_o D \cos \theta] \qquad [7]$$

where

V_{max} = the maximum measurable velocity of blood
c = the velocity of sound in tissue
f_o = the transmitted frequency of sound
D = depth of interest
θ = the intercept angle between the ultrasound beam and the direction of blood flow

If the Doppler sampling rate is not adequate, the frequency of the reflected wave is sampled only intermittently, data must be inferred, and the wave is misinterpreted as having a lower frequency, a phenomenon called *aliasing*. The phenomenon is apparent in older Western movies when the wheel of a stagecoach is perceived as rotating backwards when the stagecoach is obviously moving forwards. The movie consists of a series of stop-action photographs, which when shown one after the

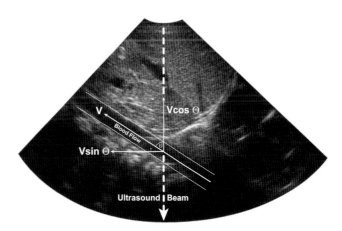

FIGURE 6.6 Angle correction for Doppler velocity assessment. The observed Doppler velocity is represented as the velocity vector parallel to the line of insonation (dotted line). This velocity is related to the true velocity, V, by the cosine of the angle, Θ, between the direction of flow and the line of insonation. For Θ > 20 degrees, the cosine function becomes significantly less than 1, and will result is significant underestimation of the true velocity, V.

other give the appearance of motion. If the stagecoach moves very fast, the wheel turns very fast and turns too great a revolutionary arc between successive photographs. The problem is solved by decreasing the time between successive photographs so the wheel turns a smaller arc between photographs (Fig. 6.7). Equation 7 demonstrates that the maximum measurable velocity of blood can be increased by decreasing the transducer frequency and/or sampling at a shallower depth. Since the latter is usually not alterable, increasing the aliasing or Nyquist limit is achieved by exchanging to a lower-frequency transducer.

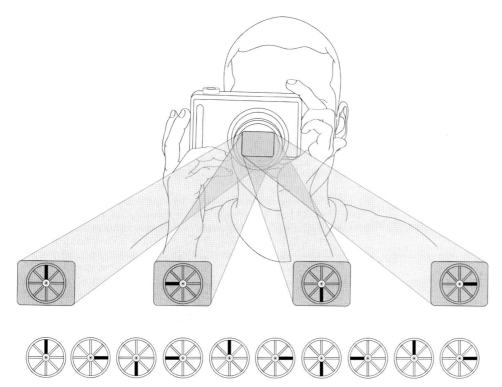

FIGURE 6.7 The principle of aliasing is similar to the phenomenon in old Western movies of a wheel of a stagecoach appearing to rotate backward when the stagecoach is obviously moving forward. The movie consists of a series of stop-action photographs, which, when placed in sequential order, give the appearance of motion. If the series of photographs are captured at too low a frequency (**top row**) any spoke on the wheel (e.g., the highlighted bold spike), will appear to be rotating backward (in this case, appearing to rotate 90 degrees counterclockwise each time an image is captured). It is only when the frequency of snapping photographs is high enough (**bottom row**), that the true forward rotation of the wheel is appreciated (in this case, rotating 90 degrees clockwise each time an image is snapped).

The phenomenon of aliasing and the value of using lower-frequency transducers for sampling higher blood velocities are also understood by contemplating the concept of pulse repetition frequency (PRF) in the context of Equation 6. Since it requires a minimum of two pulses per wave cycle to define frequency unambiguously, the minimum PRF to sample a reflected wave's frequency is twice the Doppler shift. Therefore, a more reasonable PRF is achieved by minimizing the Doppler shift. It is clear from Equation 6 that at any given blood velocity and Doppler angle, a lower Doppler shift (i.e., low f_d) is achieved only by reducing transducer frequency (i.e., low f_o).

Equation 8: The Bernoulli Equation

$$\Delta P = \tfrac{1}{2}\rho(V_2{}^2 - V_1{}^2) + \rho\int dV/dt(ds) + R(V) \qquad [8]$$

where

ΔP = the pressure difference across an obstructive orifice
V_1 = the flow velocity proximal to the obstruction
V_2 = the flow velocity distal to the obstruction
ρ = the mass density of blood = 1,060 kg/m^3
dV = change in velocity over time (dt)
ds = distance over which change in pressure occurs
R = viscous resistance in blood vessel
V = velocity of blood flow

The first term, $\tfrac{1}{2}\rho(V_2{}^2 - V_1{}^2)$, represents convective acceleration through the flow orifice. This equation becomes $4(V_2{}^2 - V_1{}^2)$ when substituting the blood density of 1,060 kg/m^3 into the equation, multiplying by $\tfrac{1}{2}$, and multiplying by the conversion factor of 0.0075, which converts kg/m/s^2 (a pascal) to mm Hg. In addition, in most clinical conditions, the proximal flow velocity is <1 m/s and is considered negligible. Thus, the first term can be simplified as $4V_2{}^2$. The second term describes energy expended to accelerate fluid at the onset of flow; clinical measurements are usually made at peak flow, and thus, this term can be assumed to be zero. The third term describes energy lost overcoming viscous friction along the walls of the vessel and is felt to be of little impact in most clinical circumstances. Therefore, the Bernoulli equation can be simplified, acknowledging the assumptions above:

$$\Delta P = 4V_2{}^2 \qquad [9]$$

It is important to understand that when the assumptions used to simplify the Bernoulli equation may not apply, the approach to estimating pressure gradients may need to be modified. A common example of such an instance is in estimation of pressure drops *where the proximal velocity (V_1) is >1 m/s* such as across an aortic coarctation, stenotic *and regurgitant* semilunar valves (where the regurgitant volume may result in an increase in V_1), multiple obstructions in series, and in the setting of high cardiac output. Viscous resistance may not be negligible in other circumstances where the obstruction is long and narrow (17) such as across Blalock-Thomas-Taussig shunts, or across tunnel-type obstructions, e.g., tubular obstruction of the left ventricular outflow tract.

THE EXAMINATION

General Considerations

Echocardiographic Windows

There are four major echocardiographic windows to the heart (Fig. 6.8): (a) parasternal, (b) apical, (c) subcostal, and

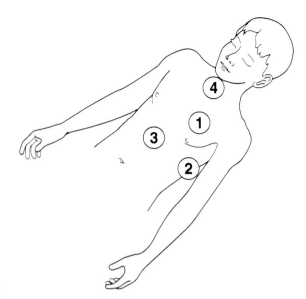

FIGURE 6.8 There are four echocardiographic windows: (1) parasternal, (2) apical, (3) subcostal, and (4) suprasternal notch. The parasternal and apical windows are obtained with the patient in a left lateral decubitus position with using a dropout mattress. Subcostal images are obtained with the patient supine and sometimes with the knees flexed. Suprasternal notch images are obtained with a roll under the shoulders so that the neck is hyperextended.

(d) suprasternal notch. (A fifth window, the right parasternal window, obtained with the patient in a right lateral decubitus position, is used for obtaining an accurate Doppler gradient in patients with aortic stenosis.) The examination usually is performed in this same order, beginning with the least noxious parasternal window and finishing with the potentially most noxious suprasternal notch window. In complex cases associated with abnormal situs or cardiac position, the examination may alternatively begin with the apical or subcostal windows so that the echocardiographer can become oriented for the other views.

Parasternal and apical imaging is performed with the patient in a left lateral decubitus position. A dropout mattress is essential for obtaining the apical view. During subcostal imaging, the patient lies supine, sometimes flexing the knees, thereby relaxing the abdominal muscles. Suprasternal imaging is performed with a roll under the shoulders to extend the neck.

Planes of the Heart and Technique of Sweeping: Thinking in Three Dimensions

Three-dimensional (3-D) imaging continues to improve (see below) but is currently not in routine clinical use. Until it is, the challenge and essence of pediatric echocardiography are and will be acquiring all the necessary 2-D images, mentally synthesizing them into a 3-D model, and conveying this 3-D representation to others by narrative or visual tools.

The spatial location of any part of an object is defined and understood by considering it in relation to the three planes (transverse [axial], sagittal, and coronal) in which the object exists (Fig. 6.9). Each of the four echocardiographic windows affords the opportunity to image the heart from one or more of these three planes. From the parasternal window, the long (sagittal) and short (axial) planes are shown. From the apical and subcostal windows, the four-chamber (coronal) and two-chamber

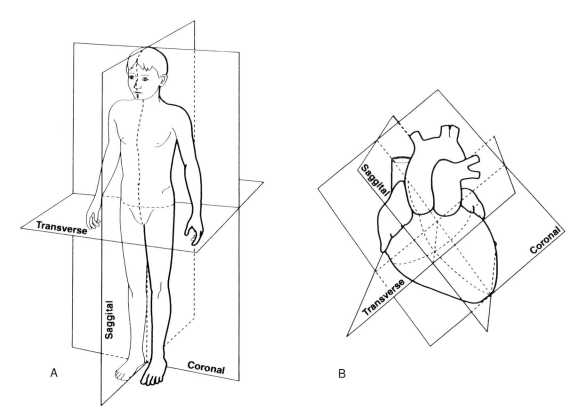

FIGURE 6.9 A: There are three imaging planes of the body: sagittal, coronal, and transverse. B: There are also three imaging planes of the heart. The cardiac imaging planes are rotated leftward and anterior because the heart's axes are rotated leftward and anterior relative to the body's.

(sagittal) planes are demonstrated. Finally, from the suprasternal notch window, the sagittal and axial axes of the upper thoracic vasculature are imaged. Sweeping the transducer through the nearly parallel planes within each of the acoustic windows mimics the ability of other imaging modalities such as magnetic resonance to obtain parallel "slices" within a given plane (Fig. 6.10). With these techniques, the spatial relationships become clear and the 3-D mental reconstruction of the heart becomes possible.

Optimizing the Doppler Examination

The robustness of Doppler echocardiography as a tool for evaluating cardiac physiology is manifested only when its practitioners exhibit precise and diligent technique. Doppler spectral envelopes need to be sharp and free of feathering. A sharp envelope is first achieved by aligning the ultrasound beam as parallel to the flow as possible. Traditionally, color Doppler is used before application of pulsed or continuous wave Doppler to determine the precise location and direction of a jet. The transducer position on the chest is then moved accordingly so that the flow is directed either exactly toward or opposite to it. The best transducer position for the Doppler examination may therefore be offset from the most ideal position for two-dimensional imaging. Second, the practitioner must be careful to avoid overgaining the spectral display, which can cause indistinct envelopes. Third, the spectral display of interest should fill as much of the screen as possible by shifting the baseline up or down and decreasing the Doppler scale. In this way, the envelope is made as large as possible, minimizing the

effect of imprecise Doppler envelope planimetry (Fig. 6.11). Fourth, tracing the Doppler envelope needs to be careful, precise, and steady. The operator must know if a trace of modal velocity (for continuity equation) or of peak velocity (for pressure gradients) is most appropriate (Fig. 6.12). Finally, the practitioner must be aware of the various Doppler modalities available to help optimize the spectral signal.

Color Flow Doppler. With its development in the 1980s, color flow Doppler revolutionized echocardiography by providing an efficient overview of flow across a relatively vast region of interest, making it extremely valuable in screening for normal and abnormal flows across valves, vessels, and septa. The color Doppler modality interrogates flow with multiple pulsed Doppler sample volumes placed successively along multiple scan lines. For each sampling gate, the baseline frequency is compared with the received frequency. Pixels in the image are assigned a color (red for flow toward the transducer and blue for flow away from the transducer) and a color intensity based on the magnitude of the mean velocity. The color Doppler scale should be actively manipulated throughout the examination—using low-velocity scales when interrogating venous flows (e.g., antegrade atrioventricular valve, atrial shunt, cavopulmonary, and systemic and pulmonary venous velocities) or flows generated from low-pressure gradients and high-velocity scales when interrogating arterial flows or flows generated from high-pressure gradients. The examiner must actively think about and anticipate expected physiology during the study so that the color scale is appropriately adjusted

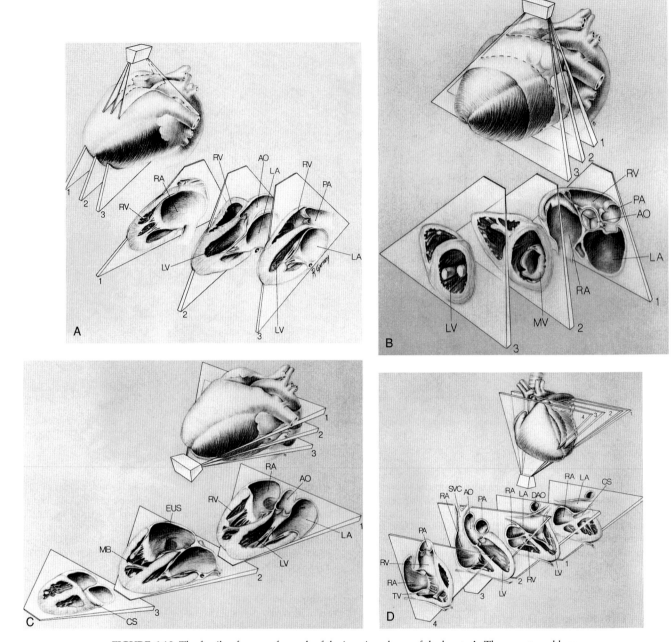

FIGURE 6.10 The family of sweeps for each of the imaging planes of the heart. **A:** The parasternal long-axis sweeps consist of the rightward tricuspid valve view (1), the standard long-axis plane (2), and the leftward pulmonary valve view (3). **B:** The parasternal short-axis sweeps consist of the superior basal view (1), the standard plane at the level of the mitral valve (2), and the inferior papillary muscle view (3). **C:** The apical sweeps consist of the anterior five-chamber view (1), the standard apical four-chamber view (2), and the posterior coronary sinus view (3). **D:** The subcostal coronal sweeps consist of the posterior coronary sinus view (1), the standard four-chamber view (2), the anterior left ventricular outflow tract view (3), and the extremely anterior right ventricular outflow tract view (4).

(Fig. 6.13). For example, in a toddler being evaluated for a suspected ventricular septal defect, interrogation of the septum with a high color Doppler scale is appropriate. However, using such a high color scale in the investigation for a ventricular septal defect in a newborn would likely miss the shunt flow since the shunt is driven by a very low pressure gradient owing to the normally elevated pulmonary vascular resistance in the newborn period. The examiner would need to interrogate the ventricular septum with a low-velocity color Doppler scale in this instance. These flows then need to be more carefully and precisely interrogated and quantitated with either pulsed or continuous wave Doppler. Because of the massive amount of data, a color Doppler sector should be kept as narrow as acceptable to improve accuracy and/or temporal resolution

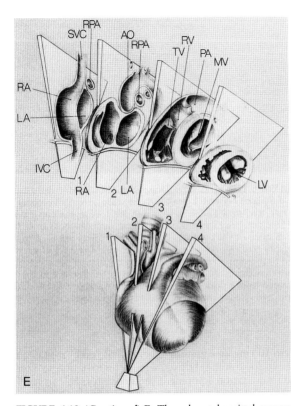

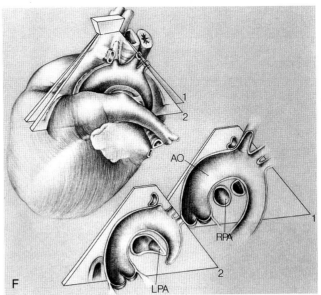

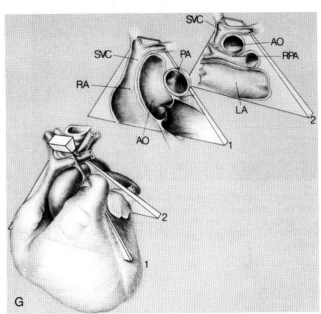

FIGURE 6.10 (*Continued*) E: The subcostal sagittal sweeps consist of the rightward systemic venous return view (1), the slightly leftward left ventricular outflow tract view (2), the leftward right ventricular outflow tract view (3), and the extremely leftward ventricular view (4). F: The suprasternal long-axis sweeps consist of the standard aortic arch view (1), the rightward superior vena caval view (not shown), and the leftward left pulmonary artery view (2). G: The suprasternal short-axis sweeps consist of the very anterosuperior strap vessels view (not shown), the anterosuperior vena cava and innominate vein view (1), the standard right pulmonary artery and left atrial view (2), and the posterior descending aorta view (not shown). AO, aorta; CS, coronary sinus; DAO, descending aorta; EUS, eustachian valve; LA, left atrium; LPA, left pulmonary artery; LV, left ventricle; MB, muscle bundle; MV, mitral valve; PA, pulmonary artery; RA, right atrium; RPA, right pulmonary artery; RV, right ventricle; SVC, superior vena cava; TV, tricuspid valve. (From Snider AR, Serwer GA, Ritter SB, eds. *Echocardiography in Pediatric Heart Disease*. 2nd ed. St. Louis, MO: Mosby–Year Book, 1997:27–52, with permission.)

(see Physics of Two-Dimensional Echocardiography, Equation 5: The Basis of Temporal Resolution).

Pulsed Wave Doppler. Pulsed wave Doppler, along with continuous wave Doppler, is the principal echocardiographic tool for evaluating cardiovascular physiology. Pulsed Doppler causes the transducer to alternately transmit and receive short ultrasound bursts. The time between transmission and reception allows calculation of the depth of the signal or range-gating, which provides the operator with the Doppler frequency shift at a specific location. A disadvantage with the technique is that the maximal detectable frequency shift is limited—the Nyquist limit (see The Basis of Aliasing: Equation 7). However, the Nyquist limit can be extended by shifting the baseline of the spectral display, exchanging to a lower-frequency transducer, or moving to a different imaging plane so that the structure of interest is at a shallower depth if possible. High-pulse repetition frequency is a technique in which volleys of pulses of ultrasound are sent before reception of prior pulses. This technique increases the Nyquist limit but causes some range ambiguity.

Continuous Wave Doppler. With the continuous wave Doppler modality, the transducer is continuously transmitting and receiving ultrasound signals. The disadvantage of this process is the absence of range-gating, but a major advantage is that the sampling rate is infinite so there is no longer a limit to the maximal frequency shift. The spectral display consists

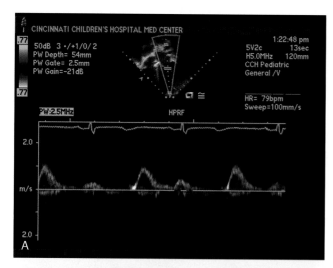

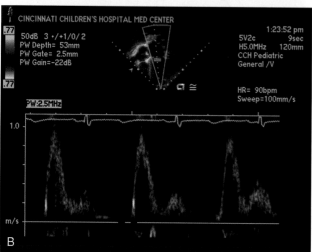

FIGURE 6.11 Mitral valve Doppler spectral profile recorded with (**A**) inappropriate and (**B**) appropriate scale and baseline shift. It is important to fill as much of the Doppler display area, thereby enlarging the Doppler spectral profile as much as possible, thus minimizing error in measurement (**B**).

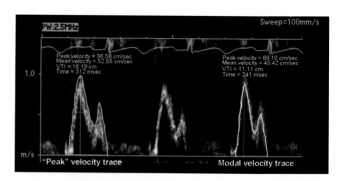

FIGURE 6.12 Mitral valve Doppler spectral profile demonstrating the difference between a peak velocity trace (green) and modal velocity trace (yellow). The peak velocity trace follows the outside edge of the Doppler spectral contour whereas the modal velocity trace follows the midline of the contour. Peak velocity traces are used to obtain pressure gradients across valves and orifices. Modal velocity traces are used in the continuity equation and in calculation of cardiac output. Note that there can be a potentially large difference in the values obtained from a peak and modal velocity trace. (e.g., 31% difference in the two velocity time integrals [VTI] in this case).

of a composite of signals with the maximal velocity representing the peak velocity at any depth in the plane of the ultrasound beam.

Approach to the Pediatric Patient

A cheerful environment is important in relieving anxiety. Bright-colored rooms filled with toys and stuffed animals capturing the environment of the patient's own bedroom can make the child feel more comfortable. Rooms should be equipped with television and DVD players so that patients can be entertained during the examination. Warm ultrasound gel also helps in reducing stress. For infants, light dimmers and an infant warmer will facilitate a comfortable environment. Formula should be available for further comforting of infants.

Even in a nonthreatening environment, patients older than 6 months and younger than 3 years of age often require sedation. Presedation guidelines delineating the fasting requirements and describing the sedation procedure need to be sent to parents before the echocardiography visit. Chloral hydrate

(75 to 100 mg/kg administered orally) or pentobarbital (5 mg/kg orally) are commonly used agents for sedation. Monitoring and resuscitation equipment should be available in each room in the event of an adverse reaction or complication.

Echocardiography: Robust Phenotyping Tool

Echocardiography represents a physiologic microscope that singularly provides phenotypic observations on an experimental preparation (the pediatric cardiovascular system) with minimal interference from external noxious influences. Therefore, unique opportunities to evaluate both cardiovascular anatomy and physiology are afforded that are not available with other imaging modalities, for example, during magnetic resonance imaging when the patient may have to endure an examination of prolonged duration or during catheterization when the heart is probed with catheters.

Defining Anatomy: Segmental Approach

The echocardiographic examination is performed, and the interpretation is presented using a segmental approach (18,19), which requires complete definition of eight features of cardiac anatomy (Table 6.1). Accurate morphology can be accomplished definitively only by imaging chamber septal structures. Next, other malformations (e.g., cardiac shunts, valve function) and physiology (biventricular function, chamber sizes, pressure estimates) are described. To ensure that no anatomy or physiology is left undescribed, it is helpful during both the performance and interpretation of the examination to imagine the course of a red blood cell traveling through the heart, beginning in the systemic veins and terminating in the systemic arteries.

Abdominal Situs and Cardiac Position

Abdominal situs is best determined from a transverse view of the abdomen below the diaphragm (Fig. 6.14). The position of the heart in the thoracic cavity is identified most easily from an apical four-chamber or subcostal coronal view. The position of the transducer on the chest from where a standard apical

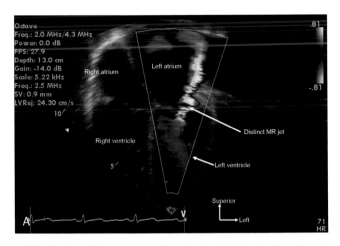

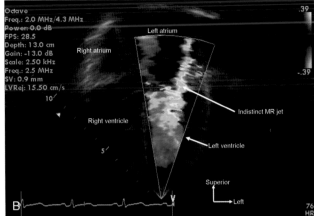

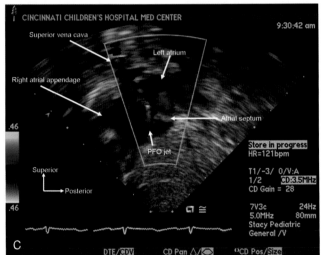

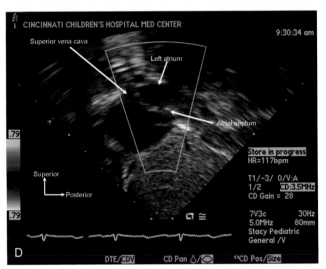

FIGURE 6.13 Series of four images demonstrating inappropriate and appropriate color aliasing limits during the echocardiographic examination. Throughout an echocardiographic examination, the echocardiographer must actively decrease and increase the color aliasing limit depending on the expected velocity of the color jet being interrogated. For example, in evaluating high-velocity jets such as mitral regurgitation (MR), color aliasing limits should be high as in the apical four-chamber view (**A**). This provides a clean, crisp and interpretable display of the mitral regurgitation flow. Inappropriate low color aliasing limit (**B**) produces an indistinct display of the mitral insufficiency jet. On the other hand, when evaluating a low-velocity color jet such as a patent foramen ovale (PFO), the color aliasing velocity should be lower to enhance recognition and display as in the subcostal image (**C**). If the aliasing velocity is set too high, detection of the low-velocity PFO jet may be impossible (**D**).

four-chamber view is obtained defines the position of the cardiac apex. From the subcostal coronal view, the side of the cardiac apex can be ascertained by tipping the transducer slightly left or right (Fig. 6.15). The normal position of the heart in the left chest is termed *levocardia*. The *mesocardiac* term refers to a cardiac position over the patient's midline. *Dextrocardia* indicates that the heart lies in the right side of the chest. There are three main categories of dextrocardia. The first is termed *dextroposition* and refers to a condition in which the heart is pushed into the right chest by either a mass in the left chest (e.g., diaphragmatic hernia) or deficiencies in right-sided chest structures. The apex remains pointed to the left; atrial situs, ventricular topology, and great vessel relationships are normal; and cardiac pathology, if any, is not complex. In the other two types of dextrocardia, termed dextroversion and mirror-image dextrocardia, the apex is pointed to

the patient's right. *Dextroversion* refers to a condition in which there is atrial situs solitus and ventricular inversion (atrioventricular discordance) and associated pathology similar to that seen in congenitally corrected transposition of the great arteries. The final type of dextrocardia is called *mirror-image dextrocardia* with atrial situs inversus. There may be major and complex pathology associated with this type of dextrocardia. However, in situs inversus totalis (a condition in which all body organs are on the contralateral side of the body from which they usually reside), the heart may be completely normal. When evaluating a patient with dextrocardia, the echocardiographer must maintain left/right conventions rather than attempting to make the image look familiar. Specifically, the echocardiographer must remain true to the established echocardiographic convention that the *right* side of the screen/monitor in the parasternal short-axis, apical

TABLE 6.1

SEGMENTAL APPROACH TO DEFINING CARDIAC ANATOMY BY ECHOCARDIOGRAPHY

Anatomic Feature	Diagnostic Possibilities
Thoracoabdominal situs	Solitus
	Inversus
	Ambiguous
Cardiac position	Levocardia
	Mesocardia
	Dextrocardia
Atria	Solitus (S)
	Inversus (I)
	Ambiguous (A)—bilateral right- and left-sidedness
Atrioventricular connection	Concordant
	Discordant
	Atresia
	Double inlet
	Common
	Straddling
	Crisscross
Ventricles	d-looped (D)
	l-looped (L)
Conus	Subpulmonic
	Subaortic
	Bilateral
	Absent or very deficient
Ventriculoarterial connection	Concordant
	Discordant
	Double outlet
	Single outlet
Great vessels	Solitus (S)
	Inversus (I)
	Transposed (D, L, A)
	Right and anterior (D)
	Left and anterior (L)
	Directly anterior (A)
	Side by side

A complete segmental description of the heart by echocardiography begins by defining these eight features, which include the three segments of the heart (shown in bold) and the two junctional segments (shown in italics). The letters in parentheses following the diagnostic possibilities for the three cardiac segments are frequently used as abbreviated three-letter descriptors of these segments: The first initial describes atrial situs, the second describes ventricular topology, and the third describes the great vessel relationship. For example, (S, D, S) describes a normal heart, whereas (I, L, I) describes mirror image dextrocardia. Following description of the morphology, intrinsic (e.g., pulmonary stenosis), myocardial (e.g., hypertrophic cardiomyopathy), septal (e.g., tetralogy of Fallot), orientation (e.g., crisscross heart), defect (e.g., ventricular septal defect or aortopulmonary window) pathology is described.

four-chamber, and subcostal coronal view is always the *left* side of the patient. This convention is maintained by the echocardiographer rotating the transducer so that the orientation mark is pointing to the patient's left in these imaging planes. There will be a tendency (which must be resisted) for the echocardiographer to rotate the transducer to an unusual or atypical position to attempt to make the image look normal.

Venous Return and Atria

Situs. The fact that an atrial chamber is on the patient's right or left or that it receives a particular venous structure does not allow a conclusion regarding atrial morphology. Atrial situs can be deduced only by evaluation of the atrial appendages and the septal structures.

The atrial appendages are consistently committed to their respective atria and are distinctly morphologically different. The right atrial appendage is short, fat, and broad based and best seen in the subcostal sagittal view (Fig. 6.16). The left atrial appendage is long, thin, and narrow based and best seen in the parasternal short axis and apical four-chamber views (Fig. 6.17). Although remaining committed to their respective atria, the atrial appendages may be juxtaposed, making their delineation more difficult.

The unique septal structures of the right atrium (RA) are the embryonic valves—eustachian and thebesian—seen in the subcostal coronal and sagittal views. The unique left atrial septal structure is the flap valve seen in the apical and subcostal coronal and sagittal views (Fig. 6.18). In heterotaxy syndrome with bilateral right- or left-sidedness and common atrium, the atrial septal structures will not be obvious and atrial situs will be indeterminate or ambiguous.

Systemic Veins and Right Atrium. The innominate veins are identified in the suprasternal short-axis view. Both innominate veins are identified and traced downstream as they join to form the right superior vena cava (SVC), which, in turn, is followed to its entrance into the heart. The left innominate vein is traced upstream to identify a possible left SVC (Fig. 6.19). These maneuvers are particularly important in any patient undergoing surgical repair using cardiopulmonary bypass and in the newborn with single-ventricle physiology (who will undergo eventual cavopulmonary anastomosis). In patients with unexplained cyanosis or systemic emboli or with absent innominate vein without dilated coronary sinus, the presence of a left SVC draining directly into the left atrium (LA) should be investigated. This may require using agitated saline contrast (see Contrast Echocardiography below).

The inferior vena cava (IVC) is identified in the subcostal abdominal and cardiac views. Anyone performing cardiac catheterization needs to be alerted for interruption of the IVC, which is usually first apparent by imaging a large venous vessel adjacent or posterior to the aorta (the azygous or hemiazygous vein) in the short-axis abdominal view (Fig. 6.20).

The RA and its appendage are best evaluated in the subcostal coronal and sagittal imaging planes. Left juxtaposition of the RA appendage is usually evident in the parasternal long and short axes, where the wall of the appendage can be seen coursing perpendicular to the atrial septum. The entrance of the coronary sinus into the RA can be seen in the subcostal coronal and the apical four-chamber views. The size and possible unroofing of the coronary sinus can be assessed in a posterior sweep from the standard apical four-chamber and parasternal long-axis views.

Atrial Septum. The atrial septum is examined in the subcostal coronal and sagittal views. The size of an atrial septal defect, as well as the degree of remaining atrial septal rim tissue for anchoring of a possible atrial septal defect (ASD) closure device and the total atrial septal length for the maximum possible diameter for said device, is best performed in both these views to give information from two mutually orthogonal planes.

Superior and inferior vena caval sinus venosus defects are best seen in the subcostal sagittal view. The transducer should

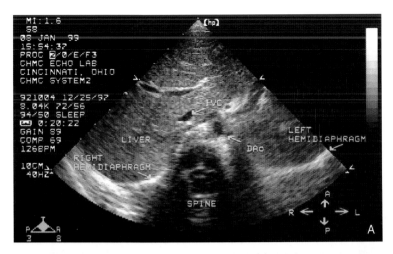

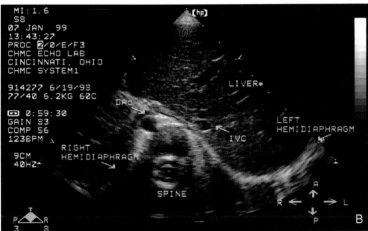

FIGURE 6.14 Subcostal transverse abdominal views in patient with abdominal situs solitus (**A**) and in a patient with abdominal situs inversus (**B**). With abdominal situs solitus, the liver is on the patient's right and the stomach is on the left. In abdominal situs inversus, the liver is on the left and the stomach is on the right. A, anterior; DAo, descending aorta; IVC, inferior vena cava; L, left; P, posterior; R, right.

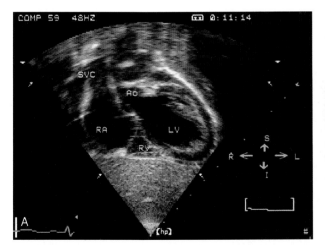

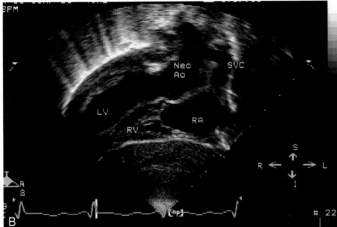

FIGURE 6.15 Subcostal coronal views of a patient with levocardia (**A**) and dextrocardia (**B**). In the patient with dextrocardia (who also had an arterial switch operation for transposition of the great arteries so that the left ventricle (LV) now gives rise to the neo-aorta (Neo Ao), the apex of the heart is pointing to the patient's right. Ao, aorta; I, inferior; L, left; R, right; RA, right atrium; RV, right ventricle; S, superior; SVC, superior vena cava.

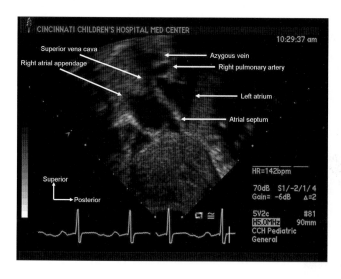

FIGURE 6.16 Subcostal sagittal view with rightward sweep demonstrating superior vena cava, left atrium, azygous vein, and right pulmonary artery. In this view the short and wide features of the right atrial appendage can be demonstrated.

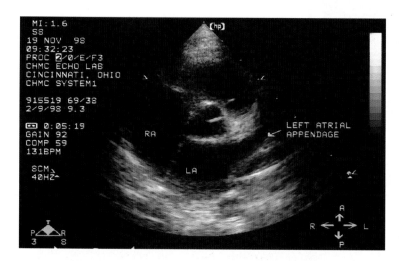

FIGURE 6.17 Parasternal short axis demonstrating the left atrial appendage, which is long and thin, distinguishing it from the right atrial appendage, which is short and broad. A, anterior; L, left; LA, left atrium; P, posterior; R, right; RA, right atrium.

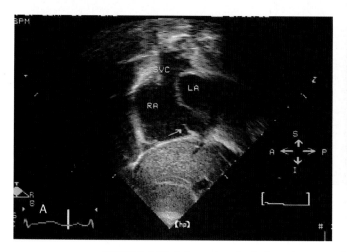

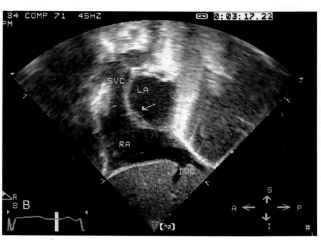

FIGURE 6.18 Subcostal sagittal views demonstrating eustachian valve (*arrow* in **A**) and flap valve (*arrow* in **B**). These unique septal structures are the most reliable method for defining the morphologic right and left atrium, respectively. A, anterior; I, inferior; IVC, inferior vena cava; LA, left atrium; P, posterior; RA, right atrium; S, superior; SVC, superior vena cava.

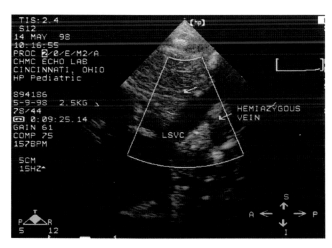

FIGURE 6.19 Hybrid suprasternal notch oblique axis view of left superior vena cava (LSVC), which is partially fed by the hemiazygous vein. A small communicating vein (*arrow*) connecting the left and right superior vena cavae is also seen. A, anterior; I, inferior; P, posterior; S, superior.

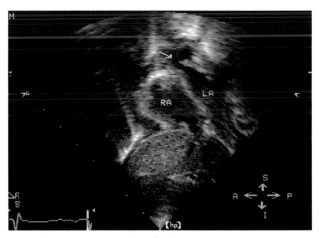

FIGURE 6.21 Subcostal sagittal view obtained by sweeping the transducer rightward from the systemic venous view consistently demonstrates the right upper pulmonary vein (*arrow*). A, anterior; I, inferior; LA, left atrium; P, posterior; RA, right atrium; S, superior.

be swept gradually and deliberately posterior and rightward to investigate for possible associated partial anomalous pulmonary venous return. Secundum atrial septal defects are best seen in the same imaging planes. The ostium primum defect is related to the crux of the heart seen in the apical view. The coronary sinus defect is visualized by sweeping the transducer posterior from the standard apical four-chamber view.

Pulmonary Veins and Left Atrium. The pulmonary veins are identified most easily from the suprasternal short-axis plane. Alternatively, the pulmonary veins can be visualized from the parasternal short axis and apical four-chamber views. An extreme rightward sweep (tilt right from the SVC, RA, IVC views) in the subcostal sagittal plane consistently reveals the right upper pulmonary vein (Fig. 6.21). Color Doppler can aid in visualizing the individual pulmonary veins (20). Anomalous

pulmonary venous pathways, the confluences from which they emanate, and the entrances of the pulmonary veins into the confluences should be investigated from the suprasternal short-axis view (supracardiac drainage), parasternal and apical views (cardiac drainage), and subcostal coronal and sagittal views (infracardiac drainage). Unlike systemic venous anomalies, in which color Doppler demonstrates flow coursing toward the heart, these anomalous pulmonary venous pathways will have color Doppler flow coursing away from the heart, often the first sign of which an echocardiographer becomes aware in this condition.

The LA is best evaluated in the apical four-chamber and the subcostal coronal and sagittal views. Membranes (e.g., supravalvar stenosing mitral ring and cor triatriatum) are identified in the apical four-chamber view. The diagnostic relationship of these membranes relative to the left atrial appendage (i.e., membrane of cor triatriatum upstream from the LA appendage orifice and membrane of supravalvar stenosing mitral ring downstream) is visualized from the apical four-chamber view.

Atrioventricular Connection

Type. The septal structures of the atrioventricular valves serve as the only consistent feature allowing morphologic diagnosis. The tricuspid valve has an intimate relationship with the ventricular septum, with multiple chordal attachments emanating from its septal leaflet, seen best in the apical four-chamber view. On the other hand, the mitral valve has no chordal attachments with the ventricular septum, and its entire attachments course to the left ventricular free wall (Fig. 6.22). In addition, the hinge point of the septal leaflet of the tricuspid valve is inferior to the hinge point of the anterior leaflet of the mitral valve. Because each atrioventricular valve is associated with its appropriate ventricle (i.e., tricuspid valve with right ventricle, mitral valve with left ventricle), the atrioventricular connection can be determined as concordant (RA to right ventricle and LA to left ventricle) or discordant (RA to left ventricle and LA to right ventricle). Atretic atrioventricular connections are easily identified in the apical and subcostal views. The relationship of the atrioventricular valves to each other in double-inlet connections are explored in the parasternal

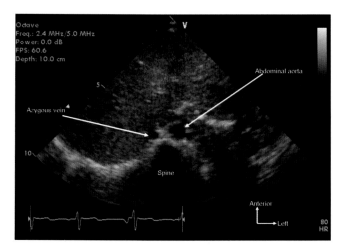

FIGURE 6.20 Subcostal transverse abdominal view demonstrating the features of interrupted inferior vena cava. There is no venous structure identified anterior to the aorta. Instead, there is a venous structure that is adjacent and slightly posterior to the aorta. The structure is also rightward of the aorta, indicating that it is an azygous continuation of interrupted inferior vena cava.

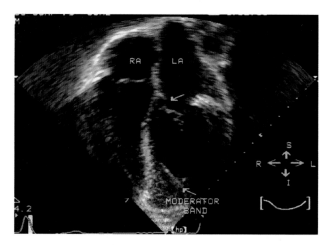

FIGURE 6.22 Apical four-chamber view in a patient with ventricular inversion with congenitally corrected transposition of the great arteries {S, L, L}. The left-sided atrioventricular valve has attachments to the ventricular septum, whereas the right-sided valve does not, allowing diagnosis of a left-sided tricuspid valve and a right-sided mitral valve. In addition, the septal hinge point of the tricuspid valve is inferior to that of the mitral valve, which is another distinguishing feature of a tricuspid valve. There is a moderator band near the apex of the left-sided ventricle, further defining this ventricle as a morphologic right ventricle. I, inferior; LA, left atrium; RA, right atrium; S, superior.

views. The five leaflets of the common atrioventricular valve (superior/anterior bridging, right superior, right mural, inferior/posterior bridging, and left mural) are best seen in a right anterior oblique subcostal view (midway between the coronal and sagittal views). In this view, the presence or absence of a tongue of tissue connecting the two bridging leaflets should be identified first to allow the establishment of a complete (absent connecting tissue) or partial (present connecting tissue) atrioventricular septal defect. Then the degree of bridging of the superior leaflet and its attachments are identified, allowing for Rastelli's classification (Fig. 6.23). Straddling and crisscross connections are seen in the apical four-chamber and subcostal

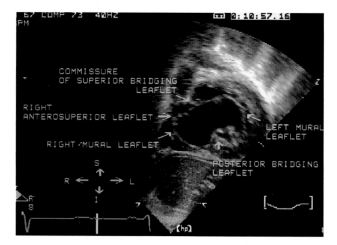

FIGURE 6.23 The subcostal oblique view (a hybrid between coronal and sagittal views) of a common atrioventricular valve. The five leaflets of the common atrioventricular valve are shown. The commissure of the superior bridging leaflet attaches to the inferior portion of the outlet septum (Rastelli type A). I, inferior; S, superior.

views. A straddling atrioventricular valve (valve attachments to contralateral ventricle) must be distinguished from mere overriding (valve annulus partially displaced over the ventricle) in these views. Crisscross atrioventricular relationships necessitate deliberate and slow sweeping of the transducer anterior and posterior in the subcostal coronal or superior and inferior in the parasternal short-axis views with careful, simultaneous observation of each valve's upstream atrium and downstream ventricle.

Tricuspid Valve. The tricuspid valve is examined in the parasternal long-axis plane (sweeping right from the standard plane), the apical four-chamber view, and the subcostal coronal and sagittal views. The septal leaflet and its attachments to the interventricular septum are best seen in the apical four-chamber view. Also, in this view, the posterior leaflet (with a slight posterior sweep) or the anterior leaflet (with a slight anterior sweep) is seen on the lateral portion of the right ventricular wall. The anterior leaflet and its attachments to the conal papillary muscle (Lancisi) are best visualized in the subcostal coronal view sweeping anteriorly.

In the evaluation of Ebstein's anomaly, the degree of atrialization of the right ventricle is assessed from the apical four-chamber view. From here, the septal attachments of the septal leaflet are appreciated. The posterior mural leaflet is seen with a slight posterior sweep from the apical four-chamber view. A portion of the anterior mural leaflet can be seen with an anterior sweep from the apical four-chamber view, but the subcostal coronal view is required to visualize the displacement of the anterior leaflet into the right ventricular outflow tract and the degree to which it obstructs it.

Mitral Valve. The mitral valve is visualized in the parasternal, apical four-chamber, and subcostal coronal and sagittal views. The size of the mitral annulus, which is important in determining suitability for biventricular repair in cases of relative left-sided hypoplasia (see Ventricles, Suitability of Left Ventricle for Biventricular Repair below), should be performed in the apical four-chamber view. The papillary muscles, important to assess for repair of complete atrioventricular septal defect and for diagnosing parachute mitral valve, are best visualized in the parasternal short-axis and subcostal sagittal views. Mitral stenosis is assessed in the parasternal long-axis and the apical four-chamber views, where the degree of leaflet excursion can be seen clearly. Mitral valve prolapse is best identified in the parasternal long-axis and apical four-chamber views. Clefting of the mitral valve and double orifice mitral valve are usually seen in the parasternal short-axis sweep.

Ventricles

Ventricular Morphology. Determination of the embryologic type of ventricular looping (d or l) first requires clear identification of ventricular morphology. The septal structures once again provide the definitive criteria for this evaluation. The first criterion is the type of atrioventricular valve entering the ventricle (see preceding section on Atrioventricular Connection, Type). The right ventricle also can be identified by its coarse, large, and extensive trabeculations along the septum and free wall. One of these trabeculations, the moderator band, is particularly prominent running transversely from free wall to septum in the inferior third of the right ventricular cavity in the apical view (Fig. 6.22). Once ventricular morphology has been established, the ventricular looping is determined. This is performed by imagining one is standing in the right ventricle facing the right ventricular face of the interventricular septum. The palm of one hand is placed against the septum. The looping is determined by establishing which of the two hands allow the thumb to point into the atrioventricular valve and the fingers to point into the outflow tract. If the right hand meets these criteria, the ventricles are d-looped. If the left hand meets these criteria, the ventricles are l-looped.

Right Ventricle. The size of the right ventricle and its relative contribution to the ventricular apex in conditions such as complete atrioventricular septal defect and pulmonary atresia with intact ventricular septum are best assessed from the apical four-chamber view. Because the three portions of the right ventricle (inlet, trabecular, and conus) do not lie in a single plane, visualization of the entire right ventricular cavity requires sweeping of the transducer through multiple planes in the subcostal coronal and sagittal views.

Ventricular Septum. The ventricular septum is composed of two components: (a) the membranous septum, which is an extremely small (5 mm in diameter in the adult heart), and superior portion wedged between the tricuspid and aortic valves; and (b) the large muscular septum. The membranous septum consists of two portions separated by the septal leaflet of the tricuspid valve: the pars atrioventricularis, where left ventricular to RA shunts occur, and the pars interventricularis, where ventricular septal defects are located. The muscular septum consists of three portions: the inlet portion, which is inferior to the membranous septum and is between the atrioventricular valves; the trabecular portion, which extends from the membranous septum to the apex; and the conal (or outlet or infundibular) septum, immediately below the pulmonary valve.

Many ventricular septal defects typically occur along embryologic fusion lines (e.g., a perimembranous outlet ventricular septal defect [VSD] is along the fusion line between the membranous and conal septa). VSDs within the membranous septum can be assessed in the parasternal long- and short-axis, apical five-chamber, and subcostal views. In the basal short-axis view where the subpulmonary and subaortic regions can be imaged simultaneously, it can be determined whether an outlet ventricular septal defect is below the crista supraventricularis (infracristal outlet VSD) or above the crista (supracristal outlet VSD, also known as subpulmonic or doubly-committed VSDs). The membranous septum is seen well in the parasternal long-axis sweep from the standard view toward the tricuspid valve. In the apical view, the transducer should be swept anteriorly so that the left ventricular outflow tract and aorta are visualized. VSDs within the conal septum are assessed in the parasternal long axis sweeping left toward the pulmonary valve, in the basal short axis, and in the subcostal coronal and sagittal views. The trabecular septum is so large that defects within it need to be localized, preferably describing their position in two orthogonal planes and in relation to nearby landmarks. One classification system assigns the VSD as anterior, midmuscular, apical, or posterior. The anterior trabecular VSDs can be missed if the echocardiographer is not interrogating consciously for them. Perhaps the best view is the parasternal long-axis view sweeping to the left. The midmuscular VSDs can be seen in the standard parasternal long- and short-axis views and apical four-chamber views. VSDs in the posterior trabecular septum are visualized best in the parasternal short-axis view or in the apical view swept posterior. Apical trabecular defects are best seen in the apical four-chamber view inferior to the moderator band. Inlet VSDs are best visualized in the short axis sweeping inferiorly toward the atrioventricular valves and in the standard apical four-chamber view at the level of the atrioventricular valves. These are distinguished from atrioventricular septal defects by close echocardiographic inspection of the hinge points of the atrioventricular valve annuli, which remain normal (i.e., mitral hinge point slightly superior to that of the tricuspid valve) with an inlet ventricular septal defect and at identical heights with an atrioventricular septal defect.

Left Ventricle. The size of the left ventricle, which is particularly important in evaluating atrioventricular septal defects and variants of hypoplastic left heart with relative left-sided hypoplasia, is evaluated in the apical four-chamber view. The left ventricular outflow tract, which is important to visualize for membranes and subvalvar stenosis, is seen by a slight anterior tilt of the transducer. Equally valuable are the parasternal long-axis view in which the left ventricular outflow tract is at a slightly shallower depth, improving imaging, or the subcostal coronal view.

Conal Morphology

The conus (or infundibulum) is the cavitary space formed by the muscular segment of the heart that connects the ventricles with the great arteries and separates the atrioventricular and semilunar valves. Abnormalities in conal development consist of variations in the presence, length, and diameters of the subpulmonary and subaortic conus. These variations can lead to (or be associated with) complex malformations, such as tetralogy of Fallot, interrupted aortic arch, transposition of the great arteries, and double-outlet right ventricle.

Subpulmonic. In the normal heart, the conus is the nearly vertical tubular outflow portion of the right ventricle, which is separated from the nearly horizontal right ventricular inflow portion by distinct muscle bands. These muscle bands form a near-circular rim formed by the parietal band anteriorly, the crista supraventricularis posteriorly, and the septal band medially and prohibit pulmonary valve to atrioventricular valve continuity. The subpulmonary conus is best identified in the subcostal views. Leftward anterior deviation of the conal septum leading to a narrowed conus and subvalvar pulmonary stenosis in tetralogy of Fallot is evident in these views. These relationships can be demonstrated in the subcostal coronal and sagittal views. Posterior deviation of the conal septum and ventricular septal defect results in left ventricular outflow tract obstruction and is associated with interrupted aortic arch. The conal septum in this lesion is best assessed from the parasternal long-axis view.

Subaortic. Persistence of the subaortic conus and involution of the subpulmonic conus is the usual conal relationship in d- (or l-) transposition of the great arteries (21). The subaortic conus is evident on the subcostal coronal and sagittal views. Persistence of subaortic conus prohibits continuity of the aortic valve to either atrioventricular valve, and involution of the subpulmonary conus allows continuity between the pulmonary valve and both atrioventricular valves in transposition of the great arteries. An extremely unusual variant of conal morphology is a subpulmonic conus in the setting of d-transposition of the great arteries (Fig. 6.24).

Bilateral. Bilateral persistence of the subarterial conus usually results in double-outlet right ventricle. Because the main goal of surgical correction of double-outlet right ventricle is to connect the aorta with the morphologic left ventricle through the ventricular septal defect, it is important to determine the conal

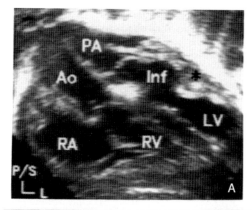

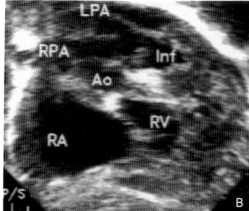

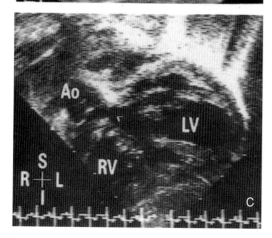

relationships with each other and with the great vessels. In double-outlet right ventricle, the relationship of the great arteries with each other is an inaccurate method by which to determine the infundibular relationships. Particularly important is to determine which conus has the interventricular septum as one of its walls, to localize the ventricular septal defect with respect to the conus, and to determine the connection of the conus to the aorta.

When two conuses are present, their relationship may be classified as either anterior/posterior or side-by-side (22). With the anterior/posterior conal relationship, the ventricular septal defect is usually subaortic; with the side-by-side relationship, the defect is usually subpulmonic. The conal relationship can be determined by subcostal coronal and sagittal imaging with anterior/posterior and left/right sweeping, respectively. With an anterior/posterior conal relationship, the outlet septum inserts

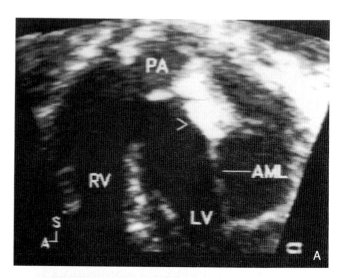

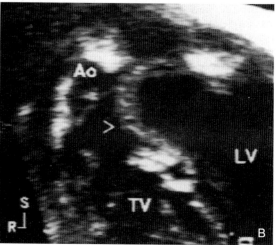

FIGURE 6.24 Subcostal view of an infant with d-transposition of the great arteries and a subpulmonic conus only. **A:** Subcostal coronal view demonstrates the posterior aorta (Ao), anterior and superior pulmonary artery (PA), and a subpulmonic infundibulum (Inf). There is ventricular arterial discordance. **B:** Subcostal coronal view swept further anteriorly demonstrating the anterior relationship of the pulmonary artery to the aorta. **C:** Subcostal oblique view showing a small subaortic ventricular septal defect (*arrowhead*). I, inferior; LPA, left pulmonary artery; lV, left ventricle; P/S, posterior/superior; RA, right atrium; RPA, right pulmonary artery; RV, right ventricle. (From Pasquini L, Sanders SP, Parness IA, et al. Conal anatomy in 119 patients with d-loop transposition of the great arteries and ventricular septal defect: an echocardiographic and pathologic study. *J Am Coll Cardiol* 1993;21:1716, with permission.)

FIGURE 6.25 Subcostal sagittal views in a patient with transposition of the great arteries with a bilateral conal relationship. **A:** Conal tissue (*arrow*) separates the pulmonary valve from the anterior leaflet of the mitral valve (AML). **B:** Conal tissue (*arrow*) separates the aortic valve (Ao) from the tricuspid valve (TV). A, anterior; LV, left ventricle; PA, pulmonary artery; RV, right ventricle; S, superior. (From Pasquini L, Sanders SJP, Parness IA, et al. Conal anatomy in 119 patients with d-loop transposition of the great arteries and ventricular septal defect: an echocardiographic and pathologic study. *J Am Coll Cardiol* 1993; 21:1714, with permission.)

anteriorly separating the anterior conus from most of the interventricular septum and, thus, the ventricular septal defect. With a side-by-side conal relationship, the outlet septum inserts near the crux of the heart separating the lateral conus from the interventricular septum and ventricular septal defect.

Bilateral conus also can be associated with d-transposition of the great arteries with VSD, a more anterior and superior location of the pulmonary root than in patients with a subaortic conus only, and discontinuity between the pulmonary and mitral valves (as well as between the aortic and tricuspid valves) (Fig. 6.25). L-transposition of the great arteries also can be associated, although rarely, with bilateral conus evident in the subcostal views.

Absent. A rare type of d-transposition can exist in the context of bilaterally deficient subarterial conus (23). This results in an unusual heart in which d-transposition of the great arteries exists with a doubly committed VSD and a posterior aorta. These relationships can be identified by parasternal and subcostal coronal and sagittal imaging (Fig. 6.26).

Ventriculoarterial Connection

Type. If the aorta arises from the left ventricle and the pulmonary artery arises from the right ventricle, the relationship is concordant. When the aorta arises from the right ventricle and the pulmonary artery from the left ventricle, the relationship is discordant. The origins of aorta and pulmonary artery are evident on the parasternal long-axis view, sweeping the transducer inferiorly from the basal short-axis view, the apical five-chamber view, and the subcostal coronal and sagittal views. The third type of ventriculoarterial connection is double outlet, almost always from the right ventricle. A great vessel should be related to a ventricle by ≤50% of its dimension to be considered committed to it. Determining the extent of commitment of a great vessel to the right ventricle is best performed in the parasternal long- and short-axis view sweeps, the apical five-chamber view, and the subcostal coronal and sagittal views.

The final type of ventriculoarterial connection is single outlet (truncus arteriosus). This entity can be diagnosed in the parasternal long axis, where a single trunk with pulmonary

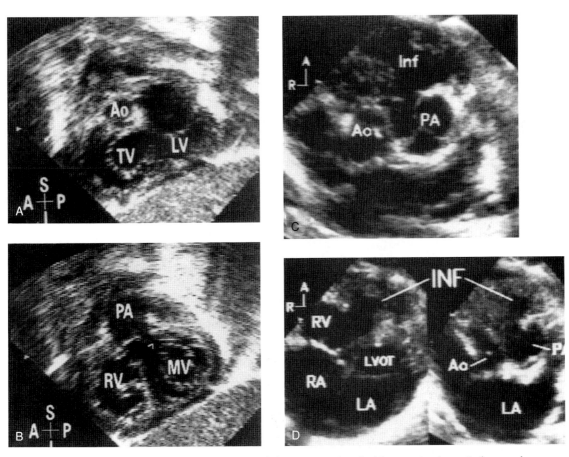

FIGURE 6.26 An infant with transposition of the great arteries, doubly committed ventricular septal defect, posterior aorta, and bilaterally deficient subarterial conus. **A:** Subcostal sagittal view demonstrating continuity between the aortic valve (Ao) and the tricuspid valve (TV). **B:** Subcostal sagittal view swept slightly leftward from **A** demonstrates continuity (*arrow*) between the pulmonary valve and the mitral valve (MV). **C:** Parasternal short-axis view showing the great vessel relationship with the aorta slightly posterior to the pulmonary artery (PA). There is an infundibular chamber (Inf) anterior to both semilunar valves. **D:** Parasternal short-axis view demonstrating the relationship of the infundibular chamber to the right ventricle and the left ventricular outflow tract (LVOT) immediately inferior to the pulmonary artery. A, anterior; I, inferior; LA, left atrium; P, posterior; S, superior. (From Pasquini L, Sanders SP, Parness IA, et al. Conal anatomy in 119 patients with d-loop transposition of the great arteries and ventricular septal defect: an echocardiographic and pathologic study. *J Am Coll Cardiol* 1993;21:1717, with permission.)

arteries arising from it can be seen. The basal short-axis view is notable for absence of a pulmonary valve; the pulmonary artery branches arising from the trunk also can be seen in this view. The subcostal coronal and sagittal views are usually diagnostic for this entity.

Great Vessels

Relationship. The aorta courses superiorly toward the thoracic inlet before coursing posteriorly, gives rise to strap vessels as it courses posteriorly, and has coronary arteries arising from its root. The pulmonary artery courses posteriorly almost immediately after it arises from the heart and bifurcates shortly after its origin. The most helpful views for identifying the great vessels are the parasternal short-axis view at the base and even more superior, the suprasternal notch long- and short-axis views and the subcostal coronal and sagittal views (Fig. 6.27).

Situs solitus of the great vessels describes the normal relative position of the aortic annulus located rightward and posterior to the pulmonary annulus. This relationship is best seen in the parasternal short-axis view, but it is also obvious in the parasternal long-axis sweeps and the subcostal coronal and sagittal views.

Situs inversus of the great vessels describes the relative position of the aortic annulus located leftward and posterior to the pulmonary valve annulus in dextrocardia. In this relationship, there is not transposition (i.e., the aorta continues to arise from the left ventricle and the pulmonary artery from the right ventricle). This relationship is evident in a right parasternal short-axis view and in the subcostal coronal and sagittal sweeps.

Transposition of the great arteries is diagnosed when there is a discordant ventriculoarterial relationship. (By definition, then, it is impossible to diagnose double-outlet right ventricle with transposition.) Instead, this is referred to as double-outlet right ventricle with malposition of the great vessels. Transposition of the great arteries can exist with the aorta right and anterior (d), left and anterior (l), and directly anterior (A) to the pulmonary artery. In addition, the aorta may exist side by side or even posterior to the pulmonary artery. These relationships are best diagnosed in the basal short-axis and subcostal coronal and sagittal views.

Main and Branch Pulmonary Arteries. The main and branch pulmonary arteries are best seen in the basal (and more superior) short-axis and subcostal coronal and sagittal views. In addition, the right pulmonary artery is best seen in the suprasternal short-axis view. The left pulmonary artery usually can be seen when sweeping the standard suprasternal long-axis view to the left.

Pulmonary valve stenosis is evident in the parasternal basal short-axis view. Frequently, continued clockwise rotation of the transducer can yield an en face view of the pulmonary valve. Supravalvar pulmonary stenosis is best visualized in this view. Aortopulmonary window is usually evident on the parasternal short-axis view and careful, deliberate sweeps

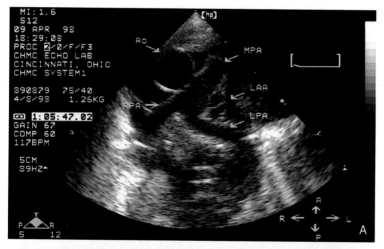

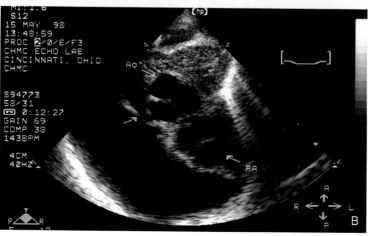

FIGURE 6.27 Parasternal short-axis images demonstrating different relationships between the great vessels. **A:** An echocardiogram from an infant with tetralogy of Fallot and pulmonary atresia demonstrates the identifying features of a pulmonary artery (MPA) with its bifurcation into right and left pulmonary arteries (RPA, LPA). The great vessels are normally related. **B:** In a patient with d-transposition of the great arteries, both semilunar valves are in cross section in the parasternal short-axis view. The aorta is identified as the rightward anterior vessel and has a right coronary artery (*arrow*) originating from the right facing sinus of Valsalva. A, anterior; Ao, aorta; LAA, left atrial appendage; P, posterior; PA, pulmonary artery.

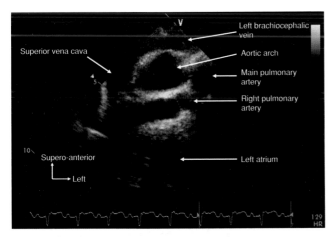

FIGURE 6.28 Suprasternal notch short-axis view demonstrating typical normal vascular anatomy. From this view the left brachiocephalic vein, superior vena cava, transverse aortic arch, main pulmonary artery, right pulmonary artery, and left atrium can all be visualized.

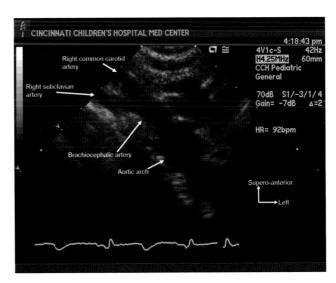

FIGURE 6.29 Suprasternal notch short-axis view swept superiorly to demonstrate the bifurcation of the brachiocephalic artery into right subclavian artery and right common carotid artery. The fact that the first strap vessel is a brachiocephalic artery that bifurcates into the right subclavian and common carotid arteries indicates that this patient has a left aortic arch.

between the aorta and main pulmonary artery in the subcostal coronal and sagittal views.

Aorta and Branch Vessels. The aorta, which lies more posterior in the center of the heart, can be visualized in many different views, including the parasternal long- and short-axis views, the apical five-chamber view, the subcostal views, and the suprasternal notch views (Fig. 6.28). The aortic arch is best seen in the subcostal oblique view and the suprasternal views.

Valve morphology in aortic stenosis can be understood by examining the parasternal views. The short-axis views allow determination of dysplasia and number of leaflets. Supravalvar stenosis and root dilation are best measured in the parasternal long-axis view.

The side of the aortic arch (important in tetralogy of Fallot, truncus arteriosus, hypoplastic left heart, vascular rings, and before tracheoesophageal fistula repair) is diagnosed by sweeping the transducer in the suprasternal long-axis view and noting the relationship of the arch to the trachea, the rings of which resemble a stack of coins. Equally important is sweeping the transducer in the suprasternal notch short-axis view from the origin of the aorta superiorly toward the arch and branch vessels and then back inferiorly and posteriorly following the descending aorta. Using this view, the transducer should also be swept superiorly to follow the course of each branch vessel arising from the arch. In a normal, left-sided aortic arch, the first branch vessel is a right brachiocephalic artery that can be shown to bifurcate into right subclavian and carotid arteries (Fig. 6.29). In a right-sided aortic arch, the first branch vessel is usually a left brachiocephalic artery, which usually bifurcates into a left subclavian and carotid arteries. In either case, the first branch vessel should be followed to its bifurcation. If no bifurcation is present, anomalous origin of the ipsilateral subclavian artery should be suspected. Likewise, superior sweeping from the origin of each of the other strap vessels upstream should be performed deliberately to completely delineate the strap vessel anatomy.

Arch hypoplasia, coarctation, and interruption are best diagnosed from the suprasternal long- and short-axis views. The proximal (the segment between brachiocephalic and common carotid artery origins) and distal (the segment between common carotid artery and subclavian artery origins) transverse arch should be imaged and measured.

Aortopulmonary collateral vessels (important in tetralogy of Fallot and single ventricle/Fontan physiology) are best seen in the suprasternal notch long- and short-axis views. The subcostal oblique view of the descending aorta also allows identification of these vessels.

Coronary Arteries. The coronary arteries are best seen in the parasternal short-axis views. The coronary arteries can also be seen in the apical four-chamber view as they course in the atrioventricular grooves. The midportion of the right coronary artery is seen in the subcostal coronal view. Frequently, the origin of the left coronary artery and the left anterior descending coronary artery are seen in the subcostal coronal view or a leftward sweep from the standard parasternal long-axis view. Anomalous origins and courses are important to delineate in transposition of the great arteries, tetralogy of Fallot, anomalous origin of the left (or more rarely, the right) coronary artery from the pulmonary artery, dilated cardiomyopathy, and exertional syncope and are seen in the parasternal short axis. If 2-D imaging in the short-axis view shows isolated dilation of a proximal coronary artery, a coronary artery fistula or anomalous origin of a coronary artery should be suspected. The entire extent of the coronary artery must be interrogated for fistulous communications from all imaging planes. The main and branch pulmonary arteries should be carefully imaged for an anomalously arising coronary artery. Simultaneous use of color Doppler is extremely helpful when investigating for coronary artery fistulae or anomalous origin of a coronary artery. Coronary cameral sinusoids, seen within high-pressure ventricles such as the right ventricle in pulmonary atresia with intact ventricular septum, are best visualized in the apical four-chamber view with simultaneous use of color Doppler. Evaluation of the coronary arteries during and following Kawasaki's disease for aneurysms and stenoses should be performed in all the aforementioned imaging planes so that almost the entire extent of the coronary artery is interrogated.

Defining Physiology

Venous Return and Atria

Characteristics of Venous Flow. Flow patterns in venous systems are demonstrated by Doppler evaluation. The characteristic venous flow is typically low velocity and triphasic, consisting of a systolic S wave, and early diastolic D wave, and an A wave during atrial systole (Fig. 6.30). Forward flow during ventricular systole corresponds to the venous S wave; during passive diastolic filling and diastasis, the forward venous D wave is produced. There is usually a small flow reversal noted at end-systole, and at end-diastole, atrial contraction produces a small reversal in venous flow; this reversal can vary in magnitude depending on physiologic conditions and the type of vein being evaluated by Doppler (see Systemic Venous Return and Pulmonary Venous Return sections below) (24,25). It is also useful to note the timing of venous flow in relation to atrioventricular valve inflow. The venous D wave occurs in conjunction with atrioventricular valve opening and concomitantly with the atrioventricular valve E wave (see Atrioventricular Valve Antegrade Doppler section). With atrial contraction, there is both forward flow across the atrioventricular valve (the atrioventricular valve A wave) as well as reverse flow into the venous system.

Technical Considerations. Venous flow velocities, in general, are relatively low (Fig. 6.30), with peak S- and D-wave velocities in the 40 to 50 cm/s range (25). As such, venous flow is best assessed using pulsed wave Doppler. Unless high-grade venous obstruction is present, flow velocities rarely exceed the Nyquist limits inherent to pulsed wave Doppler analysis. When imaging venous flow with color flow Doppler, one can often optimize the color flow map by lowering the Nyquist limit to correspond to the lower venous flow velocities. As in all Doppler analysis, interrogation should be performed as parallel to the direction of flow as possible.

Systemic Venous Return. Doppler evaluation of flow in the systemic venous system is typically performed in superior vena cava, inferior vena cava, or hepatic veins. The magnitude of

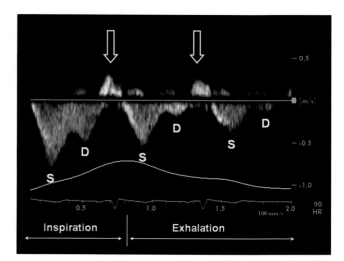

FIGURE 6.31 Hepatic flow with respirometry. Normal systemic venous flow features phasic, low-velocity flow. The venous S and D waves correspond to ventricular systole and early diastole, respectively. The venous A wave (*arrows*) consists of a flow reversal during atrial systole. Note the augmentation in venous flow velocities during inspiration.

the venous flow velocities can vary significantly—particularly in the systemic venous circulation—during the respiratory cycle. It is therefore important that Doppler recordings be obtained with respirometry tracings in addition to an electrocardiogram. A typical sample of flow in the hepatic vein is demonstrated in Figure 6.31. During inspiration, forward flow velocities of the S and D waves are increased, and with exhalation, forward flow velocities decrease.

Significant variation in the magnitude of flow reversals during the respiratory cycle is typically not seen (25). However, alterations in the pattern of systemic venous flow can be observed in the setting of right ventricular diastolic dysfunction (26), pericardial tamponade (27) (28), or constrictive pericarditis (29–31). Regardless of the cause, compromise of late right ventricular filling manifests as augmentation of the reverse flow wave during atrial systole; this reversal is often further magnified during the respiratory cycle, particularly in the setting of constrictive (during expiration) or restrictive physiology (with inhalation) (see Stage III Diastolic Dysfunction: Restrictive Physiology and Constrictive Pericarditis sections).

Although uncommon, systemic venous obstruction, e.g., related to surgical anastomoses following superior cavopulmonary anastomosis, lateral tunnel Fontan, or cannulation of the SVC during cardiopulmonary bypass, will manifest with alterations in the normal venous flow pattern. When significant venous obstruction is present, Doppler flow analysis will reveal loss of the normal phasic flow pattern with persistent, higher-velocity forward flow.

Pulmonary Venous Return. As with systemic venous flow, pulmonary venous flow is normally characterized by lower-velocity, phasic flow (Fig. 6.32). As with systemic venous Doppler, flow in the pulmonary veins consists of a systolic S wave, early diastolic D wave, and a late diastolic reversal during atrial systole (the A wave). Pulmonary venous Doppler assessment has assumed a significant role in the assessment of left ventricular diastolic function, as investigators came to

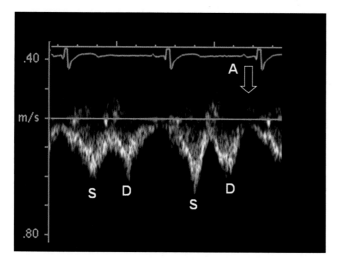

FIGURE 6.30 Pulsed Doppler flow profile in superior vena cava. Note phasic, low-velocity venous flow, with a systolic S wave, early diastolic D wave, and small atrial systolic flow reversal (A wave, *arrow*).

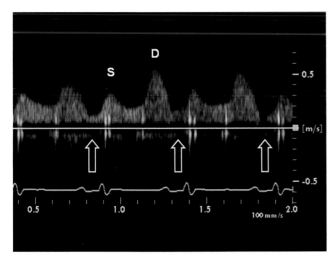

FIGURE 6.32 Normal pulmonary venous Doppler flow profile. Flow features phasic, low-velocity flow with a characteristic systolic S wave and an early diastolic D wave. Note the low-to-absent flow velocities during atrial systole (*arrows*). In the normal pediatric population, the S/D velocity ratio is often less than zero, and atrial systole is often accompanied by small pulmonary venous flow reversals.

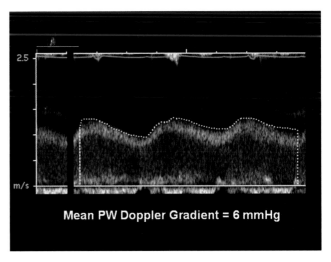

FIGURE 6.33 Pulsed Doppler flow profile in pulmonary venous obstruction. With pulmonary venous obstruction, the phasic pattern of venous flow is blunted, with persistent, higher-velocity forward flow. Digitization of the area under the Doppler velocity profile allows estimation of the mean Doppler flow gradient (6 mm Hg in this case). PW, pulsed wave.

appreciate the factors influencing atrioventricular valve inflow Doppler in the setting of diastolic dysfunction (see Pulmonary Venous Doppler Flow Analysis in Diastolic Ventricular Function below).

In addition to its importance in assessment of diastolic dysfunction, Doppler assessment of pulmonary venous flow is important in identifying pulmonary venous obstruction, which can be seen in various clinical settings. Following Mustard or Senning palliation of d-transposition of the great arteries, obstruction to the egress of pulmonary venous blood into the pulmonary venous atrium can occur (32). Obstruction can also be seen following repair of total anomalous pulmonary venous return (33). Obstruction can occur either at the level of the venous baffle—following Senning or Mustard procedure—or at the site of anastomosis of the pulmonary venous confluence to the left atrium (32). Obstruction occurs less commonly at the level of the individual pulmonary veins. In all cases, the Doppler flow pattern features a high-velocity pattern with spectral broadening and loss of the typical phasic flow pattern (Fig. 6.33) (32). Upstream of the obstruction, pulmonary venous flow can also be noted to lose its phasic characteristics. The magnitude of pulmonary venous obstruction can be quantified by digital planimetry of the Doppler flow profile, which correlates well with gradients obtained by catheter pullback in the catheterization laboratory (34).

Atrial Septum and Intra-atrial Flow. Flow across the atrial septum is dependent on the presence of an interatrial communication, most frequently either a patent foramen ovale or secundum atrial septal defect. The full spectrum of atrial septal shunts and defects is discussed in the Atrial Septum section (above). In most cases, color flow Doppler imaging is sufficient to demonstrate the size and direction of the interatrial shunt, which in most subjects is left to right. Shunting at the atrial level is determined by the relative compliances of the right and left ventricle and occurs throughout the cardiac cycle relative to differences in right and left atrial pressure (35). In most patients, lower compliance in the right ventricle produces a left-to-right shunt. With alterations in right ventricular compliance,

however, color flow Doppler should be used to evaluate the possibility of right-to-left atrial shunting. Examples of conditions producing reduced right ventricular compliance, usually in conjunction with right ventricular hypertrophy, are tetralogy of Fallot, primary pulmonary hypertension, cor pulmonale, and critical pulmonary valve stenosis. Isolated right atrial pressure elevation, as seen with congenital tricuspid valve stenosis or severe tricuspid regurgitation—e.g., Ebstein's malformation—may also produce right-to-left atrial level shunting.

Assessment of the flow gradient across the atrial septum—when the interatrial flow is from left to right atrium—can be used to estimate left atrial pressure (36,37). Estimation of the mean gradient across the interatrial shunt (mean ΔP) by digital planimetry can be performed. Left atrial pressure (*LAP*) can then be estimated from the equation:

$$LAP = \text{mean } \Delta P + RAP$$

where *RAP* is an assumed (or with the use of a central venous catheter, measured) right atrial pressure.

Estimates of left atrial pressure by this method agree well with catheter measurement when right atrial pressure is assumed to be approximately 10 mm Hg. Measurement of left atrial pressure can add physiologic information in the setting of left heart obstruction, cardiomyopathy, and in large left-to-right shunts complicated by left atrial hypertension. Similarly, the intra-atrial flow gradient across a cor triatriatum membrane can be used to assess severity of obstruction to pulmonary venous inflow into the left atrium (38). Assessments of flow gradients across the atrial septum from right to left atrium are not generally predictive of right atrial pressure. This is likely owing to the increased capacitance of the systemic venous system, which limits the degree to which right atrial hypertension can develop. This issue often arises in the setting of tricuspid valve atresia with suspected restriction at the foramen ovale, where low cardiac output is felt clinically to be caused by poor egress of blood from right to left atrium. Significant Doppler mean gradients across the atrial septum in this setting are rarely seen despite clinical improvements in patients who undergo atrial septoplasty in the catheterization laboratory. This is likely secondary to the capacitance of the systemic venous system, where increases in right atrial pressure in the setting of right atrial outflow obstruction are dampened by the ability of the systemic venous system to absorb the pressure increases in the right atrium.

Atrioventricular Valve Size and Function

Size. The tricuspid and mitral valve annuli are best measured from the apical four-chamber view. Normal values for the atrioventricular valve annuli from the newborn through young adulthood have been established (39–41). Actual measurements can be compared with these normative data and expressed as a Z value (i.e., the number of standard deviations the value lies above or below the normative mean; Z values >2 or <−2 are therefore considered abnormally large or small, respectively; see Appendices 6.1 and 6.2). Measurement of the tricuspid and mitral valve annuli are most important in the assessment of suitability of a marginal ventricle for use in a dual ventricular circulation (e.g., pulmonary atresia with intact ventricular septum, hypoplastic left heart syndrome, and variants). In addition, the annuli values are necessary when considering valvuloplasty or valve replacement so that appropriate interventional equipment (balloon catheters, dilators, prosthetic devices) is made available before intervention.

Atrioventricular Valve Antegrade Doppler. The antegrade atrioventricular valve Doppler velocity profile consists of a higher peak E (early) velocity owing to rapid ventricular filling on valve opening, a period of diastasis, or slow ventricular filling when the Doppler velocity is near zero; and a lower peak A (late) velocity owing to filling from atrial contraction. The peak E/A ratio is one of the better methods for assessing ventricular diastolic function (see Transmitral Doppler Flow Evaluation in Diastolic Ventricular Function section below). In patients with atrioventricular valve stenosis, the Doppler velocity will usually be turbulent and elevated, but conventional gradient determinations have limitations because of the confounding effects of valve area, left ventricular relaxation, and stiffness. Accordingly, it is preferable, in the case of mitral valve disease, to instead follow left atrial pressure, which can be done echocardiographically by using a combination of Doppler blood and tissue velocity measurements (42).

Another useful index of mitral stenosis is the pressure half-time (Fig. 6.34). As mitral stenosis worsens, the pressure gradient between the LA and LV persists for a greater duration of diastole. This can be quantitated by measuring the time it takes for the peak pressure gradient (peak pressure gradient $(P_{peak}) = 4v_{peak}^2$) to decrease to one half its maximal value ($\frac{1}{2}P_{peak} = \frac{1}{2}(4v_{peak}^2) = 4v_{half-time}^2$; solving for $v_{half-time} = v_{peak} \div 2^{0.5} = v_{peak}/1.4$). A pressure half-time <60 ms is normal. A pressure half-time >100 ms is indicative of significant mitral stenosis.

The atrioventricular valve antegrade Doppler velocities are also helpful in the assessment of pericardial effusions. In patients with significant pericardial effusion with impending cardiac tamponade, the atrioventricular valve velocities vary markedly with respiration; the tricuspid velocities increase (as much as 80% from baseline) and the mitral velocities decrease (25% to 40% from baseline) during inspiration (43). The mitral E wave decreases more than the A wave so that the E/A ratio decreases during inspiration in this setting.

Atrioventricular Valve Insufficiency. Assessing the degree of atrioventricular insufficiency unfortunately continues to be an inexact practice. Qualitative or semiquantitative indices include color Doppler vena contracta (area of maximal velocity

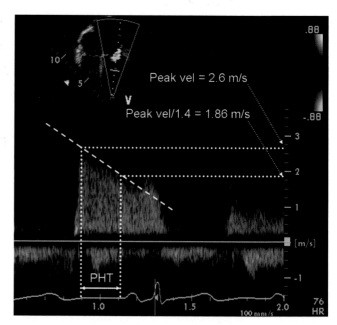

FIGURE 6.34 Example of pressure half-time (PHT) calculation in a patient with mitral stenosis. In this example the peak velocity (vel) of the mitral Doppler profile is 2.6 m/s. The initial pressure gradient is decreased by one half when the peak velocity falls to 2.6/1.4 or 1.86 m/s. The pressure half-time is the time between peak velocity and when the velocity falls to 1.86 m/s, which in this example is slightly >200 ms, which is indicative of significant mitral stenosis.

and thus maximal pressure drop and smallest flow area) width or jet length, measurement of ventricular and atrial size, and abnormal venous flow into the atrium. These indices can be affected by a myriad of factors including variations in echocardiographic equipment settings and alterations in atrial pressure. Two quantitative indices have been used with success—regurgitant fraction and effective regurgitant orifice area. The *regurgitant fraction* is the percent of antegrade blood flow in one cardiac cycle that regurgitates. The technique relies on the principle that, in the steady state, the ventricle is neither growing nor shrinking on a beat-to-beat basis. In the case of mitral insufficiency, the volume of blood in a single beat flowing into the left ventricle is the mitral valve antegrade volume and is equal to the volume ejected by the left ventricle (i.e., the antegrade aortic volume and the mitral regurgitant volume). The antegrade mitral and aortic volumes are calculated by obtaining both the area and the Doppler mean *modal* antegrade velocity of each valve. The area is obtained from a measurement of the valve diameter (d) (from the apical four-chamber view for the mitral and from the parasternal long-axis view for the aortic) and assuming that the valve area approximates a circle (area = $\pi d^2/4$). The mean *modal* velocity is obtained from a sharp pulsed wave Doppler envelope from which the time–velocity integral is obtained by tracing the *center* (rather than the peak edge as one would do for a gradient determination) of the Doppler envelope continuously for the entire duration of valve opening (Fig. 6.12). The antegrade volumes are calculated (*volume = area* × mean modal velocity). Regurgitant volume (antegrade mitral volume − antegrade aortic volume) and regurgitant fraction (regurgitant volume ÷ antegrade mitral volume) are then calculated. A regurgitant fraction of >40% is considered severe.

Calculation of the effective regurgitant orifice area (EROA) takes advantage of the proximal isovelocity surface areas

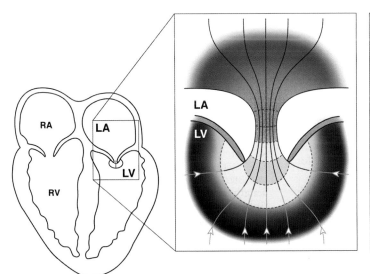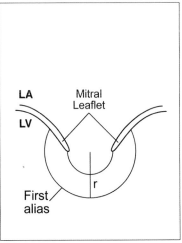

FIGURE 6.35 Diagram demonstrating the proximal isovelocity surface area (PISA) phenomenon and measurement technique in the case of mitral insufficiency. From an apical four-chamber view, proximal isovelocity surface areas created by the mitral insufficiency will be evident on the left ventricular (LV) side of the mitral valve leaflet tips (**left panel**). As the flow approaches the regurgitant orifice, the velocity accelerates along concentric hemispheres centered on the orifice evident on a two-dimensional color Doppler echocardiogram as concentric semicircles of color with increasing velocity. In the case of mitral insufficiency, the color jet will become progressively lighter blue in color as it approaches the orifice. When the flow reaches a velocity exceeding the color Doppler scale (i.e., the aliasing velocity), the color jet will alias from light blue to yellow producing a sharp concentric demarcation within the color jet evident as a distinct semicircle (**middle panel**). As the velocity continues to increase, additional smaller semicircles of color will be evident as each aliasing velocity is exceeded. In practice, the first radius (r) of the semicircle produced by the first aliasing velocity is measured to calculate regurgitant orifice area and regurgitant volume (**right panel**). Qualitatively, a higher first aliasing velocity and larger first aliasing velocity semicircle radius indicate a larger regurgitant orifice area and regurgitant volume. LA, left atrium; RA, right atrium; RV, right ventricle.

(PISA). As it converges to a constricted area, flow gradually accelerates in a uniform fashion. This acceleration is manifested on a color Doppler examination by concentric semicircles (on a three-dimensional study, concentric hemispheres) of aliasing color interfaces proximal to the regurgitant orifice (Fig. 6.35). Because of conservation of mass, the flow at any of these interfaces is equal to the flow at the orifice. Because the area of a hemisphere is $2\pi r^2$,

$$EROA = (2\pi r^2 \times V_{al}) \div V_{EROA} \qquad [11]$$

where

r = radius from the orifice to the aliasing interface
V_{al} = velocity at the aliasing interface
V_{EROA} = peak velocity of the regurgitant jet

Regurgitant volume can be calculated by multiplying the EROA by the velocity–time integral of the regurgitant jet. The EROA equation demonstrates that qualitatively on a color Doppler examination, a larger aliasing radius at a higher aliasing velocity is indicative of more severe regurgitation. Most of the limitations of this PISA technique focus on the difficulty in measuring the aliasing radius, which tends to be small and the center localization of which can be elusive. Nevertheless, the predictive power of EROA has been shown to supersede that of all other mitral regurgitant indices (44). The technique becomes even more accurate (but less practical) if the surface areas are assumed to be hemiellipses rather than hemispheres (which requires the measurement of aliasing radii in orthogonal planes).

Atrioventricular insufficiency jets provide valuable information on ventricular hemodynamics. An assumed (or simultaneously measured via central line) right atrial pressure can be added to the tricuspid insufficiency peak gradient to obtain an accurate measurement of RV pressure, a critical monitoring index in many congenital heart defects. Likewise, a mitral (in the case of the LV) or tricuspid (in the case of the RV) insufficiency jet can be digitized over the entire systole cycle to generate a continuous ventricular pressure curve when the corresponding assumed atrial pressure is added to it. This elegant technique has been used successfully to noninvasively derive tau, the time constant of ventricular relaxation (45) and noninvasively generate the systolic portion of a ventricular pressure–volume loop, probably the most robust tool in the assessment of ventricular function (see Ventricular Pressure–Volume Loops in the Systolic Ventricular Function section below).

Tricuspid and mitral regurgitant gradients should also be used to verify and ensure the accuracy of ventricular outflow gradients. For example, the outflow gradients necessarily need to be less than the sum of the regurgitant gradient and atrial pressure. The echocardiographer should always be cognizant of unique applications of the regurgitant jets. For example, in the case of a patient with aortic arch repair for coarctation or interruption who also has an aberrant origin of the usually upstream subclavian artery, an instance when the upper and lower blood extremity pressure determination would not be valuable in assessing any residual arch obstruction, the sum of the Doppler mitral insufficiency gradient and an assumed left atrial pressure can be substituted for the upstream systolic pressure. Finally, the spectral profiles of atrioventricular regurgitant jets can be digitized to obtain the peak rate of isovolumic ventricular contraction or relaxation (dP/dt, $-dP/dt$) (46,47).

Ventricles

Ventricular Morphology

Ventricular volumes. The left ventricular volume should be measured from the apical four-chamber view for a single-plane determination and from the apical four- and two-chamber views for a biplane determination. Various models for left ventricular volume determination exist, but the most reliable are those that use the modified Simpson's rule. These methods mathematically divide the left ventricle into a stack of discs from apex to base. The volume of each of these discs is calculated assuming the discs are circular for single-plane determination or ellipsoidal for biplane determination and then summed.

The modified Simpson's rule can be used with ventricles of ellipsoidal geometry. Unfortunately, many important ventricles in congenital heart disease (e.g., right ventricles and single ventricles) exhibit unusual or bizarre geometry not amenable to ellipsoidal formulae. Levine et al. (48) published a method for estimating right-ventricular volume using two orthogonal views: the apical four-chamber view of the right-ventricular inflow and body and the subcostal sagittal view of the outflow tract:

$$RV\ volume\ (\text{mL}) = 0.67 \times A_{Ap} \times L_{SC} \qquad [12]$$

where

A_{Ap} = RV area from apical four-chamber view
L_{SC} = length of outflow tract from subcostal sagittal view
   or alternatively:

$$RV\ volume\ (\text{mL}) = 0.67 \times A_{SC} \times L_{Ap} \qquad [13]$$

where

A_{SC} = area of RV outflow tract from subcostal sagittal view
L_{Ap} = length of RV from apical four chamber view

Suitability of left ventricle for biventricular repair. One of the most critical roles of the echocardiographer is assessing suitability for biventricular repair in cases of left heart hypoplasia (e.g., in critical aortic stenosis, hypoplastic left heart syndrome, unbalanced atrioventricular septal defect, total anomalous pulmonary venous return). In newborns with critical aortic stenosis, the following factors (with suggested threshold values for biventricular suitability) may be needed to support biventricular physiology: (a) mitral valve annulus diameter (>8 mm) (49), (b) mitral valve area indexed to body surface area (BSA) (>4.75 cm²/m²) (50), (c) left ventricular area >1.6 cm² (51), (d) contribution of the left ventricle to the cardiac apex or long-axis ratio (>0.8) (50), (e) left ventricular volume indexed to BSA (>20 mL/m²) (51), (f) left ventricular mass indexed to BSA (>35 g/m²) (50), (g) aortic annulus diameter (>5 mm) (49), and (h) aortic sinus of Valsalva diameter indexed to BSA (>3.5 cm/m²) (50). Rhodes et al. (50) developed a scoring system using a combination of these echocardiographic parameters for neonates with critical aortic stenosis:

$$Score = 14(BSA) + 0.943(iAo) + 4.78(LAR)$$
$$+ 0.157(iMVA) - 12.03 \qquad [14]$$

where

LAR = ratio of the long axis of the left ventricle to the long axis of the heart
$iMVA\ (\text{cm}^2/\text{m}^2)$ = mitral valve area indexed to BSA
$iAo\ (\text{cm}/\text{m}^2)$ = aortic sinus of Valsalva diameter indexed to BSA (threshold value for biventricular suitability >−0.35)

Phoon and Silverman (52) pointed out, however, that in patients with small left ventricles, these parameters in general, and left ventricular volume specifically, may not be truly hypoplastic, but rather, distorted because of left ventricular compression from right ventricular dilation. They suggest using the preoperative left ventricular circumference to calculate a predicted potential left ventricular volume. Further, Minich et al. (53) showed that structures with initially subthreshold measurements can actually grow significantly. Alternatively, the Congenital Heart Surgeon's Society has developed additional criteria for biventricular suitability (54). These include (a) degree of endocardial fibroelastosis, (b) degree of tricuspid insufficiency, (c) aortic sinus of Valsalva diameter (in centimeters from the parasternal long-axis view), (d) ascending aorta diameter (in centimeters from the parasternal long-axis view), and (e) left ventricular long-axis length (in centimeters from apical four-chamber view). The Society has created an internet-based calculator into which these data can be input to arrive at the difference in percent survival at 5 years after entry for Norwood versus biventricular pathway. This calculator can be found at: http://www.ctsnet.org/aortic_stenosis_calc/index.cfm?action=calculator.

In 2006, the Rhodes criteria were re-evaluated (54a). A new discriminant analysis was found to more accurately predict survival with a biventricular circulation than with the model using the traditional criteria. The new criteria first emphasized the need for having an adequate mitral valve by requiring the mitral valve area (calculated by assuming the morphology was that of an ellipse with radii measured from the parasternal long axis and apical 4 chamber views) to have a z score of >−2. Only then, can the new criteria be applied. These criteria consist of 1) aortic annulus z score measured from the parasternal long axis view, 2) ratio of the long axis of the left ventricle to the long axis of the heart, 3) endocardial fibroelastosis grade none, mild (affecting papillary muscles only), moderate (affecting papillary muscles and some of the endocardium), and severe (affecting papillary muscles and extensive portions of the endocardium). A new regression equation was developed:

$$Score = 10.98\ (BSA) + 0.56(\text{Aortic annulus z score})$$
$$+ 5.89\ (LAR) - 0.79\ (\text{EFE grade}) - 6.78$$

where

EFE grade = 0 for none or mild
          = 1 for moderate or severe

The threshold score for survival to be better with biventricular versus univentricular repair is >−0.65.

Left ventricular mass. In patients with left ventricular pressure overload (e.g., coarctation of the aorta, aortic stenosis, and systemic hypertension) or volume overload (e.g., aortic and mitral regurgitation), hemodynamic burden is assessed by left ventricular mass. M-mode calculation requires obtaining the LV cavity size and posterior wall thickness and septal thickness from a two-dimensionally-guided parasternal long-axis view with the M-mode cursor at the chordal-mitral valve junction. There are two conventions for measurement (Penn and American Society Echocardiography [ASE]). In the former, the endocardial thicknesses are included as part of the left ventricular end-diastolic cavity rather than as part of the septal (s_d) and posterior wall (h_d), and measurements are made at the peak of the R wave on the ECG (55). Using this method, anatomic LV mass in grams can be predicted accurately by the equation (55,56):

$$1.04\ \{[LVED + h_d + s_d]^3 - LVED^3\} - 14 \qquad [15]$$

In the ASE convention, measures are made from leading edge (relative to ultrasound beam propagation) to leading edge so that the septal endocardium is part of the LV cavity but the posterior wall endocardium is part of the posterior wall thickness. In addition, measures are made at the beginning of the QRS. This method accurately predicts LV mass through the equation (56,57):

$$0.8 \times 1.04[(LVED + h_d + s_d)^3 - LVED^3] + 0.6 \quad [16]$$

Although in large series substituting Penn and ASE conventions has had little effect on analyses (58), the existence of two conventions underscores the need for laboratories to define their protocol and remain consistent with their methods. Although the intraobserver and interobserver variability for LV mass determination is good (0.96 and 0.89, respectively, in one series (57), laboratories should assess their data reproducibility independently (59).

Some believe that although M-mode LV mass can be useful for populations, it may not be sensitive enough to detect serial changes in individuals and have suggested calculation of LV mass from two-dimensional echocardiography (60). Two-dimensional measurement of LV mass is based on either the area-length (AL) or truncated ellipse (TE) model. For both, parasternal short-axis and apical four-chamber views are required. From the former view, the epicardial and endocardial areas (A_1 and A_2, respectively) are traced at the level of the chordal-mitral junction including the papillary muscles as part of the LV cavity. From the latter view, the LV length (L) is obtained. The LV length consists of two components—the semimajor axis (a), which is the long-axis distance from the apex to the level of the widest minor axis (b); and the truncated semimajor axis (d) which is the long axis distance from the mitral annulus to b (note that $L = a + d$).

$$Mass\ AL\ (g) = 1.055\{[(5/6)(A_1)(L + t)] \\ - [(5/6)(A_2)(L)]\} \quad [17]$$

where

$$t = \text{mean wall thickness} = (A_1/\pi)^{0.5} - (A_2/\pi)^{0.5}$$

The truncated ellipse model also requires the same imaging planes (61):

$$Mass\ TE\ (g) = 1.05\pi\{(b + t)^2[2/3(a + t) \\ + d - d^3/3(a + t)^2] - b^2[2/3(a) \\ + d - d^3/3a^2]\} \quad [18]$$

where

$$b = (A_2/\pi)^{0.5}$$

Although this formula looks daunting, it requires only one more measurement than the area-length method: demarcation of a point along the long axis at the widest minor axis dimension (Fig. 6.36).

Adjusting LV mass to account for differences in age, height, and weight allows establishment and application of uniform reference values and criteria for LV hypertrophy. An index incorporating patient weight, however, may inadvertently mask the powerful and important effect of obesity on LV mass. The most ideal indexing parameter is lean body mass (62), but this is difficult to measure. Indexing LV mass by patient height raised to approximately cubic exponential power (e.g., LM mass/height$^{2.7}$) has been shown to produce the greatest reduction in LV mass variability in normal subjects older than 8 years of age, most correctly detect differences between normal and obese subjects (58), and importantly, correlate most closely to indexing by lean body mass (57,62). However, dispersion of residual variation of LV mass/height$^{2.7}$ increases with increasing height or age in children but not in adults, suggesting that other variables effect ventricular growth in children and indicating that further investigation is needed to determine the most nearly ideal

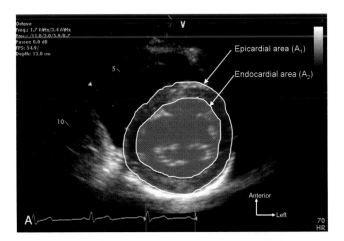

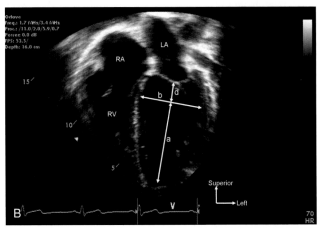

FIGURE 6.36 To calculate left ventricular mass by two-dimensional echocardiography, a parasternal short-axis view of the left ventricle at the level of the mitral valve leaflets (**A**) and an apical four-chamber view (**B**) are needed. From the parasternal short axis, the LV epicardial and endocardial area (A_1 and A_2, respectively) are measured. From the apical four-chamber view, the left ventricular length is measured from the mitral valve annulus to the cardiac apex. The left ventricular length consists of two components: the semimajor axis (a), which is the long axis distance from the apex to the level of the widest minor axis (b); and the truncated semimajor axis (d), which is the long-axis distance from the mitral annulus to (b). LA, left atrium; RA, right atrium; RV, right ventricle.

indexing parameter (63). For children 4 to 8 years old, indexing mass by height squared appears to be optimal. For children younger than 4 years of age, the most appropriate indexing technique has not been established.

Echocardiographically measured left ventricular mass is an independent risk factor for cardiovascular morbidity and mortality. For example, in patients with essential hypertension, left ventricular mass stratifies cardiovascular risk independently of and more strongly than blood pressure and other potentially reversible risk factors and may help to stratify the need for intensive treatment (64). Indeed, reducing LV mass during antihypertensive treatment results in reduced likelihood of adverse cardiac events, an effect that is additive to the effects of blood pressure lowering (65). Since it so strongly predicts cardiovascular risk, left ventricular mass has been the subject of multiple studies aimed at determining its correlates in children (66–70). For example, in obese children, the pattern of fat distribution is a more important predictor of elevated left ventricular mass than the absolute percent of body fat (68).

Mass also may be indexed by dividing by the left ventricular end-diastolic volume. The mass:volume ratio helps to determine whether the amount of hypertrophy is appropriate for the prevailing hemodynamic conditions. When the ratio is normal (0.97 ± 0.12 g/mL), hypertrophy is considered an adequate and adaptive physiologic response. Inappropriate hypertrophy is defined as a ratio of >1.1 g/mL, which may occur, for example, in some patients undergoing the Fontan operation and is associated with poorer outcome. The mass:volume ratio and the relative wall thickness ($RWT = 2h_d/LVED$) distinguish concentric from eccentric hypertrophy. *Concentric hypertrophy*, thickening toward the central axis of the chamber, is commonly a result of pressure overload (e.g., aortic stenosis, coarctation, or systemic hypertension) and is defined as increased wall thickness with normal or decreased chamber size (i.e., elevated mass:volume ratio or elevated LV mass with $RWT \geq 0.45$). *Eccentric hypertrophy*, increasing mass away from the central axis, is commonly a result of volume overload (e.g., aortic or mitral regurgitation) and is defined as hypertrophy with an increase in chamber size relative to wall thickness (i.e., decreased mass:volume ratio or elevated LV mass with $RWT < 0.45$). Although both geometric patterns are detrimental, concentric hypertrophy is associated with greater cardiovascular risk (71).

Diastolic Ventricular Function. Although Doppler methods for assessment of diastolic ventricular function enjoy widespread use in the adult population, application of these methods in pediatric echocardiography has yet to become commonplace in many centers. More recently, however, the role of diastolic function in both acquired and congenital pediatric heart disease is becoming better appreciated.

Diastolic physiology. In simple terms, ventricular diastole can be defined as the time between semilunar valve closure and atrioventricular valve closure, and consists of periods of isovolumic relaxation, rapid early filling, diastasis, and filling during atrial systole (Fig. 6.37). However, if one looks more closely at the factors affecting each phase of diastole, it becomes quickly apparent that diastole is a complex process with both active and passive components. Moreover, each phase of diastole can be impacted by multiple factors that may modify observed diastolic events during the cardiac cycle. As discussed in Chapter 27, *ventricular relaxation* is actually an active process that is dependent on the removal of Ca^{2+} from troponin C in the myocyte. Development of the sarcoplasmic reticulum and calcium handling in the myocyte is an age-dependent process that is relatively immature in the fetus and neonate. Age, an obvious variable in pediatrics, will therefore impact the rate of ventricular relaxation and the observed Doppler variables describing this phenomenon. *Passive filling* will be impacted by atrial pressure, heart rate, and elastic properties of the ventricle. The degree of ventricular filling *during atrial systole* can also be modified by variables such as ventricular compliance and atrial function. The interplay of factors impacting diastolic function is portrayed in Figure 6.38.

History of Doppler assessment. Although the echocardiographer must remain aware of the multiple factors that may influence diastolic ventricular function (and therefore confound precise Doppler characterization of the diastolic function of the ventricle), our understanding of the progression of left ventricular diastolic *dysfunction* became more clear in 1992 when Appleton and Hatle (72) described the natural history of diastolic dysfunction. Using Doppler echocardiography, this study demonstrated that diastolic dysfunction occurred in

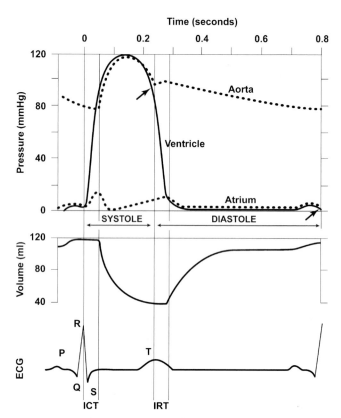

FIGURE 6.37 Physiologic tracing of left ventricular (*solid line*), left atrial (*dotted line*), and aortic (*dotted line*) pressure during the cardiac cycle. Diastole is defined as the time between aortic valve closure (*arrow*, top left) and mitral valve closure (*arrow*, bottom right). Isovolumic relaxation (IVRT) occurs between aortic valve closure and mitral valve opening. ECG, electrocardiogram; ICT, isovolumic contraction time.

progressive sequence and that stages of worsening diastolic dysfunction could be characterized by Doppler echocardiography techniques analyzing both transmitral and pulmonary venous flow profiles. Subsequent work in advanced Doppler techniques such as Doppler tissue imaging (73–75) resulted in the development of additional tools with which to refine the assessment of diastolic ventricular function.

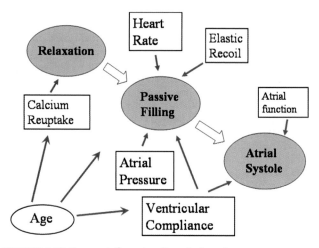

FIGURE 6.38 Factors influencing diastolic function.

Ventricular diastolic dysfunction develops along a spectrum but can be described stepwise as one of three stages of increasing severity. In mild (stage I) diastolic dysfunction, the abnormality is impaired ventricular relaxation. In moderate (stage II) diastolic dysfunction, pseudonormal function—described below—is noted. And in the most severe (stage III) diastolic dysfunction, restrictive physiology is present.

Doppler evaluation of diastolic function. Regardless of the stage of diastolic dysfunction, a standard protocol for evaluating left ventricular diastolic function in children should be used. This is usually centered around the following modalities: (a) transmitral Doppler flow, (b) pulmonary venous flow patterns, and (c) Doppler tissue imaging of the lateral mitral annulus.

TRANSMITRAL DOPPLER FLOW EVALUATION. A normal transmitral Doppler flow pattern (Fig. 6.39) features an E wave, which includes the flow profile of early ventricular filling from the end of isovolumic relaxation to the onset of atrial systole. This is followed by a transmitral A wave, which includes flow occurring during atrial systole. For a comprehensive diastolic function evaluation, the peak E- and A-wave velocities, the A-wave duration, and deceleration time should be measured. The peak E-wave/peak A-wave velocity ratio is also calculated. In addition, by sampling with pulsed wave Doppler in the left ventricular outflow tract, one is also able to obtain a simultaneous display of both mitral inflow and LV outflow. The isovolumic relaxation time can then be measured as the interval between cessation of systolic flow and onset of mitral inflow.

PULMONARY VENOUS DOPPLER FLOW ANALYSIS. As described previously, pulmonary venous flow features a lower velocity phasic flow pattern consisting of a systolic S wave, an early diastolic D wave, and a late diastolic reversal during atrial systole (the A wave). During a comprehensive diastolic function assessment, the peak S- and D-wave velocities and the duration and peak velocity of the pulmonary venous A wave are measured, and the S-wave/D-wave velocity ratio is calculated (Fig. 6.40).

DOPPLER MYOCARDIAL VELOCITY ASSESSMENT. Doppler tissue imaging (DTI) is a Doppler modality in which myocardial motion can be displayed both by color Doppler velocity maps

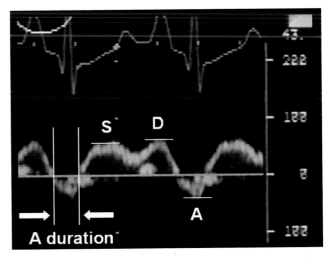

FIGURE 6.40 Measurement of pulmonary venous Doppler flow indices by pulsed wave Doppler analysis. Peak S- and D-wave velocities are measured as indicated. The duration (A duration) and peak velocity of the pulmonary venous flow reversal—or A wave—is also measured. The A wave in this example is prominent and was obtained in a patient with diastolic dysfunction and elevated left atrial pressure.

and by pulsed Doppler spectral display. Tissue motion features low velocity and high amplitude; therefore, Doppler tissue imaging presets optimize low-pass filters and lower-gain amplification to allow display of tissue velocities. This is in contrast to blood flow velocities, for which high-velocity and low-amplitude signals require different Doppler settings.

Although qualitative color Doppler velocity maps of myocardial motion can be obtained by DTI, quantitative diastolic function assessment requires pulsed wave spectral Doppler display of tissue velocity. For assessment of left ventricular diastolic function, it is conventional to use pulsed wave Doppler assessment of the lateral mitral valve annulus to obtain the spectral display necessary for diastolic function evaluation (Fig. 6.41). Typically, the peak tissue E-wave (Ea)

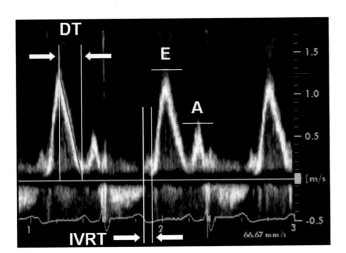

FIGURE 6.39 Normal transmitral pulsed wave Doppler pattern, featuring an early diastolic E wave, and a late diastolic A wave during atrial systole. Typical measurements are shown and include E-wave deceleration time (DT), peak E- and A-wave velocities, and isovolumic relaxation time (IVRT), measured from the cessation of left ventricular outflow to onset of the E wave.

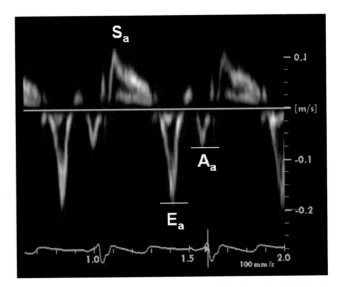

FIGURE 6.41 Pulsed wave Doppler spectral display of lateral mitral valve annular velocities. In addition to the systolic myocardial S_a wave, the peak velocities of the early diastolic E_a wave and late diastolic A_a wave are measured.

and A-wave (Aa) velocities are measured, and the peak Ea/Aa-wave velocity ratio is calculated. DTI indices can be measured at any point of the ventricular myocardium to give information on regional wall motion. Because of this feature, DTI indices are not only very useful in the assessment of diastolic function but extremely valuable in assessing ventricular dyssynchrony and response to biventricular pacing in patients with ventricular bundle branch block (76).

ESTIMATION OF LEFT ATRIAL VOLUME. Estimation of left atrial volume is becoming another important parameter in the assessment of diastolic functional status and is felt to represent the effects of chronic left ventricular diastolic dysfunction. Increased left atrial volume has been associated with increasing severity of left ventricular diastolic function (77) in hypertrophic cardiomyopathy (78) and in both adult (78) and pediatric hypertension (79). Left atrial volume has also been correlated to mortality in the setting of hypertrophic cardiomyopathy (80).

Left atrial volume can be measured using the biplane methods of discs (81), imaging the left atrium orthogonally in the apical 2- and 4-chamber views (Fig. 6.42). Echocardiographic estimates of left atrial volume correlate well with estimates by cineangiography (82) and computed tomography (83), and can be compared to published normal values (82).

Normal diastolic function. In the normal left ventricle, ventricular relaxation leads to a normal rate of fall in LV pressure during isovolumic relaxation. This leads to a normal pressure gradient in early systole between the left atrium and left ventricle (Fig. 6.43). Early diastolic flow into the left ventricle is driven by this pressure gradient, producing a normal mitral valve E-wave. During diastasis, there is minimal pressure gradient between left atrium and left ventricle; however, during atrial systole, there is again a significant left atrial-left ventricle pressure gradient producing late diastolic filling—the mitral valve A-wave.

The normal E-wave/A-wave velocity ratio in children between 3 years of age and adulthood is approximately 2.3 ± 0.6, with a mitral valve A-wave duration of approximately

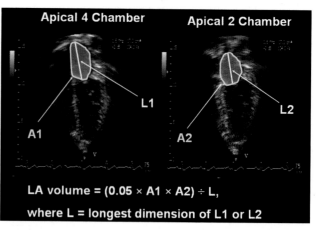

$$\text{LA volume} = (0.05 \times A1 \times A2) \div L,$$
where L = longest dimension of L1 or L2

FIGURE 6.42 Estimation of left atrial (LA) volume by two-dimensional echocardiography. The LA volume can be estimated by digital planimetry of LA area in orthogonal apical four- (A1) and two-chamber (A2) views. The longest dimension of the left atrium (either L1 or L2) is then used to estimate left atrial volume.

140 ± 21 ms (84). The normal pattern of mitral inflow is portrayed in Figure 6.44. Both isovolumic relaxation time (IVRT) and mitral E-wave deceleration time are heart rate dependent, but nomograms for deceleration time versus heart rate have been published (84). It has recently been proposed that correcting the isovolumic relaxation time for heart rate by dividing by the square root of the R to R interval (or the cardiac cycle length) identifies a normal heart rate corrected IVRT of 63 ± 7 ms in children from several months to 20 years of age (85). Reference values for normal atrioventricular valve Doppler flow indices are presented in Appendix 6.3. In infants younger than 2 months of age and in the fetus, myocardial immaturity features impaired relaxation, which will impact diastolic function parameters similar to those seen with pathologic

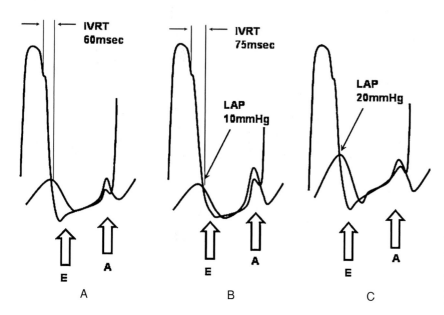

FIGURE 6.43 Physiologic left ventricle/left atrial pressure relation with normal diastolic function and two stages of diastolic dysfunction. **A:** Normal ventricular relation produces a normal rise in the pressure gradient between the left atrium and left ventricle at the conclusion of isovolumic relaxation. This results in a normal mitral E wave. Normal atrial contraction at end-diastole produces a normal mitral A wave. **B:** Impaired relaxation prolongs the isovolumic relaxation time (IVRT) and results in a diminished pressure gradient between the left atrium and left ventricle in early diastole. This results in a diminished mitral E wave, with a compensatory increase in the mitral A wave during atrial systole. **C:** rising left atrial pressure restores the early diastolic gradient between the left atrium and left ventricle, resulting in a pseudonormal E-wave velocity. LAP, left atrial pressure.

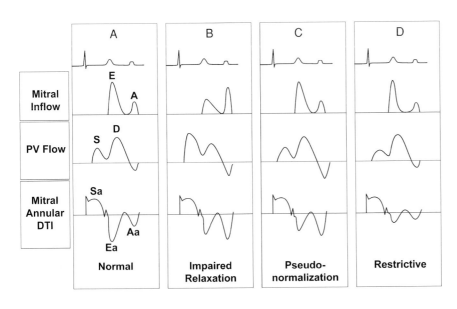

FIGURE 6.44 Progression from normal diastolic function (**A**) to early (**B** and **C**) and advanced (**D**) phases of diastolic dysfunction with demonstration of the associated changes in the mitral inflow, pulmonary venous flow, and mitral annular Doppler tissue imaging indices. DTI, Doppler tissue imaging; PV, pulmonary venous.

relaxation impairment (see Stage I Diastolic Dysfunction: Impaired Relaxation below). Thus, in the fetus and neonate, E wave/A wave ratios <1 and prolonged isovolumic relaxation times are noted; the degree to which these indices differ from normal children and adolescents is a function of myocardial maturity, and thus these changes are seen more dramatically in the fetus than in the newborn and in the newborn more than in the 2- to 3-month-old infant.

Normal pulmonary venous flow (Fig. 6.44) has typical S and D waves and usually a small atrial systolic A wave. In the pediatric population, the S-to-D velocity ratio is typically < 1, a finding that differs from the adult population for which the S/D wave velocity ratio in normal subjects is typically > 1. Studies in the pediatric age group also differ from adult studies in that a small atrial systolic flow reversal is often present (84,86). The normal pulmonary venous S wave/D wave ratio in the pediatric age group (between 3 and 17 years of age) is 0.8 ± 0.2. The pulmonary venous A-wave velocity is 21 ± 5 cm/s with a duration of approximately 130 ± 20 ms (84). Age-specific normal values for pulmonary venous Doppler flow indices are presented in Appendix 6.4.

DTI assessment of mitral annular velocities (Fig. 6.44) in the normal left ventricle reveals an Ea-wave/Aa-wave velocity ratio >1. Relaxation of the ventricle produces movement of the mitral valve annulus away from the transducer in the apical four-chamber view; atrial systole produces a mitral annular Aa wave, reflecting motion of the mitral annulus away from the transducer with late systolic ventricular filling. Normal values for both mitral and tricuspid annular velocities in children are shown in Appendix 6.5 (87–89).

Abnormalities of Left Ventricular Diastolic Function

Stage I diastolic dysfunction: impaired relaxation. In the earliest stages of diastolic dysfunction, the rate of ventricular relaxation is impaired. Delayed LV relaxation (Fig. 6.43B) results in a slower decline in left ventricular pressure. This in turn results in a diminished gradient between the left atrium and left ventricle in early diastole, in turn resulting in a diminished mitral E-wave velocity. This also results in a lengthening of the isovolumic relaxation time and a lengthening of the E-wave deceleration time. As a result of these events in early diastole, there is a compensatory increase in late filling during atrial systole, producing an augmented mitral A wave. These changes occur

in the setting where ventricular compliance and left atrial and left ventricular end-diastolic pressures are at near normal levels. These changes are summarized in Figure 6.44B.

In the pulmonary veins, delayed relaxation results in a decrement in flow during early diastole, resulting in an augmented systolic S wave and a diminished D wave. This results in an increased S-/D-wave velocity ratio. As atrial pressures are near normal at this stage of dysfunction, atrial systolic flow reversal remains absent or minimal (Fig. 6.44B).

Doppler tissue imaging of the lateral mitral annular velocities will demonstrate a decrease in the peak Ea velocity, corresponding to decrease in early diastolic ventricular relaxation. The Ea/Aa velocity ratio will therefore be <1 in this setting (Fig. 6.44B).

Stage II: pseudonormal diastolic dysfunction. Diastolic function indices in stage II dysfunction are summarized in Figure 6.44C. As diastolic dysfunction advances, ventricular compliance progressively diminishes along with continued abnormality in ventricular relaxation. This results in a compensatory increase in left atrial pressure (Fig. 6.43C). The increase in left atrial pressure has several effects: An increase in the left atrium to left ventricular pressure gradient in early diastole produces an increase in the mitral E-wave velocity and a shortening of the isovolumic relaxation time by producing early mitral valve opening. Progressive decreases in ventricular compliance result in shortening of the E-wave deceleration time.

The pulmonary venous flow profile features a decrement in the magnitude of the S wave and an increase in the D wave, resulting in a diminished S-/D-wave velocity ratio. The pulmonary venous A-wave velocity and duration will increase as ventricular compliance worsens. In adult studies, pulmonary venous A-wave velocities of >35 cm/s or pulmonary venous A-wave durations that exceed the mitral A-wave duration by ≥20 ms have been reported to distinguish normal mitral inflow profiles from pseudonormal mitral inflow profiles (90). In the pediatric population, the difference between pulmonary venous A-wave duration and mitral A-wave duration can identify children with elevated left ventricular filling pressures. However, these methods are adequately predictive only when the LV end-diastolic pressures are >18 mm Hg, which may be more applicable in the setting of restrictive physiology (see Stage III Diastolic Dysfunction: Restrictive Physiology below) (84).

The pattern of mitral annular velocities remains largely unchanged in the setting of pseudonormal dysfunction. Abnormal relaxation will again result in a diminished Ea velocity and an Ea/Aa velocity ratio of <1. Thus, Doppler tissue imaging is an important tool in distinguishing normal from pseudonormal mitral valve inflow profiles (91,92). This is particularly true when obtaining technically adequate pulmonary venous A-wave profiles on transthoracic echocardiography proves difficult, or when pseudonormal dysfunction exists in the setting of modestly elevated left atrial pressure. An additional index of diastolic function that has been correlated to elevations in ventricular filling pressures is the ratio of transmitral E wave to lateral mitral annular velocity, or the E/Ea ratio. This ratio has a close positive correlation with pulmonary capillary wedge pressures (93,94).

Stage III diastolic dysfunction: restrictive physiology. Diastolic findings with restrictive physiology are summarized in Figure 6.44. As diastolic dysfunction worsens, a restrictive pattern emerges. Left atrial pressure and left ventricular stiffness are very high. The increase in left atrial pressure results in rapid inflow of blood into the left ventricular during early diastole, producing a large E wave. Low left ventricular compliance prohibits further filling in later diastole, resulting in a small A wave and further shortening of the E wave deceleration. Transmitral Doppler findings therefore feature an increased E-/A-wave ratio, with a mitral E-/A-wave velocity ratio typically >2, and further shortening of the E-wave deceleration time, which is typically less than the 150 ms in adult studies (90). Of note, severe restrictive physiology results in a rapid rise in intraventricular pressures during diastolic filling, which will occasionally produce diastolic mitral regurgitation; these findings can be appreciated on color flow Doppler imaging (95,96).

In the pulmonary veins, there is further worsening of the trend seen in pseudonormal dysfunction, with further decreases in the fraction of systolic pulmonary venous flow and further increases in the diastolic fraction, resulting in further decreases in the S-/D-wave velocity ratio. The magnitude of the atrial systolic reversal frequently becomes quite pronounced.

Doppler tissue imaging of the lateral mitral annulus in restrictive physiology will reveal a decrease in Ea velocities (74,92). Overall, the magnitude of annular velocities—both Ea and Aa waves—is low given the combined effects of severely decreased relaxation and compliance.

Constrictive Pericarditis. Constrictive pericarditis, although uncommon in children, can manifest very similar diastolic findings to restrictive physiology. The transmitral flow pattern can be very similar and feature an increased E-/A-wave ratio and a shortened E-wave deceleration time. However, there several findings can help distinguish constrictive pericarditis from restrictive cardiomyopathy. In constrictive pericarditis, simultaneous respirometry will reveal increased variation in the mitral valve E-wave velocities (>25%). Augmentation of pulmonary venous flows during respiration, not present with restrictive physiology, are also seen (29). In addition, Doppler assessment of the hepatic venous flow will reveal increased atrial systolic flow reversals *during expiration* with constriction and *during inspiration* with restrictive physiology (97). Doppler tissue imaging in constrictive pericarditis will reveal a normal Ea velocity in comparison with restrictive physiology in which, as previously stated, the Ea velocity is quite low (92). It should be noted that these findings have not been validated in pediatric studies of constrictive and restrictive physiology.

Doppler Assessment of Right Ventricular Diastolic Function. Diastolic dysfunction of the right ventricle (either in a systemic or pulmonary position or as a single ventricle) can also be assessed by Doppler techniques. However, it is less clear what specific findings are representative of normal baseline ventricular diastolic function in these instances. There has been work describing diastolic dysfunction, for example, in the single ventricle (98,99), but it is likely that diastolic dysfunction will need to be stratified for severity within a specific diagnosis. Moreover, it is well known that variation of flow patterns with respiration are prevalent on the right side of the heart, and therefore diastolic findings will need interpretation in view of their phase of respiration.

Diastolic function of the right ventricle can be assessed by assessment of transtricuspid Doppler flow patterns, Doppler tissue imaging of the lateral tricuspid annulus, and assessment of the systemic venous inflow. Unlike the left ventricle, however, in which diastolic function indices have been validated in a large adult population, assessment of right ventricular diastolic dysfunction in children has historically been confined to assessment in several fairly heterogeneous circumstances such as postoperative tetralogy of Fallot (100–102), systemic right ventricles, and single right ventricular physiology (99,103). As such, normal diastolic function is difficult to define in these circumstances, and diastolic findings are often compared within a specific population against other clinical parameters.

Nonetheless, published normal values for both tricuspid inflow Doppler flow profiles (Appendix 6.3) (87,104,105) and tricuspid annular velocities (Appendix 6.5) (87,106) exist for the pediatric population and can be used to evaluate right ventricular diastolic function in the same way as one would assess diastolic function of the left ventricle. Both systemic venous and transtricuspid flow can vary significantly during respiration (104); diastolic assessments of the right ventricle and systemic venous inflow should therefore be standardized for phase of respiration using simultaneous respirometry. Respirometry can be particularly helpful in assessing systemic venous flow patterns, as these can often be important in distinguishing restrictive diastolic physiology from a more constrictive pattern as described above. Pulsed wave Doppler assessment of flow in the proximal pulmonary artery is also useful when right ventricular diastolic dysfunction is suspected, as antegrade flow in the main pulmonary artery during atrial systole has been associated with restrictive right ventricular physiology in postoperative tetralogy of Fallot (101,107).

Systolic Ventricular Function. Indices of ventricular systolic function evaluate one of two main characteristics of ventricular physiology—myocardial mechanics or chamber mechanics. *Myocardial mechanics* refer to the behavior of the ventricle at the myofiber level. They are based on isolated muscle experiments such as the isometric contraction experiment in which tension developed during the contraction is directly related to initial muscle length and the isotonic contraction experiment in which the velocity of myofiber shortening is inversely and exponentially related to initial load (Fig. 6.45). From an echocardiographic point of view, the indices that measure myocardial mechanics should ideally be regional and free of loading conditions, thereby more reflective of the inherent ventricular contractility.

Chamber mechanics refer to the behavior of the ventricle on the larger scale, and the indices that measure them are global in nature (e.g., ejection fraction). Most of these indices are not only dependent on contractility but also loading conditions (preload and afterload) and, therefore, reflect global

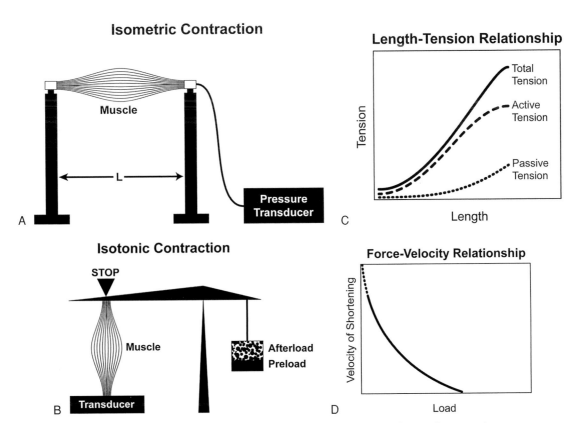

FIGURE 6.45 Chamber mechanics are based on myocardial mechanics (**A** and **B**). In the isometric contraction experiment (**A**), the tension developed during the contraction is directly related to the initial muscle length (**C**). In the isotonic contraction experiment (**B**). the velocity of myofiber shortening during a contraction is inversely and exponentially related to the initial load (**D**). The principles of chamber mechanics are extrapolated from these basic myocardial mechanical principles. The chamber mechanical equivalent to the length–tension curve is the pressure–volume loop, and the chamber mechanical equivalent to the force–velocity relationship is the wall stress–velocity of circumferential fiber-shortening relationship. Although the myocardial mechanical relationships cannot be measured in the intact heart, the chamber mechanical equivalents are readily measurable by assessing changes in ventricular chamber dimension.

ventricular performance within the context of the entire cardiovascular system. Other indices provide a more hybrid approach. These indices (e.g., pressure volume loops and the end-systolic stress–velocity relationship) use sophisticated measurements of chamber function to provide information on myocardial mechanics.

Each type of index (chamber or hybrid) is useful (108). There are times when an assessment of myocardial mechanics is the critical need, for example, in evaluating a patient with suspected adriamycin cardiotoxity or a patient with severe mitral regurgitation. In the former, the oncologist needs to know if there is inherent myocardial damage. In the latter, indices of chamber mechanics might appear quite normal because of partial ejection into the low-pressure left atrium luring the clinician into a false sense of security. In these instances, the echocardiographer needs to use those hybrid methods that use evaluation of the chamber function to attempt to assess myocardial function. There are other times when an assessment of chamber mechanics is necessary, for example, in appraising an intensive care unit patient's response to intravenous medications given to manipulate loading conditions. Here, the intensivist needs to know if global chamber performance in the context of the entire cardiovascular system improves with the manipulation. Here, the echocardiographer

should use indices of basic chamber function such as shortening fraction and ejection fraction.

Shortening fraction. Although M-mode echocardiography has the major and obvious limitation of assessing only a limited "ice pick" view of the heart, it provides fast frame rates, which enhances both temporal and spatial resolution of measurements. Left ventricular shortening fraction (SF) continues to provide a reasonable assessment of left ventricular systolic performance:

$$SF = (LVED - LVES)/LVED \qquad [19]$$

where

$LVED$ = left ventricular end-diastolic dimension
$LVES$ = left ventricular end-systolic dimension

Normal shortening fraction values range between 0.28 and 0.40.

Ejection fraction. Because ejection fraction incorporates ventricular volume (a 3-D parameter), it reflects global left ventricular performance in a more accurate manner than shortening fraction. Its echocardiographic determination relies on digitization of both left ventricular end-diastolic (LVEDV) and end-systolic

(LVESV) volumes using either biplane (apical four- and two-chamber views) or single-plane (apical four-chamber) techniques. Ejection fraction (EF) is calculated as follows:

$$EF\ (\%) = 100(LVEDV - LVESV) \div LVEDV \qquad [20]$$

Normal values of ejection fraction are 54% to 75%.

End-systolic wall stress–velocity relationship. The relationship between end-systolic wall stress and velocity of circumferential fiber shortening is one of the first and best echocardiographic measurements providing information on myocardial mechanics. According to La Place's principle, left ventricular wall stress is directly related to chamber dimension and pressure and inversely related to wall thickness. During ventricular ejection, the dimension decreases while pressure and wall thickness increase. Normally, wall stress peaks in early systole and, despite rising pressure, decreases thereafter because of decreasing chamber dimension and increasing wall thickness through the remainder of systole. Wall stress at end-systole is the force that limits further shortening. End-systolic wall stress is literally the afterload—the force the ventricle can no longer overcome to sustain further shortening, thereby causing a cessation of ejection. It is a distinctly different concept than the traditional concept of afterload, the systemic vascular resistance, which is defined by analogy to Ohm's law as the ratio of mean pressure drop to total flow across the systemic vascular bed. This concept assumes that the cardiovascular system is equivalent to an electrical circuit generating constant pressure and flow. In reality, the left ventricle is a pulsatile pump that must overcome not only an internal load consisting of pressure and geometric factors but also an external load consisting of pulsatile and nonpulsatile components. These factors are incompletely described by systemic vascular resistance, but wall stress accounts for the combined effects of peripheral loading conditions and factors internal to the heart (109).

Clinical applicability of end-systolic stress has been most useful when relating it to an ejection phase index of shortening such as the velocity of circumferential fiber shortening (110,111). The relationship is linear and inverse—as wall stress

(afterload) increases, shortening decreases. Both parameters are easily obtained from an M-mode echocardiogram of the left ventricle with simultaneous indirect carotid artery pulse trace and blood pressure determination (Fig. 6.46). Meridional (or longitudinal) end-systolic wall stress (ESWS) is derived from the formula (112–114):

Meridional ESWS $(g/cm^2) = [1.35(P_{es})(LVES)]$
$$\div\ [(4)(h_{es})(1 + h_{es}/LVES)] \qquad [21]$$

where

1.35 = conversion factor from mm Hg to g/cm^2
P_{es} = end-systolic pressure derived from linear interpolation of the dicrotic notch on the pulse trace assigning the systolic blood trace to its peak and the diastolic pressure to its nadir
LVES = left ventricular end-systolic dimension
h_{es} = left ventricular end-systolic wall thickness

Circumferential end-systolic wall stress can also be easily calculated with the addition of only one more measurement, the left ventricular long-axis end-systolic length from the mitral annulus to the left ventricular apex in the apical four-chamber view (L) (115):

Circumferential ESWS $(g/cm^2) = [(1.35)(P_{es})(LVES/2h_{es})]$
$$\times\ [1 - (LVES)^2/2(L^2)]$$

Heart rate–corrected velocity of circumferential fiber shortening (VCF_c) is derived from the following formula:

$$VCF_c\ (circ/s) = [(SF)(RR)^{0.5}] \div (ET) \qquad [22]$$

where

SF = shortening fraction
RR = R to R interval
ET = ejection time measured from the carotid pulse trace

The relationship between VCF_c and meridional ESWS is linear over the physiologic range, independent of heart rate and preload (110,116), and incorporates afterload, making it responsive

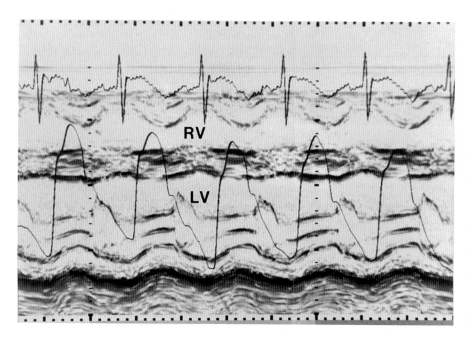

RV

LV

FIGURE 6.46 To obtain the left ventricular stress–velocity relationship, simultaneous M-mode echocardiogram of the left ventricle and indirect carotid or axillary pulse traces are obtained. Blood pressure is measured at the same time, and the pulse trace is calibrated by linear interpolation so that the end-systolic pressure (the pressure at the dicrotic notch) can be obtained. The heart rate–corrected velocity of circumferential fiber shortening and end-systolic wall stress then can be calculated. (From Kimball TR, Ralston MA, Khoury PJ, et al. The effect of ligation of patent ductus arteriosus in left ventricular performance and its determinants in premature neonates. *J Am Coll Cardiol* 1996; 27:194, with permission.)

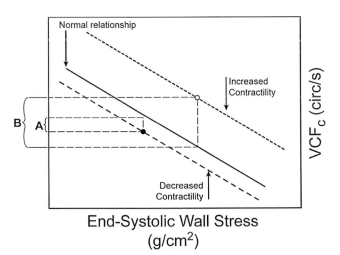

FIGURE 6.47 The relationship between heart rate–corrected velocity of circumferential fiber shortening (VCF_c) and meridional end-systolic wall stress is linear over the physiologic range, independent of heart rate and preload, and incorporates afterload, making it responsive to changes in ventricular inotropy. In the setting of enhanced contractility, the relationship undergoes a parallel shift up and to the right whereas negative inotropic changes cause the relationship to shift down and to the left. Contractility can be assessed quantitatively by calculating the difference between the measured VCF_c and the predicted VCF_c for the measured wall stress. A positive difference reflects enhanced contractility (B) and a negative difference is indicative of depressed contractility (A).

to changes in ventricular inotropy. Specifically, in the setting of enhanced contractility, the relationship undergoes a parallel shift upward and to the right, whereas negative inotropic changes cause the relationship to shift downward and to the left (Fig. 6.47). Normal values are established (Fig. 6.48) (117,118), and the relationship has proven useful in various clinical conditions. Ideally, when evaluating a patient, a series of VCFc-ESWS data pairs should be obtained by altering afterload (e.g., by administration of methoxamine or phenylephrine). However, a single data pair in the baseline state has proven not only equally useful (since the relationship shifts in a parallel manner across the physiologic range of afterload) but also more practical (69,70,119–124). Contractility can be assessed quantitatively from this relationship by calculating either the Z value or the difference between the measured VCF_c and the predicted VCF_c for the measured wall stress (VCF_c difference) (Fig. 6.47).

Midwall shortening. Experimental data indicate that myocardial shortening in the left ventricular subendocardial layers exceeds that in the subepicardial layers, producing a nonuniform pattern of wall thickening (125,126). The midwall and subepicardial fibers, therefore, migrate in an epicardial direction relative to the subendocardial fibers during ventricular systole (Fig. 6.49). Systolic ejection phase indices (e.g., shortening fraction, ejection fraction, velocity of circumferential fiber shortening) are measured at the endocardium and therefore do not reflect true shortening of myofibers in the deeper layers of the myocardium. The discrepancy between endocardial and midwall shortening increases in hearts with increased relative wall thickness or mass/volume ratios (i.e.. concentric hypertrophy). In these instances, midwall mechanics provide a more physiologically appropriate measurement of left ventricular function. These can be estimated using a two-shell cylin-

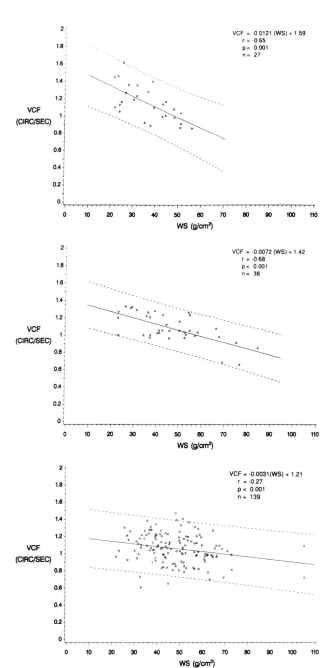

FIGURE 6.48 The stress–velocity relationship in normal children younger than 6 months of age (**top**), between 6 months and 3 years of age (**middle**), and older than 3 years of age (**bottom**). (From Kimball TR, Daniels SR, Khoury P, et al. Age-related variation in contractility estimate in patients less than or equal to 20 years of age. *Am J Cardiol* 1991;68:1385, with permission.)

drical model and assuming constant volumes of the total left ventricular wall and of its inner and outer halves during the cardiac cycle (127). With these assumptions, midwall shortening fraction (SF_{mid}) can be calculated from M-mode echocardiographic measurements:

$$SF_{mid} = [(LVED + h_d/2 + s_d/2) - LVES - mwst]/ (LVED + h_d/2 + s_d/2)$$ [23]

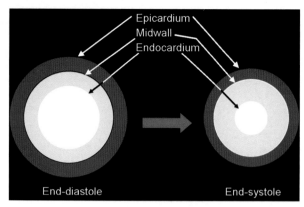

FIGURE 6.49 Parasternal short-axis images of the left ventricle at end-diastole (**left**) and at end-systole (**right**) demonstrating the mid-wall mechanics concept. The epicardium is the outermost border of the left ventricle. The endocardium is the innermost border of the left ventricle. The midwall is defined as the midpoint between the endocardium and epicardium at end-diastole. At end-systole there is a relative epicardial migration of the midwall and subepicardial fibers relative to the subendocardial fibers. Note that the midwall fibers in the diagram have contracted inward but less so than the endocardial fibers at end-systole. Since traditional systolic ejection phase indices are measured at the endocardium, they do not reflect true shortening of myofibers in the deeper layers of the myocardium. In hypertrophied hearts, midwall mechanics may provide a more physiologically appropriate measurement of left ventricular function.

where

$$LVED = \text{left ventricular end-diastolic dimension}$$
$$h_d = \text{left ventricular end-diastolic posterior wall thickness}$$
$$s_d = \text{end-diastolic septal thickness}$$
$$LVES = \text{left ventricular end-systolic dimension}$$
$$mwst = \text{left ventricular end-systolic inner shell myocardial thickness}$$
$$= \{[LVED + (h_d + s_d)/2]^3 - LVED^3 + LVES^3\}^{0.333} - LVES$$

Traditionally, midwall shortening is related to end-systolic wall stress to provide assessment of myocardial performance. Normal values for midwall shortening have been established in children (Fig. 6.50) (128).

Fiber stress. Because the left ventricle shortens in a twisting pattern similar to that of a wet towel being wrung dry, the directional vectors of left ventricular chamber contraction are intricate. However, these complex motions can be simplified into forces occurring in the three major planes only—meridional, circumferential, or radial. End-systolic wall stress is a measurement of the forces opposing shortening in the meridional and circumferential planes but neglects the radial forces, critical components acting on the myofiber. In addition, wall stress is an index of the total force per unit of myocardium and therefore includes transmitted forces and pressure exerted by more external fibers, which are negative components in its calculation, causing an underestimation in true afterload. Fiber stress,

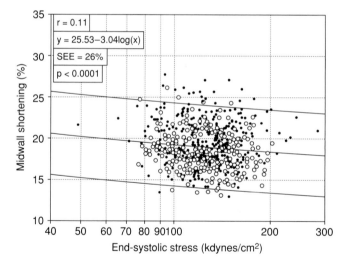

Children and Adolescents (n = 332)		Adults (n = 388)	
Equation of Regression – SEE	**r**	**Equation of Regression – SEE**	**r**
$eS = 82.20\text{-}22.60*\log[\sigma_c] - 4.26\%$	−0.47	$eS = 103.03\text{-}31.81*\log[\sigma_c] - 3.53\%$	−0.60
$mS = 24.20\text{-}2.08*\log[\sigma_c] - 2.85\%$	−0.07	$mS = 25.99\text{-}3.54*\log[\sigma_c] - 2.13\%$	−0.14
$eS = 90.13\text{-}24.89*\log[\sigma_c] \text{-}0.32 [years] - 4.16\%$	Multiple 0.51	$eS = 99.33\text{-}31.11*\log[\sigma_c] \text{-}0.05 [years] - 3.50\%$	Multiple 0.62
$mS = 30.78\text{-}3.98*\log[\sigma_c] \text{-}0.26 [years] - 2.75\%$	Multiple 0.29	$mS = 27.72\text{-}3.87*\log[\sigma_c] \text{-}0.02 [years] - 2.11\%$	Multiple 0.19

FIGURE 6.50 Normal values for the logarithmic relationship between midwall shortening versus circumferential end-systolic wall stress in normal human subjects including both children (**closed circles**) and adults (**open circles**). The Table shows the regression lines for the midwall shortening (mS) or endocardial shortening (eS) versus the end-systolic circumferential wall stress (σ_c) with and without age included in the model in both children and adults. (From de Simone G, Kimball TR, Roman MJ, et al. Relation of left ventricular chamber and midwall function to age in normal children, adolescents and adults. *Ital Heart J* 2000; 1:295–300, with permission).

on the other hand, not only accounts for radial force but also is more representative of myofiber afterload because it is the fiber pulling force per unit area excluding all pressure. In addition, whereas wall stress is dependent on both chamber shape and mass/volume ratio; fiber stress is dependent on only the former, making it a more accurate index of afterload in the setting of ventricular hypertrophy or severe dilatation (129). Fiber stress can be easily calculated from echocardiographic data (130):

$$\text{Fiber stress (g/cm}^2) = [(1.35)(P_{es})(b_m)]/(2b_{es}) \quad [24]$$

where

b_m = midwall minor semiaxis at end-systole = $h_{es}/[\ln(LVES/2 + h_{es}) - \ln(LVES/2)]$

The use of fiber stress in combination with midwall shortening indices to calculate predicted midwall fiber shortening for a measured fiber stress from the formula

$$\text{Midwall VCFc} = 0.0007(\text{fiber stress}) + 0.65 \quad [25]$$

currently provides one of the most robust and accurate echocardiographic assessments of myofiber performance (130,131).

Myocardial mechanics have also been evaluated with myocardial fiber strain and strain rate analyses. Doppler tissue imaging provides the velocity (dd/dt) of a myocardial segment of interest. The real-time spatial derivative of this velocity is the strain rate and the real-time integration over time of the strain rate is the myocardial strain (a unitless measure of regional myocardial function). Strain and strain rate are directly related to ventricular contractility (132). In patients with a Senning operation for transposition of the great arteries, right ventricular strain indices are reduced relative to control values (i.e., subpulmonary right ventricular strain indices) and correlate well with magnetic resonance–derived right ventricular ejection fraction (133). Likewise in patients undergoing closure of atrial septal defect, right and left ventricular strain indices are more globally abnormal after surgical closure than after device closure (134). In postoperative tetralogy of Fallot patients, strain analyses in both the right and left ventricles have been used to show that right ventricular systolic function is abnormal and that the left ventricular contraction is significantly asynchronous, causing poor left ventricular function (135,136). Finally, strain analyses have been used successfully to demonstrate that the Norwood procedure performed with a right ventricular to pulmonary artery conduit modification is associated with better postoperative right ventricular function than when a traditional systemic to pulmonary artery shunt is used (137).

More advanced approaches

VENTRICULAR PRESSURE–VOLUME LOOP. In the invasive cardiology laboratory, the pressure–volume loop is one of the most robust indices of ventricular function. Construction of a loop requires plotting of simultaneous paired data points throughout the cardiac cycle of ventricular pressure traditionally measured by high-fidelity catheters and ventricular volume traditionally measured by application of Simpson's rule to angiographic images or conductance catheters. However, because of improvements in echocardiographic technology, it is now possible to construct a pressure–volume loop noninvasively (138). The echocardiographic modality of automatic border detection provides a continuous, instantaneous curve of chamber area or volume (139). The technique uses ultrasonic backscatter data to differentiate pixels of tissue density from those of blood density. The interface between these two pixel types is the endocardium. In this manner, the endocardium is tracked throughout the cardiac cycle, allowing derivation of a continuous ventricular volume or area curve. In the presence of atrioventricular valve regurgitation, continuous ventricular pressure tracings can be generated (see section on atrioventricular valve insufficiency above). Plotting dimensional data from the automatic border detection technique with simultaneous pressure data derived from the atrioventricular valve regurgitation, Doppler technique yields a ventricular pressure-dimension loop (Fig. 6.51). In addition, loading conditions can be manipulated noninvasively by postural changes (e.g., those occurring on a tilt table) or abdominal compression (138) allowing production of a family of pressure–volume loops. From these loops, mechanical work (the area enclosed by the loop) (140) and end-systolic elastance (the slope of the end-systolic pressure–volume data points) can be calculated.

ASSESSING THE CARDIOVASCULAR SYSTEM. No ventricle is an island. The ventricle exists within the framework of the entire cardiovascular system with impact from both the arterial vasculature and the contralateral ventricle. In addition, the ventricles exist in a milieu that subjects them to variable activity levels, the responses to which are valuable in understanding ventricular well-being but are not evident on the traditional resting echocardiographic examination.

VENTRICULOARTERIAL COUPLING. Optimal total cardiovascular performance (i.e., pumping and delivering flow to the tissues) requires appropriate coupling of the left ventricle and the arterial system. A comprehensive assessment of left ventricular function is possible only by interpreting that assessment in the context of simultaneous assessment of arterial system function. For example, end-systolic ventricular elastance relative to arterial elastance (end-systolic pressure/stroke volume) has been used as an index of ventriculoarterial coupling to show that stroke work is maximal when ventricular and arterial elastance are equal, and that in the normal resting state, the cardiovascular system does, indeed, operate in this range (141). Many of the techniques that evaluate peripheral arterial anatomy and function are also used as surrogate measures for evaluation of the coronary arteries (see Coronary Arteries below) and can be used in conjunction with ventricular functional indices to assess ventriculoarterial coupling.

PERTURBING THE SYSTEM. Children are rarely sedentary. Yet, echocardiographic examinations are largely performed when the child is in a resting, supine state—a condition that the child is actually experiencing for only brief moments. These resting examinations shed little light on the child's typically more active physiology, which, ironically, becomes apparent only after the patient leaves our laboratory. An echocardiographic assessment with the addition of a stressing agent (exercise, dobutamine, mental, isometric, electrophysiologic) provides greater insight on the hemodynamics present during the active state typical of children.

One simple approach is the force–frequency relationship—increasing frequency of contraction induced by cardiac pacing (142) results in increased contractile force generation (as measured by ejection phase indices or by wall stress relations) with a maximal force (F_{max}) at a stimulus frequency of approximately 175 bpm (Treppe phenomenon). Thereafter, the response becomes inverted (increased frequency results in decreased force). In the chronic failing heart owing, for example, to dilated cardiomyopathy, mitral insufficiency, or diabetic cardiomyopathy, F_{max} is depressed because of decreased activity of the calcium adenosine triphosphatase in the sarcoplasmic reticulum (SERCA-2) (143). Another, similar approach is the assessment of contractile reserve. In chronic heart failure, a rise in circulating catecholamines is accompanied by decreased beta receptor density and down-regulation of receptors leading to a poor response to inotropic agents

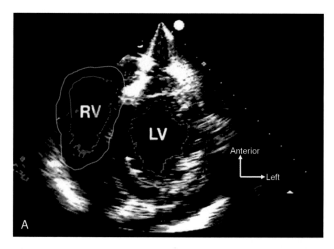

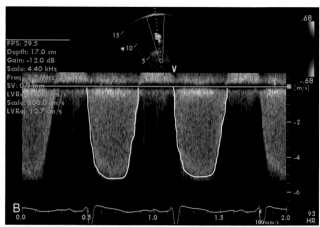

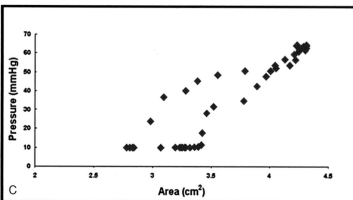

FIGURE 6.51 Using automatic border detection techniques and Doppler interrogation of AV valve insufficiency jets, a pressure–volume/area loop can be generated. In this case automatic border detection technique is used in the parasternal short-axis view to continuously and instantaneously track the right ventricular (RV) area (**A**). These data can be combined with a near-simultaneous Doppler interrogation of a tricuspid insufficiency jet (**B**) from which instantaneous and continuous right ventricular pressure data can be obtained when a right atrial pressure is assumed. The combination of the automatic border detection and the tricuspid insufficiency Doppler data yields a right ventricular pressure–volume/area loop determination (**C**).

(144). Poor contractile response to exogenous catecholamines, therefore, has prognostic value in identifying the marginal ventricle more likely to require chronic medications, assistive devices, and possibly transplant (145) and is associated with overexpression of apoptosis-related proteins (146–148). The magnitude of augmentation of cardiac performance during cardiovascular stress is termed *contractile reserve* and can be assessed noninvasively using exercise or pharmacologic stress (149–151). Whereas stress echocardiography administered to unmask occult coronary artery disease requires a large stressing dose to maximize myocardial oxygen consumption (see below), administration of stress for assessment of contractile reserve requires far less but nevertheless still substantial dosing (dobutamine at approximately 20 μg/kg/min) (152). Normal responses of left ventricular performance (shortening fraction) and contractility (VCF_c difference) to exercise and dobutamine stress have been established (Fig. 6.52) (152,153). Stress echocardiography can also be used to assess the behavior of cardiac pathology during altered activity levels. For example, the gradients in hypertrophic cardiomyopathy, coarctation, or pulmonary and aortic valvar stenosis (154); and the pulmonary artery pressure in patients with suspected pulmonary hypertension can all be evaluated with echocardiography during stress (Fig. 6.53).

Ventricular interaction. Acute and chronic alterations in loading of one ventricle influence function of the other ventricle,

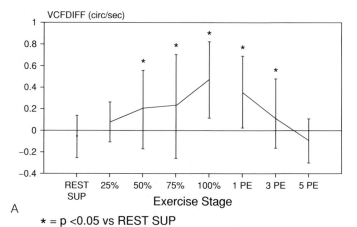

* = p <0.05 vs REST SUP

FIGURE 6.52 Normal responses to VCF difference, a quantitative measure of left ventricular contractility, in children during exercise (**A**) and during dobutamine stress (**B**). (Reprinted from The Journal of Pediatrics, Volume 122, Kimball: "Echocardiographic determination of left ventricular preload, afterload, and contractility during and after exercise", pages S92–S93, copyright 1993, with permission from Elsevier. Reprinted from Journal of the American Society of Echocardiography, Volume 16, Michelfelder: "Moderate-dose dobutamine maximizes left ventricular contractile response during dobutamine stress echocardiography in children, page144, copyright 2003, with permission from the American Society of Echocardiography.)

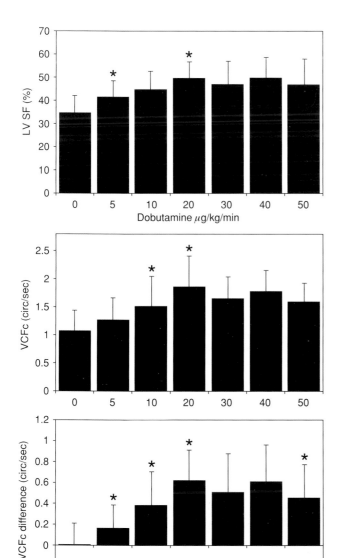

FIGURE 6.52 (*Continued*)

mitral atresia). The effects of the left ventricle either as a well-developed or even a hypoplastic ventricle on right ventricular function are unknown. Some investigations have suggested that right ventricular function can be assisted by the left ventricle in certain instances. Indeed, in an elegant isolated rabbit heart study (157), the individual effects of the (i) right ventricular free wall, (ii) left ventricular free wall, and (iii) interventricular septum on right and left ventricular function were assessed by induction of ischemia, injection of glutaraldehyde and incision into these three myocardial locations. These experiments demonstrated that right ventricular free wall function has a minimal effect on left ventricular hemodynamics but both the septum and the left ventricular free wall have profound effects on right ventricular function. In the clinical setting, the right ventricle is associated with a wide variety of left ventricular loading conditions, from decreased to increased afterload or even absence of the left ventricle. It has been suggested that in patients with chronic right ventricular hypertrophy, the presence of a left ventricle with normal pressures preserves right ventricular function (158,159). Indeed, in lambs, it has been shown that although function of the normal right ventricle is not affected by acute reductions in left ventricular pressure, similar decreases in left ventricular pressure can cause the hypertrophied right ventricle to increase cardiac output even in the face of decreased contractility, presumably by enhanced preload (160). These types of studies have important

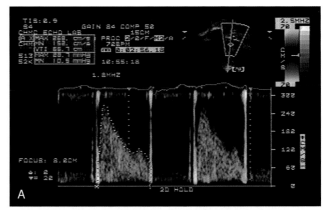

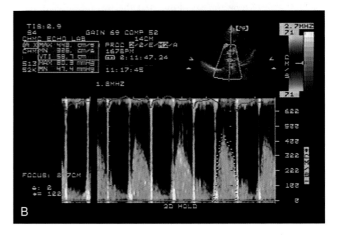

FIGURE 6.53 Mitral valve Doppler tracings from an apical four-chamber view in a 16-year-old male with a prosthetic mitral valve at baseline (**A**) and at peak exercise (**B**). The mean mitral valve gradient at baseline is 10.5 mm Hg. With exercise, the mean gradient increases to 47 mm Hg.

both because the two ventricles pump in series and are also anatomically positioned in parallel sharing the common ventricular septum. In right ventricular *volume overload*, for example, the right ventricle fills at the expense of the left ventricle as the two chambers compete for space resulting in leftward displacement of the ventricular septum during diastole and a reduction in left ventricular ejection fraction (155). Interestingly, however, the effects of volume and pressure overload are different. Right ventricular *pressure overload* has been shown to cause a systolic shift resulting in an augmentation of left ventricular shortening (156). Pathology of the right ventricle is common in several types of congenital heart disease, yet its impact on left ventricular function is largely unknown.

In many other types of congenital heart disease, the right ventricle may support the systemic circulation (e.g., in patients with congenitally corrected transposition or with an atrial-level switch for transposition of the great arteries) or may exist as the sole ventricle, responsible for providing blood flow to both the systemic and pulmonary circulations (e.g., in clinical correlates. For example, it has been shown that, in congenitally corrected transposition of the great arteries, relief of pulmonary artery stenosis (i.e., reduction in left ventricular afterload) results in right ventricular (i.e., systemic ventricular) dysfunction (161).

These studies demonstrate a clear interaction of each ventricle on the other's hemodynamics. Future echocardiographic indices and studies evaluating ventricular function may need to account for the impact of the contralateral ventricle on the subject ventricle of interest.

Assessing function of the ventricle with unusual geometry. Advances in surgical management of congenital heart disease have resulted in many patients surviving chronically with surgical palliations consisting of a univentricular heart that must support both the systemic and pulmonary circulations. In addition, assessment of right ventricular function in a biventricular circulation has become increasingly critical not only in monitoring its function as a pulmonary ventricle (e.g., in postoperative tetralogy of Fallot) but also in evaluating its performance as a systemic ventricle (e.g., postoperative atrial switch or congenitally corrected transposition of the great arteries {S, L, L}).

Unlike the normal left ventricle, which resembles a prolate ellipse, univentricular and right ventricular anatomy is not amenable to simple geometric assumptions, making functional assessment very difficult. In addition, these ventricles may be difficult to image as portions of their wall are often inaccessible. Nevertheless, investigators have developed some indices that are proving useful.

As described previously (Ventricular Morphology) echocardiographic assessment of right ventricular volume is possible, which in turn makes calculation of ejection fraction feasible when calculating the volume at both end-diastole and end-systole (48). A similar approach uses the right ventricular area and length from the apical four chamber view (162,163):

$$RV \ volume = 0.85(area)^2/length \qquad [26]$$

A fractional area change of the right ventricle from an apical four-chamber view has also been used with success (164,165). These approaches unfortunately neglect the infundibulum of the right ventricle, which may contribute significantly to right ventricular hemodynamics. However, investigators have used automatic border detection techniques to explore the contribution of the infundibulum to both right ventricular volume and stroke volume. These experiments show that the infundibulum comprises approximately 30% of the total right ventricular volume. Compared with the right ventricular body, the infundibulum exhibits significantly less but important shortening (42% for the body versus 28% for the infundibulum) and delayed activation indicating a peristalticlike contraction of the right ventricle (166).

As previously discussed, strain analyses are valuable in assessing ventricles of unusual geometry. A similar concept has been used in assessing right ventricular function with longitudinal shortening. The longitudinal function of the heart contributes to greater systolic pump effectiveness and even a suction effect in diastole. More important, most myocardial fibers in the right ventricle are oriented in the longitudinal plane coursing from the apex to the atrioventricular junction (167). A practical means of capturing right ventricular longitudinal function is through measurement of percent tricuspid valve displacement with M-mode echocardiography from an apical four-chamber view (168,169). Care must be taken to align the cursor so that it transects the annulus throughout the cardiac cycle. Surprisingly, the tricuspid parietal annulus moves to a greater extent than either the tricuspid septal annulus or even both mitral annular points, indicating greater

longitudinal function of the right ventricle relative to the left ventricle. In addition, for all valve annuli, percent displacement decreases with growth but is unaffected by heart rate. Clinically, the assessment of tricuspid valve displacement has been useful in demonstrating that right ventricular longitudinal function is increased in right ventricular volume overload and decreased in right ventricular pressure overload (168). The technique has also been useful in demonstrating that systolic function of a right ventricle in a systemic position is significantly worse than either a systemic left ventricle or a pulmonary right ventricle (169).

The myocardial performance index (MPI or Tei index, [170]) is a Doppler-derived index of ventricular function that is free of geometric constraints. It involves simultaneous (or near simultaneous at equivalent heart rates) measurement of atrioventricular inflow and ipsilateral semilunar outflow Doppler velocities (Fig. 6.54). For example, assessment of MPI for the right ventricle requires near-simultaneous Doppler sampling of the tricuspid inflow and pulmonary outflow velocities.

$$MPI = (ICT + IVRT) \div ET \qquad [27]$$

where

ICT = isovolumic contraction time
$IVRT$ = isovolumic relaxation time
ET = systolic ejection time

Alternatively, a more facile but equivalent calculation can be performed:

$$MPI = (a - ET) \div ET \qquad [28]$$

where

a = time between atrioventricular valve closure and opening

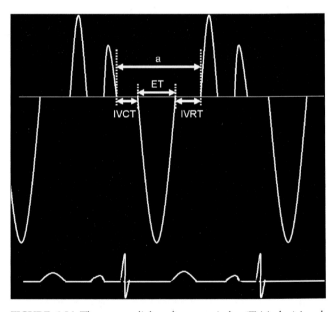

FIGURE 6.54 The myocardial performance index (Tei index) is calculated from simultaneous or near-simultaneous Doppler determination of atrioventricular valve and ipsilateral semilunar valve (i.e., mitral and aortic valves or tricuspid and pulmonary valves) inflow and outflow velocities. The myocardial performance index is equal to the sum of the isovolumic contraction time (*IVCT*) and isovolumic relaxation time (*IVRT*) divided by the ejection time (*ET*). Alternatively, the time between AV valve closure and opening (time *a*) can be measured. The Tei index is then calculated as the difference between time *a* and *ET* (a – *ET*) divided by *ET*.

The index assesses global function, and because it incorporates both systolic and diastolic components of the cardiac cycle, it is also global from a temporal perspective as well. MPI has been useful in evaluating systemic right ventricular function in patients with transposition of the great arteries remote from atrial switch operations. In this population, MPI has excellent inverse correlation with magnetic resonance–derived right ventricular ejection fraction and a value > 0.45 is generally associated with poorer ejection fraction (171,172). The index has also been used in the evaluation of the single-ventricle population. For instance, by assessing MPI, investigators have shown that univentricular function is poorer than systemic left ventricular function in a biventricular circulation but significantly improves in patients undergoing a bidirectional cavopulmonary anastomosis before 1 year of age (173,174).

The reference standard in accurate assessment of right ventricular and/or univentricular hearts may ultimately rely on three-dimensional reconstruction. This has been done using the two orthogonal views of the subcostal sagittal and coronal planes and has been useful in distinguishing normotensive from hypertensive right ventricles (175). Real-time three-dimensional imaging has been useful in demonstrating ventricular resynchronization with multisite pacing after palliation in patients with univentricular hearts (176).

Semilunar Valves and Great Vessels

Quantitative Anatomic Evaluation. Quantitative anatomic assessment of the proximal great vessels and their branches is important in a number of circumstances. It is routine to perform a quantitative evaluation of the aortic structures from the level of the valve annulus through to the distal aortic arch. Evaluation of the aortic root itself consists of 2-D assessment of the aortic annular dimension, dimension of the aorta at the level of the sinuses of Valsalva, and dimension of the sinotubular junction, ascending aorta, proximal and distal transverse aortic arch, and aortic isthmus. In general, 2-D axial resolution is superior to lateral resolution. Therefore, aortic root dimensions are best assessed in the parasternal long axis with the proximal ascending aorta and aortic root roughly perpendicular to the plane of sound. Aortic root dimensions are then determined in end-diastole as described by Roman et al. (177) (Fig. 6.55). Imaging of the transverse arch and isthmus is usually done in long-axis images of the aortic arch from the suprasternal notch window. In this window, one takes advantage of axial resolution in assessing dimension of the transverse aorta and isthmus.

Assessment of the aortic annular dimension is important in several pathologic states. Hypoplasia of the aortic annulus can be seen in various congenital heart lesions, including aortic stenosis, interruption of the aorta with ventricular septal defect (VSD) and posterior deviation of the outlet (conal) septum, and in some forms of double-outlet right ventricle. All of these conditions can be accompanied by hypoplasia of the ascending aorta and aortic arch, thus making a comprehensive evaluation of the aortic arch morphometry important in these lesions. In the setting of aortic coarctation, assessment of transverse arch dimension is often as important because transverse arch hypoplasia often accompanies a discreet juxtaductal coarctation, which may—particularly in the neonate with coarctation—result in an alteration of the surgical procedure to correct the coarctation.

Dilation of the aortic root and proximal ascending aorta can occur in various pathologic conditions, including connective tissue disorders (177–180), bicuspid aortic valve (181–183),

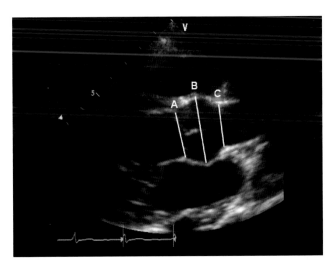

FIGURE 6.55 Aortic root dimension measurements. Standardized assessment of aortic root dimensions includes measurement of A, the aortic valve annulus; B, the aortic sinus dimension; and C, the sinotubular junction dimension. Measurements are obtained in the parasternal long axis view at end-diastole.

tetralogy of Fallot (184), following arterial switch for transposition of the great arteries (185), and following autograft replacement of the aorta with the pulmonary artery, e.g., after the Ross procedure (186–189).

Assessment of the pulmonary valve, main pulmonary artery, and branch pulmonary arteries is typically done in parasternal long- and short-axis views. Alternatively, branch pulmonary artery anatomy can be well demonstrated in a modified high parasternal short-axis view. Standard measurements include pulmonary valve annulus, annulus dimension, the sinotubular junction dimension, main pulmonary artery dimension, and proximal right and left branch pulmonary artery dimensions. Accurate assessment of the pulmonary valve annulus dimension is important in ensuring adequate annular size and also in assisting in selection of the appropriate valvuloplasty balloon when patients are undergoing pulmonary valvuloplasty in the cardiac catheterization lab. In the setting of valvar pulmonary stenosis, it is also important to make an accurate quantitative assessment of the dimension of the sinotubular junction dimension, as supravalvar narrowing of the main pulmonary artery often accompanies—or in some settings, mimics—valvar pulmonary stenosis. Main pulmonary artery dilation can accompany valvar pulmonary stenosis or connective tissue disease or occur idiopathically (190,191). Branch pulmonary artery anatomy and size are important clinical concerns in numerous disease states, including tetralogy of Fallot, and in patients with single ventricular anatomy undergoing staged surgical palliation ending in the Fontan procedure (192). Branch pulmonary hypoplasia can also be seen in various noncardiac conditions including Williams' syndrome (193,194), Alagille's syndrome (195), and following congenital rubella infection (196–198). In addition to the high parasternal short-axis view of the branch pulmonary arteries, a suprasternal notch short axis is frequently used to image the proximal and higher right pulmonary artery (199) (Fig. 6.28).

Semilunar Valve Stenosis. In the setting of semilunar valve stenosis, Doppler quantitation of the transvalvar gradient is central in determining risk and the need for intervention in these lesions. As in all Doppler assessments, interrogation of the trans-valvar flow jets should be performed with the angle of insonation as parallel to the direction of flow as possible to minimize underestimation of the valve gradient. As such, aortic valve gradients are most accurately obtained from either the apical window or from a high right parasternal window, with the plane of sound angled inferiorly toward the ascending aorta.

It is important to note the distinction between peak instantaneous pressure gradients—those measured by Doppler echocardiography using the Bernoulli equation—and peak-to-peak gradients as measured in the cardiac catheterization laboratory by catheter pullback. The peak instantaneous pressure gradient is calculated from the peak instantaneous flow velocity that occurs across the semilunar valve at a single time point in systole. When peak-to-peak gradients are measured by catheter pullback in the cardiac catheterization laboratory, the gradient is expressed as the difference between the peak pressure upstream of the valve (or point of obstruction) and peak pressure downstream of the valve, which usually do not occur simultaneously in the cardiac cycle. Measurement of transvalvar pressure gradients by Doppler therefore will frequently result in a peak instantaneous pressure gradient that is higher than the observed peak-to-peak gradient measured in the catheterization laboratory (Fig. 6.56). This does not represent an overestimation, but rather, a difference in the physiologic

data being generated by the two modalities. The mean transvalvar aortic gradient can be obtained by digitization of the transaortic flow profile and integration of the area under the velocity curve. The mean transvalvar gradients correlate well to peak-to-peak gradients obtained in the catheterization laboratory. Although it is not necessarily the intent of echocardiographers to alter their calculations to conform to catheter measurements, approximation of the peak-to-peak gradient is important in the sense that most of the large early natural history studies of heart disease were based on catheter data.

Doppler evaluation of pulmonary valve stenosis is most frequently performed in the parasternal windows where the angle of insonation is most parallel to the pulmonary stenotic flow jet. In pulmonic stenosis, a peak instantaneous pressure gradient is estimated, as the narrower pulmonary artery pulse pressure (relative to the aortic pulse pressure) should result in peak instantaneous gradient that approximates peak-to-peak gradients obtained by catheter measurement. Recently, however, use of the mean Doppler gradient across the pulmonic valve has been shown to more closely estimate catheter peak-to-peak gradients across the pulmonary valve; estimation of peak instantaneous Doppler gradients results in a consistent overestimation of peak-to-peak catheter gradients (200).

Although pulsed wave Doppler is usually adequate to assess normal flow across semilunar valves, it is frequently necessary to use continuous wave Doppler in assessing semilunar valve stenoses. This is owing to the fact that flow velocities across stenotic semilunar valves generally exceed the Doppler Nyquist limits inherent to pulsed wave Doppler echocardiography. Although continuous wave Doppler will circumvent these limits, it is important for the echocardiographer to understand that continuous wave Doppler represents a display of the peak velocity occurring anywhere along the line of insonation, and therefore one must be careful to sample the structure of interest rather than an adjacent structure that is crossed by the line of interrogation.

Calculation of Valve Areas. Estimation of valve area is an additional method of assessing severity of semilunar valve stenosis. Use of the calculated valve area to assess semilunar valve stenosis can be particularly useful when flow across the semilunar valve is either diminished—as in the setting of ventricular dysfunction—or increased. Increases in net flow across the semilunar valve can be seen in the setting of concomitant regurgitation, anemia, or left-to-right shunts. To calculate valve area, one must have an understanding of the Doppler continuity equation. This equation, based on the principle of conservation of mass, states that with no net loss of fluid from the system, the volumetric flow at area A must be equal to the volumetric flow at area B. The equation is therefore stated as:

$$A_1 V_1 = A_2 V_2$$

where

A = cross-sectional area of either position 1 or 2, and
V = mean velocity of the modal spectral profile at either position 1 or 2.

As the mean flow velocity, V, equals the velocity–time integral of flow divided by the ejection time, and as the ejection times across both areas 1 and 2 are essentially the same, the continuity equation is further simplified as follows:

$$A_1(VTI_1) = A_2(VTI_1)$$

where

VTI = velocity–time integral of flow across either area 1 or 2

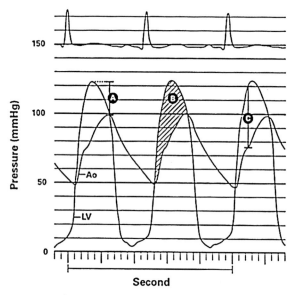

FIGURE 6.56 Simultaneous left ventricular (LV) and aortic (Ao) pressure tracings demonstrating differences in measured peak-to-peak, mean, and peak instantaneous LV-Ao gradients. **A:** measurement of peak-to-peak LV-Ao gradient, as typically measured in the catheterization laboratory, expresses the aortic valve gradient as a difference in two pressure measurements that do not occur at the same time in the cardiac cycle. The peak aortic pressure, particularly in the setting of aortic stenosis, occurs later in systole than the peak LV pressure. The peak-to-peak aortic valve gradient in this example is approximately 22 mm Hg. **B:** The mean gradient across the aortic valve can be derived either from catheter tracings, as shown, or by digitization of the transaortic Doppler flow profile. **C:** The peak instantaneous LV-Ao gradient, as measured by Doppler echocardiography, is the maximal pressure difference between LV and Ao during systole. Differential increases in LV and aortic pressure versus time will result in a larger instantaneous gradient than measured peak to peak. In this example, the peak instantaneous gradient is 44 mm Hg. (From Beekman RH, Rocchini AP, Gillon JH, et al. Hemodynamic determinants of the peak systolic left ventricular-aortic pressure gradient in children with valvar aortic stenosis. *Am J Cardiol* 1992;69:813, with permission.)

The continuity equation is most frequently used in clinical studies to estimate the effective aortic valve area in the setting of aortic stenosis. By rearranging the continuity equation, the effective valve area of a stenotic aortic valve can be solved for as follows:

$$A_{AOV} = (A_{LVOT} \times VTI_{LVOT})/VTI_{AOV} \qquad [29]$$

where

A_{AOV} = cross-sectional area of the effective aortic valve orifice
A_{LVOT} = cross-sectional area of the left ventricular outflow tract (LVOT), solved for by measuring the diameter of the LVOT in the parasternal long-axis view
VTI_{LVOT} = velocity–time integral of flow across the LVOT
VTI_{AOV} = velocity–time integral across the stenotic aortic valve

Using the continuity equation, it has been demonstrated that the aortic valve areas calculated in children by Doppler correlate well to aortic valve areas calculated by the Gorlin equation on cardiac catheterization, although Doppler methods tend to underestimate catheter areas slightly (201). In normal children and adolescents, it has been shown that aortic valve area indexed to body surface area is approximately 1.33 cm^2/m^2 (202), which is very close to values obtained in normal adults (203).

Aortic Valve Insufficiency. Isolated aortic regurgitation in the pediatric population is relatively uncommon, but it can be seen, particularly in children with bicuspid aortic valves. More often, aortic regurgitation is seen in conjunction with an abnormal aortic valve that features both aortic stenosis and insufficiency. Evaluation of neoaortic insufficiency, however, can be important following aortic valve replacement by pulmonary autograft (Ross procedure), in hypoplastic left heart syndrome following a Norwood reconstruction or following an arterial switch operation in transposition of the great arteries. In general, methods of assessing quantity of aortic regurgitation can be divided into (a) assessment of left ventricular end-diastolic and end-systolic dimensions, (b) indirect Doppler methods of assessing aortic regurgitation severity, and (c) direct estimation of aortic regurgitant volume by two-dimensional and Doppler methods.

Hemodynamically significant aortic regurgitation should result in enlargement of the left ventricle owing to the volume load imposed by the regurgitant lesion. Increases in left ventricular end-diastolic volume will be observed in the setting of moderate or greater aortic regurgitation. Because of the Starling relationship, left ventricular volume loading often results in hyperdynamic left ventricular function; therefore, the left ventricular end-systolic dimension often remains low. However, with progressing aortic regurgitation, the end-systolic dimensions (and volume) will also increase. In adult patients, it has been proposed that aortic valve replacement or repair be undertaken for end-systolic dimensions >55 mm to protect against irreversible myocardial damage and risk of sudden death (204). In children, however, no such cut point has been demonstrated, as the dimensions obviously change progressively with size and age. Clinical decisions regarding need for aortic valve replacement are therefore generally made when progressive ventricular enlargement is seen or when observed left ventricular systolic performance appears to decrement during serial follow-up.

Doppler echocardiography can also be used to indirectly evaluate the severity of aortic regurgitation. Pulsed-wave Doppler flow patterns in the distal aortic arch and descending

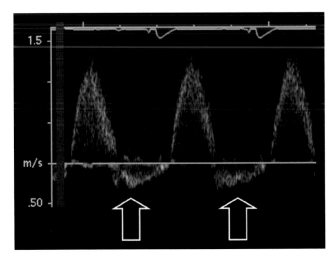

FIGURE 6.57 Holodiastolic flow reversals in the descending aorta in a patient with severe aortic regurgitation. Pulsed wave Doppler sampling of the descending aorta at the level of the diaphragm reveals prominent, holodiastolic flow reversals (*arrows*), consistent with severe aortic regurgitation.

aorta can be used to assess severity of aortic regurgitation. In the setting of significant aortic regurgitation, holodiastolic flow reversals will be noted in the distal aortic arch. As the degree of aortic regurgitation worsens, holodiastolic flow reversals can be seen in the descending aorta at the level of the diaphragm (Fig. 6.57). Holodiastolic flow reversals in the descending aorta have been positively correlated to angiographic grades 3 and 4+ aortic regurgitation (205).

Doppler interrogation of the aortic insufficiency jet itself can also be performed. This is most commonly obtained by Doppler interrogation of the insufficiency jet from the apical window. By continuous wave Doppler, the velocity profile of the aortic insufficiency jet can be displayed (Fig. 6.58). From this velocity profile, indices that describe the rate and timing of the deceleration of the insufficiency jet can be obtained. The two most commonly obtained indices are the pressure half-time and deceleration slope of aortic insufficiency velocity

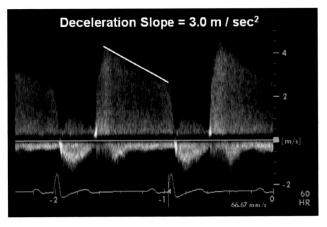

FIGURE 6.58 Continuous-wave Doppler profile of aortic regurgitation obtained in the apical four-chamber window. The aortic regurgitation deceleration slope is relatively steep (3.0 m/s^2), consistent with moderately severe (grade 3+) aortic regurgitation.

profile. Both indices reflect the rate of decrease in the diastolic pressure difference between aorta and left ventricle. The pressure half-time represents the time required for the initial peak gradient between aorta and left ventricle to decrease by half. This has been previously described in the discussion on mitral valve pressure half-time (see Atrioventricular Valve Antegrade Doppler section above). A pressure half-time of <400 ms is consistent with 3 to 4+ aortic regurgitation by angiography (206,207). The deceleration slope represents the slope of the velocity decline, measured from the peak velocity in early diastole to the shoulder of the profile at end diastole (Fig. 6.58). For both methods, it is important to ensure that the entirety of the aortic regurgitant velocity profile is obtained as partial display of the profile may result in inaccurate representations of the deceleration slope and pressure half-time. It should be noted that the degree of aortic regurgitation is not the only factor that impacts the slope of the aortic regurgitant profile. The rate of change in the velocity gradient between aorta and left ventricle can be impacted by left ventricular diastolic function (208). In general a deceleration slope >3 m/s^2 has been shown in both adult and animal studies to correlate with 3 to 4+ aortic regurgitation by angiography (206,208–210).

Severity of aortic regurgitation can also be indirectly assessed by assessment of the size of the regurgitant jet. This can be done by quantitative evaluation of the spatial distribution of the aortic regurgitant jet on color flow Doppler imaging. Several methods have been proposed, including measurements assessing the length, width, and area of the regurgitant jet. Ultimately, the width of the regurgitant jet at its origin relative to the width of the left ventricular outflow tract appears to be the best predictor of angiographic severity of aortic regurgitation (211). In general, a regurgitant jet width to LV outflow tract dimension ratio of >50% will discriminate patients with angiographic grades of aortic regurgitation of 3 to 4+ from those with milder degrees of regurgitation (211). It is important to realize, however, that regurgitant jets do not always have circular orifices, and thus the shape of the regurgitant jet should be evaluated in orthogonal imaging planes. The regurgitant jet width to LV outflow tract dimension ratio should obviously be interpreted with caution when the cross-sectional shape of the regurgitant jet is felt to be noncircular. In this setting, other direct or indirect methods in conjunction with estimates of jet width should be used to assess aortic regurgitation severity.

Regurgitant volume, regurgitant fraction, and effective regurgitant orifice area can all be directly estimated by a combination of Doppler and two-dimensional echocardiography (212,213) (see Atrioventricular Valve Insufficiency Section above). In all methods, the regurgitant volume (RV) can be determined by estimating total stroke volume (SV) and forward SV (i.e., the volume contributing to net cardiac output), and solving for regurgitant volume by the following equation:

$$RV = total\ SV - forward\ SV \qquad [30]$$

With pulsed Doppler techniques alone, the total stroke volume can be estimated by a determination of the forward flow across the aortic valve (which represents forward stroke volume plus regurgitant volume) using the cross-sectional area of the aortic valve annulus or LV outflow tract dimension and the time–velocity integral of transaortic flow. Forward stroke volume can be estimated by calculating the flow across the mitral valve using the mitral annular dimension and a time–velocity integral of flow across the mitral valve. Regurgitant fraction (RF) in all cases can be calculated by the following equation:

$$RF = RV/total\ SV \qquad [31]$$

Effective regurgitant orifice area (EROA) can be calculated by dividing the regurgitant volume by the time–velocity integral of the regurgitant velocity jet obtained by continuous wave Doppler. The use of Doppler alone to estimate these volumes requires that there be no other left-sided regurgitant lesions or intracardiac shunting, both of which will confound the estimates of regurgitant flow.

A combination of two-dimensional imaging and pulsed Doppler can also be used to calculate these volumes. The total stroke volume can be estimated by 2-D determination of the left ventricular end-diastolic and end-systolic volumes (see Ventricular Volumes above); stroke volume can then be solved as the difference between end-diastolic volume and end-systolic volume. Forward stroke volume can then be determined by pulsed Doppler using either the mitral or pulmonary valve flows as already described. This method is not confounded by the presence of aortic stenosis (which is common in children) and can also be performed in this setting of mitral regurgitation, as the difference between transaortic and transmitral flow will continue to represent the aortic regurgitant volume. Unfortunately, this method is hampered by inability to use it in the setting of intracardiac shunting.

Estimation of regurgitant volume and EROA can also be done using color flow Doppler imaging of the regurgitant jet and its proximal size of velocity surface area (PISA). This method can be performed for the aortic valve in a fashion that is described in detail (see Atrioventricular Valve Insufficiency section above). As stated previously, PISA estimation of effective regurgitant orifice areas will also be impacted by nonspherical configurations of the PISA, and therefore on orthogonal imaging, if the PISA appears to be nonspherical, this method may result in an inaccurate estimate of the regurgitation severity.

Pulmonary Regurgitation. In theory, all the techniques described above for aortic regurgitation could be used to quantitatively assess severity of pulmonic regurgitation. However, there are multiple reasons why these techniques have not gained widespread use in the pediatric population. For one, any method requiring two-dimensional estimation of RV volumes would be hampered by the significant difficulty in reliably estimating RV volumes by cross-sectional echocardiography. Second, hemodynamically significant, isolated pulmonary regurgitation rarely occurs. Significant pulmonary regurgitation is a significant issue following transannular RV outflow tract patching in postoperative tetralogy of Fallot; however, reliable measurement of the surgically altered RV outflow tract and transected pulmonary valve annulus makes reliable estimation of transpulmonary flows difficult. Severity of pulmonary regurgitation is largely assessed by semiquantitative assessment of RV dimensions (assessing the degree of volume loading of the right ventricle), qualitative impressions of the size of the regurgitant jet by color flow Doppler imaging, and by assessment of retrograde flow in the branch pulmonary arteries. In general, the presence of significant flow reversals in the distal portions of the branch pulmonary arteries is seen in the setting of grades 3 to 4+ pulmonary regurgitation.

Recently, reappraisal of Doppler methods describing the profile of the pulmonary regurgitant spectral display has suggested that short duration of the pulmonary regurgitant flow relative to the total time of diastole may be associated with greater degrees of pulmonary regurgitation as seen by angiography and as estimated by magnetic resonance imaging methods (214,215). Although not related to the assessment of pulmonary regurgitant volume, the pulmonary regurgitant spectral display can also be used to estimate pulmonary artery end-diastolic pressure. By using an assumed right ventricular end-diastolic pressure, the pulmonary artery end-diastolic pressure (PAP_{ed}) can be estimated by measuring the peak end-diastolic gradient between pulmonary artery and right ventricle (Fig. 6.59):

$$PAP_{ed} = \Delta P_{PA\text{-}RV} + 10 \text{ mm Hg} \qquad [31]$$

where

$\Delta P_{PA\text{-}RV}$ = estimated pressure gradient between pulmonary artery and right ventricle in end-diastole

The value of 10 mm Hg is the assumed right ventricular end-diastolic pressure.

Coronary Arteries

Coronary Artery Anatomy. Quantification of coronary artery caliber is reserved for various specific circumstances. Most frequently, quantitative evaluation of coronary artery size is performed in patients with suspected Kawasaki's disease. In these patients, it is routine to measure proximal, mid, and distal right coronary artery dimension; left main coronary artery dimension; proximal left anterior descending coronary artery; proximal left circumflex coronary artery; and, when possible, the posterior descending coronary artery (imaged in a posteriorly oriented apical four-chamber view. When coronary artery aneurysms are present, these are classified as either small (<5 mm internal dimension), medium (5 to 8 mm internal dimension), or giant (>8 mm internal dimension) according to the American Heart Association statement (216).

Coronary Artery Physiology. Coronary physiology can be assessed by studying peripheral arterial structure and function. These peripheral arteries serve as surrogate windows for the study of the coronary arterial anatomy because they are exposed to the same noxious influences and undergo the same pathologic processes but are more image accessible. For example, carotid intima-medial thickness is a precursor of atherosclerosis (217,218) and can be measured by high-frequency ultrasound (15 MHz). The exact technique involves examining a longitudinal section of each common carotid artery 1 cm upstream to the carotid bulb at rigorously defined insonation angles using a protractor (Fig. 6.60).

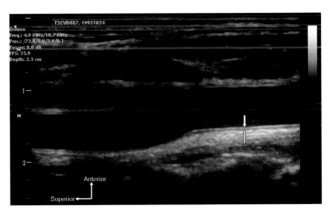

FIGURE 6.60 High-frequency ultrasound of the left common carotid artery as it branches into left internal and external carotid arteries at the bulb. The carotid intimal medial thickness (bracketed by the *arrowheads*) is then measured. This index serves as a surrogate window to the coronary arteries. Increased carotid intimal medial thickness is associated with higher cardiovascular morbidity and mortality.

Peripheral arterial endothelial function is assessed by brachial artery flow-mediated dilation. This technique involves inflating a sphygmomanometer cuff placed on the forearm or upper arm to a pressure of 100 to 150 mm Hg above the systolic pressure for 4 to 5 minutes. The brachial artery diameter immediately after cuff deflation is compared with the baseline diameter before inflation. The technique produces very subtle changes and therefore must be performed in a highly controlled environment free of extraneous influences (i.e., temperature regulation of room, consistent NPO (nothing by mouth) status of patients, and patient avoidance of exercise, smoking, and caffeine prior to the test). Both carotid intima-medial thickness and brachial artery flow-mediated dilation have been used successfully to show impairment of vascular function, and therefore presumably coronary arterial function, in children with insulin-dependent diabetes mellitus (219). Vascular function can also be assessed by applanation tonometry, a nonultrasound technique which necessitates noninvasive capture of a large artery waveform using high-fidelity transducers and from which a measurement called the augmentation index, which is associated with cardiovascular risk, can be obtained (220).

Total systemic vascular compliance can assessed by using a combination of techniques including echocardiography, Doppler echocardiography, blood pressure measurement, and acquiring an arterial waveform with applanation tonometry. Compliance can then be calculated from either of the following two formulae:

1. $Compliance$ (cm³/mm Hg) = $A_d / SVR(P_{es} - P_d)$ $\qquad$ [32]

where

A_d = area under the diastolic portion of the waveform
P_{es} = end-systolic pressure
P_d = diastolic pressure
SVR = systemic vascular resistance = [80(*mean arterial pressure*)] ÷ [(*stroke volume*)(*heart rate*)]

where stroke volume can be calculated from the Doppler measurement of the aortic valve velocity and echocardiographic measurement of aortic annulus diameter

2. $Compliance$ (cm³/mm Hg) = [(A_d)(*stroke volume*)(60)]/ [(A_t)(P_{es} − P_d)] $\qquad$ [33]

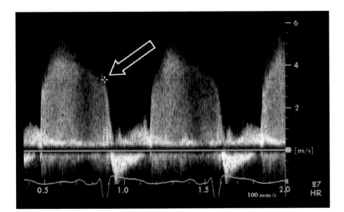

FIGURE 6.59 Continuous wave Doppler profile of pulmonary regurgitation jet in a patient with severe pulmonary hypertension. The pulmonary artery–right ventricle end-diastolic flow velocity (+ at tip of arrow) can be used to estimate pulmonary artery end-diastolic pressure (see text), which in this case is severely elevated (approximately 53 mm Hg).

where

A_t = total area under the arterial waveform

Compliance of a specific large artery can be assessed by measuring the diameter of the artery at systole and diastole along with a simultaneous blood pressure determination (221):

$$Regional\ compliance = [\pi(D_s^2 - D_d^2)] \div [4(PP)] \quad [34]$$

where

D_s = lumen diameter in systole
D_d = lumen diameter in diastole
PP = pulse pressure

The beta index is a similar measurement of regional arterial stiffness and is calculated as follows:

$$\beta\ index = [\ln(P_s/P_d)] \div [(D_s - D_d)/D_d] \quad [35]$$

where

P_s = peak systolic blood pressure

Stress Echocardiography. One of the major uses of stress echocardiography is in the assessment of coronary perfusion. When myocardial oxygen demand induced by the stressor exceeds supply, myocardial ischemia develops. Ischemia can manifest itself by angina (a relatively late manifestation evident by patient history), a metabolic abnormality (a relatively early manifestation evident by positron emission tomography), or several intermediate manifestations such as ST-segment depression on the electrocardiogram or poor radioisotope perfusion on a thallium scan. On the echocardiogram, ischemia is manifested by a new or worsening regional wall motion abnormality.

Technical aspects. In pediatrics, the usual stressors are exercise and dobutamine (222,223). Exercise is the reference standard, and most of the other stressing agents are used to mimic it. However, exercise has the disadvantages of patient movement and respiration, which impair echocardiographic imaging, and lack of threshold dosing (the entire stress dose is given without the option for early termination). Since imaging is so poor during exercise, echocardiography must be performed immediately after exercise, necessitating a hurried process to acquire images before the exercise dose dissipates (usually <60 seconds). Dobutamine infusion offers a controlled environment in which dosing can be gradually increased or terminated on the basis of immediate echocardiographic feedback. Imaging is usually excellent because there are no patient movement or deep respirations. The main disadvantage of dobutamine is that it does not duplicate exercise exactly.

For an exercise echocardiogram, imaging is performed in four echocardiographic planes (parasternal long- and short-axis, apical two-and four-chamber views) with the patient in a left lateral decubitus position before, immediately after, and 20 minutes after exercise. For a dobutamine stress echocardiogram, imaging is performed in the same four planes at rest, at each dobutamine dose, at peak heart rate, and 20 to 30 minutes after termination of dobutamine. Dobutamine is given in consecutive doses of 10, 20, 30, 40, and 50 μg/kg/min. Atropine (0.01 mg/kg) is administered to augment the heart rate, if necessary. The test is terminated if (a) target heart rate (85% of age-related maximal heart rate) is achieved, (b) adverse reactions occur, (c) the electrocardiogram shows abnormalities (e.g., significant ST-segment depression or significant dysrhythmia), (d) the patient's rating of perceived exertion is excessive (exercise), or (e) the maximum dose has been given (dobutamine).

Wall motion abnormalities. The detection of a wall motion abnormality is the most difficult part of a stress echocardiogram. It is essential that pediatric cardiologists contemplating the introduction of stress echocardiography into their laboratories receive and maintain adequate training in the interpretation of wall motion from cardiologists treating adults. In evaluating wall motion, it frequently helps to first examine the overall end-systolic cavity size. If there is little or no change at peak heart rate versus rest, abnormal wall motion is diagnosed and each segment examined in detail to detect specific regional wall motion abnormalities. In addition, an abnormality seen in one view should be verified by examination of the same or adjacent segment in another view.

CONTRAST ECHOCARDIOGRAPHY

Contrast echocardiography involves administration of one of two distinct contrast agents—agitated saline or commercially available transpulmonary contrast. Although both are administered through an intravenous line, each has a distinct purpose and use.

Agitated Saline Contrast Echocardiography

Principle

Agitation of saline produces microbubbles of gas (10 to 100 μ in diameter) that pass through the circulation until they are filtered and absorbed by transit into a capillary bed. With a systemic intravenous injection, therefore, the microbubble "cloud" will follow the downstream flow of blood, pass into the large systemic veins, and enter the right-sided cardiac structures. In the absence of right-to-left shunts, the microbubbles should not be present in the left side of the heart because of filtering and absorption in the pulmonary capillary bed. The presence of contrast in the left side of the heart after an intravenous injection of agitated saline, therefore, is a very sensitive marker for the existence of a right-to-left intrapulmonary or intracardiac shunt (224). Likewise, the presence of contrast in the right side of the heart after a left heart injection (e.g., in the operating room or cardiac intensive care unit through a left atrial line) is indicative of an intracardiac left-to-right shunt.

Technique

A stopcock to which are connected two syringes (one empty, the other filled with saline [approximately 3 mL for newborn, approximately 20 mL for adult]) is connected to the intravenous line close to its entry into the body. The addition of a small amount (0.25 to 0.5 mL) of the patient's blood will enhance contrast opacification (225). Agitation is achieved by turning the stopcock off to the patient and forcefully pushing the saline (or saline/blood mixture) alternately between the two syringes for approximately 30 seconds. The sonographer should obtain a view (usually the apical four-chamber view) in which both right and left heart structures are imaged simultaneously so that the contrast can be visualized passing through the right heart to verify that the contrast injection was indeed adequate and through the left heart if a right-to-left shunt is indeed present. The stopcock is then turned on to the patient, and the contrast is pushed rapidly into the vein. In older patients, a Valsalva maneuver may be performed to enhance the ability to detect a right-to-left shunt.

Indications

Agitated saline contrast is helpful whenever a right-to-left intrapulmonary or intracardiac shunt is suspected but cannot be detected or definitively diagnosed by standard echocardiographic modalities. These scenarios include the patient with a suspected thromboembolic stroke, unexplained cyanosis, suggestion of an intracardiac shunt on an echocardiogram with suboptimal windows, poor oxygen saturations following a Glenn or Fontan operation (226), suspected baffle leak following atrial switch procedure for transposition, suspected unroofed coronary sinus, and liver disease with suspected hepatopulmonary syndrome (227,228) (Fig. 6.61).

With intrapulmonary shunts, as seen in pulmonary arteriovenous malformations occurring in cavopulmonary connections and in the hepatopulmonary syndrome, microbubbles in the left heart usually appear three to four cardiac cycles after the contrast cloud appears in the right heart. With intracardiac shunts such as atrial or ventricular septal defects, unroofed coronary sinus, or atrial baffle leak, microbubbles appear in the left heart almost immediately on appearance in the right heart. The exact site of initial left heart microbubble appearance should also be carefully noted since the location of the right-to-left shunt can be pinpointed to either that level or upstream to it.

The site of injection should be considered beforehand. For example, an injection into a left arm vein would be appropriate for evaluation of any suspected pathology involving a left superior vena cava isolated from the right superior vena cava. Likewise, an injection in a lower-extremity vein may be more appropriate, for instance, when a leak or persistent fenestration is suspected in a Fontan conduit. Sometimes agitated saline contrast should be administered through central catheters during cardiac catheterization, for example, to pinpoint the exact location of a Fontan leak.

Diagnosis of the hepatopulmonary syndrome is one of the leading indications for agitated saline contrast. This syndrome is a well-defined cause of hypoxemia in patients with liver disease and carries an incidence as high as 29% (227). It is caused by abnormal intrapulmonary vascular dilation resulting in excess perfusion (of deoxygenated blood) for the given state of ventilation. This pathophysiology is in distinction from that occurring in the other well-recognized cardiopulmonary complication, portopulmonary hypertension, which is characterized by abnormal pulmonary vasoconstriction and obliterative vascular remodeling. Alteration in the hepatic synthesis or metabolism of vasoactive pulmonary substances, nitric oxide and possibly endothelin-1, are believed to be integral to the development of intrapulmonary vascular dilation in the hepatopulmonary syndrome (227,229). A particularly interesting congenital cause of the hepatopulmonary syndrome is the Abernethy malformation because its initial presentation is one of dyspnea and cyanosis rather than of frank liver disease (228). The malformation is owing to congenital absence of the portal vein, which results in a diversion of portal blood away from the liver and directly into the vena cava.

Transpulmonary Contrast Echocardiography

Principle

Unlike agitated saline, commercially available transpulmonary contrast agents (e.g., Albunex, Optison, Levovist, Definity) consist of a suspension of microspheres designed to pass through the pulmonary capillary bed and densely opacify the left heart structures (230). These microspheres are tenfold smaller than the microbubbles created with saline agitation (1 to 10 μ versus 10 to 100 μ) (230). The microspheres consist of an internal gas (air in the case of Albunex and Levovist and a fluorocarbon [octafluoropropane] for contrast enhancement in the case of Optison and Definity) encapsulated by an external shell (aggregated albumin in the case of Albunex and Optison, galactose in the case of Levovist, and lipid in the case of Definity). After an intravenous injection, the microspheres will follow the downstream course of the blood into the right heart and pulmonary vasculature. The microspheres are sufficiently small and, in the case of Optison and Definity, the diffusion of the inert gas is sufficiently limited by its low partition coefficient that the microspheres pass through the capillary bed into the left heart. Because the acoustic impedance of the microspheres is much lower than that of the blood, the ultrasound waves are scattered and reflected at the microsphere–blood interface.

Technique

All contrast agents are activated by suspending the microspheres through agitation of the vial (either by hand or in the case of Definity by a commercially supplied small mechanical agitator). The contrast agent can then be administered intravenously by infusion or bolus. Although pediatric dosages have not been established, 50% of the adult dose produces excellent left heart opacification without side effects (231) (Fig. 6.62). Contrast effect persists for approximately 3 to 5 minutes. The ultrasound system should be set to low power or mechanical index so that bubble destruction is minimized. With this setting, the myocardium will appear black and the contrast-filled cavity will be white. Adverse reactions have not been reported in children; in adults, adverse reactions are extremely rare and when present consist of allergic reaction, headache, flushing, and nausea. In the presence of an intracardiac shunt, the microspheres can bypass filtering by the lung

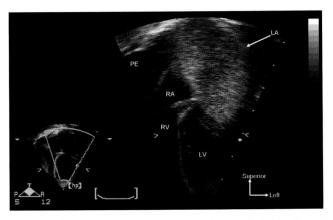

FIGURE 6.61 Apical four-chamber view during administration of agitated saline contrast in the left antecubital vein demonstrates dense opacification of the left atrium (LA) supportive of the suspected diagnosis of a left superior vena cava draining directly into the roof of the left atrium. (This patient also has a moderate pericardial effusion [PE]). LV, left ventricle; RA, right atrium; RV, right ventricle.

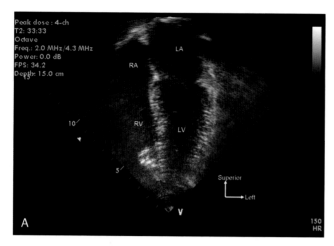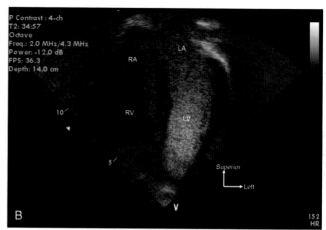

FIGURE 6.62 Apical four-chamber views at peak heart rate during dobutamine stress echocardiogram without (**A**) and with (**B**) transpulmonary contrast agent. Although the noncontrast image (**A**) is reasonably clear and most wall segments can be identified, the contrast image (**B**) makes identification of all wall segments (particularly those at the apex) particularly easy. LA, left atrium; LV, left ventricle; RA, right atrium; RV, right ventricle.

and enter the arterial circulation directly. It is believed that the larger ($\leq 32\ \mu$) microspheres, which constitute a very small percentage of the total suspension and which are normally filtered by the lungs, can pass into the left heart and produce arterial occlusions in this setting. Therefore, no transpulmonary contrast agent should ever be administered to a patient with a known or suspected intracardiac shunt.

Indications

Currently, contrast agents are approved for the use of heart opacification and endocardial visualization only. Therefore, they are indicated when traditional echocardiographic modalities yield suboptimal myocardial and endocardial visualization. Most often this is necessary during stress echocardiography when visualization of all myocardial segments is required to adequately assess integrity or compromise of coronary perfusion (231). Other instances in which contrast agents are beneficial are in the evaluation of right ventricular function since the right ventricular endocardium and myocardium can be very difficult to visualize.

An active area of research interest is the use of contrast agents to noninvasively measure myocardial perfusion (232,233). Since the microspheres enter the left heart, they will also pass through the coronary arteries into the myocardium. Measurement of myocardial perfusion involves alternately first destroying these myocardial bubbles with a pulse of ultrasound and then immediately imaging for return of myocardial contrast enhancement owing to new microspheres transiting the coronary circulation. Although the technique is arduous, it has shown promise. In the pediatric population, investigators have used a variation of the technique intraoperatively during cardiopulmonary bypass with cardioplegia to demonstrate that myocardial inflammation may occur during cardioplegia delivery (234).

An extremely exciting potential use of contrast agents is for gene transfer (235,236). Despite the great promise of gene therapy in treating a wide variety of diseases, safe and tissue-specific delivery remains one of its major limitations. For example, viruses are efficient delivery systems but are associated with serious problems of immunogenicity and cytotoxicity. Delivery with plasmid DNA is safer, but the efficiency is poor. Microbubble ultrasound has been shown to enhance gene transfer most likely through production of small, transient, nonlethal cell membrane pores (sonoporation). Microbubbles act as cavitation nuclei that focus ultrasound energy and potentiate bioeffects including sonoporation. Microbubbles can be targeted to tissues by incorporating ligands such as antibodies or peptides. A transgene can be either mixed with or complexed to microbubbles, thus increasing the probability of genes entering specific cells.

TRANSESOPHAGEAL ECHOCARDIOGRAPHY

In 1991, Ritter (237) reported initial experience of biplane transesophageal echocardiography to evaluate congenital heart disease in patients as small as 2.4 kg without complications, and it later became clear that intraoperative echocardiography allowing immediate revision of initial repair improved patient outcome (238). In addition, transesophageal echocardiography has become standard for guidance of defect-closure devices during interventional catheterization procedures (239), guidance of balloon atrial septostomy, and evaluation for thrombi (240).

Approach

The probe should be inspected carefully for any defects before it is inserted into the oropharynx. Probe size should be chosen on the basis of the patient's weight. Esophageal intubation can be enhanced with the neck slightly flexed and the patient in a slight left lateral decubitus position. Under no circumstances should the probe be forced into the posterior pharynx; sometimes direct visualization with a laryngoscope for difficult intubations is necessary.

Probe manipulation consists of the transesophageal equivalents of transthoracic sweeps: sliding the transducer superiorly and inferiorly within the esophagus, rotating the transducer left and right at the patient's mouth, and changing the plane from transverse to longitudinal (or intermediate planes in the case of a multiplane transducer) (Fig. 6.63). The examination should proceed in a segmental manner with identification of the systemic venous return moving the transducer superiorly and inferiorly in the esophagus in the longitudinal and transverse views. The atrial septum should be examined in these same views. The tricuspid valve is best visualized in the transverse four-chamber view and the longitudinal plane with rightward rotation. The interventricular septum is visualized in the transverse four-chamber view, sweeping the longitudinal view from left to right, and in the transgastric views. The right ventricular outflow tract and pulmonary valve are seen in a superior transverse view, in the longitudinal view swept leftward from the aorta, and in the longitudinal gastric view. Pulmonary veins are best seen in the transverse plane with

sweeping right and left. The mitral valve is investigated from the transverse four-chamber view and the longitudinal plane with a far leftward sweep. The left ventricular outflow tract and the aorta are evaluated in a slightly superior sweep from the transverse four-chamber view and in the longitudinal view between the SVC and the pulmonary artery.

Complications from transesophageal echocardiography are rare; however, there are reports of upper-airway obstruction secondary to esophageal hematoma (241), compression of an aberrant right subclavian artery (242), accidental endotracheal tube extubation, and esophageal burns and tears resulting from defective or improperly maintained probes.

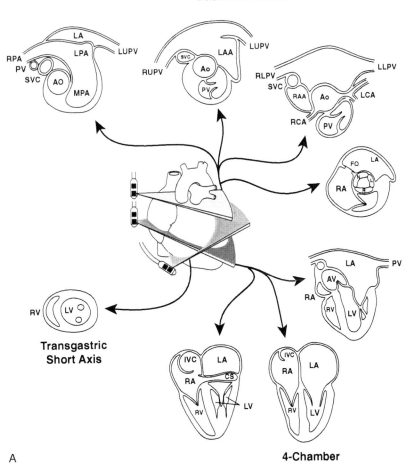

FIGURE 6.63 There are two basic imaging planes used in pediatric transesophageal echocardiography: the horizontal imaging plane (**A**) and the vertical imaging plane (**B**). Omniplane probes can image at planes intermediate between these two. Imaging can be performed in three basic esophageal positions: the midesophagus, the upper esophagus at the base of the heart, and transgastrically. Horizontal-plane imaging in the midesophagus provides the four-chamber view, coronary sinus view, and pulmonary vein view. Horizontal imaging in the higher esophagus provides views of the base of the heart, including the aorta, coronary arteries, pulmonary valve, branch pulmonary arteries, pulmonary veins, and superior vena cava. Horizontal imaging in the transgastric view yields a short-axis view of the ventricles. Vertical imaging in the midesophagus provides views of the left ventricular outflow tract and the mitral valve. Vertical imaging in the higher esophagus provides views of the right ventricular outflow tract, main pulmonary artery, branch pulmonary arteries, left ventricular outflow tract, aorta, superior vena cava, and atrial septum. Transgastric vertical plane imaging provides images of the left ventricular and right ventricular outflow tracts. A, aorta; AO, aorta; AV, aortic valve; CS, coronary sinus; FO, foramen ovale; IVC, inferior vena cava; LA, left atrium; LAA, left atrial appendage; LCA, left carotid artery; LLPV, left lower pulmonary valve; LPA, left pulmonary artery; LPV, left pulmonary valve; LUPV, left upper pulmonary valve; LV, left ventricle; MPA, main pulmonary artery; PV, pulmonary valve; RA, right atrium; RAA, right atrial appendage; RCA, right coronary artery; RPA, right pulmonary artery; RUPV, right upper pulmonary valve; RV, right ventricle; SVC, superior vena cava.

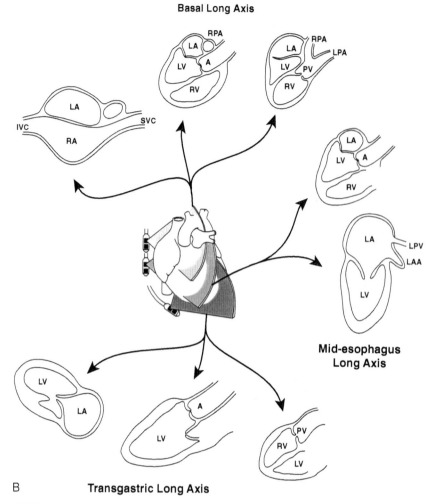

FIGURE 6.63 (*Continued*)

Intraoperative Transesophageal Echocardiography

The value of intraoperative transesophageal echocardiography is in evaluating residual problems relating to ventricular outflow tract obstruction, semilunar valve insufficiency, septal defects, atrioventricular valve insufficiency and stenosis, ventricular function, and wall motion abnormalities. Stevenson et al. (243) reported that reoperation occurred in 7.5% of cases as a result of residual findings on intraoperative transesophageal echocardiography. Ungerleider et al. (238) showed a similarly low rate of reoperation but also demonstrated a significant impact on length of stay and hospital costs for patients undergoing immediate reoperation because of intraoperative echocardiographic findings. In addition, the knowledge that a repair is satisfactory helps guide bypass weaning and immediate postoperative care. Although intraoperative imaging can confirm adequate surgical repair/palliation, findings can evolve postoperatively owing to changing hemodynamics, loading conditions, or other factors, which may make repeat imaging necessary or advisable. For example, the degree of mitral regurgitation seen on predischarge echocardiography agrees with the intraoperative transesophageal findings in only approximately 50% of studies in patients following repair of atrioventricular septal defects (244).

Guidance of Transcatheter Device Deployment

Transesophageal echocardiography has been of immense value in guiding interventional catheterization procedures (Fig. 6.64), in particular, device closure of atrial septal defect. The echocardiographer can guide the interventionalist in (a) placing the deployment sheath across the defect into the LA, (b) proper deployment of the LA and RA components of the device, (c) release of the device, and (d) evaluation of residual shunts. Particularly important is ensuring that the device straddles the atrial septum, does not occlude systemic and pulmonary venous returns, and does not interfere with atrioventricular valve function (Fig. 6.65). Transesophageal echocardiography also facilitates transcatheter closure of a ventricular septal defect (239) and has been used to assist atrial septoplasty, particularly in the setting of hypoplastic left heart syndrome with highly restrictive atrial septum (245).

Evaluation for Thrombi and Complications of Endocarditis

Consideration of performing transesophageal echocardiography should be given when there is suspicion of thrombi (i.e., because of neurologic changes, dysrhythmias, spontaneous

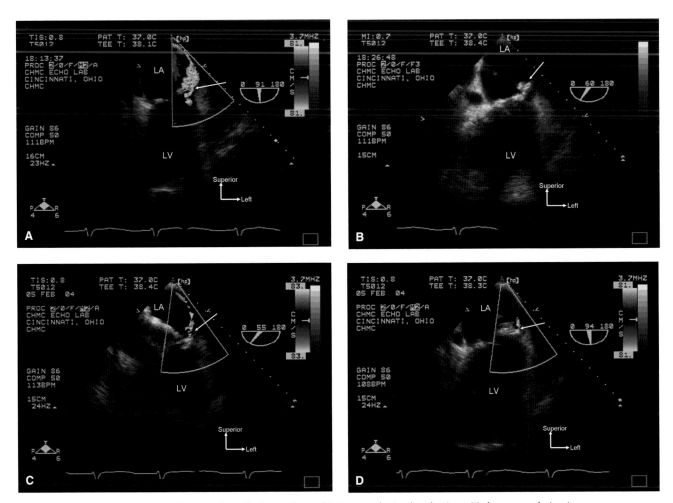

FIGURE 6.64 Transesophageal echocardiographic images obtained with 60- to 90-degree angulation in a 14-year-old male with a perivalvular abscess of the mitral valve following mitral valve replacement. In **A**, there is a moderate to severe perivalvar leak (*arrow*). In **B**, the catheter is seen crossing the atrial septum and coursing into the left atrium (LA). At the tip of the catheter (*arrow*) is a patent ductus arteriosus (PDA) closure device that is being positioned in the perivalvar leak. In **C**, the device has not yet been released from the catheter. Nevertheless, there is a marked decrease in the size of the perivalvar color jet. In **D**, the device has been released and there is a trivial perivalvar leak (*arrow*). LV, left ventricle.

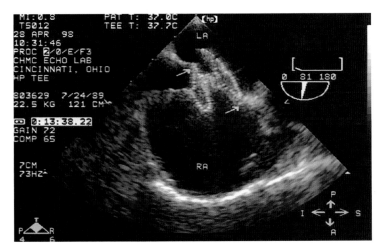

FIGURE 6.65 Near-vertical imaging plane view of the atrial septum in a patient undergoing closure of an atrial septal defect with Amplatzer's device. The left atrial (LA) and right atrial (RA) disks have been deployed, but the device remains securely attached to the catheter coursing from the inferior vena cava. There is some torque on the device, causing some displacement of the atrial septum out of a vertical orientation. Careful imaging demonstrates the atrial septum coursing between the two disks (*arrows*). A, anterior; I, inferior; P, posterior; S, superior.

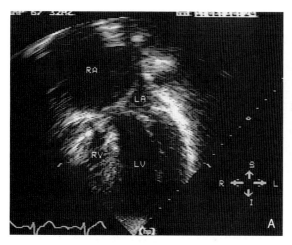 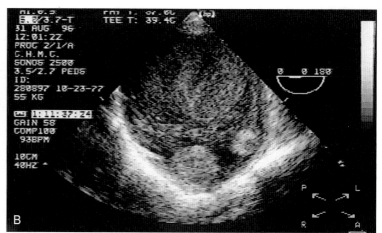

FIGURE 6.66 A: Transthoracic apical four-chamber view in an adolescent patient with pulmonary atresia and intact ventricular septum who had previously undergone a classic Fontan procedure with the right atrium (RA) directly anastomosed to the pulmonary artery. The electrocardiogram shows atrial fibrillation/flutter. The patient was being evaluated for the possibility of thrombi before DC cardioversion. This echocardiogram revealed no obvious thrombi. In particular, the RA appeared free of thrombus. **B:** Transesophageal echocardiogram of the right atrium in the horizontal plane. There is marked spontaneous contrast indicative of a thrombogenic milieu. In addition, there are two large thrombi on the RA free wall. Further imaging revealed thrombi in the midcavity of the RA and at the inferior vena cava orifice. Transthoracic echocardiography may lead to false-negative results, and transesophageal echocardiography is often necessary to evaluate for thrombi, particularly in patients with classic Fontan operation. A, anterior; I, inferior; LA, left atrium; LV, left ventricle; P, posterior; RV, right ventricle.

contrast on the transthoracic echocardiogram). Patients with the Fontan procedure, particularly those with an atriopulmonary anastomosis, are at high risk for developing thrombi in the RA, IVC, or pulmonary artery (240) (Fig. 6.66).

Transesophageal echocardiography (TEE) may have utility in the evaluation of suspected infective endocarditis in children but may not be necessary when transthoracic imaging is adequate (246,247). Although TEE has been shown to be significantly more sensitive that transthoracic echo in diagnosing valvular vegetations and abscesses in adults with suspected endocarditis (248–250), higher-quality acoustic windows in the pediatric population in general may negate the improvements in diagnostic sensitivity seen with use of TEE in adults (246,247). Moreover, the use of TEE in children is generally performed under conditions of endotracheal intubation and deep sedation/anesthesia, making the performance of TEE more invasive in this population. Therefore, TEE should be performed in any patient with suspected endocarditis in whom the transthoracic study is negative or inconclusive owing to technical inadequacies. Alternatively, in the patient with confirmed endocarditis, TEE may be useful in more fully delineating the cardiac sequelae, such as perivalvar abscess and extent of vegetations (247).

THREE-DIMENSIONAL ECHOCARDIOGRAPHY

The goal of the echocardiographic examination is to create and convey a 3-D reconstruction of the heart. Currently, 3-D reconstruction is a mental process. This can be vastly improved on by an actual reconstruction. Three-dimensional images can be produced with any medical imaging technique, but echocardiography is uniquely qualified because images are

tomographic, are acquired at a relatively high rate, can be triggered to an appropriate phase of the electrocardiogram, and can be acquired from any angle.

Evolution of current three-dimensional ultrasound systems progressed from static to dynamic, and ultimately, to real-time 3-D imaging. Static 3-D images were initially obtained from a single volume of voxels—a volume of pixels—by sweeping the ultrasound transducer through the area of interest. Although this can be achieved by sweeping the ultrasound probe through the area of interest by linear, fanlike, or rotational sweeps, the most common method ultimately became rotational acquisition (251,252). Dynamic 3-D imaging is also possible, but portrayal of the heart in motion was dependent on reconstruction algorithms that were in turn dependent on 2-D image quality and were often deemed impractical owing to the long and tedious nature of data acquisition and data analysis. The current state of the art in 3-D imaging is represented by real-time 3-D imaging. Several recently developed ultrasound systems (253) feature matrix-array transducers that allow acquisition of high-quality, pyramidal image volumes in real time.

Research indicates that right ventricular volumes can be measured accurately (254–256). This information may be helpful in evaluating right ventricular size in patients with relative right ventricular hypoplasia (e.g., in pulmonary atresia with intact ventricular septum) and evaluating right ventricular function (e.g., in cardiomyopathy, tetralogy of Fallot, and transposition of great vessels with Senning and Mustard operation). Recently, Altmann et al. (257) showed that 3-D echocardiographic measurements of single ventricular volume and mass are also accurate and suggest that this technique will be valuable in planning palliation with the Fontan procedure. With 3-D echocardiography, anatomy can be viewed from unique perspectives, for example, that of the surgeon (258)

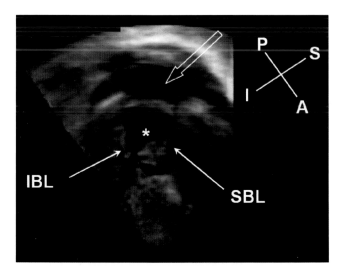

FIGURE 6.67 Three-dimensional imaging of an atrioventricular septal defect. Three-dimensional image processing of this apical view has removed the right atrial and ventricular free walls and allows visualization of the right atrial and right ventricular septal surface, including imaging of the primum atrial septal defect (*open arrow*) and inlet ventricular septal defect (*asterisk*). The superior (SBL) and inferior (IBL) bridging leaflets of the common atrioventricular valve can also be seen. S, superior; I, inferior; A, anterior; P, posterior. (Image courtesy of Dr. Girish Shirali, Medical University of South Carolina.)

(Fig. 6.67). In addition, particularly complex anatomy may be better visualized (259). This may be specifically useful in determining the relation of the ventricular septal defect to the great vessels in double-outlet right ventricle. Advances in three-dimensional ultrasound processing and faster computing times have currently made real-time three-dimensional imaging possible (260), which is likely to lead to its more widespread use in the future.

DIGITAL ECHOCARDIOGRAPHY

The analogue laboratory of our immediate past collects nondiscrete, analogue waveform signals of varying voltage that are stored to videotape, conforming to the National Television Standards set in the 1940s. Benefits of digital technology include the ability to preserve image quality, simplify and speed access to studies for analysis and comparison, and generate reports with embedded images.

Digital technology stores the gray scale of each of the pixels of the echocardiographic image into a series of binary digits. The depth of binary storage dictates the resolution. For example, an 8-bit depth binary system stores the image as series of eight digits (e.g., 00000000, 00000001, and so on) providing for 2^8, or 256, shades of gray. This level is more than sufficient when one considers that the human eye can distinguish only 50 shades of gray. The digital image has almost complete fidelity to the true real-time image.

However, digital imaging comes with a considerable storage burden. Typically, a freeze-frame ultrasound image has 512 lines of information with 512 samples per line, resulting in approximately 262,000 pixels per frame. Each pixel is described by an 8-bit binary system, resulting in approximately 2 million bits of data to describe a single frame. At ultrasound frame rates of 45 frames per second, it therefore

requires 283 megabytes of storage to save a single 3-second (approximately five-beat) sweep. A typical study of 60 to 80 clips and a few still frames approaches 20 to 25 gigabytes of data! Guidelines for the management of this massive amount of digital echocardiographic data have been developed by the American Society of Echocardiography (261).

Compression of digital data aids in practical storage and transmission. There are two types of compression: lossless and lossy. Lossless compression ensures that no data are lost but provides only a modest 3:1 reduction in data storage. Lossy compression (e.g., Joint Photography Expert Group method) reduces data storage by 20:1, allowing transmission of video through computer networks and without loss of image quality compared with super VHS video (262). The Motion Picture Expert Group (MPEG) method is a second compression process that uses a motion picture prediction algorithm exploiting redundancy between preceding and subsequent images, thereby offering better motion-image quality, higher compression ratios (e.g., 1,500:1), and easier integration into a computer network. Disadvantages to MPEG compression are that it is not yet validated for echocardiography, is not standardized within DICOM (the Digital Imaging and Communications in Medicine standard), and has inferior still-frame image quality (263,264).

Despite the large amount of data created with digital echocardiographic image acquisition, image management has been relatively facile and has indeed improved efficiency in the pediatric echocardiography laboratory (265). As computer technology continues its steady improvements in data management efficiency, digital echocardiography techniques will become even more sophisticated with teaching and research images existing as part of web-based journal articles (266) and clinical images transferred easily through web-based networks and onto personal digital devices.

RESEARCH ECHOCARDIOGRAPHY

Because of its ease of use, portability, low cost, absence of side effects, and high diagnostic accuracy; echocardiography is a robust research tool. Echocardiography has been used successfully to provide mechanistic insights on disease processes and therapeutic outcomes, to provide both cross-sectional and longitudinal data in large epidemiologic studies, and to measure functional and structural changes now considered to be end points. The Framingham Heart Study was the first epidemiologic study to use echocardiographic measurements (267). The single largest application of echocardiography in epidemiologic studies has been the measurement of left ventricular mass and its change with antihypertensive therapy (65,79,268–270). Recently, the use of echocardiography has been expanded to clinical trials investigating cardiac resynchronization therapy for congestive heart failure (271–274). In addition, echocardiography is the major tool for providing detailed phenotypes for large human genetic studies (275).

The use of echocardiography for any research purpose necessitates establishing methods to limit measurement variability. Intraobserver and interobserver variability needs to be measured and repeated periodically. Protocols for training qualification need to be developed. A minimum number of sonographers and readers should be used to limit the effects of interobserver variability. Only contemporary equipment should be used. Digital archiving should be established to

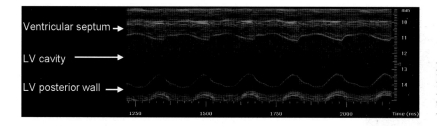

FIGURE 6.68 An M-mode echocardiogram of the left ventricle of a mouse using a high-frequency (40 MHz) transducer demonstrates excellent resolution of the ventricular septum, left ventricular cavity, and left ventricular posterior wall.

provide a bioinformatic data bank of echocardiographic images. These practices are best established by the creation of a core research laboratory (276,277).

Echocardiography has also been instrumental in animal research, most notably in the phenotyping of transgenic mice (278–283). Previous phenotyping methods (Langendorf preparation, histologic examination) necessitated sacrifice of the animal. This prohibited not only acquisition of longitudinal data and but also further breeding. Mouse echocardiography is performed using high-frequency transducers (≤15 MHz) while the animal is anesthetized with 2% inhaled isoflurane and kept warm on a heated examination table. Parasternal and apical images are obtained, and quantitative data include left ventricular dimensions, function, mass, and aortic and mitral valve Doppler velocities (Fig. 6.68). If the animal has undergone microcatheterization of the left ventricle or a systemic artery, pressure data can be coupled with simultaneous echocardiographic left ventricular dimensional data to create pressure–dimension loops or end-systolic wall stress data, powerful indices of ventricular function (see above) (Fig. 6.69) (283).

Recently, the development of high-frequency ultrasound transducers (30 to 70 MHz) has allowed imaging of hearts in mouse pups or even mouse embryos (284–290). This echocardiographic technique, more appropriately called ultrasound biomicroscopy, involves mounting the anesthetized pup or pregnant ewe on a microscope stage embedded with heating elements to keep the animal warm and which can be moved spatially in x, y, and z planes using three micromanipulator knobs just as when using a microscope. Embryonic mice imaging is extremely valuable since many transgenic mice models are embryonic lethal. Doppler signals are apparent as early as the eighth embryonic day, essentially the heart tube stage (gestational age of mouse, 18.5 days). Four chambers can be identified with echocardiography at embryonic day 11.5, and septation is evident by ultrasound at embryonic day 13.5. Resolution has improved significantly with these higher-frequency transducers such that it will now be possible to phenotype transgenic mice models targeted for maldevelopment of the cardiac valves.

HAND-CARRIED ULTRASOUND DEVICES

Because of continued miniaturization of computer and ultrasound equipment, hand-carried ultrasound devices have been used for medical diagnostics. Most of these devices now have the capabilities of even the most technologically advanced ultrasound systems but are the size of a laptop computer or less and weigh between 5 to 10 pounds. Using such devices, echocardiographers can provide point-of-service care more effectively. More important, these devices expand the community that can now receive and benefit from the diagnostic power of echocardiography. In addition, the devices improve diagnostic accuracy by complementing the cardiac physical.

Although auscultation has been the traditional foundation of the cardiac physical examination, many primary care physicians and even some cardiologists have imperfect auscultatory skills. For example, diagnostic accuracy of current resident physicians using auscultation alone is notoriously poor (291–293). It is likely that these skills will continue to decline as resident physicians cope with the competing forces of having to learn vast amounts of newer medical information within the time constraints imposed by resident work-hour regulations. Hand-carried ultrasound devices extend the diagnostic accuracy of echocardiography from the ultrasound lab-

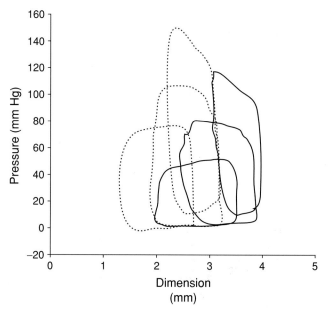

FIGURE 6.69 Left ventricular pressure-dimension loops in control mice (*thin lines*) and hypothyroid mice (*thick lines*) derived from simultaneous M-mode echocardiography and catheterization of the left ventricle. Afterload was manipulated with phenylephrine and nitroprusside infusion to create a family of pressure–dimension loops from which end-systolic relations can be measured. At any given end-systolic dimension, the end-systolic pressure is less in the hypothyroid mice versus the control mice, indicating depressed contractility in the hypothyroid mice. (From Williams RV, Lorenz JN, Witt SA, et al. End-systolic stress-velocity and pressure-dimension relationships by transthoracic echocardiography in mice. *Am J Physiol* 1998;274 (pt 2):H1828–H1835.)

oratory to the time and place of the physical examination. By complementing stethoscope use with a handheld system, an examiner can not only *hear* the heart but *see* it as well, thereby improving diagnostic accuracy (294). Implementation of a hand-carried ultrasound device program into the medical school curriculum significantly increases the diagnostic accuracy of the physical examination performed by medical students (295). Even the accuracy of the cardiovascular examination performed by board-certified cardiologists is enhanced by their use of a hand-carried device (296,297). In pediatrics, handheld ultrasound has been shown to have similar diagnostic accuracy as traditional ultrasound systems, and its use is speculated to only increase (298).

The increased availability of echocardiography made possible by hand-carried devices has tempted other noncardiac specialists to practice cardiac ultrasound (299,300). Although this has the potential benefit of enhancing overall patient care by improving diagnostic accuracy, it also emphasizes the need for responsible practice of ultrasound. It is the duty of the echocardiography community to develop standards for the practice of hand-carried ultrasound and ensure that they are met. The situation is similar to stethoscope use. Most physicians who use a stethoscope are not cardiologists, the diagnostic accuracy of the stethoscope varies according to its user, and cardiologists have greater expertise in its use. Likewise, the future of hand-carried ultrasound devices will certainly involve broad usage by various health care providers, many not cardiologists. However, as with the stethoscope, it would be expected and need to be indoctrinated as standard of care, that when a noncardiologist identified a patient with suspected pathology using a handheld device, the patient would be referred to a cardiologist for further evaluation.

The development and expansion of handheld ultrasound devices speaks to us as physicians, specifically, to the reasons as to why many of us chose medicine as our career. We have a powerful, robust tool in echocardiography; a tool with which we can do much good by providing very advanced medical care to an even vaster population. There is great value in the fact that handheld devices allow us to provide increased availability to our tertiary care populations at surrounding satellite clinics, improving medical care by obviating the need for lengthy, stressful, and time-consuming journeys to the central facility. But there is perhaps greater value and meaning in the fact that handheld devices allow us to spread echocardiographic technology to those patients who would otherwise never benefit from it—the patients using the underserved urban and rural health clinics and the patients in developing countries (301–303). As investigators from the Cedars Sinai Medical Center state, it is this use of echocardiography that truly makes "an impossible mission possible" (302).

APPENDIX 6.1

Nomograms for newborn annular diameter versus patient weight for the tricuspid valve (**A**), pulmonary valve (**B**), mitral valve from the apical view (**C**), the mitral valve from the long axis view (**C**), and the aortic valve (**D**) as a function of newborn patient weight. (From Tacey TA, Vermillion PR, Ludomirsky A. Range of normal valve annulus size in neonates. *Am J Cardiol* 1995;75:542, with permission.)

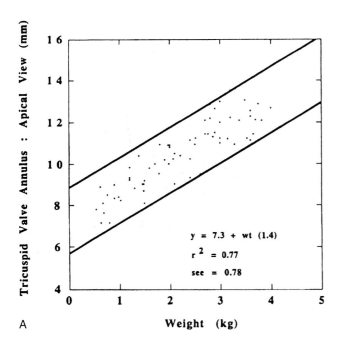

$$y = 7.3 + wt\ (1.4)$$
$$r^2 = 0.77$$
$$see = 0.78$$

A

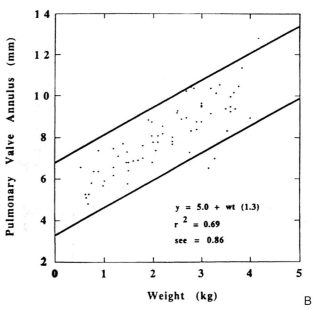

$$y = 5.0 + wt\ (1.3)$$
$$r^2 = 0.69$$
$$see = 0.86$$

B

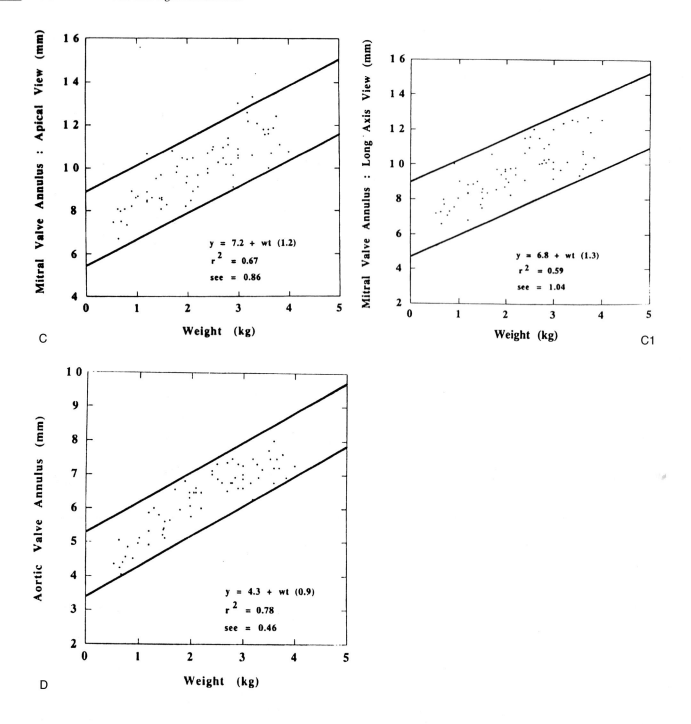

C

C1

D

APPENDIX 6.2

Nomograms for infant and children echocardiographic dimensional indices versus body surface area from which z-values (y-axis of each figure) can be obtained. Definitions of each index and the echocardiographic view from which they were obtained are shown in the first Table. An exact Z value can be calculated from the equation:

$$Z = [ln(measured\ structure) - ln(mean\ normal\ value)] \div (root\ mean\ square\ error)$$

where

$$ln(mean\ normal\ value) = intercept + (multiplier)(ln\ BSA)$$

and the intercept, multiplier, and root mean square error are obtained for each echocardiographic index from the second table. (From Daubeney PEF, Blackstone EH, Weintraub RG, et al. Relationship of the dimension of cardiac structures to body size: an echocardiographic study in normal infants and children. *Cardiol Young* 1999;9:402–410, with permission.)

TABLE 1

SUMMARY OF CARDIAC DIMENSIONS MEASURED, ECHOCARDIOGRAPHIC VIEWS USED AND THE DEFINITIONS OF EACH MEASUREMENT

Cardiac Dimension	Echocardiographic View	Definition
Tricuspid valve	Apical four chamber	Distance between 'hinge points' of leaflets at level of annulus
RV inflow	Apical four chamber	Ventricular length from midpoint of plane of tricuspid valve annulus to apex of RV
RV outflow	Subcostal parasagitcal	Length from diaphragmatic surface of RV to midpoint of pulmonary valve
RV area	Apical four chamber	Maximal area bordered by RV endocardium
RV-pulmonary junction	Parasternal short axis	Distance between 'hinge points' of attachment of the valve
Pulmonary crunk	Parasternal short axis	Diameter of pulmonary trunk halfway between pulmonary valve and bifurcation
Right pulmonary artery	Parasternal short axis	Diameter immediately beyond bifurcation
Left pulmonary artery	Parasternal short axis	Diameter immediately beyond bifurcation
Mitral valve (antero-posterior)	Parasternal long axis	Distance between 'hinge points' of leaflets at level of annulus
Mitral valve (lateral)	Apical four chamber	Distance between 'hinge points' of leaflets at level of annulus
LV inflow	Apical four chamber	Ventricular length from midpoint of place of mitral valve annulus to apex of LV
LV area	Apical four chamber	Maximal area bordered by LV endocardium
LV-aortic junction	Parasternal long axis	Distance between 'hinge points' of attachment of the valve
Sinuses of Valsalva	Parasternal long axis	Maximum antero-posterior diameter of aortic root at level of sinuses of Valsalva
Sinotubular junction	Parasternal long axis	Maximum antero-posterior diameter of aortic root at level of sinotubular junction

LV, left ventricular; RV, right ventricular.

TABLE 2

REGRESSION EQUATIONS RELATING CARDIAC DIMENSION AND BODY SURFACE AREA ARE SHOWN, AS WELL AS THE REGRESSION COEFFICIENT, ROOT MEAN SQUARE ERROR, AND THE COMPLETE VARIANCE-COVARIANCE MATRIX

Structure	n	Intercept	Multiplier	Root-mean Square Error	Variance 10^4 (intercept)	Variance 10^4 (multiplier)	Covariance* 10^4	Correlation Coefficient
Tricuspid valve	120	1.084	0.4945	0.08121	0.8031	1.144	0.5386	0.97
RV inflow	119	1.823	0.4962	0.1086	1.451	2.052	0.9709	0.95
RV outflow	101	1.943	0.6185	0.1009	1.696	2.327	1.265	0.97
RV area	116	2.795	0.9566	0.1753	3.821	5.484	2.537	0.97
RV-pulmonary junction	105	0.6367	0.5028	0.1143	1.909	2.429	1.271	0.95
Pulmonary trunk	80	0.6067	0.4941	0.1430	4.503	4.918	3.095	0.93
Right pulmonary artery	81	0.1396	0.5495	0.1294	3.774	4.087	2.642	0.95
Left pulmonary artery	112	0.2024	0.6039	0.1446	3.075	3.844	2.155	0.94
Mitral valve (antero-posterior)	124	0.9445	0.5022	0.09403	1.017	1.538	0.6836	0.96
Mitral valve (lateral)	124	0.9651	0.4658	0.09167	0.9664	1.452	0.6475	0.96
LV inflow	121	1.893	0.4936	0.09847	1.164	1.713	0.7878	0.96
LV area	120	3.141	1.020	0.1806	3.956	5.778	2.673	0.97
LV-aortic junction	122	0.5183	0.5347	0.06726	0.5248	0.7887	0.3484	0.98
Sinuses of Valsalva	122	0.7224	0.5082	0.07284	0.6154	0.9250	0.4086	0.98
Sinotubular junction	85	0.5417	0.5490	0.08656	1.439	1.7260	0.9437	0.98

LV, left ventricular; RV, right ventricular.
The form of the equation is: *ln (mean normal value of structure = intercept + multiplier · ln (BSA)*; where ln (*) is the natural logarithm and BSA is body surface area (m²). The structures are expressed in cm or cm². Z can then be calculated: Z = (In [measured structure] − ln (mean normal value)])/root-mean square error.

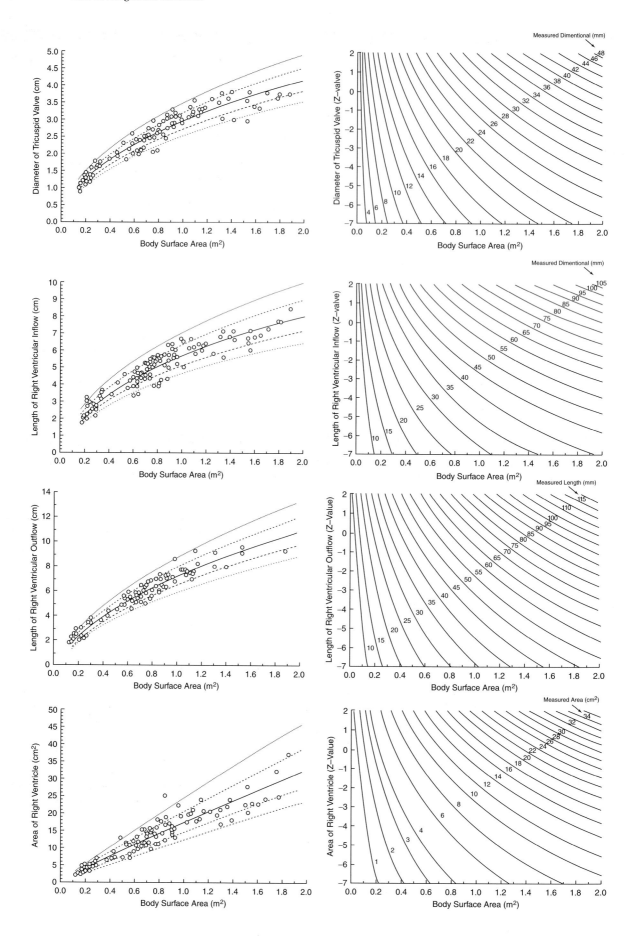

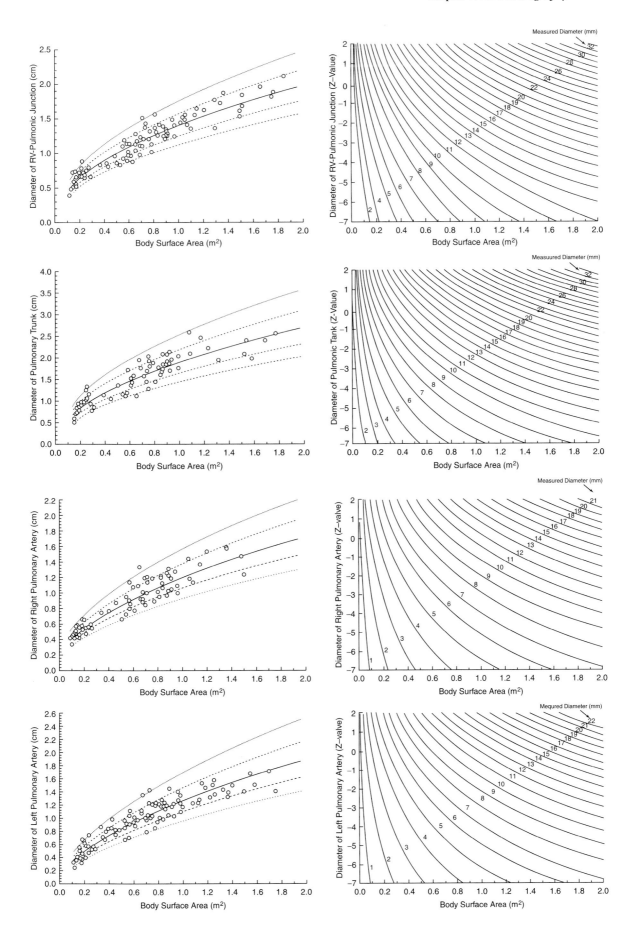

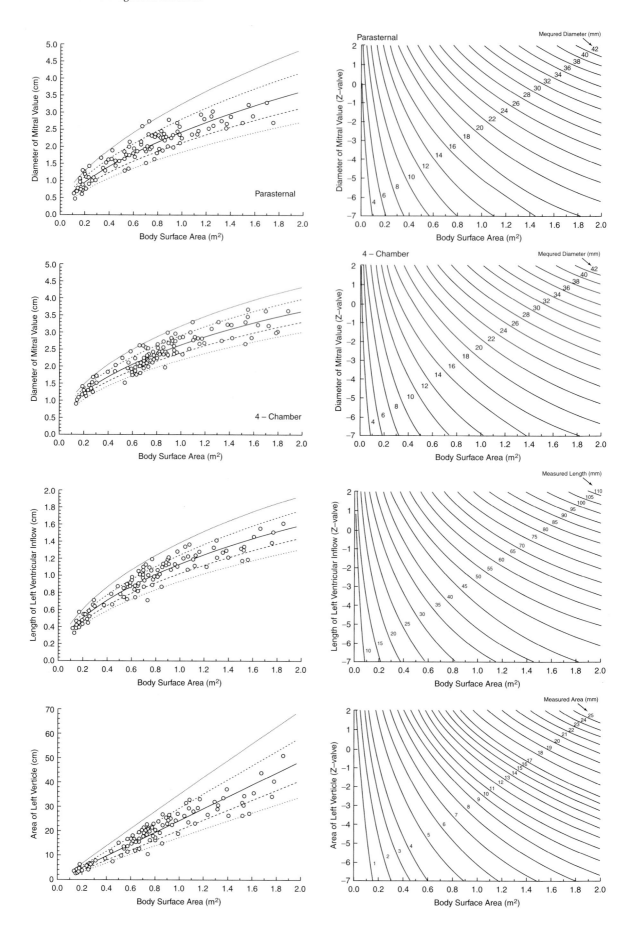

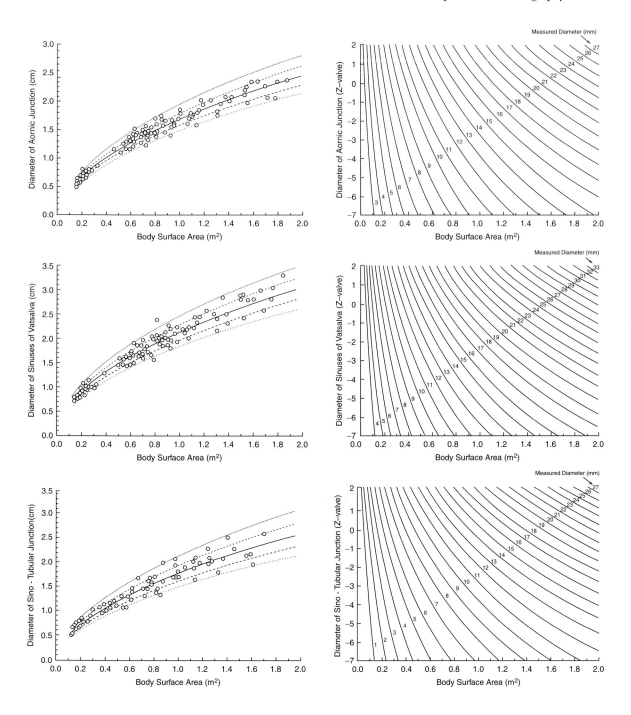

APPENDIX 6.3 ■ REFERENCE RANGES FOR ATRIOVENTRICULAR VALVE DOPPLER INDICES BY AGE

Reference	Age Range (y)	MV E Velocity (cm/s)	MV A Velocity (cm/s)	MV E/A Velocity Ratio	MV E-Wave DT (ms)	LV IVRT (ms)	TV E Velocity (cm/s)	TV A Velocity (cm/s)	TV E/A Velocity Ratio
O'Leary et al. (1998)	3–8	92 ± 14	42 ± 11	2.4 ± 0.7	145 ± 18	62 ± 10			
	9–12	86 ± 15	41 ± 9	2.2 ± 0.6	157 ± 19	67 ± 10			
	13–17	88 ± 14	39 ± 8	2.3 ± 0.6	172 ± 22	74 ± 13			
Eidem et al. (2004)	<1	80 ± 19	65 ± 13	1.2 ± 0.3			53 ± 12	53 ± 13	1.0 ± 0.4
	1–5	95 ± 20	61 ± 12	1.6 ± 0.5			62 ± 13	48 ± 12	1.3 ± 0.3
	6–9	94 ± 15	49 ± 13	2.0 ± 0.5			61 ± 14	42 ± 11	1.5 ± 0.4
	10–13	95 ± 16	50 ± 14	2.0 ± 0.6			60 ± 11	39 ± 11	1.6 ± 0.5
	14–18	90 ± 18	46 ± 13	2.1 ± 0.7			60 ± 11	35 ± 11	1.9 ± 0.6

MV, mitral valve; DT, deceleration time; LV IVRT, left ventricle isovolumic relaxation time; TV, tricuspid valve.

APPENDIX 6.4 ■ REFERENCE VALUES FOR PULMONARY VENOUS DOPPLER FLOW INDICES BY AGE

Reference	Age Range (y)	PV S Velocity (cm/s)	PV D Velocity (cm/s)	PV S/D Velocity Ratio	PV A Velocity (cm/s)	PV A Duration (ms)
O'Leary et al. (1998)	3–8	46 ± 9	59 ± 8	0.8 ± 0.2	21 ± 4	130 ± 20
	9–12	45 ± 9	54 ± 9	0.8 ± 0.2	21 ± 5	125 ± 20
	13–17	41 ± 10	59 ± 11	0.7 ± 0.2	21 ± 7	140 ± 28
Eidem et al. (2004)	<1	45 ± 10	46 ± 10		16 ± 6	
	1–5	48 ± 9	55 ± 11		21 ± 4	
	6–9	51 ± 11	53 ± 11		20 ± 4	
	10–13	49 ± 11	58 ± 12		21 ± 5	
	14–18	48 ± 7	58 ± 15		20 ± 5	

PV, pulmonary venous.

APPENDIX 6.5 ■ REFERENCE RANGES FOR LONGITUDINAL ANNULAR VELOCITY INDICES BY AGE

Reference	Age Range (y)	MV E_a Velocity (cm/s)	MV A_a Velocity (cm/s)	LV ICT (ms)	LV IVRT (ms)	MV E/E_a Ratio	TV E_a Velocity (cm/s)	TV A_a Velocity (cm/s)	RV ICT (ms)	RV IVRT (ms)	TV E/E_a Ratio
Frommelt et al. (2002)	<1						12 ± 4	10 ± 2	38 ± 14	30 ± 29	
	>1						18 ± 3	10 ± 3	57 ± 13	24 ± 20	
Swaminathan et al. (2003)	1–3	17 ± 3	8 ± 2				15 ± 2	10 ± 2			
	4–6	20 ± 3	8 ± 2				16 ± 3	10 ± 2			
	7–9	19 ± 4	7 ± 2				16 ± 3	8 ± 2			
	10–12	18 ± 2	7 ± 2				15 ± 2	8 ± 2			
	13–15	19 ± 3	7 ± 2				15 ± 2	8 ± 2			
	16–18	18 ± 2	7 ± 2				16 ± 3	9 ± 2			
Eidem et al. 2004	<1	10 ± 3	6 ± 2	77 ± 18	57 ± 15	8.8 ± 2.7	14 ± 8	10 ± 2	69 ± 18	52 ± 13	4.4 ± 2.3
	1–5	15 ± 3	7 ± 2	77 ± 16	62 ± 13	6.5 ± 2.0	17 ± 4	11 ± 3	78 ± 15	59 ± 14	3.8 ± 1.1
	6–9	17 ± 4	7 ± 2	78 ± 19	63 ± 12	5.8 ± 1.9	17 ± 3	10 ± 3	92 ± 22	59 ± 18	3.6 ± 0.8
	10–13	20 ± 3	6 ± 2	77 ± 16	63 ± 12	4.9 ± 1.3	17 ± 3	10 ± 3	98 ± 22	62 ± 20	3.5 ± 1.4
	14–18	21 ± 4	7 ± 2	79 ± 17	70 ± 16	4.7 ± 1.3	17 ± 3	10 ± 3	102 ± 20	63 ± 19	3.7 ± 1.0

MV, mitral valve; LV ICT, left ventricle isovolumic contraction time; IVRT, isovolumic relaxation time; TV, tricuspid valve; RV, right ventricle.

References

1. Tworetzky W, et al. Echocardiographic diagnosis alone for the complete repair of major congenital heart defects. *J Am Coll Cardiol* 1999;33(1):228–233.

2. Kelves BH. Looking through women: The development of ultrasound and mammography. In: *Naked to the Bone: Medical Imaging in the Twentieth Century*. Reading, MA: Addison-Wesley; 1997:228–250.

3. Goldberg BB, Kimmelman BA. *Medical Diagnostic Ultrasound: A Retrospective on its 40th Anniversary*. Rochester, NY: Eastman Kodak Company; 1988:2–19.

4. Goldberg SJ, Allen HD, Sahn DJ. Pediatric and Adolescent Echocardiography: A Handbook. Chicago, IL: Year Book Medical Publishers; 1975.

5. Baylen B, et al. Left ventricular performance in the critically ill premature infant with patent ductus arteriosus and pulmonary disease. *Circulation* 1977;55(1):182–188.

6. Snider AR, et al. Congenital left ventricular inflow obstruction evaluated by two-dimensional echocardiography. *Circulation* 1980;61(4):848–855.

7. Clyman RI, et al. Prenatal administration of betamethasone for prevention of patent ductus arteriosus. *J Pediatr* 1981;98(1):123–126.

8. Snider AR, et al. Doppler evaluation of left ventricular diastolic filling in children with systemic hypertension. *Am J Cardiol* 1985;56(15):921–926.

9. Snider AR. Two-dimensional and Doppler echocardiographic evaluation of heart disease in the neonate and fetus. *Clin Perinatol* 1988;15(3):523–565.

10. Bierman FZ, Williams RG. Subxiphoid two-dimensional imaging of the interatrial septum in infants and neonates with congenital heart disease. *Circulation* 1979;60(1):80–90.

11. Bierman FZ, Williams RG. Prospective diagnosis of d-transposition of the great arteries in neonates by subxiphoid, two-dimensional echocardiography. *Circulation* 1979;60(7):1496–1502.

12. Bierman FZ, Fellows K, Williams RG. Prospective identification of ventricular septal defects in infancy using subxiphoid two-dimensional echocardiography. *Circulation* 1980;62(4):807–717.

13. van Doesburg NH, Bierman FZ, Williams RG. Left ventricular geometry in infants with d-transposition of the great arteries and intact interventricular septum. *Circulation* 1983;68(4):733–739.

14. Stevenson JG, Kawabori I, Guntheroth WG. Noninvasive detection of pulmonary hypertension in patent ductus arteriosus by pulsed Doppler echocardiography. *Circulation* 1979;60(2):355–359.

15. Stevenson JG, et al. Pulsed Doppler echocardiographic evaluation of ventricular septal defect patches. *Circulation* 1984;70(3 Pt 2):I38–I46.

16. Hedrick WR, Hykes DL, Starchman DE. Ultrasound Physics and Instrumentation. St. Louis, MO: Mosby-Year Book; 1995:1–90.

17. Yoganathan AP, et al. Review of hydrodynamic principles for the cardiologist: Applications to the study of blood flow and jets by imaging techniques. *J Am Coll Cardiol* 1988;12(5):1344–1353.

18. Angelini P, Lopez-Velarde P, Leachman RD. Ventriculoarterial discordance revisited: Angiographic presentation and discussion of a typical case. *Tex Heart Inst J* 1988;15(3):174–182.

19. Kovalchin JP, et al. Echocardiographic determinants of clinical course in infants with critical and severe pulmonary valve stenosis. *J Am Coll Cardiol* 1997;29(5):1095–1101.

20. Kimball TR, et al. Color flow mapping to document normal pulmonary venous return in neonates with persistent pulmonary hypertension being considered for extracorporeal membrane oxygenation. *J Pediatr* 1989;114(3):433–437.

21. Van Praagh R, et al. Transposition of the great arteries with posterior aorta, anterior pulmonary artery, subpulmonary conus and fibrous continuity between aortic and atrioventricular valves. *Am J Cardiol* 1971;28(6):621–631.

22. de la Cruz MV, et al. The infundibular interrelationships and the ventriculoarterial connection in double outlet right ventricle. Clinical and surgical implications. *Int J Cardiol* 1992;35(2):153–164.

23. Pasquini L, et al. Conal anatomy in 119 patients with d-loop transposition of the great arteries and ventricular septal defect: An echocardiographic and pathologic study. *J Am Coll Cardiol* 1993;21(7):1712–1721.

24. Ahmetoglu A, et al. Hepatic vein flow pattern in children: Assesment with Doppler sonography. *Eur J Radiol* 2005;53(1):72–77.

25. Appleton CP, Hatle LK, Popp Rl. Superior vena cava and hepatic vein Doppler echocardiography in healthy adults. *J Am Coll Cardiol* 1987;10(5):1032–1039.

26. Klein AL, et al. Comprehensive Doppler assessment of right ventricular diastolic function in cardiac amyloidosis. *J Am Coll Cardiol* 1990;15(1):99–108.

27. Borganelli M, Byrd BF, 3rd. Doppler echocardiography in pericardial disease. *Cardiol Clin* 1990;8(2):333–348.

28. Zhang S, Kerins DM, Byrd BF, 3rd. Doppler echocardiography in cardiac tamponade and constrictive pericarditis. *Echocardiography* 1994;11(5):507–521.

29. Klein AL, et al. Differentiation of constrictive pericarditis from restrictive cardiomyopathy by Doppler transesophageal echocardiographic measurements of respiratory variations in pulmonary venous flow. *J Am Coll Cardiol* 1993;22(7):1935–1943.

30. Gomes Ferreira SM, et al. Constrictive chronic pericarditis in children. *Cardiol Young* 2001;11(2):210–213.

31. Abdalla IA, et al. Reversal of the pattern of respiratory variation of Doppler inflow velocities in constrictive pericarditis during mechanical ventilation. *J Am Soc Echocardiogr* 2000;13(9):827–831.

32. Smallhorn JF, et al. Pulsed Doppler echocardiographic assessment of the pulmonary venous pathway after the Mustard or Senning procedure for transposition of the great arteries. *Circulation* 1986;73(4):765–774.

33. Minich LL, et al. Abnormal Doppler pulmonary venous flow patterns in children after repaired total anomalous pulmonary venous connection. *Am J Cardiol* 1995;75(8):606–610.

34. Vick GW, 3rd, et al. Pulmonary venous and systemic ventricular inflow obstruction in patients with congenital heart disease: Detection by combined two-dimensional and Doppler echocardiography. *J Am Coll Cardiol* 1987;9(3):580–587.

35. Lin FC, et al. Doppler atrial shunt flow patterns in patients with secundum atrial septal defect: Determinants, limitations, and pitfalls. *J Am Soc Echocardiogr* 1988;1(2):141–149.

36. Goldfarb A, Chinitz LA, Kronzon I. High flow velocity across a complicated atrial septal defect: Doppler findings and hemodynamic correlations. *J Am Soc Echocardiogr* 1988;1(5):348–350.

37. Kronzon I, et al. Echocardiographic and hemodynamic characteristics of atrial septal defects created by percutaneous valvuloplasty. *J Am Soc Echocardiogr* 1990;3(1):64–71.

38. Mori K, Dohi T. Mitral and pulmonary vein blood flow patterns in cor triatriatum. *Am Heart J* 1989;117(5):1167–1169.

39. Tacy TA, Vermilion RP, Ludomirsky A. Range of normal valve annulus size in neonates. *Am J Cardiol* 1995;75(7):541–543.

40. Daubeney PE, et al. Relationship of the dimension of cardiac structures to body size: An echocardiographic study in normal infants and children. *Cardiol Young* 1999;9(4):402–410.

41. Gutgesell HP, Rembold CM. Growth of the human heart relative to body surface area. *Am J Cardiol* 1990;65(9):662–668.

42. Diwan A, et al. Doppler estimation of left ventricular filling pressures in patients with mitral valve disease. *Circulation* 2005;111(24):3281–3289.

43. Leeman DE, Levine MJ, Come PC. Doppler echocardiography in cardiac tamponade: Exaggerated respiratory variation in transvalvular blood flow velocity integrals. *J Am Coll Cardiol* 1988;11(3):572–578.

44. Enriquez-Sarano M, et al. Quantitative determinants of the outcome of asymptomatic mitral regurgitation. *N Engl J Med* 2005;352(9):875–883.

45. Nishimura RA, et al. Noninvasive measurement of rate of left ventricular relaxation by Doppler echocardiography. Validation with simultaneous cardiac catheterization. *Circulation* 1993;88(1):146–155.

46. Chen C, et al. Continuous wave Doppler echocardiography for noninvasive assessment of left ventricular dP/dt and relaxation time constant from mitral regurgitant spectra in patients. *J Am Coll Cardiol* 1994;23(4):970–976.

47. Chen C, et al. Noninvasive measurement of the time constant of left ventricular relaxation using the continuous-wave Doppler velocity profile of mitral regurgitation. *Circulation* 1992;86(1):272–278.

48. Levine RA, et al. Echocardiographic measurement of right ventricular volume. *Circulation* 1984;69(3):497–505.

49. Iannettoni MD, et al. Improving results with first-stage palliation for hypoplastic left heart syndrome. *J Thorac Cardiovasc Surg* 1994;107(3):934–940.

50. Rhodes LA, et al. Predictors of survival in neonates with critical aortic stenosis. *Circulation* 1991;84(6):2325–2335.

51. Hammon JW, Jr., et al. Predictors of operative mortality in critical valvular aortic stenosis presenting in infancy. *Ann Thorac Surg* 1988;45(5):537–540.

52. Phoon CK, Silverman NH. Conditions with right ventricular pressure and volume overload, and a small left ventricle: "Hypoplastic" left ventricle or simply a squashed ventricle? *J Am Coll Cardiol* 1997;30(6):1547–1553.

53. Minich LL, et al. Possibility of postnatal left ventricular growth in selected infants with non-apex-forming left ventricles. *Am Heart J* 1997;133(5):570–574.

54. Sugiyama H, et al. The relation between right ventricular function and left ventricular morphology in hypoplastic left heart syndrome: Angiographic and pathological studies. *Pediatr Cardiol* 1999;20(6):422–427.

54a. Colan SD, McElhinney DB, Crawford EC, et al. Validation and Re-Evaluation of a Discriminant Model Predicting Anatomic Suitability for Biventricular Repair in Neonates With Aortic Stenosis. *J Am Coll Cardiol* 2006;47:1858–1865.

55. Devereux RB, Reichek N. Echocardiographic determination of left ventricular mass in man. Anatomic validation of the method. *Circulation* 1977;55(4):613–618.

56. Devereux RB, et al. Echocardiographic assessment of left ventricular hypertrophy: Comparison to necropsy findings. *Am J Cardiol* 1986;57(6):450–458.

57. Daniels SR, et al. Echocardiographically determined left ventricular mass index in normal children, adolescents and young adults. *J Am Coll Cardiol* 1988;12(3):703–708.

58. de Simone G, et al. Relation of left ventricular hypertrophy, afterload, and contractility to left ventricular performance in Goldblatt hypertension. *Am J Hypertens* 1992;5(5 Pt 1):292–301.

59. de Simone G, et al. Assessment of left ventricular function by the midwall fractional shortening/end-systolic stress relation in human hypertension. *J Am Coll Cardiol* 1994;23(6):1444–1451.

60. Bouchard A, et al. Noninvasive assessment of cardiomyopathy in normotensive diabetic patients between 20 and 50 years old. *Am J Med* 1989;87(2):160–166.

61. Schiller NB, et al. Canine left ventricular mass estimation by two-dimensional echocardiography. *Circulation* 1983;68(1):210–216.

62. Daniels SR, et al. Indexing left ventricular mass to account for differences in body size in children and adolescents without cardiovascular disease. *Am J Cardiol* 1995;76(10):699–701.

63. de Simone G, et al. Midwall left ventricular performance in salt-loaded Dahl rats: Effect of AT1 angiotensin II inhibition. *J Hypertens* 1995;13(12 Pt 2):1808–1812.

64. Koren MJ, et al. Relation of left ventricular mass and geometry to morbidity and mortality in uncomplicated essential hypertension. *Ann Intern Med* 1991;114(5):345–352.

65. Devereux RB, et al. Prognostic significance of left ventricular mass change during treatment of hypertension. *JAMA* 2004;292(19):2350–2356.

66. Mitsnefes, MM, et al. Left ventricular mass and systolic performance in pediatric patients with chronic renal failure. *Circulation* 2003;107(6):864–868.

67. Amin RS, et al. Left ventricular hypertrophy and abnormal ventricular geometry in children and adolescents with obstructive sleep apnea. *Am J Respir Crit Care Med* 2002;165(10):1395–1399.

68. Daniels SR, et al. Association of body fat distribution and cardiovascular risk factors in children and adolescents. *Circulation* 1999;99(4):541–545.

69. Kimball TR, et al. Relation of left ventricular mass, preload, afterload and contractility in pediatric patients with essential hypertension. *J Am Coll Cardiol* 1993;21(4):997–1001.

70. Kimball TR, et al. Cardiovascular status in young patients with insulin-dependent diabetes mellitus. *Circulation* 1994;90(1):357–361.

71. Muiesan ML, et al. Left ventricular concentric geometry during treatment adversely affects cardiovascular prognosis in hypertensive patients. *Hypertension* 2004;43(4):731–738.

72. Appleton CP, Hatle LK. The natural history of left ventricular filling abnormalities: Assessment by two-dimensional and Doppler echocardiography. *Echocardiography* 1992;9:438–457.

73. Garcia MJ, et al. An index of early left ventricular filling that combined with pulsed Doppler peak E velocity may estimate capillary wedge pressure. *J Am Coll Cardiol* 1997;29(2):448–454.

74. Garcia MJ, Thomas JD, Klein AL. New Doppler echocardiographic applications for the study of diastolic function. *J Am Coll Cardiol* 1998;32(4):865–875.

75. Swaminathan S, et al. Usefulness of tissue Doppler echocardiography for evaluating ventricular function in children without heart disease. *Am J Cardiol* 2003;91(5):570–574.

76. Pham PP, et al. Impact of conventional versus biventricular pacing on hemodynamics and tissue Doppler imaging indexes of resynchronization postoperatively in children with congenital heart disease. *J Am Coll Cardiol* 2005;46(12):2284–2289.

77. Pritchett AM, et al. Diastolic dysfunction and left atrial volume: A population-based study. *J Am Coll Cardiol* 2005;45(1):87–92.

78. Mattioli AV, et al. Regression of left ventricular hypertrophy and improvement of diastolic function in hypertensive patients treated with telmisartan. *Int J Cardiol* 2004;97(3):383–388.

79. Daniels SR, et al. Left atrial size in children with hypertension: The influence of obesity, blood pressure, and left ventricular mass. *J Pediatr* 2002;141(2):186–190.

80. Yang H, et al. Enlarged left atrial volume in hypertrophic cardiomyopathy: A marker for disease severity. *J Am Soc Echocardiogr* 2005;18(10):1074–1082.

81. Sauter HJ, et al. The relationship of left atrial pressure and volume in patients with heart disease. *Am Heart J* 1964;67:635–642.

82. Hofstetter R, et al. Determination of left atrial area and volume by cross-sectional echocardiography in healthy infants and children. *Am J Cardiol* 1991;68(10):1073–1078.

83. Kircher B, et al. Left atrial volume determination by biplane two-dimensional echocardiography: Validation by cine computed tomography. *Am Heart J* 1991;121(3 Pt 1):864–871.

84. O'Leary PW, et al. Diastolic ventricular function in children: A Doppler echocardiographic study establishing normal values and predictors of increased ventricular end-diastolic pressure. *Mayo Clin Proc* 1998;73(7):616–628.

85. Schmitz L, Schneider MB, Lange PE. Isovolumic relaxation time corrected for heart rate has a constant value from infancy to adolescence. *J Am Soc Echocardiogr* 2003;16(3):221–222.

86. de Marchi SF, et al. Pulmonary venous flow velocity patterns in 404 individuals without cardiovascular disease. *Heart* 2001;85(1):23–29.

87. Eidem BW, et al. Impact of cardiac growth on Doppler tissue imaging velocities: A study in healthy children. *J Am Soc Echocardiogr* 2004;7(3):212–221.

88. Mori K, et al. Left ventricular wall motion velocities in healthy children measured by pulsed wave Doppler tissue echocardiography: Normal values and relation to age and heart rate. *J Am Soc Echocardiogr* 2000;13(11):1002–1011.

89. Rychik J, Tian ZY. Quantitative assessment of myocardial tissue velocities in normal children with Doppler tissue imaging. *Am J Cardiol* 1996;77(14):1254–1257.

90. Rakowski H, et al. Canadian consensus recommendations for the measurement and reporting of diastolic dysfunction by echocardiography: From the Investigators of Consensus on Diastolic Dysfunction by Echocardiography. *J Am Soc Echocardiogr* 1996;9(5):736–760.

91. Sohn DW, et al. Assessment of mitral annulus velocity by Doppler tissue imaging in the evaluation of left ventricular diastolic function. *J Am Coll Cardiol* 1997;30(2):474–480.

92. Rajagopalan N, et al. Comparison of new Doppler echocardiographic methods to differentiate constrictive pericardial heart disease and restrictive cardiomyopathy. *Am J Cardiol* 2001;87(1):86–94.

93. Nagueh SF, et al. Doppler estimation of left ventricular filling pressure in sinus tachycardia. A new application of tissue doppler imaging. *Circulation* 1998;98(16):1644–1650.

94. Sundereswaran L, et al. Estimation of left and right ventricular filling pressures after heart transplantation by tissue Doppler imaging. *Am J Cardiol* 1998;82(3):352–357.

95. Appleton CP, Hatle LK, Popp RL. Demonstration of restrictive ventricular physiology by Doppler echocardiography. *J Am Coll Cardiol* 1988;11(4):757–768.

96. Appleton CP, Hatle LK, Popp RL. Relation of transmitral flow velocity patterns to left ventricular diastolic function: New insights from a combined hemodynamic and Doppler echocardiographic study. *J Am Coll Cardiol* 1988;12(2):426–440.

97. Oh JK, et al. Diagnostic role of Doppler echocardiography in constrictive pericarditis. *J Am Coll Cardiol* 1994;23(1):154–162.

98. Vitarelli A, et al. Quantitative assessment of systolic and diastolic ventricular function with tissue Doppler imaging after Fontan type of operation. *Int J Cardiol* 2005;102(1):61–69.

99. Border WL, et al. Color M-mode and Doppler tissue evaluation of diastolic function in children: Simultaneous correlation with invasive indices. *J Am Soc Echocardiogr* 2003;16(9):988–994.

100. Brili S, et al. Tissue Doppler imaging and brain natriuretic peptide levels in adults with repaired tetralogy of Fallot. *J Am Soc Echocardiogr* 2005;18(11):1149–1154.

101. Gatzoulis MA, et al. Right ventricular diastolic function 15 to 35 years after repair of tetralogy of Fallot. Restrictive physiology predicts superior exercise performance. *Circulation* 1995;91(6):1775–1781.

102. Gatzoulis MA, Norgard G, Redington AN. Biventricular long axis function after repair of tetralogy of Fallot. *Pediatr Cardiol* 1998;19(2):128–132.

103. Olivier M, et al. Serial Doppler assessment of diastolic function before and after the Fontan operation. *J Am Soc Echocardiogr* 2003;16(11):1136–1143.

104. Riggs TW, Snider AR. Respiratory influence on right and left ventricular diastolic function in normal children. *Am J Cardiol* 1989;63(12):858–861.

105. Zoghbi WA, Habib GB, Quinones MA. Doppler assessment of right ventricular filling in a normal population. Comparison with left ventricular filling dynamics. *Circulation* 1990;82(4):1316–1324.

106. Frommelt PC, et al. Usefulness of Doppler tissue imaging analysis of tricuspid annular motion for determination of right ventricular function in normal infants and children. *Am J Cardiol* 2002;89(5):610–613.

107. Cullen S, Shore D, Redington A. Characterization of right ventricular diastolic performance after complete repair of tetralogy of Fallot. Restrictive physiology predicts slow postoperative recovery. *Circulation* 1995;91(6):1782–1789.

108. Walley KR, Lewis TH, Wood LD. Acute respiratory acidosis decreases left ventricular contractility but increases cardiac output in dogs. *Circ Res* 1990;67(3):628–635.

109. Lang RM, et al. Systemic vascular resistance: An unreliable index of left ventricular afterload. *Circulation* 1986;74(5):1114–1123.

110. Colan SD, Borow KM, Neumann A. Left ventricular end-systolic wall stress-velocity of fiber shortening relation: A load-independent index of myocardial contractility. *J Am Coll Cardiol* 1984;4(4):715–724.

111. Borow KM, et al. Left ventricular end-systolic stress-shortening and stress-length relations in human. Normal values and sensitivity to inotropic state. *Am J Cardiol* 1982;50(6):1301–1308.

112. Grossman W, Jones D, McLaurin LP. Wall stress and patterns of hypertrophy in the human left ventricle. *J Clin Invest* 1975;56(1):56–64.

113. Borow KM, Newburger JW. Noninvasive estimation of central aortic pressure using the oscillometric method for analyzing systemic artery pulsatile blood flow: Comparative study of indirect systolic, diastolic, and mean brachial artery pressure with simultaneous direct ascending aortic pressure measurements. *Am Heart J* 1982;103(5):879–886.

114. Colan SD, et al. Noninvasive determination of systolic, diastolic and end-systolic blood pressure in neonates, infants and young children: Comparison with central aortic pressure measurements. *Am J Cardiol* 1983;52(7):867–870.

115. Quinones MA, et al. Echocardiographic determination of left ventricular stress-velocity relations. *Circulation* 1975;51(4):689–700.

116. Borow KM, et al. Effects of simultaneous alterations in preload and afterload on measurements of left ventricular contractility in patients with dilated cardiomyopathy: Comparisons of ejection phase, isovolumetric and end-systolic force-velocity indexes. *J Am Coll Cardiol* 1992;20(4):787–795.

117. Kimball TR, et al. Age-related variation in contractility estimate in patients less than or equal to 20 years of age. *Am J Cardiol* 1991;68(13):1383–1387.

118. Colan SD, et al. Developmental modulation of myocardial mechanics: age- and growth-related alterations in afterload and contractility. *J Am Coll Cardiol* 1992;19(3):619–629.

119. Albanna II, et al. Diastolic dysfunction in young patients with insulin-dependent diabetes mellitus as determined by automated border detection. *J Am Soc Echocardiogr* 1998;11(4):349–355.

120. Kimball TR, et al. Relation of symptoms to contractility and defect size in infants with ventricular septal defect. *Am J Cardiol* 1991;67(13):1097–1102.

121. Kimball TR, et al. Effect of digoxin on contractility and symptoms in infants with a large ventricular septal defect. *Am J Cardiol* 1991;68(13):1377–1382.

122. Kimball TR, et al. Effect of ligation of patent ductus arteriosus on left ventricular performance and its determinants in premature neonates. *J Am Coll Cardiol* 1996;27(1):193–197.

123. Lipshultz SE, Grenier MA, Colan SD. Doxorubicin-induced cardiomyopathy. *N Engl J Med* 1999;340(8):653–655.

124. Colan SD, et al. Status of the left ventricle after arterial switch operation for transposition of the great arteries. Hemodynamic and echocardiographic evaluation. *J Thorac Cardiovasc Surg* 1995;109(2):311–321.

125. Gallagher KP, et al. Nonuniformity of inner and outer systolic wall thickening in conscious dogs. *Am J Physiol* 1985;249(2 Pt 2):H241–H248.

126. Sabbah HN, Marzilli M, Stein PD. The relative role of subendocardium and subepicardium in left ventricular mechanics. *Am J Physiol* 1981;240(6):H920–H926.

127. Shimizu G, et al. Left ventricular midwall mechanics in systemic arterial hypertension. Myocardial function is depressed in pressure-overload hypertrophy. *Circulation* 1991;83(5):1676–1684.

128. de Simone G, et al. Relation of left ventricular chamber and midwall function to age in normal children, adolescents and adults. *Ital Heart J* 2000;1(4):295–300.

129. Regen DM. Calculation of left ventricular wall stress. *Circ Res* 1990;67(2):245–252.

130. Gentles TL, Colan SD. Wall stress misrepresents afterload in children and young adults with abnormal left ventricular geometry. *J Appl Physiol* 2002;92(3):1053–1057.

131. Gentles TL, Sanders SP, Colan SD. Misrepresentation of left ventricular contractile function by endocardial indexes: Clinical implications after coarctation repair. *Am Heart J* 2000;140(4):585–595.

132. Greenberg NL, et al. Doppler-derived myocardial systolic strain rate is a strong index of left ventricular contractility. *Circulation* 2002;105(1):99–105.

133. Eyskens B, et al. Regional right and left ventricular function after the Senning operation: An ultrasonic study of strain rate and strain. *Cardiol Young* 2004;14(3):255–264.

134. Di Salvo G, et al. Comparison of strain rate imaging for quantitative evaluation of regional left and right ventricular function after surgical versus percutaneous closure of atrial septal defect. *Am J Cardiol* 2005;96(2):299–302.

135. Solarz DE, et al. Right ventricular strain rate and strain analysis in patients with repaired tetralogy of Fallot: Possible interventricular septal compensation. *J Am Soc Echocardiogr* 2004;17(4):338–344.

136. Abd El Rahman MY, et al. Detection of left ventricular asynchrony in patients with right bundle branch block after repair of tetralogy of Fallot using tissue-Doppler imaging-derived strain. *J Am Coll Cardiol* 2005;45(6):915–921.

137. Hughes ML, et al. Improved early ventricular performance with a right ventricle to pulmonary artery conduit in stage 1 palliation for hypoplastic left heart syndrome: Evidence from strain Doppler echocardiography. *Heart* 2004;90(2):191–194.

138. Senzaki H, et al. Assessment of cardiovascular dynamics by pressure-area relations in pediatric patients with congenital heart disease. *J Thorac Cardiovasc Surg* 2001;122(3):535–547.

139. Perez JE, et al. On-line assessment of ventricular function by automatic boundary detection and ultrasonic backscatter imaging. *J Am Coll Cardiol* 1992;19(2):313–320.

140. Kim IS, et al. Prognostic value of mechanical efficiency in ambulatory patients with idiopathic dilated cardiomyopathy in sinus rhythm. *J Am Coll Cardiol* 2002;39(8):1264–1268.

141. Little WC, Cheng CP. Left ventricular-arterial coupling in conscious dogs. *Am J Physiol* 1991;261(1 Pt 2):H70–H76.

142. Khoury SF, et al. Effects of thyroid hormone on left ventricular performance and regulation of contractile and Ca(2+)-cycling proteins in the baboon. Implications for the force-frequency and relaxation-frequency relationships. *Circ Res* 1996;79(4):727–735.

143. Mulieri LA, et al. Altered myocardial force-frequency relation in human heart failure. *Circulation* 1992;85(5):1743–1750.

144. Fowler MB, et al. Assessment of the beta-adrenergic receptor pathway in the intact failing human heart: Progressive receptor down-regulation and subsensitivity to agonist response. *Circulation* 1986;74(6):1290–1302.

145. Pratali L, et al. Prognostic significance of the dobutamine echocardiography test in idiopathic dilated cardiomyopathy. *Am J Cardiol* 2001;88(12):1374–1378.

146. Ho YL, et al. The correlation between expression of apoptosis-related proteins and myocardial functional reserve evaluated by dobutamine stress echocardiography in patients with dilated cardiomyopathy. *J Am Soc Echocardiogr* 2003;16(9):931–936.

147. Paraskevaidis IA, Adamopoulos S, Kremastinos DT. Dobutamine echocardiographic study in patients with nonischemic dilated cardiomyopathy and prognostically borderline values of peak exercise oxygen consumption: 18-month follow-up study. *J Am Coll Cardiol* 2001;37(6):1685–1691.

148. Naqvi TZ, et al. Myocardial contractile reserve on dobutamine echocardiography predicts late spontaneous improvement in cardiac function in patients with recent onset idiopathic dilated cardiomyopathy. *J Am Coll Cardiol* 1999;34(5):1537–1544.

149. Klewer SE, et al. Dobutamine stress echocardiography: A sensitive indicator of diminished myocardial function in asymptomatic doxorubicin-treated long-term survivors of childhood cancer. *J Am Coll Cardiol* 1992;19(2):394–401.

150. De Wolf D, et al. Dobutamine stress echocardiography in the evaluation of late anthracycline cardiotoxicity in childhood cancer survivors. *Pediatr Res* 1996;39(3):504–512.

151. Suarez WA, et al. Preclinical cardiac dysfunction in transfusion-dependent children and young adults detected with low-dose dobutamine stress echocardiography. *J Am Soc Echocardiogr* 1998;11(10):948–956.

152. Michelfelder EC, et al. Moderate-dose dobutamine maximizes left ventricular contractile response during dobutamine stress echocardiography in children. *J Am Soc Echocardiogr* 2003;16(2):140–146.

153. Kimball TR, et al. Echocardiographic determination of left ventricular preload, afterload, and contractility during and after exercise. *J Pediatr* 1993;122(6):S89–S94.

154. Cyran SE, et al. Aortic "recoarctation" at rest versus at exercise in children as evaluated by stress Doppler echocardiography after a "good" operative result. *Am J Cardiol* 1993;71(11):963–970.

155. Lin SS, et al. Right ventricular volume overload results in depression of left ventricular ejection fraction. Implications for the surgical management of tricuspid valve disease. *Circulation* 1994;90(5 Pt 2):II209–II213.

156. Louie EK, et al. Pressure and volume loading of the right ventricle have opposite effects on left ventricular ejection fraction. *Circulation* 1995;92(4):819–824.

157. Li KS, Santamore WP. Contribution of each wall to biventricular function. *Cardiovasc Res* 1993;27(5):792–800.

158. Bjarke BB, Kidd BS. Congenitally corrected transposition of the great arteries. A clinical study of 101 cases. *Acta Paediatr Scand* 1976;65(2):153–160.

159. Cochrane AD, Karl TR, Mee RB. Staged conversion to arterial switch for late failure of the systemic right ventricle. *Ann Thorac Surg* 1993;56(4):854–862.

160. Leeuwenburgh BP, et al. Effects of acute left ventricular unloading on right ventricular function in normal and chronic right ventricular pressure-overloaded lambs. *J Thorac Cardiovasc Surg* 2003;125(3):481–490.

161. Sano T, et al. Intermediate-term outcome after intracardiac repair of associated cardiac defects in patients with atrioventricular and ventriculoarterial discordance. *Circulation* 1995;92(9 Suppl):II272–II278.

162. Ritchie M, et al. Echocardiographic characterization of the improvement in right ventricular function in patients with severe pulmonary hypertension after single-lung transplantation. *J Am Coll Cardiol* 1993;22(4):1170–1174.

163. Clark SJ, Yoxall CW, Subhedar NV. Measurement of right ventricular volume in healthy term and preterm neonates. *Arch Dis Child Fetal Neonatal Ed* 2002;87(2):F89–F94.

164. Zornoff LA, et al. Right ventricular dysfunction and risk of heart failure and mortality after myocardial infarction. *J Am Coll Cardiol* 2002;39(9):1450–1455.

165. Burgess MI, et al. Comparison of echocardiographic markers of right ventricular function in determining prognosis in chronic pulmonary disease. *J Am Soc Echocardiogr* 2002;15(6):633–639.

166. Geva T, et al. Evaluation of regional differences in right ventricular systolic function by acoustic quantification echocardiography and cine magnetic resonance imaging. *Circulation* 1998;98(4):339–345.

167. Rushmer RF, Crystal DK, Wagner C. The functional anatomy of ventricular contraction. *Circ Res* 1953;1(2):162–170.

168. Arce OX, et al. Longitudinal motion of the atrioventricular annuli in children: Reference values, growth related changes, and effects of right ventricular volume and pressure overload. *J Am Soc Echocardiogr* 2002; 15(9):906–916.

169. Derrick GP, et al. Abnormalities of right ventricular long axis function after atrial repair of transposition of the great arteries. *Heart* 2001;86(2): 203–206.

170. Tei C. New non-invasive index for combined systolic and diastolic ventricular function. *J Cardiol* 1995;26(2):135–136.

171. Morhy SS, et al. Non-invasive assessment of right ventricular function in the late follow-up of the Senning procedure. *Cardiol Young* 2005;15(2): 154–159.

172. Salehian O, et al. Assessment of systemic right ventricular function in patients with transposition of the great arteries using the myocardial performance index: Comparison with cardiac magnetic resonance imaging. *Circulation* 2004;110(20):3229–3233.

173. Williams RV, et al. Quantitative assessment of ventricular function in children with single ventricles using the Doppler myocardial performance index. *Am J Cardiol* 2000;86(10):1106–1110.

174. Mahle WT, et al. Quantitative echocardiographic assessment of the performance of the functionally single right ventricle after the Fontan operation. *Cardiol Young* 2001;11(4):399–406.

175. Marcus EN, et al. Echocardiographic assessment of the right ventricular response to hypertension in neonates on the basis of average-shaped contraction models. *J Am Soc Echocardiogr* 2002;15(10 Pt 1):1145–1153.

176. Bacha EA, et al. Ventricular resynchronization by multisite pacing improves myocardial performance in the postoperative single-ventricle patient. *Ann Thorac Surg* 2004;78(5):1678–1683.

177. Roman MJ, et al. Two-dimensional echocardiographic aortic root dimensions in normal children and adults. *Am J Cardiol* 1989;64(8):507–512.

178. Hwa J, et al. The natural history of aortic dilatation in Marfan syndrome. *Med J Aust* 1993;158(8):558–562.

179. Roman MJ, et al. Aortic root dilatation as a cause of isolated, severe aortic regurgitation. Prevalence, clinical and echocardiographic patterns, and relation to left ventricular hypertrophy and function. *Ann Intern Med* 1987;106(6):800–807.

180. Wenstrup RJ, et al. Prevalence of aortic root dilation in the Ehlers-Danlos syndrome. *Genet Med* 2002;4(3):112–117.

181. Nistri S, et al. Aortic root dilatation in young men with normally functioning bicuspid aortic valves. *Heart* 1999;82(1):19–22.

182. Gurvitz M, et al. Frequency of aortic root dilation in children with a bicuspid aortic valve. *Am J Cardiol* 2004;94(10):1337–1340.

183. Dore A, et al. Progressive dilation of the diameter of the aortic root in adults with a bicuspid aortic valve. *Cardiol Young* 2003;13(6):526–531.

184. Niwa K, et al. Progressive aortic root dilatation in adults late after repair of tetralogy of Fallot. *Circulation* 2002;106(11):1374–1378.

185. Hutter PA, et al. Fate of the aortic root after arterial switch operation. *Eur J Cardiothorac Surg* 2001;20(1):82–88.

186. Tantengco MV, et al. Aortic root dilation after the Ross procedure. *Am J Cardiol* 1999;83(6):915–920.

187. Simon-Kupilik N, et al. Dilatation of the autograft root after the Ross operation. *Eur J Cardiothorac Surg* 2002;21(3):470–473.

188. David TE, et al. Dilation of the pulmonary autograft after the Ross procedure. *J Thorac Cardiovasc Surg* 2000;119(2):210–220.

189. Savoye C, et al. Echocardiographic follow-up after Ross procedure in 100 patients. *Am J Cardiol* 2000;85(7):854–857.

190. Ugolini P, et al. Idiopathic dilatation of the pulmonary artery: Report of four cases. *Magn Reson Imaging* 1999;17(6):933–937.

191. Chang RY, et al. Idiopathic dilatation of the pulmonary artery. A case presentation. *Angiology* 1996;47(1):87–92.

192. Fontan F, et al. The size of the pulmonary arteries and the results of the Fontan operation. *J Thorac Cardiovasc Surg* 1989;98(5 Pt 1):711–724.

193. Zalzstein E, et al. Spectrum of cardiovascular anomalies in Williams-Beuren syndrome. *Pediatr Cardiol* 1991;12(4):219–223.

194. Kim YM, et al. Natural course of supravalvar aortic stenosis and peripheral pulmonary arterial stenosis in Williams' syndrome. *Cardiol Young* 1999;9(1):37–41.

195. McElhinney DB, et al. Analysis of cardiovascular phenotype and genotype-phenotype correlation in individuals with a JAG1 mutation and/or Alagille syndrome. *Circulation* 2002;106(20):2567–2574.

196. Ellis JG, Kuzman WJ. Pulmonary artery stenosis, a frequent part of the congenital rubella syndrome. *Calif Med* 1966;105(6):435–439.

197. Hastreiter AR, et al. Cardiovascular lesions associated with congenital rubella. *J Pediatr* 1967;71(1):59–65.

198. Celermajer JM, Varghese PJ, Rowe RD. Cardiovascular lesions in rubella embryopathy with special emphasis on pulmonary arterial disease. *Isr J Med Sci* 1969;5(4):568–571.

199. Snider AR, et al. Two-dimensional echocardiographic determination of aortic and pulmonary artery sizes from infancy to adulthood in normal subjects. *Am J Cardiol* 1984;53(1):218–224.

200. Silvilairat S, et al. Outpatient echocardiographic assessment of complex pulmonary outflow stenosis: Doppler mean gradient is superior to the maximum instantaneous gradient. *J Am Soc Echocardiogr* 2005;18(11): 1143–1148.

201. Bengur AR, et al. Doppler evaluation of aortic valve area in children with aortic stenosis. *J Am Coll Cardiol* 1991;18(6):1499–1505.

202. Gutgesell HP, French M. Echocardiographic determination of aortic and pulmonary valve areas in subjects with normal hearts. *Am J Cardiol* 1991; 68(8):773–776.

203. Davidson Jr. WR, Pasquale MJ, Fanelli C. A Doppler echocardiographic examination of the normal aortic valve and left ventricular outflow tract. *Am J Cardiol* 1991;67(6):547–549.

204. Bonow RO. Asymptomatic aortic regurgitation: Indications for operation. *J Card Surg* 1994;9(2 Suppl):170–173.

205. Tani LY, et al. Doppler evaluation of aortic regurgitation in children. *Am J Cardiol* 1997;80(7):927–931.

206. Ishii M, et al. What is the validity of continuous wave Doppler grading of aortic regurgitation severity? A chronic animal model study. *J Am Soc Echocardiogr* 1998;11(4):332–337.

207. Teague SM, et al. Quantification of aortic regurgitation utilizing continuous wave Doppler ultrasound. *J Am Coll Cardiol* 1986;8(3):592–599.

208. Beyer RW, et al. Correlation of continuous-wave Doppler assessment of chronic aortic regurgitation with hemodynamics and angiography. *Am J Cardiol* 1987;60(10):852–856.

209. Labovitz AJ, et al. Quantitative evaluation of aortic insufficiency by continuous wave Doppler echocardiography. *J Am Coll Cardiol* 1986;8(6): 1341–1347.

210. Masuyama T, et al. Noninvasive evaluation of aortic regurgitation by continuous-wave Doppler echocardiography. *Circulation* 1986;73(3): 460–466.

211. Perry GJ, et al. Evaluation of aortic insufficiency by Doppler color flow mapping. *J Am Coll Cardiol* 1987;9(4):952–959.

212. Enriquez-Sarano M, et al. Quantitative Doppler assessment of valvular regurgitation. *Circulation* 1993;87(3):841–848.

213. Enriquez-Sarano M, et al. Effective regurgitant orifice area: A noninvasive Doppler development of an old hemodynamic concept. *J Am Coll Cardiol* 1994;23(2):443–451.

214. Lei MH, et al. Reappraisal of quantitative evaluation of pulmonary regurgitation and estimation of pulmonary artery pressure by continuous wave Doppler echocardiography. *Cardiology* 1995;86(3):249–256.

215. Li W, et al. Doppler-echocardiographic assessment of pulmonary regurgitation in adults with repaired tetralogy of Fallot: Comparison with cardiovascular magnetic resonance imaging. *Am Heart J* 2004;147(1): 165–172.

216. Newburger JW, et al. Diagnosis, treatment, and long-term management of Kawasaki disease: A statement for health professionals from the Committee on Rheumatic Fever, Endocarditis and Kawasaki Disease, Council on Cardiovascular Disease in the Young, American Heart Association. *Circulation* 2004;110(17):2747–2771.

217. Davis PH, et al. Increased carotid intimal-medial thickness and coronary calcification are related in young and middle-aged adults. The Muscatine Study. *Circulation* 1999;100(8):838–842.

218. Davis PH, et al. Carotid intimal-medial thickness is related to cardiovascular risk factors measured from childhood through middle age: The Muscatine Study. *Circulation* 2001;104(23):2815–2819.

219. Singh TP, Groehn H, Kazmers A. Vascular function and carotid intimal-medial thickness in children with insulin-dependent diabetes mellitus. *J Am Coll Cardiol* 2003;41(4):661–665.

220. Nurnberger J, et al. Augmentation index is associated with cardiovascular risk. *J Hypertens* 2002;20(12):2407–2414.

221. Tounian P, et al. Presence of increased stiffness of the common carotid artery and endothelial dysfunction in severely obese children: A prospective study. *Lancet* 2001;358(9291):1400–1404.

222. Pahl E, et al. Feasibility of exercise stress echocardiography for the follow-up of children with coronary involvement secondary to Kawasaki disease. *Circulation* 1995;91(1):122–128.

223. Kimball TR, Witt SA, Daniels SR. Dobutamine stress echocardiography in the assessment of suspected myocardial ischemia in children and young adults. *Am J Cardiol* 1997;79(3):380–384.

224. Thanigaraj S, et al. Comparison of transthoracic versus transesophageal echocardiography for detection of right-to-left atrial shunting using agitated saline contrast. *Am J Cardiol* 2005;96(7):1007–1010.

225. Fan S, et al. Superiority of the combination of blood and agitated saline for routine contrast enhancement. *J Am Soc Echocardiogr* 1999;12(2): 94–98.

226. Chang RK, et al. Bubble contrast echocardiography in detecting pulmonary arteriovenous shunting in children with univentricular heart after cavopulmonary anastomosis. *J Am Coll Cardiol* 1999;33(7): 2052–2058.

227. Hoeper MM, Krowka MJ, Strassburg CP. Portopulmonary hypertension and hepatopulmonary syndrome. *Lancet* 2004;363(9419):1461–1468.

228. Alvarez AE, et al. Abernethy malformation: One of the etiologies of hepatopulmonary syndrome. *Pediatr Pulmonol* 2002;34(5):391–394.

229. Ashrafian H, Swan L. The mechanism of formation of pulmonary arteriovenous malformations associated with the classic Glenn shunt (superior cavopulmonary anastomosis). *Heart* 2002;88(6):639.

230. Christiansen C, et al. Physical and biochemical characterization of Albunex, a new ultrasound contrast agent consisting of air-filled albumin microspheres suspended in a solution of human albumin. *Biotechnol Appl Biochem* 1994;19(Pt 3):307–320.

231. Zilberman MV, Witt SA, Kimball TR. Is there a role for intravenous transpulmonary contrast imaging in pediatric stress echocardiography? *J Am Soc Echocardiogr* 2003;16(1):9–14.

232. Vogel R, et al. The quantification of absolute myocardial perfusion in humans by contrast echocardiography: Algorithm and validation. *J Am Coll Cardiol* 2005;45(5):754–762.

233. Tsutsui JM, et al. Safety of dobutamine stress real-time myocardial contrast echocardiography. *J Am Coll Cardiol* 2005;45(8):1235–1242.

234. Sheil ML, et al. Contrast echocardiography: Potential for the in-vivo study of pediatric myocardial preservation. *Ann Thorac Surg* 2003;75(5):1542–1549.

235. Wang X, et al. Gene transfer with microbubble ultrasound and plasmid DNA into skeletal muscle of mice: Comparison between commercially available microbubble contrast agents. *Radiology* 2005;237(1):224–229.

236. Li T, Tachibana K, Kuroki M. Gene transfer with echo-enhanced contrast agents: Comparison between Albunex, Optison, and Levovist in mice—initial results. *Radiology* 2003;229(2):423–428.

237. Ritter SB. Transesophageal real-time echocardiography in infants and children with congenital heart disease. *J Am Coll Cardiol* 1991;18(2):569–580.

238. Ungerleider RM, et al. Intraoperative echocardiography during congenital heart operations: Experience from 1,000 cases. *Ann Thorac Surg* 1995;60(6 Suppl):S539–S542.

239. van der Velde ME, et al. Transesophageal echocardiographic guidance of transcatheter ventricular septal defect closure. *J Am Coll Cardiol* 1994;23(7):1660–1665.

240. Fyfe DA, et al. Transesophageal echocardiography detects thrombus formation not identified by transthoracic echocardiography after the Fontan operation. *J Am Coll Cardiol* 1991;18(7):1733–1737.

241. Saphir JR, et al. Upper airway obstruction after transesophageal echocardiography. *J Am Soc Echocardiogr* 1997;10(9):977–978.

242. Bensky AS, O'Brien JJ, Hammon JW. Transesophageal echo probe compression on an aberrant right subclavian artery. *J Am Soc Echocardiogr* 1995;8(6):964–966.

243. Stevenson JG, et al. Transesophageal echocardiography during repair of congenital cardiac defects: Identification of residual problems necessitating reoperation. *J Am Soc Echocardiogr* 1993;6(4):356–365.

244. Lee HR, et al. Usefulness of intraoperative transesophageal echocardiography in predicting the degree of mitral regurgitation secondary to atrioventricular defect in children. *Am J Cardiol* 1999;83(5):750–753.

245. Walayat M, Cooper SG, Sholler GF. Transesophageal echocardiographic guidance of blade atrial septostomy in children. *Catheter Cardiovasc Interv* 2001;52(2):200–202.

246. Humpl T, McCrindle BW, Smallhorn JF. The relative roles of transthoracic compared with transesophageal echocardiography in children with suspected infective endocarditis. *J Am Coll Cardiol* 2003;41(11):2068–2071.

247. Ayres NA, et al. Indications and guidelines for performance of transesophageal echocardiography in the patient with pediatric acquired or congenital heart disease: Report from the task force of the Pediatric Council of the American Society of Echocardiography. *J Am Soc Echocardiogr* 2005;18(1):91–98.

248. Lowry RW, et al. Clinical impact of transesophageal echocardiography in the diagnosis and management of infective endocarditis. *Am J Cardiol* 1994;73(15):1089–1091.

249. Shively BK, et al. Diagnostic value of transesophageal compared with transthoracic echocardiography in infective endocarditis. *J Am Coll Cardiol* 1991;18(2):391–397.

250. Pedersen WR, et al. Value of transesophageal echocardiography as an adjunct to transthoracic echocardiography in evaluation of native and prosthetic valve endocarditis. *Chest* 1991;100(2):351–356.

251. Roelandt J, et al. Precordial three-dimensional echocardiography with a rotational imaging probe: Methods and initial clinical experience. *Echocardiography* 1995;12(3):243–252.

252. Ludomirsky A, et al. Transthoracic real-time three-dimensional echocardiography using the rotational scanning approach for data acquisition. *Echocardiography* 1994;11(6):599–606.

253. Wang XF, et al. Live three-dimensional echocardiography: Imaging principles and clinical application. *Echocardiography* 2003;20(7):593–604.

254. Jiang L, et al. Three-dimensional echocardiography. In vivo validation for right ventricular volume and function. *Circulation* 1994;89(5):2342–2350.

255. Jiang L, et al. Three-dimensional echocardiographic reconstruction of right ventricular volume: In vitro comparison with two-dimensional methods. *J Am Soc Echocardiogr* 1994;7(2):150–158.

256. Wang J, et al. Evaluation of right ventricular volume and systolic function by realtime three-dimensional echocardiography. *J Huazhong Univ Sci Technolog Med Sci* 2005;25(1):94–96, 99.

257. Altmann K, et al. Comparison of three-dimensional echocardiographic assessment of volume, mass, and function in children with functionally single left ventricles with two-dimensional echocardiography and magnetic resonance imaging. *Am J Cardiol* 1997;80(8):1060–1065.

258. Vogel M, et al. Three-dimensional echocardiography can simulate intraoperative visualization of congenitally malformed hearts. *Ann Thorac Surg* 1995;60(5):1282–1288.

259. Salustri A, et al. Transthoracic three-dimensional echocardiography in adult patients with congenital heart disease. *J Am Coll Cardiol* 1995;26(3):759–767.

260. Bu L, et al. Rapid full volume data acquisition by real-time 3-dimensional echocardiography for assessment of left ventricular indexes in children: A validation study compared with magnetic resonance imaging. *J Am Soc Echocardiogr* 2005;18(4):299–305.

261. Thomas JD, et al. Guidelines and recommendations for digital echocardiography. *J Am Soc Echocardiogr* 2005;18(3):287–297.

262. Karson TH, et al. Digital storage of echocardiograms offers superior image quality to analog storage, even with 20:1 digital compression: Results of the Digital Echo Record Access Study. *J Am Soc Echocardiogr* 1996;9(6):769–778.

263. Thomas JD. Digital storage and retrieval: The future in echocardiography. *Heart* 1997;78(Suppl 1):19–22.

264. Thomas JD, Main ML. Digital echocardiographic laboratory: Where do we stand? *J Am Soc Echocardiogr* 1998;11(10):978–983.

265. Mathewson JW, et al. Conversion to digital technology improves efficiency in the pediatric echocardiography laboratory. *J Am Soc Echocardiogr* 2002;15(12):1515–1522.

266. Feigenbaum H. Journal of the american society of echocardiography case reports with digital images. *J Am Soc Echocardiogr* 2005;18(6):619.

267. Savage DD, et al. The spectrum of left ventricular hypertrophy in a general population sample: The Framingham Study. *Circulation* 1987;75(1 Pt 2):I26–I33.

268. Gardin JM, et al. Relation of echocardiographic left ventricular mass, geometry and wall stress, and left atrial dimension to coronary calcium in young adults (the CARDIA study). *Am J Cardiol* 2005;95(5):626–629.

269. Lonn E, et al. Effects of ramipril on left ventricular mass and function in cardiovascular patients with controlled blood pressure and with preserved left ventricular ejection fraction: A substudy of the Heart Outcomes Prevention Evaluation (HOPE) Trial. *J Am Coll Cardiol* 004;43(12):2200–2206.

270. Daniels SR, et al. Effect of lean body mass, fat mass, blood pressure, and sexual maturation on left ventricular mass in children and adolescents. Statistical, biological, and clinical significance. *Circulation* 1995;92(11):3249–3254.

271. Penicka M, et al. Improvement of left ventricular function after cardiac resynchronization therapy is predicted by tissue Doppler imaging echocardiography. *Circulation* 2004;109(8):978–983.

272. Pitzalis MV, et al. Cardiac resynchronization therapy tailored by echocardiographic evaluation of ventricular asynchrony. *J Am Coll Cardiol* 2002;40(9):1615–1622.

273. Sogaard P, et al. Tissue Doppler imaging predicts improved systolic performance and reversed left ventricular remodeling during long-term cardiac resynchronization therapy. *J Am Coll Cardiol* 2002;40(4):723–730.

274. Yu CM, et al. A novel tool to assess systolic asynchrony and identify responders of cardiac resynchronization therapy by tissue synchronization imaging. *J Am Coll Cardiol* 2005;45(5):677–684.

275. Cripe L, et al. Bicuspid aortic valve is heritable. *J Am Coll Cardiol* 2004;44(1):138–143.

276. Hole T, et al. Differences between echocardiographic measurements of left ventricular dimensions and function by local investigators and a core laboratory in a 2-year follow-up study of patients with an acute myocardial infarction. *Eur J Echocardiogr* 2002;3(4):263–270.

277. Gottdiener JS, et al. American Society of Echocardiography recommendations for use of echocardiography in clinical trials. *J Am Soc Echocardiogr* 2004;17(10):1086–1119.

278. Wilkins BJ, et al. Calcineurin/NFAT coupling participates in pathological, but not physiological, cardiac hypertrophy. *Circ Res* 2004;94(1):110–118.

279. Schultz Jel J, et al. Accelerated onset of heart failure in mice during pressure overload with chronically decreased SERCA2 calcium pump activity. *Am J Physiol Heart Circ Physiol* 2004;286(3): H1146–H1153.

280. Bueno OF, et al. Calcineurin Abeta gene targeting predisposes the myocardium to acute ischemia-induced apoptosis and dysfunction. *Circ Res* 2004;94(1):91–99.

281. Schultz Jel J, et al. TGF-beta1 mediates the hypertrophic cardiomyocyte growth induced by angiotensin II. *J Clin Invest* 2002;109(6):787–796.

282. Sussman MA, et al. Hypertrophic defect unmasked by calcineurin expression in asymptomatic tropomodulin overexpressing transgenic mice. *Cardiovasc Res* 2000;46(1):90–101.

283. Williams RV, et al. End-systolic stress-velocity and pressure-dimension relationships by transthoracic echocardiography in mice. *Am J Physiol* 1998;274(5 Pt 2): H1828–H1835.

284. Phoon CK, et al. Embryonic heart failure in NFATc1-/- mice: Novel mechanistic insights from in utero ultrasound biomicroscopy. *Circ Res* 2004; 95(1):92–99.

285. Phoon CK, Turnbull DH. Ultrasound biomicroscopy-Doppler in mouse cardiovascular development. *Physiol Genomics* 2003;14(1):3–15.

286. Ji RP, et al. Onset of cardiac function during early mouse embryogenesis coincides with entry of primitive erythroblasts into the embryo proper. *Circ Res* 2003;92(2):133–135.

287. Phoon CK, Aristizabal O, Turnbull DH. Spatial velocity profile in mouse embryonic aorta and Doppler-derived volumetric flow: A preliminary model. *Am J Physiol Heart Circ Physiol* 2002;283(3): H908–H916.

288. Zhou YQ, et al. Abnormal cardiac inflow patterns during postnatal development in a mouse model of Holt-Oram syndrome. *Am J Physiol Heart Circ Physiol* 2005;289(3):H992–H1001.

289. Zhou YQ, et al. Comprehensive transthoracic cardiac imaging in mice using ultrasound biomicroscopy with anatomical confirmation by magnetic resonance imaging. *Physiol Genomics* 2004;18(2):232–244.

290. Zhou YQ, et al. Applications for multifrequency ultrasound biomicroscopy in mice from implantation to adulthood. *Physiol Genomics* 2002;10(2):113–126.

291. Mangione S, Nieman LZ. Cardiac auscultatory skills of internal medicine and family practice trainees. A comparison of diagnostic proficiency. *JAMA* 1997;278(9):717–722.

292. Mangione S. Cardiac auscultatory skills of physicians-in-training: A comparison of three English-speaking countries. *Am J Med* 2001;110(3):210–216.

293. Gaskin PR, et al. Clinical auscultation skills in pediatric residents. *Pediatrics* 2000;105(6):1184–1187.

294. Kobal SL, Atar S, Siegel RJ, Hand-carried ultrasound improves the bedside cardiovascular examination. *Chest* 2004;126(3):693–701.

295. Decara JM, et al. Use of hand-carried ultrasound devices to augment the accuracy of medical student bedside cardiac diagnoses. *J Am Soc Echocardiogr* 2005;18(3):257–263.

296. Spencer KT, et al. Physician-performed point-of-care echocardiography using a laptop platform compared with physical examination in the cardiovascular patient. *J Am Coll Cardiol* 2001;37(8):2013–2018.

297. Kobal SL, et al. Usefulness of a hand-carried cardiac ultrasound device to detect clinically significant valvular regurgitation in hospitalized patients. *Am J Cardiol* 2004;93(8):1069–1072.

298. Li X, et al. Will a handheld ultrasound scanner be applicable for screening for heart abnormalities in newborns and children? *J Am Soc Echocardiogr* 2003;16(10):1007–1014.

299. Spurney CF, et al. Use of a hand-carried ultrasound device by critical care physicians for the diagnosis of pericardial effusions, decreased cardiac function, and left ventricular enlargement in pediatric patients. *J Am Soc Echocardiogr* 2005;18(4):313–319.

300. Kirkpatrick JN, et al. Effectiveness of echocardiographic imaging by nurses to identify left ventricular systolic dysfunction in high-risk patients. *Am J Cardiol* 2005;95(10):1271–1272.

301. Kobal SL, et al. Hand-carried cardiac ultrasound enhances healthcare delivery in developing countries. *Am J Cardiol* 2004;94(4):539–541.

302. Kobal SL, et al. Making an impossible mission possible. *Chest* 2004;125 (1):293–296.

303. Kirkpatrick JN, et al. Hand-carried cardiac ultrasound as a tool to screen for important cardiovascular disease in an underserved minority health care clinic. *J Am Soc Echocardiogr* 2004;17(5):399–403.

CHAPTER 7 ■ MAGNETIC RESONANCE IMAGING

TAL GEVA, MD, AND ANDREW J. POWELL, MD

Since publication of the previous edition of this textbook, the field of cardiovascular magnetic resonance imaging (CMR) has continued to experience rapid evolution in technology and clinical applications. During the past decade, developments in hardware design, computer sciences, and imaging sequences have led to a marked expansion of the clinical utility of CMR in patients with congenital and acquired pediatric heart disease. CMR is rarely used as the first or the sole diagnostic imaging test. It complements echocardiography, provides a noninvasive alternative to x-ray angiography, and overcomes many of the limitations of these modalities. For example, in contrast to echocardiography, acoustic windows and body size do not limit CMR, and, unlike cardiac catheterization, CMR does not use ionizing radiation. In today's clinical practice, CMR is increasingly used in concert with other imaging modalities (most commonly echocardiography) for assessment of cardiac anatomy and function, measurements of blood flow, tissue characterization, and, more recently, for evaluation of myocardial perfusion and viability. This chapter reviews common CMR techniques and discusses the clinical applications of CMR in patients with congenital and acquired pediatric heart disease.

INDICATION FOR MAGNETIC RESONANCE IMAGING EVALUATION OF CONGENITAL HEART DISEASE

The indications for CMR in patients with congenital heart disease (CHD) continue to expand. Given that CMR has been shown to provide helpful diagnostic information in most types of CHD, it is not practical to list individual anomalies in which the test is indicated. In general, the clinical reasons for a CMR examination fall into one or more of the following categories:

1. When transthoracic echocardiography cannot provide the required diagnostic information
2. When clinical assessment and other diagnostic tests are inconsistent
3. As an alternative to diagnostic cardiac catheterization with its associated risks and higher cost
4. To obtain diagnostic information for which CMR offers unique advantages

TABLE 7.1

PRIMARY REFERRAL DIAGNOSES IN 1,119 CONSECUTIVE PATIENTS WITH CONGENITAL AND ACQUIRED PEDIATRIC HEART DISEASE

Referral Diagnosis		Number of Studies (%)
Tetralogy of Fallot		256 (22.9%)
Anomalies of the Aorta		182 (16.3%)
Coarctation	112	
Other	70	
Complex two-ventricle		144 (12.9%)
TGA	75	
S/P arterial switch operation	47	
S/P atrial switch operation	28	
Single ventricle		110 (9.8%)
Ventricular function		81 (7.2%)
R/O arrhythmogenic RV cardiomyopathy		52 (4.6%)
Pulmonary veins		49 (4.4%)
Valve regurgitation		47 (4.2%)
Septal defects		39 (3.5%)
ASD	32	
VSD	7	
R/O vascular ring		29 (2.6%)
PA/IVS		21 (1.9%)
Congenital coronary anomaly		21 (1.9%)
Vascular anomalies		17 (1.5%)
Cardiac tumor		11 (1%)
Other		60 (5.4%)

TGA, transposition of the great arteries; S/P, status post; R/O, rule out; RV, right ventricle; ASD, atrial septal defect; VSD, ventricular septal defect; PA/IVS, pulmonary atresia with intact ventricular septum.

In clinical practice, CMR is typically ordered after other imaging studies have been performed and additional diagnostic information is required. Table 7.1 summarizes the primary reasons for CMR in 1,119 consecutive patients evaluated at Children's Hospital Boston in 2002–2003, illustrating the wide range of cardiovascular anomalies evaluated.

It is worth noting that the role of CMR in infants and toddlers is more limited than that in older patients. Because poor acoustic windows are less common in infants, echocardiography can provide the necessary diagnostic information in most patients, and CMR under sedation or anesthesia is reserved for those in whom additional information is necessary. A review of 99 consecutive CMR examinations in patients younger than 1 year of age during a 4-year period (January 1999 through December 2002) at Children's Hospital Boston found that delineation of the thoracic vasculature was the most common indication (55%), followed by assessment of airways compression (25%) and evaluation of cardiac tumors (6%) (1). In the future, CMR will likely assume a greater role in this age group, primarily as an alternative to diagnostic cardiac catheterization. Examples of such scenarios include delineation of sources of pulmonary blood supply in tetralogy of Fallot with pulmonary atresia and preoperative assessment of candidates for a bidirectional Glenn shunt.

MAGNETIC RESONANCE IMAGING TECHNIQUES

Background

In MRI, magnetic fields and radiofrequency energy are used to stimulate nuclei in selected regions of the body to emit radio waves that are then processed to construct images. The primary source of signals used to construct MR images is derived from hydrogen protons (^{1}H). The ^{1}H protons are often referred to as *spins* because their angular momentum results in a precession (spinning) around the axis of the primary magnetic field. The highest concentrations of ^{1}H protons are in water and fat. Through the use of a strong static magnetic field, much weaker but rapidly varying magnetic field gradients, and short pulses of radiofrequency (RF) energy, the ^{1}H protons (spins) in selected regions of the body are stimulated to emit RF waves. These RF waves are then used to construct MR images (Fig. 7.1). The strength of the static magnetic field in most clinical scanners used for CMR is 1.5 Tesla (T) (1 Tesla = 10,000 gauss [G]; the strength of earth's magnetic field at its surface is approximately 0.5 G). More recently, MRI scanners with a static field strength of 3 T have become commercially available.

As with any other diagnostic modality, an in-depth knowledge of the underlying MRI physics is essential for maximizing its utility and understanding its pitfalls and limitations. This, in turn, enhances the quality of the interpretation of the imaging data. A detailed discussion of MRI physics is beyond the scope of this chapter and can be found in other sources (2,3). Selected imaging sequences commonly used in CMR are described together with their clinical applications later in this chapter.

Cardiac and Respiratory Gating

Because most CMR techniques acquire data over multiple heartbeats, cardiac and respiratory motions during image acquisition result in image blurring. Several techniques have been developed to overcome this problem. The most common approach to compensate for cardiac motion is to synchronize image acquisition with the cardiac cycle. The cardiac cycle is tracked using either electrocardiographic (ECG) gating or a pulse oximetry trace (called *peripheral gating*) (Fig. 7.2). Electrocardiographic gating can be accomplished with a high-quality standard ECG trace or with a vectorcardiogram (VCG) signal (4). Recently, a new technique called *self-gating*, which relies on cardiac motion and avoids the use of ECG triggering altogether, has been described (5). Blurring owing to respiratory motion can be avoided either by having the patient hold his or her breath for periods of 5 to 10 seconds during data acquisition or by synchronizing image data acquisition to the respiratory as well as to the cardiac cycle. Another approach that reduces blurring from respiratory motion is to repeat the image acquisition several times and average the data. Respiratory motion can be tracked either by a bellows device placed around the abdomen or by a MR navigator pulse that concurrently tracks the position of the diaphragm or cardiac border (Fig. 7.3) (6).

A more desirable approach to avoid motion-induced image blurring is to acquire the MR data fast enough so that cardiac and respiratory motions are adequately resolved. Recent advances in gradient coil performance, parallel acquisition techniques, and image display methods have allowed real-time CMR at 20 to 24 frames per second, albeit at the expense of

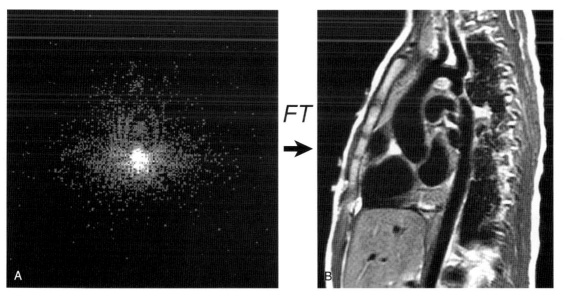

FIGURE 7.1 From signal to image. **A:** The raw magnetic resonance (MR) signal is stored as an array of numbers called *k-space*. By applying Fourier transformation (FT), the raw MR data stored in k-space are translated into an image (**B**).

spatial resolution (7–10). This technology, which is now commercially available on some clinical scanners, may obviate the need for ECG and respiratory triggering.

SEDATION AND MONITORING

Patients undergoing CMR examinations must remain still in the scanner bore for up to 60 minutes to minimize motion artifact during image acquisition and allow planning of successive imaging sequences. Accordingly, the need for performing the examination under sedation or anesthesia and an assessment of the risk/benefit ratio for proceeding under these circumstances should be determined well before the examination date. Multiple factors are taken into account when deciding whether a patient should have an examination without sedation, including the length of the anticipated examination protocol, the child's developmental age and maturity, the child's experience with prior procedures, and the parents' opinion of their child's capability to cooperate with the examination. True claustrophobia

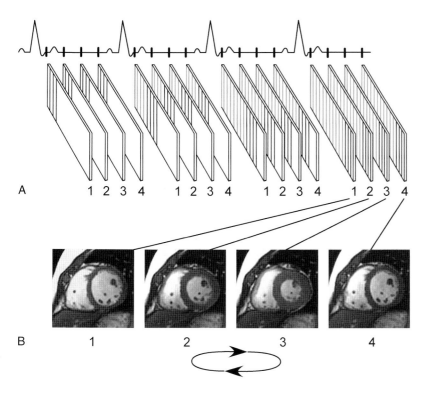

FIGURE 7.2 Cine MRI. **A:** Schematic representation of image data acquisition. Using the ECG signal, the cardiac cycle is divided into multiple equally spaced acquisition windows. Several lines of k-space are acquired during each acquisition window (a technique called *segmented k-space*). Over several heartbeats, a series of images spanning the cardiac cycle is reconstructed and viewed in cine loop mode (**B**).

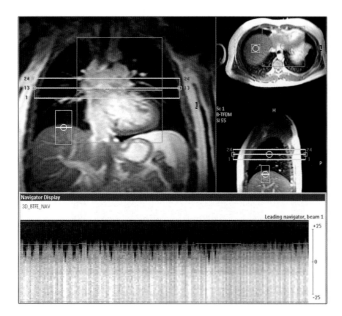

FIGURE 7.3 Respiratory navigator. The navigator beam is positioned over the right hemidiaphragm and includes lung and liver tissues (**top**). The motion of the right hemidiaphragm is continuously displayed (**bottom**) along with the acceptance window (*horizontal lines*). Only data acquired when the position of the right hemidiaphragm is registered within the acceptance window are used for image reconstruction.

in the pediatric age group is rare. In general, most children 7 years of age and older can cooperate sufficiently for a good-quality CMR study. Parents should be provided with a detailed description of the examination and asked to discuss it with their child in an age-appropriate manner in advance to increase the likelihood of a successful study. After proper screening, parents can be allowed into the scanner room to help their child complete the examination. Allowing patients to listen to music or watch movies through a specialized MRI-compatible audiovisual system may reduce anxiety and improve patient cooperation.

Strategies for sedation and anesthesia in CMR vary and often depend on institutional preference and resources such as availability of qualified pediatric anesthesiologists. Although it is possible to wait for young children to fall into a natural sleep, this approach may be time consuming and complicated by early awakening. Sedation can be achieved with various medications (e.g., pentobarbital, propofol, fentanyl, midazolam, chloral hydrate) and is a reasonable approach (11–16). Its principal drawbacks are an unprotected airway and reliance on spontaneous respiratory effort with the associated risks of aspiration, airway obstruction, and hypoventilation. In addition, because images are often acquired over several seconds, respiratory motion will degrade image quality. This motion artifact can be reduced by synchronizing image data acquisition to the respiratory cycle tracked by either a bellows device around the abdomen or by navigator echoes that concurrently image the position of the diaphragm or heart. An alternative strategy to reduce respiratory motion artifacts is to acquire multiple images at the same location and average them, thereby minimizing variations from respiration. The principal limitations of both these strategies are prolonged scan times and incomplete elimination of respiratory motion that can lead to reduced image quality.

Because of these safety and image quality concerns, we and others frequently prefer to perform CMR examinations under

general anesthesia in children who cannot undergo an awake examination (17,18). This approach, described in detail elsewhere (1,19), is safe, consistently achieves adequate sedation, protects the airway, and offers control of ventilation. Respiratory motion artifact can be completely eliminated by suspending ventilation in conjunction with neuromuscular blockade. Breath-hold periods of 30 to 60 seconds are typically well tolerated and allow multiple locations to be scanned efficiently.

When using either sedation or anesthesia, is it important that both nurses and physicians have sufficient experience with these procedures in children with cardiovascular disorders. Continuous monitoring of the electrocardiogram, pulse oximetry, end-tidal carbon dioxide, anesthetic gases, and blood pressure with a MRI compatible physiologic monitoring system is required. MRI-compatible anesthesia machines are available that can be located in the scanner room and connected to the patient's endotracheal tube by an extended breathing circuit. To maximize patient safety and examination quality, it is recommended that different health care providers be responsible for supervising the imaging and sedation/anesthesia aspects of the study and that they communicate closely with each other.

PATIENT PREPARATION

Prior to bringing the patient into the scanner room, the physician and technologists should review the patient's history, safety screening form, and the most recent chest radiograph to identify implanted devices that may be hazardous in the MRI environment or produce image artifact. A detailed discussion on MRI safety can be found in the next section and elsewhere (20–25).

Following safety screening, physiologic monitoring devices and hearing protection (for both awake and anesthetized patients) are put in place. A high-quality electrocardiogram signal is essential for optimum image quality in cardiac-gated sequences. The signal should be checked both when the patient is outside and then inside the scanner bore. In patients with dextrocardia, electrocardiogram leads are best placed on the right chest. Because young children dissipate body heat faster than adults, the scanner room temperature should be adjusted and prewarmed blankets applied to minimize heat loss.

The imaging coil should be chosen to maximize the signal-to-noise ratio over the entire body region to be examined. Because congenital heart disease often involves abnormalities of the thoracic vasculature, the coil should be large enough to cover the entire thorax rather than just the heart. Adult head or knee coils are often appropriate for infants weighing <10 kg, and adult cardiac coil for medium-sized children weighing between 10 and 40 kg. Adequate coil coverage and placement should be confirmed early in the examination by reviewing the localizing images.

SAFETY

Standard clinical imaging scanners present no known hazards to biologic materials. Guidelines set by the Food and Drug Administration (FDA) keep the strength of the magnetic fields and the deposition of radiofrequency energy well below levels that could cause significant biologic effects. Animal studies evaluating the influence of static magnetic fields have not demonstrated significant biologic effects for fields of up to 2 T (26). Millions of patients have undergone MRI studies without any noticeable immediate or long-term sequelae. Pregnancy was

TABLE 7.2

SAFETY CONSIDERATIONS AND IMAGE ARTIFACTS OWING TO IMPLANTED DEVICES USED IN PATIENTS WITH CONGENITAL HEART DISEASE

Device	Safety[a]	Image Artifact[b]	Comment
Pacemaker	RC	2	The assertion that presence of a pacemaker/
AICD	RC	2	defibrillator is an absolute contraindication to MRI has been challenged (22).
Permanent pacemaker lead—no generator	RC	1	Experiments in animal models found heating of permanent pacemaker leads (277).
Temporary pacemaker lead—no generator	OK	1	
Sternal wire	OK	2	
Hemostatic vascular clips	OK	1–2	
Stent	*		
Stainless steel	OK	2	
Nonferromagnetic or minimally ferromagnetic	OK	1	
Vascular occluding coil	*		
Stainless steel	OK	3	
Platinum	OK	1	Compared with stainless steel coils, platinum coils are more expensive and less thrombogenic.
Occluding devices	*		
Rashkind occluder	OK	3	
Clamshell	OK	3	
CardioSEAL	OK	2	
STARFlex	OK	2	
Amplatzer	OK	2	
Prosthetic heart valves	OK	2	

CI, contraindication; AICD, automatic implantable cardioverter defibrillator; RC, relative contraindication; OK, no known adverse events related to clinical MRI.

[a]Safety grade in a 1.5T scanner with commercially available imaging sequences.

[b]Extent of image artifact: 1, none or trivial; 2, small on standard gradient echo sequences (GRE) and minimal on spin echo sequences; 3, large (several centimeters) on standard gradient echo sequences (GRE) and remains substantial on spin echo sequences.

*Some centers advocate avoiding MRI for an arbitrary period of time after implantation (usually for several weeks), but such practice is not supported by conclusive published data. A decision to perform MRI examination shortly after cardiac surgery or implantation of a biomedical device must weigh the risk/benefit ratio for the individual patient (27).

considered a relative contraindication to MRI studies, although the magnetic field levels used in clinical imagers have no known effects on the embryo. Many women have undergone MRI imaging during all trimesters of pregnancy without reported ill effect on the mother, fetus, or resultant infant. When maternal and fetal health considerations necessitate diagnostic studies, MRI is preferable to methods that use x-rays, such as computed tomography or standard angiography.

Implanted metallic objects are of particular concern in the MR environment since they could potentially undergo undesirable movements if the magnetic field were sufficiently strong and if they contained sufficient ferromagnetic material (Table 7.2). Fortunately, surgical clips and sternotomy wires implanted in the chest and abdomen are typically only weakly ferromagnetic. Furthermore, these devices quickly become immobilized by surrounding fibrous tissue, and MRI can safely be used to study patients with these implants. The wires and clips, however, may cause localized image artifact. Similarly, MRI can be used to image patients with implanted intravascular coils, stents, and occluding devices once the implants are believed to be immobile. Many centers choose to avoid exposing these patients to MRI for an arbitrarily chosen period of time after implantation (usually for several weeks), but such practice is not supported by conclusive published data. A decision to perform MRI examination shortly after cardiac surgery or implantation of a biomedical device must weigh the risk/benefit ratio for the individual patient (27).

Several devices are considered either relative or absolute contraindications to using MRI (24,27–31). Presence of an intracranial, intraocular, or intracochlear metallic object is considered a contraindication to MRI. The presence of a cardiac pacemaker is also considered a contraindication to MRI (32), although some reports have suggested that scanning patients who have modern pacemakers may be possible (22,33,34).

Because MRI scanners attract ferromagnetic objects, extreme caution should be used in approaching magnets with objects containing iron or other ferromagnetic materials. Only specially designed MRI-compatible physiologic monitoring equipment should be used in conjunction with MRI studies. There have been several reported cases of patient burns resulting from the use of MRI-incompatible pulse oximeters and electrocardiographic monitoring devices.

EXAM SUPERVISION AND INTERPRETATION

Detailed pre-examination planning is crucial given the wide array of imaging sequences available and the often-complex nature of the clinical, anatomic, and functional issues in patients with CHD. The importance of a careful review of the patient's medical history, including details of all cardiovascular surgical procedures, interventional catheterizations, findings of previous diagnostic tests, and current clinical status, cannot be overemphasized. As with echocardiography and cardiac catheterization, CMR examination of CHD is an interactive diagnostic procedure that requires on-line review and interpretation of the data by the supervising physician. The unpredictable nature of the anatomy and hemodynamics often require adjustment of the examination protocol, modification of imaging planes, changing sequences, and adjustment of imaging parameters. Reliance on standardized protocols and postexamination review alone in these patients may result in incomplete or even erroneous interpretation.

CLINICAL APPLICATIONS

CMR Examination Techniques

The building blocks of any MRI examination are called *pulse sequences* (Fig. 7.4). An MRI pulse sequence describes the way the magnetic field gradients and RF pulses are applied to produce images with particular characteristics. Some of the pulse sequences used in CMR practice are described below together with their clinical applications. During the course of a CMR examination, the examiner selects the pulse sequences and prescribes imaging locations and planes to acquire the image data to address specific clinical questions.

Assessment of Cardiovascular Anatomy

Evaluation of cardiovascular anatomy and function in patients with CHD is often inseparable. Several MRI sequences can be

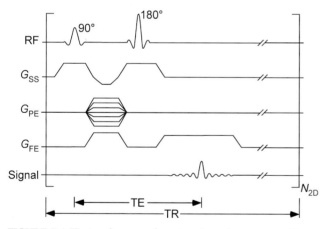

FIGURE 7.4 Timing diagram of a spin echo pulse sequence. The x-axis represents time. The first step is the simultaneous applications of a 90-degree radiofrequency (RF) pulse and a slice-selective gradient (G_{SS}) pulse. The next step is the application of a slice-selective 180-degree RF pulse to refocus the transverse magnetization that lost phase coherence owing to inhomogeneities in the magnetic field. To locate the MR signal in space (spatial localization), multiple frequency-encoding (G_{PE}) and a single phase-encoding (G_{FE}) gradients are applied. The time at which the MR signal (echo) is recorded is called *echo time*, or TE. This sequence results in the acquisition of one line of k-space data. The sequence is repeated N_{2D} times, each with a different phase-encoding value, until all lines of k-space are collected and a 2-D image is reconstructed. The time from onset of one sequence to the next is called *repletion time*, or TR.

used for anatomic delineation; each provides particular information. In practice, the anatomy in question is often assessed by more than one imaging sequence, yielding overlapping information that increases diagnostic confidence.

Spin Echo

The MR signal is produced by applying a brief RF pulse that tips the spins 90 degrees relative to the axis of the main magnetic field, followed by a 180-degree refocusing RF pulse (Fig. 7.4). Because of the relatively long time interval between spin excitation and data sampling, flowing blood will leave the image plane by the time the signal is sampled. The result is an image in which flowing blood appears black whereas more stationary tissues produce MR signals displayed in varying shades of gray or white ("black blood" imaging) (Fig. 7.5A). Other features of spin echo (SE) pulse sequences include a single image per cardiac cycle (static imaging), high tissue contrast, and, compared with gradient echo pulse sequences, relative insensitivity to inhomogeneities in the magnetic field. In clinical practice, such inhomogeneities are mostly owing to ferromagnetic implants such as sternal wires, prosthetic heart valves, stents, coils, or other implants. SE sequences can also be modified to alter tissue contrast and characterize abnormal structures (e.g., T1 and T2 weighting) (Fig. 7.5B). Standard SE requires several minutes (usually 2 to 4 minutes depending on heart rate and imaging parameters) to acquire an image dataset. Fast or turbo spin echo (FSE or TSE) requires a much shorter image acquisition time because, instead of acquiring a single phase encoding line for each 90-degree RF pulse, multiple phase encoding lines are acquired in rapid succession (called *echo train*). As a result, image acquisition can be completed during 10 to 15 seconds of breath holding. In the FSE or TSE sequence, the blood signal is nulled by an inversion pulse (called *double inversion recovery*) rather than relying on blood flow alone.

Standard SE was the work horse of CMR during the 1980s. In today's clinical practice, standard SE has been largely replaced by FSE or TSE with double inversion recovery (2). Examples of clinical applications include assessment of tissue characteristics (e.g., cardiac tumors, arrhythmogenic right ventricular dysplasia, myocardial noncompaction, and ventricular aneurysm), vessel wall imaging (e.g., aortic dissection), evaluation of the pericardium, and anatomic imaging in patients with metallic implants.

Gradient Echo Cine MRI

Gradient echo MR is a class of pulse sequences that produce bright blood images. The fundamental difference between SE and gradient echo sequences is that in the latter the initial RF pulse tips the spins at an angle (called *flip angle*) <90 degrees. Gradient echo sequences are generally faster than SE sequences because the time between spin excitation and signal detection (called *echo time* or TE) is much shorter. The signal from stationary or relatively slow-moving tissues (such as the myocardium) is gray because the spins within the selected slice are partially saturated by the rapid repetition of the RF pulse. This is because the spins do not have sufficient time to return to their original unexcited state during the short interval between RF pulses, which results in a relatively weak signal. On the other hand, blood that flows into the slice contains unsaturated spins that produce relatively strong signals, hence the term "bright blood" imaging (Fig. 7.6). An important feature of gradient echo sequences is high imaging speed, which allows reconstruction of multiple images during the cardiac cycle that can be displayed in cine loop format. Compared with SE techniques, gradient echo sequences have a relatively low

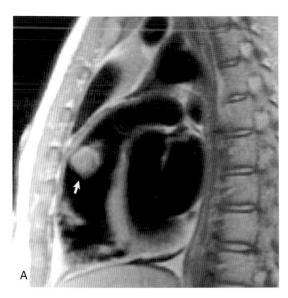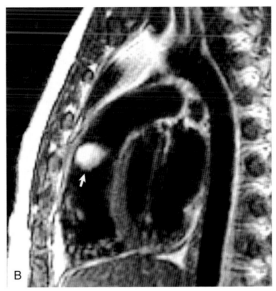

FIGURE 7.5 Short-axis fast (turbo) spin echo image in a patient with hemangioma of the right ventricular outflow tract. **A:** T1-weighted image showing a slightly hyperintense globular tumor (*arrow*). **B:** T2-weighted image showing the tumor is markedly hyperintense, consistent with a vascular tumor.

tissue contrast and are more susceptible to inhomogeneities within the magnetic field.

ECG- or VCG-triggered steady-state free precession (SSFP) is currently the most commonly used cine MRI technique for assessment of cardiovascular anatomy and ventricular function. This sequence relies on the ratio of T2-to-T1 relaxations with a resultant high contrast between the blood pool ($T2/T1 = 360/1200 = 0.3$) and the myocardium ($T2/T1 = 75/880 = 0.085$), which clearly depicts the boundaries of cardiovascular structures (Fig. 7.6) (35). This sequence is known by several proprietary names, including true fast imaging with steady pre-

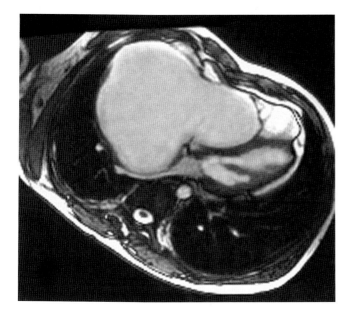

FIGURE 7.6 ECG-triggered steady-state free precession image in the four-chamber plane in a patient with Ebstein anomaly. Note the apical displacement of the tricuspid valve, "atrialization" of the right ventricular inflow, and the markedly dilated right atrium.

cession (TrueFISP), balanced fast field echo (bFFE), and fast imaging employing steady state acquisition (FIESTA). The acquisition time of SSFP cine MRI is short, typically requiring 4 to 10 seconds for each location depending on heart rate, spatial resolution, and other acquisition parameters. Use of parallel imaging techniques such as sensitivity encoding (SENSE) allows even shorter acquisition times. The SSFP sequence, however, is highly sensitive to inhomogeneities in the magnetic field such as those induced by implanted metallic devices.

A segmented *k*-space fast (turbo) gradient recalled echo (fast GRE) sequence was used extensively during the 1990s, and its accuracy and reproducibility in measuring ventricular dimensions and function have been validated (36–38). Compared with SSFP, the distinction between blood and myocardium on fast GRE images is less sharp, the contrast-to-noise ratio and the temporal resolution are lower, image acquisition time is longer, and images are more susceptible to blood flow effects. On the other hand, fast GRE is less susceptible to inhomogeneities in the magnetic field than SSFP. Therefore, in patients with image artifacts caused by implanted devices, the use of a fast GRE sequence offers an advantage over SSFP.

In clinical practice, an ECG-gated gradient echo cine MRI sequence is prescribed across the anatomy of interest to yield a stack of contiguous cross-sectional slices that can be displayed on a computer workstation in a multilocation, multiphase (cine loop) format. ECG-gated segmented *k*-space SSFP cine MRI is currently the sequence of choice for evaluation of cardiac anatomy and function because of its excellent blood–myocardium contrast, high spatial and temporal resolutions, and short acquisition time. The SSFP sequence allows detailed imaging of the cardiac chambers, the atrioventricular and semilunar valves, the papillary muscles and chordae tendineae, the membranous septum, septum primum, and blood vessels (Fig. 7.6). The SSFP sequence, however, is relatively insensitive to flow disturbances due to stenotic or regurgitant jets and is highly sensitive to inhomogeneities in the magnetic field. Alternatively, a segmented *k*-space fast (turbo) gradient echo sequence can be prescribed when further delineation of abnormal flow jets is desirable

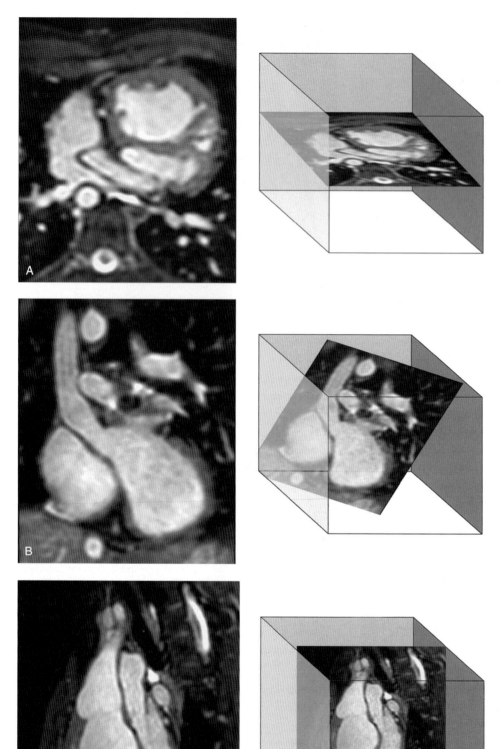

FIGURE 7.7 Free-breathing (navigator-gated), ECG-triggered, isotropic, 3-D steady-state free precession imaging in a patient with Mustard palliation of transposition of the great arteries. The 3-D data volume is reformatted off-line in multiple user-defined planes. **A:** Transverse view of the pulmonary venous pathway. **B:** Oblique view depicting the superior vena cava pathway. **C:** Oblique sagittal view of the left and right ventricular outflow tracts.

or when implanted metallic devices produce severe imaging artifacts.

Isotropic Three-Dimensional Steady-State Free Precession MRI

This recently described cardiac-triggered steady-state free precession (SSFP) technique acquires a three-dimensional image volume over a period of 4 to 7 minutes of free breathing (39). The motion of the diaphragm is tracked with a navigator pulse, and image data are accepted only when the position of the diaphragm lies within a narrow window defined by the operator, thus avoiding artifacts from respiratory motion. The volume elements (voxels) of the image dataset are isotropic, which allows off-line reformatting of the image volume in any arbitrary plane. This imaging technique does not require administration of contrast agents and provides high-resolution static imaging of both intracardiac and extracardiac anatomy (Fig. 7.7).

Coronary Artery Imaging

The origin and course of the epicardial coronary arteries can be evaluated by several MRI techniques. Most of the published experience with MRI evaluation of the coronary arteries is based on a cardiac-triggered, navigator-gated free-breathing three-dimensional (3-D) magnetic resonance angiography (MRA) sequence (40). This technique has been used successfully in patients with various congenital anomalies of the coronary arteries (Fig. 7.8) and in Kawasaki disease (41–45).

Contrast-Enhanced Three-Dimensional MRA

Gadolinium (Gd)-enhanced 3-D MRA is ideally suited for imaging of extracardiac vascular anatomy. Examples of common clinical applications include imaging of the aorta and its branches, pulmonary arteries, pulmonary veins, systemic

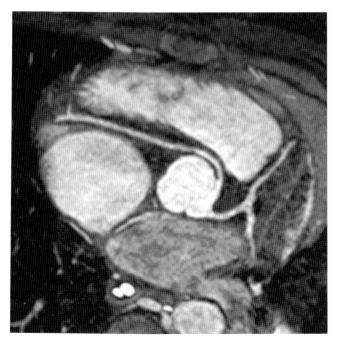

FIGURE 7.8 Free-breathing (navigator-gated), ECG-triggered, coronary magnetic resonance angiography (MRA) showing anomalous origin of the right coronary artery from the left aortic sinus of Valsalva.

veins, aortopulmonary and venous–venous collateral vessels, systemic-to-pulmonary artery shunts, conduits, and vascular grafts (12,46). Although this technique is mostly used for imaging of extracardiac anatomy, we have also found it useful in the evaluation of intra-atrial systemic and pulmonary baffles (e.g., Mustard or Senning operations and Fontan palliation), as well as for imaging of the outflow tracts (e.g., repaired tetralogy of Fallot [TOF] and the arterial switch operation). In addition, Gd-enhanced 3-D MRA clearly delineates the spatial relationships between vascular structures, the tracheobronchial tree, chest wall, spine, and other landmarks that may be useful for planning interventional catheterization or surgical procedures (Fig. 7.9). More recently, time-resolved 3-D MRA has been introduced, but its clinical utility awaits further study given the trade-offs between spatial and temporal resolutions.

In practice, the contrast (e.g., gadopentetate dimeglumine 0.2 to 0.3 mmol/kg) is infused through a peripheral intravenous cannula either by hand (in patients weighing <8 to 10 kg) or by a power injector at a rate of 2 to 2.5 mL/s. Patients are instructed to take several deep breaths before image acquisition. The time delay between the start of contrast injection and data acquisition is determined either by the best estimate method or, more recently, by a magnetic resonance fluoroscopic method that allows real-time visualization of the arrival of the contrast bolus to the heart. Two or more sequential 3-D MRA data acquisitions are usually obtained 10 to 15 seconds apart during which patients are being asked to hold their breath. In patients under anesthesia, ventilation is suspended during imaging.

Ventricular Function

Technique. ECG- or VCG-triggered steady-state free precession (SSFP) is currently the most commonly used cine MRI technique for assessment of ventricular function. In patients in whom image artifacts from metallic implants obscure the ventricles, a fast (turbo) GRE sequence can be used because it is less susceptible to inhomogeneities in the magnetic field (47). ECG-triggered SSFP cine MRI is acquired during short periods of breath holding. Depending on heart rate and image acquisition parameters (matrix size, number of k-space lines per segment, and the scanner's gradient system capabilities), high-resolution acquisition may last 7 to 10 seconds per slice. A modest decrease in spatial and temporal resolutions will lower the acquisition time to 4 to 5 seconds while producing diagnostically acceptable images. The use of sensitivity encoding (SENSE) technology allows shorter acquisitions time by a factor of 2 to 4 (at the expense of reduced signal-to-noise ratio), an increase in spatial or temporal resolutions while maintaining the same acquisition time, or a combination of the two. Patients are instructed to hold their breath at end-expiration to minimize variations in the position of the diaphragm and, consequently, the heart. In patients who are incapable of holding their breath, images are acquired during free breathing either with multiple signal averages, with respiratory triggering, or with real-time MR fluoroscopy (48,49).

Quantitative evaluation of ventricular function is achieved by obtaining a series of contiguous SSFP cine MRI slices that cover the ventricles in short-axis views (Fig. 7.10). This involves the following steps:

a. *Two-chamber plane (also known as long axial oblique and vertical long-axis planes):* A slice is prescribed parallel to the plane of the interventricular septum based on previously obtained scout images in the axial (transverse) plane (Fig. 7.10A). In patients with a biventricular heart and a systemic left ventricle (LV), the slice extends from the center of the

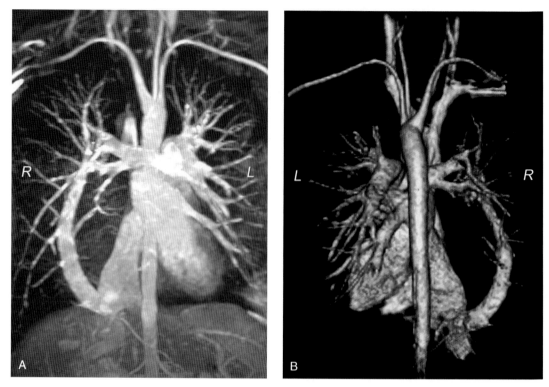

FIGURE 7.9 Gadolinium-enhanced 3-D MRA of scimitar syndrome. **A:** Subvolume maximal intensity projection. **B:** Three-dimnensional volume rendering (posterior view). L, left; R, right.

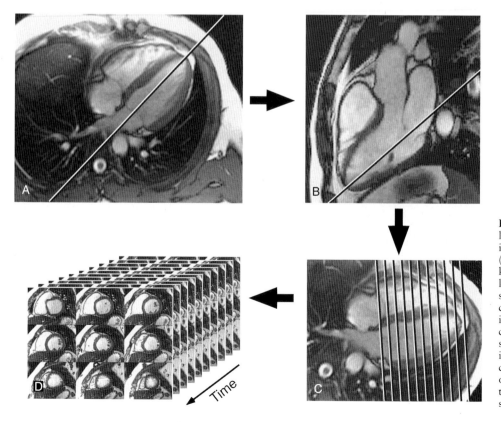

FIGURE 7.10 Evaluation of ventricular volumes and mass. **A:** Using a localizing image obtained in the axial (transverse) plane, a two-chamber (also known as long axial oblique or vertical long-axis) plane is prescribed as shown. **B:** Prescription of the four-chamber plane from an end-diastolic image of the previous two-chamber cine sequence; **C:** Prescription of the short-axis plane from an end-diastolic image of the previous four-chamber cine sequence extending from the plane of the atrioventricular (AV) valves through the cardiac apex; **D:** The short-axis stack is viewed in cine mode.

mitral valve to the LV apex. In patients with a systemic right ventricle (RV) (e.g., atrial switch operation for transposition of the great arteries), it is advantageous to place the slice between the center of the tricuspid valve and the RV apex. In patients with a single ventricle, the slice is placed between the center of the atrioventricular (AV) valve(s) to the ventricular apex. This acquisition accounts for the orientation of the ventricles in the transverse plane of the chest.

b. *Four-chamber plane (also known as horizontal long-axis plane)*: A stack of slices is prescribed from an end-diastolic image of a slice acquired perpendicular the previous two-chamber cine sequence (Fig. 7.10B). This acquisition accounts for the superior-inferior orientation of the ventricles in the chest.

c. *Short-axis plane*: Multiple equidistant slices are prescribed from an end-diastolic image of the previous 4-chamber cine sequence covering the ventricles from the plane of the AV valve(s) to the cardiac apex (Fig. 7.10C). The first slice is placed at the level of the AV annuli by connecting the right coronary artery (seen in cross section in the right AV groove) with the left circumflex coronary artery (seen in the left AV groove). Subsequent slices are positioned in equidistance through the cardiac apex (Fig. 7.10D). In most patients, 12 slices will cover the ventricles from base to apex with adjustment of slice thickness between 4 and 8 mm and the interslice spacing from 0 to 2 mm. Using these guidelines, the range of ventricular lengths covered is 4.8 to 12 cm. In some infants, the number of slices can be reduced, whereas in older patients with markedly dilated ventricles, the number of slices may need to be increased. We prefer not to increase the slice thickness >8 mm and interslice spacing >2 mm to avoid partial volume effect and to minimize extrapolation of interslice data.

Image Analysis. Accurate determination of ventricular volume requires clear depiction of the blood–myocardial boundary. Adjustment of the image brightness and contrast on the computer screen can facilitate visualization of that boundary. By tracing the blood–endocardium boundary, the slice's blood pool volume is calculated as the product of its cross-sectional area and thickness (which is prescribed by the operator). The left ventricular papillary muscles and the major trabeculations of the right ventricle (e.g., septal and moderator bands) are excluded from the blood pool and are considered part of the myocardium. Ventricular volume is then determined by summation of the volumes of all slices. The process can be repeated for each frame in the cardiac cycle to obtain a continuous time–volume loop or may be performed only on end-diastolic (maximal area) and end-systolic (minimal area) frames to calculate diastolic and systolic volumes. From these data one can calculate left and right ventricular ejection fractions and stroke volumes. Since the patient's heart rate at the time of image acquisition is known, one can calculate left and right ventricular outputs. Ventricular mass is calculated by tracing the epicardial borders and calculating the epicardial volume, subtracting the endocardial volume, and multiplying the resultant muscle volume by the specific gravity of the myocardium (1.05 g/mm^3).

Most manufacturers of MRI scanners and some third party companies offer software packages that automatically perform the above calculations. Development of algorithms for automatic border detection has facilitated the application of these techniques, but further refinements are required to improve its accuracy (50–53).

Potential Sources of Errors in Determining Ventricular Volumes by MRI. Translational motion of the ventricles in the base-to-apex direction is most prominent at the base of the heart. Given that the prescribed short-axis slices are fixed in space, there is significant through-plane motion in the basal slices during the cardiac cycle. As a result, the first (and sometimes also the second) most basal slices may contain atrial blood pool during part of the cardiac cycle because the atrioventricular junction has moved out of the imaging plane during systole. To avoid erroneous inclusion of the atrial blood pool in the calculation of ventricular volume, the image dataset is examined to distinguish between ventricular and atrial structures. In general, when a slice contains a ventricular chamber throughout the cardiac cycle, the chamber's cross-sectional area decreases in systole and its wall thickness increases. In contrast, in a slice containing ventricular myocardium in diastole and atrial blood pool in systole, the chamber's cross-sectional area increases and wall thickness decreases.

Another potential source of error in measurements of ventricular volumes is when the left ventricular papillary muscles and the right ventricular trabeculations are traced in an inconsistent fashion during systole and diastole. For example, exclusion of the papillary muscles from the blood pool in diastole but not in systole will lead to underestimation of end-systolic volume, stroke volume, and ejection fraction.

Inconsistent position of the diaphragm during breath holding can lead to spatial variations in the location of the ventricles during acquisition of the short-axis images. This source of error in volume calculation can be minimized by instructing the patient to hold breath at end-expiration (54,55).

Accuracy, Reproducibility, and Reference Values of Ventricular Volumes and Function by CMR. The combination of a three-dimensional dataset, clear distinction between the blood pool and the myocardium, and high spatial and temporal resolutions allow for accurate measurements of any cardiac chamber regardless of its morphology and without geometric assumptions. Much research was performed in the late 1980s and early 1990s on *in vitro* phantoms, animal models, and in human subjects to validate the accuracy of CMR measurements of ventricular volumes and mass (56–62). More recently, attention has focused on investigating the test characteristics of CMR assessment of chamber dimensions and function and on comparison of its accuracy and reproducibility with those of echocardiography and radionuclide techniques (63–66). Germain et al. (67), in a study of 20 patients with "good echocardiographic windows." found that the mean (±SD) interstudy variability of CMR measurement of left ventricular mass was 6.75 ± 3.8% compared with 11 ± 6.4% for M-mode echocardiography. Bellenger et al. (68) calculated that the sample size required to detect changes in left ventricular volumes, ejection fraction, and mass by CMR in patients with heart failure was substantially smaller compared with published values for two-dimensional echocardiography. For example, to detect a 10-mL change in end-diastolic volume (with 90% power and $p <0.05$), 12 subjects must be studied by CMR versus 121 patients examined by 2-D echocardiography; a 3% change in ejection fraction requires 15 CMR versus 102 echocardiograms, and a 10-g change in mass requires 9 CMR versus 273 echocardiograms. Ioannidis et al. (69) compared the accuracy of single photon emission computed tomography (SPECT) for assessment of left ventricular volumes and ejection fraction with that of CMR. Although the two modalities correlated well, compared with CMR, there was a substantial variation in individual measurements by SPECT. Half of the SPECT ejection fraction determinations deviated by at least 5% from CMR-obtained values, and one in four deviated by at least 10%.

Since CMR techniques are evolving rapidly, different sequences may lead to differing measurements of ventricular dimensions and function. Several studies have compared the normal range of left and right ventricular mass, volume, and ejection fraction measured by SSFP cine MRI with values obtained by the fast (turbo) GRE cine technique. Plein et al. (70) found that compared with fast GRE, SSFP values of LV end-diastolic and end-systolic volumes were 8.8% and 17.8% higher, respectively. LV mass was 13.8% lower, and the ejection fraction was not significantly different between the two techniques. Importantly, both intraobserver and interobserver variations were lower with SSFP measurements compared with fast GRE. In another study, Alfakih et al. (71) demonstrated that RV end-diastolic and end-systolic volumes measured by SSFP were 7.4% and 15.6% higher than by fast GRE, respectively. As for the LV, measurements of RV dimension and ejection fraction by SSFP were more reproducible than by fast GRE. The range of SSFP-based left and right ventricular volumes, mass, and ejection fraction in 60 healthy subjects ranging in age from 20 to 65 years published by Alfakih et al. (72) is summarized in Table 7.3. It should be noted that SSFP-based normal values of ventricular dimensions in children have not been published.

Assessment of Myocardial Function

Although ejection fraction and other ejection phase indices such as shortening fraction and velocity of circumferential fiber shortening are useful markers of ventricular function and provide valuable prognostic information, they are influenced by preload, afterload, heart rate, and the contractile state of the myocardium. Moreover, load-dependent ejection phase indices such as ejection fraction can be normal despite depressed contractility and, conversely, can be depressed despite having normal contractility. Therefore, assessment of ventricular function by load-independent indexes provides useful information on the contractile state of the myocardium. A detailed discussion of ventricular mechanics is beyond the scope of this chapter and can be found elsewhere (73,74).

Assessment of the contractile state of the myocardium by CMR has been investigated by Setser et al. (75) using normalized maximal ventricular power. An alternative approach is to adjust ejection phase variables such as ejection fraction, velocity of fiber shortening, or wall strain to end-systolic stress. With knowledge of left ventricular end-systolic volume, mass,

and pressure (estimated based on mean arterial blood pressure measured by sphygmomanometry), end-systolic stress can be estimated as follows (74):

$$P = (2/3)\sigma_p (\ln V_0 - \ln V_c)$$

where

V_c is cavity volume
V_0 is chamber volume (cavity volume + myocardial volume)
σ_p is average of orthogonal fiber stresses $(\sigma_{p\phi} + \sigma_{p\theta})/2$.

It should be noted that experience with this method in CMR is lacking.

Analysis of Regional Wall Motion

A simple qualitative approach is to visually evaluate segmental ventricular wall motion and thickening imaged from long- and short-axis gradient echo (SSFP or fast GRE) cine MRI. The left ventricle is divided into 17 segments, as recommended by the American Heart Association (Fig. 7.11) (76), and the right ventricle is divided into 9 segments as described by Klein et al. (77) (Fig. 7.12). Ventricular wall motion is classified as normal (appropriate systolic wall motion normal to the local wall segment accompanied by myocardial thickening indicative of fiber shortening), hypokinesis (reduced systolic motion and wall thickening), akinesis (no appreciable systolic wall motion and no change in wall thickness), or dyskinesis (outward systolic wall motion without myocardial thickening). A more objective approach is to define the endocardial and epicardial boundaries of the ventricles throughout the cardiac cycle, and, using commercially available software, quantitatively analyze wall motion and myocardial thickening (78). The main drawback of this approach is that it is time consuming, which hinders its acceptance into routine clinical practice. However, improvements in automatic border detection can shorten the process and may lead to increased use of this technique.

Analysis of Myocardial Strain and Stress

Analysis of myocardial strain provides information on regional myocardial function. Although myocardial strain can be calculated from velocity information obtained by phase-velocity

TABLE 7.3

NORMAL VALUES OF SSFP-BASED LV AND RV VOLUMES, MASS, AND EJECTION FRACTION IN 60 SUBJECTS RANGING IN AGE FROM 20 TO 65 YEARS

	Male ($n = 30$) Mean ± SD (range[a])	Female ($n = 30$) Mean ± SD (range[a])
LV EDV index (mL/m²)	82.3 ± 14.7 (53–112)	77.7 ± 10.8 (56–99)
LV ejection fraction (%)	64.2 ± 4.6 (55–73)	64.0 ± 4.9 (54–74)
LV mass index (g/m²)	64.7 ± 9.3 (46–83)	52.0 ± 7.4 (37–67)
RV EDV index (ml/m²)	86.2 ± 14.1 (58–114)	75.2 ± 13.8 (48–103)
RV ejection fraction	55.1 ± 3.7 (48–63)	59.8 ± 5.0 (50–70)

SD, standard deviation; LV, left ventricle; EDV, end-diastolic volume; RV, right ventricle.
[a]−2 SD to +2 SD.
Adapted from Alfakih K, Plein S, Thiele H, et al. Normal human left and right ventricular dimensions for MRI as assessed by turbo gradient echo and steady-state free precession imaging sequences. *J Magn Reson Imaging* 2003;17(3):323–329 with permission.

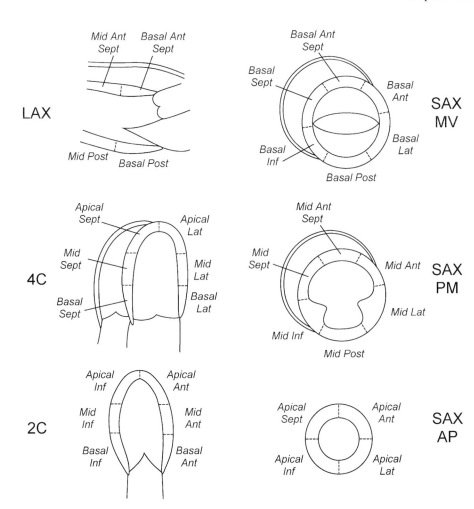

FIGURE 7.11 Left ventricular wall segments. Ant, anterior; Inf, inferior; Lat, lateral; LV, left ventricle; MV, mitral valve; PM, papillary muscles; Post, posterior; RV, right ventricle; SAX, short-axis; Sept, septal. (Adapted and modified from Cerqueira MD, Weissman NJ, Dilsizian V, et al. Standardized myocardial segmentation and nomenclature for tomographic imaging of the heart: a statement for healthcare professionals from the Cardiac Imaging Committee of the Council on Clinical Cardiology of the American Heart Association. *Circulation* 2002;105:539–542, with permission.)

cine MRI technique (similar to tissue Doppler imaging), most investigators favor a technique called *myocardial tagging* using spatial modulation of magnetization (SPAMM) (79). This technique is a modification of cine gradient echo MRI that allows tracking of myocardial motion in two or three spatial dimensions over time. Using a preparatory radiofrequency pulse, saturation bands or "tags" that appear as dark lines or stripes are applied across the image at end-diastole (Fig. 7.13). On subsequent images, the stripes (tags) will remain unchanged on stationary tissue such as the chest wall and spine but will change their position on moving tissues such as ventricular myocardium. As the myocardium moves during the cardiac cycle, the tags follow it and their rotation, translation, and

deformation can be tracked allowing for calculation of myocardial strain and strain rate (80). This analysis can be done during systole or diastole and in two or three dimensions (81). Early studies with myocardial tagging were mostly done by manually tracking the tags, a time-consuming process that hindered the clinical use of this technique. A recently described technique for the analysis of myocardial tagging data, harmonic phase imaging (HARP), greatly shortens analysis time because it does not require manual tracing of the tags (82). This technique relies on automatic analysis of the raw MRI data for changes in phase between images. With recent advances in automatic analysis of the tag data and fast image acquisition and display techniques, it is now possible to evaluate myocardial strain in real time (10).

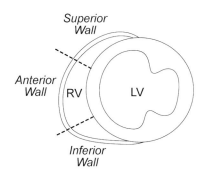

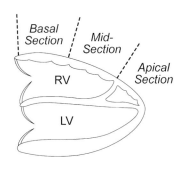

FIGURE 7.12 Right ventricular wall segments. (Adapted and modified from Klein SS, Graham TP Jr, Lorenz CH. Noninvasive delineation of normal right ventricular contractile motion with magnetic resonance imaging myocardial tagging. *Ann Biomed Eng* 1998;26:756–763, with permission.)

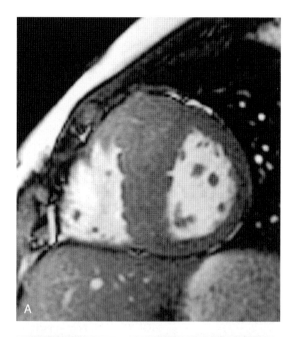

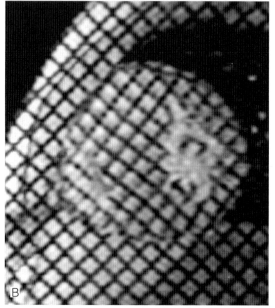

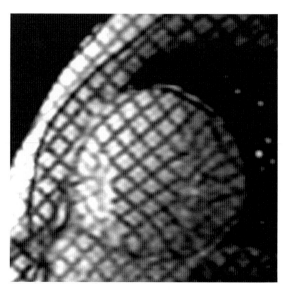

FIGURE 7.13 Myocardial tagging in a patient with hypertrophic cardiomyopathy. **A:** ECG-triggered, breath-hold steady-state free precession image showing asymmetric septal hypertrophy. **B:** Diastolic frame showing the undistorted tags before the onset of systole. **C:** Systolic frame showing distortion of the myocardial tags over the left ventricular free wall with little distortion of the tags over the septum, indicating reduced septal myocardial strain.

Myocardial tagging has been shown to be an important tool in the study of normal left (83–97) and right ventricular mechanics in healthy volunteers (77,98). In the clinical arena, analysis of wall strain by myocardial tagging has provided useful information in patients with ischemic and valvular heart disease (99–110). In a study of 211 patients with chest pain, Kuijpers et al. (111) demonstrated that myocardial tagging detects more segments with regional wall motion abnormalities by dobutamine stress CMR than by visual assessment alone. Evaluating patients with congenital heart disease, Fogel et al. (112–115) used myocardial tagging to characterize patterns of wall motion and strain in patients with functionally single ventricles. As new fast MRI techniques coupled with automatic analysis of myocardial tagging become more widely available, the clinical application of ventricular strain analysis will likely expand. Further research is necessary to determine

the clinical implications of the strain data and how they can be used to assess prognosis and guide patient management.

Stress CMR

There is a growing body of literature on the use of dobutamine stress CMR in the evaluation of myocardial ischemia in adults with coronary artery disease (see discussion in the section on myocardial ischemia below). Several studies have evaluated the use of stress CMR in patients with congenital heart disease. Tulevski et al. (116,117) used low-dose (15 μg/kg/min) dobutamine to evaluate the functional reserve of the left and right ventricles in asymptomatic and minimally symptomatic patients with repaired transposition of the great arteries, physiologically corrected transposition of the great arteries, and pulmonary outflow obstruction. Compared with controls, patients with systemic right ventricles had decreased functional reserve. In another study from the same group, Dodge-Khatar et al. (118) showed that the functional reserve of the systemic ventricle is comparable in healthy adults and in patients with unoperated physiologically corrected transposition of the great arteries. Roest et al. (119) demonstrated the feasibility of assessing biventricular dimensions and function by CMR during supine exercise, a method that provides an alternative to pharmacologic stress.

Diastolic Function

Diastole is a complex process during which the force of the myofibers is restored (120). A detailed discussion of diastolic ventricular mechanics is beyond the scope of this chapter and can be found elsewhere in this text. Researchers have used various modalities and a wide array of parameters to assess diastolic function, such as changes in pressure and chamber dimensions, wall thinning, myocardial velocities and strain, and a wide range of flow-derived variables obtained by Doppler interrogation of the AV valves and pulmonary veins. With the exception of direct pressure measurements, MRI can evaluate all of the above variables (121–135). For example, Helbing et al. (128) used CMR to measure blood flow through the tricuspid and pulmonary valves as well as changes in right ventricular dimensions to assess diastolic function after tetralogy of Fallot repair. Although the data derived from analysis of blood flow and chamber dimensions by MRI are not fundamentally different from similar data obtained by other techniques, MRI offers an advantage in terms of its ability to track tissue motion and deformation during the cardiac cycle using tissue tagging techniques (131,133–136). Fogel et al. (131) used myocardial tagging to study left ventricular diastolic strain in 11 infants with structurally normal hearts. They demonstrated inhomogeneities in both circumferential lengthening (E_2) and radial thinning (E_1). Another investigation using a canine model demonstrated that measurements of the velocity of myocardial untwisting and recoil rate assessed by MRI using tissue tagging correlated closely with the time constant of relaxation or tau (τ) ($r = -0.86$), was unaffected by left atrial pressure, and that τ but not loading conditions was an independent predictor of the recoil rate (134). Thus, the rate of recoil of torsion derived by tissue tagging may provide a noninvasive preload-independent isovolumic phase measure of ventricular relaxation.

Flow Analysis

Quantitative and qualitative assessment of blood flow is frequently used in functional MR evaluation of congenital and acquired pediatric heart disease (137). Qualitative evaluation of abnormal flow patterns is used to visualize turbulent flow jets related to stenotic or regurgitant valves or abnormal communications between cardiac chambers or blood vessels (e.g., septal defects, patent ductus arteriosus, systemic-to-pulmonary shunts, etc.). Site-specific quantification of flow rate, flow velocity, stroke volume, and minute flow can, in principal, be measured across any blood vessel within the central cardiovascular system.

Technique. An ECG-gated velocity-encoded cine (VEC) MRI sequence, a type of gradient echo sequence, can be used to measure blood flow velocity and quantify blood flow rate (137,138). The VEC MRI technique is based on the principle that the signal from hydrogen nuclei (such as those in blood) flowing through specially designed magnetic field gradients accumulates a predictable phase shift that is proportional to its velocity. Multiple phase images are constructed across the cardiac cycle in which the signal amplitude (intensity) of each voxel is proportional to mean flow velocity within that voxel. Using specialized software, regions of interest around a vessel are defined, and the flow rate is automatically calculated as the product of the mean velocity and the cross-sectional area (Fig. 7.14).

In practice, an imaging plane is prescribed perpendicular to the vessel of interest and two sets of multiphase images are reconstructed following a VEC MRI acquisition: a set of *magnitude images* that provide anatomic information and a set of *phase images* in which the velocity information is encoded. For each acquisition, the operator prescribes the field of view, matrix size, and slice thickness, which, in turn, determine spatial resolution. Greil et al. (139), in an *in vitro* study using a pulsatile flow model, found that spatial resolution is important for accurate measurements of flow rate by VEC MRI with an optimal number of pixels within the cross section of the vessel of interest ≥16. Other variables such as the angle between the prescribed imaging plane and flow direction, velocity encoding range, flip angle, and slice thickness must also be considered. Other known caveats of quantitative assessment of blood flow by VEC MRI include flow aliasing and dephasing secondary to turbulent flow. Aliasing can be avoided by prescribing a velocity encoding range higher than the maximal velocity within the target vessel. Avoiding dephasing secondary to turbulent blood flow can be achieved by shortening the echo time, prescribing a thinner slice thickness, or repositioning the imaging slice proximal or distal to the turbulent jet.

Accuracy of Blood Flow Measurements by MRI. VEC MRI flow calculations have been shown to be accurate and reproducible by *in vitro* and *in vivo* studies (139–148). *In vitro* studies have demonstrated that measurements of continuous flow are accurate within 5% of reference standard (149,150). Greil et al. (139) demonstrated that the accuracy and reproducibility of *in vitro* pulsatile flow measurements by VEC MRI is 0.8 ± 1.5%. Evans et al. (146) found a strong correlation ($r^2 = 0.99$) with a 95% confidence interval of ±0.07 L/min over a range of flow rates of 0.125 to 1.9 L/min. Powell et al. (141) used a phantom model that mimics flow conditions in the aorta of a child (flow rates 1.25 to 3.5 L/min) and found a similarly strong correlation, close agreement (bias = −0.045 L/min), and 95% limits of agreement of −0.19 to 0.1 L/min.

The accuracy of *in vivo* VEC MRI measurements of blood flow has been demonstrated by numerous studies. Investigators have used ventricular stroke volume, thermodilution, Fick principle, indicator dilution, and flow probe measurements as reference standards, showing strong correlations with VEC MRI (141,151–159). Hundley et al. (157) found that ascending aorta flow in 23 adults was within 4% of flow measurements by the Fick method and within 5% measured by thermodilution. Evans et al. (146), in a study of ten adult subjects, demonstrated an average difference between pulmonary (Qp) and systemic (Qs) flow ratio of 5%. Powell et al. (141), in a study of 20 volunteers, found that Qp/Qs closely approximated unity (mean ± SD = 0.99 ± 0.1, range 0.85 to 1.19). Beerbaum et al. (140), in a study of 50 children with atrial or ventricular septal defects who underwent concomitant cardiac catheterization, reported a mean difference between VEC MRI and oximetry of 2% (2 SD = −20% to +26%). Powell et al. (160), in a study of 20 patients with atrial septal defect, found a mean difference between VEC MRI and oximetry of 2.3% with a reproducibility of repeat VEC MRI flow measurements of 1.1 ± 4.2% in the main pulmonary artery and 0.7 ± 5.4% in the ascending aorta (Fig. 7.15).

Clinical Applications. Measurements of blood flow are an integral element of functional assessment by MRI in a wide

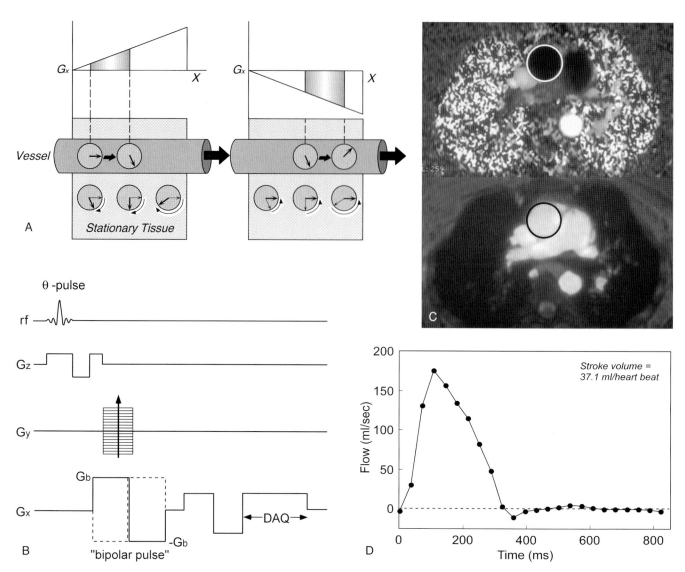

FIGURE 7.14 Flow velocity cine MRI. **A:** Schematic representation of phase-velocity encoding. **Left panel:** A magnetic field gradient (Gx) is briefly applied in the velocity-encoding direction (x) causing phase variations to develop. **Right panel:** The gradient is then reversed so that it has equal magnitude and duration but opposite polarity. In stationary tissue, there is no net phase shift because the reversal of the gradient field cancels the effect of the initial gradient application. In contrast, flowing blood in the vessel is now in a different location and is therefore exposed to a different gradient strength (*shaded region*). Consequently, a net phase shift will result that is proportional to flow velocity. **B:** A typical phase-velocity cine MRI pulse sequence diagram (rf, radiofrequency; Gz, slice select gradient; Gy, frequency select gradient; Gx, -encoding gradient; DAQ, data acquisition window). **C:** Transverse (axial) view of phase-velocity cine MRI perpendicular to the ascending aorta. **Top panel:** Phase-sensitive image. The signal intensity in this image is linearly proportional to flow velocity. Flow direction is encoded in black (inferior to superior) or white (superior to inferior). **Bottom panel:** Magnitude image reconstructed based on the amplitude of the tissue signal intensity. To measure the flow in the ascending aorta, a region of interest (*circle*) is placed using off-line computer software. **D:** Flow–time curve. Instantaneous flow rates are calculated multiple times during the cardiac cycle by integrating the flow velocities across the vessel cross-sectional area. The area under the curve represents the stroke volume. Minute flow is calculated by multiplying the stroke volume by the heart rate.

range of clinical scenarios. Examples include measurement of cardiac output (157,161), pulmonary-to-systemic flow ratio in patients with intracardiac and extracardiac shunts (140–142, 160,162,164), regional flow to selected organs or vascular beds (e.g., patients with vascular malformations) (164–166), valvular regurgitation in patients with native and postoperative lesions (e.g., pulmonary regurgitation after tetralogy of Fallot repair) (167–181), differential lung perfusion (e.g., branch pulmonary artery stenosis) (182–184), AV valve inflow (128), and estimation of pressure gradient (180,185,186).

Keeping in mind the known limitations of VEC MRI (137,139,187), site-specific quantification of flow rate, flow velocity, stroke volume, and minute flow can provide useful hemodynamic information in a wide range of clinical scenarios.

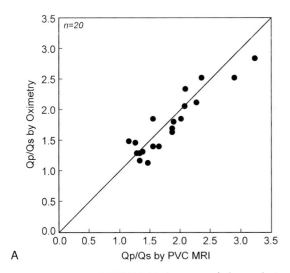

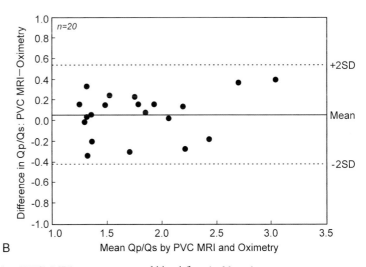

A   B

FIGURE 7.15 Accuracy of phase-velocity cine (PVC) MRI measurements of blood flow in 20 patients with interatrial shunt. **A:** Mean pulmonary-to-systemic (Qp/Qs) flow ratio by oximetry versus mean Qp/Qs by PVC MRI. **B:** The difference in Qp/Qs versus mean Qp/Qs by PVC MRI and oximetry. The mean difference was 0.06 L/min (*solid line*) and ±2 standard deviations (SD) from the mean (95% limits of agreement) were −0.42 and 0.54 L/min (*dashed lines*). (From Powell AJ, Tsai-Goodman B, Prakash A, et al. Comparison between phase-velocity cine magnetic resonance imaging and invasive oximetry for quantification of atrial shunts. *Am J Cardiol* 2003;91:1523–1525, with permission.)

Pharmacologic stress can be used to provide additional information on functional reserve (188). For example, by using either dipyridamole or adenosine for vasodilation of the coronary vascular bed, coronary flow reserve can be assessed (189). An inherent strength of functional assessment by MRI is the ability to measure the same variable by different methods, thus allowing for internal validation of the functional data. For example, in a patient with an atrial septal defect, the pulmonary-to-systemic flow ratio can be assessed based on (i) flow measurements in the main pulmonary artery and ascending aorta; (ii) flow measurements through the tricuspid and mitral valves (typically obtained in a single acquisition perpendicular to the plane of the AV valves); and (iii) LV and RV stroke volumes obtained by short-axis cine MR. Although standard VEC MRI techniques require 2 to 4 minutes of data acquisition in each site, recent developments of faster imaging strategies (e.g., segmented *k*-space acquisition and parallel processing) have greatly shortened the acquisition time (163,190–192). Although these techniques allow data acquisition during a short period of breath holding (10 to 14 seconds), the physiologic effects of suspended respiration may alter intrathoracic pressure and affect flow measurements. Sakuma et al. (193) demonstrated that flow measurements during large lung volume breath holding significantly underestimated cardiac output (4.47 ± 0.63 versus 6.09 ± 0.49 L/min) whereas cardiac output measurements during small lung volume breath holding were similar to those obtained during free breathing. Development of real-time velocity encoded techniques has a potential utility analogous to color Doppler in echocardiography (176). This technique has recently proved valuable in providing unique physiologic information in patients with Fontan circulation (194).

The preceding discussion focused on through-plane flow measurements. When velocity information is measured in the three orthogonal planes (anterior-posterior, superior-inferior, and through plane), multidimensional flow imaging and shear stress calculation can be accomplished (195–198). Three-dimensional flow vector mapping is a useful adjunct to cine flow imaging because it provides dynamic 3-D flow maps that can readily detect abnormal flow patterns (Fig. 7.16).

Myocardial Perfusion and Viability

Compared with the adult population, myocardial ischemia owing to coronary artery disease is uncommon in infants and children. In the pediatric population, ischemia may be associated with congenital coronary abnormalities such as anomalous origin of a coronary artery from the pulmonary artery or from the opposite sinus of Valsalva, or acquired conditions,

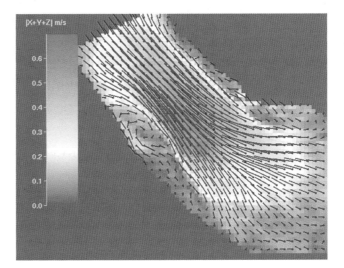

FIGURE 7.16 Three-dimensional flow vector mapping in the aortic root and proximal ascending aorta in a patient with Marfan syndrome. The origin of the flow is depicted as a *blue dot*, and the *red line* represents the direction and velocity of the flow.

most notably Kawasaki disease. Alternatively, the coronary circulation may be compromised in postoperative patients, especially those whose procedure involved relocation of the coronary arteries (e.g., arterial switch operation). Patients who have undergone heart transplantation are also at risk for the development of accelerated coronary artery disease and abnormalities of the coronary microvasculature.

In comparison with nuclear techniques, cardiac MRI is a relatively young tool for detection of myocardial ischemia and viability. As a result, one should remember during the subsequent discussion that the available data on its clinical utility and applicability are considerably smaller than for the more established techniques. This limitation is perhaps offset by the fact that data specific to children and young adults are scarce for all of the noninvasive techniques. The feasibility of assessing myocardial perfusion and viability by CMR in children and patients with congenital heart disease has been demonstrated with encouraging early results (199).

Myocardial Ischemia. Currently, the two most widely used CMR techniques to detect ischemia are dobutamine stress CMR and first-pass myocardial perfusion. Dobutamine stress CMR is performed using a protocol similar to dobutamine stress echocardiography with increasing doses of dobutamine up to 40 to 50 μg/kg/min and the addition of atropine if necessary to reach the target heart rate. The goal of the test is to detect ventricular myocardium supplied by a stenotic coronary artery. At rest, the myocardial blood supply/demand ratio may be sufficient to allow normal wall motion and thickening. However, with increasing metabolic demand under pharmacologic stress, ischemia may be induced and wall motion is impaired. Imaging is usually performed with breath-hold cine SSFP MRI, thereby providing high-quality images of left ventricular wall motion and thickening. Nagel et al. (200) compared the sensitivity and specificity of dobutamine stress CMR (DSMR) with that of dobutamine stress echocardiography (DSE) in 208 patients for the detection of >50% coronary artery stenosis determined by coronary angiography. Compared with DSE, DSMR was more sensitive (86.2% versus 74.3%) and had a higher specificity (85.7% versus 69.8%) and better accuracy (86% versus 72.7%) (p <0.05 for all). CMR has a particular advantage over echocardiography in patients who have poor acoustic windows (≤15% of studies in adults).

First-pass myocardial perfusion CMR can also be used to diagnose myocardial ischemia. After intravenous injection of a gadolinium-based contrast agent, the enhancement pattern of the myocardium is evaluated during the first transit of the bolus through the heart. The appearance of contrast will be attenuated, both in amplitude and rate, in regions of compromised coronary blood flow (Fig. 7.17). In practice, contrast

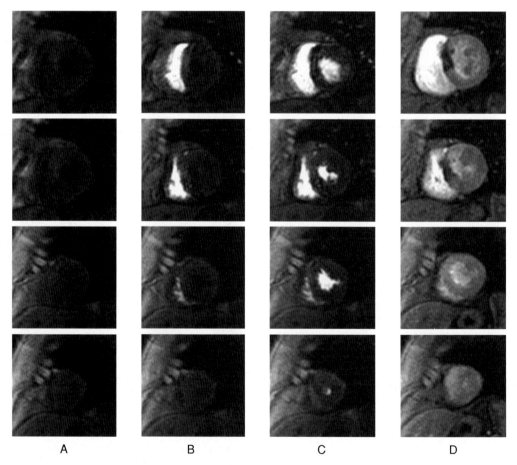

A   B   C   D

FIGURE 7.17 First-pass myocardial perfusion in a patient with anterior septal myocardial infarction. **A:** Four short-axis slices (top frame, basal slice; bottom frame, apical slice) before arrival of the contrast. **B:** The contrast enters the right ventricle. **C:** The contrast enters the left ventricle but not the coronary arteries (note the bright signal from the blood pool but not from the myocardium). **D:** Segments with well-perfused myocardium show a bright signal whereas the hypoperfused anterior septal segment remains dark.

(e.g., gadopentetate dimeglumine 0.05 to 0.1 mmol/kg) is infused through a large-bore cannula using a power injector at a rate of 3 to 5 mL/s. With the patient holding his or her breath, the heart is rapidly imaged in multiple planes for approximately 30 seconds using a cardiac-triggered fast gradient hybrid echo-planar (or SSFP) pulse sequences. An inversion preparation pulse is also used, which minimizes the signal from myocardium and thus enhances the relative increase in signal intensity produced by the T1-shortening effects of the contrast agent. Because exercise stress cannot be readily done in the MRI scanner, most perfusion studies are performed with vasodilators such as adenosine or dipyridamole. Both qualitative and quantitative analysis have been reported; the latter is done typically by constructing time–intensity curves of myocardial regions and calculating a perfusion reserve index (201,202).

Myocardial Viability. In addition to detection of ischemia, CMR can also be used to differentiate viable from nonviable myocardium. Myocardial delayed enhancement (MDE) imaging has become the dominant MRI technique to assess viability. It is based on the observation that the washout kinetics of standard gadolinium-based intravenous MRI contrast agents is delayed in necrotic myocardium and in areas where the myocardium is replaced by collagen (e.g., scar tissue). Consequently, nonviable myocardium appears bright or hyperenhanced compared with viable myocardium when imaged with a segmented inversion recovery fast gradient echo sequence after contrast injection (Fig. 7.18). In practice, MDE imaging is performed 10 to 20 minutes after administration of 0.1 to 0.2 mmol/kg of gadolinium-based contrast. MDE is first done using several inversion times to select the one that best nulls the myocardium. Using this inversion time, MDE is then performed in short- and long-axis planes.

Several studies in both animals and humans have shown that this technique is effective at identifying the presence, location, and size of acute and chronic myocardial infarction (203–212). Klein et al. (213) found close agreement between MDE imaging and PET scar size measurements in 31 patients with ischemic heart failure. Because of its superior spatial resolution, MDE is more sensitive than SPECT in patients with small or subendocardial infarctions (214). Most important, the transmural extent of MDE can be used to predict improvement in contractile function after revascularization in patients with acute and chronic coronary artery disease (215–218). Another promising clinical application of MDE imaging is detection of myocardial fibrosis in patients with hypertrophic cardiomyopathy (219). Kim and Judd (220) recently demonstrated that the extent of myocardial fibrosis assessed by MDE can be used to stratify risk in these patients. In pediatric and congenital heart disease patients, Prakash et al. (199) studied 30 patients with a median age of 13 years (range 0.3 to 40 years) whose diagnoses included repaired congenital heart disease in 15, cardiomyopathy in 6, cardiac tumor in 3, dysplastic LV in 2, congenital coronary anomaly in 2, and coronary artery aneurysm following Kawasaki disease in 2. They found good agreement between MRI evaluation of myocardial perfusion and viability and analysis of segmental wall motion as well as coronary angiography (*n* = 10) and single photon emission computed tomography (*n* = 6). Further studies are needed to validate and expand this initial experience.

Tissue Characteristics

Assessment of the myocardium, pericardium, blood vessel walls, and extracardiac tissue for pathologic changes can be valuable in various clinical circumstances. MRI offers a distinct advantage over other modalities when it comes to evaluation of soft tissues because of its ability to discern even minor changes in tissue composition. By manipulations of T1 and T2 weightings and by applying various prepulses or suppression of signals from specific tissue elements such as fat or water, tissue composition can be evaluated. Clinical applications include assessment of myocardial architecture (e.g., myocardial noncompaction [221,222] and ventricular aneurysm [223]), evaluation of cardiac and pericardial tumors (Fig. 7.19) (224), vessel

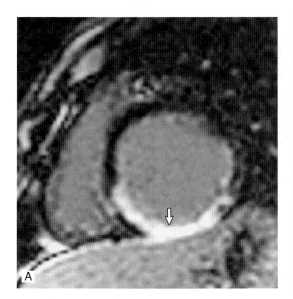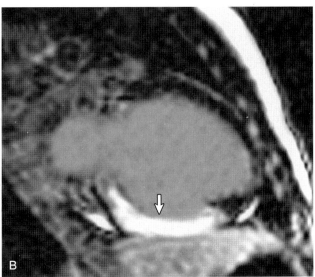

FIGURE 7.18 Myocardial delayed enhancement imaging in a 4-year-old patient with Kawasaki disease complicated by coronary artery aneurysms and occlusion of the left circumflex coronary artery. **A:** Short-axis view showing enhancement of the inferior wall (*arrow*), consistent with transmural myocardial infarction. **B:** Long-axis view showing the base-to-apex extent of the infarct.

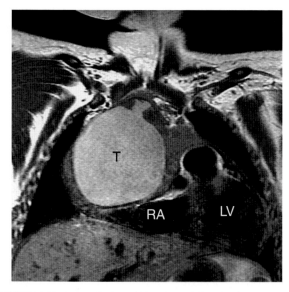

FIGURE 7.19 Coronal plane T1-weighted fast (turbo) spin echo image in a patient with pericardial teratoma (T). Note the compressed right atrium (RA). LV, left ventricle.

wall imaging (e.g., aortic dissection [225,226]), assessment of the myocardium for fatty infiltration or other pathologic changes (e.g., arrhythmogenic right ventricular cardiomyopathy [227,228]), evaluation of the pericardium (e.g., constrictive pericardium [229,230]), and assessment of myocardial iron load (231).

In practice, MRI assessment of tissue characteristics is based on the use of several imaging sequences. Standard or fast spin echo are used for morphologic imaging of the myocardium, pericardium, blood vessel walls, and extracardiac structures. Manipulations of image contrast (T1, T2, or proton density weighting) and the addition of prepulses (e.g., triple inversion recovery, T2 preparation, and fat or water saturation) result in highlighting or suppression of specific tissue characteristics. Gradient echo sequences provide information on signal intensity and, more important, on motion of the tissue in question. First-pass myocardial perfusion, early- and late-enhancement after intravenous administration of gadolinium-based contrast, and myocardial tagging can provide additional diagnostic information about tissue characteristics.

EXAMPLES OF CLINICAL APPLICATIONS OF CMR

Shunt Lesions

Atrial Septal Defect

CMR can be helpful in selected patients with a known or suspected atrial septal defect (ASD), usually adolescents and adults with inconclusive clinical and echocardiographic findings. For example, CMR provides a noninvasive alternative to transesophageal echocardiography and to diagnostic catheterization in patients with right ventricular (RV) volume overload in whom transthoracic echocardiography cannot demonstrate the source of the left-to-right shunt (232–236). CMR can visualize different types of atrial-level defects, including secundum, primum, sinus venosus, and coronary sinus septal defects. In patients with sinus venosus defect, CMR can provide all the necessary information required for surgical planning. The goals of the CMR examination include delineation of the location and size of the ASD, its relations to key neighboring structures, its size, suitability for transcatheter versus surgical closure, and functional assessment of the hemodynamic burden, including pulmonary-to-systemic flow ratio and RV size and function.

Although spin echo sequences have been used to diagnose ASDs, thin structures such as septum primum may not be

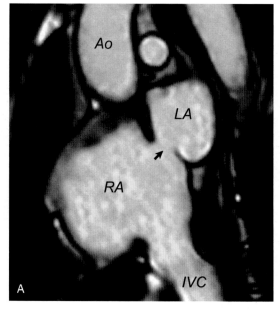

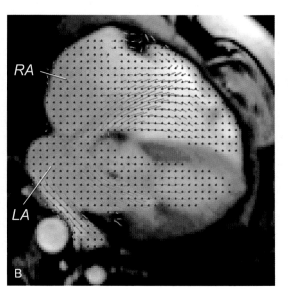

FIGURE 7.20 Secundum atrial septal defect. **A:** Oblique sagittal steady-state free precession image showing a centrally located defect (*arrow*). **B:** Three-dimensional flow vector mapping showing flow from the left atrium (LA) to the right atrium (RA). Ao, aorta; IVC, inferior vena cava.

clearly demonstrated, leading to an overestimation of the defect's size or to a false-positive diagnosis. A SSFP sequence is capable of providing high-quality cine imaging of the atrial septum and the adjacent anatomic structures, including the vena cavae, pulmonary veins, and the AV valves. The atrial septum is imaged in at least two planes by obtaining a stack of ECG-triggered multiphase SSFP images, a stack in the axial or four-chamber planes, and a stack in an oblique sagittal plane (Fig. 7.20). Additional cine SSFP imaging is performed in the short-axis plane across the ventricles to quantify LV and RV volumes and function. This stack also allows qualitative assessment of RV systolic pressure based on the configuration of the interventricular septum. The septal geometry is concave toward the RV when the RV/LV pressure ratio is low and assumes a flat configuration, or even a concave shape, toward the LV as the RV/LV pressure ratio increases. Interpretation of the hemodynamic significance of septal configuration may be confounded by factors such as inhomogeneous contraction of the RV, intraventricular conduction delay (e.g., right or left bundle branch block, pre-excitation), and a high LV pressure.

Measurement of the pulmonary-to-systemic flow ratio (Qp/Qs) is clinically helpful in patients with ASD. Several studies have shown that flow measurements in the main pulmonary artery (Qp) and ascending aorta (Qs) using VEC MRI agree closely with catheterization-based oximetry (140,237–239). In the absence of AV valve regurgitation or an additional shunt, Qp/Qs can also be measured by VEC MRI in the ventricular short-axis plane perpendicular to the mitral (Qs) and tricuspid valve (Qp) inflows. A third option is to compare the RV and LV stroke volumes obtained by the short-axis cine SSFP. In clinical practice, it is recommended to measure the Qp/Qs ratio by more than one method to evaluate the data for internal consistency.

The non–ECG-triggered Gd-enhanced 3-D MRA sequence is not ideally suited for evaluation of secundum ASDs because of blurring of thin intracardiac structures. However, this sequence is helpful in the evaluation of sinus venosus septal defects, especially since these defects invariably involve the pulmonary veins (Fig. 7.21).

Ventricular Septal Defect

CMR is rarely used primarily for the evaluation of a ventricular septal defect (VSD). In our experience, only 7 of 1,119 CMR examinations (0.6%) were requested for evaluation of VSD, primarily for assessment of ventricular dimensions and function and Qp/Qs measurement in patients with inadequate or inconsistent echocardiographic data. Many other CMR studies, however, were performed for other indications in patients in whom a VSD was present.

VSDs can be imaged by gradient echo (preferably SSFP) or spin echo sequences obtained in any combination of planes (Fig. 7.22). The four-chamber plane provides a base-to-apex view of the septum whereas the short-axis plane images the interventricular septum from anterior-superior to posterior-inferior. Additional imaging in other planes should be performed if the location of the defect and its relation to neighboring key structures (e.g., atrioventricular or semilunar valves) is not demonstrated by imaging in standard planes. Measurement of ventricular dimensions and function is a key element of the CMR evaluation in a patient with VSD. Quantification of Qp/Qs provides additional hemodynamic information and can be achieved either by VEC MRI flow measurements in the ascending aorta and main pulmonary artery, across the mitral and tricuspid valves, or by comparison of the LV and RV stroke volumes. In the presence of additional

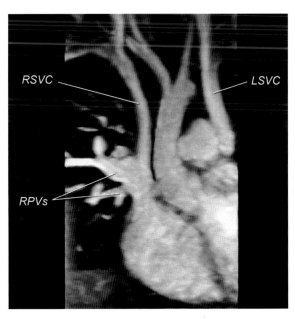

FIGURE 7.21 Maximal intensity projection Gd-enhanced 3-D MRA showing drainage of right pulmonary veins (RPVs) to the cardiac end of the right superior vena cava (RSVC) in a patient with sinus venosus defect. LSVC, left superior vena cava.

shunts (e.g., ASD or PDA) or valve regurgitation, calculation of Qp/Qs must be adjusted to account for the hemodynamic effect of the additional flow.

Patent Ductus Arteriosus

CMR is seldom requested primarily for assessment of an isolated patent ductus arteriosus (PDA). In several types of complex CHD, evaluation of the ductus arteriosus is an important element of the examination. For example, in patients with tetralogy of Fallot and pulmonary atresia, the ductus arteriosus can be an important source of pulmonary blood supply (240,241). Gd-enhanced 3-D MRA is a particularly helpful imaging technique in these patients because it allows accurate delineation of all sources of pulmonary blood supply, including a PDA, aortopulmonary collateral vessels, and the central pulmonary arteries (242). Another clinical circumstance in which MRI evaluation of a PDA may be requested is the adult with CHD in whom limited acoustic windows can hamper echocardiographic evaluation. Imaging of a PDA can be accomplished by several MRI sequences (Fig. 7.23). If a PDA is detected, it is vital to also evaluate the direction of flow across the duct by VEC MRI, to assess the hemodynamic burden by measurements of ventricular volumes and function, to measure the Qp/Qs, and to assess RV pressure by septal position in the short-axis plane.

Anomalies of the Aorta

Coarctation of the Aorta

The use of MRI to image anomalies of the aortic arch dates back to the early 1980s (243). Whereas those studies provided mostly static anatomic information, the advent of new imaging sequences has greatly expanded the diagnostic capabilities of CMR to include comprehensive anatomic and functional

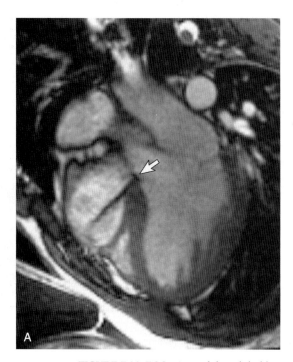

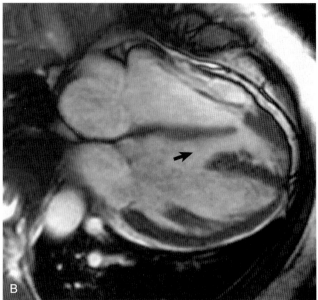

FIGURE 7.22 ECG-triggered, breath-hold, cine steady-state free precession imaging of ventricular septal defect. **A:** Small membranous ventricular septal defect (*arrow*). **B:** Large muscular ventricular septal defect (*arrow*).

evaluation. In adults with CHD, Thierrin et al. (244) have shown that the combination of clinical assessment and MRI provides a better cost-effective yield compared with a combination that relies on echocardiography as the primary imaging modality. Others have shown the utility of CMR in infants and children with coarctation and other anomalies of the

FIGURE 7.23 Maximal intensity projection Gd-enhanced 3-D magnetic resonance angiogram showing patent ductus arteriosus (PDA). DAo, descending aorta.

aortic arch (285,245,246). In our practice, CMR evaluation of coarctation accounts for approximately 10% of the studies (Table 7.1).

The objectives of the CMR evaluation of suspected or repaired aortic coarctation include (i) detailed imaging of the aorta including the proximal brachiocephalic arteries and the descending aorta to the level of the renal arteries; (ii) imaging of blood flow throughout the thoracic aorta to detect high-velocity flow jets suggestive of stenosis; (iii) detection of collateral vessels that bypass the coarctation site; (iv) assessment of left ventricular mass, volumes and function; and (v) detection of any associated lesions.

Much of the anatomic information is gleaned from the Gd-enhanced 3-D MRA, including the anatomy of the aorta, imaging of collateral vessels, and cross-sectional measurements of the aorta in various locations (Fig. 7.24). A spin echo sequence with double inversion recovery provides high-resolution imaging of the aortic wall. This may be particularly important in cases with discrete coarctation comprised of a thin "shelf" that protrudes into the aortic lumen and in patients with atypical location of the coarctation such as in the abdomen (Fig. 7.25). Gradient echo sequences are helpful for detection of signal void owing to high-velocity turbulent jets.

Evaluation of the hemodynamic significance of coarctation is an important element of the CMR examination. Several investigations compared the anatomic features and the extent of collateral blood flow with coarctation diameter measured by x-ray angiography (245,246), blood pressure measurements by sphygmomanometry (247), and Doppler assessment of flow velocity (248). Riquelme et al. (249) showed a correlation coefficient of 0.99 between gradient echo cine MRI measurement of coarctation diameter and angiography. Simpson et al. (245) and Mendelson et al. (246) reported correlation coefficients of 0.9 and 0.91, respectively. Other groups have focused on the percent increase in descending aorta flow from collateral vessels to assess coarctation severity. Steffens et al. (250) reported

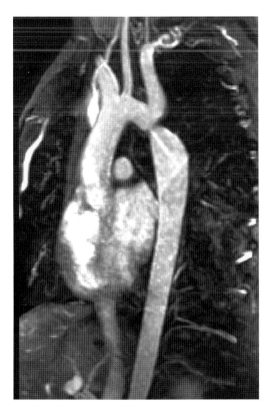

FIGURE 7.24 Maximal intensity projection Gd-enhanced 3-D MRA in a patient with severe aortic coarctation.

that the percent increase in flow correlated with the diameter of the coarctation segment ($r = 0.94$), with arm-to-leg blood pressure difference ($r = 0.84$), and with Doppler gradient ($r = 0.76$). More recently, Araoz et al. (247) demonstrated that the percent increase in descending aorta flow in 19 patients with repaired coarctation more accurately reflected the degree of

narrowing than arm-to-leg blood pressure measurements. We have developed a CMR-based model to predict the probability of hemodynamically significant coarctation defined as a pressure gradient ≥20 mm Hg measured by catheterization (251). The combination of the smallest cross-sectional area of the aorta (measured from the Gd-enhanced 3-D MRA) and the heart rate–adjusted mean deceleration of flow in the descending aorta (measured by VEC MRI distal to the coarctation) (Fig. 7.26) predicted coarctation severity group with 95% sensitivity, 82% specificity, 90% positive and negative predictive values, and an area under the receiver–operator characteristics curve of 0.94.

Aortic Aneurysm and/or Dissection

Severe dilation, aneurysm formation, and dissection can complicate the course of some congenital cardiac defects such as bicommissural aortic valve and tetralogy of Fallot and are common in patients with Marfan syndrome and other connective tissue disorders. CMR is an ideal modality for longitudinal noninvasive assessment of the aorta, especially in adolescents and adults in whom the echocardiographic windows are often limited. In contrast to computed tomography, CMR does not expose the patients to the risks of ionizing radiation and can also provide functional information such as measuring aortic regurgitation fraction and left ventricular dimensions and function. In patients with suspected acute dissection who may require emergent intervention, CT angiography might be more readily available.

The imaging strategy for assessment of aortic aneurysm is modified from the protocol used for aortic coarctation. Both spin and gradient echo sequences are acquired in planes perpendicular and parallel to the long axis of the aorta (Fig. 7.27A). The branch vessels of the aorta are also examined to determine for extension of an aneurysm, dissection, or obstruction. A stack of thin-sliced ECG-triggered SSFP cine is acquired perpendicular to the aortic root and ascending aorta. This sequence allows accurate measurements of orthogonal dimensions of the dilated aortic segment during systole. In addition, the aortic

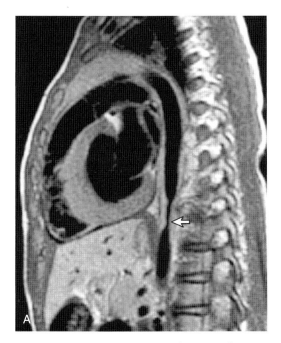

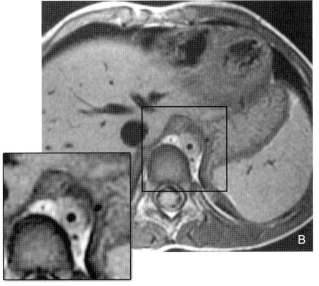

FIGURE 7.25 Fast (turbo) spin echo imaging showing severe long-segment abdominal coarctation in a 5-year-old patient with Takayasu arteritis. **A:** Sagittal view. **B:** Axial (transverse) view showing marked thickening of the aortic wall.

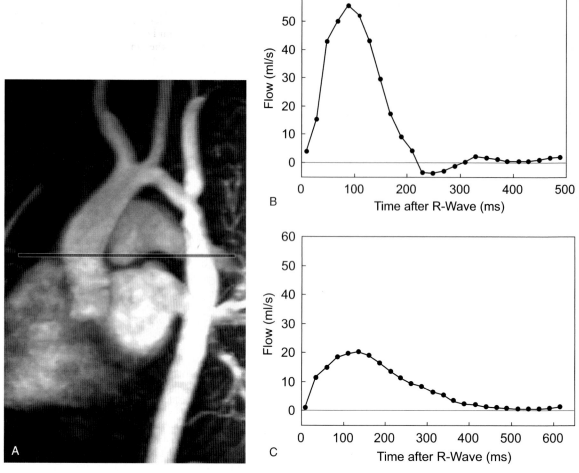

FIGURE 7.26 Evaluation of coarctation severity based on flow pattern in the descending aorta and the smallest cross-sectional area of the coarctation segment (276). **A:** Imaging plane for flow measurements in the ascending and descending aorta. **B:** Descending aorta flow pattern in a patient with repaired coarctation and no residual obstruction. Note the sharp upstroke and short deceleration phase. **C:** Descending aorta flow pattern in a patient with severe coarctation. Note the shallow upstroke and prolonged deceleration. **D:** Evaluation of smallest aortic cross-sectional area based on subvolume maximal intensity projection Gd-enhanced 3-D MRA.

wall is examined in detail for evidence of dissection and VEC MRI is used to evaluate aortic valve function. This technique can also be used to distinguish between flow in the true and false lumen of aortic dissection. Gd-enhanced MRA is particularly helpful for evaluation of tortuous aortic segments and branch vessels (Fig. 7.27B).

Vascular Rings and Pulmonary Artery Sling

Vascular rings constitute an uncommon form of congenital vascular anomaly in which the trachea and esophagus are surrounded completely by vascular structures. Rings are formed by abnormal persistence and/or regression of components of the aortic arch complex. MRI is ideally suited for evaluation of vascular rings and LPA sling because it provides good visualization of the airways and the vasculature, imaging can be performed in any plane, and there is no exposure to ionizing radiation. The main drawback of MRI is the need for sedation given that most patients with vascular rings are too young to

cooperate. Although vascular rings account for fewer than 1% of patients with CHD, they account for 2.6% of all CMR examinations in our laboratory and for 10% of studies in patients younger than 1 year of age. Although multirow detector CT with contrast can provide excellent imaging of the airways and vasculature, this technique is associated with a significant exposure to ionizing radiation. On the other hand, the potential ability of CT to obtain good-quality images without general anesthesia and endotracheal intubation is advantageous.

MRI evaluation of vascular rings and left pulmonary artery sling can be accomplished by a combination of spin echo and Gd-enhanced 3-D MRA (Fig. 7.28A). Thin (2 to 3 mm) contiguous fast spin echo with double inversion recovery slices provide excellent visualization of the trachea, main stem bronchi, and the vasculature. In addition to the axial plane, imaging of the trachea in oblique coronal and sagittal planes parallel to its long axis can be helpful. Occasionally, fast spin echo imaging may not be able to distinguish stenotic from atretic aortic segments with confidence. Gd-enhanced 3-D

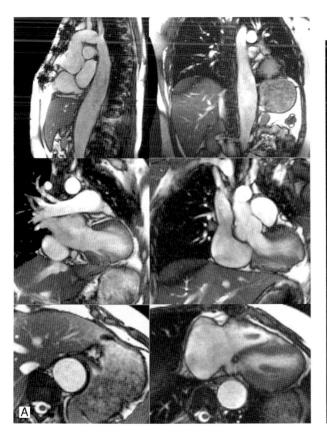
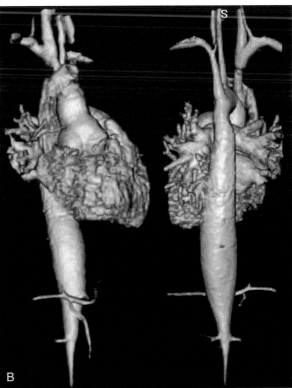

FIGURE 7.27 Large aneurysm of the descending aorta in a patient with connective tissue disorder who underwent replacement of the ascending aorta and transverse arch. A: Steady-state free precession cine MRI in multiple planes. B: Volume rendered reconstruction of Gd-enhanced 3-D MRA. The *left panel* shows an anterior view, and the *right panel* shows a posterior view.

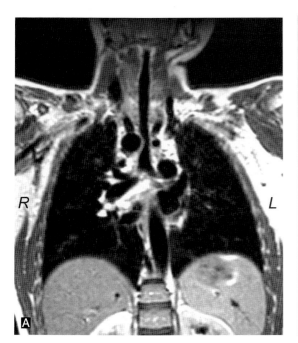
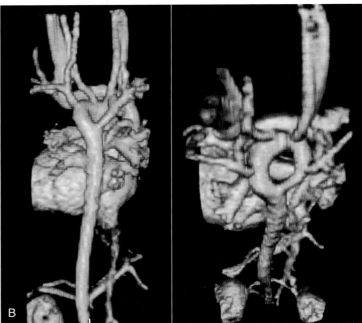

FIGURE 7.28 Vascular ring consisting of a double aortic arch. A: Fast (turbo) spin echo with double inversion recovery sequence in the coronal plane showing tracheal compression and cross sections of the larger right and the smaller left arches. B: Volume rendered reconstruction of Gd-enhanced 3-D MRA. The *left panel* shows a posterior view, and the *right panel* shows a superior view.

MRA can be used to determine if any segment of the vascular ring does not have luminal continuity and is ideally suited for 3-D reconstruction (Fig. 7.28B).

Pulmonary Artery Anomalies

Most anomalies of the pulmonary arteries occur in association with other CHD. For example, stenosis, hypoplasia, and/or discontinuity of the branch pulmonary arteries are commonly associated with tetralogy of Fallot. Congenitally absent branch pulmonary artery without additional CHD is a rare anomaly. It is characterized by absence of the mediastinal pulmonary artery on the opposite side of the aortic arch in most cases (Fig. 7.29) (252). A ligamentum arteriosum can usually be found between the base of the subclavian artery and peripheral pulmonary arteries at the hilum of the ipsilateral lung. Early diagnosis and establishment of vascular continuity between the main pulmonary artery and the peripheral branches on the affected side may promote growth of the pulmonary vascular bed and reduce the likelihood of complications. Another condition where a branch pulmonary artery is absent is agenesis of the corresponding lung. In contrast to congenitally absent branch pulmonary artery without associated anomalies, in agenesis of a lung the ipsilateral pulmonary veins are absent as well. Other rare anomalies of the branch pulmonary arteries include origin from the ascending aorta (so-called hemitruncus) and crossed pulmonary arteries.

Spin and gradient echo cine sequences can be used to assess the central pulmonary arteries, but these techniques may have a limited ability to depict very small and tortuous vessels, especially in infants (see discussion on MRI evaluation of preoperative TOF). Gd-enhanced 3-D MRA provides excellent depiction of the pulmonary arterial tree, including the second-

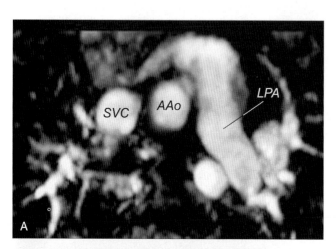

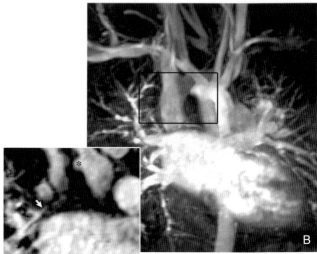

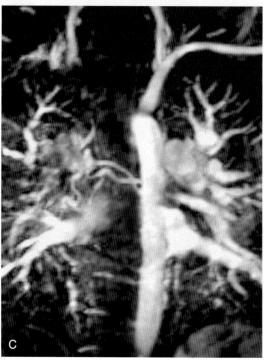

FIGURE 7.29 Congenitally absent right pulmonary artery. **A:** Axial (transverse) view of a cine MRI showing a dilated left pulmonary artery (LPA) and absence of a right pulmonary artery behind the ascending aorta (AAo) and superior vena cava (SVC). **B:** Subvolume maximal intensity projection Gd-enhanced 3-D MRA in the coronal plane. Note the ductal dimple at the base of the right innominate artery (*) and the markedly hypoplastic distal right pulmonary artery at the hilum of the right lung (*arrow*). **C:** Aortopulmonary collateral vessels to the right lung.

and third-generation branches. This sequence has been shown to image pulmonary arterial branches as small as 1 mm even in the absence of antegrade blood flow, as is the case in congenitally absent branch pulmonary artery without associated anomalies (Fig. 7.29) (242).

Systemic and Pulmonary Venous Anomalies

Although referral to CMR primarily for evaluation of the pulmonary veins accounts for only 4.4% of cases in our hospital, evaluation of the systemic and pulmonary veins is integral to a comprehensive CMR evaluation in patients with CHD. Venous anomalies are often associated with other CHD, and unsuspected but clinically important abnormalities can be detected on exams performed for other indications. Gd-enhanced 3-D MRA is particularly helpful for anatomic evaluation of systemic and pulmonary venous anomalies (Fig. 7.30) (46). Gradient echo sequences can be used to depict an abnormal blood flow pattern such as a turbulent jet. A fast (turbo) spin echo sequence can be used to provide high-resolution imaging of vessel wall, such as in patients with pulmonary veins stenosis. VEC MRI is used to measure blood flow in selected vessels to assess regional blood flow. Applications include the fractional flow to each lung in patients with pulmonary veins stenosis and the direction of flow in the azygos vein in a patient with narrowing of the superior vena cava.

Tetralogy of Fallot

Tetralogy of Fallot (TOF) is the most frequent diagnosis among patients referred for CMR evaluation at Children's

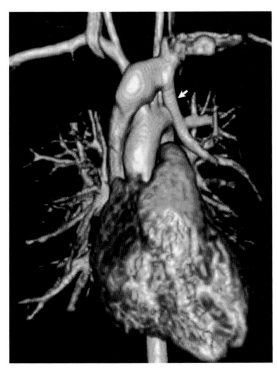

FIGURE 7.30 Volume rendered reconstruction of Gd-enhanced 3-D MRA in a patient with partially anomalous pulmonary venous connection of the left upper pulmonary vein (*arrow*) to the left innominate vein.

Hospital Boston (Table 7.1). Unlike infants in whom echocardiography generally provides all the necessary diagnostic information for surgical repair (241,253), MRI assumes an increasing role in adolescents and adults with TOF in whom the acoustic windows are frequently limited (167). CMR is useful in both preoperative and postoperative assessment of TOF, but the focus of the examination is different.

Preoperative MRI

In most patients with unrepaired TOF, the central question for the CMR examination is to delineate all sources of pulmonary blood flow—pulmonary arteries, aortopulmonary collateral vessels, and the ductus arteriosus. Several studies have shown that spin echo and 2-D gradient echo cine MRI techniques provide excellent imaging of the central pulmonary arteries and major aortopulmonary collaterals (240,254–256). However, these MRI techniques require relatively long scan times for complete anatomic coverage, and small vessels (<2 mm) may not be detected. Furthermore, these two-dimensional techniques are not optimal for imaging long and tortuous blood vessels. Gd-enhanced 3-D MRA is ideally suited to image these vessels (Fig. 7.31). Compared with conventional x-ray angiography, MRA has been shown to be highly accurate in depicting all sources of pulmonary blood supply in patients with complex pulmonary stenosis or atresia, including infants with multiple small aortopulmonary collaterals (242).

Gradient echo cine MRI, preferably SSFP, is used to assess ventricular dimensions and function, the right ventricular outflow tract, as well as dynamic flow imaging of valve function. When the origins and proximal course of the left and right coronary arteries are not known from other imaging studies, they should be imaged either by a gradient echo sequence designed for coronary imaging or by a fast spin echo sequence in the axial or four-chamber planes. Particular attention is paid to the exclusion of a major coronary artery crossing the right ventricular outflow tract.

Postoperative MRI

CMR has been used extensively for assessment of postoperative TOF patients of all ages, but its greatest clinical utility is in adolescents and adults (167,175). Many studies have shown that the degree of pulmonary regurgitation measured by VEC MRI is closely associated with the degree of RV dilation (155,257–259). Another factor that affects RV function is the presence and extent of an aneurysm in the RVOT (260). Quantitative assessment of RV and LV dimensions and function is a key element of CMR evaluation in patients with repaired TOF (Fig. 7.32). The degree of RV dysfunction is an important determinant of clinical status late after TOF and is also closely associated with LV function, likely through ventricular-ventricular interaction (261). Taken together with clinical assessment and electrophysiologic data, information derived from CMR on pulmonary regurgitation fraction, RV and LV dimensions and function, presence and extent of a RVOT aneurysm, and presence of branch pulmonary artery stenosis is used to direct clinical care in patients with repaired TOF.

The goals of the CMR examination, therefore, include quantitative assessment of left and right ventricular volumes, mass, stroke volumes, and ejection fraction; imaging the anatomy of the right ventricular outflow tract, pulmonary arteries, aorta, and aortopulmonary collaterals; quantification of pulmonary regurgitation, tricuspid regurgitation, cardiac output, pulmonary-to-systemic flow ratio; and detection of scar tissue, especially in the right ventricular outflow tract.

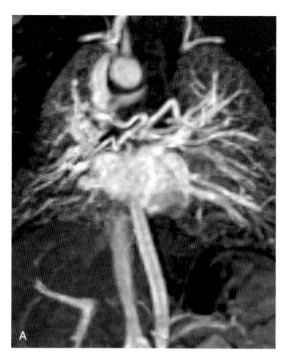

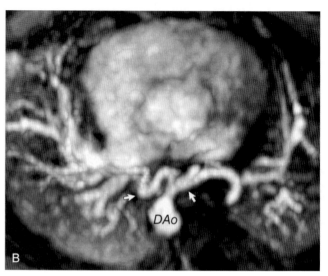

FIGURE 7.31 Subvolume maximal intensity projection Gd-enhanced 3-D MRA showing aortopulmonary collateral vessels (*arrows*) in a newborn with tetralogy of Fallot and pulmonary atresia. **A:** Coronal plane. **B:** Axial (transverse) plane.

Transposition of the Great Arteries

CMR is seldom requested for preoperative assessment of infants with D-loop transposition of the great arteries (TGA) because echocardiography usually provides all necessary diagnostic information (262). In postoperative TGA, CMR assumes an increasing role because of its ability to noninva-

sively evaluate most clinically relevant issues (116,117, 263–269).

Postoperative Atrial Switch (Senning or Mustard operation)

The goals of CMR evaluation of postoperative atrial switch include (i) quantitative evaluation of the size and function of

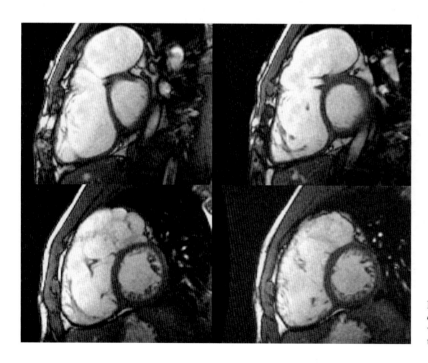

FIGURE 7.32 Short-axis ECG-triggered, breath-hold, cine steady-state free precession imaging in a patient with tetralogy of Fallot, severe pulmonary regurgitation, and markedly dilated right ventricle.

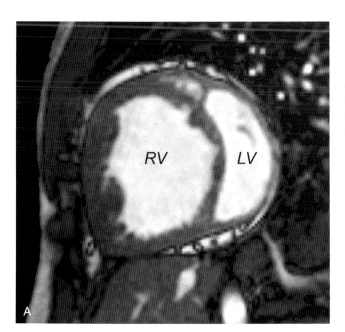

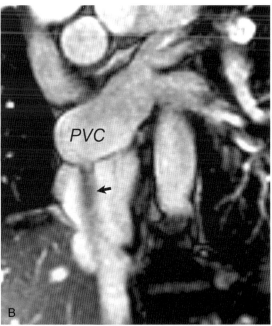

FIGURE 7.33 ECG-triggered, breath-hold, cine steady-state free precession imaging in a patient with Mustard palliation of transposition of the great arteries. A: Short-axis view showing the dilated and hypertrophied right ventricle (RV), which compresses the thin-walled left ventricle (LV). B: Baffle leak (*arrow*) from the pulmonary venous chamber (PVC) to the systemic venous chamber.

the systemic RV (Fig. 7.33A) (264); (ii) imaging of the systemic and pulmonary venous pathways for obstruction and/or baffle leak(s) (Fig. 7.33B); (iii) assessment of tricuspid valve regurgitation; (iv) evaluation of the left and right ventricular outflow tracts for obstruction; (v) detection of aortopulmonary collateral vessels and other associated anomalies; (vi) evaluation of the coronary arteries (270); and (vii) detection of myocardial fibrosis and/or scar tissue (271,272). The response of the systemic RV to pharmacologic stress (dobutamine) or to exercise can be tested by CMR, but the clinical utility of this information awaits further study (117,269).

Postoperative Arterial Switch

The long-term concerns in patients after the arterial switch operation (ASO) relate primarily to the technical challenges of the operation—transfer of the coronary arteries from the native aortic root to the neoaortic root (native pulmonary root) and the transfer of the pulmonary arteries anterior to the neoascending aorta. Consequently, the goals of CMR evaluation of postoperative arterial switch include (i) evaluation of global and regional LV and RV size and function; (ii) evaluation of the left and right ventricular outflow tracts for obstruction; (iii) qualitative estimation of RV systolic pressure based on the configuration of the interventricular septum; (iv) imaging of the great vessels with emphasis on evaluation of the pulmonary arteries for stenosis and the aortic root for dilation (Fig. 7.34); (v) detection of aortopulmonary collateral vessels and other associated anomalies; and (vi) detection of myocardial fibrosis and/or scar tissue. It is recognized that the role of myocardial perfusion and viability imaging in this population deserves further study, especially with regard to the sensitivity,

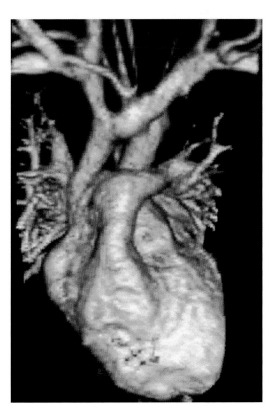

FIGURE 7.34 Volume rendered reconstruction of Gd-enhanced 3-D MRA in a patient with arterial switch operation for transposition of the great arteries. Note the relationship between the pulmonary arteries and the ascending aorta (Lecompte maneuver).

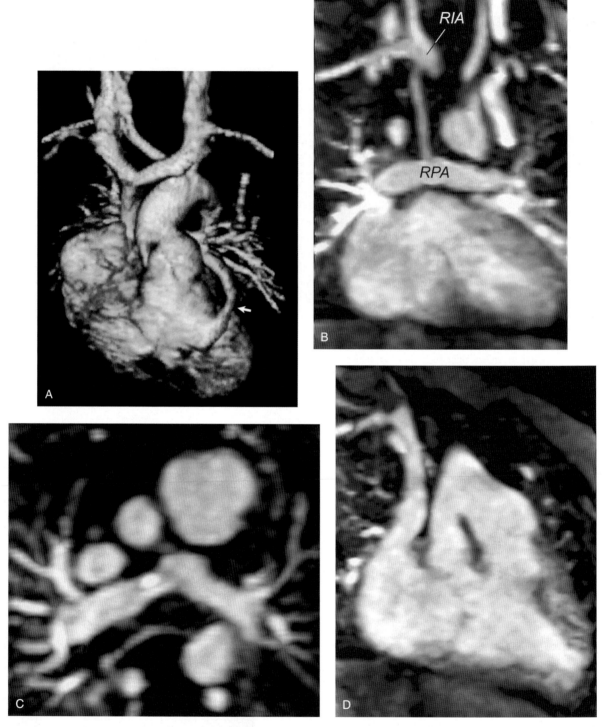

FIGURE 7.35 MRI evaluation of hypoplastic left heart syndrome after stage I palliation. **A:** Volume rendered reconstruction of Gd-enhanced 3-D MRA showing the right ventricle–to–pulmonary artery conduit (*arrow*) and the arterial anastomoses. **B:** Maximal intensity projection of a modified right Blalock-Thomas-Taussig shunt. **C:** Maximal intensity projection image in the axial (transverse) plane showing the branch pulmonary arteries. **D:** Maximal intensity projection image showing the anastomosis between the main pulmonary artery and the native ascending aorta.

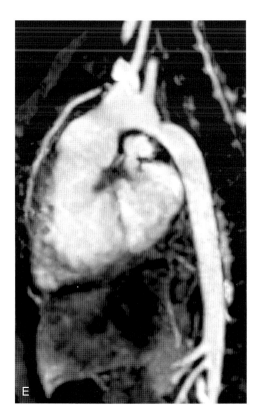

FIGURE 7.35 (*Continued*) E: Maximal intensity projection image of the reconstructed aorta. RIA, right innominate artery; RPA, right pulmonary artery.

specificity, and predictive values of these technique for detection of myocardial ischemia and the prognostic implications of myocardial fibrosis and/or scar tissue detected by delayed myocardial enhancement.

Single Ventricle and Fontan

Before Stage I Palliation

CMR has an important role in the diagnostic evaluation and follow-up of patients with anatomic and functional single ventricle. Echocardiography is the primary imaging tool during the initial evaluation since most patients present in the newborn period or early infancy and their acoustic windows are typically adequate. CMR is used before the first palliative procedure only in selected cases, usually to evaluate incompletely diagnosed extracardiac anatomy such as anomalies of the aortic arch, pulmonary arteries, and venous anomalies.

Before Stage II Palliation

The role of CMR increases after the first palliative surgical procedure. CMR may be requested to assess potential complications or sequelae of the first operation such as residual or recurrent aortic arch obstruction, stenosis or compression of branch pulmonary arteries or pulmonary veins, aortopulmonary or ventriculopulmonary shunts, airway compression, and others. In patients who are candidates for a bidirectional Glenn shunt or a hemi-Fontan procedure (second-stage palliation), CMR may have an important role as a substitute for routine diagnostic catheterization (272). Evidence from two retrospective studies suggests that in a substantial number of patients who are candidates for a second-stage palliation cardiac catheterization data do not change the surgical plan (273,274). Although some of these patients undergo a concomitant transcatheter intervention (e.g., balloon dilation of coarctation or coil occlusion of aortopulmonary collaterals), the indications for and the clinical benefits from such procedures are not clearly defined. Whereas echocardiography can provide much of the anatomic and functional information in these patients, there are circumstances in which parts of the anatomy may not be fully defined and additional quantitative functional data may be desired. CMR can potentially fulfill these goals (Fig. 7.35). The results of an ongoing prospective randomized trial comparing routine diagnostic catheterization with CMR in patients who are candidates for a second-stage palliation may shed light on the role of CMR in these patients. The goals of the CMR examination in patients who are candidates for a second-stage palliation include the following: (i) anatomy of the systemic and pulmonary veins; (ii) anatomy of the branch pulmonary arteries; (iii) anatomy of the thoracic aorta with an emphasis on exclusion of arch obstruction; (iv) presence and distribution of aortopulmonary and venous collaterals; (v) quantitative assessment of systemic ventricular function; (vi) quantitative assessment of valve regurgitation; (vii) evaluation of the atrial septum for restriction; and (viii) detection of myocardial fibrosis or scar tissue (275).

Before and After Fontan Palliation

Several reports have used CMR as an investigational tool to study blood flow dynamics within the Fontan pathways and to delineate the distribution of inferior and superior caval flow to each lung (182,183,194,195). Myocardial tagging has proved an important investigational tool in the evaluation of myocardial mechanics in patients with functional single ventricle and Fontan circulation, demonstrating asynchrony and impaired regional wall motion (113). The clinical utility of CMR in patients with the Fontan circulation increases as these patients grow and their acoustic windows become more restricted. The goals of the MRI examination in patients with the Fontan circulation include (i) assessment of the pathways from the systemic veins to the pulmonary arteries for obstruction and for a thrombus (Fig. 7.36); (ii) detection of Fontan baffle fenestration or leaks; (iii) evaluation of the pulmonary veins for compression; (iv) evaluation of systemic ventricular volumes, mass, and function; (v) imaging of the systemic ventricular outflow tract for obstruction; (vi) quantitative assessment of the atrioventricular and semilunar valve(s) for regurgitation; (vii) imaging the aorta for obstruction or an aneurysm; and (viii) detection of aortopulmonary, systemic venous, or systemic-to-pulmonary venous collateral vessels.

An important limitation of CMR in patients with a Fontan circulation is the frequent presence of metallic implants (e.g., coils, stents, occluding devices) that produce image artifacts. Garg et al. (47) reviewed the CMR studies of 120 consecutive CMR examinations and found that artifacts owing to metallic implants were present in 54% of the studies. Major artifacts (mostly caused by stainless steel coils) were present in 36% of patients, and in 20% the artifact precluded complete volumetric assessment of the ventricle. CT can be used as an alternative to CMR in patients with large image artifacts as well as in those with contraindications (e.g., pacemaker).

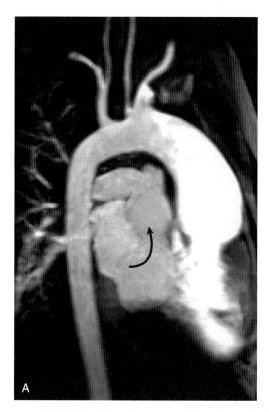 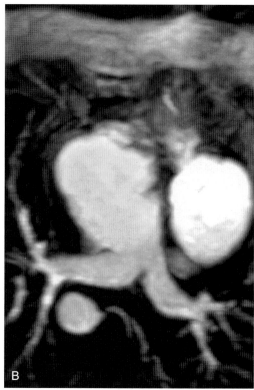

FIGURE 7.36 Subvolume maximal intensity projection image of Fontan pathway in a patient with atrio-pulmonary anastomosis. **A:** Oblique sagittal view showing the atriopulmonary anastomosis (*curved arrow*). **B:** Oblique transverse view showing the pulmonary anastomosis and branch pulmonary arteries.

References

1. Tsai-Goodman B, Geva T, Odegard KC, et al. Clinical role, accuracy, and technical aspects of cardiovascular magnetic resonance imaging in infants. *Am J Cardiol* 2004;94:69–74.
2. Mulkern RV, Chung T. From signal to image: Magnetic resonance imaging physics for cardiac magnetic resonance. *Pediatr Cardiol* 2000;21(1):5–17.
3. Axel L. Physics and technology of cardiovascular MR imaging. *Cardiol Clin* 1998;16(2):125–133.
4. Chia JM, Fischer SE, Wickline SA, et al. Performance of QRS detection for cardiac magnetic resonance imaging with a novel vectorcardiographic triggering method. *J Magn Reson Imaging* 2000;12(5):678–688.
5. Larson AC, White RD, Laub G, et al. Self-gated cardiac cine MRI. *Magn Reson Med* 2004;51(1):93–102.
6. Spuentrup E, Buecker A, Stuber M, et al. Navigator-gated coronary magnetic resonance angiography using steady-state-free-precession: Comparison to standard T2-prepared gradient-echo and spiral imaging. *Invest Radiol* 2003;38(5):263–268.
7. Wetzel SG, Lee VS, Tan AG, et al. Real-time interactive duplex MR measurements: Application in neurovascular imaging. *AJR Am J Roentgenol* 2001;177:703-707.
8. Buecker A, Adam GB, Neuerburg JM, et al. Simultaneous real-time visualization of the catheter tip and vascular anatomy for MR-guided PTA of iliac arteries in an animal model. *J Magn Reson Imaging* 2002;16(2):201–208.
9. Plein S, Smith WH, Ridgway JP, et al. Measurements of left ventricular dimensions using real-time acquisition in cardiac magnetic resonance imaging: Comparison with conventional gradient echo imaging. *Magma* 2001;13(2):101–108.
10. Sampath S, Derbyshire JA, Atalar E, et al. Real-time imaging of two-dimensional cardiac strain using a harmonic phase magnetic resonance imaging (HARP-MRI) pulse sequence. *Magn Reson Med* 2003;50(1):154–163.
11. Gutierrez FR. Magnetic resonance imaging of congenital heart disease. *Top Magn Reson Imaging* 1995;7(4):246–257.
12. Masui T, Katayama M, Kobayashi S, et al. Gadolinium-enhanced MR angiography in the evaluation of congenital cardiovascular disease pre- and postoperative states in infants and children. *J Magn Reson Imaging* 2000;12(6):1034–1042.
13. Schlesinger AE, Hernandez RJ. Magnetic resonance imaging in congenital heart disease in children. *Tex Heart Inst J* 1996;23(2):128–143.
14. Fogel MA, Donofrio MT, Ramaciotti C, et al. Magnetic resonance and echocardiographic imaging of pulmonary artery size throughout stages of Fontan reconstruction. *Circulation* 1994;90:2927–2936.
15. Beekman RP, Hoorntje TM, Beek FJ, et al. Sedation for children undergoing magnetic resonance imaging: Efficacy and safety of rectal thiopental. *Eur J Pediatr* 1996;155(9):820–822.
16. Didier D, Ratib O, Beghetti M, et al. Morphologic and functional evaluation of congenital heart disease by magnetic resonance imaging. *J Magn Reson Imaging* 1999;10(5):639–655.
17. Baker E. What's new in magnetic resonance imaging? *Cardiol Young* 2001;11(4):445–452.
18. Holmqvist C, Larsson EM, Stahlberg F, et al. Contrast-enhanced thoracic 3D-MR angiography in infants and children. *Acta Radiol* 2001;42(1):50–58.
19. Odegard KC, DiNardo JA, Tsai-Goodman B, et al. Anaesthesia considerations for cardiac MRI in infants and small children. *Paediatr Anaesth* 2004;14(6):471–476.
20. Ahmed S, Shellock FG. Magnetic resonance imaging safety: Implications for cardiovascular patients. *J Cardiovasc Magn Reson* 2001;3(3):171–182.
21. Shellock FG, O'Neil M, Ivans V, et al. Cardiac pacemakers and implantable cardioverter defibrillators are unaffected by operation of an extremity MR imaging system. *AJR Am J Roentgenol* 1999;172:165–170.
22. Martin ET, Coman JA, Shellock FG, et al. Magnetic resonance imaging and cardiac pacemaker safety at 1.5-Tesla. *J Am Coll Cardiol* 2004;43:1315–1324.

23. Shellock FG. Prosthetic heart valves and annuloplasty rings: Assessment of magnetic field interactions, heating, and artifacts at 1.5 Tesla. *J Cardiovasc Magn Reson* 2001;3(4):317–324.

24. Shellock FG, Shellock VJ. Cardiovascular catheters and accessories: Ex vivo testing of ferromagnetism, heating, and artifacts associated with MRI. *J Magn Reson Imaging* 1998;8(6):1338–1342.

25. Shellock FG, Morisoli SM. Ex vivo evaluation of ferromagnetism and artifacts of cardiac occluders exposed to a 1.5-T MR system. *J Magn Reson Imaging* 1994;4(2):213–215.

26. Wolff S, James TL, Young GB, et al. Magnetic resonance imaging: Absence of in vitro cytogenetic damage. *Radiology* 1985;155(1):163–165.

27. Shellock FG. Metallic surgical instruments for interventional MRI procedures: Evaluation of MR safety. *J Magn Reson Imaging* 2001;13(1):152–157.

28. Sawyer-Glover AM, Shellock FG. Pre-MRI procedure screening: Recommendations and safety considerations for biomedical implants and devices. *J Magn Reson Imaging* 2000;12(1):92–106.

29. Rutledge JM, Vick GW 3rd, Mullins CE, et al. Safety of magnetic resonance imaging immediately following Palmaz stent implant: A report of three cases. *Catheter Cardiovasc Interv* 2001;53(4):519–523.

30. Jagannathan NR. Magnetic resonance imaging: Bioeffects and safety concerns. *Indian J Biochem Biophys* 1999;36(5):341–347.

31. Edwards MB, Taylor KM, Shellock FG. Prosthetic heart valves: Evaluation of magnetic field interactions, heating, and artifacts at 1.5 T. *J Magn Reson Imaging* 2000;12(2):363–369.

32. Ordidge RJ, Shellock FG, Kanal E. A Y2000 update of current safety issues related to MRI. *J Magn Reson Imaging* 2000;12(1):1.

33. Hofman MB, de Cock CC, van der Linden JC, et al. Transesophageal cardiac pacing during magnetic resonance imaging: Feasibility and safety considerations. *Magn Reson Med* 1996;35(3):413–422.

34. Gimbel JR, Johnson D, Levine PA, et al. Safe performance of magnetic resonance imaging on five patients with permanent cardiac pacemakers. *Pacing Clin Electrophysiol* 1996;19:913–919.

35. Carr JC, Simonetti O, Bundy J, et al. Cine MR angiography of the heart with segmented true fast imaging with steady-state precession. *Radiology* 2001;219:828–834.

36. Bax JJ, Lamb H, Dibbets P, et al. Comparison of gated single-photon emission computed tomography with magnetic resonance imaging for evaluation of left ventricular function in ischemic cardiomyopathy. *Am J Cardiol* 2000;86:1299–1305.

37. Bellenger NG, Marcus NJ, Davies C, et al. Left ventricular function and mass after orthotopic heart transplantation: A comparison of cardiovascular magnetic resonance with echocardiography. *J Heart Lung Transplant* 2000;19(5):444–452.

38. Bellenger NG, Burgess MI, Ray SG, et al. Comparison of left ventricular ejection fraction and volumes in heart failure by echocardiography, radionuclide ventriculography and cardiovascular magnetic resonance; are they interchangeable? *Eur Heart J* 2000;21:1387–1396.

39. Sorensen TS, Korperich H, Greil GF, et al. Operator-independent isotropic three-dimensional magnetic resonance imaging for morphology in congenital heart disease: A validation study. *Circulation* 2004;110:163–169.

40. Manning WJ, Stuber M, Danias PG, et al. Coronary magnetic resonance imaging: Current status. *Curr Probl Cardiol* 2002;27(7):275–333.

41. Greil GF, Stuber M, Botnar RM, et al. Coronary magnetic resonance angiography in adolescents and young adults with kawasaki disease. *Circulation* 2002;105:908–911.

42. Taylor AM, Thorne SA, Rubens MB, et al. Coronary artery imaging in grown up congenital heart disease: Complementary role of magnetic resonance and x-ray coronary angiography. *Circulation* 2000;101:1670–1678.

43. Aydogan U, Onursal E, Cantez T, et al. Giant congenital coronary artery fistula to left superior vena cava and right atrium with compression of left pulmonary vein simulating cor triatriatum—diagnostic value of magnetic resonance imaging. *Eur J Cardiothorac Surg* 1994;8(2):97–99.

44. Danias PG, Stuber M, McConnell MV, et al. The diagnosis of congenital coronary anomalies with magnetic resonance imaging. *Coron Artery Dis* 2001;12:621–626.

45. Boxer RA, LaCorte MA, Singh S, et al. Noninvasive diagnosis of congenital left coronary artery to right ventricle fistula by nuclear magnetic resonance imaging. *Pediatr Cardiol* 1989;10(1):45–47.

46. Greil GF, Powell AJ, Gildein HP, et al. Gadolinium-enhanced three-dimensional magnetic resonance angiography of pulmonary and systemic venous anomalies. *J Am Coll Cardiol* 2002;39:335–341.

47. Garg R, Powell AJ, Sena L, et al. Effects of metallic implants on magnetic resonance imaging evaluation of Fontan palliation. *Am J Cardiol* 2005;95:688–691.

48. Kaji S, Yang PC, Kerr AB, et al. Rapid evaluation of left ventricular volume and mass without breath-holding using real-time interactive cardiac magnetic resonance imaging system. *J Am Coll Cardiol* 2001;38:527–533.

49. Schalla S, Nagel E, Lehmkuhl H, et al. Comparison of magnetic resonance real-time imaging of left ventricular function with conventional magnetic resonance imaging and echocardiography. *Am J Cardiol* 2001;87(1):95–99.

50. Fu JC, Chai JW, Wong ST. Wavelet-based enhancement for detection of left ventricular myocardial boundaries in magnetic resonance images. *Magn Reson Imaging* 2000;18:1135–1141.

51. Makowski P, Sorensen TS, Therkildsen SV, et al. Two-phase active contour method for semiautomatic segmentation of the heart and blood vessels from MRI images for 3D visualization. *Comput Med Imaging Graph* 2002;26(1):9–17.

52. Zimmer Y, Akselrod S. An automatic contour extraction algorithm for short-axis cardiac magnetic resonance images. *Med Phys* 1996;23:1371–1379.

53. Yezzi A Jr, Kichenassamy S, Kumar A, et al. A geometric snake model for segmentation of medical imagery. *IEEE Trans Med Imaging* 1997;16(2):199–209.

54. Holland AE, Goldfarb JW, Edelman RR. Diaphragmatic and cardiac motion during suspended breathing: Preliminary experience and implications for breath-hold MR imaging. *Radiology* 1998;209(2):483–489.

55. Raichura N, Entwisle J, Leverment J, et al. Breath-hold MRI in evaluating patients with pectus excavatum. *Br J Radiol* 2001;74:701–708.

56. Ostrzega E, Maddahi J, Honma H, et al. Quantification of left ventricular myocardial mass in humans by nuclear magnetic resonance imaging. *Am Heart J* 1989;117(2):444–452.

57. Maddahi J, Crues J, Berman DS, et al. Noninvasive quantification of left ventricular myocardial mass by gated proton nuclear magnetic resonance imaging. *J Am Coll Cardiol* 1987;10:682–692.

58. Keller AM, Peshock RM, Malloy CR, et al. In vivo measurement of myocardial mass using nuclear magnetic resonance imaging. *J Am Coll Cardiol* 1986;8:113–117.

59. Katz J, Milliken MC, Stray-Gundersen J, et al. Estimation of human myocardial mass with MR imaging. *Radiology* 1988;169(2):495–498.

60. Florentine MS, Grosskreutz CL, Chang W, et al. Measurement of left ventricular mass in vivo using gated nuclear magnetic resonance imaging. *J Am Coll Cardiol* 1986;8:107–112.

61. Caputo GR, Tscholakoff D, Sechtem U, et al. Measurement of canine left ventricular mass by using MR imaging. *AJR Am J Roentgenol* 1987;148:33–38.

62. Koch JA, Poll LW, Godehardt E, et al. In vitro determination of cardiac ventricular volumes using MRI at 1.0 T in a porcine heart model. *Int J Cardiovasc Imaging* 2001;17(3):237–242.

63. Semelka RC, Tomei E, Wagner S, et al. Interstudy reproducibility of dimensional and functional measurements between cine magnetic resonance studies in the morphologically abnormal left ventricle. *Am Heart J* 1990;119:1367–1373.

64. Semelka RC, Tomei E, Wagner S, et al. Normal left ventricular dimensions and function: Interstudy reproducibility of measurements with cine MR imaging. *Radiology* 1990;174(pt 1):763–768.

65. Doherty NE 3rd, Fujita N, Caputo GR, et al. Measurement of right ventricular mass in normal and dilated cardiomyopathic ventricles using cine magnetic resonance imaging. *Am J Cardiol* 1992;69:1223–1228.

66. Doherty NE 3rd, Seelos KC, Suzuki J, et al. Application of cine nuclear magnetic resonance imaging for sequential evaluation of response to angiotensin-converting enzyme inhibitor therapy in dilated cardiomyopathy. *J Am Coll Cardiol* 1992;19:1294–1302.

67. Germain P, Roul G, Kastler B, et al. Inter-study variability in left ventricular mass measurement. Comparison between M-mode echography and MRI. *Eur Heart J* 1992;13:1011–1019.

68. Bellenger NG, Davies LC, Francis JM, et al. Reduction in sample size for studies of remodeling in heart failure by the use of cardiovascular magnetic resonance. *J Cardiovasc Magn Reson* 2000;2(4):271–278.

69. Ioannidis JP, Trikalinos TA, Danias PG. Electrocardiogram-gated single-photon emission computed tomography versus cardiac magnetic resonance imaging for the assessment of left ventricular volumes and ejection fraction: A meta-analysis. *J Am Coll Cardiol* 2002;39:2059–2068.

70. Plein S, Bloomer TN, Ridgway JP, et al. Steady-state free precession magnetic resonance imaging of the heart: Comparison with segmented k-space gradient-echo imaging. *J Magn Reson Imaging* 2001;14:230–236.

71. Alfakih K, Thiele H, Plein S, et al. Comparison of right ventricular volume measurement between segmented k-space gradient-echo and steady-state free precession magnetic resonance imaging. *J Magn Reson Imaging* 2002;16(3):253–258.

72. Alfakih K, Plein S, Thiele H, et al. Normal human left and right ventricular dimensions for MRI as assessed by turbo gradient echo and steady-state free precession imaging sequences. *J Magn Reson Imaging* 2003;17(3):323–329.

73. Colan SD. Assessment of ventricular and myocardial performance. In: Fyler DC, ed. *Nadas' Pediatric Cardiology*. Philadelphia: Hanley & Belfus, 1992:225–248.

74. Regen DM. Calculation of left ventricular wall stress. *Circ Res* 1990;67(2):245–252.

75. Setser RM, Sayre K, Flacke S, et al. Assessment of ventricular contractility during cardiac magnetic resonance imaging examinations using normalized maximal ventricular power. *Ann Biomed Eng* 2001;29:974–982.

76. Cerqueira MD, Weissman NJ, Dilsizian V, et al. Standardized myocardial segmentation and nomenclature for tomographic imaging of the heart: A

statement for healthcare professionals from the Cardiac Imaging Committee of the Council on Clinical Cardiology of the American Heart Association. *Circulation* 2002;105:539–542.

77. Klein SS, Graham TP Jr, Lorenz CH. Noninvasive delineation of normal right ventricular contractile motion with magnetic resonance imaging myocardial tagging. *Ann Biomed Eng* 1998;26:756–763.

78. Lamb HJ, Singleton RR, van der Geest RJ, et al. MR imaging of regional cardiac function: Low-pass filtering of wall thickness curves. *Magn Reson Med* 1995;34(3):498–502.

79. Reichek N. MRI myocardial tagging. *J Magn Reson Imaging* 1999;10(5): 609–616.

80. Fogel MA. Assessment of cardiac function by magnetic resonance imaging. *Pediatr Cardiol* 2000;21(1):59–69.

81. Haber I, Metaxas DN, Axel L. Three-dimensional motion reconstruction and analysis of the right ventricle using tagged MRI. *Med Image Anal* 2000;4(4):335–355.

82. Garot J, Bluemke DA, Osman NF, et al. Fast determination of regional myocardial strain fields from tagged cardiac images using harmonic phase MRI. *Circulation* 2000;101:981–988.

83. Kuijer JP, Marcus JT, Gotte MJ, et al. Simultaneous MRI tagging and through-plane velocity quantification: A three-dimensional myocardial motion tracking algorithm. *J Magn Reson Imaging* 1999;9(3):409–419.

84. Fonseca CG, Oxenham HC, Cowan BR, et al. Aging alters patterns of regional nonuniformity in LV strain relaxation: A 3D MR tissue tagging study. *Am J Physiol Heart Circ Physiol* 2003;285(2):H621–630.

85. Oxenham HC, Young AA, Cowan BR, et al. Age-related changes in myocardial relaxation using three-dimensional tagged magnetic resonance imaging. *J Cardiovasc Magn Reson* 2003;5(3):421–430.

86. Tustison NJ, Davila-Roman VG, Amini AA. Myocardial kinematics from tagged MRI based on a 4-D B-spline model. *IEEE Trans Biomed Eng* 2003;50:1038–1040.

87. McVeigh ER, Atalar E. Cardiac tagging with breath-hold cine MRI. *Magn Reson Med* 1992;28(2):318–327.

88. Azhari H, Weiss JL, Shapiro EP. Distribution of myocardial strains: An MRI study. *Adv Exp Med Biol* 1995;382:319–328.

89. Matter C, Nagel E, Stuber M, et al. Assessment of systolic and diastolic LV function by MR myocardial tagging. *Basic Res Cardiol* 1996;91(suppl 2):23–28.

90. Moulton MJ, Creswell LL, Downing SW, et al. Myocardial material property determination in the in vivo heart using magnetic resonance imaging. *Int J Card Imaging* 1996;12(3):153–167.

91. Park J, Metaxas D, Axel L. Analysis of left ventricular wall motion based on volumetric deformable models and MRI-SPAMM. *Med Image Anal* 1996;1(1):53–71.

92. Dong SJ, Hees PS, Huang WM, et al. Independent effects of preload, afterload, and contractility on left ventricular torsion. *Am J Physiol* 1999; 277(pt 2):H1053–1060.

93. Wyman BT, Hunter WC, Prinzen FW, et al. Mapping propagation of mechanical activation in the paced heart with MRI tagging. *Am J Physiol* 1999;276(pt 2):H881–891.

94. O'Dell WG, McCulloch AD. Imaging three-dimensional cardiac function. *Annu Rev Biomed Eng* 2000;2:431–456.

95. Osman NF, Prince JL. Visualizing myocardial function using HARP MRI. *Phys Med Biol* 2000;45:1665–1682.

96. Ozturk C, McVeigh ER. Four-dimensional B-spline based motion analysis of tagged MR images: Introduction and in vivo validation. *Phys Med Biol* 2000;45:1683–1702.

97. Power TP, Kramer CM, Shaffer AL, et al. Breath-hold dobutamine magnetic resonance myocardial tagging: Normal left ventricular response. *Am J Cardiol* 1997;80:1203–1207.

98. Haber I, Metaxas DN, Geva T, et al. Three-dimensional systolic kinematics of the right ventricle. *Am J Physiol Heart Circ Physiol* 2005;289: H1826–1833.

99. Marcus JT, Gotte MJ, Van Rossum AC, et al. Myocardial function in infarcted and remote regions early after infarction in man: Assessment by magnetic resonance tagging and strain analysis. *Magn Reson Med* 1997; 38:803–810.

100. Chin BB, Esposito G, Kraitchman DL. Myocardial contractile reserve and perfusion defect severity with rest and stress dobutamine (99m)Tc-sestamibi SPECT in canine stunning and subendocardial infarction. *J Nucl Med* 2002;43(4):540–550.

101. Saito I, Watanabe S, Masuda Y. Detection of viable myocardium by dobutamine stress tagging magnetic resonance imaging with three-dimensional analysis by automatic trace method. *Jpn Circ J* 2000;64(7):487–494.

102. Nagel E, Fleck E. Functional MRI in ischemic heart disease based on detection of contraction abnormalities. *J Magn Reson Imaging* 1999;10 (3):411–417.

103. Mankad R, McCreery CJ, Rogers WJ Jr, et al. Regional myocardial strain before and after mitral valve repair for severe mitral regurgitation. *J Cardiovasc Magn Reson* 2001;3(3):257–266.

104. Ungacta FF, Davila-Roman VG, Moulton MJ, et al. MRI-radiofrequency tissue tagging in patients with aortic insufficiency before and after operation. *Ann Thorac Surg* 1998;65:943–950.

105. Geskin G, Kramer CM, Rogers WJ, et al. Quantitative assessment of myocardial viability after infarction by dobutamine magnetic resonance tagging. *Circulation* 1998;98:217–223.

106. Kramer CM, Rogers WJ, Geskin G, et al. Usefulness of magnetic resonance imaging early after acute myocardial infarction. *Am J Cardiol* 1997;80:690–695.

107. Kramer CM, Rogers WJ, Theobald TM, et al. Dissociation between changes in intramyocardial function and left ventricular volumes in the eight weeks after first anterior myocardial infarction. *J Am Coll Cardiol* 1997;30:1625–1632.

108. Kraitchman DL, Wilke N, Hexeberg E, et al. Myocardial perfusion and function in dogs with moderate coronary stenosis. *Magn Reson Med* 1996;35:771–780.

109. Azhari H, Weiss JL, Rogers WJ, et al. A noninvasive comparative study of myocardial strains in ischemic canine hearts using tagged MRI in 3-D. *Am J Physiol* 1995;268(pt 2):H1918–1926.

110. Setser RM, White RD, Sturm B, et al. Noninvasive assessment of cardiac mechanics and clinical outcome after partial left ventriculectomy. *Ann Thorac Surg* 2003;76:1576–1585; discussion 1585–1576.

111. Kuijpers D, Ho KY, van Dijkman PR, et al. Dobutamine cardiovascular magnetic resonance for the detection of myocardial ischemia with the use of myocardial tagging. *Circulation* 2003;107:1592–1597.

112. Fogel MA, Weinberg PM, Fellows KE, et al. A study in ventricular-ventricular interaction. Single right ventricles compared with systemic right ventricles in a dual-chamber circulation. *Circulation* 1995;92:219–230.

113. Fogel MA, Gupta KB, Weinberg PM, et al. Regional wall motion and strain analysis across stages of Fontan reconstruction by magnetic resonance tagging. *Am J Physiol* 1995;269(pt 2):H1132–1152.

114. Fogel MA, Weinberg PM, Chin AJ, et al. Late ventricular geometry and performance changes of functional single ventricle throughout staged Fontan reconstruction assessed by magnetic resonance imaging. *J Am Coll Cardiol* 1996;28:212–221.

115. Fogel MA, Weinberg PM, Gupta KB, et al. Mechanics of the single left ventricle: A study in ventricular-ventricular interaction II. *Circulation* 1998;98:330–338.

116. Tulevski II, van der Wall EE, Groenink M, et al. Usefulness of magnetic resonance imaging dobutamine stress in asymptomatic and minimally symptomatic patients with decreased cardiac reserve from congenital heart disease (complete and corrected transposition of the great arteries and subpulmonic obstruction). *Am J Cardiol* 2002;89:1077–1081.

117. Tulevski II, Lee PL, Groenink M, et al. Dobutamine-induced increase of right ventricular contractility without increased stroke volume in adolescent patients with transposition of the great arteries: Evaluation with magnetic resonance imaging. *Int J Card Imaging* 2000;16(6):471–478.

118. Dodge-Khatami A, Tulevski II, Bennink GB, et al. Comparable systemic ventricular function in healthy adults and patients with unoperated congenitally corrected transposition using MRI dobutamine stress testing. *Ann Thorac Surg* 2002;73:1759–1764.

119. Roest AA, Kunz P, Lamb HJ, et al. Biventricular response to supine physical exercise in young adults assessed with ultrafast magnetic resonance imaging. *Am J Cardiol* 2001;87:601–605.

120. Grossman W. Diastolic function and heart failure: An overview. *Eur Heart J* 1990;11(Suppl C):2–7.

121. Mohiaddin RH, Amanuma M, Kilner PJ, et al. MR phase-shift velocity mapping of mitral and pulmonary venous flow. *J Comput Assist Tomogr* 1991;15(2):237–243.

122. Suzuki J, Chang JM, Caputo GR, et al. Evaluation of right ventricular early diastolic filling by cine nuclear magnetic resonance imaging in patients with hypertrophic cardiomyopathy. *J Am Coll Cardiol* 1991;18 (1):120–126.

123. Hartiala JJ, Mostbeck GH, Foster E, et al. Velocity-encoded cine MRI in the evaluation of left ventricular diastolic function: Measurement of mitral valve and pulmonary vein flow velocities and flow volume across the mitral valve. *Am Heart J* 1993;125:1054–1066.

124. Hoff FL, Turner DA, Wang JZ, et al. Semiautomatic evaluation of left ventricular diastolic function with cine magnetic resonance imaging. *Acad Radiol* 1994;1(3):237–242.

125. Schwammenthal E, Wichter T, Joachimsen K, et al. Detection of regional left ventricular asynchrony in obstructive hypertrophic cardiomyopathy by magnetic resonance imaging. *Am Heart J* 1994;127:600–606.

126. Dendale PA, Franken PR, Waldman GJ, et al. Regional diastolic wall motion dynamics in anterior myocardial infarction: Analysis and quantification with magnetic resonance imaging. *Coron Artery Dis* 1995;6:723–729.

127. Mohiaddin RH, Hasegawa M. Measurement of atrial volumes by magnetic resonance imaging in healthy volunteers and in patients with myocardial infarction. *Eur Heart J* 1995;16(1):106–111.

128. Helbing WA, Niezen RA, Le Cessie S, et al. Right ventricular diastolic function in children with pulmonary regurgitation after repair of tetralogy of Fallot: Volumetric evaluation by magnetic resonance velocity mapping. *J Am Coll Cardiol* 1996;28:1827–1835.

129. Kudelka AM, Turner DA, Liebson PR, et al. Comparison of cine magnetic resonance imaging and Doppler echocardiography for evaluation of left ventricular diastolic function. *Am J Cardiol* 1997;80:384–386.

130. Eroglu AG, Sarioglu A, Sarioglu T. Right ventricular diastolic function after repair of tetralogy of Fallot: Its relationship to the insertion of a 'transannular' patch. *Cardiol Young* 1999;9(4):384–391.

131. Fogel MA, Weinberg PM, Hubbard A, et al. Diastolic biomechanics in normal infants utilizing MRI tissue tagging. *Circulation* 2000;102:218–224.

132. Kroft LJ, Simons P, van Laar JM, et al. Patients with pulmonary fibrosis: Cardiac function assessed with MR imaging. *Radiology* 2000;216(2):464–471.

133. Lorenz CH, Flacke S, Fischer SE. Noninvasive modalities. Cardiac MR imaging. *Cardiol Clin* 2000;18:557–570.

134. Dong SJ, Hees PS, Siu CO, et al. MRI assessment of LV relaxation by untwisting rate: A new isovolumic phase measure of tau. *Am J Physiol Heart Circ Physiol* 2001;281:H2002–2009.

135. Paelinck BP, Lamb HJ, Bax JJ, et al. Assessment of diastolic function by cardiovascular magnetic resonance. *Am Heart J* 2002;144:198–205.

136. Young AA, Cowan BR, Occleshaw CJ, et al. Temporal evolution of left ventricular strain late after repair of coarctation of the aorta using 3D MR tissue tagging. *J Cardiovasc Magn Reson* 2002;4(2):233–243.

137. Powell AJ, Geva T. Blood flow measurement by magnetic resonance imaging in congenital heart disease. *Pediatr Cardiol* 2000;21(1):47–58.

138. Pelc NJ, Herfkens RJ, Shimakawa A, et al. Phase contrast cine magnetic resonance imaging. *Magn Reson Q* 1991;7(4):229–254.

139. Greil G, Geva T, Maier SE, et al. Effect of acquisition parameters on the accuracy of velocity encoded cine magnetic resonance imaging blood flow measurements. *J Magn Reson Imaging* 2002;15(1):47–54.

140. Beerbaum P, Korperich H, Barth P, et al. Noninvasive quantification of left-to-right shunt in pediatric patients: Phase-contrast cine magnetic resonance imaging compared with invasive oximetry. *Circulation* 2001;103:2476–2482.

141. Powell AJ, Maier SE, Chung T, et al. Phase-velocity cine magnetic resonance imaging measurement of pulsatile blood flow in children and young adults: In vitro and in vivo validation. *Pediatr Cardiol* 2000;21(2):104–110.

142. Hundley WG, Li HF, Lange RA, et al. Assessment of left-to-right intracardiac shunting by velocity-encoded, phase-difference magnetic resonance imaging. A comparison with oximetric and indicator dilution techniques. *Circulation* 1995;91:2955–2960.

143. Papaharilaou Y, Doorly DJ, Sherwin SJ. Assessing the accuracy of two-dimensional phase-contrast MRI measurements of complex unsteady flows. *J Magn Reson Imaging* 2001;14:714–723.

144. Robertson MB, Kohler U, Hoskins PR, et al. Quantitative analysis of PC MRI velocity maps: Pulsatile flow in cylindrical vessels. *Magn Reson Imaging* 2001;19:685–695.

145. Wise RG, Newling B, Gates AR, et al. Measurement of pulsatile flow using MRI and a Bayesian technique of probability analysis. *Magn Reson Imaging* 1996;14:173–185.

146. Evans AJ, Iwai F, Grist TA, et al. Magnetic resonance imaging of blood flow with a phase subtraction technique. In vitro and in vivo validation. *Invest Radiol* 1993;28(2):109–115.

147. Zananiri FV, Jackson PC, Goddard PR, et al. An evaluation of the accuracy of flow measurements using magnetic resonance imaging (MRI). *J Med Eng Technol* 1991;15(4–5):170–176.

148. Steinman DA, Frayne R, Zhang XD, et al. MR measurement and numerical simulation of steady flow in an end-to-side anastomosis model. *J Biomech* 1996;29(4):537–542.

149. Firmin DN, Nayler GL, Kilner PJ, et al. The application of phase shifts in NMR for flow measurement. *Magn Reson Med* 1990;14:230–241.

150. Ku DN, Biancheri CL, Pettigrew RI, et al. Evaluation of magnetic resonance velocimetry for steady flow. *J Biomech Eng* 1990;112(4):464–472.

151. Sondergaard L, Thomsen C, Stahlberg F, et al. Mitral and aortic valvular flow: Quantification with MR phase mapping. *J Magn Reson Imaging* 1992;2(3):295–302.

152. Firmin DN, Nayler GL, Klipstein RH, et al. In vivo validation of MR velocity imaging. *J Comput Assist Tomogr* 1987;11:751–756.

153. Kondo C, Caputo GR, Semelka R, et al. Right and left ventricular stroke volume measurements with velocity-encoded cine MR imaging: In vitro and in vivo validation. *AJR Am J Roentgenol* 1991;157:9–16.

154. Rebergen SA, van der Wall EE, Doornbos J, et al. Magnetic resonance measurement of velocity and flow: Technique, validation, and cardiovascular applications. *Am Heart J* 1993;126:1439–1456.

155. Rebergen SA, Chin JG, Ottenkamp J, et al. Pulmonary regurgitation in the late postoperative follow-up of tetralogy of Fallot. Volumetric quantitation by nuclear magnetic resonance velocity mapping. *Circulation* 1993;88(pt 1):2257–2266.

156. Rebergen SA, Ottenkamp J, Doornbos J, et al. Postoperative pulmonary flow dynamics after Fontan surgery: Assessment with nuclear magnetic resonance velocity mapping. *J Am Coll Cardiol* 1993;21:123–131.

157. Hundley WG, Li HF, Hillis LD, et al. Quantitation of cardiac output with velocity-encoded, phase-difference magnetic resonance imaging. *Am J Cardiol* 1995;75:1250–1255.

158. Matsumura K, Nakase E, Haiyama T, et al. Determination of cardiac ejection fraction and left ventricular volume: Contrast-enhanced ultrafast cine MR imaging vs IV digital subtraction ventriculography. *AJR Am J Roentgenol* 1993;160:979–985.

159. Pelc LR, Pelc NJ, Rayhill SC, et al. Arterial and venous blood flow: Noninvasive quantitation with MR imaging. *Radiology* 1992;185:809–812.

160. Powell AJ, Tsai-Goodman B, Prakash A, et al. Comparison between phase-velocity cine magnetic resonance imaging and invasive oximetry for quantification of atrial shunts. *Am J Cardiol* 2003;91:1523–1525, A1529.

161. Hundley WG, Meshack BM, Willett DL, et al. Comparison of quantitation of left ventricular volume, ejection fraction, and cardiac output in patients with atrial fibrillation by cine magnetic resonance imaging versus invasive measurements. *Am J Cardiol* 1996;78:1119–1123.

162. Brenner LD, Caputo GR, Mostbeck G, et al. Quantification of left to right atrial shunts with velocity-encoded cine nuclear magnetic resonance imaging. *J Am Coll Cardiol* 1992;20:1246–1250.

163. Beerbaum P, Korperich H, Gieseke J, et al. Rapid left-to-right shunt quantification in children by phase-contrast magnetic resonance imaging combined with sensitivity encoding (SENSE). *Circulation* 2003;108:1355–1361.

164. Buonocore MH. Estimation of total coronary artery flow using measurements of flow in the ascending aorta. *Magn Reson Med* 1994;32:602–611.

165. Kolbitsch C, Lorenz IH, Hormann C, et al. The impact of increased mean airway pressure on contrast-enhanced MRI measurement of regional cerebral blood flow (rCBF), regional cerebral blood volume (rCBV), regional mean transit time (rMTT), and regional cerebrovascular resistance (rCVR) in human volunteers. *Hum Brain Mapp* 2000;11(3):214–222.

166. Sommer G, Noorbehesht B, Pelc N, et al. Normal renal blood flow measurement using phase-contrast cine magnetic resonance imaging. *Invest Radiol* 1992;27(6):465–470.

167. Geva T, Sahn DJ, Powell AJ. Magnetic resonance imaging of congenital heart disease in adults. *Prog Pediatr Cardiol* 2003;17:21–39.

168. Holmqvist C, Oskarsson G, Stahlberg F, et al. Functional evaluation of extracardiac ventriculopulmonary conduits and of the right ventricle with magnetic resonance imaging and velocity mapping. *Am J Cardiol* 1999;83:926–932.

169. Walker PG, Houlind K, Djurhuus C, et al. Motion correction for the quantification of mitral regurgitation using the control volume method. *Magn Reson Med* 2000;43:726–733.

170. Walker PG, Oyre S, Pedersen EM, et al. A new control volume method for calculating valvular regurgitation. *Circulation* 1995;92:579–586.

171. Globits S, Higgins CB. Assessment of valvular heart disease by magnetic resonance imaging. *Am Heart J* 1995;129:369–381.

172. Reid SA, Walker PG, Fisher J, et al. The quantification of pulmonary valve haemodynamics using MRI. *Int J Cardiovasc Imaging* 2002;18(3):217–225.

173. Dohmen PM, Hotz H, Lembcke A, et al. Magnetic resonance imaging of stentless xenografts for reconstruction of right ventricular outflow tract. *Semin Thorac Cardiovasc Surg* 2001;13(4 suppl 1):24–27.

174. Kuehne T, Saeed M, Reddy G, et al. Sequential magnetic resonance monitoring of pulmonary flow with endovascular stents placed across the pulmonary valve in growing Swine. *Circulation* 2001;104:2363–2368.

175. Helbing WA, de Roos A. Clinical applications of cardiac magnetic resonance imaging after repair of tetralogy of Fallot. *Pediatr Cardiol* 2000;21(1):70–79.

176. Nayak KS, Pauly JM, Kerr AB, et al. Real-time color flow MRI. *Magn Reson Med* 2000;43:251–258.

177. Arrive L, Najmark D, Albert F, et al. Cine MRI of mitral regurgitation in planes angled along the intrinsic cardiac axes. *J Comput Assist Tomogr* 1994;18:569–575.

178. Ohnishi S, Fukui S, Kusuoka H, et al. Assessment of valvular regurgitation using cine magnetic resonance imaging coupled with phase compensation technique: Comparison with Doppler color flow mapping. *Angiology* 1992;43:913–924.

179. Nishimura F. Oblique cine MRI for the evaluation of aortic regurgitation: Comparison with cineangiography. *Clin Cardiol* 1992;15(2):73–78.

180. Mitchell L, Jenkins JP, Watson Y, et al. Diagnosis and assessment of mitral and aortic valve disease by cine-flow magnetic resonance imaging. *Magn Reson Med* 1989;12:181–197.

181. Metcalfe MJ, Jones RA, Redpath TW, et al. Low-field cine magnetic resonance imaging in aortic valve disease. *Br J Radiol* 1989;62:1063–1066.

182. Fogel MA, Weinberg PM, Rychik J, et al. Caval contribution to flow in the branch pulmonary arteries of Fontan patients with a novel application of magnetic resonance presaturation pulse. *Circulation* 1999;99:1215–1221.

183. Fratz S, Hess J, Schwaiger M, et al. More accurate quantification of pulmonary blood flow by magnetic resonance imaging than by lung perfusion scintigraphy in patients with fontan circulation. *Circulation* 2002;106:1510–1513.

184. Henk CB, Schlechta B, Grampp S, et al. Pulmonary and aortic blood flow measurements in normal subjects and patients after single lung transplantation at 0.5 T using velocity encoded cine MRI. *Chest* 1998;114:771–779.

185. Rupprecht T, Nitz W, Wagner M, et al. Determination of the pressure gradient in children with coarctation of the aorta by low-field magnetic resonance imaging. *Pediatr Cardiol* 2002;23(2):127–131.

186. Ebbers T, Wigstrom L, Bolger AF, et al. Estimation of relative cardiovascular pressures using time-resolved three-dimensional phase contrast MRI. *Magn Reson Med* 2001;45:872–879.

187. van der Geest RJ, Reiber JH. Quantification in cardiac MRI. *J Magn Reson Imaging* 1999;10(5):602–608.

188. Pennell DJ, Firmin DN, Burger P, et al. Assessment of magnetic resonance velocity mapping of global ventricular function during dobutamine infusion in coronary artery disease. *Br Heart J* 1995;74(2):163–170.

189. Schwitter J, DeMarco T, Kneifel S, et al. Magnetic resonance-based assessment of global coronary flow and flow reserve and its relation to left ventricular functional parameters: A comparison with positron emission tomography. *Circulation* 2001;101:2696–2702.

190. Shibata M, Sakuma H, Isaka N, et al. Assessment of coronary flow reserve with fast cine phase contrast magnetic resonance imaging: Comparison with measurement by Doppler guide wire. *J Magn Reson Imaging* 1999;10(4):563–568.

191. Rodriguez-Gonzalez AO. Arterial flow determined with half Fourier echoplanar imaging. *Arch Med Res* 2000;31(5):470–485.

192. Thompson RB, McVeigh ER. Fast measurement of intracardiac pressure differences with 2D breath-hold phase-contrast MRI. *Magn Reson Med* 2003;49:1056–1066.

193. Sakuma H, Kawada N, Kubo H, et al. Effect of breath holding on blood flow measurement using fast velocity encoded cine MRI. *Magn Reson Med* 2001;45:346–348.

194. Hjortdal VE, Emmertsen K, Stenbog E, et al. Effects of exercise and respiration on blood flow in total cavopulmonary connection: A real-time magnetic resonance flow study. *Circulation* 2003;108:1227–1231.

195. Be'eri E, Maier SE, Landzberg MJ, et al. In vivo evaluation of Fontan pathway flow dynamics by multidimensional phase-velocity magnetic resonance imaging. *Circulation* 1998;98:2873–2882.

196. Kohler U, Marshall I, Robertson MB, et al. MRI measurement of wall shear stress vectors in bifurcation models and comparison with CFD predictions. *J Magn Reson Imaging* 2001;14(5):563–573.

197. Oyre S, Ringgaard S, Kozerke S, et al. Accurate noninvasive quantitation of blood flow, cross-sectional lumen vessel area and wall shear stress by three-dimensional paraboloid modeling of magnetic resonance imaging velocity data. *J Am Coll Cardiol* 1998;32:128–134.

198. Morgan VL, Roselli RJ, Lorenz CH. Normal three-dimensional pulmonary artery flow determined by phase contrast magnetic resonance imaging. *Ann Biomed Eng* 1998;26:557–566.

199. Prakash A, Powell AJ, Krishnamurthy R, et al. Magnetic resonance imaging evaluation of myocardial perfusion and viability in congenital and acquired pediatric heart disease. *Am J Cardiol* 2004;93:657–661.

200. Nagel E, Lehmkuhl HB, Bocksch W, et al. Noninvasive diagnosis of ischemia-induced wall motion abnormalities with the use of high-dose dobutamine stress MRI: Comparison with dobutamine stress echocardiography. *Circulation* 1999;99:763–770.

201. Nagel E, Klein C, Paetsch I, et al. Magnetic resonance perfusion measurements for the noninvasive detection of coronary artery disease. *Circulation* 2003;108:432–437.

202. Schwitter J, Nanz D, Kneifel S, et al. Assessment of myocardial perfusion in coronary artery disease by magnetic resonance: A comparison with positron emission tomography and coronary angiography. *Circulation* 2001;103:2230–2235.

203. Dendale P, Franken PR, Block P, et al. Contrast enhanced and functional magnetic resonance imaging for the detection of viable myocardium after infarction. *Am Heart J* 1998;135(pt 1):875–880.

204. Kim RJ, Fieno DS, Parrish TB, et al. Relationship of MRI delayed contrast enhancement to irreversible injury, infarct age, and contractile function. *Circulation* 1999;100:1992–2002.

205. Gerber BL, Garot J, Bluemke DA, et al. Accuracy of contrast-enhanced magnetic resonance imaging in predicting improvement of regional myocardial function in patients after acute myocardial infarction. *Circulation* 2002;106:1083–1089.

206. Perin EC, Silva GV, Sarmento-Leite R, et al. Assessing myocardial viability and infarct transmurality with left ventricular electromechanical mapping in patients with stable coronary artery disease: Validation by delayed-enhancement magnetic resonance imaging. *Circulation* 2002;106:957–961.

207. Motoyama S, Kondo T, Anno H, et al. Relationship between thrombolytic therapy and perfusion defect detected by Gd-DTPA-enhanced fast magnetic resonance imaging in acute myocardial infarction. *J Cardiovasc Magn Reson* 2001;3(3):237–245.

208. Sandstede JJ, Lipke C, Beer M, et al. Analysis of first-pass and delayed contrast-enhancement patterns of dysfunctional myocardium on MR imaging: Use in the prediction of myocardial viability. *AJR Am J Roentgenol* 2000;174:1737–1740.

209. Lauerma K, Niemi P, Hanninen H, et al. Multimodality MR imaging assessment of myocardial viability: Combination of first-pass and late contrast enhancement to wall motion dynamics and comparison with FDG PET-initial experience. *Radiology* 2000;217:729–736.

210. Kim RJ, Hillenbrand HB, Judd RM. Evaluation of myocardial viability by MRI. *Herz*. 2000;25(4):417–430.

211. Bax JJ, de Roos A, van Der Wall EE. Assessment of myocardial viability by MRI. *J Magn Reson Imaging* 1999;10(3):418–422.

212. Kim RJ, Chen EL, Lima JA, et al. Myocardial Gd-DTPA kinetics determine MRI contrast enhancement and reflect the extent and severity of myocardial injury after acute reperfused infarction. *Circulation* 1996;94:3318–3326.

213. Klein C, Nekolla SG, Bengel FM, et al. Assessment of myocardial viability with contrast-enhanced magnetic resonance imaging: Comparison with positron emission tomography. *Circulation* 2002;105:162–167.

214. Wagner A, Mahrholdt H, Holly TA, et al. Contrast-enhanced MRI and routine single photon emission computed tomography (SPECT) perfusion imaging for detection of subendocardial myocardial infarcts: An imaging study. *Lancet* 2003;361:374–379.

215. Kim RJ, Wu E, Rafael A, et al. The use of contrast-enhanced magnetic resonance imaging to identify reversible myocardial dysfunction. *N Engl J Med* 2000;343:1445–1453.

216. Choi KM, Kim RJ, Gubernikoff G, et al. Transmural extent of acute myocardial infarction predicts long-term improvement in contractile function. *Circulation* 2001;104:1101–1107.

217. Knuesel PR, Nanz D, Wyss C, et al. Characterization of dysfunctional myocardium by positron emission tomography and magnetic resonance: Relation to functional outcome after revascularization. *Circulation* 2003;108:1095–1100.

218. Beek AM, Kuhl HP, Bondarenko O, et al. Delayed contrast-enhanced magnetic resonance imaging for the prediction of regional functional improvement after acute myocardial infarction. *J Am Coll Cardiol* 2003;42:895–901.

219. Wilson JM, Villareal RP, Hariharan R, et al. Magnetic resonance imaging of myocardial fibrosis in hypertrophic cardiomyopathy. *Tex Heart Inst J* 2002;29(3):176–180.

220. Kim RJ, Judd RM. Gadolinium-enhanced magnetic resonance imaging in hypertrophic cardiomyopathy: In vivo imaging of the pathologic substrate for premature cardiac death? *J Am Coll Cardiol* 2003;41:1568–1572.

221. Bax JJ, Atsma DE, Lamb HJ, et al. Noninvasive and invasive evaluation of noncompaction cardiomyopathy. *J Cardiovasc Magn Reson* 2002;4(3):353–357.

222. Hamamichi Y, Ichida F, Hashimoto I, et al. Isolated noncompaction of the ventricular myocardium: Ultrafast computed tomography and magnetic resonance imaging. *Int J Cardiovasc Imaging* 2001;17(4):305–314.

223. Frances CD, Shlipak MG, Grady D. Left ventricular pseudoaneurysm: Diagnosis by cine magnetic resonance imaging. *Cardiology* 1999;92(3):217–219.

224. Kiaffas MG, Powell AJ, Geva T. Magnetic resonance imaging evaluation of cardiac tumor characteristics in infants and children. *Am J Cardiol* 2002;89:1229–1233.

225. Sakuma H, Bourne MW, O'Sullivan M, et al. Evaluation of thoracic aortic dissection using breath-holding cine MRI. *J Comput Assist Tomogr* 1996;20(1):45–50.

226. Moore NR, Parry AJ, Trottman-Dickenson B, et al. Fate of the native aorta after repair of acute type A dissection: A magnetic resonance imaging study. *Heart* 1996;75(1):62–66.

227. van der Wall EE, Kayser HW, Bootsma MM, et al. Arrhythmogenic right ventricular dysplasia: MRI findings. *Herz* 2000;25(4):356–364.

228. Midiri M, Finazzo M. MR imaging of arrhythmogenic right ventricular dysplasia. *Int J Cardiovasc Imaging* 2001;17(4):297–304.

229. Breen JF. Imaging of the pericardium. *J Thorac Imaging* 2001;16(1):47–54.

230. White CS. MR evaluation of the pericardium. *Top Magn Reson Imaging* 1995;7(4):258–266.

231. Mollet NR, Dymarkowski S, Volders W, et al. Visualization of ventricular thrombi with contrast-enhanced magnetic resonance imaging in patients with ischemic heart disease. *Circulation* 2002;106:2873–2876.

232. Baur LH, Vliegen HW, van der Wall EE, et al. Imaging of an aneurysm of the sinus of Valsalva with transesophageal echocardiography, contrast angiography and MRI. *Int J Card Imaging* 2000;16(1):35–41.

233. Taylor AM, Stables RH, Poole-Wilson PA, et al. Definitive clinical assessment of atrial septal defect by magnetic resonance imaging. *J Cardiovasc Magn Reson* 1999;1(1):43–47.

234. Holmvang G. A magnetic resonance imaging method for evaluating atrial septal defects. *J Cardiovasc Magn Reson* 1999;1(1):59–64.

235. Dinsmore RE, Wismer GL, Guyer D, et al. Magnetic resonance imaging of the interatrial septum and atrial septal defects. *AJR Am J Roentgenol* 1985;145:697–703.

236. Holmvang G, Palacios IF, Vlahakes GJ, et al. Imaging and sizing of atrial septal defects by magnetic resonance. *Circulation* 1995;92:3473–3480.

237. Powell AJ, Tsai-Goodman B, Prakash A, et al. Comparison between phase-velocity cine magnetic resonance imaging and invasive oximetry for quantification of atrial shunts. *Am J Cardiol* 2003;91:1523–1525.

238. Sieverding L, Jung WI, Klose U, et al. Noninvasive blood flow measurement and quantification of shunt volume by cine magnetic resonance in congenital heart disease. Preliminary results. *Pediatr Radiol* 1992;22(1):48–54.

239. Rebergen SA, van der Wall EE, Helbing WA, et al. Quantification of pulmonary and systemic blood flow by magnetic resonance velocity mapping in the assessment of atrial-level shunts. *Int J Card Imaging* 1996;12(3):143–152.

240. Powell AJ, Chung T, Landzberg MJ, et al. Accuracy of MRI evaluation of pulmonary blood supply in patients with complex pulmonary stenosis or atresia. *Int J Card Imaging* 2000;16(3):169–174.

241. Mackie AS, Gauvreau K, Perry SB, et al. Echocardiographic predictors of aortopulmonary collaterals in infants with tetralogy of fallot and pulmonary atresia. *J Am Coll Cardiol* 2003;41:852–857.

242. Geva T, Greil GF, Marshall AC, et al. Gadolinium-enhanced 3-dimensional magnetic resonance angiography of pulmonary blood supply in patients with complex pulmonary stenosis or atresia: Comparison with x-ray angiography. *Circulation* 2002;106:473–478.

243. Amparo EG, Higgins CB, Shafton EP. Demonstration of coarctation of the aorta by magnetic resonance imaging. *AJR Am J Roentgenol* 1984;143:1192–1194.

244. Therrien J, Thorne SA, Wright A, et al. Repaired coarctation: A "cost-effective" approach to identify complications in adults. *J Am Coll Cardiol* 2000;35:997–1002.

245. Simpson IA, Chung KJ, Glass RF, et al. Cine magnetic resonance imaging for evaluation of anatomy and flow relations in infants and children with coarctation of the aorta. *Circulation* 1988;78:142–148.

246. Mendelsohn AM, Banerjee A, Donnelly LF, et al. Is echocardiography or magnetic resonance imaging superior for precoarctation angioplasty evaluation? *Cathet Cardiovasc Diagn* 1997;42(1):26–30.

247. Araoz PA, Reddy GP, Tarnoff H, et al. MR findings of collateral circulation are more accurate measures of hemodynamic significance than arm-leg blood pressure gradient after repair of coarctation of the aorta. *J Magn Reson Imaging* 2003;17(2):177–183.

248. Mohiaddin RH, Kilner PJ, Rees S, et al. Magnetic resonance volume flow and jet velocity mapping in aortic coarctation. *J Am Coll Cardiol* 1993;22:1515–1521.

249. Riquelme C, Laissy JP, Menegazzo D, et al. MR imaging of coarctation of the aorta and its postoperative complications in adults: Assessment with spin-echo and cine-MR imaging. *Magn Reson Imaging* 1999;17:37–46.

250. Steffens JC, Bourne MW, Sakuma H, et al. Quantification of collateral blood flow in coarctation of the aorta by velocity encoded cine magnetic resonance imaging. *Circulation* 1994;90:937–943.

251. Nielsen J, Powell AJ, Gauvreau K, et al. Magnetic resonance imaging predictors of the hemodynamic severity of aortic coarctation. *J Am Coll Cardiol* 2004;43:24A.

252. Ten Harkel AD, Blom NA, Ottenkamp J. Isolated unilateral absence of a pulmonary artery: A case report and review of the literature. *Chest* 2002;122:1471–1477.

253. Need LR, Powell AJ, del Nido P, et al. Coronary echocardiography in tetralogy of fallot: Diagnostic accuracy, resource utilization and surgical implications over 13 years. *J Am Coll Cardiol* 2000;36:1371–1377.

254. Vick GW 3rd, Wendt RE 3rd, Rokey R. Comparison of gradient echo with spin echo magnetic resonance imaging and echocardiography in the evaluation of major aortopulmonary collateral arteries. *Am Heart J* 1994;127:1341–1347.

255. Holmqvist C, Hochbergs P, Bjorkhem G, et al. Pre-operative evaluation with MR in tetralogy of fallot and pulmonary atresia with ventricular septal defect. *Acta Radiol* 2001;42(1):63–69.

256. Beekman RP, Beek FJ, Meijboom EJ. Usefulness of MRI for the pre-operative evaluation of the pulmonary arteries in Tetralogy of Fallot. *Magn Reson Imaging* 1997;15:1005–1015.

257. Roest AA, Helbing WA, Kunz P, et al. Exercise MR imaging in the assessment of pulmonary regurgitation and biventricular function in patients after tetralogy of fallot repair. *Radiology* 2002;223(1):204–211.

258. Niezen RA, Helbing WA, van Der Wall EE, et al. Left ventricular function in adults with mild pulmonary insufficiency late after Fallot repair. *Heart* 1999;82:697–703.

259. Niezen RA, Helbing WA, van der Wall EE, et al. Biventricular systolic function and mass studied with MR imaging in children with pulmonary regurgitation after repair for tetralogy of Fallot. *Radiology* 1996;201(1):135–140.

260. Davlouros PA, Kilner PJ, Hornung TS, et al. Right ventricular function in adults with repaired tetralogy of Fallot assessed with cardiovascular magnetic resonance imaging: Detrimental role of right ventricular outflow aneurysms or akinesia and adverse right-to-left ventricular interaction. *J Am Coll Cardiol* 2002;40:2044–2052.

261. Geva T, Sandweiss BM, Gauvreau K, et al. Factors associated with impaired clinical status in long-term survivors of tetralogy of Fallot repair evaluated by magnetic resonance imaging. *J Am Coll Cardiol* 2004;43:1068–1074.

262. Blume ED, Altmann K, Mayer JE, et al. Evolution of risk factors influencing early mortality of the arterial switch operation. *J Am Coll Cardiol* 1999;33:1702–1709.

263. Chung KJ, Simpson IA, Glass RF, et al. Cine magnetic resonance imaging after surgical repair in patients with transposition of the great arteries. *Circulation* 1988;77(1):104–109.

264. Lorenz CH, Walker ES, Graham TP Jr, et al. Right ventricular performance and mass by use of cine MRI late after atrial repair of transposition of the great arteries. *Circulation* 1995;92(suppl):II233–239.

265. Hardy CE, Helton GJ, Kondo C, et al. Usefulness of magnetic resonance imaging for evaluating great-vessel anatomy after arterial switch operation for D-transposition of the great arteries. *Am Heart J* 1994;128(2):326–332.

266. Beek FJ, Beekman RP, Dillon EH, et al. MRI of the pulmonary artery after arterial switch operation for transposition of the great arteries. *Pediatr Radiol* 1993;23(5):335–340.

267. Theissen P, Kaemmerer H, Sechtem U, et al. Magnetic resonance imaging of cardiac function and morphology in patients with transposition of the great arteries following Mustard procedure. *Thorac Cardiovasc Surg* 1991;(39 suppl 3):221–224.

268. Rees S, Somerville J, Warnes C, et al. Comparison of magnetic resonance imaging with echocardiography and radionuclide angiography in assessing cardiac function and anatomy following Mustard's operation for transposition of the great arteries. *Am J Cardiol* 1988;61:1316–1322.

269. Roest AA, Lamb HJ, van der Wall EE, et al. Cardiovascular response to physical exercise in adult patients after atrial correction for transposition of the great arteries assessed with magnetic resonance imaging. *Heart* 2004;90(6):678–684.

270. Taylor AM, Dymarkowski S, Hamaekers P, et al. MR coronary angiography and late-enhancement myocardial MR in children who underwent arterial switch surgery for transposition of great arteries. *Radiology* 2005;234(2):542–547.

271. Babu-Narayan SV, Goktekin O, Moon JC, et al. Late gadolinium enhancement cardiovascular magnetic resonance of the systemic right ventricle in adults with previous atrial redirection surgery for transposition of the great arteries. *Circulation* 2005;111:2091–2098.

272. Muthurangu V, Taylor AM, Hegde SR, et al. Cardiac magnetic resonance imaging after stage I Norwood operation for hypoplastic left heart syndrome. *Circulation* 2005;112:3256–3263.

273. Brown DW, Gauvreau K, Moran AM, et al. Clinical outcomes and utility of cardiac catheterization prior to superior cavopulmonary anastomosis. *J Thorac Cardiovasc Surg* 2003;126(1):272–281.

274. McMahon CJ, Eidem BW, Bezold LI, et al. Is cardiac catheterization a prerequisite in all patients undergoing bidirectional cavopulmonary anastomosis? *J Am Soc Echocardiogr* 2003;16:1068–1072.

275. Tworetzky W, del Nido PJ, Powell AJ, et al. Usefulness of magnetic resonance imaging of left ventricular endocardial fibroelastosis in infants after fetal intervention for aortic valve stenosis. *Am J Cardiol* 2005;96:1568–1570.

276. Nielsen JC, Powell AJ, Gauvreau K, et al. Magnetic resonance imaging predictors of coarctation severity. *Circulation* 2005;111:622–628.

277. Luechinger R, Zeijlemaker VA, Pedersen EM, et al. In vivo heating of pacemaker leads during magnetic resonance imaging. *Eur Heart J* 2005;26(4):376–383; discussion 325–377.

CHAPTER 8 ■ CARDIAC COMPUTED TOMOGRAPHY IN CHILDREN WITH CONGENITAL HEART DISEASE

FREDERICK R. LONG, MD, JOHN J. WHELLER, MD, AND JOACHIM G. EICHHORN, MD

Cardiac computed tomography (CT) has several advantages over other imaging modalities that account for its increasing popularity in imaging children with congenital heart disease (CHD). In comparison with CT, cardiac catheterization and digital angiography (DA), long considered the gold standards for morphology and function, are two-dimensional (2-D) modalities with a restricted field of view that is more invasive, requires longer sedation times, and exposes the patient to higher doses of ionizing radiation (1). Echocardiography with Doppler, the first-line imaging modality owing to its noninvasive nature and accessibility, is also limited by field of view, which affects especially visualization of extracardiac structures. Last, cardiac MRI, although not limited by field of view and not requiring ionizing radiation exposure, requires longer sedation and examination times, is less accessible, has poorer spatial resolution, and is unable to visualize well such hardware as vascular stents owing to its susceptibility to artifact from metallic-induced inhomogeneities in the magnetic field (2).

The first articles describing the use of CT in congenital heart disease were mainly descriptive. They were performed using electron beam or single-slice CT technology (3–5). Single-slice CT technology lacks sufficient spatial and temporal resolution to rival MRI and conventional angiography. In recent years, the rapid development and adoption of multidetector spiral computed tomography (MDCT) has resulted in a renaissance for cardiac CT applications (6–11), which include evaluation of the pulmonary arteries, great vessels, coronary arteries, and intracardiac structures (Fig. 8.1). The number of detector rows that can be simultaneously used, resulting in greater speed and resolution in MDCT scanners, has rapidly evolved from 4 in 1998 to 8 (2001), 16 (2002), and 64 (2004). The latest 64-detector MDCT scanners are able to acquire volumetric images with true isotropic resolution of 0.35 mm across 40 mm of anatomy during a <0.4-second gantry rotation (12). This remarkable engineering achievement has been made possible by the exponential growth in computing power, capable of processing data arising from 64 helical datasets consisting of 888 detector elements that are spinning at <0.4 seconds per rotation. The increased speed and resolution is reflected by the fact that a 64-MDCT scanner can image a 2-year-old's chest in 1 second compared with 6 seconds using a similar pitch on an 8-MDCT scanner with double the resolution. Because of their superior temporal and spatial resolution (13), 64-MDCT scanners are marketed and sold for imaging coronary arteries noninvasively, but they are also ideal for depicting the small cardiac and vascular structures in neonates and infants (Fig. 8.2).

METHODS AND TECHNIQUE

Contrast Enhancement

CT requires intravenous contrast enhancement to image the heart and great vessels. Although MRI can image flowing blood without intravenous contrast, most cardiac MRI examinations also use intravenous contrast to improve depiction of the heart and great vessels, particularly for complex anatomy and in small children. Because of their speed, MDCT scanners offer the opportunity to achieve a greater level and uniformity of contrast enhancement by capturing the narrow temporal window of the peak of a rapid bolus of contrast. This opportunity exists for both adults and children, although it is more difficult in children, who have smaller and more tenuous intravenous access, limiting the speed at which intravenous contrast can be safely injected. In infants, venous access may consist of only a hand, foot, or scalp vein. Thus, for practical reasons, contrast enhancement is usually achieved in infants by manual injection at a rate of approximately 1 to 2 mL per second.

The optimal timing for initiation of scanning to capture the peak of contrast enhancement is more challenging in children owing to the smaller amount of contrast injected, which is determined on a per weight basis (2 mL/kg). There is a shorter window of time that both the right and left sides of the heart, the pulmonary arteries, and veins are well opacified before the contrast bolus dilutes. When manually injecting a small dose of contrast, the delay from the start of injection to start of scanning is approximated by a circulation time of approximately 12 to 15 seconds (14). In general, this translates to being able to start the scan right after the manual injection of contrast and saline flush. The use of automated contrast bolus tracking software would be ideal, and is helpful in adults, but in general is not robust enough to be practical to use in infants and young children in whom one is attempting to visualize a small intravenous bolus of contrast in the setting of a fast circulation time.

Sedation and Controlling Respirations

Motion of any kind creates artifacts and blurring that degrade images. In infants and young children, the inability to hold still and to breath-hold may significantly degrade image quality for both MRI and CT imaging. Image degradation can be severe in children if they move, are crying, or just suddenly take in a big breath, such as during contrast injection. Faster scan speeds

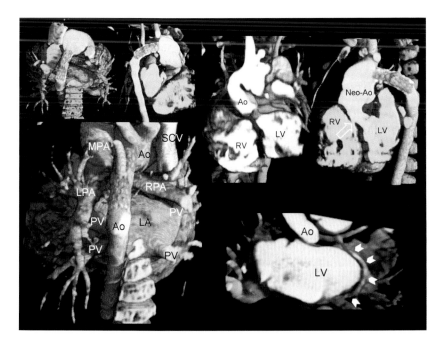

FIGURE 8.1 Eight-month-old boy with type B interrupted aortic arch after Damus-Kaye-Stansel anastomosis, aortic arch repair, pulmonary homograft, and aortic stent placement (two "overlapping" stents in *blue*). Three-dimensional volume-rendered images shown were acquired during controlled ventilation with deep conscious sedation on an eight-slice multidetector computed tomography (MDCT) following 25 mL contrast by hand injection. The 6-second scan demonstrates in a single shot the following relevant information (in order from **top** to **bottom**, **left** to **right**): correct position of the stent, mild left subclavian artery stenosis, left ventricle (LV) outflow tract to the native aorta, LV outflow tract to the neoaorta (Neo-Ao) (appreciate the small ventricular septal defect marked by the *arrow*) and coronary arteries (*small arrows*). Ao, aorta; LA, left atrium; LPA, left pulmonary artery; MPA, main pulmonary artery; PV, pulmonary vein; RPA, right pulmonary artery; RV, right ventricle; SVC, superior vena cava.

cannot compensate for such gross movements. The motion occurring during quiet resting breathing is amenable to improvement with faster scanning. This is of greater importance for younger children, who have faster resting respiratory and heart rates and who have smaller anatomic structures that blur more easily. For imaging the extracardiac vasculature,

there may be no need for sedation to control respirations, even in a small child, when using fast scan speeds. In this way, MDCT scanners can decrease the need for sedation, which represents a major advantage over MRI (Figs. 8.3 and 8.4).

On the other hand, it is unpredictable whether a child who is too young to cooperate with breath-holding will manage to

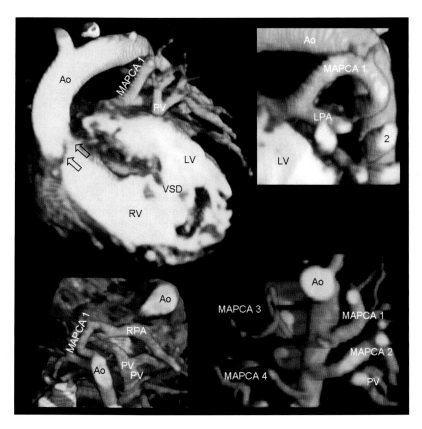

FIGURE 8.2 Newborn with heterotaxia transposition, pulmonary atresia, and total anomalous pulmonary venous drainage to the portal vein. Three-dimensional volume-rendered images obtained on a 64-slice multidetector computed tomography (MDCT) scanner (GE Volume CT) following hand injection of 6 mL of contrast in the umbilical venous catheter. Images (**right** to **left** and **top** to **bottom**) show the aortic valve (*arrows*) and ventricular septal defect (VSD) as well as multiple aortopulmonary collaterals (MAPCAs) arising from the aorta (Ao) to supply the lung and the left and right pulmonary arteries (LPA and RPA). LV, left ventricle; RV, right ventricle.

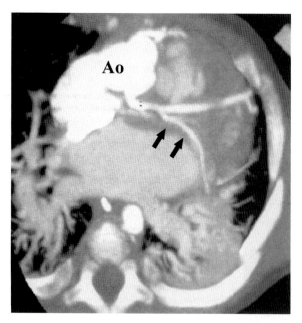

FIGURE 8.3 Axial image of aortic root in a 3-month-old boy with heart rate of 111 acquired in 3 seconds using ECG gating without sedation on a 64-slice multidetector computed tomography (MDCT) scanner (GE Volume CT). Ao, aorta. (Images courtesy of Dr Hauschield, San Diego Children's Hospital.)

hold still and quietly breathe during an examination. For practical reasons, sedation may be an attractive option to ensure completion of an exam. If sedation is used, there is also the opportunity to use respiratory control and to inflate the lungs during imaging, both of which further enhance image quality. Although such enhancements in image quality may not always be necessary, especially with higher resolution and

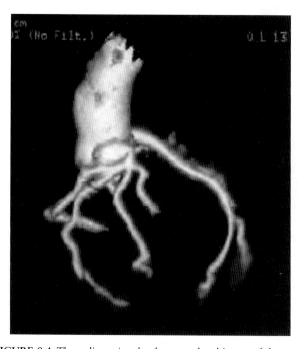

FIGURE 8.4 Three-dimensional volume-rendered image of the coronaries in same patient as in Figure 8.3.

faster MDCT scanners, it can be advantageous in the smallest children.

In many children's hospitals, sedation can be accomplished in several ways: by dedicated sedation nurses, intensivists, or anesthesiologists. In Children's Hospital Radiology Departments, sedation is achieved commonly with either oral chloral hydrate or intravenous pentobarbital administered by dedicated sedation nurses under the supervision of a radiologist (15,16). A disadvantage of chloral hydrate and pentobarbital is that the duration of sedation is much longer than needed for a CT exam but may not be long enough to accomplish all that would be desired in a cardiac MR exam (17). Sedation done by an anesthesiologist is attractive in children with complex congenital heart disease because they are at a higher risk for an untoward event during sedation. Anesthesia assistance has several other advantages. One is improved and more tolerable acquisition of IV access, which is often difficult in children with CHD. Most children come from home without an IV in place for their CT scan. With anesthesia assistance, the IV can be placed after inhalation induction, typically with a short-acting agent such as sevuflurane (18), which has the benefit of having a vasodilatory effect. Another benefit to anesthesia assistance for CT imaging is the ability to use short-acting agents (sevoflurane, propofol, and remifentanil), which are better suited for the short duration of a CT scan (18,19).

When using deep conscious sedation, respiratory motion-free images can be achieved for CT imaging using a method called controlled ventilation (20), which does not require endotracheal tube intubation and which has a good safety profile (21,22). In general, if a child can be sedated, controlled ventilation can be performed. The technique does require dedicated personnel, who are respiratory therapists at our institution (22). The controlled ventilation method involves positive-pressure face mask hyperventilation to induce a transient respiratory pause. Using this method, a short series of augmented breaths at 25-cm water pressure timed to spontaneous respirations creates sufficient hypocarbia to induce transient apnea. During the respiratory pause, the lungs can be inflated with steady positive pressure for inspiratory imaging, typically at 25-cm water pressure, which corresponds to a breath-hold near total lung capacity; or the lungs can be allowed to rest at end-exhalation near functional residual capacity for expiratory imaging. The duration of the pauses is sufficient for imaging: approximately 10 to 25 seconds at full inflation and 5 to 10 seconds at expiration (21).

Radiation Exposure

One of the chief limitations of CT when compared with MR is exposure to ionizing radiation. In infants and children, this is of particular concern because of their greater sensitivity to radiation (23). The optimal radiation dose settings for performing cardiac CT in infants and pediatric patients are still being worked out. Preliminary work indicates that diagnostically adequate cardiac CT scans can be obtained at much lower radiation doses than commonly quoted in the literature (14). The radiation dose received is proportional to the square root of the kilovolt potential (kVp) and is directly related to tube current or milliamps (mA) times the duration of exposure (seconds). Routine settings for an adult body CT scan would be 120 kVp and 200 mA (24). Because of the reduced x-ray attenuation secondary to lower body mass in children, the exposure settings can be reduced without loss in image quality (Fig. 8.5). When intravenous contrast is used, a lower kVp is advantageous in that it accentuates the beam absorption properties of the high atomic weight of iodine (14,24).

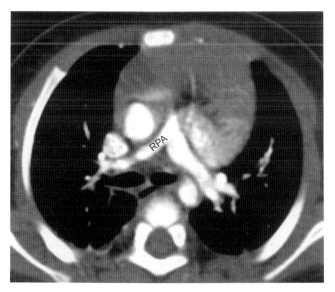

FIGURE 8.5 Six-month-old boy with history of pulmonary atresia and small right pulmonary artery (RPA). A 1.25-mm axial image obtained during controlled ventilation with deep conscious sedation on an eight-slice MDCT following 15 mL contrast by hand injection at 120 kVp and 40 mAs (effective dose estimate of 150 mrem).

Recently described cardiac CT protocols for small children use a kVp of either 80 or 100 with mA values between 25 and 65 (Figs. 8.6 and 8.7). Such protocols result in considerable reduction in radiation dose. The average effective dose was estimated to be 1.8 mSv for cardiac CT studies in a group of 41 children (ages 3 months to 12 years; median 3.5 years) with transcatheter-placed stents (25). In this study, an eight-slice MDCT scanner was used with 1.25 mm collimation, a

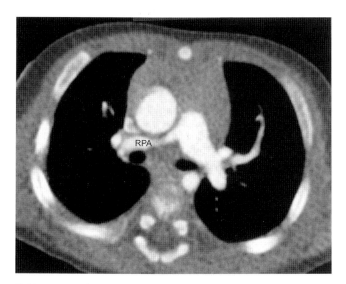

FIGURE 8.6 Three-month-old boy with hypoplastic right heart syndrome and small right pulmonary artery (RPA). A 1.25-mm axial image obtained during controlled ventilation with deep conscious sedation on an eight-slice multidetector computed tomography (MDCT) following 10 mL contrast by hand injection at 80 kVp and 20 mAs (effective dose estimate 28 mrem). The radiation dose was decreased 80% compared with example shown in Figure 8.5 without loss of diagnostic quality.

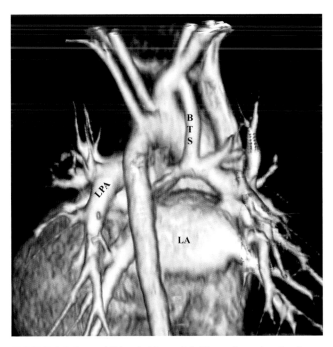

FIGURE 8.7 Same child as in Figure 8.5. Three-dimensional volume-rendered coronal image (posterior view) obtained at 80 kVp and 20 mAs. Note Blalock-Thomas-Taussig shunt (BTS), left pulmonary artery (LPA), and pulmonary veins entering the left atrium (LA).

median kVp of 120, median mAs of 40, and 13.5-mm table speed per rotation. The effective dose of 1.8 mSv corresponds favorably to the mean natural background radiation of 3 mSv in the United States for a year and reported effective dose for diagnostic catheterization of 4.6 mSv in a similar patient group (1). There has been some concern as to whether lowering the kVp may result in beam hardening artifacts in the upper chest around the shoulders (24). This has not been our experience, particularly if the arms are raised above the head for the scan.

Electrocardiograph Gating

With the fast temporal resolution of MDCT, electrocardiographic (ECG) gating is possible. ECG gating is necessary for a comprehensive evaluation of the coronary arteries and allows CT to perform functional analyses typically in the domain of MRI, including ventricular wall motion, ventricular ejection fraction, and motion of the cardiac valves. With a 64-MDCT system, this can be accomplished within approximately five heart beats. There are limitations in successfully gating if the heart rate is too fast, which depends on the particular scanner used, with an upper limit of approximately 110 beats per minute on a 64-slice scanner. Few studies have compared MRI and CT in functional assessment. One such study found no difference between MRI with CT in assessing RV function in adults with tetralogy of Fallot (26). However, there is a significant increase in radiation exposure if ECG gating is performed, estimated at 11 mSv for coronary artery imaging in adults (9). When using ECG gating for noncoronary cardiac imaging, lower doses could be used, making it feasible for pediatric patients. The required dose, optimal protocol, and benefits of using ECG gating for noncoronary pediatric cardiac imaging are under investigation.

INDICATIONS

Echocardiography with Doppler is the primary imaging modality for the initial evaluation and follow-up of CHD. In many instances, such as the assessment of acyanotic CHD, including solitary septal defects and pulmonic stenosis, no additional imaging is necessary. In cases of complex congenital lesions where surgical intervention is required or where the best course of management is unclear, digital angiography (DA) is performed to assess the function of the ventricles and valves and to characterize the nature of the hemodynamic problems leading to heart failure or cyanosis. DA also delineates clearly aortopulmonary collateral arteries. As already mentioned, however, ultrasound (US) and DA are limited in their field of view and are susceptible to difficulties in resolving overlapping arterial and venous flow. Because they are inherently 2-D modalities, they also have less ability to demonstrate the dimensions and spatial relationships of cardiac structures and their extracardiac connections, which may be important in planning therapy.

MDCT excels in 3-D modeling by acquiring an isotropic volumetric dataset whereby the anatomy can be displayed with the same resolution in any conceivable imaging plane. In optimally depicting the relevant anatomy, which is oriented obliquely and perpendicular to the axial imaging plane, multiplanar 2-D and 3-D reconstructions can be considered almost a necessity. MRI cannot acquire an isotropic volumetric dataset, in part owing to set limitations in how fast gradients can be switched on and off without causing serious side effects.

The enhanced diagnostic information available from 3-D MDCT can in some cases replace the need for diagnostic catheterization before surgery: for example, in patients considered for Glenn shunt procedures. MDCT could be used as a supplement to US in problematic cases, precluding diagnostic

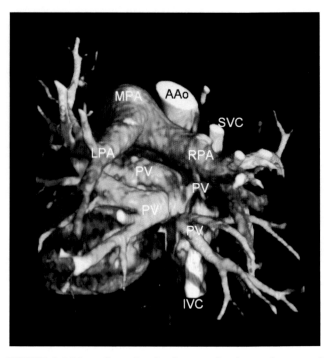

FIGURE 8-9 Three-dimensional volume-rendered posterior coronal image of the same child as in Figure 8.8. MPA, main pulmonary artery; RPA, right pulmonary artery; LPA, left pulmonary artery; PV, pulmonary vein; LA, left atrium; AAo, ascending aorta; SVC, superior vena cava; IVC, inferior vena cava.

catheterization when no catheter intervention is considered. In one recent study of 75 children (mean age of 9 months) MDCT replaced DA in 31 (41%) for surgical planning or to exclude a vascular anomaly. In an additional 29 patients, radiation dose and sedation time in the interventional lab could be reduced (27).

One of the major indications for performing 3-D MDCT is a comprehensive evaluation of the pulmonary arteries and veins (Figs. 8.8 and 8.9). US is limited in the assessment of the pulmonary arteries. The creation and maintenance of good pulmonary blood flow is a central theme in the management of CHD and is the goal of several common surgical procedures used to treat CHD: modified Blalock-Thomas-Taussig shunt, Glenn shunt, and Fontan procedure. Problems with the pulmonary arteries often occur postoperatively, such as with the arterial switch procedure, or are prevalent in certain conditions, such as tetralogy of Fallot.

Transcatheter balloon dilation with stent placement has become a common nonoperative way to treat pulmonary artery stenoses (28,29). Three-dimensional MDCT is helpful in planning optimal stent placement by showing the orientation and extent of stenoses (Figs. 8.10 and 8.11). MDCT is surprisingly free of artifacts from the metallic component of stents (Fig. 8.12) such that the lumen of the stent can be assessed for intimal hyperplasia causing in-stent stenosis, a common complication of stent therapy (29). The ability to diagnose in-stent stenosis by MDCT was evaluated in a study of children with pulmonary artery and aortic stents who also underwent DA (25). MDCT correlated well with DA ($r = 0.89$) for all grades of stenosis. Using a threshold of approximately $\geq 20\%$ stenosis, the sensitivity and specificity of MDCT exceeded 95% (25). Restenosis following catheter therapy can also be caused by stent fracture or segmental defor-

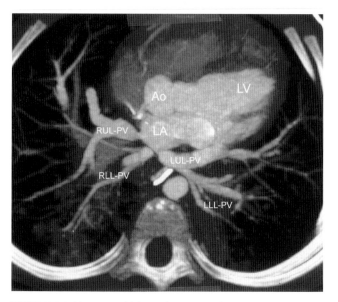

FIGURE 8.8 Two-year-old boy who presented with right-sided heart failure. A 1.25-mm axial image obtained during controlled ventilation with deep conscious sedation on an eight-slice multidetector computed tomography (MDCT) scanner at 100 kVp and 40 mAs shows stenoses of the pulmonary veins at their insertions into left atrium. Ao, aorta; LA, left atrium; LLL-PV and RLL-PV, left and right lower lung–pulmonary vein; LUL-PV and RUL-PV, left and right upper lung–PV; LV, left ventricle.

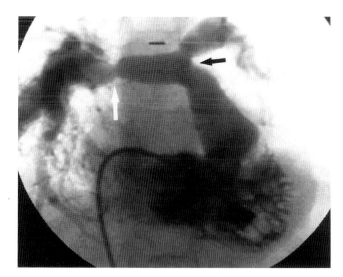

FIGURE 8.10 Two-year-old boy with history of tetralogy of Fallot status after complete repair. Digital angiography spot film following injection of the right ventricle shows bilateral pulmonary artery stenoses (*white arrow*, right pulmonary artery; *black arrow*, left pulmonary artery).

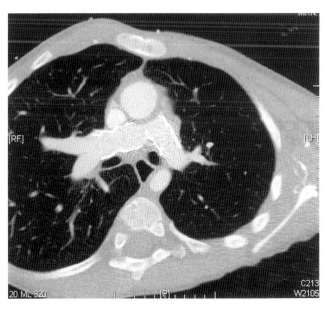

FIGURE 8.12 Same child as in Figure 8.10. A 1.25-mm axial image obtained during controlled ventilation with deep conscious sedation on an eight-slice multidetector computed tomography (MDCT) scanner following angioplasty and placement of bilateral pulmonary artery stents. Note lack of major stent artifacts.

mity, which may be difficult to appreciate at DA (Fig. 8.13). CT has a clear advantage over MRI in stent evaluation as the metallic struts cause significant signal dephasing and signal loss owing to inhomogeneities induced in the magnetic field (2). The use of MDCT as a supplement for US in screening children with pulmonary or aortic stents should decrease

rather than increase overall radiation exposure by resulting in a net decrease in the number and/or length of diagnostic cardiac catheterizations.

It is well known that in children with CHD, enlargement of cardiac chambers and pulmonary arteries and veins, as well as abnormal vascular connections, may compress the trachea (Fig. 8.14) or bronchi resulting in atelectasis or air trapping that may complicate the overall management of CHD (30). CHD is also associated with tracheomalacia and bronchomalacia (31). MDCT is excellent at depicting the airways and a combination of inspiratory and expiratory images can be used to diagnose airway malacia and air trapping. The ability of MDCT not only to assess the heart but also to make a rapid global assessment of the entire body, in particular the lungs, is an important and unique advantage of CT in very ill patients, very small patients, or in complex clinical cases.

FUTURE DIRECTIONS

The rapid evolution of MDCT technology, with its ability to generate routinely submillimeter volumetric cardiac CT datasets, should yield new insights into the management of children with CHD. Increases in computing power coupled with the availability of high-quality 3-D CT datasets will allow us to develop new indices and refine with greater accuracy standard measures to assess and follow CHD. More quantitative approaches to diagnosis and management should result. For example, computer-assisted calculation of differential lung and blood volumes could easily be performed today. To take advantage of this new quantitative power, thought must be given to establishing normative data and acquiring examinations in a reproducible, standardized manner.

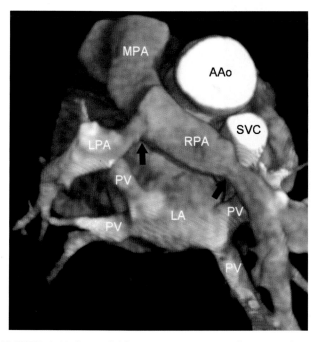

FIGURE 8.11 Same child as in Figure 8.10. The 3-D volume-rendered image of heart (posterior view) obtained during controlled ventilation with deep conscious sedation on an eight-slice multidetector computed tomography (MDCT) depicts the nature and extent of bilateral pulmonary artery stenoses (*arrows*) more clearly. MPA, main pulmonary artery; RPA, right pulmonary artery; LPA, left pulmonary artery; PV, pulmonary vein; LA, left atrium; AAo, ascending aorta; SVC, superior vena cava.

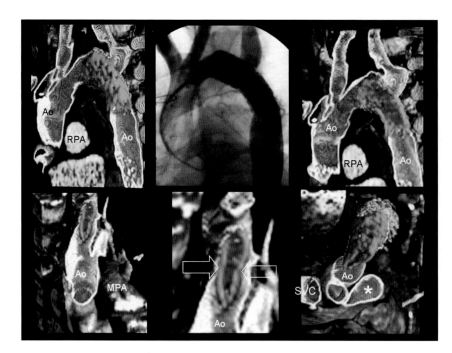

FIGURE 8.13 Seven-year old girl with history of aortic coarctation postangioplasty and aortic stent placement (*green*). Multiple volume-rendered images from an eight-slice multidetector computed tomography (MDCT) obtained during a voluntary breath-hold of the aortic arch show inward collapse of lumen of stent (*arrows*) on coronal projection not seen on sagittal views or on digital angiogram (**top middle**). MPA, main pulmonary artery; RPA, right pulmonary artery; Ao, aorta.

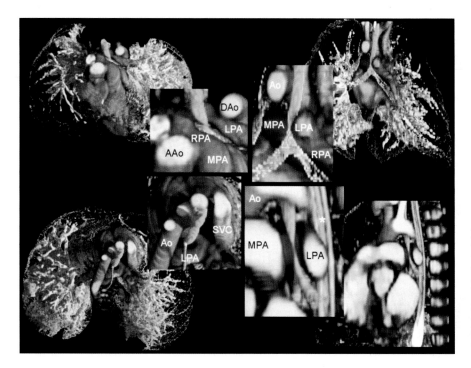

FIGURE 8.14 A 3½-month-old baby boy with pulmonary artery sling. Multiple volume-rendered images show compression of trachea (*green*) by the anomalous course of the left pulmonary artery (LPA). Note virtual bronchograms of lungs (*turquoise*) highlighting the capability of CT to simultaneously assess both heart and lungs. MPA, main pulmonary artery; RPA, right pulmonary artery; LPA, left pulmonary artery; Ao, aorta; DAo descending aorta.

CONCLUSION

This chapter describes the expanding role of cardiac CT in the management of children with CHD, which is directly related to the rapid evolution of MDCT scanners. A 3-D submillimeter evaluation of the heart and great vessels can be achieved routinely in a matter of seconds with little respiratory motion, potentially without sedation, and with much less radiation exposure than previously thought. This technologic advance should have the greatest impact in the smallest, youngest, and most critically ill children with congenital heart disease.

References

1. Bacher K, Bogaert E, Lapere R, et al. Patient-specific dose and radiation risk estimation in pediatric cardiac catheterization. *Circulation* 2005;111:83–89.
2. Maintz D, Tombach B, Juergens KU, et al. Revealing in-stent stenoses of the iliac arteries: Comparison of multidetector CT with MR angiography and digital radiographic angiography in a Phantom model. *AJR Am J Roentgenol* 2002;179:1319–1322.
3. Westra SJ, Hill JA, Alejos JC, et al. Three-dimensional helical CT of pulmonary arteries in infants and children with congenital heart disease. *AJR Am J Roentgenol* 1999;173:109–115.
4. Lee JJ, Kang D. Feasibility of electron beam tomography in diagnosis of congenital heart disease: comparison with echocardiography. *Eur J Radiol* 2001;38:185–190.
5. Kawano T, Ishii M, Takagi J, et al. Three-dimensional helical computed tomographic angiography in neonates and infants with complex congenital heart disease. *Am Heart J* 2000;139:654–660.
6. Chandran A, Fricker FJ, Schowengerdt KO, et al. An institutional review of the value of computed tomographic angiography in the diagnosis of congenital cardiac malformations. *Cardiol Young* 2005;15:47–51.
7. Gilkeson RC, Markowitz AH, Ciancibello L. Multisection CT evaluation of the reoperative cardiac surgery patient. *Radiographics* 2003;23 Spec No:S3–17.
8. Goo HW, Park IS, Ko JK, et al. CT of congenital heart disease: Normal anatomy and typical pathologic conditions. *Radiographics* 2003;23 Spec No:S147–165.
9. Deibler AR, Kuzo RS, Vohringer M, et al. Imaging of congenital coronary anomalies with multislice computed tomography. *Mayo Clin Proc* 2004;79: 1017–1023.
10. Bean MJ, Pannu H, Fishman EK. Three-dimensional computed tomographic imaging of complex congenital cardiovascular abnormalities. *J Comput Assist Tomogr* 2005;29:721–724.
11. Hong C, Woodard PK, Bae KT. Congenital coronary artery anomaly demonstrated by three dimensional 16 slice spiral CT angiography. *Heart* 2004;90:478.
12. Schubert S. *What is Volume Computed Tomography?* Advanced CT: A GE healthcare publication; 2004:49–51.
13. Lawler LP, Pannu HK, Fishman EK. MDCT evaluation of the coronary arteries, 2004: How we do it—data acquisition, postprocessing, display, and interpretation. *AJR Am J Roentgenol* 2005;184:1402–1412.
14. Siegel MJ. Multiplanar and three-dimensional multi-detector row CT of thoracic vessels and airways in the pediatric population. *Radiology* 2003;229:641–650.
15. Beebe DS, Tran P, Bragg M, et al. Trained nurses can provide safe and effective sedation for MRI in pediatric patients. *Can J Anaesth* 2000;47:205–210.
16. Bluemke DA, Breiter SN. Sedation procedures in MR imaging: Safety, effectiveness, and nursing effect on examinations. *Radiology* 2000;216:645–652.
17. Malviya S, Voepel-Lewis T, Tait AR, et al. Pentobarbital vs chloral hydrate for sedation of children undergoing MRI: Efficacy and recovery characteristics. *Paediatr Anaesth* 2004;14:589–595.
18. Johr M, Berger TM. Paediatric anaesthesia and inhalation agents. *Best Pract Res Clin Anaesthesiol* 2005;19:501–522.
19. Grundmann U, Uth M, Eichner A, et al. Total intravenous anaesthesia with propofol and remifentanil in paediatric patients: A comparison with a desflurane-nitrous oxide inhalation anaesthesia. *Acta Anaesthesiol Scand* 1998;42:845–850.
20. Long FR, Castile RG, Brody AS, et al. Lungs in infants and children: Improved thin-section CT with a noninvasive controlled-ventilation technique-initial experience. *Radiology* 1999;212:588–593.
21. Long FR, Castile RG. Technique and clinical applications of full-inflation and end-exhalation controlled-ventilation chest CT in infants and young children. *Pediatr Radiol* 2001;31:413–422.
22. Long FR. High-resolution CT of the lungs in infants and young children. *J Thorac Imaging* 2001; 16:251–258.
23. Brenner DJ, Elliston CD, Hall EJ, et al. Estimates of the cancer risks from pediatric CT radiation are not merely theoretical: Comment on "point/counterpoint: In x-ray computed tomography, technique factors should be selected appropriate to patient size against the proposition". *Med Phys* 2001;28:2387–2388.
24. Cody DD, Moxley DM, Krugh KT, et al. Strategies for formulating appropriate MDCT techniques when imaging the chest, abdomen, and pelvis in pediatric patients. *AJR Am J Roentgenol* 2004;182:849–859.
25. Eichhorn J, Long F, Hill S, et al. Assessment of in-stent stenosis in small children with congenital heart disease using multi-detector computed tomography—a validation study. *Catheter Cardio Interv* 2006;68:11–20.
26. Raman SV, Cook SC, McCarthy B, et al. Usefulness of multidetector row computed tomography to quantify right ventricular size and function in adults with either tetralogy of Fallot or transposition of the great arteries. *Am J Cardiol* 2005;95:683–686.
27. Eichhorn JG, Fink C, Long F, et al. Multidetector CT for the diagnosis of congenital vascular anomalies and associated complications in newborns and infants [in German]. *Rofo* 2005;177:1366–1372.
28. Holzer R, Hijazi ZM. Interventional approach to congenital heart disease. *Curr Opin Cardiol* 2004;19:84–90.
29. Hoffmann R, Mintz GS, Dussaillant GR, et al. Patterns and mechanisms of in-stent restenosis. A serial intravascular ultrasound study. *Circulation* 1996;94:1247–1254.
30. Kussman BD, Geva T, McGowan FX. Cardiovascular causes of airway compression. *Paediatr Anaesth* 2004;14:60–74.
31. Chen SJ, Lee WJ, Wang JK, et al. Usefulness of three-dimensional electron beam computed tomography for evaluating tracheobronchial anomalies in children with congenital heart disease. *Am J Cardiol* 2003;92:483–486.

CHAPTER 9 ■ CARDIAC CATHETERIZATION AND ANGIOGRAPHY

RONALD G. GRIFKA, MD

Cardiac catheterization has a long and illustrious history, beginning in 1929 when Werner Forssmann, a surgical resident and future urologist, performed the first cardiac catheterization from an arm vein—on himself (1). In the 1950s, the catheterization laboratory (cath lab) was used to understand the physiology of congenital heart defects. By the 1960 to 1970s, advances in cardiac surgery required more detailed anatomic information, which was addressed using axial angiography (2,3). In the 1980s, two-dimensional (2-D) echocardiography made it possible for some patients to be diagnosed and treated without cardiac catheterization. In the 1990s, transesophageal echocardiography and magnetic resonance imaging produced various cardiac images, decreasing the need for diagnostic cardiac catheterization. However, as more complex cardiac repairs are undertaken, more detailed physiologic data are necessary for the evaluation and treatment of children with congenital or acquired heart defects. This chapter will discuss the acquisition of hemodynamic data and angiographic images.

DIAGNOSTIC CARDIAC CATHETERIZATION AND ANGIOGRAPHY

Indications

A thorough cardiac catheterization provides complete physiologic and anatomic data. With the appropriate team, the risk of cardiac catheterization is low—usually less than the risk associated with clinical decisions based on inadequate information. The three major indications for performing a cardiac catheterization are the following:

1. A complete anatomic diagnosis or necessary hemodynamic information cannot be obtained by noninvasive methods.
2. Clinical signs and symptoms are not consistent with a patient's diagnosis.
3. A patient's clinical course is not progressing as expected.

Common indications for diagnostic cardiac catheterization are listed in Table 9.1.

Techniques

Planning the Study

The probability of acquiring complete and accurate information from cardiac catheterization increases directly with the cardiologist's understanding of the specific question(s) to be answered. Anticipatory preparation for all catheterizations must include a complete history, review of all previous cardiac catheterizations and surgeries, physical examination, and review of all pertinent noninvasive studies. Studies obtained prior to catheterization may include a chest x-ray view, 15-lead electrocardiogram, and a complete blood count. Other laboratory studies should be obtained as indicated by the clinical findings, including electrolytes in patients taking diuretics; blood urea nitrogen and creatinine if there is concern for renal insufficiency; and drug levels of antiarrhythmic or immunosuppressive agents. Increasingly, patients referred for cardiac catheterization are severely ill or marginally compensated (e.g., unstable postoperative condition, cardiomyopathy, pulmonary hypertension). In these patients and patients with other special needs (airway abnormalities, pulmonary parenchymal disease, internal jugular or subclavian venous access), consultation with a pediatric cardiac anesthesiologist is helpful.

For patients who weigh <10 kg who will have a transseptal puncture or an interventional procedure, one unit of packed red blood cells is prepared. When a patient is anemic, transfusion prior to cardiac catheterization can optimize the baseline hemodynamic condition. In patients with a hematocrit (Hct) >65%, a partial exchange transfusion may be performed prior to catheterization to lower the hematocrit to 60%, using the following formula:

Exchange volume (mL)

$$= \frac{(\text{initial Hct} - \text{desired Hct}) \times (\text{weight in kg}) \times (70)}{\text{Initial Hct}}$$

Premedication, Sedation, and Anesthesia

Physicians and institutions vary in their approaches to premedication, sedation, and anesthesia. Management is influenced by the diversity of cardiac defects and the expertise of the cardiologist and anesthesiologist. The goals of premedication and sedation or anesthesia are to decrease anxiety, facilitate parental separation, ensure comfort, promote amnesia, and facilitate the safe and efficient performance of the procedure. The potential for hemodynamic compromise and airway-related complications is increasing as a greater percentage of "hemodynamically stable" patients go to surgery without cardiac catheterization, leaving the patients with "less stable" complex cardiac defects or who require jugular or subclavian vein access for catheterization. For any cardiac catheterization other than a routine low-risk procedure, there should be a person other than the primary physician who is responsible for sedation and airway monitoring. This may require a cardiac anesthesiologist, especially for patients who

TABLE 9.1

GUIDELINES FOR DIAGNOSTIC CARDIAC CATHETERIZATION

Cardiac lesion	Diagnostic issues requiring cardiac catheterization[a]	Comments
Atrial septal defect	Usually none. In older patients, pulmonary hypertension may need to be evaluated	Catheterization may be performed for defect closure.
Aortic stenosis	Measurement of peak-to-peak gradient, cardiac index, and left ventricular end-diastolic pressure; angiographic assessment of aortic insufficiency, if present; exclusion by hemodynamic measurement and angiography of other sites of left-sided obstruction	Catheterization may be performed for valve dilation. In some cases, all necessary information may be obtained noninvasively.
Coarctation of the aorta	Often none; if catheterization is performed, measurement is made of peak-to-peak gradient, cardiac index, and left ventricular end-diastolic pressure; other sites of left-sided obstruction are excluded	Arch anatomy can be assessed by magnetic resonance imaging, if not well seen by echocardiography. Catheterization may be indicated for balloon angioplasty or stenting.
Complete AV septal defect	Usually none	Usually, definition of atrioventricular valve anatomy and relative size of the two ventricles is clear by noninvasive assessment. Catheterization may be indicated if elevated pulmonary vascular resistance is suspected.
Functional single ventricle lesions, preshunt or preband	Variable, depending on specific lesion. In some cases (e.g., tricuspid atresia with normally related great arteries and severe pulmonic stenosis, or hypoplastic left heart syndrome), catheterization is not necessary. Issues that may need to be addressed at cardiac catheterization in other lesions include degree of pulmonic stenosis, presence or absence of subaortic obstruction, anatomy of the branch pulmonary arteries, presence or absence of aortopulmonary collaterals, and presence or absence of right ventricular dependent coronary circulation	
Functional single ventricle lesions, pre-Glenn or pre-Fontan	Measurement of pulmonary artery pressure, pulmonary vascular resistance, and ventricular end-diastolic pressure; angiographic assessment of pulmonary artery and pulmonary and systemic venous anatomy	Interventions such as pulmonary artery dilation or stenting or coil embolization of aortopulmonary collateral vessels or unwanted venous connections may be indicated prior to surgery.
Patent ductus arteriosus	None	Catheterization may be performed for transcatheter closure.
Pulmonic stenosis	None	Catheterization may be performed for pulmonary valve dilation.
Tetralogy of Fallot	A complete anatomic diagnosis is usually possible with echocardiography or MRI. Indications for catheterization include uncertainty regarding coronary artery anatomy, pulmonary artery anatomy, or presence of multiple ventricular septal defects, mitral stenosis, or aorto-pulmonary collateral vessels	
Pumonary atresia with ventricular septal defect	Pulmonary atresia, ventricular septal defect. Angiographic definition of aorto-pulmonary collateral vessels and pulmonary artery anatomy	Catheterization may also be performed for pulmonary artery dilation and/or coil embolization of aortopulmonary collaterals.
Totally anomalous pulmonary venous return	Usually none	In most cases, a complete diagnosis can be made noninvasively.
Transposition of the great arteries	Often none; diagnostic indications include uncertainty regarding coronary artery anatomy or presence of multiple ventricular septal defects	Catheterization may be performed for balloon atrial septostomy.
Isolated conoventricular ventricular septal defect	Usually, none; uncertainty about multiple ventricular septal defects is an indication for catheterization	Catheterization may be indicated if elevated pulmonary vascular resistance is suspected.
Multiple muscular ventricular septal defects	Angiographic definition of number, location, and size of defects as a supplement to echocardiographic definition	Catheterization may be performed for transcatheter VSD closure.

[a]Where no catheterization is indicated, it is assumed that the anatomic diagnosis made noninvasively is complete, and that the clinical findings are consistent with the anatomic diagnosis.
AV, arteriovenous; VSD, ventricular septal defect.

have elevated pulmonary vascular resistance or depressed myocardial function.

Prior to the catheterization, patients cannot have solid food or milk for 6 hours and clear fluids for 2 hours. Certain patients should have an intravenous line placed in an upper extremity before arriving in the cath lab; this facilitates administering IV fluid (to ensure hydration) and sedation, especially in cyanotic or polycythemic patients. Premedications can be administered orally, intravenously, or intramuscularly. Some children are best treated with mask induction. The periprocedure management should be individualized for each patient and his or her cardiac defects.

Local anesthesia is administered prior to starting percutaneous access. Lidocaine is the usual anesthetic, which is painful when initially injected. Premedication diminishes the discomfort to lidocaine infiltration, as does buffering the lidocaine with sodium bicarbonate, pretreatment with a topical anesthetic cream (lidocaine 2.5% and prilocaine 2.5%), and use of a small needle (25 gauge) to infiltrate the skin prior to infiltrating deeper tissues. The dose of lidocaine should not exceed 6 mg/kg, as an excessive dose or accidental IV administration can cause seizures.

Effective sedation and analgesia can be maintained during the procedure using various intravenous medications, including morphine, fentanyl, midazolam, ketamine, and propofol. Systemic vasodilators (e.g., propofol) must be used cautiously or avoided in patients with right-to-left shunts. Conversely, ketamine can increase the systemic vascular resistance. When administering sedative medications, it is important to observe any changes in heart rate, blood pressure, and pulse oximetry and to have someone in the cath lab who is capable of maintaining airway patency and adequate ventilation. The equipment and medications necessary for emergent endotracheal intubation must be immediately available in the cath lab. Sedation protocols are influenced by individual preference, experience, and institutional policies regarding conscious sedation.

Vascular Access

Vascular access is a crucial part of the cardiac catheterization procedure. The manner in which it is achieved affects this and all future cardiac catheterizations.

Umbilical Approach

Umbilical venous access is generally possible until the third day of life. The umbilical artery may be cannulated up to 1 week of age. It is best to avoid maneuvering a wire through the umbilical vessels. Often, infants arrive in the cath lab with umbilical lines in place. An indwelling umbilical vein catheter with its tip in the right atrium can be exchanged over a 0.018- to 0.021-inch guide wire for a sheath and dilator; the sheath should be long enough to cross the ductus venosus and just enter the right atrium, but not so long as to puncture the right atrium. An indwelling umbilical arterial line may be exchanged over a wire; however, the circuitous course of this vessel makes catheter exchanges difficult. The use of a sheath in the umbilical artery is optional.

Catheter manipulation is difficult from the umbilical vessels. An umbilical venous catheter is directed toward the roof of the left atrium. Directing it to any other location will probably require use of a deflecting wire. With an umbilical arterial catheter, the initial inferior loop (that the umbilical artery takes before joining the internal iliac artery), limits the ability to manipulate the catheter. The newborn heart is very thin, especially in the atria, and there is little distance in the heart to manipulate the catheter. The catheter can stretch the heart, resulting in bradycardia or hypotension. Thus, it is necessary to use gentle technique, purposefully guiding the catheter using small movements. Since small sheaths and catheters (3 and 4 French) can be placed in the femoral vessels, the benefits of improved catheter manipulation make a femoral approach preferable in most cases, even when the umbilical vessels are available.

Femoral Approach

Atraumatic percutaneous entry of the femoral vessels should be possible in nearly all pediatric patients. This requires knowledge of the anatomy, attention to detail, excellent technique, and patience. Several percutaneous access techniques are used. The most common approach, using a plain beveled needle, is described here (4).

The patient is positioned on the catheterization table with the hips elevated slightly, and the legs restrained in a straight or slightly inward rotation. Conversely, some physicians prefer to have the legs rotated outward in a more "frog-legged" position; this displaces the femoral vessels to a more lateral position. The anatomic landmarks are identified both before and after draping the patient. The pertinent landmarks for determining the site of vessel entry are the anterior superior iliac spine, the pubic tubercle, the inguinal ligament, and the femoral pulse. In small patients, the inguinal ligament is palpable. The femoral vessels should be entered 1 to 2 cm below the inguinal ligament to ensure reliable hemostasis at the completion of the procedure. Vessel entry above the inguinal ligament is likely to result in a labial or scrotal hematoma or retroperitoneal bleeding. Often, the inguinal crease is assumed to be the appropriate site for percutaneous entry; however this may be incorrect. The area is anesthetized with lidocaine. In small patients, lidocaine should be used sparingly to avoid distortion of the landmarks and compression of the vein within the vascular sheath.

The right femoral vein is preferable (to the left), as it is more of a straight course into the right atrium, which improves catheter maneuverability. In patients who have situs inversus, the left femoral vein may be preferable. Usually, the femoral vein is accessed before the artery, except in neonates, where insertion of a femoral venous sheath may distort or obscure access to the femoral artery. In infants, the femoral vein is entered 1 cm below the inguinal ligament; if the vein is entered distally, wire passage is difficult. The vein is medial to the artery, and in infants it is close to the pulse. Vessel entry should be achieved "on the way in" without aspiration on the needle. The angle between the needle and the skin is ≤45 degrees. The needle should be inserted using an "advance and wait" technique, observing for backflow of blood between 1- to 2-mm advances. If no backflow of blood occurs, once the needle is advanced to the bone, it should be withdrawn slowly, with or without gentle aspiration with a syringe. Once there is backflow of venous blood, the needle is stabilized with the left hand, and the soft end of a wire is advanced through the needle with the right hand. A straight wire is used in infants and small children; a J-wire may be used in older patients. If the needle tip is centered in the vessel, the wire advances easily. If any resistance is felt, the wire is withdrawn and the needle adjusted; the needle is withdrawn slightly or depressed into a more horizontal plane to help center the tip in the vessel. Using fluoroscopic guidance, the wire is advanced above the diaphragm into the right atrium to ensure that the wire is in the vein (not in a right-sided descending aorta). The needle is removed, a small skin incision is made using a pointed blade, then the sheath and dilator are advanced over the wire using a screwing motion (which facilitates sheath and dilator insertion through the subcutaneous tissue). Once the sheath is in the vessel several centimeters, the dilator is held stationary and the sheath is advanced over the dilator and wire. The dilator and wire are removed, and the sheath is allowed to bleed back (or is gently aspirated) through the sidearm and stopcock, then flushed with heparinized saline.

Arterial access is obtained using the same technique. When the needle is centered in the artery, there is brisk, pulsatile blood flow. Initially, an 18- or 20-gauge catheter is placed in the artery for pressure monitoring and blood gas sampling. If a retrograde catheterization is needed, the monitoring catheter is later exchanged for a sheath, minimizing the time the sheath remains in the artery. With the small sheath sizes available (3 and 4 French), arterial sheaths are used for nearly all retrograde catheterizations.

Subclavian Approach

The subclavian vein is posterior to the clavicle, superficial and inferior to the subclavian artery, and lies partly on the pleura. Complications of subclavian vein access include pneumothorax, hemothorax, and intravascular air. Complications are more likely to occur when there is pulmonary parenchymal disease, pulmonary hypertension, or anatomic thoracic abnormalities (including previous surgery). The patient is positioned with a small roll under the shoulders. Airway adequacy is verified before proceeding. Important landmarks to identify, prior to draping the patient and again before vessel entry, are the suprasternal notch and the depression at the lateral third of the clavicle. In the usual anatomy with a right superior vena cava and left innominate vein, left subclavian vein access is preferred. In the region of clavicular depression, the skin, subcutaneous tissues, and clavicular periosteum are infiltrated with lidocaine. The needle, with attached syringe, enters the skin and is advanced gently until it contacts the clavicle, then it is "walked" under the clavicle. The needle must be oriented anteriorly to avoid entering the subclavian artery or the apex of the lung. Once under the clavicle, the needle is advanced slowly with constant gentle aspiration until a steady venous blood return is obtained. Using fluoroscopic guidance, the soft end of a wire is advanced into the right atrium (or the pulmonary artery in a cavopulmonary anastomosis). Due to negative intrathoracic pressure, air will be sucked into the vein if the needle is left open to air or if there is a mismatch between the size of the needle lumen and the wire diameter. Because of the risk of intravascular air, a sheath with a bleedback valve is always used.

Internal Jugular Approach

The internal jugular vein is used to perform right heart catheterizations and right ventricle endomyocardial biopsies; it is also used when the femoral veins are not accessible. The internal jugular vein is entered outside the thorax, decreasing the risk of pneumothorax or intravascular air. However, the patient's head must remain turned to one side; thus in a sedated patient (particularly an infant), the airway may be compromised. A visible, although tiny, puncture scar may occur. The right internal jugular vein is preferred (to the left) because it offers a more direct course into the right atrium, and the apex of the lung is lower on the right side. The patient is positioned with the neck hyperextended and the head turned to the left. Landmarks to be identified before and after draping the patient are the carotid pulse and the two divisions of the sternocleidomastoid muscle. The right internal jugular

vein lies below the sternocleidomastoid muscle, anterior and lateral to the carotid artery.

There are three approaches to accessing the internal jugular vein. Using the central approach, the needle enters the skin at the apex of the triangle formed by the convergence of the sternal and clavicular heads of the sternocleidomastoid muscle. Using the anterior approach, the needle enters at the anterior border of the sternocleidomastoid muscle, half the distance from the mastoid process to its sternal insertion. For both approaches, the needle is aimed toward the ipsilateral nipple, with 30 to 45 degrees of posterior angulation to avoid entering the carotid artery. Using the posterior approach, the needle enters the skin posterior to the sternocleidomastoid muscle, one-third its length above the clavicular insertion, just posterior to the external jugular vein, aiming for the sternal notch. With all approaches, the needle is advanced with constant gentle aspiration with a syringe until a steady venous blood return is obtained. Using fluoroscopic guidance, a guide wire is passed through the needle, then into the right atrium (or pulmonary artery in a cavopulmonary anastomosis).

Internal jugular vein cannulation is facilitated by using a small ultrasonic imaging device designed specifically for this technique. Patient landmarks are identified, then the internal jugular vein and common carotid artery are imaged by ultrasound while the percutaneous puncture is performed. The internal jugular vein is distinguished from the carotid artery as gentle pressure with the transducer compresses the vein, and the artery has obvious pulsations with the heart rate.

Catheter Manipulation

Although comprehensive discussion of catheter manipulation is beyond the scope of this chapter, several points deserve mentioning. In the neonate and infant, cardiac tissue is thin. Perforation can occur easily, especially in the atrial appendages, right ventricular outflow tract, left ventricular apex, and aortic valve cusps. The risk of perforation can be decreased by gentle catheter manipulation, using small movements, the use of balloon catheters, and a thorough understanding of the cardiac anatomy and the desired catheter route and destination. The importance of reviewing *all* previous imaging studies *before* the catheterization cannot be overemphasized. If a catheter is too straight to manipulate to the desired location (e.g., across the tricuspid valve), it may be safely curved outside the body, in a hepatic vein, or using a tip-deflecting wire, rather than within the heart. The small catheters used in infants and children can be damaged by vigorous manipulation. Thin-walled catheters, such as pigtails, should be advanced over a wire. Large catheter loops in the atrium or right ventricular outflow tract can cause hemodynamic instability owing to reflex bradycardia or tricuspid valve insufficiency. A common operator error is to concentrate on the position of the catheter tip without regard for the loops of catheter behind it.

Collection of Hemodynamic Data

The purpose of a diagnostic heart catheterization is to collect data that will be used to define the patient's condition and make management decisions. Inaccurate catheterization data result in suboptimal patient management. During data collection, the child's condition must be continually assessed. Oxygen saturations and pressure measurements must be evaluated as they are obtained. Thus, the operator is constantly

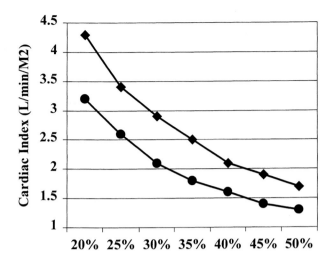

Difference in arterial-venous oxygen saturation

FIGURE 9.1 Graph displaying the relationship between cardiac index and varying arteriovenous oxygen saturations. Note the greater cardiac index with a hemoglobin of 12 g/dL (*squares*) compared with 16 g/dL (*circles*). The assumed oxygen consumption is 140 mL/min/m².

aware of the patient's hemodynamic state, and inconsistencies in the data must be clarified before the catheters are removed. The practice of collecting data in the cath lab and deferring all interpretation until after the procedure is unacceptable.

Oxygen saturations in the superior vena cava and aorta should be obtained at the beginning of the procedure. These data immediately inform the operator of the patient's initial hemodynamic status, which is a crucial aspect of the procedure. Children with a superior vena cava saturation <60% or arterial saturation <70% have limited cardiac reserve. All factors influencing their condition (i.e., body temperature, ventilatory status, acid: base balance, volume status) should be assessed at the start of the procedure and continually during the procedure. Although this is stating the obvious, all catheterization procedures should be completed as expeditiously as possible.

Any abnormal data must be verified in the cath lab. If a pulmonary vein sample is desaturated, one must ascertain if the catheter sampling port(s) was positioned in the pulmonary vein, not in the atrium or coronary sinus. If pulmonary artery saturation is elevated, one must ascertain if the catheter was partially wedged or if there is a left-to-right shunt.

After collection of all saturations and pressures, and before proceeding to angiography, it is important to assess the pulmonary and systemic flows, resistances, and flow ratios. Systemic flow index is estimated using the observation that a "normal" arterial-venous (A-V) saturation difference of 20% to 25% corresponds to a cardiac index of approximately 3.5 L/min/m². For a given A-V O₂ difference, the higher the hemoglobin level, the lower the flow index (Fig. 9.1). The flow index and resistance calculations will be discussed in a later section.

Measurement of Hemodynamic Variables

Oxygen in the Blood

Oxygen is carried in the blood attached to hemoglobin and dissolved in plasma. As room air is breathed, the vast majority of oxygen in the blood is bound to hemoglobin. The amount

of oxygen dissolved in plasma is determined by the solubility coefficient of oxygen, the temperature, and the partial pressure of oxygen. At 37°C (body temperature), the amount of oxygen dissolved in blood is 0.03 mL/mm Hg/L. Thus, in arterial blood with an oxygen tension of 100 mm Hg, there is 3 mL of dissolved oxygen per liter. This amount of oxygen is so small compared with the amount of oxygen bound to hemoglobin; it is usually ignored in hemodynamic calculations. However, if the patient is receiving supplemental oxygen, with the partial pressure of O₂ (pO₂) >100 mm Hg, then the dissolved oxygen must be considered in calculating the total oxygen content. The amount of oxygen bound to hemoglobin is influenced by the amount and type of hemoglobin, temperature, partial pressure of oxygen, hydrogen ion concentration, partial pressure of carbon dioxide, and levels of 2,3-DPG. The amount of oxygen that can be taken up by hemoglobin in blood is referred to as the oxygen capacity. The maximum oxygen capacity is 1.36 mL O₂/g of hemoglobin. Thus, for a given patient, the oxygen capacity (mL O₂/L) is:

$$\text{(Hemoglobin in g/dL)} \times \text{(1.36 mL O}_2\text{/g of hemoglobin)} \times \text{(10 dL/L)}$$

The oxygen content is the total amount of oxygen present in a sample of blood. It includes both dissolved oxygen and oxygen bound to hemoglobin. The oxygen content is:

$$\text{(Oxygen capacity)} \times \text{(oxygen saturation)} + \text{(PaO}_2\text{)} \times \text{(0.03 mL/mm Hg)}$$

For example, if the hemoglobin is 11.5 g/dL, the femoral artery oxygen saturation is 99%, and the PaO₂ is 106 mm Hg, the oxygen content is:

$$\text{(11.5 g/dL)} \times \text{(1.36 mL/g)} \times \text{(10 dL/L)} \times \text{(0.99)} + \text{(106 mm Hg)} \times \text{(0.03 mL/mm Hg)}$$
$$= 155 + 3.3 = 158$$

If the femoral artery PaO₂ is 566 and the oxygen saturation is 100%, the oxygen content is 156 + 17 = 173.

Oxygen saturation is measured spectrophotometrically. Oxidized hemoglobin and reduced hemoglobin have different spectral absorptions at 650 nm but similar ones at 805 nm. Oximeters measure the absorption at 650 nm to represent the amount of oxidized hemoglobin and the absorption at 805 nm to represent total hemoglobin; the ratio of these two numbers is the oxygen saturation. The method is accurate at oxygen saturations between 60% and 95%, if there are no other substances in the blood that affect the spectral absorption (e.g., carboxyhemoglobin). The oxygen saturation also may be derived by using the pH, partial pressure of CO₂ (pCO₂), and pO₂, using the oxygen dissociation curve. However, factors that affect the affinity of oxygen for hemoglobin (i.e., temperature, hydrogen ion, fetal hemoglobin, and levels of 2,3-DPG) are difficult to measure accurately, which makes this method inaccurate in neonates and cyanotic children.

Cardiac Output

Cardiac output can be measured using the indicator dilution technique described by Fick (5). The indicators most commonly used to measure cardiac output are oxygen or cold saline (thermodilution) (6). Various models have been used to describe the concept of the Fick principle, including wood chips dumped in a river. When flow cannot be measured directly, as is the case of a river, it can be measured indirectly by using an indicator. In the river analogy, wood chips are dumped at a known, constant rate into a flowing river. When the river flows swiftly (analogous to high cardiac output), the chip concentration is dilute; when the river flows sluggishly (analogous to low cardiac output), the chip concentration is dense. In quantitative terms:

A fluid flows at an unknown rate (mL/min).

An indicator is present in the fluid in a measurable concentration (mg/mL).

The indicator is added or removed at a known rate (mg/min).

Measurement of the change in concentration (mg/mL) allows one to calculate flow:

Rate of addition or removal (mg/min)

Change in concentration (mg/mL) = flow (mL/min)

Oxygen Method. When cardiac output is calculated using the Fick method, the indicator is oxygen. The rate of change of the indicator is the oxygen consumption. It is assumed that measurements are taken at a steady-state condition, thus oxygen consumption by the tissues equals oxygen uptake by the lungs. Oxygen consumption may be measured or assumed.

There are two widely used methods of measuring oxygen consumption: the Douglass bag and the polarographic method. The Douglass bag method requires collection of a timed sample of expired air. During the collection period, the patient's nose is clipped shut, and he or she breathes entirely through a mouthpiece. Room air (with a known oxygen concentration) is inhaled, and expired air is collected in the bag. For obvious reasons, this technique is rarely applied in the pediatric cath lab.

The polarographic method uses a metabolic rate meter (7). The patient's head is placed in a plastic hood. Room air (which has a known oxygen concentration) is drawn into the hood, and the expired gases, diluted with room air, are withdrawn from the hood at a fixed rate. The concentration of oxygen in the collected gas mixture is measured using a polarographic sensor cell. With the rate of flow of the gas (determined by the apparatus and the patient's ventilatory rate) and the change in concentration of oxygen (measured in the inhaled and exhaled air), the rate of change of oxygen can be calculated. This is the oxygen consumption. Accurate measurements depend on meticulous attention to the procedure. If there is a leak of exhaled gas out of the hood, oxygen consumption will be underestimated.

Because of the difficulty (in some cases impossibility) of measuring oxygen consumption in the cath lab, assumed values are frequently used, based on the formulas of Lafarge and Meittinen (8). The formulas are derived from measurements made in 879 patients using the Douglass bag method. Values for patients 3 to 18 years of age and at various heart rates are listed in Table 9.2.

There are specific equations for applying the Fick principle to the calculation of the systemic and pulmonary flow. The systemic flow (Qs) is equal to the oxygen consumption divided by the change in oxygen content across the body (oxygen content of the aorta minus the superior vena cava).

$$Q_s = O_2 \text{ consumption}/(1.36) \times (10) \times (Hgb)$$
$$\times (\text{aorta sat} - \text{SVC sat})$$

Similarly, the pulmonary flow (Qp) is equal to the oxygen consumption divided by the change in oxygen content across the lungs (oxygen content of the pulmonary vein minus oxygen content of the pulmonary artery).

$$Q_p = O_2 \text{ consumption}/(1.36) \times (10) \times (Hgb)$$
$$\times (\text{pulmonary vein sat} - \text{pulmonary art sat})$$

Possible sources of error include inaccuracy of the value used for oxygen consumption, inaccurate sample for the mixed venous saturation, and absence of a steady-state condition. For pediatric catheterization procedures, flows are indexed to body surface area. Inaccurate measurements of patient length, especially in infants, may be another source of error.

Thermodilution Method. With the thermodilution method, the indicator is temperature. A double-lumen thermodilution catheter is used. A bolus of cold saline (room temperature, approximately 21°C) is injected through the proximal port (positioned in the right atrium). A thermistor for measuring temperature is located near the catheter tip (positioned in the pulmonary artery). The cold saline cools the blood as they mix together. The degree of cooling of the blood is inversely proportional to the magnitude of flow and directly proportional to several factors: the amount of "cold" injected (a function of the volume injected), the temperature difference between the injectate and the blood, and the specific heats of the injectate and the blood. The thermodilution cardiac output measurement is an automated system (except for the hand injection of cold saline), and the calculations are performed by a laptop computer. To minimize error, three to five sequential injections of cold saline are performed over 1 to 2 minutes. The technique is simple, precise, and easily allows serial measurements to compare interventions in the cath lab or intensive care unit. The thermodilution method (as with any indicator dilution method) requires complete mixing; thus it is most accurate when there is a mixing chamber proximal to the thermistor. The thermodilution method is used in patients who do not have intracardiac or great vessel level shunts. Possible sources of error include inconsistent volume of injectate, variable temperature of the blood or injectate, apposition of the thermistor to a vessel wall, and inadequate mixing. Thorough mixing is problematic in venous systems with low flow (e.g., bidirectional cavopulmonary anastomosis, Fontan operation).

Pressure Measurements

In most cath labs, pressures are measured using fluid-filled catheters connected to pressure-sensitive transducers. The change in pressure (force/unit area) in the cardiac chamber or vessel being measured is transmitted along a column of incompressible fluid (saline or blood) contained within a nonexpansile tube (catheter) to a transducer. The transducer contains a diaphragm that moves a small distance (in a linear fashion) in response to change in pressure. The movement of the diaphragm is transmitted to an electronic strain gauge. The strain gauge converts pressure-induced changes into voltage changes. The voltage changes are converted into an electric signal, which is amplified and displayed on an oscilloscope and recorded on paper. Systolic and diastolic pressures are measured in a continuous, instantaneous manner. A mean pressure is obtained by electronic damping of the signal over several cardiac cycles. The system is calibrated to an arbitrarily assigned zero point, the center of the heart. It is important to understand potential sources of error and artifact in the pressure tracings obtained. Two important concepts are frequency response (the ratio of output amplitude to input amplitude over the range of frequencies of the input pressure wave) and damping (the dissipation of the energy of oscillation of a pressure measurement system). Inaccurate pressure waveforms frequently are related to deterioration of the frequency response, or to overdamping or underdamping. Other references contain a more complete discussion of these principles (9). Eight practical guidelines for avoiding artifact and error are listed below:

TABLE 9.2

OXYGEN CONSUMPTION

Age (yr)	Heart rate (bpm)	VO$_2$, boys[a]	VO$_2$, girls[b]	Age (yr)	Heart rate (bpm)	VO$_2$, boys[a]	VO$_2$, girls[b]
3	80	156	150	11	80	141	127
	100	163	157		100	148	135
	120	171	165		120	156	143
	140	178	172		140	163	150
	160	186	180		160	171	158
4	80	152	145	12	80	140	126
	100	160	152		100	147	134
	120	168	160		120	155	141
	140	175	167		140	162	149
	160	183	175		160	170	156
5	80	150	141	13	80	139	125
	100	157	148		100	146	132
	120	165	156		120	154	140
	140	173	164		140	162	147
	160	180	171		160	169	155
6	80	148	138	14	80	138	123
	100	155	145		100	146	131
	120	163	153		120	153	138
	140	170	160		140	161	146
	160	178	168		160	168	154
7	80	146	135	15	80	137	122
	100	154	143		100	145	130
	120	161	150		120	152	137
	140	169	158		140	160	145
	160	176	165		160	167	152
8	80	144	133	16	80	136	121
	100	152	140		100	144	129
	120	160	148		120	152	136
	140	167	156		140	159	144
	160	175	163		160	167	151
9	80	143	131	17	80	136	120
	100	151	138		100	143	128
	120	158	146		120	151	135
	140	166	154		140	158	143
	160	173	161		160	166	150
10	80	142	129	18	80	135	119
	100	149	137		100	143	127
	120	157	144		120	150	134
	140	165	152		140	158	142
	160	172	159		160	165	149

[a]For boys, VO$_2$ = 138.1 − 11.49 In(age) + 0.378 (heart rate).
[b]For girls, VO$_2$ = 138.1 − 17.04 In(age) + 0.378 (heart rate).
VO$_2$, oxygen consumption.

1. Loose connections in the system: These usually result in an overdamped tracing. Backup of blood into the transducer tubing is an indication of a loose connection.
2. Air in the system: This is probably the most common cause of measurement error. Air may be introduced into the system at any of the connections, or dissolved air may come out of the saline used to flush the system. The presence of air (which is compressible) in the system lowers the frequency response. As a result, information inherent in the applied pressure wave is lost, producing what is commonly referred to as a damped tracing. Another indication of air in the system is the amplification of high-frequency input, producing overshoot or "fling" in the tracing. The appearance of a small amount of blood with obvious pulsatility in the transducer tubing is an indication that there is air in the system.
3. Inaccurate calibration or baseline drift: Even if the transducers are properly calibrated at the beginning of the procedure, movement of either the patient or the transducers, or electric drift of the baseline, may result in inaccurate pressure recordings. It is a useful to check crucial measurements

by switching the transducers (i.e., by connecting the venous pressure line to the arterial transducer and vice versa). Although small errors in calibration may be inconsequential in arterial recordings, they can make a huge impact in the measurement of venous pressures and pulmonary vascular resistance (this will be discussed further).

4. Partial catheter obstruction: This is usually the result of the catheter clotting or kinking. This usually occurs when small or thin-walled catheters are used. If blood is allowed to remain in the catheter lumen for any length of time, deposition of fibrin or platelets will reduce the lumen size, hence the frequency response.

5. Catheter "fling": The appearance of fling (a tall, narrow spike) on a pressure recording has many causes. Overshoot, produced by air in the system, has been discussed. Rapid movement of the catheter tip, which may occur if the tip lies in a turbulent jet, can result in superimposition of high-frequency oscillations on the pressure recording. If the catheter is contacted by a cardiac structure (such as the mitral valve), the superimposed oscillation can alter the waveform dramatically. At times, these conditions are unavoidable. To minimize this error, use the mean systolic pressure rather than the peak systolic pressure (if an option), or inject a small amount blood or contrast media in the tubing to intentionally damp the system.

6. End-hole artifact: When a column of blood stops suddenly against an end-hole catheter, kinetic energy is transformed into pressure energy, and the recorded pressure is falsely elevated. Similarly, when a column of blood is moving away from an end-hole catheter, the pressure recorded will be less than the true intravascular pressure, in proportion to the velocity of flow. This explains why the pressure in a stenotic proximal pulmonary artery has a lower peak systolic pressure than the distal larger vessel (which appears to violate the rule that water flows downhill).

7. Peripheral pulse wave amplification: Both the peak systolic pressure and the pulse pressure are amplified with increasing distance from the aortic valve. This phenomenon is demonstrating by recording the pressure tracing during a pullback around the aortic arch, where the systolic pressure increases from the ascending to descending aorta. When comparing the ascending aorta systolic pressure with the femoral or radial artery systolic pressure, failure to take into account pulse wave amplification will result in underestimation of a pressure gradient across an aortic valve or coarctation of the aorta. Interestingly, although the peak systolic pressure and pulse pressures are higher in the descending aorta than in the ascending aorta, the mean pressures are the same.

8. Catheter entrapment: An end-hole catheter placed in a small or heavily trabeculated ventricle can trap a small volume of fluid, resulting in an exaggerated pressure elevation during systole. To eliminate this error, slightly withdraw of the catheter or deflate the balloon (if a balloon-tipped catheter is used). If these maneuvers are not possible, the pressure should be recorded using a side-hole (multipurpose) catheter.

Right Heart Catheterization

Characteristic right heart waveforms are shown in Figure 9.2. There are three characteristic waves in the right atrial tracing; the a, c, and v waves. The a wave occurs just after the P wave on the electrocardiogram (ECG). The a wave represents atrial systole. The c wave is due to either right ventricular contrac-

tion or tricuspid valve closure, and the v wave results from filling of the right atrium against a closed tricuspid valve. The decrease in pressure after the a wave is the x descent, which is due to atrial relaxation. The decrease in pressure after the v wave is the y descent, which represents the opening of the tricuspid valve in early diastole.

Normally, the right atrial a wave exceeds the v wave by 2 to 3 mm Hg, neither wave exceeds 8 mm Hg, and both waves are within 5 mm Hg of the mean right atrial pressure. An elevated a wave is seen in tricuspid stenosis, pulmonic stenosis, pulmonary atresia, pulmonary hypertension, or a noncompliant right ventricle (hypertrophy, diastolic dysfunction). Also, cannon a waves may be seen with certain arrhythmias, when atrial contraction occurs after right ventricular contraction has closed the tricuspid valve. Elevated v waves are found with tricuspid insufficiency, Ebstein anomaly, or a left ventricular–to–right atrial shunt. The right atrium and venae cavae are compliant structures and can accept a large volume of blood with minimal change in pressure; thus, the absence of high v waves does not rule out any of the aforementioned conditions. Elevation of the mean pressure is seen with any condition that elevates the a wave or v wave, or with myocardial failure. Low right atrial pressure (<1 to 2 mm Hg) suggests hypovolemia. Marked variability of the a wave and mean pressure may be seen with atrioventricular dissociation or with obstructive airway disease.

The right ventricular pressure tracing has a rapid upstroke during isovolumic contraction, a plateau during systolic ejection, a decline to near zero during isovolumic relaxation, and a slow rise to the end-diastolic pressure during diastolic filling. Normally, the peak systolic pressure is <30 mm Hg, and the end diastolic pressure is <8 mm Hg; the end diastolic pressure corresponds to (and should be equal to) the right atrial a wave. With a large ventricular septal defect, the right and left ventricular pressures are equal. Also, right ventricular outflow tract obstruction will increase the systolic pressure. Other causes of elevated right ventricular pressure are discussed with the causes of pulmonary hypertension.

The normal pulmonary artery systolic pressure is equal to the right ventricular systolic pressure (<30 mm Hg), and the mean pressure is <20 mm Hg. Increased pulmonary artery pressure occurs with peripheral pulmonary stenosis, pulmonary arteriolar obstruction, pulmonary thromboembolism, pulmonary venous obstruction, left atrial hypertension, and left ventricular failure. Also, elevated pulmonary artery pressure occurs with communications between the aorta and pulmonary artery or between the right and left ventricles (if no pulmonic stenosis). In the presence of pulmonary hypertension, a pulse pressure of <40% of the peak systolic pressure suggests a fixed resistance, whereas a wide pulse pressure (>60% of the peak systolic pressure) suggests high flow and low resistance.

Systolic pressure gradients between right ventricle and pulmonary artery are due to right ventricular outflow tract obstruction, although gradients of 5 mm Hg may be normal. Gradients ≤10 mm Hg may be seen with structurally normal pulmonary valves and increased blood flow, as with a large atrial septal defect.

The pulmonary artery wedge pressure is usually a good reflection of the left atrial and left ventricular end-diastolic pressures because of the absence of valves in the pulmonary circulation. The wedged catheter position is confirmed by observation of the characteristic left atrial waveform or by withdrawal of fully saturated blood. When small catheters are used, it may not be possible to withdraw a blood sample from the wedged position. To confirm that the catheter is wedged, a

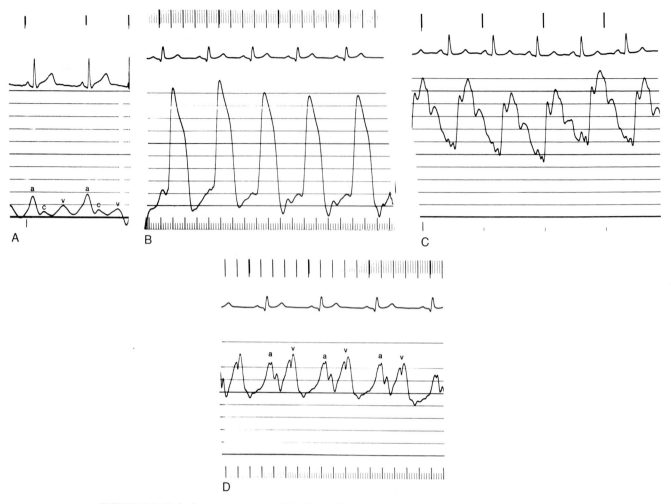

FIGURE 9.2 Right heart pressures (each horizontal line = 2 mm Hg). A: Right atrium: a wave = 3, c wave = 1, v wave = 2. B: Right ventricle: 20/0,2. C: Pulmonary artery: 22/10. D: Pulmonary capillary wedge: a wave = 14, v wave = 16.

small injection of contrast is performed after recording the pressure. Interpretation of the wedge pressure must be guided by an understanding of the anatomy. The pulmonary artery wedge pressure does not reflect the left ventricular end-diastolic pressure when there is pulmonary vein stenosis, cor triatriatum, mitral stenosis, or anomalous pulmonary venous return. When the wedge pressure is elevated, these lesions must be confirmed or ruled out by direct measurement of the left atrial or left ventricular end-diastolic pressure.

Left Heart Catheterization

Characteristic left heart waveforms are shown in Figure 9.3. The normal left atrial mean pressure is 6 to 10 mm Hg (depending on age), which is several mm Hg higher than the right atrial mean pressure. The v wave is usually higher than the a wave (which differs from the right atrium), and neither is >5 mm Hg above the mean pressure. An elevated a wave is seen with defects resulting in left atrial outflow obstruction (mitral stenosis, supravalve mitral membrane) or with diseases

that impair left ventricular compliance (aortic stenosis, coarctation of the aorta). The a wave may be dominant with an atrial septal defect or diseases that elevate the right atrial a wave, and a large atrial septal defect allows transmission of pressure across the septum. Elevated v waves occur with mitral insufficiency. Elevation of the left atrial mean pressure (and the a and v waves) may be encountered with large left-to-right shunts at the ventricle or great vessel level or as a sign of left ventricular failure. If the end-diastolic pressures in the left atrium and left ventricle are not equal, some form of mitral valve obstruction is present; higher gradients (>8 to 10 mm Hg) suggest structural mitral stenosis, whereas lower gradients suggest a relative stenosis owing to increased blood flow, as seen with a large ventricular septal defect.

The normal left ventricular systolic pressure varies according to age, ranging from 50 to 60 mm Hg in a neonate or infant to 120 mm Hg in an adolescent. The left ventricular tracing is more rectangular (than that of the right ventricle), with a longer and flatter plateau at maximum systolic pressure. The normal end-diastolic pressure may be as high as 8 to 12 mm Hg in children. The end-diastolic pressure is increased

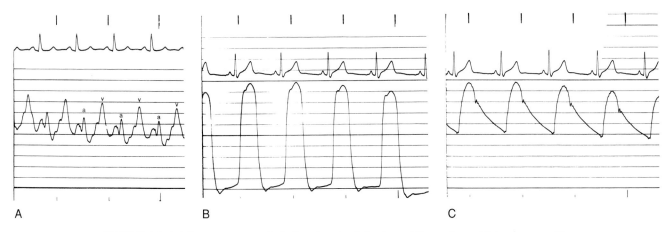

FIGURE 9.3 Left heart pressures. **A:** Left atrium (each horizontal line = 2 mm Hg): a wave = 13, v wave = 16. **B:** Left ventricle (each horizontal line = 10 mm Hg): 98/0,6. **C:** Aorta (each horizontal line = 10 mm Hg): 98/50.

with a large left-to-right shunt, heart failure, and restrictive pericardial or myocardial disease. Identification of the end-diastolic pressure from the left ventricular pressure tracing can be difficult, at times requiring a simultaneous left atrial tracing. At end-diastole, the upstroke of the ventricular tracing crosses the atrial tracing.

The peak systolic pressure in the left ventricle should be equal to or up to 5 mm Hg greater than the peak systolic pressure in the ascending aorta. The aortic pressure is a reflection of the cardiac output and systemic vascular resistance. Near the aortic valve, the arterial waveform displays a relatively slow upstroke, a broad peak, and a near-linear drop to end-diastole. In the distal arteries, the peak becomes sharper, the dicrotic notch more obvious, and pulse wave amplification occurs.

The pulse pressure in the ascending aorta is usually 25 to 50 mm Hg, or <50% of the peak systolic aortic pressure. Increased pulse pressure and low diastolic pressure may be seen with aortic insufficiency, a ruptured sinus of Valsalva, or conditions in which there is a low-resistance diastolic runoff, such as patent ductus arteriosus, aortopulmonary shunt, aortopulmonary window, truncus arteriosus, and systemic AV fistula. A gradient between the ascending and descending aorta is present in coarctation of the aorta. A narrow pulse pressure may be encountered in pericardial tamponade or low cardiac output states.

Derived Hemodynamic Variables

Intracardiac Shunts

Ideally, the oxygen saturation in the superior vena cava, right atrium, right ventricle, and pulmonary artery would all be equal. Similarly, the oxygen saturation in the pulmonary veins, left atrium, left ventricle, and aorta and its branches would all be equal. An increase in oxygen saturation between different sites of the right heart would give precise information on the location and magnitude of left-to-right shunts, whereas a decrease in saturation between successive chambers of the left heart would define a right-to-left shunt.

To evaluate possible intracardiac shunts in the cath lab, it is necessary to understand four assumptions inherent in these calculations and to be certain they are applicable. The first assumption is that the patient is at steady state. This is true if the patient is asleep or resting quietly; if conditions change during the measurements, errors may be introduced. The second assumption is that an oxygen saturation sample is an accurate representation of the chamber or vessel. This is often the case, but oxygenation sampling is fraught with difficulty; scattered areas of pulmonary parenchymal disease or atelectasis (owing to cardiomegaly) may lead to inhomogeneous oxygenation of pulmonary artery flow. Similarly, the right atrium is a difficult site for obtaining a representative sample because of streaming from the highly saturated renal vein, the less saturated hepatic vein, and the very low saturated coronary sinus. The third assumption is that the sample is not "contaminated" by blood from a distal chamber. This may not be true when there is atrioventricular or semilunar valve regurgitation, or a right ventricle saturation may be falsely elevated when there is pulmonary regurgitation and a patent ductus arteriosus. The fourth assumption is that the patient's hemodynamic state in the cath lab represents the baseline hemodynamic state. This is probably the most difficult assumption to support; at one end of the spectrum, inadequate sedation results in a terrified or combative child, while at the other end of the spectrum is general anesthesia. Neither condition represents a normal physiologic state. The best an operator can do is to establish the conditions of the cardiac catheterization, then maintain these same conditions until a complete set of measurements has been obtained.

Qualitative Assessment of Shunts

The normal variation between oxygen samples throughout the right heart was investigated in nearly 1,000 catheterizations in children with aortic or pulmonic stenosis who had no intracardiac shunts (confirmed by dye curves or angiography) (10). The mean oxygen saturations were similar in the superior vena cava, right atrium, right ventricle, and pulmonary artery. The oxygen saturation sample in the proximal chambers was subtracted from the pulmonary artery sample to determine the variability in the absence of a left-to-right shunt. The standard deviation of the pulmonary artery–superior vena cava difference was 2.9%, the pulmonary artery–right atrium difference was 1.8%, and the pulmonary artery–right ventricle difference was 1.8%. Thus, in the absence of a shunt, a step-up of >6% at the atrial level, 4% at the ventricular level, and 4% at the great vessel level will occur <5% of the time (i.e., twice the standard deviation). Variations of >9%, 6%, and 6%, respectively (i.e., three times the standard deviation), would be expected no more than 1% of the time, thus would be highly unlikely in the absence of intracardiac shunting.

The sample in the superior vena cava is taken in the midportion, superior to the entrance of the azygous vein. A high saturation may be seen in a high-output state, partial or total anomalous pulmonary venous return to the superior vena cava or innominate vein, or an arteriovenous fistula. Occasionally, a subclavian vein sample may be elevated without explanation; it can be ignored. A low saturation may be present when the systemic arterial saturation is low (pulmonary venous desaturation, right-to-left shunt) or with a low cardiac output state (high tissue extraction).

The right atrial sample should be obtained at the lateral midatrial wall to avoid the low saturation stream from the coronary sinus and to facilitate mixing from the inferior and superior venae cavae streams. A step-up of >9% is highly suggestive of a left-to-right shunt from an atrial septal defect, anomalous pulmonary venous connection, a left ventricle-to-right atrium shunt, a ventricular septal defect with tricuspid insufficiency, or a shunt from the aorta (ruptured sinus of Valsalva aneurysm, coronary artery fistula).

The right ventricular saturation should be approximately equal to that in the right atrium; a step-up of >6% suggests a left-to-right shunt. A step-up at the ventricular level may be seen with a low atrial septal defect, a ventricular septal defect, a ruptured sinus of Valsalva aneurysm, a coronary AV fistula draining into the right ventricle, or a left-to-right shunt at the great vessel level with pulmonary insufficiency.

A step-up of >6% at the pulmonary artery level is seen with a high ventricular septal defect, patent ductus arteriosus, aortopulmonary window, coronary artery fistula (into the pulmonary artery), anomalous origin of the coronary artery from the pulmonary artery, or an aortopulmonary connection (congenital or surgical).

Similar data for the qualitative detection of right-to-left shunts are not available. If the aortic saturation is <92% (sea level, normal ventilation) or if there is >3% decrease in oxygen saturation on the left side of the heart, a right-to-left shunt is likely present. Pulmonary vein desaturation results most commonly from hypoventilation (sedation), pulmonary parenchymal disease, or pulmonary edema. Administering 100% oxygen will increase the pulmonary vein saturation and the systemic artery saturation. The right-to-left shunt from an intrapulmonary arteriovenous malformation causes left heart desaturation that does not improve with supplemental oxygen.

Left atrium desaturation, with normal pulmonary vein saturation, usually results from a right-to-left shunt through an atrial septal defect or patent foramen ovale. This is a necessary shunt with tricuspid atresia, and is seen frequently with tricuspid stenosis, Ebstein's anomaly of the tricuspid valve, pulmonary atresia or severe pulmonic stenosis, or severe pulmonary vascular disease. However, it may be seen with any disease that markedly decreases right ventricular compliance or leads to right ventricular failure. Occasionally, right-to-left atrial shunting can occur even in the presence of normal right-sided pressures and resistances. An interesting condition, orthodeoxia platypnea (cyanosis and dyspnea), occurs as one changes position from supine to sitting, owing to right-to-left shunting across a patent foramen ovale (PFO). A rare congenital defect, a persistent left superior vena cava to the left atrium, also can cause left atrial desaturation.

Left ventricular desaturation may occur with any lesion that produces desaturation in the pulmonary veins or left atrium. Right-to-left shunting at the ventricular level occurs when the right ventricular systolic pressure is equal to or greater than left ventricular systolic pressure (e.g., a ventricular septal defect and right ventricular outflow tract obstruction). Right-to-left shunting can occur during diastole if the right ventricular end-diastolic pressure is elevated, even if the right ventricular systolic pressure is less than that of the left ventricle. Occasionally, the streaming effect of a right-to-left shunt through a ventricular septal defect is such that the desaturation is not detected at the ventricular level but is detected in the ascending aorta (e.g., tetralogy of Fallot).

A decrease in oxygen saturation between the left ventricle and aorta requires both a communication between the aorta and the pulmonary artery and increased pulmonary vascular resistance. Typically, this is a patent ductus arteriosus or aortopulmonary window, combined with either pulmonary vascular obstructive disease or peripheral pulmonary stenosis. A decrease in saturation from the ascending to the descending aorta occurs with the combination of a patent ductus arteriosus and coarctation of the aorta; this right-to-left shunt from the pulmonary artery to the descending aorta causes pink upper extremities and cyanotic lower extremities (differential cyanosis).

Equal oxygen saturations in the aorta and pulmonary artery occur with lesions that cause complete mixing at any level. Occasionally, even when complete mixing is expected, different saturations may be found in the pulmonary artery and aorta. Most patients with truncus arteriosus have preferential streaming, resulting in lower saturation in the pulmonary artery and higher saturation in the aorta.

In children who have transposition of the great arteries with intact ventricular septum, the pulmonary artery saturation is always higher than the aortic saturation. This defines transposition physiology, higher pulmonary artery saturation than aortic saturation. This physiology is found in several anatomic lesions. With transposition of the great arteries and a large ventricular septal defect, there may be complete mixing, thus equal saturations in the pulmonary artery and aorta. If the saturation in the descending aorta is higher than that in the ascending aorta, the child has transposition of the great arteries with a patent ductus arteriosus and coarctation of the aorta (or interrupted aortic arch), causing cyanotic upper extremities and pink lower extremities (reversed differential cyanosis).

Quantitative Assessment of Shunts

Use of the Fick principle to calculate pulmonary flow (Q_p) and systemic flow (Q_s) has been discussed. To calculate left-to-right and right-to-left shunts requires understanding the concept of effective pulmonary flow (Q_{ep}) and the effective systemic flow (Q_{es}). The Q_{ep} is the volume of systemic venous return (i.e., "blue" blood) that flows to the lungs to be oxygenated. The Q_{ep} is calculated by using the oxygen saturation in the "red" blood flowing out of the lungs (pulmonary vein) minus the "blue" blood flowing into the lungs (superior vena cava) using the following equation:

$$Q_{ep} = O_2 \text{ consumption}/(1.36) \times (10) \times (Hgb) \times (\text{pulmonary vein sat} - \text{SVC sat})$$

The Q_{es} is the volume of pulmonary venous return (i.e., "red" blood) that flows to the body. In all patients:

$$Q_{ep} = Q_{es}$$

Simply stated, the amount of "blue" blood that flows to the lungs is equal to the amount of "red" blood that flows to the body.

If there is no left-to-right shunt, all of the blood flowing to the lungs (Q_p) is "blue" blood (Q_{ep}). That is:

$$Q_p = Q_{ep}$$

When there is a left-to-right shunt, some oxygenated blood recirculates through the lungs, thus $Q_p > Q_{ep}$. The volume of a left-to-right shunt is the difference between the total pulmonary flow (Q_p) and the effective pulmonary flow (Q_{ep}):

$$Q_{L\text{-}R} = Q_p - Q_{ep}$$

When there is a right-to-left shunt, some of the deoxygenated ("blue") blood bypasses the lungs and is pumped directly to the body, thus $Q_s > Q_{es}$. The volume of a right-to-left shunt is the difference between the total systemic flow (Q_s) and the effective systemic flow (Q_{es}):

$$Q_{R\text{-}L} = Q_s - Q_{es}$$

Since $Q_{ep} = Q_{es}$

$$Q_{R\text{-}L} = Q_s - Q_{ep}$$

Mathematically, the ratio of pulmonary flow to systemic flow is Q_p/Q_s. Calculating the Q_p/Q_s is simple, since the oxygen consumption (which is difficult to measure) is in the numerator of both the Q_p and Q_s equations, it cancels out, leaving the following equation:

$$Q_p/Q_s = \text{systemic AV saturation difference/}$$
$$\text{pulmonary AV saturation difference}$$

Stated in terms of oxygen saturation samples:

$$Q_p/Q_s = \text{aorta sat} - \text{superior vena cava sat/}$$
$$\text{pulmonary vein sat} - \text{pulmonary artery sat}$$

When the pulmonary blood flow is markedly increased (e.g., pulmonary artery saturation 89%), the difference in pulmonary vein–pulmonary artery saturation is small (e.g., 99% − 89%), so the normal error that occurs with each measurement (±2%–3%) becomes significant. Thus, when there is a large left-to-right shunt, the Q_p/Q_s is simply reported as "greater than 3:1."

Vascular Resistance

One of the most common indications for cardiac catheterization in children is to assess the pulmonary vascular resistance. Thus, it is crucial that the data used for this calculation are collected meticulously, the calculations are performed correctly, and the limitations of the resultant value are appreciated. The assessment of vascular resistance is based on laws of Poiseuille and Ohm. Poiseuille's law relates the constant flow (Q) in rigid tubes to the pressure drop across the tube, the cross-sectional area and length of the tube, and the viscosity of the fluid:

$$Q = (\pi) \times (\Delta P) \times (r^4)/(8) \times (\mu) \times (l)$$

where Q = flow
ΔP = inflow pressure − outflow pressure
r = radius of the tube
μ = fluid viscosity
l = length of the tube.

In the vascular system, fluid viscosity and tube length are assumed to be constant.

Combining these two constants with the other two constants (π and 8), the equation simplifies to:

$$Q = (\text{constant}) \times (\Delta P) \times (r^4)$$

Rearranging and further simplifying the equation,

$$r^4 \approx Q/(\Delta P)$$

This demonstrates that the flow divided by the change in pressure is proportional to the radius^4. This is consistent with hemodynamic calculations, where the cross-sectional area of the vascular bed is proportional to the flow divided by the change in pressure.

Vascular resistance may be conceptualized in terms of Ohm's law:

$$V = IR$$

where V = difference in electrical potential (analogous to change in pressure)
I = current (analogous to flow)
R = resistance
Rearranging the equation:

$$R = V/I$$

Adapting the equation to physiologic conditions:

$$\text{Resistance} = \text{pressure/flow}$$

In hemodynamic calculations, the vascular resistance is defined as the change in pressure across a vascular bed divided by the blood flow through that vascular bed. Combining this equation with $r^4 \approx Q/(\Delta P)$ reveals that the vascular resistance is inversely proportional to the cross-sectional area of the vascular bed.

Obviously, neither concept is an ideal description of a biologic system. Blood flow is pulsatile (not constant) and not laminar, vascular walls are distensible (not rigid), and blood is not a homogeneous fluid. In addition, vascular resistance is not a fixed entity. Rather, it is a dynamic set of blood vessels changing in response to numerous mechanical and neurohormonal factors. For example, if a sedated patient in the cath lab is hypoventilated, hypercarbia and acidosis develop, causing an elevated pulmonary vascular resistance. Another important factor affecting pulmonary resistance is pulmonary capillary recruitment, or a minimal distending pressure. When there is decreased pulmonary flow or pressure (e.g., tetralogy of Fallot, restrictive aortopulmonary shunt, cavopulmonary anastomosis), there is derecruitment of capillaries in the pulmonary vasculature, resulting in an elevated resistance (11). There is no method to predict if (and how much) the pulmonary resistance will decrease with increased flow or pressure. Nevertheless, the concept of vascular resistance is very important in managing patients with congenital heart defects. The pulmonary (R_p) and systemic (R_s) vascular resistance equations are:

$$R_p = \Delta\text{pulmonary pressure/pulmonary blood flow}$$

where Δpulmonary pressure = pulmonary artery mean pressure − left atrial mean pressure

$$R_s = \Delta\text{systemic pressure/systemic blood flow}$$

where Δsystemic pressure = systemic arterial mean pressure − right atrial mean pressure

When assessing the pulmonary vascular reactivity to various medications, a drop in pulmonary pressure may be related to the medicine decreasing the systemic resistance. Thus, calculating the relative resistances of the pulmonary and systemic vasculature may be useful information:

$$R_p/R_s = \text{pulmonary vascular resistance/}$$
$$\text{systemic vascular resistance}$$

This "hybrid" vascular resistance unit, the Wood unit, is defined in mm Hg/L/min; it is used for pediatric hemodynamic calculations. Because of the considerable size range of pediatric patients, Wood units are indexed to body surface area (mm Hg/L/min/m^2). In adult Cardiology, the metric unit of resistance (dyne·s/cm^5) is used, which requires a conversion factor of 80:

$$\text{Resistance (dyne·s/cm}^5) = \text{Wood units} \times 80$$

When calculating the pulmonary vascular resistance in patients with normal pulmonary artery pressures, the numerator (i.e., Δpressure) is a small number (4 to 10 mm Hg), similar in magnitude to the denominator (i.e., the pulmonary blood flow, 2 to 8 L/min). Thus, a 1- to 2-mm Hg error in pressure measurement can result in a large error in the calculated R_p. Thus, it is crucial to make sure the pulmonary artery and left atrial pressures are measured accurately. If there is concern for measurement error, recalibrate or change transducers to verify the pressures obtained. The normal range for indexed pulmonary resistance is 1 to 3 Wood units·m^2 (80 to 240 dyne·s/cm^5). The normal range for indexed systemic resistance is 20 to 28 Wood units·m^2 (1,600 to 2,240 dyne·s/cm^5).

Valve Area

The pressure gradient across a valve is a function of both the flow across the valve and valve orifice size. At normal flow rates, cardiac valves offer little resistance to flow. As the flow increases, a small pressure gradient may develop across a normal valve (e.g., a large left-to-right shunt through a ventricular septal defect resulting in a flow gradient across a normal pulmonary valve). Conversely, at low flow rates (e.g., shock), there may be little pressure gradient across a severely obstructed valve (e.g., neonatal critical aortic stenosis). Adult cardiologists describe valve stenosis in terms of the valve area (not the pressure gradient), as the valve area calculation includes flow. Most pediatric cardiologists describe valve gradients in terms of the peak pressure gradient across the valve. However, these pressure gradients are meaningful only when considered in conjunction with the transvalvar flow.

In 1951, Gorlin and Gorlin reported a method to calculate the valve area based on the physical properties of flow through a circular orifice and the relationship between the pressure gradient and velocity of flow (12). The valve area is calculated from the flow across the valve, the mean pressure gradient across the valve, and a constant (Table 9.3).

Flow across a valve is not continuous throughout the cardiac cycle. Flow occurs in systole for the aortic and pulmonary valves, and in diastole for the mitral and tricuspid valves. The systolic ejection time is the period during which the aortic valve is open and blood is flowing across the valve. The systolic ejection time is determined from simultaneous pressure tracings of the left ventricle and ascending aorta. The two boundaries of the systolic ejection time are the points at which the ventricular tracing crosses the aortic tracing. The diastolic filling period is the time during which the mitral valve is open, and blood is flowing across the valve. The diastolic filling period is determined from simultaneous pressure tracings of the left atrium and left ventricle; the two boundaries of the diastolic filling period are the points at which the left ventricular tracing crosses the left atrial tracing. More commonly, there are simultaneous pressure tracings of the left ventricle and the pulmonary artery capillary

TABLE 9.3

CALCULATION OF VALVE AREAS USING THE GORLIN FORMULA

Calculation of the aortic valve area:
  Determine cardiac output (in mL), systolic ejection time (in seconds/beat), and R-R interval (in seconds).
  Calculate systolic flow:

$$\text{Systolic flow} = \frac{\text{cardiac output} \times \text{R-R interval}}{60 \times \text{systolic ejection time}}$$

  Determine mean aortic valve gradient (mm Hg, by planimetry):

$$\text{Aortic valve area (cm}^2) = \frac{\text{systolic flow}}{44.5 \times \sqrt{\text{mean systolic gradient}}}$$

Calculation of mitral valve area:
  Determine cardiac output (in mL), diastolic filling time (in seconds/beat), and R-R interval (in seconds).
  Calculate diastolic flow:

$$\text{Diastolic flow} = \frac{\text{cardiac output} \times \text{R-R interval}}{60 \times \text{diastolic filling time}}$$

  Determine mean mitral valve gradient (mm Hg, by planimetry):

$$\text{Mitral valve area} = \frac{\text{Diastolic flow}}{37.8 \times \sqrt{\text{mean diastolic gradient}}}$$

wedge. These tracings must be realigned to compensate for the time delay of the pulmonary wedge tracing. In adult patients (who have slower heart rates), the wedge tracing is delayed by 50 to 70 ms; in pediatric patients (who have faster heart rates), the wedge tracing is moved to the left so that the v wave is bisected by or just precedes the downstroke of the left ventricular tracing. Once the appropriate ejection or filling period is determined, flow across the valve is calculated from the Gorlin equation:

Aortic valve flow = (cardiac output) × (R-R interval)/(60)
  × (systolic ejection time)

Mitral valve flow = (cardiac output) × (R-R interval)/(60)
  × (diastolic filling period)

In patients with congenital heart defects, determining the valve area is challenging, as the flow may be different across each valve. For example, with a ventricular septal defect, there is greater flow across the mitral valve. When the flow across a valve cannot be accurately determined, the valve area cannot be calculated; the mitral valve flow cannot be determined when there are both atrial and ventricular septal defects, and the aortic valve flow cannot be determined when there is bidirectional flow across a patent ductus arteriosus.

The mean aortic valve gradient is most accurately determined by planimetry of the area between the left ventricular and aortic tracings during the systolic ejection time. The mean mitral valve gradient is most accurately determined by planimetry of the area between the left ventricular and the left atrial (or pulmonary capillary wedge) tracings during the diastolic filling period. Previously, planimetry was done by manual tracing or averaging multiple parallel lines; now computer programs easily perform planimetry.

ANGIOCARDIOGRAPHY

Basic Concepts

This section discusses basic cardiac angiography issues, including contrast agents, radiation exposure, catheters, and camera angles. Angiographic imaging of selected defects is discussed.

Contrast Media

Contrast media are either ionic (high osmolality) or nonionic (low osmolality) compounds. Both types yield excellent image quality and contain various concentrations of iodine.

There is extensive literature discussing the advantages and disadvantages of ionic versus nonionic contrast media (13). Ionic media cause more physiologic derangement than nonionic media, including the following: a rapid shift of interstitial and intracellular fluid into the vascular space, binding serum calcium, increasing pulmonary artery and left atrial pressures, reflex tachycardia, a sensation of intense heat or pain, coughing (pulmonary artery injection), and exacerbation of pulmonary hypertension. For these and other reasons, ionic media should not be used in pediatric patients. Nonionic media are safer, well tolerated, but more expensive. To prevent blood from clotting in contrast media, heparin is added to obtain a concentration of 2 to 5 units heparin/mL of contrast.

Radiation Dose and Exposure

Compared with other diagnostic procedures performed in pediatric patients, cardiac catheterization produces a relatively large dose of radiation. In adults, the cardiac catheterization radiation dose is about 600 times the dose of a chest x-ray view (14). Pediatric patients undergoing complex diagnostic evaluation or therapeutic cardiac catheterization are exposed to longer fluoroscopy times, thus a higher radiation dose. Also, an increasingly aggressive approach to treat certain complex lesions (e.g., pulmonary atresia) has resulted in an increased number of catheterizations at an earlier age. It is difficult to quantitate the patient's risk from the radiation exposure in the cath lab. It is assumed to be greater in pediatric patients than in adults. Factors that affect the radiation dose include the duration of exposure, the body surface area exposed, and the current (mA) and voltage (kV) used to generate the image. Although the patient's risk associated with the radiation exposure should be less than that associated with untreated congenital heart defects or incomplete diagnosis, the cardiologist must be cognizant of issues that affect both the patient and staff exposure to radiation and do everything possible to minimize the exposure.

Patient Dose. Cineangiography is associated with a markedly higher radiation dose per unit time than fluoroscopy, with 1 second of cineangiography at 60 frames per second equivalent to approximately 20 seconds of fluoroscopy. Thus, in a simple diagnostic catheterization, cineangiography accounts for most of the radiation exposure. However, in lengthy interventional cases, fluoroscopy time contributes significantly to the total radiation dose. Biplane imaging (both fluoroscopy and cineangiography) doubles the radiation dose compared with single-plane imaging. Similarly, the radiation dose increases with frame rate; pulsed fluoroscopy at 30 frames per second is twice the dose of pulsed fluoroscopy at 15 frames per second. By selecting the lowest frame rate necessary (fluoroscopy and

cineangiography) and judiciously minimizing the use of biplane imaging, the cardiologist can significantly reduce the radiation dose to the patient and cath lab personnel.

Recent improvements in cath lab equipment have reduced the radiation dosage. In particular, digital flat panel imaging systems can decrease the radiation dosage from 25% to 50% compared with conventional film systems. Also, these digital flat panel systems do not increase the radiation dosage at higher levels of magnification, which is particularly important for pediatric studies.

Collimation of the x-ray beam is another important factor in reducing radiation exposure. Collimate the beam to the smallest area necessary to view the pertinent catheter and cardiovascular structures. This reduces the volume of patient tissue exposed, reduces scatter radiation to personnel, and improves image quality. Collimators should provide various shapes and sizes, particularly in a pediatric cath lab. Also, wedge filters should be positioned in the corners of the radiographic field to further reduce unnecessary radiation exposure and improve image quality.

When creating a radiographic image, three parameters are selected: milliamperes (tube current), kilovoltage, and milliseconds of exposure (pulse width). Some of these parameters are set automatically; others can be adjusted by the operator. Usually, the pulse width is selected by the operator (and occasionally the milliamperage); then the kilovoltage is determined by the equipment's automatic brightness control. One should choose the pulse width and milliamperage that result in a kilovoltage of 65 to 75 kV; higher kilovoltage degrades image quality, and lower kilovoltage results in excessive patient exposure.

Cath Lab Personnel Exposure. Much of the previous discussion of radiation exposure was relevant to both patient and cath lab staff. The following considerations apply to the protection of cath lab staff.

Scatter of the x-ray beam is the major source of personnel exposure in the cath lab. X-ray scatter increases with increasing patient size, increasing field size, and angled views. It is approximately 20 times greater with cineangiography than with fluoroscopy. Lead shielding and increased distance from the patient provide the best protection against exposure from x-ray scatter; the radiation dose decreases rapidly as one moves away from the patient ($1/r^2$) (14).

All staff working in the cardiac cath lab must wear "lead" aprons. New aprons, which are not made of lead, can be as much as 50% lighter than a lead apron, making them more comfortable to wear and producing less fatigue. They are made from several layers of very light fabric; each layer absorbs a different wavelength of radiation but covers the same radiation spectrum as a lead apron. Those personnel likely to have their backs to the patient during the procedure (e.g., staff obtaining equipment, performing transesophageal echocardiography) should wear lead aprons that completely wrap around them. A thyroid collar reduces the exposure risk to the thyroid by approximately one half. Wraparound leaded eyeglasses reduce ocular exposure by approximately one fifth. Regular eyeglasses with glass lenses provide some protection; eyeglasses with plastic lenses provide virtually no protection. For personnel who may have their hands near the x-ray field, lead-equivalent gloves are available.

Catheters

Catheters used for angiography are thin walled and have multiple side holes to allow rapid delivery of contrast media at relatively high pressures without catheter recoil (Fig. 9.4). In certain

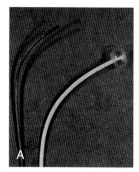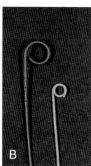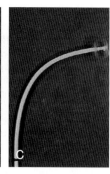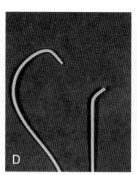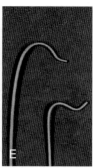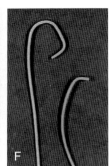

FIGURE 9.4 A: Angiographic catheters, the NIH catheter (USCI, Billerica, MA) and the Berman angiographic catheter (Arrow, Reading, PA). These two catheters have side holes but no end hole. The Berman catheter is soft and balloon tipped; it can be flow directed but cannot be effectively torqued. The NIH is a stiffer catheter, without a balloon and with an angled tip; it responds well to torque maneuvering. B: Pigtail catheters (Medi-Tech, Watertown, MA; and UMI, Ballston Spa, NY). These are thin-walled catheters that have both end and side holes, designed to deliver a large volume of contrast quickly for ventriculography. They may be angled and may have radio-opaque markers to facilitate making measurements. Note the smaller diameter curve on the right catheter, which is better for neonates and infants. C: Pulmonary wedge catheter (Arrow). This is an end-hole, balloon-tipped catheter that is not used for angiographic purposes; however, it is used for balloon-occlusion hand injections in various situations. D: End-hole catheters. There are many preformed end-hole catheters designed for selective entry of non-coronary vessels. The catheters are required for selective angiography (by hand injection) and coil embolization. Pictured are Cobra and Berenstein (Medi-Tech) catheters. E,F: Coronary artery catheters. These catheters are designed for selective hand injection of normally originating right and left coronary arteries. Pictured are the Amplatz left and right (E) and the Judkins left and right (F) (Cook, Bloomington, IN) coronary catheters.

situations, hand injections are performed using specially configured end-hole catheters. The French size of a catheter is the outer circumference in millimeters. Thus, a 5 French catheter is 5 mm in circumference and has an outer diameter of 1.67 mm. If the catheter's French size is known, the catheter may be used as a reference to determine the x-ray magnification, allowing absolute measurements to be made from the angiogram. More accurate measurements may be obtained using a marker catheter, which has radio-opaque bands placed 1 or 2 cm apart (compared with a catheter that may be only 1 to 3 mm in diameter); the x-ray beam must be perpendicular to the catheter to avoid foreshortening, which causes a calibration error.

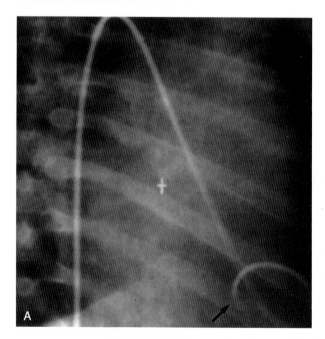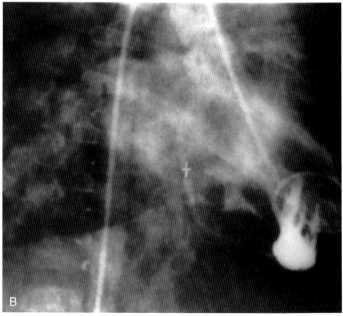

FIGURE 9.5 A: Retrograde catheter positioned for a left ventriculogram, right anterior oblique projection. Note that the pigtail catheter is partially uncurled (arrow), suggesting that the tip of the catheter is not free in the ventricle. B: Following the injection, a left ventricular stain (resulting from intramyocardial injection of contrast) is seen.

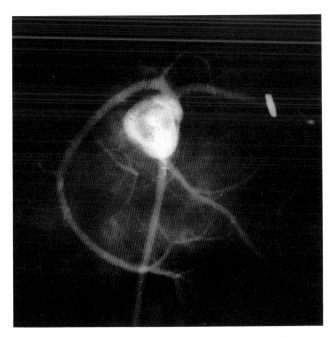

FIGURE 9.6 Caudally angulated, balloon-occlusion, ascending aortogram in transposition of the great arteries, demonstrating the left anterior descending and right coronary arteries arising from the anterior cusp and the circumflex artery arising from the posterior cusp.

Thin-walled angiographic catheters, especially the smaller French sizes, can kink with catheter manipulation; they should be advanced over a wire. Ventriculography of the systemic ventricle may be performed antegrade using the venous approach or retrograde using the arterial approach. The retrograde approach avoids catheter-induced atrioventricular valve insufficiency but requires placing a sheath in the artery. When crossing the aortic valve using the retrograde approach, it is preferable to cross the valve with a loop of wire, followed by the catheter, rather than with the tip of the wire. This prevents inadvertent wire entry into a coronary artery or perforation of a valve leaflet. A pigtail catheter should not be pushed across the aortic valve without a wire, as the catheter may become kinked. Once a catheter is positioned in the ventricle and before performing a power injection, it is necessary to ascertain that the catheter tip is not wedged in the myocardium or entangled posteriorly in the atrioventricular valve apparatus (Fig. 9.5). When positioned in a ventricle, a balloon-tipped angiographic catheter may cause less ectopy than other catheters.

Angled Views

The importance of angled views for imaging congenital heart lesions was described by Taussig in the 1940s (15). In 1977, several manuscripts were published describing the use of angled views (axial angiography) in the cardiac cath lab (2,3). Increasingly complicated surgical and transcatheter interventional techniques required more sophisticated angled views. Implementation of the arterial switch operation led to the development of the balloon occlusion ascending aortogram with caudal angulation for definition of the coronary artery origins and course (16) (Fig. 9.6). An exhaustive discussion of the use of angled views in congenital heart disease is beyond the scope of this chapter. Basic imaging of the biventricular heart, and several other common defects, is discussed.

Imaging of the Biventricular Heart

Position of the Camera, Image Intensifier, and Radiographic Source. Figure 9.7 shows a biplane catheterization laboratory with the radiographic tubes in the straight frontal (0-degree) and lateral (90-degree) positions, and the cranially angulated (25-degree) frontal camera for a sitting up view. Images acquired in those views are shown in Figure 9.8. As viewed from the image intensifier, the image plane is perpendicular to a line drawn between the x-ray tube and the image intensifier.

Right Ventricle and Pulmonary Arteries. Usually, the right ventricle is imaged in the frontal and straight lateral views. Occasionally, 0 to 25 degrees of cranial angulation is added to the frontal image intensifier. Note the following:

1. Neither view displays the interventricular septum well. The right ventricle wraps around the left ventricle. The interventricular septum should be imaged from a left ventricle injection (unless there is simple transposition of the great arteries).
2. The right ventricular outflow tract and main pulmonary artery takes a posterior course from the heart. Without cranial angulation (Fig. 9.7A), these structures are poorly imaged. The cranially angulated frontal view (Fig. 9.7C) displays the bifurcation of the pulmonary arteries, and the lateral view displays the infundibulum (Fig. 9.7B and D).
3. The right pulmonary artery courses posterior to the ascending aorta and travels laterally into the right chest, alongside of and anterior to the right bronchus (the epiarterial bronchus). It is well seen in the frontal view and almost completely foreshortened in the lateral view.
4. The left pulmonary artery courses posteriorly in the chest, anterior to the descending aorta, over and behind the left bronchus (the hyparterial bronchus). Its most proximal portion may not be well seen in either the frontal or straight lateral view; the distal portion can be seen well in the lateral view but is foreshortened in the frontal view.

Left Ventricle and Aorta. The left ventricle is imaged in the right anterior oblique (RAO) and long axial oblique (LAO) views (Fig. 9.9). The frontal image intensifier has 20 to 30 degrees of rightward angulation, whereas the lateral image intensifier has 60 to 70 degrees of leftward angulation with 20 to 30 degrees of cranial angulation. Images created with these projections are shown in Figure 9.10B and C; compare these images with that of the left ventricle as seen in the straight lateral view (Fig. 9.9D). Note the following:

1. The RAO view displays the anterior portion of the interventricular septum (between the arrowheads in Fig. 9.9B). An anterior muscular ventricular septal defect or a defect arising from conal septal hypoplasia would be displayed in this view as a jet of contrast coursing superiorly into the right ventricular outflow tract. The mitral valve is visualized, and mitral insufficiency (if present) would be noted.
2. The LAO view displays the membranous, midmuscular, and apical portions of the ventricular septum. A qualitative assessment of left ventricular function can be performed in this view.
3. Neither view optimally profiles the inlet portion of the ventricular septum.
4. The coronary arteries are displayed. The right coronary artery can be seen in the RAO and LAO views, outlining the position of the tricuspid valve. The left main coronary

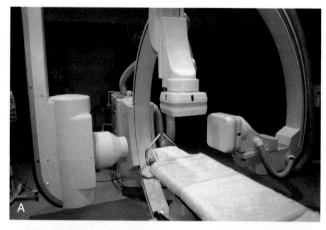

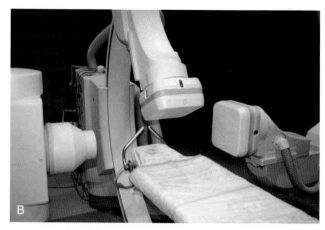

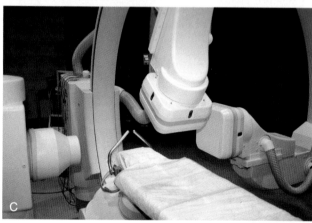

FIGURE 9.7 A: Biplane cardiac catheterization laboratory with cameras positioned for frontal and lateral projections. The frontal flat panel detector is above the table at 0 degrees, with the x-ray source below the table. The lateral flat panel detector is at 90 degrees on the patient's left, with the x-ray source to the patient's right. **B:** Frontal flat panel detector positioned for a "sitting up" view, with 25 degrees of cranial angulation. **C:** Frontal flat panel detector positioned for "laid back" view, with 30 degrees of caudal angulation.

artery is seen in the LAO view coursing posteriorly from the aortic root, bifurcating into the left anterior descending branch anteriorly and the circumflex branch posteriorly.

5. The aortic valve is imaged well (Fig. 9.10). When the left and right coronary cusps are fused, a narrow antegrade jet is seen in the RAO view (Fig. 9.10A). With fusion of the right and noncoronary cusps, the valve is seen as a straight line in the RAO view, and the narrow antegrade jet is seen in the LAO view.

For atrioventricular septal defects and posterior muscular ventricular septal defects, visualization of the inlet portion of the ventricular septum is required. This requires more cranial and more vertical angulation (than the LAO view), best displayed in the hepatoclavicular view (Fig. 9.11). The lateral image intensifier has 40 degrees of leftward angulation and 40 degrees of cranial angulation, whereas the frontal camera has 30 degrees of rightward angulation (Fig. 9.12).

Specific Techniques

Ventriculography with Abnormal Segmental Anatomy

In transposition of the great arteries with atrioventricular discordance (S,L,L), the ventricular septum is oriented more sagitally than with atrioventricular concordance (S,D,S). An angiogram performed in the (right-sided) left ventricle in a frontal projection with a small amount of oblique and cranial angulation profiles the septum well (Fig. 9.13).

Central Pulmonary Arteries. In some patients, particularly those who have tetralogy of Fallot, it is not possible to obtain sufficient cranial angulation to display the pulmonary artery bifurcation. This is true prior to and after (surgical or transcatheter) intervention. In such cases, extreme caudal angulation may display the central pulmonary artery bifurcation. The catheter must be positioned beyond the right ventricular outflow tract, as contrast in the right ventricle will obscure the pulmonary arteries (Fig. 9.14). Alternatively, RAO and LAO projections, both with cranial angulation, may display the proximal right and left branch pulmonary arteries respectively.

Left Superior Vena Cava or Venous Collateral Vessels. Definition of the venous drainage of the upper body is necessary prior to a cavopulmonary anastomosis or Fontan operation. An angiogram in the left innominate vein will display a left superior vena cava or venous collateral vessels, if they are present. The angiogram may be performed using either a side-hole angiographic catheter positioned at the junction of the left internal jugular and subclavian veins or balloon-occlusion technique using an end-hole catheter. The balloon catheter is positioned in the innominate vein just medial to the left jugular vein, the balloon is inflated (occluding the innominate vein), 2 to 5 mL of contrast is hand injected, then the balloon

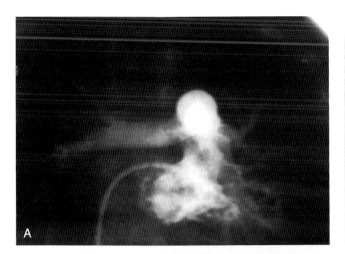

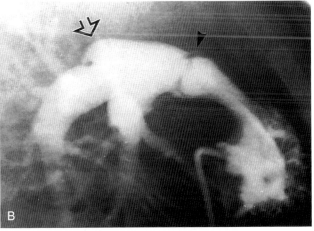

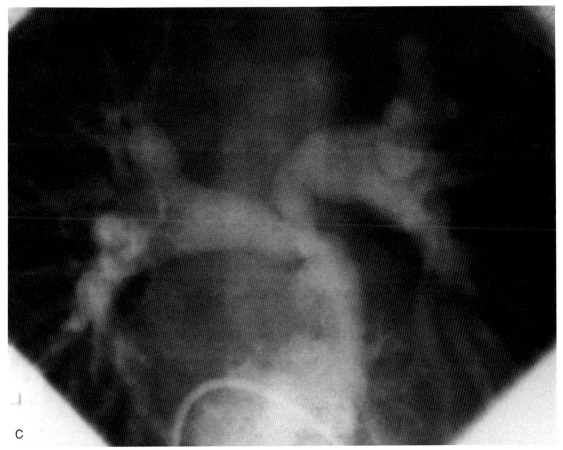

FIGURE 9.8 A,B: Right ventricle angiogram in a child with pulmonary valve stenosis. In the frontal projection (**A**), the right pulmonary artery is seen well, but the left, which courses posteriorly, is foreshortened. The lateral projection (**B**) displays the thickened, doming pulmonary valve (*arrowhead*). Most of the left pulmonary artery is seen well in this view, but the right pulmonary artery is foreshortened. There is a prominent ductus diverticulum (*open arrow*). **C:** Right ventriculogram in a child with tetralogy of Fallot. This cranially angulated projection displays the pulmonary artery bifurcation.

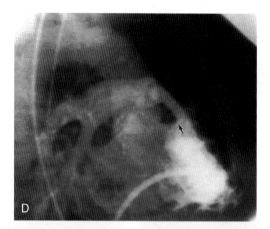

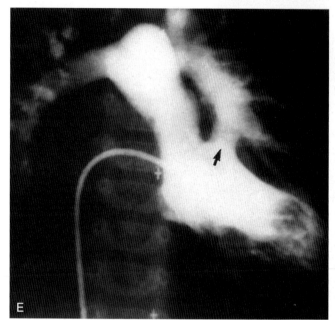

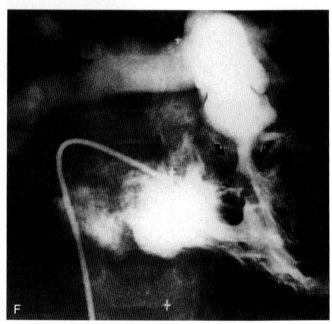

FIGURE 9.8 (*Continued*) **D:** Right ventriculogram in a child with tetralogy of Fallot. The lateral projection displays the anteriorly displaced infundibular septum (*arrow*) and associated infundibular narrowing. **E:** Left ventricular injection in a child with double-inlet single left ventricle and transposition of the great arteries. The frontal projection profiles the ventricular septal defect (bulboventricular foramen, *arrow*) with flow into the hypoplastic right ventricle. **F:** Right ventricle angiogram in a child with double-chambered right ventricle. In the frontal projection, the anomalous muscle bundles and severe narrowing of the os infundibulum are shown (*arrows*).

is deflated, allowing the contrast to drain via the right superior vena cava into the heart (Fig. 9.15).

Pulmonary Angiography through a Modified Blalock–Thomas–Taussig Shunt

Often, the pulmonary arteries can be imaged without crossing the shunt (Fig. 9.16). A balloon-tipped angiographic catheter is advanced antegrade through the heart into the subclavian artery, distal to the origin of the shunt. The balloon is inflated, occluding the distal subclavian artery, while a power injection of 1 mL/kg of contrast is performed. Positioning the side holes directly over the shunt origin prevents dense filling of the aorta, which would obscure the pulmonary arteries. In certain patients, it may be necessary to cross a modified Blalock–Thomas–Taussig

shunt to directly measure pulmonary artery pressure or for a selective pulmonary artery injection. The use of soft-tipped, floppy, 0.014- to 0.018-inch wires and 3 or 4 French soft-tipped catheters facilitates this procedure and minimizes negative hemodynamic effects. As discussed previously, to image the pulmonary artery bifurcation may require cranial or RAO/LAO angulation.

Pulmonary Vein Wedge Angiography

When the pulmonary arteries cannot be imaged by direct injection or by injection of an aortopulmonary shunt or aortopulmonary collateral, pulmonary vein wedge angiography may be necessary (17). An end-hole catheter is advanced antegrade into the pulmonary vein. A 5- to 12-mL syringe is

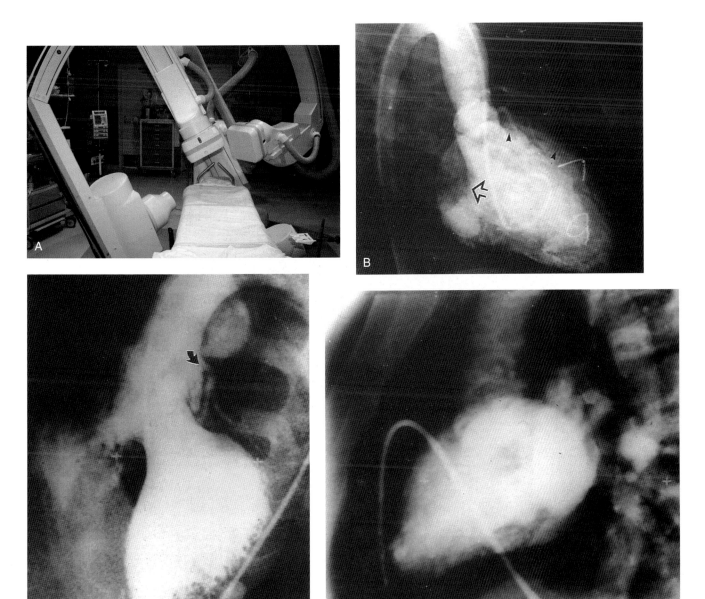

FIGURE 9.9 A: Biplane cardiac catheterization laboratory with the c-arms positioned for right anterior oblique and long axial oblique projections. The frontal flat panel detector has 20 degrees of rightward angulation, while the lateral flat panel detector has 70 degrees of leftward and 25 degrees of cranial angulation. **B:** Retrograde left ventriculogram, right anterior oblique projection. The anterior muscular septum is indicated by the two *arrowheads*; a ventricular septal defect in this region would appear as a superiorly directed contrast jet. The mitral valve is indicated by the *open arrow*, and mitral insufficiency would be seen in the view. **C:** Retrograde left ventriculogram, long axial oblique projection, in a child with a perimembranous ventricular septal defect. The defect appears to be partially covered by tricuspid valve tissue. The interventricular septum is well profiled, ruling out additional ventricular septal defects. Note that the left main coronary artery and its bifurcation into the left anterior descending and circumflex arteries are seen in this view (*arrow*). **D:** The left ventricle in a straight lateral projection, as seen on the return phase of a right ventricular injection. Note that in this projection, neither the ventricular septum nor the left ventricular outflow tract is seen well.

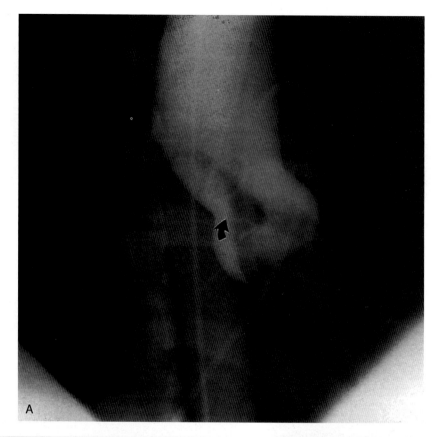

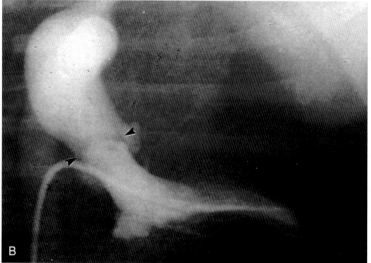

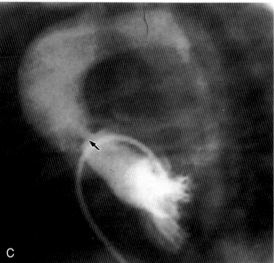

FIGURE 9.10 A: Retrograde ascending aortogram, right anterior oblique view, in a patient with aortic stenosis. The valve is bicuspid, with fusion of the left and right coronary cusps. In this view, the narrow antegrade jet emerges between the noncoronary cusp (*arrow*) and the fused coronary cusps. **B,C:** Retrograde left ventriculogram, right anterior oblique view (**B**) and long axial oblique view (**C**) in different child with aortic stenosis. There is fusion of the noncoronary and right coronary cusps. The valve is seen as a curved line (between *small arrowheads*) in the right anterior oblique view. The narrow antegrade jet (*arrow*) is seen in the long axial oblique view, emerging between the left coronary cusp and the fused cusps. Note that the valve leaflets are thickened and there is poststenotic dilation of the ascending aorta.

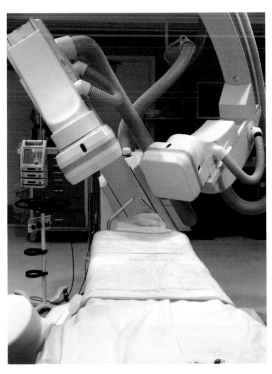

FIGURE 9.11 Biplane catheterization laboratory with c-arms positioned in the hepatoclavicular projection. The frontal flat panel detector has 30 degrees of rightward angulation, while the lateral flat panel detector has 40 degrees of and 40 degrees of cranial angulation.

held in vertical position with the plunger on top; 4 to 8 mL of saline are drawn into the syringe, followed by slowly drawing up 1 to 4 mL of nonionic contrast (0.3 mL/kg, maximum 4 mL). The contrast forms a separate layer in the syringe below the saline—as long as the syringe remains in a vertical position to avoid mixing the saline and contrast. The pulmonary vein is occluded by advancing the catheter or inflating the balloon, then the contrast and saline are slowly hand injected to backfill the pulmonary capillary bed and pulmonary artery (Fig. 9.17). If the contrast is injected too rapidly, the capillaries may rupture into the airways, causing coughing and respiratory distress. If there is significant flow to that pulmonary artery from an aortopulmonary collateral vessel, it may be necessary to balloon-occlude the collateral vessel during the injection.

Selective Coronary Arteriography

In some pediatric patients, adequate imaging of the coronary arteries is achieved with an aortic root injection, or even a left ventriculogram. Indications for selective coronary angiography include a coronary artery fistula (including pulmonary atresia with intact ventricular septum), Kawasaki's disease, heart transplant, and coronary ischemia (Figs. 9.18 and 9.19). Coronary catheter size refers to the diameter of curvature of its preformed distal end: A JL-2 catheter is a Judkins shaped tip preformed to access the left coronary artery with a 2-cm diameter of curvature of the distal tip. The proper size catheter is a function of the aortic root diameter. Some pediatric patients who require selective coronary angiography (e.g., previous arterial switch procedure, heart transplant)

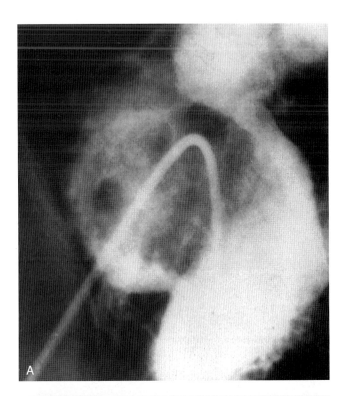

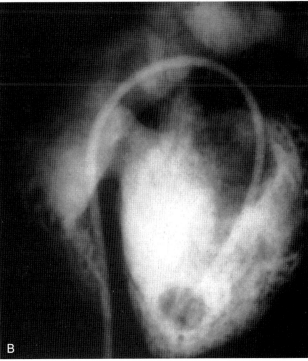

FIGURE 9.12 A: Left ventriculogram in a child with a complete common atrioventricular septal defect, hepatoclavicular view. The left ventricle is densely opacified, and contrast has crossed a large ventricular septal defect to outline the common atrioventricular valve. The right ventricle is not yet opacified in this frame. **B:** Left ventriculogram in a child with tricuspid atresia, hepatoclavicular view. The ventricular septal defect and moderately hypoplastic right ventricle are well seen.

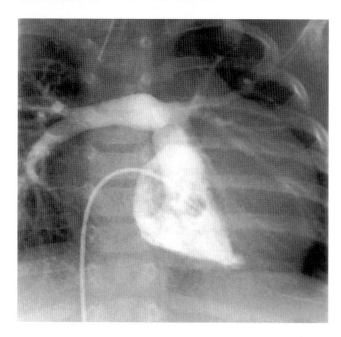

FIGURE 9.13 Left ventriculogram in a child with atrioventricular and ventriculoarterial discordance (congenitally corrected transposition). The orientation of the ventricular septum is almost in a straight sagittal plane. This patient has undergone a pulmonary artery banding procedure in preparation for a "double-switch" operation.

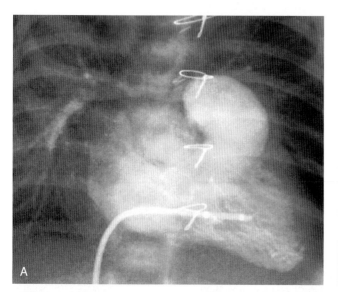

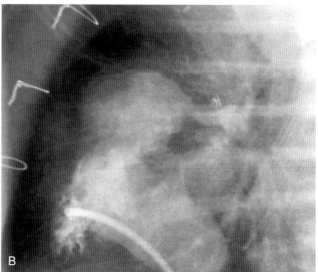

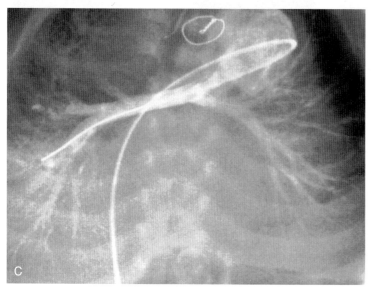

FIGURE 9.14 A: Right ventriculogram, frontal view with cranial angulation. The aneurysm of the right ventricular outflow patch overlaps the bifurcation of the pulmonary arteries, obscuring their origins. B: Right ventriculogram, lateral view. Obstruction of the distal main pulmonary artery is demonstrated, but the pulmonary artery bifurcation is not imaged. C: Proximal right pulmonary artery angiogram (over a wire). The caudally angulated view demonstrates the pulmonary artery bifurcation and the main right and left pulmonary arteries.

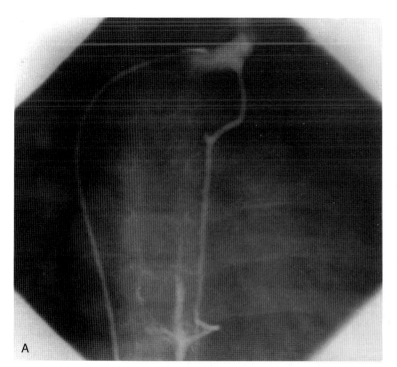
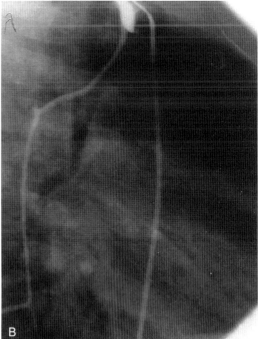

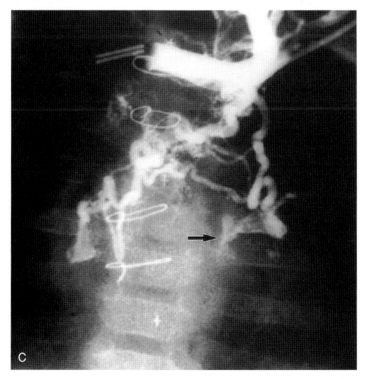

FIGURE 9.15 Balloon-occlusion angiography to define systemic venous drainage. **A,B:** Frontal projection (**A**), with the balloon occluded in the proximal left innominate vein, a left superior vena cava is ruled out. However, a prominent superior intercostal vein is seen. The lateral projection (**B**) confirms the posterior course of the vessel. **C:** After a bidirectional cavopulmonary anastomosis, a balloon-occlusion left innominate vein angiogram demonstrated a complex network of venous collaterals. One portion of this network drains directly into the left atrium (*arrow*), which is a potential source of cyanosis.

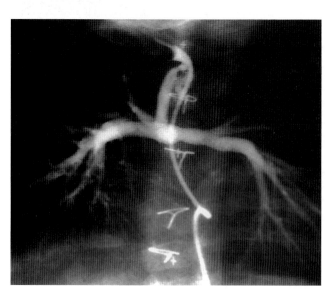

FIGURE 9.16 Imaging of the pulmonary arteries through a modified right Blalock–Thomas-Taussig shunt, using a balloon-occlusion injection in the right subclavian artery. (See text for details.)

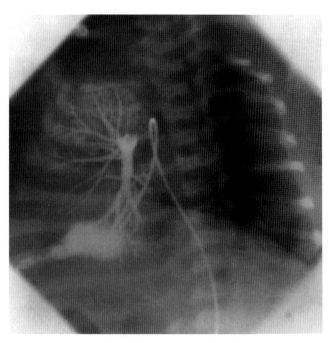

FIGURE 9.17 A right pulmonary vein wedge angiogram displaying the right pulmonary artery in an infant with congenital discontinuity of the pulmonary arteries and a thrombosed right-sided modified Blalock–Thomas-Taussig shunt. The right upper lobe is not opacified owing to a thrombus. The atelectasis of the right lung results in displacement of the heart into the right chest.

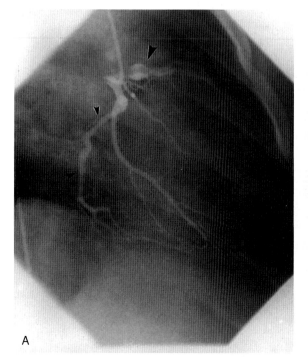

A

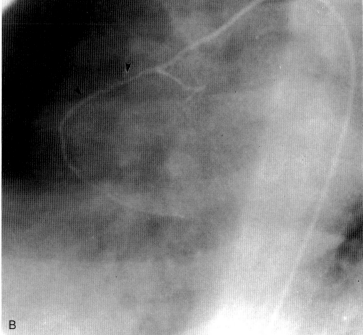

B

FIGURE 9.18 Selective coronary artery angiography in a patient with Kawasaki's disease. **A:** Left main coronary artery angiogram, right anterior oblique projection. Aneurysms are seen in the left main coronary artery extending into the left anterior descending artery (*large arrowheads*) as well as in the circumflex artery (between *small arrowheads*). **B:** Right coronary artery angiogram, left anterior oblique view with caudal angulation. An irregular, beaded area is seen in the middle third of the right coronary artery (*small arrowheads*).

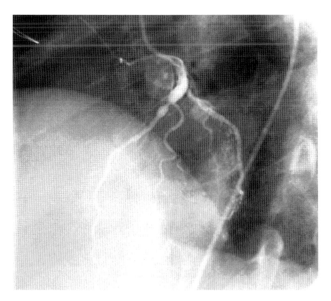

FIGURE 9.19 Selective coronary angiogram. Severe, diffuse coronary artery disease 1 year after orthotopic heart transplant. Note the stenotic lesions in the proximal right and left anterior descending arteries.

have atypical locations of the coronary artery origins (Fig. 9.20). Successful cannulation of the coronary arteries requires an understanding of the anatomy and choosing the appropriate catheter for this anatomy; a right coronary catheter may easily enter the left coronary orifice. Initially, an aortic root injection may be necessary to display the coronary artery origins. Occasionally, when there is a ventricular septal defect (including tetralogy of Fallot) or the aorta arises from the right ventricle (transposition of the great arteries), antegrade selective coronary angiography can be performed.

Imaging of a Subaortic Membrane

The LAO projection displays the left ventricular outflow tract. A subaortic membrane may be displayed by including 20 to 25 degrees of caudal angulation to the right anterior oblique projection.

Definition of Aortopulmonary Collateral Vessels

In patients with obstructed pulmonary flow (tetralogy of Fallot, pulmonary atresia, complex single ventricle), accurate definition of the collateral supply to the pulmonary arteries is crucial prior to surgical or transcatheter intervention. Initially, an aortogram is performed to display all aortopulmonary collateral vessels. In an infant, this is best accomplished by an antegrade balloon-occlusion injection in the descending aorta, with the balloon inflated just below the diaphragm. This is followed by selective injections in the subclavian arteries and in the collateral vessels (Fig. 9.21). When a pulmonary lobar segment is supplied by more than one source (e.g., a native pulmonary artery and a collateral vessel, or two collateral vessels), temporary balloon occlusion of the collateral vessel along with simultaneous injection in the other vessel may be necessary to accurately define the pulmonary anatomy. Aor-

topulmonary collateral or dilated bronchial vessels can occur in patients with transposition of the great arteries, although in most cases they are of no physiologic significance; a descending aortogram should identify these vessels (18).

Imaging the Aortic Arch in Critical Left-Sided Heart Obstruction

Many infants with left heart obstruction undergo surgery without a heart catheterization. When angiographic definition of the arch anatomy is required, a left ventriculogram or ascending aortogram can be performed. Alternatively, a balloon angiographic catheter can be advanced antegrade through the right heart, across the patent ductus arteriosus into the descending aorta. A balloon-occlusion angiogram is performed as the retrograde filling displays the aortic arch (Fig. 9.22).

Complications

Although patients referred for cardiac catheterization are now smaller and have more complex cardiac abnormalities, the procedure has become safer. Cassidy et al. (19) reported the complication rate in >1,000 procedures; there were 885 diagnostic studies and a median age of 15.6 months. Two deaths were complications of the catheterization, for a mortality of 0.2%; two other deaths that occurred shortly after the procedure were attributed to the underlying disease. There were 26 serious complications (2.4%) (10).

Patient with Pulmonary Vascular Disease

There is an increased risk associated with cardiac catheterization of children who have elevated pulmonary vascular resistance (20). The periprocedural mortality has been reduced markedly by advances in pharmacologic management of pulmonary hypertension, and by using a team of experienced pediatric cardiologists and cardiac anesthesiologists. Indications for catheterization include hemodynamic evaluation, assessment of the disease severity, and pulmonary reactivity using pharmacologic agents. In most cases, pulmonary artery angiography should be avoided, as it could precipitate acute pulmonary artery vasoconstriction, which could be fatal. If pulmonary angiography is necessary, the use of nonionic contrast media and selective pulmonary artery injections or pulmonary artery wedge injections are recommended. In patients with severe right-sided heart failure caused by pulmonary hypertension who do not have an intracardiac shunt as a "pop-off," any elevation in pulmonary vascular resistance (e.g., acidosis, contrast injection) may result in systemic hypotension. Also, they may become bradycardic and hypotensive with rapid infusion of small volumes of fluid into the right atrium or ventricle (e.g., during thermodilution cardiac output measurements).

Arrhythmias

Arrhythmias during cardiac catheterization are common. Preprocedural evaluation of electrolytes and drug levels and ensuring adequate ventilation during the procedure are important. Typically, arrhythmias result from catheter impact on the myocardium and usually resolve with repositioning the catheter. However, bradyarrhythmias or tachyarrhythmias of brief duration can have serious consequences in the child who has little hemodynamic reserve. In children who have a supraventricular arrhythmia or atrial enlargement, it is prudent

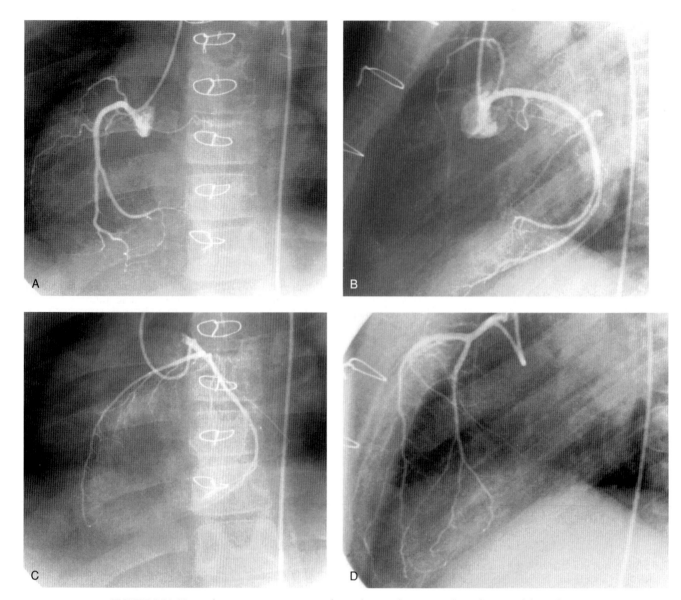

FIGURE 9.20 Unusual coronary artery pattern after orthotopic heart transplant of a normal donor heart into a child with heterotaxy syndrome. The heart was implanted using venous anastomoses. Straight posteroanterior and lateral views. In **A** and **B**, the right coronary artery originates posteriorly and courses posteriorly and rightward. In **C** and **D**, the left main coronary artery arises anteriorly and bifurcates into the left anterior descending and circumflex arteries.

to avoid stretching the atrium. Careful catheter manipulation, and in some lesions using tip-deflector wires or balloon-tipped catheters to diminish irritation of the myocardium, are helpful in avoiding arrhythmias. In children with severe or critical aortic stenosis, pretreatment with lidocaine prior to entering the left ventricle may decrease the risk of ventricular arrhythmias. Catheter-induced atrioventricular block can easily occur in children with atrioventricular discordance (S, L, L), but can also occur in children with d-transposition of the great arteries (S, D, D) and tetralogy of Fallot, particularly during passage of a catheter from the right ventricle to the aorta. Children with baseline ECG evidence of bifascicular block are at increased risk for complete complete heart block during retrograde passage of a catheter from the aorta into the left ventricle. For these

patients, it is prudent to have a pacing catheter and a stimulator readily available prior to placement of any catheters in the heart.

Cardiac Perforation

Improved catheter technology and better noninvasive definition of the cardiac anatomy have resulted in fewer complications, including cardiac perforation. Pushing a wire or Brockenbrough needle through the wall of the heart usually does not cause a problem owing to the small size of the puncture. Passage of anything larger (e.g., dilator, catheter, sheath) through the atrial wall is likely to require surgical repair. Perforations in the ventricle are more likely to seal over without

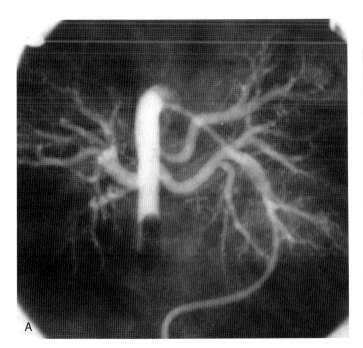
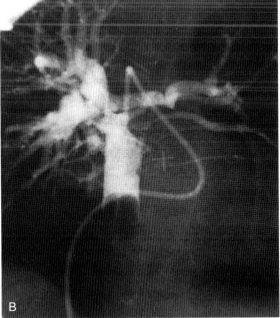
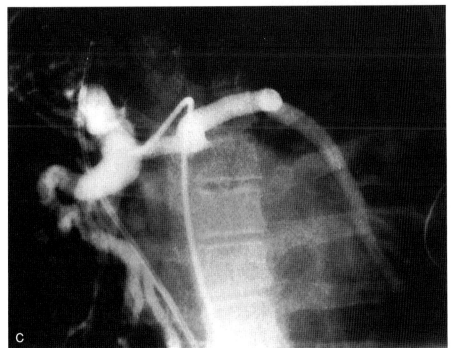

FIGURE 9.21 Definition of aortopulmonary collaterals in an infant with pulmonary atresia, ventricular septal defect. **A:** Antegrade balloon-occlusion decending aortogram. No central pulmonary arteries are seen. There are three collateral vessels. **B:** In a different infant with this same defect, antegrade balloon-occlusion decending aortogram reveals continuous pulmonary arteries supplied by a right-sided collateral vessel from the descending aorta. **C:** A selective injection into an aortopulmonary collateral vessel displays small but continuous pulmonary arteries.

needing surgery. The most common sites of cardiac perforation are the atrial appendages (especially if the heart is viewed in only one plane), the right ventricular outflow tract of small infants, the right ventricle during endomyocardial biopsy, the left ventricular apex, and the aortic valve cusps. When hypotension occurs during or shortly after cardiac catheteri-

zation, cardiac perforation resulting in tamponade must be considered. An echocardiogram should be obtained immediately. While in the cath lab, there are two fluoroscopic clues to alert the staff about a pericardial effusion: An enlarged cardiac silhouette and absence of movement of the cardiac silhouette; this exemplifies the importance of knowing the

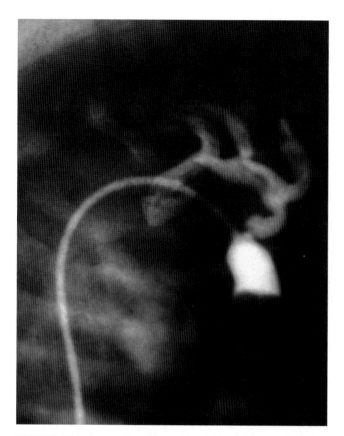

FIGURE 9.22 Antegrade catheter course through a patent ductus arteriosus to perform a balloon-occlusion aortogram. This demonstrates a severe coarctation of the aorta and hypoplastic arch just proximal to origin of the ductus arteriosus.

cardiac size, shape, and motion prior to starting the catheterization. When cardiac perforation occurs, initial treatment includes removal of the catheter, and observation. If clinically indicated, pericardiocentesis is performed. By connecting a stopcock and sterile intravenous (IV) tubing to the pericardial drain, the drained blood can be reinfused into a venous catheter (this may exacerbate a coagulopathy). If there is continued accumulation of pericardial blood, packed red blood cells and plasma are indicated while surgical repair is arranged.

Hypotension

Children with congenital heart defects have multiple possible causes for hypotension during cardiac catheterization. In addition to intracardiac catheter manipulation, pericardial effusion, and arrhythmias (previously discussed), other causes of hypotension include the following: Blood loss, hypothermia, contrast reaction, hypoventilation (acidosis), hyperventilation or oxygen administration (with a large left-to-right shunt), and certain anesthetic agents (decrease in peripheral vascular resistance, myocardial depressants).

Peripheral Vascular Injury

Factors contributing to peripheral vascular injury include small vessel size (in infants), large catheter or sheath size, multiple previous entries into the vessel, multiple catheter exchanges, and improper technique for achieving vascular

access or hemostasis. Measures that reduce the incidence and severity of peripheral vascular injury include the following: Skilled percutaneous access (not cutdown), the use of a small IV catheter in the artery (until a sheath is needed to perform angiography or intervention), use of finely tapered sheaths and dilators over appropriate-sized wires, systemic heparinization, antegrade left-sided heart catheterization through a patent foramen ovale, and efficient execution of the procedure minimizing the time catheters are in the vessel (21). At the end of the procedure, the catheters and sheaths should be aspirated to remove any thrombus, and then they are removed, allowing the vessel to bleed back briefly. Hemostasis is achieved by applying pressure with one or two fingers cephalad to the site of percutaneous entry, which should be at the site of entry into the vessel. Just enough pressure is needed to prevent bleeding from the vessel, not necessarily completely occluding all flow through the vessel. While holding pressure, the pedal pulses should be palpated often to ensure adequate perfusion. It is wrong to place a large gauze bandage over the entry site, then lean heavily on it, as this does not prevent bleeding from the vessel into the surrounding tissues, it does not allow the entry site to be monitored visually, and this excessive pressure may result in vessel thrombosis. The routine use of sandbags or mechanical devices to apply pressure to percutaneous sites is contraindicated in pediatric catheterization procedures.

After a diagnostic catheterization, pulse loss is rare. Even in small infants, the use of a 3 French pigtail catheter tapered to a 0.021-inch wire should allow a safe retrograde arterial catheterization (although the catheter flow rate is low). When loss of a pulse occurs, heparin is continuously infused until the pulse returns or for 12 to 24 hours. There is likely a component of arterial spasm, and heparin may prevent thrombus formation at the site of spasm. If the pulse does not return, treatment with streptokinase or tPA may be instituted unless contraindications are present (22,23).

Hypoventilation

The combination of pharmacologic sedation and physical immobilization during cardiac catheterization fosters hypoventilation. In addition, the conditions imposed by jugular or subclavian access can increase the risk of airway compromise. Infants with Down syndrome are at increased risk for airway obstruction. Infants receiving a prostaglandin infusion frequently become apneic, which can be exacerbated after receiving sedation. Prevention of hypoventilation requires constant attention to the status of the airway, including movement of the chest wall and the diaphragm (by fluoroscopy), and to the sound of the respirations, and continuous pulse oximetry arterial saturation monitoring. Many diagnostic cardiac catheterizations can be performed safely using conscious sedation. Elective intubation should be considered in the presence of high-risk characteristics, such as marginal cardiac function, airway abnormality, gastroesophageal reflux with aspiration, moderately to severely elevated pulmonary vascular resistance, a prostaglandin infusion, or the need for internal jugular venous access in a small infant.

Embolism

Although pulmonary or systemic emboli are rare during cardiac catheterization in children, the potential for an embolic event is real, and the results can be devastating. Air, thrombus, and broken wires or catheters can embolize. Conditions that increase the risk of an embolic event include the use of large sheath size (particularly when placed in the left heart or with a right-to-left shunt), cyanosis with polycythemia or anemia, and prolonged catheter manipulation in the ascending aorta or transverse arch. Precautions that decrease the risk of an embolism include systemic heparinization (50 to 100 U/kg), frequent aspiration and flushing of catheters, use of carbon dioxide to inflate balloon catheters, and positioning the arterial catheter distal to the brachiocephalic vessels.

Hypercyanotic Episode

Despite appropriate precautions (hydration, sedation, careful catheter manipulation), infants and children with tetralogy of Fallot and some forms of double-outlet single ventricle are at risk for a hypercyanotic episode ("tet spell") during or shortly after cardiac catheterization. This complication occurs more frequently in small, cyanotic infants. There are no data to predict which patients are likely to have a "spell." When cardiac catheterization is indicated, it should be carried out as expeditiously as possible, with awareness on the part of everyone involved that the patient's condition places him or her at increased risk for a serious complication. Often, thorough echocardiographic assessment will have determined much of the anatomy, leaving one or more specific remaining questions (e.g., coronary artery anatomy, distal pulmonary artery anatomy, additional ventricular septal defects, collateral vessels, mitral stenosis); these unanswered questions should be answered first. A left ventriculogram provides much anatomic information (the ventricular septum, right ventricular outflow tract, coronary arteries), and may be the first angiogram performed; subsequent angiograms (pulmonary artery, ascending aorta) are obtained to complete the evaluation. Increasing cyanosis, hyperpnea, fluctuating arterial oxygen saturation, progressive hypoxemia, and metabolic acidosis can be indications of an impending hypercyanotic episode. Appropriate treatment includes administration of volume (saline, then red blood cells if needed), morphine sulfate, phenylephrine or other peripheral vasoconstrictors, sodium bicarbonate (for acidosis), and intubation (if not already performed). General anesthesia can be helpful, but it will not "break" a hypercyanotic episode.

Latex Allergy

Latex allergy can result in a wide range of symptoms, from contact urticaria to life-threatening anaphylaxis. Overwhelming anaphylaxis generally occurs during surgery and results from patient exposure to surgical latex gloves. This problem has occurred in patients who previously had minor symptoms caused by contact with latex [24]. There have been no reports of anaphylaxis owing to use of intravascular latex catheter balloons. For any patient with any history of latex allergy undergoing cardiac catheterization, standard institutional protocols for latex precautions should be observed. Specific questioning regarding a history of latex allergy is prudent, especially in patients with spina bifida and myelomeningocele, in whom latex hypersensitivity is prevalent.

The author wishes to acknowledge previous authors of this chapter, Drs. Nancy D. Bridges, Martin P. O'Laughlin, Charles E. Mullins, and Michael P. Freed. Many of their contributions remain as core information in this chapter.

Textbook References That Exclusively Discuss Cardiac Catheterization, Angiography, and Intervention

1. Mullins CE. *Cardiac Catheterization in Congenital Heart Disease: Pediatric and Adult*. Malden, MA: Blackwell Publishing, 2006.
2. Lock JE, Keane JF, Perry SB. *Diagnostic and Interventional Catheterization in Congenital Heart Disease*. 2nd ed. New York: Springer Publishing, 2000.
3. Freedom RM, Mawson JB, Yoo SJ, et al. *Congenital Heart Disease: Textbook of Angiocardiography*. Malden, MA: Blackwell Publishing, 1997.
4. Baim D. *Grossman's Cardiac Catheterization, Angiography, and Intervention*. 7th ed. Philadelphia: Lippincott Williams & Wilkins, 2005.

References

1. Forssmann W. Die sondierung des rechten herzen. *Klin Wochenschr* 1929;8:2085–2087.
2. Bargeron LM, Elliot LP, Soto B, et al. Axial cineangiography in congenital heart disease. I and II. Concept, technical and anatomic considerations, specific lesions. *Circulation* 1977;56:1075–1093.
3. Fellows KE, Keane JF, Freed MD. Angled views in cineangiography of congenital heart disease. *Circulation* 1977;56:485–490.
4. Lock JE, Keane JF, Fellows KE. Diagnostic and interventional catheterization in congenital heart disease. Boston: Martinus Nijhoff, 1987:11–13.
5. Fick A. Uber die messung des blutquantums in den herzventrikeln. *Sitz der Physik-Med Ges Wurtzberg* 1870:16.
6. Ganz W, Donoso R, Marcus HS, et al. A new technique for measurement of cardiac output by thermodilution in man. *Am J Cardiol* 1971;27:392–396.
7. Lister G, Hoffman JIE, Rudolph AM. Oxygen uptake in infants and children: A simple method for measurement. *Pediatrics* 1974;53:656–661.
8. Lafarge CG, Miettinen OS. The estimation of oxygen consumption. *Cardiovasc Res* 1970;4:23–30.
9. Yang SS, Bentivoglio L, Maranhao V, et al. *From Cardiac Catheterization Data to Hemodynamic Parameters*. 2nd ed. Philadelphia: FA Davis Co, 1978:8–24.
10. Freed MD, Miettinen OS, Nadas AS. Oximetric detection of intracardiac left-to-right shunts. *Br Heart J* 1979;42:690–694.
11. Wafner WW. Capillary recruitment in the pulmonary microcirculation. *Chest* 1988;93:85S–88S.
12. Gorlin R, Gorlin G. Hydraulic formula for calculation of area of stenotic mitral valve, other cardiac valves, and central circulatory shunts. *Am Heart J* 1951;41:1–29.
13. Bettman MA. Radiographic contrast agents: A perspective. *N Engl J Med* 1987;317:891–893.
14. Moore RJ. *Imaging Principles of Cardiac Angiography*. Queenstown, MD: Aspen, 1990:207–239.
15. Taussig HB. *Congenital Malformations of the Heart*. New York: The Commonwealth Fund, 1947:24–29.
16. Mandell VS, Lock JE, Mayer JE, et al. The "laid-back" aortogram: An improved angiographic view for demonstration of coronaries in transposition of the great arteries. *Am J Cardiol* 1990;65:1379–1383.
17. Nihill MR, Mullins CE, McNamara DG. Visualization of the pulmonary arteries in pseudotruncus by pulmonary vein wedge angiography. *Circulation* 1978;58:140–147.
18. Wernovsky G, Bridges ND, Mandell VS, et al. Persistent bronchial collaterals following early repair of transposition of the great arteries. *J Am Coll Cardiol* 1993;21:465–470.
19. Cassidy SC, Schmidt KG, van Hare GF, et al. Complications of pediatric cardiac catheterization: A three-year study. *J Am Coll Cardiol* 1992;19:1285–1293.
20. Keane JF, Fyler DC, Nadas AS. Hazards of cardiac catheterization in children with primary pulmonary vascular obstruction. *Am Heart J* 1978;96:556–558.
21. Freed MD, Keane JF, Rosenthal A. The use of heparinization to prevent arterial thrombosis after percutaneous cardiac catheterization in children. *Circulation* 1974;50:565–569.
22. Wessel DL, Keane JF, Fellows KE, et al. Fibrinolytic therapy for femoral arterial thrombosis after cardiac catheterization in infants and children. *Am J Cardiol* 1986;58:347–351.
23. Carlson KM, Rutledge JM, Parker BR, et al. Use of tissue plasminogen activator for femoral artery thrombosis following transcatheter coil occlusion of patent ductus arteriosus. *Pediatr Cardiol* 2005;26(1):83–86.
24. Sussman GL, Tarlo S, Dolovich J. The spectrum of IgE-mediated responses to latex. *JAMA* 1991;265:2844–2847.

CHAPTER 10 ■ DEVELOPMENT AND FUNCTION OF THE CARDIAC CONDUCTION SYSTEM

ARTHUR S. PICKOFF, MD

In this chapter, current concepts regarding the development and function of the cardiac conduction system will be summarized, including information concerning the expression of genetic markers of the developing cardiac conduction system and emerging information concerning transcriptional regulation of the specialized cardiac conduction system (1). Functional properties and electrophysiologic characteristics of the developing conduction system are discussed in conjunction with morphologic considerations.

INITIATION OF THE HEARTBEAT

Rhythmic contraction of the heart is present very early in embryonic life, appearing first in the bulboventricular portion of the primitive, unlooped heart tube. This led to the belief that the first electrical pacemaker to be manifest in the embryo was at a bulboventricular site, with atrialization of the pacemaker site later during development. Subsequent microelectrode studies, however, suggested that atrial pacemaker sites, not ventricular, are the first to be expressed in the chick embryo (2). More recent studies using voltage-sensitive dyes that detect spontaneous electrical depolarization have demonstrated that pacemaker activity in the chick embryo can be identified in both atrial and bulboventricular portions of the heart as early as the seventh somite stage, prior to any contractile activity (at about the tenth somite stage). By the early to mid ninth somite stage, pacemaker activity is virtually confined to atrial regions. Pacemaker activity at this early embryonic stage appears to result from the activity of a circular aggregate of approximately 100 cells (3). That contraction in the embryonic heart appears first within the ventricle and only later in the atrium is now believed to be due to differences in regional maturation of contractile elements, rather than to a shift of pacemaker activity from ventricle to atrium.

The factors that determine the cardiac pacemaker rates throughout development are complex and incompletely understood. It is known that tissue culture explants of precardiac mesenchymal tissue, destined to form specific regions of the heart, differentiate into cells with characteristic, preprogrammed beating rates. Sinoatrial-destined cell lines have intrinsic rates that are higher than those for mesenchyme destined to form ventricle or conus. These differences in intrinsic rate are thought to be the result of genetically determined differences in ion channel and ion pump activity, and of yet unidentified regional cues (4). There are few data regarding developmental changes in the ionic currents responsible for spontaneous membrane depolarization. Very early in embryonic life, prior to the development of true pacemaker ionic current(s), shuttling of calcium in and out of the sarcoplasmic reticulum, through an inositol triphosphate dependent mechanism, may be responsible for pacemaker activity at the earliest stages of development (5). Clusters of murine embryonic stem cells that in vitro demonstrate spontaneous depolarization (pacemaker nodes) emit calcium signals to adjacent contractile cells and are characterized by the expression of the genetic molecular marker GATA6 (7). With maturation, both a decline in an outward potassium current and activation of an inward ion current (probably involving calcium) are likely responsible for spontaneous depolarization. Another inward cationic current, termed If, identified in hyperpolarized sinus node cells, also may contribute to pacemaker activity of the sinus node.

Looping of the embryonic heart may be an important process in the development of the sinoatrial pacemaker. Contact between differentiated atrial muscle cells and undifferentiated noncardiac mesenchyme that occurs as a result of the looping process may, in itself, contribute to the induction and organization of the sinoatrial pacemaker (6,8).

It is just after looping that the sinus node is first morphologically identified in the human embryo (Carnegie stage 15, 5 weeks of age) (6,9). The sinus node occupies a subepicardial position at the lateral junction of the superior vena cava and right atrium (Fig. 10.1). The node is characteristically horseshoe shaped in the fetus and usually assumes more of a spindle shape with development. It is larger, relative to the atrium, in the fetus than in the adult. By light microscopy, the cells of the sinus node are morphologically distinct from the surrounding atrial myocardium; they are smaller, more compact, and contained within a fibrous matrix (10) (Fig. 10.2). A tail of transitional cells extends inferiorly from the sinus node to the terminal crest of the atrium. Malposition of the sinus node may occur in conditions in which normal atrial arrangement is lacking. These entities include left juxtaposition of the atrial appendages, where anterior displacement of the sinus node is observed; right atrial isomerism, where bilateral sinus nodes are formed; and left atrial isomerism, where a sinus node may not be identifiable (Fig. 10.3).

PROPAGATION OF THE ELECTRICAL IMPULSE FROM THE SINUS NODE TO THE ATRIOVENTRICULAR NODE

Specialized conduction pathways within the atrium have been proposed as a basis for preferential conduction of the cardiac impulse from the sinus node, through the atrium, to the atrioventricular (AV) node. In the human heart, three such

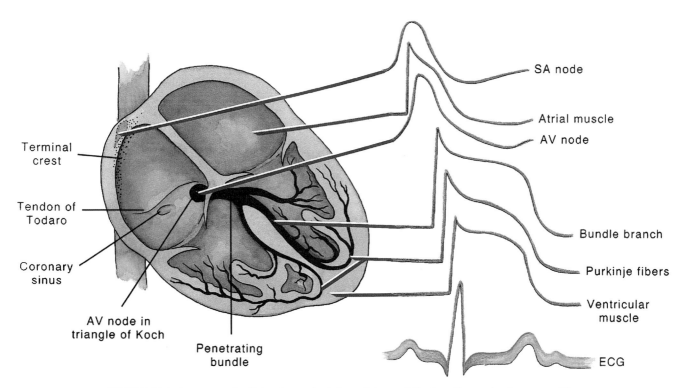

FIGURE 10.1 Anatomy and cellular electrophysiology of the specialized cardiac conduction system. The sinus (SA) node is the normal site of impulse formation in the heart. Automaticity is the result of slow depolarization of the cell from its resting membrane potential of −50 to −60 mV to its threshold potential (phase 4 depolarization). The action potential of the sinus node is characterized by a slow maximum upstroke velocity (1 to 10 V/s). Propagation of the impulse then occurs through the atrial myocardium. Atrial action potentials have a resting membrane potential of −80 to −90 mV, a maximum upstroke velocity of 100 to 200 V/s, and an abbreviated plateau phase. The atrioventricular (AV) node is located in the right atrium in the triangle of Koch. Action potentials from the midregion of the AV node have resting membrane potentials of −60 to −70 mV and a slow maximum upstroke velocity of 5 to 15 V/s. Refractoriness of AV nodal cells is both voltage and time dependent. These AV node characteristics result in slowing of conduction between atrium and ventricle and filtering of rapid or closely coupled beats. From the AV node, the penetrating bundle (or His bundle) arises and then divides into the right and left bundle branches. Purkinje fibers are characterized by action potentials with a low resting membrane potential (−90 mV), a rapid maximum upstroke velocity (500 to 700 V/s), and, therefore, a rapid conduction velocity. Action potential durations are longest in the Purkinje system (300 to 500 ms). Ventricular muscle cell action potentials are characterized by a resting membrane potential, maximum upstroke velocity, and duration that are slightly less than those for Purkinje fibers. (Illustrations are modified from Netter FH, illus. The CIBA collection of medical illustrations. Vol. 5. Heart. Summit, NJ: CIBA Publications, 1969, with permission. Action potential values are from Moak JP. Cardiac electrophysiology. In: Garson A Jr, Bricker T, McNamara DG, eds. *The Science and Practice of Pediatric Cardiology.* Vol 1. Philadelphia: Lea & Febiger, 1990:294–317, with permission.)

internodal pathways have been proposed: one running along the terminal crest of the atrium and one each along the anterior and posterior aspects of the interatrial septum (11). Earlier demonstrations of such pathways are most compelling in studies of the developing heart (12,13). More recently, in the human heart, Gittenberger-deGroot identified three internodal pathways connecting the sinus node and atrioventricular node following incorporation of the sinus venosus into the atrium. These studies, which used the HNK1 antibody to track development of the cardiac conduction system, suggested that these internodal tracks (as well as portions of the posterior left atrial wall surrounding the pulmonary veins) are derivatives of the embryonic sinoatrial ring (14). Despite these observations, the lack of light or electron microscopic evidence of true specialized cell types, or of insulation from surrounding atrial

myocardium, have been cited as evidence against specialized internodal conduction pathways (15). Electrophysiologic studies of impulse propagation in the dog atrium and rabbit atrium in the past have largely failed to find evidence of discrete, specialized conduction pathways connecting the sinus and AV nodes (16). In contrast, more recent studies of the input pathways to the canine AV node have claimed identification of three discrete bundles of myocardial fibers linking the inferior aspects of the right atrium, and possibly the sinus node, to the AV node (17,18).

Whether or not true specialized internodal conduction pathways exist, conduction within the atrium occurs as waves of excitation that propagate along specific bands of atrial myocardium. Interestingly, these bands of myocardium correspond roughly to the locations of two of the internodal

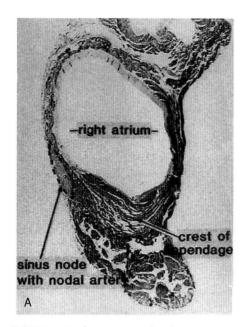
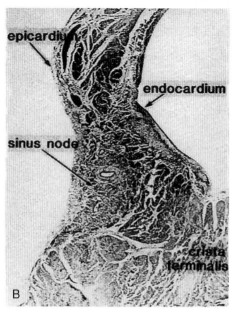

FIGURE 10.2 Photomicrographs of the sinus node. A: Section at the junction of the superior vena cava and right atrium demonstrating a spindle-shaped appearance of the node. B: The sinus node viewed in a plane perpendicular to A. (From Anderson RH, Ho SY. Cardiac conduction system in normal and abnormal hearts. In: Roberts NK, Gelband H, eds. *Cardiac Arrhythmias in the Neonate, Infant, and Child.* 2nd ed. Norwalk, CT: Appleton-Century-Crofts, 1983:1–35; with permission.)

pathways (terminal crest and anterior septum) (16). Preferential conduction along these bands may be related simply to a more uniform, longitudinal geometric arrangement of atrial myocardial cells at these sites, rather than the presence of true, specialized internodal pathways. Compared with other regions in the atrium, atrial myocardial cells in the terminal

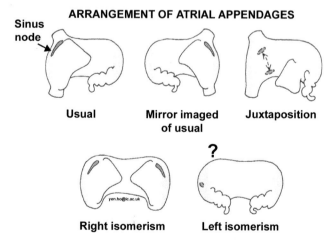

FIGURE 10.3 Localization of the sinus node in variations of arrangement of the atrial appendages. In the usual arrangement (atrial situs solitus), the sinus node is located at the junction of the superior vena cava and right atrium. The reverse occurs in atrial situs inversus (mirror imaged). In juxtaposition of the atrial appendages, the sinus node becomes displaced along the right atrial anterior wall. In right isomerism there are bilateral sinus nodes. In left atrial isomerism the sinus node is highly variable, being absent, displaced, and/or hypoplastic. (From Ho SY. Clinical pathology of the cardiac conduction system. In: Chadwick DJ, Goode J, eds. *Novartis Foundation Symposium 250. Development of the Cardiac Conduction System.* Chichester, UK: John Wiley and Sons, 2003:210–226).

crest and anterior atrial septum tend to be more uniform in alignment and less random in orientation. Because cell-to-cell conduction can be quite orientation dependent, preferential conduction along these bands of atrial myocardium may be the result of this more favorable cell alignment (19).

Age-related changes in the functional and cellular electrophysiologic properties of the atrium have been described. In rat atrial myocardium, action potentials recorded in newborn animals are characterized by a shorter plateau and duration than in older animals (20). Increasing action potential plateau and duration as a function of age have also been observed in human atrial myocardium (21). Maturation of ionic currents responsible for the plateau phase of the action potential, and maturation of currents responsible for repolarization, likely account for the changes noted in action potential duration with age. Shorter action potential durations in the immature atrium account for the shorter atrial refractory periods reported in newborn animals and human infants (22,23) (Fig. 10.4). These shorter refractory periods may facilitate the conduction of very closely coupled impulses and could render the newborn atrium more susceptible to intra-atrial re-entry (22) (Fig. 10.4). This may partly explain the occurrence of atrial arrhythmias such as atrial flutter in the otherwise healthy fetus or newborn infant (22).

In addition to a general increase in atrial action potential duration, regional age-related differences in atrial action potential morphology have been noted. In the adult dog, atrial action potential durations decrease as recordings are made at sites more distant from the sinus node (24). This regional variation in action potential duration is not noted in the atrium of newborn dogs, where repolarization is more uniform throughout the right atrium (24). Age-related changes in regional action potential morphology and in the "complex multidimensional propagation events at a microscopic and macroscopic scale" that characterize conduction in the atrium (25) probably result in differences in atrial

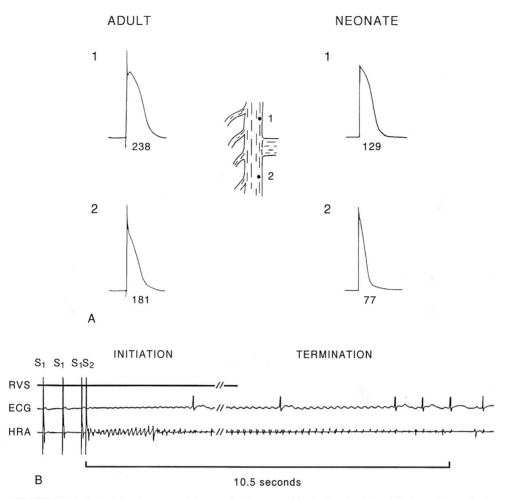

FIGURE 10.4 A: Atrial action potentials recorded from roughly similar sites (*1* and *2*) along the terminal crest in adult and newborn dogs. In contrast to the adult, neonatal atrial action potentials have little or no plateau phase and are significantly shorter in duration (durations in milliseconds noted beneath each action potential). (Modified from Spach MS, Dolber PC, Anderson PAW. Multiple regional differences in cellular properties that regulate repolarization and contraction in the right atrium of adult and newborn dogs. *Circ Res* 1989;65:1594–1611, with permission.) **B:** Introduction of a premature extrastimulus (S₂) to the right atrium of a newborn dog (during gentle vagal stimulation, RVS) results in the induction of a long train of atrial fibrillation/flutter. Similar but shorter runs of atrial fibrillation/flutter can be induced in the atrium of the neonate in the absence of vagal stimulation. Such repetitive responses become less common at older ages. HRA, high right atrium; RVS, right vagal stimulation train; ECG, electrocardiogram lead II; S₁, S₂, paced stimuli. (Modified from Pickoff AS, Stolfi A. Modulation of electrophysiological properties of neonatal canine heart by tonic parasympathetic stimulation. *Am J Physiol* 1990;258: H38–H44, with permission.)

conduction that are of clinical importance but that remain to be fully defined.

ATRIOVENTRICULAR CONDUCTION

Anatomy and Histology

The AV conduction system consists of the AV node, the penetrating bundle (or bundle of His), and the specialized conduction system of the ventricles (i.e., the right and left bundle branches). The AV node is located at the apex of the triangle of Koch (Fig. 10.1). Two sides of this triangle are formed by the septal leaflet of the tricuspid valve and the tendon of Todaro. The coronary sinus roughly defines the base of the triangle. Histologically, the AV node appears in cross section as a half-oval in adult hearts and more globular in infant hearts (26). The AV node consists of a loose transitional zone of cells that blend and extend into the surrounding atrial myocardium and, adjacent to the central fibrous body, a compact zone of closely grouped specialized cells that are smaller than atrial myocardial cells (26) (Fig. 10.5). Two posterior extensions from the compact zone have been described that extend toward the annuli of the mitral and tricuspid valves (26). The penetrating bundle, or bundle of His, arises from the compact zone of the AV node. A change in cellular appearance is noticeable as the bundle emerges from the AV node, with cells

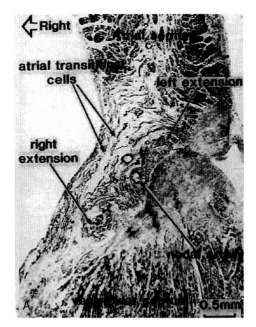

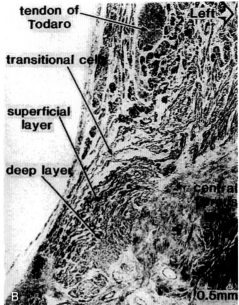

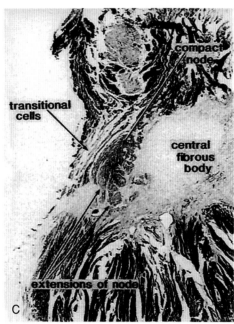

FIGURE 10.5 Photomicrographs of the atrioventricular (AV) node. **A** and **B:** The AV node consists of a loose, or transitional, zone and a compact zone that has a superficial and a deep layer. From the compact zone of the AV node, the penetrating bundle arises and pierces the central fibrous body. **C:** In the infant heart, in addition to the penetrating bundle, strands of conduction tissue extend from the compact zone of the AV node into the central fibrous body. (From Anderson RH, Ho SY. Cardiac conduction system in normal and abnormal hearts. In: Roberts NK, Gelband H, eds. *Cardiac Arrhythmias in the Neonate, Infant, and Child.* 2nd ed. Norwalk, CT: Appleton-Century-Crofts, 1983:1–35, with permission.)

gradually becoming larger and more aligned along their longitudinal axis (26). The penetrating bundle is so named because it penetrates the central fibrous body of the heart, beneath the insertion of the tendon of Todaro. The bundle migrates leftward to emerge in a subaortic position within the left ventricular outflow tract. In infant hearts, in addition to the penetrating bundle, a fine network consisting of strands of specialized conduction tissue can also be observed extending from the compact zone of the AV node well into the central fibrous body (26) (Fig. 10.5). These strands within the central fibrous body of the infant heart have been cited as representing a possible anatomic substrate for electrical instability and a cause of sudden death (27). The true functional significance of these strands, if any, is not known.

Branching of the AV conduction system into the right and left bundle branches occurs at the crest of the muscular portion of the interventricular septum, beneath the membranous septum (Fig. 10.6). The left bundle branch courses as a wide, fan-like structure rather than as discrete anterior and posterior fascicles. It courses in a subendocardial position, from the crest of the muscular septum over the left aspect of the septum, and has multiple distal interconnections (10). The right bundle branch courses within the myocardium after the take-off of the left bundle branch and emerges beneath the medial papillary muscle of the right ventricle. It then descends as a cordlike structure through the trabecula septomarginalis, along the moderator band, and then to the apex of the right ventricle. By light microscopy, the cells of both the right and left bundle branches are slightly larger than the surrounding myocardial cells. So-called Purkinje cells (large, clear cells) are not characteristically observed in the conduction system of the neonate or young infant (10).

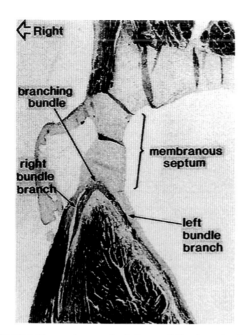

FIGURE 10.6 Photomicrograph of the specialized conduction tissue positioned at the crest of the muscular interventricular septum and dividing into the right and left bundle branches. (From Anderson RH, Ho SY. Cardiac conduction system in normal and abnormal hearts. In: Roberts NK, Gelband H, eds. *Cardiac Arrhythmias in the Neonate, Infant, and Child.* 2nd ed. Norwalk, CT: Appleton-Century-Crofts, 1983:1–35; with permission.)

Formation of the Atrioventricular Conduction System

Diverse, species-dependent genetic markers of the developing cardiac conduction system and the developing working myocardium have been reported (1). Although the functional significance of many of these genetic markers remains to be determined, they have served as useful tools for tracking the development of the conduction system. By tracking the

expression of such genetic markers, it is becoming increasingly accepted that the AV conduction system develops from cardiomyogenic precursor cells (cells capable of differentiating into either cells of the working myocardium or cells of the specialized conduction system). The sinus node, atrioventricular node, and bundle of His are derivatives of the embryonic primary myocardium, whereas the distal ramifications of the conduction system, or bundle branches, are formed from derivatives of embryonic secondary myocardium, specifically, the prechamber trabecular myocardium, a transcriptional domain that is distinct from the adjacent embryonic compact myocardium (Fig. 10.7) (1,28). Derivatives of the secondary myocardium are characterized by the expression of atrial natriuretic factor (ANF), connexin 40, and connexin 43, a genetic program not present in derivatives of the embryonic primary myocardium (28). Cardiomyogenic precursor cells may be induced by regional cues to express genetic programs that promote differentiation into cells of the specialized cardiac conduction system. These regional cues or inducers may include neural crest cells, which are known to migrate during development into the region of the central cardiac conduction system, as well as epicardium-derived cells, which may influence the differentiation of the more distal ramifications of the Purkinje network (29,30). Mounting evidence points to endothelin −1 as a candidate for the crucial signaling molecule governing the transformation of cardiomyogenic precursor cells into cells of the specialized cardiac conduction system (29,31).

The transcriptional regulation governing the differentiation of cardiomyogenic precursor cells into cells of the specialized cardiac conduction system is the subject of intense investigation. Several transcription factors, including the homeodomain transcription factor Nkx2.5, the zinc finger factor GATA6, members of the T-Box family (Tbx2, Tbx3, and Tbx5), and most recently Hop (homeodomain only protein, which acts downstream from Nkx2.5) appear to be critical in the differentiation, formation, and function of the specialized cardiac conduction system (32–34). Nkx2.5 is preferentially expressed in the developing cardiac conduction system. Mutations of this transcription factor in humans result in congenital heart defects as well as conduction disturbances and arrhythmias (35,36). In transgenic mouse models, Nkx2.5-insufficient mice develop conduction and electrophysiologic abnormalities that are in part the result of the marked hypoplasia of the AV node,

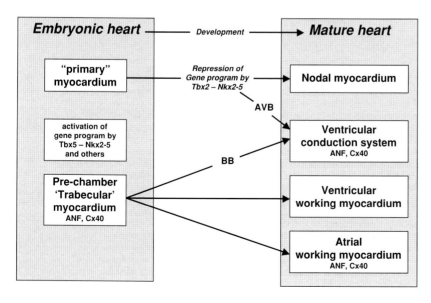

FIGURE 10.7 Scheme of cardiac development. The primary myocardium of the primitive heart tube is inherently nodal in phenotype. The sinus node, atrioventricular node, and bundle of His are derived from the embryonic primary myocardium. The ventricular conduction system (bundle branches) and ventricular myocardium are derived from the embryonic prechamber trabecular myocardium. Note expression of ANF and Cx40 in elements of the conduction system formed via the trabecular or secondary myocardium. Expression of ANF and Cx40 is repressed by Tbx and Nkx2.5 in components of the conduction system derived from the primary myocardium. AVB, His bundle; BB, bundle branches. (From Moorman AFM, Christoffels VM. Development of the cardiac conduction system: a matter of chamber development. In: Chadwick DJ, Goode J, eds. *Novartis Foundation Symposium 250. Development of the Cardiac Conduction System.* Chichester, UK John Wiley and Sons, 2003:25–43, with permission.)

His-Purkinje system noted in these haploinsufficient mice (37). How expression of the aforementioned transcription factors directs differentiation of cardiomyogenic precursor cells toward specialized conduction system cells and away from working myocardial cells is not precisely known. What is known is that ANF is a highly specific marker for the developing working myocardium. Furthermore, the promotor region of the ANF gene contains multiple binding sites for cardiac transcription factors important in the development and function of the cardiac conduction system, including Nkx2.5, GATA, and Tbx (37). It is hypothesized that chamber-specific, working myocardium gene expression is repressed secondary to an inhibition of ANF expression, as a result of the binding of these cardiac transcription factors to the ANF promotor region (35,39).

One particular monoclonal antibody directed against one of the molecular markers of the cardiac conduction system has allowed the tracking of a single region of the developing human heart as the precursor of the entire human AV conduction system (40). The monoclonal antibody is one raised against a neural tissue protein antigen derived from the ganglion nodosum of the chick, termed GLN (or G1N2). In the early human embryo (Carnegie stage 14, 31 to 35 days), a single ring of GLN-staining tissue is identified. The ring is confined to the region surrounding the primary interventricular foramen, which connects the primitive left and right ventricles. The ring, derived from the trabeculated ventricular myocardium, extends fully from the crest of the developing interventricular septum inferiorly to the lower part of the AV canal superiorly (Fig. 10.8). At this stage of development, the

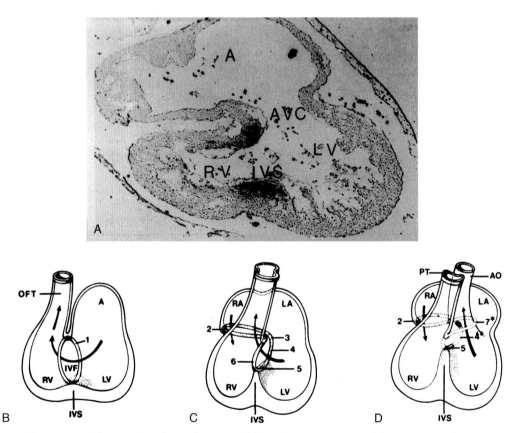

FIGURE 10.8 A: Immunohistochemical staining of the embryonic precursor of the atrioventricular conduction system in a Carnegie stage 14 human heart. A single ring of tissue is stained for the GLN antigen. It is confined to, and surrounds, the interventricular foramen. From this single ring will form the AV node, the His bundle, and the right and left bundle branches. AVC, atrioventricular canal; A, atrium; LV, left ventricle; RV, right ventricle; IVS, interventricular septum. B–D: Formation of the conduction system. B: The single GLN ring surrounds the interventricular foramen (IVF), as shown in the photomicrograph in A. At this stage the primitive atrium (A) connects solely with the LV. OFT, outflow tract. C: At Carnegie stages 15 to 17, rightward expansion of the GLN ring is observed, forming the tricuspid orifice and thereby connecting the right atrium with the right ventricle. Note the interventricular septum (IVS) rising from the floor of the ventricles. The AV node will form at site 3, the His bundle at site 4, and the bundle branches at site 5. LA, left atrium; RA, right atrium. D: At a slightly later stage of development (Carnegie stages 18 to 23), there is further development of the IVS. Involution of much of the original GLN ring then occurs, leaving the newly formed conduction system. Ao, aorta; PT, pulmonary trunk. (From Wessels A, Vermeulen JLM, Verbeek FJ, et al. Spatial distribution of "tissue-specific" antigens in the developing human heart and skeletal muscle: III. An immunohistochemical analysis of the distribution of the neural tissue antigen G1N2 in the embryonic heart; implications for the development of the atrioventricular conduction system. *Anat Rec* 1992;232:97–111, with permission.)

atrium is connected solely to the primitive left ventricle. In Carnegie stages 15 to 17 (35 to 44 days), rightward expansion of the AV canal occurs, establishing a direct connection between the atrium and the right ventricle. As a consequence of this expansion, GLN-positive tissue is now observed encircling the rightward portion of the AV canal with no staining of the leftward portion of the canal (Fig. 10.8). Thus, through development, GLN staining outlines the paths of blood flow into the right ventricle, beginning with the ventricular foramen and extending to the right AV connection. Through later stages of development (44 to 60 days), growth of the interventricular septal mass raises the GLN-stained crest of the septum toward the lesser curve, and septation is completed. Prominent staining along the left and right septal surfaces is evident. A leftward extension of the anterior aspect of the GLN ring is also noted as the subaortic outflow tract becomes positioned over the left ventricle (Fig. 10.8). According to this model, the AV node (which ultimately becomes sandwiched between endocardial cushion tissue and ingrowth of the AV sulcus) and the proximal AV bundle are formed at the most medial and posterior aspects of the rightward extension of the GLN ring (sites 3 and 4, Fig. 10.8). This position is in close approximation to the crest of the interventricular septum and, thus, to the remaining distal conduction system. The model, therefore, accounts for the formation of the entire AV conduction system from a single ring of genetically distinct tissue in the developing fetus. The model also adequately accounts for the histologic observation of islands of specialized conduction tissue that can be identified along the right (but not the left) AV ring postnatally. These represent persistent elements of the original rightward extension of the GLN ring that somehow survive maturation of the distal atrial myocardium and separation of atrium from ventricle by formation of the annulus fibrosus (41). A third branch of the AV bundle, the so-called dead-end tract, which is described in some hearts, also can be viewed as a remnant of the original GLN ring, the anterior portion that is carried into the left ventricular outflow tract during development (site 7, Fig. 10.8).

Thus, the AV conduction system develops in the embryo from a single ring of tissue surrounding the primary ventricular foramen and extending rightward with normal development of the right AV orifice. This provides a basis for understanding the localization of the conduction system in certain congenital heart defects (42). Underdevelopment of the apical trabecular portion of the right ventricle, as seen in tricuspid atresia, double-inlet left ventricle, and straddling tricuspid valve, can be viewed as representing a defect related to maldevelopment of the inflow portion of the right ventricle or to incomplete rightward expansion of the AV orifice. In these defects, the AV conduction system always forms at the junction of the posterior aspect of the interventricular septum (where the distal conduction bundle and bundle branches form) and the AV junction (where the AV node and proximal bundle form). The position of the AV node and proximal bundle is thus determined by the degree of formation and the relative positions of the right and left ventricles and the degree of expansion of the right AV ring. A similar analysis applies to the formation of the conduction system in septation defects and other malformations (Fig. 10.9).

Physiology of the Developing Atrioventricular Conduction System

Contraction delay between the atrium and ventricle of the early embryonic chick heart is observed as early as 50 hours postincubation (20th somite stage), prior to the development of the AV node or AV bundle. Action potentials recorded from the AV canal region of the 45-hour-old chick embryo exhibit a characteristic slow rate of rise and long duration, electrophysiologic characteristics that would favor slowing of conduction (43). Thus, AV canal cells are likely responsible for the AV delay observed in the early chick embryo (43). By electrophysiologically tracking the development of the AV junction, it can be shown that although AV canal cells provide the substrate for AV delay in the early chick embryo, different cells form the actual AV node in later development (44). AV delay (including Wenckebach's periodicity) also has been described in the prelooped mammalian (rat) heart, prior to formation of the AV conduction system (45). A cholinergic mechanism may be linked to the AV delay observed at these early developmental stages. In preinnervated embryonic and fetal rat hearts, acetylcholinesterase can be detected in the myocardium adjacent to the endocardial cushions but not in the free walls of the atrium and ventricle (46). In the working myocardium of the ventricles (and atrium), emulation of His–Purkinje system function becomes evident (45). Synchronization of ventricular free wall motion is observed after the process of looping is completed. The apparent conduction velocity in these looped hearts is estimated to be more than ten times faster than in prelooped hearts (45). These changes in electromechanical function of the early embryonic heart are highly correlated with an increase in the expression of myocardial gap junction proteins, such as connexin 43, and the expression of single, chamber-specific (atrial or ventricular) myosin isoforms (47,48). Gap junctions are highly specialized protein channels that connect adjacent myocytes (Fig. 10.10) (49). Gap junctions allow the passage of electrical current via a low-resistance pathway from one cell to the next, as well as the exchange of macromolecules between cells. Expression of different connexin isoforms result in gap junctions with differing electrical and functional properties. Tightly regulated changes in the expression of connexin isoforms occur throughout development (50). In the murine heart, connexin 40 is expressed throughout the heart until day 40, when it becomes localized within the atrium. In contrast, connexin 43 becomes preferentially expressed in the ventricle (47,51). A third isoform, connexin 45, is preferentially expressed in the specialized cardiac conduction system. (Fig. 10.10) Similar patterns of connexin expression have been reported in the developing human heart (52,53). The critical role of connexin expression during development for normal conduction is demonstrated by the abnormal, often lethal, cardiac conduction disturbances observed in transgenic mice with deficiencies of specific connexin isoforms (54,55).

In the developing embryo, the new regions of fast conduction remain flanked by persisting zones of slow conduction, such as in the AV canal region and the outflow tract. These regions are characterized by continued coexpression of both atrial and ventricular myosin heavy chain isoforms and very scarce gap junctional protein (1). With completion of septation, ventricular activation in the chick embryo changes from an immature base-to-apex activation pattern, to the mature apex-to-base activation pattern (56). In contrast, in the mammalian heart, the completion of septation may not be associated with such a transition in ventricular activation sequence (57).

In the developing chick and rat heart, cellular electrophysiologic changes in myocyte action potential characteristics promote an increase in conduction velocity with maturation. Increases in the maximum upstroke velocity (V_{max}) and amplitude of the action potential have been noted in both species during embryonic development (58,59). Because conduction

TRICUSPID ATRESIA

AV node is positioned on the floor of the blind right atrium. The conduction system extends onto the crest of the muscular interventricular septum, coursing posterior to the rim of the VSD.

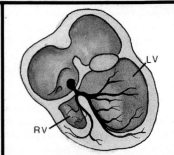

DOUBLE INLET LEFT VENTRICLE

AV node and conduction system are positioned anteriorly, at the site where the right atrioventricular ring is in contact with the crest of the muscular interventricular septum. This septum separates the left ventricle from the outlet chamber, or right ventricle.

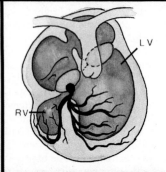

STRADDLING TRICUSPID VALVE

AV node and conduction system are positioned at a posterior site along the right atrioventricular ring where contact occurs with the interventricular septum.

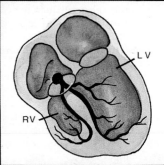

ATRIOVENTRICULAR SEPTAL DEFECT

AV node and conduction system are positioned at the site of contact of the atrioventricular junction and the posterior aspect of the interventricular septum. The central fibrous body is absent. The position of the AV node is shifted inferiorly with respect to the coronary sinus.

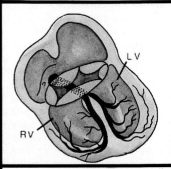

CONGENITALLY CORRECTED TRANSPOSITION OF THE GREAT VESSELS

AV node is positioned near the atrial septum along the anterior aspect of the atrioventricular ring. The conduction axis is relatively long and related to the pulmonary outflow tract, passing anterior to the rim of a VSD, if present.

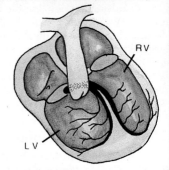

FIGURE 10.9 Conduction system in abnormal hearts. LV, left ventricle; RV, right ventricle.

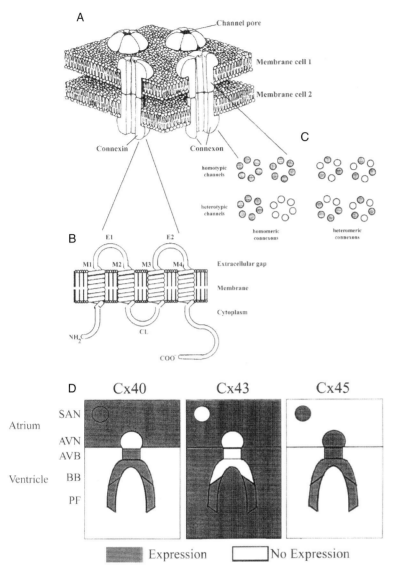

FIGURE 10.10 Ultrastructure of cardiac gap junctions. Gap junctions are arranged as plaques of intercellular channels. **A** and **B:** Section of a gap junction plaque showing four intercellular channels or pores (two complete and two sectioned in half) connecting two adjacent cell membranes (membrane cell 1 and cell 2). Each cell contributes half of the channel structure (the connexon). Each connexon contains six connexin proteins. **C:** Secondary structure of connexin. Connexons that are formed from similar connexin isoforms are termed homomeric. Those that form from different connexin isoforms are termed heteromeric. When combined to form intercellular channels, either a homotypic or heterotypic channel is formed. **D:** Expression of the major connexin isoforms (Cx40, Cx43, and Cx45) in the mammalian myocardium and specialized cardiac conduction system. SAN, sinus node; AVN, atrioventricular node; AVB, His bundle; BB, bundle branches; PF, Purkinje fibers. (From van Veen TA, van Rijen HVM, Opthof T, et al. Cardiac gap junction channels: modulation of expression and channel properties. *Cardiovasc Res* 2001;51:217–229, with permission.)

velocity is related to the maximum upstroke velocity of the action potential, higher conduction velocities result as V_{max} increases. The basis for the increase in V_{max} in these embryonic hearts appears to be twofold. First, within 8 days postincubation, the ionic channels responsible for generation of the upstroke of the action potential in the chick heart switch from slow sodium (or possibly calcium) channels to fast sodium channels (60). Second, resting membrane potential increases with development, which also contributes to a higher action potential upstroke velocity. The increase in resting membrane potential is believed to be based on increases in intracellular potassium activity and membrane permeability that occur with development.

The electrophysiologic characteristics of the specialized ventricular conduction system of the developing canine have been studied from the time of implantation to birth (61). Age-dependent increases in action potential upstroke velocity, amplitude, resting membrane potential, and duration have been described. Unlike in early embryonic chick myocardium, however, slow (calciumlike) action potentials are not observed

in this species. In addition to changes in action potential characteristics, changes in the ultrastructure of the developing canine Purkinje fiber—including changes in cell shape, increases in cross-sectional area, and the development of cell-to-cell contacts (intercalated discs and desmosomes)—undoubtedly contribute to the increase in conduction velocity noted with maturation (Fig. 10.11) (61–63). Very limited data exist concerning maturation of the electrophysiologic characteristics of the developing human heart. In the human fetus, action potentials recorded from atrial and ventricular myocardium at 12 weeks gestation are comparable with those in the adult, and conduction velocities are only slightly slower than those in the adult by midgestation (64,65).

Postnatal age-related changes in the physiology of the AV specialized conduction system have been described. The conduction velocity of Purkinje fibers from young (8-week-old) canines is significantly slower compared with adult Purkinje fibers (62). In the newborn canine heart, the first site of activation of ventricular myocardium by the specialized conduction system is the apex of the right ventricle rather than the left septal surface, as in

Myocytes

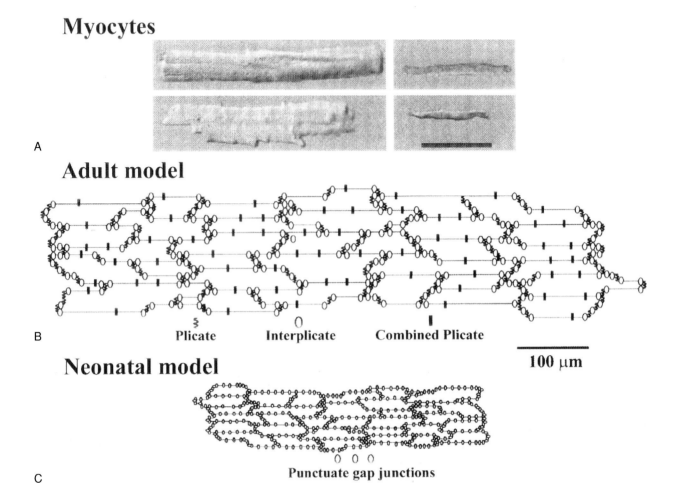

A

Adult model

B

Plicate   Interplicate   Combined Plicate

Neonatal model

100 μm

C

Punctuate gap junctions

FIGURE 10.11 Ventricular myocytes and distribution of gap junctions in the adult and newborn canine heart. **A:** Morphology of adult versus neonatal ventricular myocytes. Adult myocytes (*left*) are larger than neonatal myocytes (*right*). **B:** Multicellular model of adult ventricular myocytes and gap junction morphology and distribution. There are three morphologies recognized (interplicate, plicate, and combined). Note that most of the gap junctions are located at the ends of the ventricular myocytes. **C:** Multicellular model of newborn ventricular myocytes. Gap junctions are diffusely located, both at the ends and sides of individual cells. (From Spach MS, Heidlage JF, Dolber PC, et al. Electrophysiologic effects of remodeling cardiac gap junctions and cell size: experimental and model studies of normal cardiac growth. *Circ Res* 2000;86:302–311, with permission of The American Heart Association.)

the adult (66). Antegrade AV refractory periods are typically shorter, and intact retrograde (ventriculoatrial) conduction is more common in the young heart (23,67,68).

There has been considerable interest in the capability of the newborn AV conduction system to act as an effective filter of very rapid or premature beats. In the calf, goat, and pig, the newborn AV node lacks the ability to function as an effective filter, and conduction of very rapid impulses is possible, with resultant ventricular fibrillation and death (69–71). In contrast, in the newborn canine, the AV node does seem to act as an effective filter and has a longer refractory period than the distal conduction system (67). Cellular electrophysiologic studies of the AV node in neonatal and adult rabbits also have shown no significant differences in action potential characteristics, resting AV nodal conduction times, or Wenckebach intervals between the two age groups (72). In the human, no significant differences in the PR interval are detected by magnetocardiography in the fetus between the 20th and 42nd

gestational week, and there are no differences in AV nodal conduction times in young children when compared with adults (73,74). Therefore, species differences may exist in the degree of postnatal maturation of AV nodal function. Protection against rapid ventricular rates also may depend in part on electrophysiologic properties of the specialized conduction system at sites distal to the AV node. In the adult canine, action potential durations increase along the length of the Purkinje system, with the longest duration occurring just proximal to the subendocardial free-wall insertion. This site, therefore, acts as a physiologic gate that offers protection against closely coupled impulses (75). However, this electrophysiologic gate is not functional in the newborn heart, because near-uniform action potential durations are recorded along the entire length of the newborn Purkinje system (75) (Fig. 10.12). This could render the neonatal ventricular myocardium vulnerable to closely coupled impulses that might arise distal to the AV node.

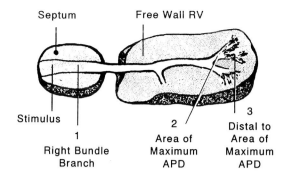

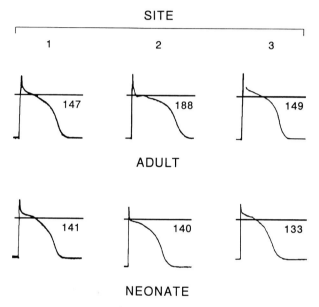

FIGURE 10.12 Action potentials recorded at three separate sites along the ventricular specialized conduction system of the newborn and adult dog. Site 1 corresponds to the proximal right bundle branch, site 2 just proximal to the distal ramifications of the conduction system, and site 3 within the distal ramifications. Note that in the adult dog, the longest action potential duration (APD) (188 ms) is recorded at site 2. This abrupt increase in action potential duration at site 2 functions as a physiologic gate, capable of blocking the conduction of closely coupled impulses to the ventricles. This abrupt increase in action potential duration is not observed in the neonate (i.e., the physiologic gate is absent). (Diagram of right bundle branch and right ventricle (RV) free wall is from Myerburg RJ, Stewart JW, Hoffman BF. Electrophysiological properties of the canine peripheral A-V conducting system. *Circ Res* 1970;26:361–378; with permission. Action potentials are modified from Untereker WJ, Danilo P Jr, Rosen MR. Developmental changes in action potential duration, refractoriness, and conduction in the canine ventricular conducting system. *Pediatr Res* 1984;18:53–58, with permission.)

References

1. Moorman AFM, de Jong F, Denyn MMFJ, et al. Development of the cardiac conduction system. *Circ Res* 1998;82:629–644.
2. Van Mierop LHS. Location of pacemaker in chick embryo heart at the time of initiation of heartbeat. *Am J Physiol* 1967;212:407–415.
3. Kamino K, Komuro H, Sakai T, et al. Functional pacemaking area in the early embryonic chick heart assessed by simultaneous multiple-site optical recording of spontaneous action potentials. *J Gen Physiol* 1988;91:573–591.
4. Satin J, Fujii S, DeHaan RL. Development of cardiac beat rate in early chick embryos is regulated by regional cues. *Dev Biol* 1988;129:103–113.
5. Mery A, Aimond F, Menard C, et al. Initiation of embryonic cardiac pacemaker activity by inositol 1,4,5-triphosphate-dependent calcium signaling. *Mol Biol Cell* 2005;16:2414–2423.
6. Viragh SZ, Challice CE. The development of the conduction system in the mouse embryo heart: III. The development of sinus muscle and sinoatrial node. *Dev Biol* 1980;80:28–45.
7. White SM, Claycomb WC. Embryonic stem cells form an organized, functional cardiac conduction system in vitro. *Am J Physiol Heart Circ Physiol* 2005;288:H670–679.
8. Tucker DC, Snider C, Woods WT Jr. Pacemaker development in embryonic rat heart cultured in oculo. *Pediatr Res* 1988;23:637–642.
9. Anderson RH, Ho SY, Becker AE, et al. The development of the sinoatrial node. In: Bonke FIM, ed. *The Sinus Node: Structure, Function and Clinical Relevance*. The Hague: Martinus Nijhoff, 1978:166–182.
10. Ho SY, Anderson RH. Embryology and anatomy of the normal and abnormal conduction system. In: Gillette PC, Garson A Jr, eds. *Pediatric Arrhythmias: Electrophysiology and Pacing*. Philadelphia: WB Saunders, 1990:2–27.
11. James TN. The connecting pathways between the sinus node and A-V node and between the right and the left atrium in the human heart. *Am Heart J* 1963;66:498–508.
12. Obrucnik M, Lichnovsky V, Machan B. Development of the conduction system of human embryonic and fetal heart: Differentiation of internodal connection. *Acta Univ Palacki Olomuc Fac Med* 1982;102:39–46.
13. Ikeda T, Iwasaki K, Shimokawa I, et al. Leu-7 immunoreactivity in human and rat embryonic hearts, with special reference to the development of the conduction tissue. *Anat Embryol (Berl)* 1990;182:553–562.
14. Blom NA, Gittenberger-de Groot AC, DeRuiter MC, et al. Development of the cardiac conduction tissue in human embryos using HNK-1 antigen expression: Possible relevance for understanding abnormal atrial automaticity. *Circulation* 1999;99:800–806.
15. Anderson RH, Ho SY, Smith A, et al. The internodal atrial myocardium. *Anat Rec* 1981;201:75–82.
16. Spach MS, Lieberman M, Scott JG, et al. Excitation sequences of the atrial septum and the AV node in isolated hearts of the dog and rabbit. *Circ Res* 1971;29:156–172.
17. Racker DK. Atrioventricular node and input pathways: A correlated gross anatomical and histological study of the canine atrioventricular junctional region. *Anat Rec* 1989;224:336–354.
18. Racker DK. Sinoventricular transmission in 10 mM K+ by canine atrioventricular nodal inputs: Superior atrionodal bundle and proximal atrioventricular bundle. *Circulation* 1991;83:1738–1753.
19. Spach MS, Miller WT III, Barr RC, et al. Electrophysiology of the internodal pathways: Determining the difference between anisotropic cardiac muscle and a specialized tract system. In: Little RC, ed. *Physiology of Atrial Pacemakers and Conductive Tissues*. Mt Kisco, NY: Futura, 1980:367–380.

20. Cavoto FV, Kelliher GJ, Roberts J. Electrophysiological changes in the rat atrium with age. *Am J Physiol* 1974;226:1293–1297.

21. Escande D, Loisance D, Planche C, et al. Age-related changes of action potential plateau shape in isolated human atrial fibers. *Am J Physiol* 1985;249:H843–H850.

22. Pickoff AS, Singh S, Flinn CJ, et al. Atrial vulnerability in the immature canine heart. *Am J Cardiol* 1985;55:1402–1406.

23. DuBrow IW, Fisher EA, Amat-y-Leon F, et al. Comparison of cardiac refractory periods in children and adults. *Circulation* 1975;51:485–491.

24. Spach MS, Dolber PC, Anderson PAW. Multiple regional differences in cellular properties that regulate repolarization and contraction in the right atrium of adult and newborn dogs. *Circ Res* 1989;65:1594–1611.

25. Spach MS, Dolber PC, Heidlage JF. Interaction of inhomogeneities of repolarization with anisotropic propagation in dog atria: A mechanism for both preventing and initiating reentry. *Circ Res* 1989;65:1612–1631.

26. Anderson RH, Ho SY. Cardiac conduction system in normal and abnormal hearts. In: Roberts NK, Gelband H, eds. *Cardiac Arrhythmias in the Neonate, Infant, and Child.* 2nd ed. Norwalk, CT: Appleton-Century-Crofts, 1983:1–35.

27. James TN. Sudden death in babies: New observations in the heart. *Am J Cardiol* 1968;22:479–506.

28. Moorman AFM, Christoffels VM, Anderson RH. Anatomic substrates for cardiac conduction. *Heart Rhythm* 2005;2:875–886.

29. Gittenberger-de Groot AC, Blom NM, Aoyama N, et al. The role of neural crest and epicardium-derived cells in conduction system formation. In: Chadwick DJ, Goode J, eds. *Novartis Foundation Symposium 250. Development of the Cardiac Conduction System.* Chichester, UK: John Wiley and Sons, 2003:125–141.

30. Gourdie RG, Harris BS, Bond J, et al. His-Purkinje lineages and development. In: Chadwick DJ, Goode J, eds. *Novartis Foundation Symposium 250. Development of the Cardiac Conduction System.* Chichester, UK: John Wiley and Sons, 2003:110–124.

31. Kanzawa N, Poma CP, Takebayashi-Suzuki K, et al. Competency of embryonic cardiomyocytes to undergo Purkinje fiber differentiation is regulated by endothelin receptor expression. *Development* 2002;129:3185–3194.

32. Edwards AV, Davis DL, Juraszek AL, et al. Transcriptional regulation in the mouse atrioventricular conduction system. In: Chadwick DJ, Goode J, eds. *Novartis Foundation Symposium 250. Development of the Cardiac Conduction System.* Chichester, UK: John Wiley and Sons, 2003:177–193.

33. Ismat FA, Zhang M, Kook H, et al. Homeobox protein Hop functions in the adult cardiac conduction system. *Circ Res* 2005;96:898–903.

34. Jay PY, Berul CI, Tanaka M, et al. Cardiac conduction and arrhythmia: Insights from Nkx2.5 mutations in mouse and humans. In: Chadwick DJ, Goode J, eds. *Novartis Foundation Symposium 250. Development of the Cardiac Conduction System.* Chichester, UK: John Wiley and Sons, 2003:227–241.

35. Harris BS, Jay PY, Rackley MS, et al. Transcriptional regulation of cardiac conduction system development: 2004 FASEB cardiac conduction system minimeeting, Washington, DC. *Anat Rec A Discov Mol Cell Evol Biol* 2004;280:1036–1045.

36. Benson DW. The genetic origin of atrioventricular conduction disturbances in humans. In: Chadwick DJ, Goode J, eds. *Novartis Foundation Symposium 250. Development of the Cardiac Conduction System.* Chichester, UK: John Wiley and Sons, 2003:242–259.

37. Jay PY, Harris BS, Buerger A, et al. Function follows form: Cardiac conduction system defects in Nkx2.5 mutation. *Anat Rec A Discov Mol Cell Evol Biol* 2004;280:966–972.

38. Nemer G, Nemer M. Regulation of heart development and function through combinatorial interactions of transcription factors. *Ann Med* 2001;33:604–410.

39. Moorman AFM, Christoffels VM. Development of the cardiac conduction system: A matter of chamber development. In: Chadwick DJ, Goode J, eds. *Novartis Foundation Symposium 250. Development of the Cardiac Conduction System.* Chichester, UK: John Wiley and Sons, 2003:25–43.

40. Wessels A, Vermeulen JLM, Verbeek FJ, et al. Spatial distribution of "tissue-specific" antigens in the developing human heart and skeletal muscle: III. An immunohistochemical analysis of the distribution of the neural tissue antigen G1N2 in the embryonic heart; implications for the development of the atrioventricular conduction system. *Anat Rec* 1992;232:97–111.

41. Anderson RH, Ho SY. The morphologic substrates for pediatric arrhythmias. *Cardiol Young* 1991;1:159–176.

42. Ho SY. Clinical pathology of the cardiac conduction system. In: Chadwick DJ, Goode J, eds. *Novartis Foundation Symposium 250. Development of the Cardiac Conduction System.* Chichester, UK: John Wiley and Sons, 2003:210–226.

43. Arguello C, Alanis J, Pantoja O, et al. Electrophysiological and ultrastructural study of the atrioventricular canal during the development of the chick embryo. *J Mol Cell Cardiol* 1986;18:499–510.

44. Arguello C, Alanis J, Valenzuela B. The early development of the atrioventricular node and bundle of His in the embryonic chick heart: An electrophysiological and morphological study. *Development* 1988;102:623–637.

45. Lloyd TR, Baldwin HS. Emulation of conduction system functions in the hearts of early mammalian embryos. *Pediatr Res* 1990;28:425–428.

46. Lamers WH, te Kortschot A, Los JA, et al. Acetylcholinesterase in prenatal rat heart: A marker for the early development of the cardiac conductive tissue? *Anat Rec* 1987;217:361–370.

47. van Kempen MJA, Fromaget C, Gros D, et al. Spatial distribution of connexin43, the major cardiac gap junction protein, in the developing and adult rat heart. *Circ Res* 1991;68:1638–1651.

48. de Jong F, Opthof T, Wilde AAM, et al. Persisting zones of slow impulse conduction in developing chicken hearts. *Circ Res* 1992;71:240–250.

49. van Veen TA, van Rijen HVM, Opthof T. Cardiac gap junction channels: Modulation of expression and channel properties. *Cardiovasc Res* 2001;51:217–229.

50. Veenstra RD, Wang HZ, Westphale EM, et al. Multiple connexins confer distinct regulatory and conduction properties of gap junctions in developing heart. *Circ Res.* 1992;71:1277–1283.

51. Gourdie RG, Green CR, Severs NJ, et al. Immunolabeling patterns of gap junction connexins in the developing and mature rat heart. *Anat Embryol* 1992;185:363–378.

52. Kaba RA, Coppen SR, Dupont E, et al. Comparison of connexin 43,40 and 45 expression patterns in the developing human and mouse hearts. *Cell Commun Adhes* 2001;8(4–6):339–343.

53. Coppen SR, Kaba RA, Halliday D, et al. Comparison of connexin expression patterns in the developing mouse heart and human foetal heart. *Mol Cell Biochem* 2003;242(1–2):121–127.

54. Kirchhoff S, Kim JS, Hangendorff A, et al. Abnormal cardiac conduction and morphogenesis in connexin 40 and connexin 43 double deficient mice. *Circ Res* 2000;87:399–405.

55. Gutstein DE, Morley GE, Tamaddon H, et al. Conduction slowing and sudden arrhythmic death in mice with cardiac-restricted inactivation of connexin 43. *Circ Res* 2001;88:333–339.

56. Watanabe M, Chuck ET, Rothenberg F, et al. Developmental transitions in cardiac conduction. In: Chadwick DJ, Goode J, eds. *Novartis Foundation Symposium 250. Development of the Cardiac Conduction System.* Chichester, UK: John Wiley and Sons, 2003:68–79.

57. Rothenberg F, Nikolski VP, Watanabe M, et al. Electrophysiology and anatomy of embryonic rabbit hearts before and after septation. *Am J Physiol Heart Circ Physiol* 2005;288(1):H344–H351.

58. Sperelakis N, Shigenobu K. Changes in membrane properties of chick embryonic hearts during development. *J Gen Physiol* 1972;60:430–453.

59. Couch JR, West TC, Hoff HE. Development of the action potential of the prenatal rat heart. *Circ Res* 1969;24:19–31.

60. Shigenobu K, Sperelakis N. Development of sensitivity to tetrodotoxin of chick embryonic hearts with age. *J Mol Cell Cardiol* 1971;3:271–286.

61. Danilo P Jr, Reder RF, Binah O, et al. Fetal canine cardiac Purkinje fibers: Electrophysiology and ultrastructure. *Am J Physiol* 1984;246:H250–H260.

62. Rosen MR, Legato MJ, Weiss RM. Developmental changes in impulse conduction in the canine heart. *Am J Physiol* 1981;240:H546–H554.

63. Legato MJ, Weintraub M, McCord GM, et al. The morphology of the developing canine conducting system: bundle branch and Purkinje cell architecture from birth to week 12 of life. *J Mol Cell Cardiol* 1991;23:1063–1076.

64. Tuganowski W, Cekanski A. Electrical activity of a single fibre of the human embryonic heart. *Pflugers Arch* 1971;323:21–26.

65. Gennser G, Nilsson E. Excitation and impulse conduction in the human fetal heart. *Acta Physiol Scand* 1970;79:305–320.

66. Myerburg RJ, Gelband H, Bassett AL. Physiology of the ventricular specialized conduction system. In: Roberts NK, Gelband H, eds. *Cardiac Arrhythmias in the Neonate, Infant, and Child.* East Norwalk, CT: Appleton-Century-Crofts, 1977:55–90.

67. McCormack J, Gelband H, Xu H, et al. Atrioventricular nodal function in the immature canine heart. *Pediatr Res* 1988;23:99–103.

68. Pickoff AS, Singh S, Flinn CJ, et al. Maturational changes in ventriculoatrial conduction in the intact canine heart. *J Am Coll Cardiol* 1984;3:162–168.

69. Preston JB, McFadden S, Moe GK. Atrioventricular transmission in young mammals. *Am J Physiol* 1959;197:236–240.

70. Moore EN. Atrioventricular transmission in newborn calves. *Ann N Y Acad Sci* 1965;127:113–126.

71. Gough WB, Moore EN. The differences in atrioventricular conduction of premature beats in young and adult goats. *Circ Res* 1975;37:48–58.

72. Hewett KW, Gaymes CH, Noh C-I, et al. Cellular electrophysiology of neonatal and adult rabbit atrioventricular node. *Am J Physiol* 1991;260:H1674–H1684.

73. Kahler C, Schleussner E, Grimm B, et al. Fetal magnetocardiography: development of the fetal cardiac time intervals. *Prenat Diagn* 2002;22(5):408–414.

74. Gillette PC, Reitman MJ, Gutgesell HP, et al. Intracardiac electrography in children and young adults. *Am Heart J* 1975;89:36–44.

75. Untereker WJ, Danilo P Jr, Rosen MR. Developmental changes in action potential duration, refractoriness, and conduction in the canine ventricular conducting system. *Pediatr Res* 1984;18:53–58.

CHAPTER 11 ■ THE NORMAL ELECTROCARDIOGRAM

GEORGE F. VAN HARE, MD, AND ANNE M. DUBIN, MD

In this era of easily available high resolution techniques, does electrocardiography (ECG) still have a place in the diagnosis and management of children with congenital heart disease? Certainly, for the noninvasive diagnosis of arrhythmias and cardiac conduction disorders, there is no substitute for careful analysis of the ECG. In addition to the assessment of arrhythmias, the ECG is important in the diagnosis and management of heart disease in children. Although rarely diagnostic of the type of congenital heart disease, the ECG should be thought of in the same way as the physical examination. It provides clues to the likely diagnosis, provides information about the severity of the condition, and may be indicative of other associated problems. Additionally, review of the ECG may identify important discrepancies as compared with the patient's presumed diagnosis, prompting further testing or a more careful review of the exiting data. Most experienced pediatric cardiologists consider a cardiology consultation incomplete without a review of the ECG.

THE HISTORY OF ELECTROCARDIOGRAPHY

Although Augustus Waller was the first to record an ECG in a human (1), Willem Einthoven of The Netherlands is considered the father of electrocardiography. In 1901, Einthoven published a description of the string galvanometer, a device ideally suited for recording the rapidly changing and weak currents of cardiac electrical activity present on the body surface (2). During subsequent work, Einthoven identified the major waveforms of the ECG, initially named A, B, C, and D. He subsequently changed the naming system to P, Q, R, S, and

T waves (Fig. 11.1), leaving room at either end of the alphabet for naming of new, as yet undiscovered, waves (as later came to pass when the U wave was described). The string galvanometer proved useful for the study of the ECG. The investigations of Einthoven and Sir Thomas Lewis dominated the early years of ECG studies, and they are credited with bringing the ECG to the bedside (3). This was not anticipated by Waller: "I certainly had no idea that the electrical signs of the heart's action could ever be utilized for clinical investigation" (1). Recordings in children followed, and Ziegler (4) reviewed the early reports on the use of the ECG in children. In 1913, Hecht published a "comprehensive" study, evaluating all three standard bipolar leads (I, II, III) in ECG tracings from hundreds of premature infants, term infants, and children with normal and abnormal hearts. By the late 1930s, the distinctive developmental changes that occur in the ECGs of normal infants and children had been described (4).

PRINCIPLES AND TECHNICAL CONSIDERATIONS IN RECORDING THE ELECTROCARDIOGRAM

The Scalar Electrocardiogram

The heart is an electrically active organ, and the current flows that result in cardiac contraction can be recorded from the body surface. How these electrical events are transmitted to the body surface is a complex topic and involves characteristics both of the heart as a current source as well as of the chest, which acts as a conductor (5,6). These characteristics change in the presence of congenital defects and other forms of cardiac disease as well as with normal growth and development.

The basic concept of the ECG is that electrical potentials generated by the heart can be accounted for by considering these electrical events to be equivalent to those generated by a dipole source in a homogeneous volume conductor (the equivalent dipole model). This concept has the limitation of seriously oversimplifying these events, especially in the assumption of homogeneity of conduction through the chest. The scalar ECG can be thought of as the record of voltage variation of this dipole with respect to time, in the particular orientation of the lead recorded. Cardiac electrical activity, of course, generates potentials in three dimensions, so any particular lead provides a very small amount of the potentially available information that can be recorded. For this reason, the conventional ECG includes 12 or 15 leads, arranged to give recordings along a variety of lead orientations to better represent the cardiac activity in three dimensions. The choice

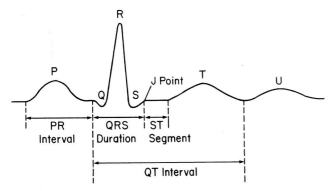

FIGURE 11.1 Scalar ECG showing P, Q, R, S, T, and U waves. The J point as well as standard intervals, including the PR interval, QRS duration, ST segment, and QT interval, are shown.

of these leads evolved as studies of the ECG progressed and, in retrospect, may not represent the best of all possible lead systems. However, these particular leads are deeply entrenched in modern cardiology practice.

Electrocardiographic interpretation begins with artifact-free ECG recordings. In addition to accurate electrode placement, cleaning of the skin with alcohol or acetone is essential to lower the skin resistance. ECG recordings in active infants and toddlers can be a technical challenge.

The standard ECG record consists of 12 leads recorded from nine body surface locations with the patient in the supine position (7). The ideal recorder should have the capability of displaying 3 to 12 leads simultaneously. The standard configuration usually is modified in children and adults with congenital heart disease, to record additional right (V3R, V4R) and left (V7) chest leads. Interpretation of rhythm disturbances is facilitated by viewing a rhythm strip with 3 or, better, 12 simultaneously recorded leads.

Electrocardiograms can be recorded at various paper speeds and at various voltage standardizations. Paper speeds of 12.5, 25, and 50 mm/s have been used, but 25 m/s is standard. Standard ECG recording paper has major time divisions at 5-mm intervals and minor time divisions at 1-mm intervals. Therefore, at a paper speed of 25 mm/s, each large block corresponds to 0.20 seconds (200 ms), and one second is represented by five large blocks. Each small block represents 0.04 seconds (40 ms). In terms of voltage, full standardization refers to 1.0 mV/10 mm in vertical deflection on the recording, whereas half standardization refers to 0.5 mV/10 mm. It is important that the ECG reader always checks standardization prior to interpreting the ECG because the use of half standardization is common when large voltages cause overlap between leads. With the exception of the signal-averaged ECG, it is uncommon to discuss or report ECG voltages in terms of millivolts. It is much more common to discuss them in terms of millimeters of amplitude at full standardization. Therefore, for the remainder of this chapter, millimeters at full standardization will be used rather than millivolts.

Vectorcardiography

Vectorcardiography was developed to correct some basic limitations of the conventional lead system and to display the data obtained by the ECG in a potentially more useful format. The dipole varies in magnitude and direction with time. The scalar ECG allows the presentation of the magnitude only, as it varies with time, and one needs to infer the direction of forces from the lead chosen. Each instant, the heart generates a force that has both magnitude and direction. This vector force changes with time and traces a loop during the duration of the QRS complex, which occupies all three dimensions. The vectorcardiography lead system allows a reasonably faithful representation of this three-dimensional loop as two-dimensional frontal, sagittal, and horizontal planes (Fig. 11.2). Several lead systems have been used. They each have their advantages and disadvantages. The Frank system has been the most widely used, but the McFee system also has been used (8). The QRS vectorcardiogram, then, consists of a loop that starts at the beginning of the QRS, ends with the end of the QRS, and is displayed on paper in three planes.

Because of the need for special equipment, technical expertise, and the inconvenience of multiple leads, vectorcardiograms rarely are obtained in modern pediatric cardiology practice. Also, because of high-quality echocardiography, vectorcardiography has limited utility. Still, the best electrocardiographers

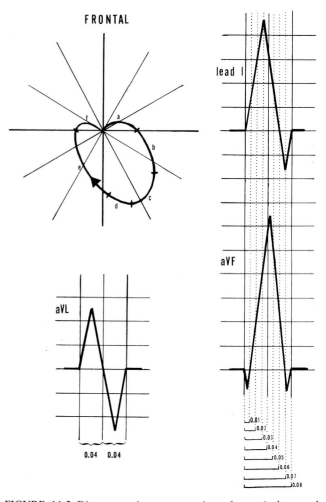

FIGURE 11.2 Diagrammatic representation of a typical normal frontal plane vector loop (**top left**) with corresponding scalar ECG leads I, aVL, and aVF. The loop is clockwise in the frontal plane and lasts for 0.08 seconds. Each lettered segment corresponds to a portion of the QRS interval: a, 0 to 0.01 seconds; b, 0.01 to 0.03 seconds; c, 0.03 to 0.04 seconds; d, 0.04 to 0.055 seconds; e, 0.055 to 0.07 seconds; f, 0.07 to 0.08 seconds.

think in terms of vectors even when interpreting the scalar ECG. Rather than memorizing patterns of QRS morphology and axis, they view the standard scalar ECG as a representation of the vector forces that vary with time, and perhaps understand the ECG better than those who simply "pattern read."

Body Surface Mapping

A natural extension of the technique of ECG and vectorcardiography is the use of body surface mapping. To obtain the spatial-temporal representation of cardiac electrical potentials on the body surface, simultaneous measurement of potentials are needed at a number of sites (from 24 to 200) on the anterior and posterior torso. Several excellent reviews have addressed the specific details, including number and location of electrodes (9), electrode type (10), sample rate (11), digital collection and processing of ECG signals (12,13), and construction of maps (13). These techniques are investigational and require specialized equipment and a high level of computerization.

They have shown promise in the noninvasive evaluation of cardiac conduction abnormalities such as Wolff–Parkinson–White (WPW) syndrome and other electrical abnormalities of the heart.

Esophageal Electrocardiography

Because the esophagus normally is behind the left atrium and is in close proximity to the heart, an electrode placed in the esophagus will record atrial activity more locally than the standard ECG leads (14). This is especially useful in evaluating cardiac rhythm disturbances, particularly in situations where the P wave is difficult to find on the surface ECG (3). For example, when there is atrial flutter with 2:1 atrioventricular (AV) conduction, flutter waves may not be obvious on the surface ECG. Even if one observes atrial activity on the surface ECG, it may not be apparent that there are twice as many atrial deflections as ventricular deflections. Esophageal ECG solves this problem by recording atrial electrograms that are as large as or larger than the simultaneously recorded ventricular electrograms.

To obtain artifact-free esophageal ECGs, a soft bipolar electrode that has widely spaced large electrodes is used. Several are commercially available from 7 to 10 French in size. The catheter is positioned at the proper site and the signal filtered, usually employing band-pass filtering at 10 to 1,000 Hz, to eliminate the low-frequency respiratory artifact (14). Electrode placement is similar to nasogastric tube placement. The insertion depth for recording the maximum atrial deflection can be estimated from the patient's height (15,16). The ideal position is the site at which the atrial electrogram is about equal to the ventricular electrogram amplitude, and both are as large as possible. Positioning too distally will yield a large ventricular electrogram and a small atrial electrogram, and positioning too proximally will yield low amplitudes of both electrograms.

Signal-Averaged Electrocardiography

Under normal circumstances, the amplitude of P waves and ST segments is <2.5 mm, and T waves do not exceed 10 mm in the precordial leads. On the other hand, precordial R and S waves may have amplitudes of 30 to 40 mm. Interest in low-level potentials has led to the development of the signal-averaged ECG as a way of eliminating noise, which may exceed 0.03 mV peak to peak.

The principal interest in the signal-averaged ECG has been to identify small high-frequency potentials either during the PR interval or during late QRS and ST segment (17). High-frequency potentials during the ST segment may result from areas of slow conduction that have been observed in myocardial infarction and associated ventricular arrhythmias (18). Interest in high-frequency potentials during the PR interval has focused on detecting depolarization within the His-Purkinje system.

The basic principle is that averaging a periodic, repetitive signal will reduce random noise to <0.001 mV, thereby enhancing the detection of low-amplitude signals. The signals are recorded at very high gain and are band-pass filtered. Waveforms usually are averaged over several minutes. Sensitivity and specificity of the technique for predicting adult patients at risk for ventricular arrhythmias have been reported. Reports of this technique for pediatric patients have

been limited (19), but it has been used to identify patients with arrhythmogenic right ventricular dysplasia (20)

24-Hour Ambulatory Electrocardiography

Named for Dr. N. J. Holter (21), the 24-hour ambulatory ECG, or Holter ECG, is an important tool in the diagnostic armamentarium of the pediatric cardiologist. It is used for various indications and is, perhaps, the most effective method to diagnose transient events such as AV block and other conduction disorders.

Modern Holter equipment records two or three channels of the ECG for 24 hours, either onto a cassette tape or digitally into a flash memory card in the recorder (22). The digital recording system has the advantage of being smaller and lighter and avoids the mechanical problems of cassette tape drag and damaged tapes. The ECG leads chosen for recording generally are modified chest leads and most closely resemble leads V1 and V5. The ECG is obtained using chest leads that are applied after adequate skin preparation, and the chest is often wrapped in an elastic bandage. The recorder can be worn on the belt, placed in a backpack, or suspended from a strap. The recorders have a digital clock for linking events with actual times, as well as a patient-activated event marker that allows the patient to annotate episodes of cardiac symptoms.

The recording is scanned using a computerized analysis system that provides both a full disclosure of the entire recording, as well as summary data regarding average, maximum, and minimum heart rates. Computerized algorithms allow the identification, characterization, and enumeration of premature atrial and ventricular contractions, as well as higher grades of ectopy and episodes of abnormal tachycardia. The patient keeps a diary of events while wearing the Holter recorder, and any such episodes of interest can be printed out and evaluated as part of the scanning process. The algorithms for arrhythmia diagnosis are limited in their applicability to pediatric patients, and the technician who scans and prints the report must be experienced in pediatric Holter scanning and supervised by a pediatric cardiologist (23–25).

Transtelephonic Event Recording

One limitation of Holter monitoring is that to record a transient symptomatic event, the event must occur spontaneously during the period that the patient is wearing the recorder. Thus, Holter monitoring often fails to record such events when they do not occur many times per day. Accordingly, to capture a symptomatic event, transtelephonic event recording allows longer periods of monitoring in a cost-effective manner (26,27). Several types of recorders are available. The simplest is a small device that records a single ECG channel for 30 to 60 seconds into the memory of the device when a button is pushed. It can be attached to the patient by several ECG electrodes or by wrist electrodes. Another such recorder has the electrodes incorporated into the recorder itself and is used by placing the recorder on the chest so that the electrodes make contact with the skin directly. These recorders have the disadvantage that the episode must be long enough for the recorder to be applied. This problem can be minimized by using a recorder that resembles a wristwatch, does not require additional electrodes, and can be worn continuously. An alternative to this simple type of recorder is the so-called memory-loop recorder. This recorder resembles a small Holter recorder, is attached to the patient by means of chest electrodes, and is worn continuously. Rather than recording and storing all the ECG data while worn, the device temporarily stores about 60 seconds of ECG data. When the patient experiences a symptom, he or she presses a button on the unit, causing it to store the 30 seconds of data that occurred prior to pressing the button as well as a short amount of data following the episode.

The recorder stores the episode as an oscillatory audio signal. After an episode is captured by the recorder, the patient or a parent can transmit the ECG by playing back the stored audio signal over the telephone to the monitoring center, where the ECG is converted back to an ECG waveform and printed out for interpretation.

Recently, implantable event recorders have been developed. These devices are implanted in the subcutaneous tissue on the chest wall and are active for at least 13 months. The device incorporates a continuous loop recording of the heart rhythm that is stored when the device is activated by the patient or parent. There is also an auto-activation component that allows the device to automatically record rhythms that are out of a preset range. This device is useful for pediatric patients with syncope and/or palpitations (28).

HOW TO READ A PEDIATRIC ELECTROCARDIOGRAM

An organized approach to evaluating the ECG is important to avoid failure to consider each characteristic of the ECG. Many advise that these characteristics be evaluated in a particular order, for example, by assessing the P wave first, the QRS second, and so on. The order, of course, is less important than a careful review of all the aspects of the recording (Table 11.1). Often pediatric ECGs are interpreted in light of extensive knowledge of the patient's condition. Clearly, the more information the reader has about the patient's condition, the more relevant the ECG interpretation will be. However, one often reads ECGs with no clinical information except the patient's age. For this reason, the ECG is considered a laboratory test. ECG attributes (e.g., intervals, voltages) are distributed within a population. Thus, the prevalence of an abnormality depends on the normal cutoff points one picks. Just as the presence of a murmur does not necessarily mean that a patient has valvar stenosis, an "abnormal" ECG does not necessarily mean that the patient has heart disease. An example of this pitfall is the pres-

TABLE 11.1

CHARACTERISTICS FOR EVALUATION OF THE ELECTROCARDIOGRAM

Rate and rhythm
Ventricular rate
Origin of the pacemaker
Atrioventricular conduction
Atrial enlargement/hypertrophy
Ventricular depolarization
QRS axis deviation
Bundle branch blocks
Pre-excitation
Hypertrophy
Initial forces
Ventricular repolarization
QT interval
ST segment, T wave, and U waves

ence of a chest deformity (e.g., pectus excavatum or scoliosis) about which the ECG reader may not have information and needs to interpret the ECG. Even if the reader knows about the deformity, he or she may not know what constitutes normal for such a situation.

Pediatric ECG features are age dependent (Table 11.2). The PR interval, ST segment, and T wave are heart rate dependent as well. The most comprehensive tabulation of age- and heart rate–dependent ECG measures was provided by Davignon et al. (29,30)

The zero-voltage baseline, which is the reference level for ECG voltage measurements, is based on the fact that no potential differences exist on the body surface at that instant. At slow heart rates, the T-P or U-P interval is a good approximation of the voltage baseline. At faster heart rates, the P wave may be superimposed on the previous T-U wave. In this situation, the PR segment is the best alternative. When measuring a large deflection, choice of baseline selection is relatively unimportant. However, when measuring a low-level potential (e.g., ST segment), or attempting to determine onset of a waveform (e.g., QRS), choice of the baseline is critical—maybe as important as the measurement of interest.

Detailed descriptions of arrhythmia diagnosis are found elsewhere in this text. Likewise, the ECG patterns characterizing various forms of complex congenital heart disease are addressed in the chapters dealing with those diseases.

Rate and Rhythm

Ventricular Rate

Heart rate is determined by measuring the R-R interval. It often is more useful to think of cycle length than heart rate, because on the standard ECG there seldom is an entire minute's worth of heartbeats to count. Cycle length and heart rate have a reciprocal relationship. Cycle length (in milliseconds) is measured directly as the R-R interval. Heart rate is calculated by dividing the measured cycle length by 60,000 ms/min. Heart rate is highly dependent on age, body temperature, autonomic tone, and physical activity. For example, in a 14-year-old, a resting heart rate (cycle length) of 150 beats per minute (400 ms) would be abnormally high. However, it might be a perfectly normal rate for an apprehensive toddler during ECG recording. Similarly, a resting heart rate of 50 beats per minute (1,200 ms) in a healthy adolescent would be normal, whereas the same heart rate in an infant would signify bradycardia.

Origin of the Pacemaker

On most ECGs, there will be normal AV conduction with P waves preceding each QRS complex. It is important to determine if the P wave originates from the sinus node or elsewhere. The vector of a sinus P wave is from top to bottom and right to left (positive in leads I, II, and aVF). The P wave in sinus rhythm is biphasic in lead V1, initially being upright followed by a brief downward deflection. If the P wave does not have these characteristics, it does not originate from the sinus node and has an "ectopic" location. One must ascertain its origin For example, a rhythm in which the P wave is inverted in leads I and aVL is termed a left atrial rhythm, whereas a P wave that is inverted in leads II, III, and aVF is termed a low right atrial rhythm (also known as a coronary sinus rhythm).

The rhythm may be regular, irregular, or regular with intermittent but predictable phases of irregularity. The last would be a description of phasic sinus arrhythmia, which results

TABLE 11.2

NORMAL ECG STANDARDS FOR CHILDREN BY AGE

	0–1 d	1–3 d	3–7 d	7–30 d	1–3 mo	3–6 mo	6–12 mo	1–3 y	3–5 y	5–8 y	8–12 y	12–16 y
Heart rate per minute	94–155 (122)	91–158 (122)	90–166 (128)	06–182 1 (149)	120–179 (149)	105–185 (141)	108–169 (131)	89–152 (119)	73–137 (109)	65–133 (100)	62–130 (91)	60–120 (80)
Frontal plane QRS axis (degrees)	59–189 (135)	64–197 (134)	76–191 (133)	0–160 (109)	30–115 (75)	7–105 (60)	6–98 (55)	7–102 (55)	6–104 (56)	10–139 (65)	6–116 (60)	9–128 (59)
PR lead II (s)	0.08–0.16 (0.107)	0.08–0.14 (0.108)	0.07–0.15 (0.102)	0.07–0.14 (0.100)	0.07–0.13 (0.098)	0.07–0.15 (0.105)	0.07–0.16 (0.106)	0.08–0.15 (0.113)	0.08–0.16 (0.119)	0.09–0.16 (0.123)	0.09–0.17 (0.128)	0.09–0.18 (0.135)
QRS duration, V5 (s)	0.02–0.07 (0.05)	0.02–0.07 (0.05)	0.02–0.07 (0.05)	0.02–0.08 (0.05)	0.02–0.08 (0.05)	0.02–0.08 (0.05)	0.03–0.08 (0.05)	0.03–0.08 (0.06)	0.03–0.07 (0.06)	0.03–0.08 (0.06)	0.04–0.09 (0.06)	0.04–0.09 (0.07)
P-wave amplitude, lead II	0.5–2.8 (1.6)	0.3–2.8 (1.6)	0.7–2.9 (1.7)	0.7–3.0 (1.9)	0.7–2.6 (1.5)	0.4–2.7 (1.6)	0.6–2.5 (1.6)	0.7–2.5 (1.5)	0.3–2.5 (1.4)	0.4–2.5 (1.4)	0.3–2.5 (1.4)	0.3–2.5 (1.4)
Q-wave amplitude, aVF	0.1–3.4 (1.0)	0.1–3.3 (1.0)	0.1–3.5 (1.1)	0.1–3.5 (1.2)	0.1–3.4 (0.9)	0–3.2 (0.9)	0–3.3 (1.0)	0–3.2 (0.9)	0–2.9 (0.6)	0–2.5 (00.6)	0–2.7 (0.5)	0–2.4 (0.4)
Q-wave amplitude, V6	0–1.7 (0.1)	0–2.2 (0.1)	0–2.8 (0.1)	0–2.8 (0.4)	0–2.6 (0.3)	0–2.6 (0.3)	0–3.0 (0.4)	0–2.8 (0.6)	0.1–3.3 (0.8)	0.1–4.6 (0.8)	0.1–2.8 (0.6)	0–2.9 (0.4)
R amplitude, V1	5–26 (13)	5–27 (15)	3–25 (12)	3–12 (10)	3–19 (10)	3–20 (10)	2–20 (9)	2–18 (8)	1–18 (8)	1–14 (7)	1–12 (5)	1–10 (4)
S amplitude, V1	1–23 (8)	1–20 (9)	1–17 (7)	0–11 (4)	0–13 (5)	0–17 (6)	1–18 (7)	1–21 (8)	2–22 (10)	3–23 (12)	3–25 (12)	3–22 (11)
R amplitude, V6	0–12 (4)	0–12 (5)	1–12 (5)	3–16 (8)	5–21 (12)	6–22 (13)	6–23 (13)	6–23 (13)	8–25 (15)	8–26 (16)	9–25 (16)	7–23 (14)
S amplitude, V6	0–10 (4)	0–9 (3)	0–10 (4)	0–10 (3)	0–7 (3)	0–10 (3)	0–8 (2)	0–7 (2)	0–6 (2)	0–4 (1)	0–4 (1)	0–4 (1)
R/S ratio, V1	0.1–9.9 (2.2)	0.1–6 (2.0)	0.1–9.8 (2.8)	1.0–7.0 (2.9)	0.3–7.4 (2.2)	0.1–6.0 (2.3)	0.1–4.0 (1.8)	0.1–4.3 (1.4)	0.03–2.7 (0.9)	0.02–2.0 (0.8)	0.02–1.9 (0.6)	0.02–1.8 (.5)
R/S ratio, V6	0.1–9 (2)	0.1–12 (3)	0.1–10 (2)	0.1–12 (4)	0.2–14 (5)	0.2–18 (7)	0.2–22 (8)	0.3–27 (10)	0.6–30 (11)	0.9–30 (12)	1.5–33 (14)	1.4–39 (15)

All values are 2nd percentile to 98th percentile (mean). All amplitudes of waves are given in millimeters at full standardization, i.e., 1 mm = 10 mV.
Derived from percentile charts in Davignon A, Rautaharju P, Boisselle E, et al. Normal ECG standards for infants and children. *Pediatr Cardiol* 1979;1:123–152, with permission.

from normal vagally mediated accelerations and decelerations of the sinus node in response to respiration. One also may observe tachyarrhythmias such as atrial tachycardia or AV reciprocating tachycardia rather than sinus rhythm.

Atrioventricular Conduction

One assesses both conduction time by measurement of the PR interval and the relationship of P waves to QRS complexes. The PR interval is age, activity, and heart rate dependent. Impaired AV conduction is described as first-, second-, or third-degree AV block. Abbreviated conduction, manifested by a short PR interval, occurs in WPW syndrome, glycogen storage disease, and the presence of a low atrial pacemaker located closer to the AV node.

Atrial Enlargement and Hypertrophy

The right atrium is to the right, superior, and anterior to the left atrium. During normal sinus rhythm, the right atrium begins to depolarize before the left atrium, so that the first 0.04 to 0.06 seconds of the P wave are due mostly to right atrial activation. Thus, effects of atrial enlargement may be manifested early, to the left and inferior (right atrial) or late and posterior (left atrial) portion of the P wave. If sinus rhythm is not present, for example, with an ectopic atrial rhythm or an electronic atrial pacemaker, these criteria are not applicable. The ECG criterion for right atrial enlargement is the presence of a peaked, tall P wave in lead II (Fig. 11.3). The upper limit of normal for the P wave amplitude is 2.5 mm over the age of 6 months, and 3.0 mm from 0 to 6 months (Table 11.2). This can be accompanied by a biphasic or tall P wave in lead V1. The criteria for left atrial enlargement include a broad notched P wave in lead II (P-wave duration >0.10 to 0.12 seconds) and/or a deep, slurred biphasic P wave in V1, particularly when the terminal negative component is broad and deep. Biatrial enlargement is considered to be present when signs of both right and left atrial enlargement are present.

Ventricular Depolarization

Normally, ventricular depolarization occurs virtually simultaneously at many sites, resulting in a QRS of brief duration. QRS duration is age dependent (Table 11.2). It is <80 ms from infancy through age 8 years, and less than 90 ms throughout childhood and early adolescence. QRS duration is an objective measure that can be determined reliably using computerized ECG recording systems. QRS duration may be prolonged by right or left bundle branch block (LBBB), ventricular pre-excitation, or a ventricular pacemaker. The term *intraventricular conduction delay* is reserved for those situations when QRS is prolonged but does not fit any of the above categories.

Axis Deviation

Axis is an ECG measurement derived from the equivalent dipole model. The electrical axis is the direction of the predominant vector of a wavefront in the frontal plane. It is a physiologic abstraction and an oversimplification because it does not take into account the time-dependent changes in vector forces that occur during atrial and ventricular depolarization. Still, it has been a popular ECG measure, and some prefer to call the axis the main frontal plane vector. The simplest way to present the concept is to represent leads I and aVF on a Cartesian system (Fig. 11.4), designating lead I as 0 (left) to 180 degrees (right) and lead aVF as 90 (inferior) to degrees 270 (superior), with the other limb leads corresponding to other angles in the frontal plane. The axis can be calculated for all three waves of the ECG. For example, using the system shown in Figure 11.4, one first determines a quadrant by looking at leads I and aVF. Once the quadrant is established, the frontal lead, which is most isoelectric, is identified. The mean QRS axis is perpendicular to this lead.

QRS and P axes are measured reliably by automated ECG interpretation systems, and normal values have been tabulated

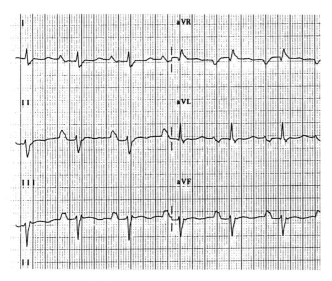

FIGURE 11.3 Six limb leads in an adolescent patient with right atrial enlargement following a Fontan procedure, at full standardization. Note that the P wave is not only tall but is broad as well.

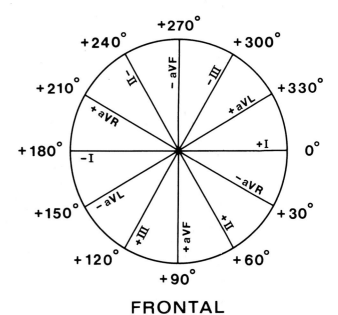

FIGURE 11.4 Reference frame for the frontal plane according to Einthoven's equilateral triangle. The lines are drawn through the center to the negative terminus of each lead. Thus, the 360 degrees are divided into multiple 30-degree sections.

(4,28,29). However, the same concepts can be applied to the ST segment, initial part of the QRS complex, and so on.

Frontal plane QRS axis deviation is age dependent. Right axis deviation is present when the QRS axis is more positive than normal, and left axis deviation is present when the QRS axis is less than normal. Right axis deviation is a criterion for right ventricular hypertrophy (RVH), albeit a very poor one. In pediatric patients, left axis deviation is not a criterion for left ventricular hypertrophy (LVH). The QRS axis is *superior* when it is between −60 and −100 degrees. The axis is *indeterminate* (neither left nor right or northwest) when it is between −100 and +210 degrees.

The most important pattern in pediatric patients is the so-called abnormally superior vector or abnormally superior axis. This occurs in patients with AV septal defects. The main QRS axis is superior, but the initial forces are inferior, so that leads II, III, and aVF inscribe a small r wave followed by a large S wave. This pattern of initial forces separates the abnormally superior vector from other causes of axis deviation.

Bundle Branch Block

Bundle branch block exists when there is prolongation of the QRS. Because the distal conduction system is divided into left and right bundle branches, which depolarize the left and right ventricles respectively, block in one of the bundle branches will lead to delayed activation of the corresponding ventricle. Thus, the diagnosis is based on knowledge of anatomy and analysis of the terminal vector forces of the QRS complex. For example, because the right ventricle is to the right, anterior and superior in relation to the left ventricle, right bundle branch block (RBBB) will give rise to terminal forces that are rightward, anterior, and superior. Furthermore, the left bundle normally divides into two fanlike sheets of specialized conduction tissue: The anterior and posterior fascicles. Delay or block in either fascicle will result in a characteristic ECG pattern.

In practice, it is not always possible to differentiate bundle branch block from severe ventricular hypertrophy. This is because severe hypertrophy can result in a prolonged QRS that mimics bundle branch block. In the hypertrophied heart, endocardial activation is presumed to be on time, but epicardial activation is delayed owing to prolonged conduction time through the hypertrophied ventricular wall.

Right Bundle Branch Block. In RBBB, the QRS complex is wide and has a characteristic morphology of a rapid initial deflection followed by a slurred slower portion of the QRS. This reflects the rapid depolarization of the left ventricle followed by the slower depolarization of the right ventricle through ventricular muscle. The criteria for complete right bundle branch includes a QRS above the upper limit for age in combination with normal initial forces and terminal conduction delay that is directed anteriorly, to the right and superior (wide and slurred S in leads I, V5, and V6; slurred R waves in leads aVR, V1, and V2; and wide and slurred S in leads II, III, and aVF) (Fig. 11.5).

The most common cause of RBBB is surgical closure of ventricular septal defects, especially in tetralogy of Fallot. When the ECG demonstrates RBBB, it is not possible to diagnose RVH. The usual markers of ischemia also are lost because of associated ST- and T-wave abnormalities.

"Incomplete" Right Bundle Branch Block. An RSR prime pattern in lead V1 with a normal or slightly prolonged QRS duration has been termed incomplete right bundle branch block. However, this pattern of ventricular conduction occurs in normal children. Further complicating matters, this pattern commonly occurs with right ventricular overload and frequently is present in patients with secundum atrial septal defects. Because of the prevalence of this pattern in normal children, it is perhaps better to refer to this as minor right ventricular conduction delay and not necessarily abnormal.

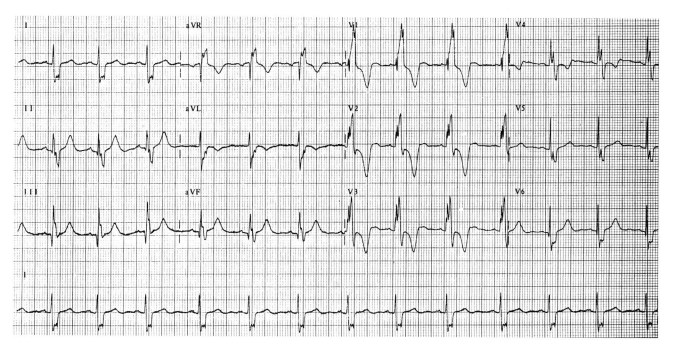

FIGURE 11.5 Twelve-lead ECG at full standardization in a 9-year-old patient with right bundle branch block, following repair of tetralogy of Fallot. Note that the initial QRS vector is normal, so left anterior hemiblock does not coexist.

Left Bundle Branch Block. Just as delay or block in the right bundle branch results in RBBB, delay or block in the main left bundle branch results in late activation of the left bundle and LBBB. The QRS is prolonged, slurred, and directed leftward, posteriorly, and inferiorly. The criteria for LBBB include an abnormally prolonged QRS duration, absent normal initial forces (no Q waves in leads aVL and V6), and notched slurred QRS complexes that are directed leftward and posteriorly (QS or rS in lead V1 and a tall notched R wave in lead V6).

Left bundle branch block is uncommon in children. It is usually the result of surgery on the left ventricular outflow tract. It also occurs with hypertrophic cardiomyopathy, myocarditis, or dilated cardiomyopathy (Fig. 11.6). As with RBBB, it is difficult, if not impossible, to assess hypertrophy and ischemic changes when LBBB is present.

Left Anterior Hemiblock. Normally, the left anterior fascicle is responsible for activation of the anterior and superior portion of the left ventricle, which occurs just ahead of activation of the posterior-inferior region by way of the left posterior fascicle. Block in the left anterior fascicle results in sequential activation of the left ventricle. The posterior-inferior region of the left ventricle is activated prior to the anterior-superior region. This causes abnormal QRS activation, with two sequential vectors: The initial forces are directed inferiorly and then spread in an anterior and superior fashion. This produces marked left axis deviation (< −30 degrees) with an rS in the inferior limb leads (II, III, and aVF). The QRS is normal or only minimally prolonged.

This conduction abnormality is relatively rare in children without congenital heart disease. It can occur with myocarditis, ischemia, or after cardiac surgery on the left ventricular outflow tract or ventricular septal defect closure. Tricuspid atresia and AV septal defects have ECG findings consistent with left anterior hemiblock (abnormally superior vector or axis) (31,32). However, these conditions do not have a true conduction defect, but rather, are related to the abnormal development of the conduction system.

Left Posterior Hemiblock. The activation sequence in left posterior hemiblock is the opposite of that seen with anterior hemiblock. The left ventricle depolarizes first in the anterior and superior region and then in the posterior and inferior portion. This produces an axis that is oriented rightward and inferiorly (120 degrees) with a normal QRS duration. Initial forces are directed superiorly (Q waves in leads II, III, and aVF). Left posterior hemiblock can be difficult to diagnose because most infants will have a rightward axis; this diagnosis should be reserved for a sudden change in axis between serial ECGs. It can result from surgical trauma and myocarditis.

Bifascicular Block. Right bundle branch block in combination with left anterior hemiblock occurs most commonly following repair of tetralogy of Fallot (10% of such patients). The ECG reflects the combination of these two conduction abnormalities. The initial forces, which in RBBB reflect only the left ventricle, initially are directed inferiorly and subsequently superiorly owing to left anterior hemiblock. The rest of the QRS complex reflects the characteristic terminal rightward and superior slurring of RBBB.

Right bundle branch block and left posterior hemiblock is rare and difficult to diagnose by ECG. It is characterized by RBBB with initial rightward forces. Because most children who develop RBBB following surgery have pre-existing RVH, it is difficult to distinguish RBBB with left posterior hemiblock from pre-existing RVH.

Pre-excitation

Pre-excitation describes an abnormal depolarization of the ventricle prior to normal conduction through the His–Purkinje system. This takes place because of activation via an accessory connection between the two chambers.

Wolff–Parkinson–White Pattern. Wolff–Parkinson–White syndrome results from the presence of an accessory pathway that connects the atria directly to ventricular muscle. Conduction occurs both across the normal conduction system (AV node and His–Purkinje system) and across the accessory pathway. The ECG has a characteristic appearance of a short PR interval and a wide QRS complex (see Chapters 13 and 14). A delta wave or slurred upstroke of the QRS, indicating conduction from atrial to ventricular muscle, is characteristic of the syndrome. The terminal part of the complex may be wide or narrow, depending on the degree of conduction via the AV node. Children who have this finding are subject to episodes of reciprocating AV tachycardia. To diagnose WPW syndrome, a patient must have both the characteristic pattern of pre-excitation as well as episodes of supraventricular tachycardia or atrial fibrillation. Therefore, the electrocardiographer should read the ECG as showing a "WPW pattern" or "pre-excitation."

Mahaim's Pathway. The Mahaim pathway is a particular type of accessory pathway that inserts into the right bundle branch or right ventricle and incorporates AV node–like tissue. There are several types. The most common is the atriofascicular pathway, with nodofascicular and fasciculoventricular pathways being less common (33). A Mahaim pattern of pre-excitation is one in which there is a widened QRS with an appearance similar to that in WPW, but in which there is a normal PR interval.

Lown–Ganong–Levine Syndrome. This entity exists when there is a short PR interval without a QRS abnormality in association with episodes of abnormal tachycardia. With the advent of invasive electrophysiologic testing, this entity has essentially disappeared from the literature, most likely owing to the fact that there does not seem to be a clear electrophysiologic correlate to the so-called Lown–Ganong–Levine syndrome. Most of these patients, in fact, were adults who had atrial fibrillation with fast AV node conduction. When there is a short PR interval with a normal QRS morphology and duration, one should simply read the ECG as showing a short PR interval rather than the Lown–Ganong–Levine pattern.

Hypertrophy

Criteria for ECG determination of ventricular hypertrophy rely largely on whether QRS voltages in specific leads exceed normal values. The criteria were derived empirically, based on studies of normal infants or on comparison of ECG measurements with findings at cardiac catheterization, surgery, or autopsy. Interpretation of criteria for hypertrophy depends on the assumption that cardiac-torso geometry is normal or near normal and the ventricular depolarization sequence is normal (i.e., no bundle branch block). Because of the proximity effect, the closer the heart is to a particular precordial lead, the greater the observed voltage, regardless of the underlying cardiac pathology. Limb leads give rise to little or no proximity effect (6). This effect is particularly important in infants who have relatively thin chests. Consequently, some leads are better for determining certain types of hypertrophy. Still, if one approaches the problem of ventricular hypertrophy by thinking in terms of the vector forces involved, combined with the

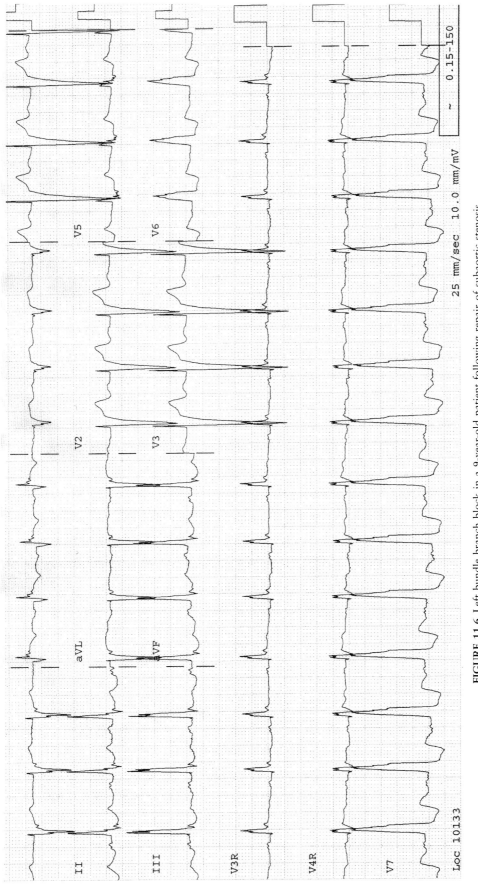

FIGURE 11.6 Left bundle branch block in a 9-year-old patient following repair of subaortic stenosis with dilated cardiomyopathy.

261

knowledge of cardiac anatomy and the relative positions of the right and left ventricle in the chest, the criteria for RVH and LVH will not seem entirely arbitrary. That is, the right ventricle is to the right, anterior, and superior, so that increased forces to the right, anterior, and superior suggest RVH. Likewise, the left ventricle is to the left, inferior, and posterior, and increased forces directed to the left, inferior, and posterior suggest LVH. Leads V5 and V6 may be used to judge left-right forces, leads V1 and V2 can be used for judging anterior-posterior forces, and aVF is the best lead for judging inferior-superior forces.

Left Ventricular Hypertrophy. In general, criteria for LVH are based on QRS voltage criteria and repolarization criteria. The voltage criteria involve voltage increase, and the repolarization criteria refer to the shift of the T-wave axis in the direction opposite to the QRS. Voltage criteria involve R and S waves in leads V1, V6, and aVF and Q wave amplitude in lead V6. These measurements are compared with known normal standards that vary with age. The repolarization criteria refer to T-wave negativity in the lateral precordial leads and the angle (>100 degrees) between the frontal plane QRS and T axis.

R-wave amplitude greater than the 98th percentile for age in lead V6 and S-wave amplitude greater than the 98th percentile in lead V1 have been used to predict LVH. Unfortunately, hypertrophy may be present with normal left-sided forces, and normal children can have R waves in lead V6 that are above the 98th percentile. The large S wave in lead V1 owing to increased posterior forces is a much better criterion for LVH (Fig. 11.7).

Patients with LVH usually have increased inferior forces manifesting a tall R wave in aVF, but this also may occur in RVH. In the absence of RVH, this criterion is helpful in supporting a diagnosis of LVH, particularly in a patient with prominent midprecordial voltages because the limb leads are not prone to proximity effect.

In newborns, if an adult pattern of R-wave progression is evident, rather than the neonatal pattern, LVH is likely. That is, when a newborn manifests small R waves and deep S waves over the right precordium progressing to tall R waves and small S waves in the left lateral precordium, it suggests that there is left ventricular dominance. This corresponds to the vectorcardiographic finding of a wide-open counterclockwise loop in the horizontal plane.

T-wave abnormalities are the most reliable indication of LVH. A so-called strain pattern consists of inverted T waves in the inferior leads (II, III, and aVF) and left precordial leads (V5 and V6). One can compare the frontal plane T-wave axis with the QRS axis, and the difference between these is the QRS-T angle. Normally it is very small, and a wide QRS-T angle of >100 degrees is supportive of the diagnosis of LVH but is not specific. T-wave abnormalities in LVH sometimes can be associated with depression of the ST segment. T-wave inversion also may be a sign of ischemia or myocardial inflammation; thus, these causes must be excluded prior to the diagnosis of LVH being made.

Left axis deviation is supportive of the diagnosis of LVH, especially in infancy. Left anterior hemiblock also may cause left axis deviation.

Abnormally prominent Q waves in the left lateral precordium (leads V5 and V6) may result from hypertrophy of the left ventricular portion of the interventricular septum, or perhaps from abnormal position of the left relative to the right ventricle owing to hypertrophy. A dilated volume-loaded left ventricle, which occurs with aortic valve insufficiency or patent ductus arteriosus, tends to produce deep Q wave in the lateral leads. On the other hand, with severe LVH, as might be seen with severe pressure loading, small or absent Q waves occur.

Right Ventricular Hypertrophy. Criteria for RVH are more specific than for LVH and include voltage and repolarization criteria. Because of normal right ventricular predominance in

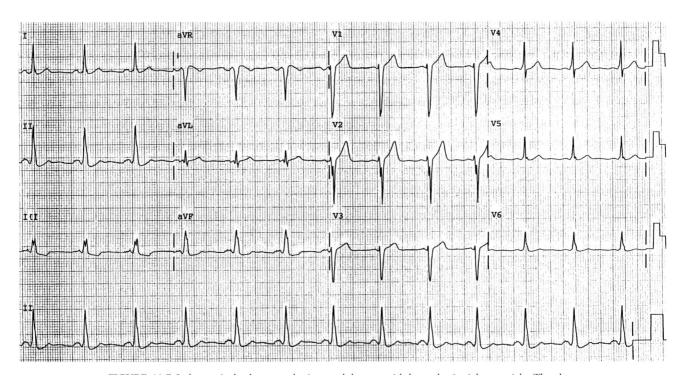

FIGURE 11.7 Left ventricular hypertrophy in an adolescent with hypoplastic right ventricle. The chest leads are half standard. Note that the S wave in V1 is very large and broad, whereas the R wave in V6 is not.

the neonate and the rapid changes in T-wave vectors in the first 2 weeks of life, the ECG interpretation of RVH in infants may be difficult.

R-wave amplitude in lead V1 that is greater than the 98th percentile for age is a very specific finding for RVH beyond the neonatal period. It has been used to estimate right ventricular pressure in isolated pulmonary stenosis using the following formula: Peak systolic right ventricular pressure = R-wave height, in mm × 5 (34). An R wave in V1 that is >20 mm correlates with a right ventricular pressure that is at least systemic.

An abnormally deep S wave in V6 (>98th percentile) is a very sensitive indicator of RVH. It often occurs in patients with increased right ventricular pressure secondary to chronic lung disease. When this pattern occurs with right atrial enlargement, it is characteristic of cor pulmonale. This criterion is less specific than the R wave in lead V1 because of the possibility of posterobasal LVH, in which large terminal superior and rightward forces result from hypertrophy of this late-activating portion of the left ventricle.

The R/S ratio is well established for various ages. If it is abnormally increased in lead V1, or abnormally decreased in lead V6, RVH is likely. However, it is rare for an abnormal R/S ratio to occur as an isolated finding, and this criterion should, therefore, be applied in conjunction with other findings of RVH.

T-wave orientation changes with age. Normally, it is upright until 4 to 7 days of age. Between 1 week of age and adolescence it is negative, and reverts to upright again in many individuals in adolescence and adulthood. An upright T wave after 7 days of age but before adolescence is a sensitive indicator of increased right ventricular pressure. The sensitivity of this measure increases when R-wave amplitude also is considered. Mild RVH is manifested by normal R-wave amplitude but an upright T wave. Moderate RVH is manifested by increased R-wave amplitude and an upright T wave, whereas severe RVH is manifested by an increased R-wave amplitude and inversion of the T wave.

A qR pattern also can be indicative of RVH, especially in conjunction with a tall R wave (typically >10 mm). It also occurs with l-looping of the ventricles (abnormal septal depolarization), anterior myocardial infarction, and WPW syndrome.

An RSR prime pattern can be associated with right ventricular volume overload, as seen with atrial septal defects, but also may be a normal finding. It should be used to diagnose RVH only when the R prime amplitude is large.

Right axis deviation alone is not a criterion for RVH, but can be used to support other findings suggestive of RVH. Another cause of right axis deviation is left posterior hemiblock.

As in LVH, the R-wave progression across the precordial leads may be helpful. The neonatal pattern, consisting of tall R waves and small S waves in the right precordium, progressing to small R waves and deep S waves in the left lateral precordium, suggests right ventricular dominance (Fig. 11.8). When this pattern occurs in older children, rather than the normal adult-type R-wave progression, it suggests severe RVH. This corresponds to a completely clockwise loop in the horizontal plane.

Biventricular Hypertrophy. The diagnosis of biventricular hypertrophy (BVH) is made most easily when there are clear criteria present for both RVH and LVH. This often is manifest by normal R-wave progression across the precordium, but with increased voltages, so that there are both large R and S waves in leads V1 and V6. Proximity effect may produce prominent voltages in normal children in the midprecordial leads (V3 to V5) without increases in leads V1 or V6 or any of the limb leads. In this situation, one should not diagnose hypertrophy, but should instead note the presence of prominent midprecordial voltage. However, if the total voltage (R plus S) in lead V4 is >60 mm, BVH is likely (the Katz–Wachtel criterion).

Some electrocardiographers diagnose BVH when there are clear criteria for hypertrophy of one chamber and normal voltages arising from the other chamber (e.g., >98th percentile R in V6 with greater than mean S in V6). They reason that the predominance of one chamber cancels or masks voltage from the other chamber, and therefore normal voltages could reflect hypertrophy. Although this approach makes some sense, in practice it seems to be dependent on the magnitude of the hypertrophy involved (i.e., it is more likely to be true if one chamber is severely hypertrophied). This criterion also suffers from the oversimplified viewpoint that R and S waves arise from one chamber only. For example, it would be

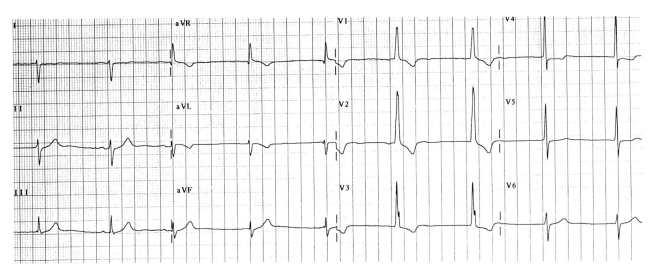

FIGURE 11.8 Right ventricular hypertrophy in a 15-year-old with d-transposition and a Mustard procedure. Twelve-lead ECG at full standardization. Note the reversed or neonatal-type R wave progression as well as the very tall and broad R wave in leads V1 and V2.

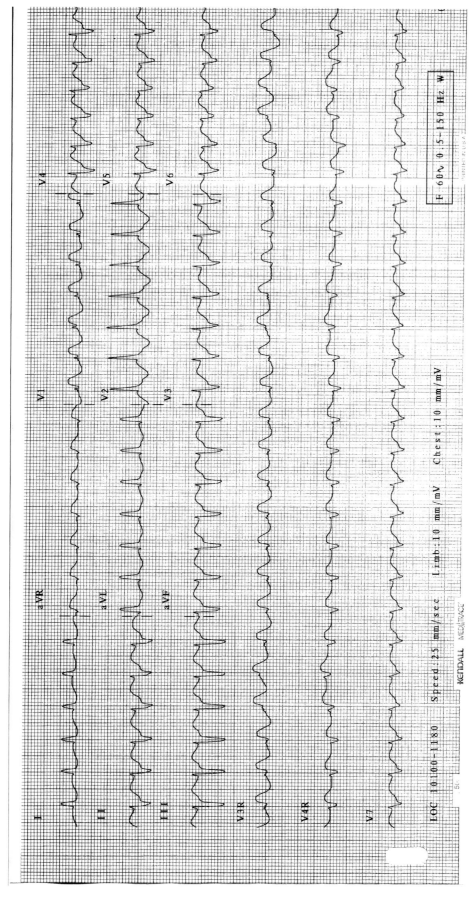

FIGURE 11.9 Low-voltage QRS complexes with ST-segment elevation and depression in a 3-year-old patient with acute myocarditis.

incorrect to believe that for patients with LVH, the S wave in V6 and the S wave in lead aVF reflect only right ventricular forces, because the posterobasal portion of the left ventricle depolarizes later than the rest of the left ventricle. LVH also may include the posterobasal portion of the left ventricle, with normal to increased S waves in leads V6 or aVF without BVH.

Low QRS Voltage. Reduced QRS voltage is a nonspecific finding that may occurs with various conditions, including myocarditis, pericardial effusion, and generalized edema. Low voltage is present when the QRS amplitude is <5 mm in all limb leads and <10 mm in all precordial leads. When associated with ST-segment change, it is characteristic of myocarditis (Fig. 11.9).

Initial Forces

The Q wave occurs at the beginning of the QRS complex. One normally finds a small (<4 mm) Q wave in leads V5 and V6, and aVF. This is because normal initial depolarization, made up of several different areas of endocardial activation including the septum, is rightward, superior, and anterior. There are only a few specific situations when the presence or absence of certain types of Q waves may be of clinical significance. If the QRS duration is prolonged, no specific significance can be attached to Q waves. For the diagnosis of myocardial infarction, Q-wave duration should be ≥40 ms (35). Q-wave amplitude is lead dependent but in all cases should exceed 4 mm. A qR pattern in lead V1 signifies RVH, and deep Q waves in leads II, III, aVF, V5, and V6 are indicative of left septal hypertrophy, usually as part of LVH. Finally, in patients with congenitally corrected transposition of the great arteries and ventricular inversion, initial forces are posterior and to the left, producing a small Q wave in V1 or a qS complex, with absence of the normal Q wave in leads V5 and V6.

Ventricular Repolarization

Considered from the standpoint of a single cardiac cell action potential, repolarization is simply defined and begins immediately following depolarization. However, viewed from the perspective of the whole heart, repolarization is more difficult to characterize (36). In the normal heart, the subendocardium depolarizes before the subepicardium, but the subepicardium repolarizes before the subendocardium. This figures prominently in ECG features during the ST segment and T wave. There is an age-dependent overlap between the end of depolarization and the onset of repolarization. In childhood, repolarization potentials appear an average of 10 ms before the end of ventricular depolarization (J point) (37).

QT Interval

There has been considerable debate regarding the best way to measure the rest and exercise QT interval. In supine patients at rest, the technical difficulty is determination of the end of the T wave, which may be fused with the U wave as it gradually blends with the baseline (37,38). Furthermore, Davignon et al. (29) demonstrated that the QT interval is both age and heart rate dependent. Attempts to correct for heart rate usually involve Bazett's formula (QTc = QT interval divided by the square root of the preceding R-R interval, where QTc is the corrected QT interval). However, this may be inaccurate at low heart rates, often seen in adolescents. An alternative proposal has been made that the predicted QT (in milliseconds) be estimated by the following formula: 656/[(1 + 0.1)(heart rate)] (39). Technical problems are compounded during exercise

because of the difficulty in identifying the ECG baseline. They also are complicated by variations in the RR interval that occur in children due to sinus arrhythmia. The choice of RR interval to be measured is critical in calculating the corrected QT interval. Garson (40) has suggested measuring the shortest RR interval. Calculating the QTc from that interval, he found that a cutoff of 460 ms for QTc identifies 98.4% of known long QT syndrome patients but only 3.8% of normal control subjects.

The QT interval may be prolonged on a congenital basis (41,42) or as the result of antiarrhythmic drugs or electrolyte imbalance (43). The significance of a prolonged QT interval in an asymptomatic child is unknown. There seems to be little disagreement that a QT of 400 ms is normal and a QT of 480 ms is abnormal. However, there is disagreement as to the significance of intermediate values, especially in asymptomatic patients. Even in patients with pathologic prolongation of the QT interval, no ECG feature has been identified (not even the QT interval) that predicts which patients will develop symptoms or torsades de pointes (44).

ST Segment, T Waves, and U Waves

ST Segment. Identifying the true baseline is extremely important when analyzing the ST segment. This is an important practical problem when the heart rate is increased as during exercise or with fever. ST segments >1 mm are said to be elevated. and ST segments <−0.5 mm are considered depressed. However, in an analysis of average (0 to 50 ms) ST-segment potentials, the maximum and minimum potentials were age dependent. Maximum potentials (1.1 to 3.7 mm) occurred during adolescence. Minimum ST-segment potentials (0.4 to 1.2 mm) occurred during childhood (37,38). Interpretation of apparent ST-segment abnormalities requires careful attention to the clinical situation and important age-dependent and technical limitations.

T Waves. The sequence of ventricular depolarization, as characterized by the time difference between the earliest and latest area to depolarize, is an important determinant of the T wave (i.e., asynchronous depolarization influences the ECG patterns). Abnormalities of depolarization have a direct effect on repolarization. Therefore, T-wave abnormalities may be entirely owing to QRS abnormalities. Such abnormalities are termed secondary T-wave abnormalities as opposed to primary T-wave abnormalities, which reflect actual abnormalities of repolarization not simply caused by changes in the QRS (45).

U Waves. Little is known about the source or significance of U waves. They are quite common in young people, but Spach et al. (37,38) did not find them in children <8 years of age. U waves usually are apparent in the midprecordial leads (V2 to V5), and they often overlap the T wave, resulting in TU fusion. The latter feature may complicate measurement of the QT interval. The amplitude of U waves is about 10% that of T waves (range 4% to 28%). The U-wave amplitude is heart rate sensitive. When U waves are large and difficult to separate from the T wave, they may indicate prolonged QT syndrome.

Specific Abnormalities Affecting the ST Segment, T Wave, and U Wave

Early Repolarization. Early repolarization usually occurs in adolescents and is associated with ST-segment elevation. This is seen best in the anterior and midprecordial leads (V2 to V4) (Fig. 11.10). Because repolarization normally begins before depolarization ends, this term is a misnomer. Elevation of the ST segment may be explained by the normal age-dependent changes of ST-segment potentials. It can mimic

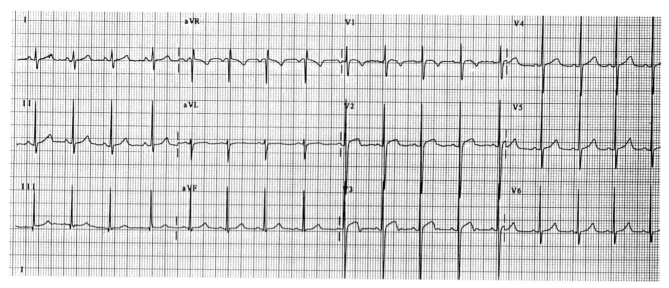

FIGURE 11.10 Early repolarization in a 6-year-old seen on a 12-lead ECG at full standardization. Note the 2-mm ST-segment elevation in leads V2 and V3.

changes associated with pericarditis and may be confusing in the evaluation of adolescents with chest pain. With early repolarization, J-point elevation often disappears with exercise. Serial ECGs may be helpful in separating early repolarization from the typical evolution of ST- and T-wave abnormality in pericarditis.

Pericarditis and Pericardial Effusions. Pericarditis is the most common cause of ST-segment elevation in children. There are a series of changes that occur as pericarditis evolves. Initially the ST segment is elevated with a normal T wave, thought to be secondary to subepicardial myocarditis. The ST segment then returns to normal, but the T wave becomes flat and then inverted. Characteristically, these findings differ from ischemic changes in that they involve all leads (46). Pericardial effusions can result in diminished QRS voltages and, rarely, electrical alternans (alternating QRS amplitude).

Myocarditis. Myocarditis usually results in flattened or inverted T waves and low-voltage QRS patterns. The QT interval may be prolonged. AV block and intraventricular conduction delay also can occur.

Ischemia. Myocardial ischemia is rare in children, but there are certain situations in which it must be considered. These include Kawasaki's disease and congenital coronary artery abnormalities. Myocardial ischemia initially presents as distortion of the T wave, which becomes tall and peaked in the leads near the affected myocardial segment. The ST segment may be affected. If ischemia is promptly reversed, these changes will resolve. If ischemia persists, however, the myocardium will progress to the injury stage. The ECG may show deviation in the ST segments. The ST segments may become elevated or depressed depending on whether the injury is endocardial or epicardial. Reversal of ischemia may reverse these changes. Further injury will result in infarction, which appears on the ECG as a decrease in R-wave voltage and appearance of abnormal Q waves facing the infarcted segment (35).

Myocardial ischemia in an infant is caused by congenital coronary abnormalities, the most common being anomalous origin of the left coronary from the pulmonary artery. These infants usually present with ischemia or infarction of the anterior and septal areas (distribution of the left anterior descending coronary artery). They have deep Q waves in leads I, aVL, and V3 to V6. There also is loss of the midprecordial R wave with a normal R wave in V1 and V6.

Kawasaki's disease is the most common acquired cause of myocardial infarction in children. The ECG is characterized initially by low QRS voltages and nonspecific T-wave changes typical of myocarditis. These may progress to a myocardial infarction pattern.

Potassium Imbalance. Hyperkalemia produces tall peaked T waves. However, this finding is nonspecific and insensitive because normal children may have peaked T waves, and those with hyperkalemia may not have peaked T waves. As the potassium level increases, the T waves become more peaked and an intraventricular conduction delay results in a widened QRS along with PR prolongation. The resultant ECG may resemble a sine wave or wide ventricular tachycardia. At concentrations of 9 mEq/L atrial standstill, AV bloc and ventricular fibrillation can occur.

Hypokalemia is associated with decreased T-wave amplitude. As potassium levels decrease, a U wave becomes apparent and the ST segment becomes depressed. Hypokalemia will enhance the arrhythmogenic effects of digoxin.

Calcium and Magnesium Imbalance. Hypercalcemia shortens the QT interval by shortening the ST segment. It also produces sinus rate slowing and sinoatrial block. Hypocalcemia lengthens the QT interval by prolonging the ST segment. A low magnesium level may enhance the effects of a low calcium level. In some infants the ECG will normalize only after calcium and magnesium both are corrected.

THE NORMAL ELECTROCARDIOGRAM

Developmental Changes

The hallmark of the ECG changes in the normal infant and child are the age-related transitions of QRS morphology, QRS duration, and the pattern of the ST segment and T wave (29,47–49). During normal development, there is a gradual decrease in heart rate and an increase in P-wave duration, PR interval, and QRS duration. Compared with those at older ages, the QRS voltages are low during the first several months of life. The mean QRS axis in the frontal plane moves in a direction from right to left. Although one might hypothesize that the observed increase in PR interval and QRS duration are related to changes in the size of the heart or the AV node, this hypothesis has not been borne out in studies in large animals.

The right ventricular dominance of the infant was one of the first age-dependent ECG changes to be recognized. The changes in depolarization of the ventricles during the first year of life occur in an orderly progression. In the newborn, the principal QRS potentials result from the right ventricle. The transition of the ECG from right ventricular dominance at birth to the pattern of left ventricular dominance lags behind hemodynamic changes. Loss of right ventricular dominance starts at about 1 month of age, and left ventricular dominance is well established by 1 year. These changes are appreciated best by the R-wave progression in the precordial leads during the first year of life. At birth and for the first several weeks of life there are tall R waves and small S waves in the right and anterior precordium (V3R, V4R, and V1), and deep S waves and small R waves in the left precordium (V6 and V7). This corresponds to a clockwise vector loop in the horizontal plane. With the establishment of left ventricular dominance, the precordial leads progress to a more adult pattern by 2 months of age, with deeper S waves in the right and anterior precordium and taller S waves in the left precordium, corresponding to a counterclockwise vector loop in the horizontal plane. At this age, however, there is still a prominent R wave in V1. By 1 year of age, the precordial R-wave progression is similar to that in the adult, with small R waves and deep S waves in the right and anterior precordium.

T waves change in a characteristic way, but the age-related patterns of repolarization are more difficult to interpret than the depolarization changes. The changes in right ventricular pressure that occur rapidly in the first days of life in normal infants have very little effect on the P wave or the QRS complex but have a great effect on the T wave. In the first minutes after birth, the T-wave vector is anterior and to the left (upright in V1 and V6). The T-wave vector may swing rightward in the next several hours, producing flattening or inversion of the T wave in the left lateral leads. Over the next 7 days, the T-wave vector moves posterior and leftward, producing an inverted T wave in V1 and an upright T wave in V6. Finally, the T wave becomes upright again in V1 after 7 or 8 years of age, but may remain inverted throughout adolescence (so-called juvenile T-wave pattern).

Preterm Infant

Compared with the ECG of term infants, the initial ECG of the premature infant is notable for its shorter QRS duration. The PR interval and QT interval also are shorter. The ECG of the premature infant is characterized by less right ventricular dominance at birth than the ECG of the full-term infant (50,51). At 1 year of age, the heart rate of the premature infant exceeds that of the term infant. Furthermore, precordial voltages are lower in the 1-year-old infant who was premature (51). The reduced precordial voltages may occur in the absence of bronchopulmonary dysplasia. Whether these differences are related to intrinsic myocardial differences of the premature versus term infant or to altered cardiac-torso geometry is unknown.

The Athlete

Athletes can have unusual ECG findings. For example, Oakley and Oakley (52) evaluated ten athletes with ECGs with voltage criteria for LVH (seven patients), nonspecific ST-segment and T-wave changes (three patients), and Q-wave changes suggestive of anterior myocardial infarction. No cardiac abnormalities were found after extensive evaluation. Balady et al. (53) reported QRS duration ≥100 ms in 60% of athletes, and 13% had ST-segment and T-wave changes that mimicked acute ischemia. Atrial enlargement was rare. Bjornstad et al. (54) reported athletes with sinus bradycardia and prolonged PR and QT intervals. They suggested that different criteria for ventricular hypertrophy were warranted for athletes.

Gender and Racial Differences

There are gender and racial ECG differences (55–57). The racial differences usually are not apparent until the preteen (ages 6 to 10) years. By 11 to 14 years of age, both sex and race differences are noted. It is important to know that the widely used normal standards published by Davignon were based on 2,141 white children (29). In general, voltages in both limb and precordial leads are increased in males when compared with females and in blacks as compared with whites. Differences are not noted between black and white females. There are differences in left ventricular posterior wall thickness among males (56). Similar findings occur in children with hypertension. It may be that the larger voltages on the ECG represent an early sign of increased left ventricular mass (58).

GUIDELINES AND INDICATIONS

The Committee on Electrocardiography of the Task Force on Assessment of Diagnostic and Therapeutic Cardiovascular Procedures has published guidelines for the use of the ECG (59). The guidelines relate to three patient groups: (i) patients with known cardiovascular disease, (ii) subjects with suspected cardiovascular disease, and (iii) subjects with normal hearts. Within groups, the guidelines are extended to (a) baseline or initial evaluation, (b) response to therapy, (c) follow-up, and (d) preoperative (noncardiac) evaluation. Within each of the subcategories, guidelines are divided as class I, or conditions for which there is general agreement regarding use of ECG; class II, or conditions for which there are divergent views regarding use of ECG; and class III, or conditions for which there is agreement that ECG is of little or no use.

In children, the primary uses of ECG include initial evaluation of patients with suspected cardiovascular disease and serial evaluation of the patient with known cardiovascular disease. The ECG is indispensable for evaluation of the patient with known or suspected disorders of rhythm and conduction, including patients with palpitations and syncope. ECGs also are indicated for determining the response to antiarrhythmic drugs or drugs with potential cardiac effects (e.g., tricyclic antidepressants). There appears to be little rationale for routine ECG screening of asymptomatic, ostensibly normal young patients ≤ age 40 years. This argument applies to routine well-child examination as well as to preoperative screening.

References

1. Burchell HB. A centennial note on Waller and the first human electrocardiogram. *Am J Cardiol* 1987;59:979–983.
2. Fournier M. Willem Einthoven—the electrophysiology of the heart. *Medicamundi* 1976;21:65–70.
3. Fisch C. Evolution of the clinical electrocardiogram. *J Am Coll Cardiol* 1989;14:1127–1138.
4. Ziegler RF. Electrocardiographic *Studies in Normal Infants and Children*. Springfield, IL: Charles C Thomas Publisher, 1951:3–9.
5. Barr RC. The electrocardiogram and its relationship to excitation of the heart. In: Sperelakis N, ed. *Physiology and Pathophysiology of the Heart*. Boston: Kluwer Academic Publishers, 1989:175–194.
6. Plonsey R. The biophysical basis for electrocardiography. In: Liebman J, Plonsey R, Gillette PC, eds. *Pediatric Electrocardiography*. Baltimore: Williams & Wilkins, 1982:1–14.
7. Bailey JJ, Berson AS, Garson A Jr, et al. Recommendations for standardization of leads and of specifications for instruments in electrocardiography and vector cardiography: Report of the Committee on Electrocardiography and Cardiac Electrophysiology of the Council on Clinical Cardiology, American Heart Association. *Circulation* 1990;81:730–739.
8. Frank E. An accurate, clinically practical system for spatial vector cardiography. *Circulation* 1956;13:737–749.
9. Barr RC, Spach MS, Herman-Giddings GS. Selection of the number and positions of measuring locations for electrocardiography. *IEEE Trans Biomed Eng* 1971;18:125–138.
10. Kavuru MS, Vesselle H, Thomas CW. Advances in body surface potential mapping (BSPM) instrumentation. In: Liebman J, Plonsey R, Rudy Y, eds. *Pediatric and Fundamental Electrocardiography*. Boston: Martinus Nijhoff, 1987:315–326.
11. Barr RC, Spach MS. Sampling rates required for digital recording of intracellular and extracellular cardiac potentials. *Circ Res* 1977;55:40–48.
12. Thomas CW, Lee D. Methodology in constructing body surface potential maps. In: Liebman J, Plonsey R, Rudy Y, eds. *Pediatric and Fundamental Electrocardiography*. Boston: Martinus Nijhoff, 1987:329–346.
13. Barr RC, Spach MS. Construction and interpretation of body surface maps. *Prog Cardiovasc Dis* 1983;26:33–42.
14. Barold SS. Filtered bipolar esophageal electrocardiography. *Am Heart J* 1972;83:431.
15. Benson DW Jr, Sanford M, Dunnigan A, et al. Transesophageal atrial pacing threshold: Role of interelectrode spacing, pulse width and catheter insertion depth. *Am J Cardiol* 1984;53:63–67.
16. Benson DW Jr. Transesophageal electrocardiography and cardiac pacing: State of the art. *Circulation* 1987;75(pt 2):III86–92.
17. Simson MB. Use of signals in the terminal QRS complex to identify patients with ventricular tachycardia after myocardial infarction. *Circulation* 1981;64:235–242.
18. Boineau JP, Cox JL. Slow ventricular activation in acute myocardial infarction: A source of re-entrant ventricular contractions. *Circulation* 1978; 45:702–713.
19. Zimmermann M, Friedli B, Adamec R, et al. Frequency of ventricular late potentials and fractionated right ventricular electrograms after operative repair of tetralogy of Fallot. *Am J Cardiol* 1987;13:737–749.
20. Blomstrom-Lundqvist C, Hirsch I, Olsson SB, et al. Quantitative analysis of the signal-averaged QRS in patients with arrhythmogenic right ventricular dysplasia. *Eur Heart J* 1988;9(3):301–312.
21. Holter J. Radioelectrocardiography: A new technique for cardiovascular studies. *Ann N Y Acad Sci* 1957;65:913–923.
22. Knoebel SB, Crawford MH, Dunn MI, et al. Guidelines for ambulatory electrocardiography: Report of ACC/AHA task force on assessment of diagnostic and therapeutic cardiovascular procedures. *Circulation* 1989;79:206–215.
23. Southall DP, Johnston F, Shinebourne EA, et al. A 24-hour ECG study of heart rate and rhythm patterns in a population of healthy children. *Br Heart J* 1981;45:281–291.
24. Dickinson DF, Scott O. Ambulatory electrocardiographic monitoring in 100 healthy teenage boys. *Br Heart J* 1984;51:179–183.
25. Southall DP, Richards JM, Mitchell P, et al. Study of cardiac rhythm in healthy newborn infants. *Br Heart J* 1980;43:14–20.
26. Dick M, McFadden D, Crowley D, et al. Diagnosis and management of cardiac rhythm disorders by transtelephonic electrocardiography in infants and children. *J Pediatr* 1979;94:612–615.
27. Goldstein MA, Hesslein P, Dunnigan A. Efficacy of transtelephonic electrocardiographic monitoring in pediatric patients. *Am J Dis Child* 1990;144: 178–182.
28. Rossano J, Bloemers B, Sreeram N, et al. Efficacy of implantable loop recorders in establishing symptom-rhythm correlation in young patients with syncope and palpitations. *Pediatrics* 2003;112(pt 1):e228–233.
29. Davignon A, Rautaharju P, Barselle E, et al. Normal ECG standards for infants and children. *Pediatr Cardiol* 1979/80;1:123–134.
30. Liebman J. Tables of normal standard. In: Liebman J, Plonsey R, Gillette PC, eds. *Pediatric Electrocardiography*. Baltimore: Williams & Wilkins, 1982:82–133.
31. Dick M, Fyler DC, Nadas AS. Tricuspid atresia: The clinical course in 101 patients. *Am J Cardiol* 1975;36:327–337.
32. Campbell RM, Dick M II, Hees P, et al. Epicardial and endocardial activation in patients with endocardial cushion defects. *Am J Cardiol* 1983;51: 277–281.
33. Sallee D, Van Hare GF. Preexcitation secondary to fasciculoventricular pathways in children: A report of three cases. *J Cardiovasc Electrophysiol* 1999;10(1):36–42.
34. Cayler GG, Onley P, Nadas AS. Relation of systolic pressure in the right ventricle to the electrocardiogram. *N Engl J Med* 1958;258:979–982.
35. Towbin JA, Bricker JT, Garson A Jr. Electrocardiographic criteria for diagnosis of acute myocardial infarction in childhood. *Am J Cardiol* 1992;69: 1545–1548.
36. Spach MS, Barr RC. Origin of epicardial ST-T wave potentials in the intact dog. *Circ Res* 1976;39:475–487.
37. Spach MS, Barr RC, Benson DW Jr, et al. Body surface low-level potentials during ventricular repolarization with analysis of the ST segment. *Circulation* 1979;59:822–836.
38. Spach MS, Barr RC, Warren RB, et al. Isopotential body surface mapping in subjects of all ages: Emphasis on low-level potentials with analysis of the method. *Circulation* 1979;59:805–821.
39. Rautaharju PM, Warren JW. Estimation of QT prolongation: A persistent, avoidable error in computer electrocardiography. *J Electrocardiol* 1990; 23(suppl):111–117.
40. Garson A Jr. How to measure the QT interval—what is normal? *Am J Cardiol* 1993;72:14B–16B.
41. Moss AL, Schwartz PJ, Crampton RS, et al. The long QR syndrome: Prospective longitudinal study of 328 families. *Circulation* 1991;84: 1135–1144.
42. Keating M. Linkage analysis and long QT syndrome. *Circulation* 1992; 85:1973–1986.
43. Singh BN. When is QT prolongation antiarrhythmic and when is it proarrhythmic? *Am J Cardiol* 1989;63:867–869.
44. Benhorin J, Merri M, Alberti M, et al. Long QT syndrome: New electrocardiographic characteristics. *Circulation* 1990;82:521–527.
45. Surawicz B. The pathogenesis and clinical significance of primary T wave abnormalities. In: Schlant RC, Hurst JW, eds. *Advances in Electrocardiography*. New York: Grune & Stratton, 1972:377–421.
46. Spodick DH. Electrocardiogram in acute pericarditis. *Am J Cardiol* 1974; 33:470–474.
47. Liebman J. The normal electrocardiogram. In: Liebman J, Plonsey R, Gillette PC, eds. *Pediatric Electrocardiography*. Baltimore: Williams & Wilkins, 1982:144–171.
48. Walsh Z. The electrogram during the first week of life. *Br Heart J* 1963;25:784–794.
49. Hait G, Gasul BM. The evolution and significance of T wave changes in the normal newborn during the first seven days of life. *Am J Cardiol* 1963; 12:494–504.
50. Sreenivasan V, Fisher BJ, Liebman J, et al. Longitudinal study of the standard electrocardiogram in the healthy premature infant during the first year of life. *Am J Cardiol* 1973;31:57–63.
51. Walsh EP, Long P, Ellison RC, et al. Electrocardiograms of the premature infant at 1 year of age. *Pediatrics* 1986;77:353–356.
52. Oakley DM, Oakley CM. Significance of abnormal electrocardiograms in highly trained athletes. *Am J Cardiol* 1982;50:985–989.
53. Balady GJ, Cadigan JB, Ryan TJ. Electrocardiogram of the athlete: An analysis of 289 professional football players. *Am J Cardiol* 1984;53:1339–1343.
54. Bjornstad H, Storstein L, Meen HD, et al. Electrocardiographic findings in athletic students and sedentary controls. *J Cardiol* 1991;79:290–305.
55. Rao PS. Racial differences in electrocardiograms and vectorcardiograms between black and white adolescents. *J Electrocardiol* 1985;18:309–313.
56. Hashida E, Nishi T. Constitutional and echocardiographic variability of the normal electrocardiogram in children. *J Electrocardiol* 1988;21:231–237.
57. Rao PS, Thapar MK, Harp RJ. Racial variations in electrograms and vectorcardiograms between black and white children and their genesis. *J Electrocardiol* 1984;17:239–252.
58. Aristimuno GG, Foster TA, Berenson GS, et al. Subtle electrocardiographic changes in children with high levels of blood pressure. *Am J Cardiol* 1984;54:1272–1276.
59. Schlant RC, Adolph RJ, DiMarco JP, et al. Guidelines for electrocardiography: A report of the American College of Cardiology/American Heart Association Task Force on Assessment of Diagnostic and Therapeutic Cardiovascular Procedures (Committee on Electrocardiography). *J Am Coll Cardiol* 1992;19:473–481.

CHAPTER 12 ■ SYNCOPE AND ASSESSMENT OF AUTONOMIC FUNCTION IN CHILDREN

TONY REYBROUCK, PhD, AND HUGO ECTOR, MD, PhD

Fainting or syncope can be a disabling condition, and these patients frequently seek medical attention. In the Framingham study the incidence of adults reporting at least one syncopal event during their lifetime was estimated at 3% (1). For children and adolescents the incidence of patients reporting a syncopal event in a U.S. registry was 71 per 100,000 (0.07%) and 126/100,000 (0.126%) for two 5-year observational periods (2). The incidence was higher in female than in male patients, with a peak at the age range of 15 to 19 years. In the same series the mortality and long-time survival of patients with syncope was not different from a general population.

CLASSIFICATION OF THE HEMODYNAMIC RESPONSE TO TILT TESTING IN NEURALLY MEDIATED SYNCOPE

Neurally mediated syncope can be classified according to the response to a tilt table test. Originally the response to tilt table testing was classified according to isolated or combined changes of heart rate and blood pressure. Sutton's first definition referred to (i) a vasodepressor type, reflecting mainly a drop in blood pressure at the time of syncope without changes in heart rate; (ii) a cardioinhibitory type with a decrease in heart rate and/or asystole; and finally (iii) a mixed type reflecting both a decrease in heart rate and blood pressure (3). Recently a new classification has been proposed by the European Task Force on Syncope (4). Four hemodynamic types of syncope have now been described.

Type 1: Mixed type. Heart rate falls at the time of syncope but does not fall to <40 beats per minute for >10 seconds with or without asystole for <3 seconds. Blood pressure falls before heart rate falls.

Type 2A: Cardioinhibition without asystole. Heart rate falls to a ventricular rate <40 beats per minute for >10 seconds but asystole of >3 seconds does not occur. Blood pressure falls before the heart rate falls.

Type 2B: Cardioinhibition with asystole. Asystole occurs for >3 sec. Blood pressure fall coincides with or occurs before the heart rate fall.

Type 3: Vasodepressor. Heart rate does not fall >10 % from its peak at the time of syncope.

Two exceptions have been described:

Exception 1: Chronotropic incompetence. A <10% increase of heart rate during tilt testing.

Exception 2: Excessive heart rate rise. An excessive heart rate rise (i.e., >130 beats per minute) both at the onset of upright position and throughout its duration before syncope.

These different hemodynamic patterns reflect the complexity of the mechanisms behind the clinical picture of neurally mediated syncope. Moreover, the hemodynamic type of syncope may vary from one moment to another (5).

Although this classification was originally defined for hemodynamic type of syncope in adults, in children the same classification is used. However, in contrast to adults, in young patients different types of neurally mediated syncope have been observed. Some investigators reported a combination of bradycardia and hypotension (mixed type of syncope) at the onset of syncope (6–9) as being most common whereas others reported mainly vasodepressor response in young patients (10).

MECHANISMS AND PATHOPHYSIOLOGY OF SYNCOPE IN CHILDREN AND ADOLESCENTS

It has been estimated that the critical cerebral blood flow in young healthy persons is 60 mL/min/100 g tissue or about 11.4 mL of oxygen, assuming a normal hemoglobin value of 14 g/100 mL blood. Cerebral blood flow is maintained by autoregulation over a wide range of perfusion pressures. With a critical reduction in PO_2 or an elevation of PCO_2, reflexive cerebral vasodilation occurs. Syncope may occur with a transient failure in this reflexive mechanism, which protects the cerebral blood perfusion for some 8 to 10 seconds. Also, other factors such as dehydration may induce syncope (11).

Syncope typically is characterized by a sudden fall in arterial blood pressure, which is associated with light-headedness, dizziness, and loss of consciousness. A common explanation is the sudden pooling of blood in the splanchnic system or in the peripheral blood vessels, which leads to a dramatic reduction of the venous return to the heart. This induces vigorous ventricular contractions. The stretching of the myocardial C-fibers owing to inadequate ventricular filling sends an afferent signal to the brain. The brainstem may respond with a paradoxical cardioinhibitory or vasodilatory response (12). However, the complexity of this phenomenon is illustrated by the fact that neurally mediated syncope also occurs in patients who have had orthotopic heart transplantation in which cardiac afferent and efferent nerves are no longer intact. This shows that the cardiac mechanoreceptor theory (the so called Bezold-Jarisch reflex) is not the exclusive etiologic factor, although it probably is an important contributory factor.

SYNCOPE EVALUATION

Causes of Syncope

The causes of syncope in children are comparable with causes in adults. The most common cause is a functional disturbance in the baroreflex control of the arterial blood pressure. The abnormal reflex activity is characterized by a sympathetic withdrawal and excessive vagal tone. This leads to a critical impairment of cerebral blood flow. Other types of syncope, owing to structural heart disease, will not be discussed in this chapter. The reader is referred to other textbooks that deal with these issues (13).

During neurally mediated syncope, afferent signals initiate a series of autonomic events in the medullary control areas that induce inappropriate vasodilatory, bradycardic, and in some instances, even asystolic responses. The resulting hemodynamic abnormalities can be classified according to a *cardioinhibitory*, a *vasodilatory*, or a *mixed* type of response for heart rate and blood pressure as has been defined above. The pattern of response is not always reproducible because some patients may develop another type of syncope on a subsequent tilt test (5).

Many adults and children may experience a syncopal event during their lifetime. Syncope occurs more frequently during adolescence than in earlier childhood (13). Some patients may have recurrent syncope. Thus, certain individuals are more susceptible to syncope.

A number of triggers have been shown to cause syncope (Table 12.1). However, the evoking factors are similar for children and adults.

General Overview of Diagnostic Tools

The starting point of the evaluation of patients with a history of fainting is to carefully seek the underlying cause. This will require a detailed medical history. For pediatric patients the medical history should include an interview of the child as well as the parents or relatives of the child. During the initial physical examination, blood pressure measurements should be performed in the supine and standing position to identify orthostatic hypotension. A 12-lead electrocardiogram is reasonable to exclude arrhythmia as a cause of syncope.

According to the guidelines of the European Society of Cardiology, further cardiac evaluation is recommended in patients with clinical symptoms that are suggestive of cardiac types of syncope. These features include the presence of structural heart disease, exercise-induced syncope, syncope preceded by palpitations, and or a family history of sudden death. Also, ECG abnormalities that suggest a cardiac cause of syncope may require further investigation. These may include, among others, atrioventricular block, intraventricular block, sinus bradycardia (even asymptomatic), pre-excitation, and prolonged QT interval.

The recommended diagnostic tests are echocardiography, prolonged electrocardiographic monitoring, Holter monitoring, and exercise testing. Tilt testing also is considered a first-line diagnostic test, particularly in young (pediatric) patients.

Tilt Table Testing Methodology with Special Reference to Children and Adolescents

Tilt table testing is feasible in children as young as 6 years of age. One difficulty in young children is anxiety, which may occur when safety belts are applied. For adult patients a passive tilt test is 45 minutes at a tilt angle of 60 degrees (Westminster protocol) (14). For children, the same time is used. For children with neurally mediated syncope, the number of positive responders was different than that for adults at a tilt duration of 20 minutes but not at 30 minutes (15). Therefore, it could be that the orthostatic stress during tilt testing is different in children as compared with adults (11). The longer duration of the tilt as used in adults (45 minutes) may reduce the specificity of the test in children. For this reason, in pediatric patients shorter time periods could be recommended.

No uniform tilt table protocol exists. Some investigators use pharmacologic provocation for eliciting the susceptibility to neurally mediated syncope, whereas others use only a passive tilt. A considerable number of investigators have used isoproterenol infusion to decrease the duration of the tilt test protocol. However, although the use of pharmacologic stimulation increases the sensitivity of the test, the large number of false-positive responders decreases its specificity. Nitroglycerin also has been used (11).

TABLE 12.1

TRIGGERS OF NEURALLY MEDIATED REFLEX SYNCOPE IN THE YOUNG

- Emotional circumstances and pain, such as venipunctures, immunizations
- Prolonged motionless standing, especially in combination with warm temperature, confined spaces, crowded rooms ("church syncope")
- Fasting, lack of sleep, fatigue, menstruation, illness with fever
- Micturition
- Postexercise (i.e., after termination of long runs or vigorous bursts of activity during competitive sports)
- Hyperventilation and straining (self-induced syncope)
- Stretching
- Coughing
- Standing up quickly or arising from squatting
- Pronounced weight loss
- Certain medications, alcohol, and drugs (these need to be distinguished from intoxicated states, which can also cause loss of consciousness)

From Wieling W, Ganzeboom K, Janousek J. Syncope and other causes of loss of consciousness in children, teenagers, and adolescents. In: Benditt DG, Blanc JJ, Brignole M, et al., eds. *The Evaluation and Treatment of Syncope.* New York: Futura Publishing, 2003:163–178, with permission.

ASSESSMENT OF THE AUTONOMIC SYSTEM

In children and adolescents with neurally mediated syncope, it may be useful to assess cardiovascular autonomic function because syncope may be the result of a transient autonomic dysfunction (12,16,17). A considerable number of autonomic function tests have been proposed (13) (Table 12.2). In most of the tests, modulations of heart rate and/or blood pressure are assessed during provocative maneuvers. Some investigators have found it useful to assess the slope of heart rate versus blood pressure changes (16,17).

Beat-to-beat changes of heart rate are a complex interaction of respiration, vasomotor tone, body temperature, and central stimulation. Therefore, heart rate variability has been

TABLE 12.2

EXAMPLES OF CARDIOVASCULAR AUTONOMIC NERVOUS SYSTEM TESTS

	Measurement of interest	Normal response	Interpretation of abnormal response
Baroreflex sensitivity (graded phenylephrine boluses)	Slope of R-R intervals + corresponding systolic BP	log (reflex sensitivity slope) = 2.47 − (0.0164 × age)- (0.086 × mean arterial BP)	Defect in reflex arc involving SNS α-receptors, carotid and aortic arch baroreceptors, brain-stem, cardiac vagal efferents
Cold pressor test	BP rise HR rise	20 mm Hg systolic BP rise 10 beats/min HR rise	Defect in reflex arc involving sensory nerves, spinothalamic tracts, suprapontine and intra thalamic relays, descending SNS α-receptors, cardiac SNS efferents, and β-receptors
Cuff occlusion test	BP drop	Systolic BP drop by <10 mm Hg	Defect in reflex response involving cardiac chamber volume sensors and carotid and aortic arch baroreceptors, brainstem, efferent SNS nerves, and α receptors
Isoproterenol test (graded boluses)	HR rise	25 beats/min rise after 1 μg (adolescent response)	Hypersensitive response, reduced circulating catecholamines β-receptor up-regulation
			Reduced response (β-receptor down-regulation)
Neuronal norepinephrine store (graded tyramine boluses)	BP rise	<20 mm Hg systolic BP rise after 1 g	If reduced response, neuronal stores of NE reduced by drugs or peripheral SNS neuronal destruction
		>25 mm Hg systolic BP rise after 6 g (usual adult response: 25 mm Hg rise after 2–3 g)	Exaggerated response if excessive neuronal NE stores (pheochromocytoma)
Sinus arrhythmia (control led breathing for 1 min)	HR variation	>15 beats/min	Dysfunction of vagus nerve, thoracic afferent fibers, or the vasomotor center
Valsalva maneuver	Phase IV/II RR ratio	>1.2	Defect in baroreceptor, brainstem, cardiac vagal efferent (IV) reflex, or cardiac SNS efferent or β-receptor (II) reflex
	Phase II HR rise	>20 beats/min	Defect in baroreceptor, brainstem, or cardiac SNS efferent or β-receptor
	Phase IV HR drop		Defect in baroreceptor, brainstem, or cardiac vagal efferent
	Phase IV BP rise	>10 mm Hg (mean)	SNS dysfunction as in CHF

SNS, sympathetic nervous system; BP, blood pressure; HR, heart rate; NE, norepinephrine; CHF, congestive heart failure.
Phase I: transient rise in blood pressure and fall in heart rate; phase II: fall in blood pressure early in the phase with recovery later in phase (accompanied by an increase in heart rate); phase III: fall in blood pressure and increase in heart rate occur with cessation of expiration; phase IV: increase in blood pressure above baseline (overshoot). From Freeman R. Noninvasive evaluation of heart rate variability. The time domain. In: Low PA, ed. *Clinical Autonomic Disorders*. Philadelphia: Lippincott–Raven Publishers, 1997, reprinted with permission.
Modified from Robertson D. Assessment of autonomic function. In: Baughman KL, Green BM, eds. Clinical diagnosis manual for the house officer. Baltimore: Williams & Wilkins, 1981, with permission; Kanter RJ. Syncope and sudden death. In: Garson A Jr, Bricker JT, Fisher DJ, et al., eds. *The Science and Practice of Pediatric Cardiology*. Baltimore: Williams & Wilkins, 1998:2169–2199, with permission; and Low PA, ed. *Clinical Autonomic Disorders*. Philadelphia: Lippincott–Raven Publishers, 1997, with permission.

proposed as a tool to assess the reflex changes of the cardiovascular system (16,17). Similar to measurements in adults, heart rate variability with time and frequency domain analysis has been applied to children (18). In adult patients with cardiovascular disease, attenuated heart rate variability is an indicator of morbidity and mortality. However, in children and adolescents this has not been shown, probably because ischemic cardiovascular disease is uncommon in children. For a more detailed description of autonomic function tests and heart rate variability, the reader is referred to specialized reviews (13,16,17). Specific standards for heart rate variability in the pediatric age group have been published (13).

The application of autonomic function testing for children and adolescents is very limited. Similar to observations in adults, spectral analysis of heart rate and blood pressure studies during tilt testing in pediatric patients with syncope also shows a decline in low-frequency heart rate and blood pressure power at the time of syncope (e.g., during long standing in hot crowded environments).

TREATMENT OF PATIENTS WITH NEURALLY MEDIATED SYNCOPE

General Treatment Issues

Before any medical treatment is started, the patients and/or their parents should be reassured and educated about the benign nature and excellent prognosis of syncope. The patients also should be advised to avoid situations that may trigger syncope (e.g., long standing, hot crowded environments; other mechanisms have included hot showers, hair dryers, hair combing, urinating while standing, and in church [see Table 12.1]).

Medical Treatment

The complexity of the pathophysiology of neurally mediated syncope is illustrated by the wide variety of medical treatments that have been proposed. A review of the proposed therapeutic options for adults is presented in Table 12.3. These therapeutic options include vagolytic drugs, beta blocking agents, fludrocortisone (to enhance plasma volume), serotonin reuptake inhibitors, and alpha agonists. These agents frequently have

been prescribed as an initial treatment (11,13). However, the multitude of therapeutic options illustrate the unpredictable and unsatisfactory therapeutic results. These different therapeutic options are generally the same in children and adults. However, short-term and long-term follow-up of patients with neurally mediated syncope, treated by pharmacotherapy, has shown that a considerable number of patients continued to have syncope. Many trials have demonstrated that these drugs frequently are ineffective and, in addition, have important side effects (4,10,13). In a review of the literature, Benditt et al. (19) observed ≤56% recurrence of syncope in adult patients treated with pharmacotherapy during a follow-up period of 18.5 months. Similarly, children have had a recurrence rate of 32% for a 3.5-year follow-up period (20). The recurrence rate was similar for patients with either a positive or a negative tilt test and also for both treated and untreated patients. Thus, medical treatment is unsatisfactory in many cases.

Nonpharmacologic Methods

Since pharmacological treatment may have important side effects in children, other treatment methods are preferred. Moreover, in children the compliance to a prescribed therapeutic regime may be problematic. Therefore, nonpharmacologic therapy should be chosen as first-line therapy. The parents and children must be educated about hygienic measures to prevent syncope. These include an increase of the daily amount of water intake (4,31,32). The intake of salt or salty or sweet liquids without caffeine should be encouraged. Patients should be instructed to perform orthostatic maneuvers to improve venous return.

- Orthostatic maneuvers to improve venous return: Several maneuvers can abort syncope in children and adolescents. The patients and the parents can be instructed to learn these maneuvers that prevent the pooling of blood in the venous capacitance system. Syncope can be aborted if the patients cross their legs, stand on their toes, tense their leg muscles (34), or perform isometric arm exercises (35). Squatting can prevent the onset of loss of consciousness (34). It is helpful for the children and/or their parents learn these maneuvers.
- Electrolyte and water intake: Another preventive measure is to increase water, salt, and electrolyte intake. Studies in adult patients with orthostatic hypotension (36) have

---

TABLE 12.3

THERAPEUTIC OPTIONS IN THE TREATMENT OF NEURALLY MEDIATED SYNCOPE

Neurally mediated syncope therapeutic options	
Disopyramide	Salt and fluid supplement
Metoprolol, atenolol	Prevent hypoglycemia
Fludrocortisone	Blood pressure raising
Theophylline, etilefrine	Maneuvers: Coughing
Ephedrine, etilefrine	Leg crossing, squatting
Serotonin reuptake inhibitors: Fluoxetine, sertraline	Muscle contraction
Midodrine	Endurance training
Cardiac pacing	Avoid static position
	Sleeping in head-up bed
	Tilt training

shown that increased water intake (0.5 L/day) is effective for preventing syncope. Water drinking induces a pressor response that may be effective in the treatment of orthostatic hypotension. The same benefits can be expected in children and adolescents. The effect of water drinking can be enhanced by increasing the sodium content of the fluids (e.g., sport drinks), which have a volume-expanding effect.

- Exercise training: Because moderate exercise training increases plasma volume, it can be speculated that exercise training may have a beneficial effect in the management of patients with neurally mediated syncope. However, some studies have shown that reduced orthostatic tolerance in athletes was due to an excessive vagal tone (39).

Studies in adults with neurally mediated syncope have used aerobic exercise training as a treatment. In normal volunteers, Mtinangi and Hainsworth (37) demonstrated that exercise training increased orthostatic tolerance. Hachul et al. (38) compared three groups of patients with neurally mediated syncope treated with exercise training, tilt training, and pharmacotherapy. In this study, 40% of the patients treated with exercise training reported syncope recurrence versus 23.5% of the patients treated with pharmacotherapy (beta blockers, fludrocortisone, and selective serotonin reuptake inhibitors [SSRI]). No recurrence of syncope was reported in the patients treated with tilt training.

Decreased orthostatic tolerance has been shown in physically inactive bedridden patients on one end of the spectrum and in competitive athletes on the other end. Exercise training has only a beneficial role when patients change from an inactive to a moderately active lifestyle.

Tilt Training

In an earlier study by Morillo et al. (21), a reduction in syncope was observed in patients who underwent repeated tilt tests. This study included a crossover design with oral disopyramide treatment and placebo. Sheldon et al. (22) reported a reduction in syncope after the performance of repeated diagnostic tilt tests. This suggests that together with conditioning of the baroreflex activity, a combination of factors such as natural history, counseling, and adoption of appropriate maneuvers will prevent syncope. However, these authors never used repeated tilt testing (tilt training) as a treatment for neurally mediated syncope. It was postulated that the frequency of syncope decreased in these studies because after several tilt tests, patients learned to recognize prodromal symptoms of syncope and could avoid situations that triggered syncope.

We also have observed that patients who have had repeated diagnostic tilt tests showed spontaneous improvement of tilt tolerance both during tilt table testing and during daily life. Therefore, we initiated a tilt training program (23). The patients were tilted daily on a tilt table to a 60-degree position (Westminster protocol). The patients had serial tilt tests (one per day) until syncope or signs of severe orthostatic intolerance occurred. At the onset of orthostatic weakness or syncope, the patients were immediately placed in the recumbent position and closely monitored until full recovery. In all patients, the target was to obtain two consecutive negative tilt tests. Orthostatic tolerance was considered normal if the patients could sustain the test for at least 45 minutes. Thereafter, the patients were discharged from the hospital and had to continue training at home. For safety reasons, it is recommended that patients start the therapy in a clinical setting with monitoring of the ECG and blood pressure. One limitation of this therapy, particularly in children and adolescents, may be the low compliance to the tilt training schedule (4). Therefore, it is mandatory that patients have ongoing evaluation at an outpatient clinic.

For standing training at home, the patients were instructed to stand with their feet 15 cm away from the wall and lean with the upper back against the wall. During the first 6 weeks, intensive tilt training therapy was required for two sessions per day. After 6 weeks, a tilt test was performed during an outpatient clinic visit. If this test was negative (normal duration of 45 minutes), the patients had to continue the therapy at home, but the frequency of the tilt training was reduced to one session per day. Other outpatient clinic visits with tilt tests were planned 3 months after the first outpatient test and then 6 months and 1 year after the first tilt training session. After 1 year of tilt training therapy, the frequency of tilt training was reduced (24).

In the field of cardiovascular rehabilitation, the treatment of neurally mediated syncope by repeated tilt testing is a new and fascinating therapy with promising results. In our cumulative experience of 222 patients who underwent tilt training therapy for neurally mediated syncope, we obtained a negative tilt test in every patient after an average of 2.9 ± 1.3 (median 2) sessions (25). Only 25% of the patients remained tilt positive and required three or more sessions. However, a negative response to tilt table testing could be obtained eventually in all patients. This was found in all types of neurally mediated syncope. Also, patients with the cardioinhibitory type of syncope, with long periods of asystole (mean 19.4 ± 15, minimum 5, maximum 60 s) became tilt-negative during consecutive tilt training. Therefore, it may be prudent to avoid pacemaker therapy in patients with neurally mediated syncope.

For 31 of 38 patients (82%) followed for an average of 43 ± 7.8 months, no syncope recurrence was reported (23). Syncope recurrence was observed only in patients who had discontinued the therapy. Nevertheless, there was a remarkable improvement in the clinical condition of the patients who became symptomatic again after early discontinuation of the tilt training therapy. When the patients reported recurrence of syncope, we simply advised them to resume the tilt training program and syncope disappeared again.

Pacemaker Therapy

In adult patients with the cardioinhibitory type of syncope, pacemaker therapy has been used to prevent the asystole. A reduction of syncope was found in several studies (26–29), but many patients still developed recurrence of syncope (27,28). This was ascribed to the vasodepressor component of this disorder. Similarly, in children with the cardioinhibitory type of syncope, beneficial effects of pacemaker therapy have been shown in some studies, but recurrence of syncope also has been observed in several studies (30–32). However, because in many instances a vasodepressor component is also present, pacemaker therapy may not always be effective (33). Therefore, pacemaker implantation should not be considered as a first-line therapy in children with syncope.

PROGNOSIS

In adults who experienced a syncopal event, long-term follow-up studies have shown that syncope recurs at a rate of about 30% during a 30-month period. (11,40). Similarly, in a long-term follow-up study of children and adolescents with neurally mediated syncope, a recurrence rate of about 32% has been reported during a 46-month follow-up period (7). This recurrence rate was similar for patients with a positive or a negative tilt test and for both treated and untreated patients. The highest recurrence rate was found in patients with the most prior syncopal spells.

Although in patients with neurally mediated syncope and without structural heart disease the prognosis is benign, syncope recurrence can be harmful because it may lead to injuries, and it induces anxiety and loss of self-confidence. In patients with a cardiac cause of syncope, sudden death has been reported (11). Excess mortality has been found in patients with ventricular tachyarrhythmias and in patients with structural heart disease and malignant syncope. Moreover, excess mortality also has been found in patients with severe aortic stenosis and hypertrophic cardiomyopathy.

References

1. Savage D, Corwin L, McGee D, et al. Epidemiologic features of isolated syncope: The Framingham Study. *Stroke* 1985;16:626–629.
2. Driscoll D, Jacobsen S, Porter CJ, et al. Syncope in children and adolescents. *J Am Coll Cardiol* 1997;29:1039–1045.
3. Sutton R, Peterson M, Brignole M, et al. Proposed classification of tilt induced vasovagal syncope. *Eur J Card Pacing Electrophysiol* 1992;2:180–183.
4. Brignole M, Alboni P, Benditt D, et al. Guidelines on management (diagnosis and treatment) of syncope. *Eur Heart J* 2001;22:1256–1306.
5. Ector H. Neurocardiogenic vasovagal syncope. *Eur Heart J* 1999;20:1686–1687.
6. Mc Leod K. Dysautonomia and neurcardiogenic syncope. Curr Opin Cardiol 2001;16:92–96.
7. Kouakam C, Vaksmann G, Lacroix D, et al. Value of the tilt test in the management of syncope in children and adolescents [in French]. *Arch Mal Coeur* 1997;90:679–686.
8. Pongiglione G, Fish FA, Strasburger JF, et al. Heart rate and blood pressure response to upright tilt in young patients with unexplained syncope. *J Am Coll Cardiol* 1990;16:165–170.
9. Alehan D, Lenk M, Ozme S, et al. Comparison of sensitivity and specificity of tilt protocols with and without isoproterenol in children with unexplained syncope. *Pacing Clin Electrophysiol* 1997;20:1769–1776.
10. Lewis DA, Dhala A. Syncope in the pediatric patient. The cardiologist's perspective. *Pediatr Clin North Am* 1999;46:205–219.
11. Benditt DG. Syncope. In: Topol EJ, ed. *Textbook of Cardiovascular Medicine*. Philadelphia: Lippincott–Raven Publishers, 1998:1807–1831.
12. Ross B, Grubb BP. Syncope in the child and adolescents. In: Grubb BP, Olshansky B, eds. *Syncope: Mechanisms and Management*. Armonk, NY: Futura Publishing, 1998:305–316.
13. Kanter RJ. Syncope and sudden death. In: Garson A Jr, Bricker JT, Fisher DJ, et al., eds. *The Science and Practice of Pediatric Cardiology*. Baltimore: Williams & Wilkins, 1998:2169–2191.
14. Fitzpatrick AP, Theodorakis G, Vardas P, et al. Methodology of head-up tilt testing in patients with unexplained syncope. *J Am Coll Cardiol* 1991;17:125–130.
15. Berkowitz JB, Auld P, Hulse JE, et al. Tilt table evaluation for control patients: Comparison with symptomatic patients. *Clin Cardiol* 1995;18:521–525.
16. Hohnloser SH, Klingenheben T. Basic autonomic tests. In: Malik M, ed. *Clinical Guide to Cardiac Autonomic Tests*. Dordrecht, Netherlands: Kluwer Academic Publishers, 1998:51–66.
17. Moak JP, Bailey JJ, Makhlouf FT, et al. Simultaneous heart rate and blood pressure. Variability analysis: Insight in mechanisms underlying neurally mediated cardiac syncope in children. *J Am Coll Cardiol* 2002;40:1466–1474.
18. Sehra R, Hubbard JE, Straka SP, et al. Autonomic changes and heart rate variability in children with neurocardiogenic syncope. *Pediatr Cardiol* 1999;20:242–247.
19. Benditt DG, Fahey GJ, Lurie KG, et al. Pharmacotherapy of neurally mediated syncope. *Circulation* 1999;100:1242–1248.
20. Kouakam C, Vaksmann G, Pachy E, et al. Long-term follow-up of children and adolescents with syncope. Predictor of syncope recurrence. *Eur Heart J* 2001;22:1618–1625.
21. Morillo CA, Leith JW, Yee R, et al. A placebo-controlled trial of intravenous and oral disopyramide for prevention of neurally mediated syncope induced by head-up tilt. *J Am Coll Cardiol* 1993;22:1843–1848.
22. Sheldon R, Rose S, Flanagan P, et al. Risk factors for syncope recurrence after a positive tilt test in patients with syncope. *Circulation* 1996;93:973–981.
23. Reybrouck T, Heidbüchel H, Ector H, et al. Tilt training: A treatment for malignant and recurrent neurocardiogenic syncope. *Pacing Clin Electrophysiol* 2000;23:493–498.
24. Reybrouck T, Heidbüchel H, Ector H, et al. Long-term follow-up results of tilt training therapy in patients with recurrent neurocardiogenic syncope. *Pacing Clin Electrophysiol* 2002;25:144–146.
25. Ector H, Willems R, Reybrouck T, et al. Repeated tilt testing in patients with tilt positive neurally mediated syncope. *Europace* 2005;7:628–633.
26. Connolly SJ, Sheldon R, Roberts RS, et al. The North American Vasovagal Pacemaker Study (VPS). A randomised trial of permanent pacing for the prevention of vasovagal syncope. *J Am Coll Cardiol* 1999;33:16–20.
27. Sutton R, Brignole M, Menozzi C, et al. Dual chamber pacing in the treatment of neurally mediated tilt-positive cardio-inhibitory syncope. *Circulation* 2000;102:294–295.
28. Connolly SJ, Sheldon R, Thorpe KE, et al. VPS II Investigators. Pacemaker therapy for prevention of syncope in patients with recurrent severe vasovagal syncope: Second Vasovagal Pacemaker Study (VPS II): A randomized trial. *JAMA* 2003;289:2224–2229.
29. Ammirati F, Coivicchi F, Santini M. Syncope Diagnosis and Treatment Study Investigators. Permanent cardiac pacing versus medical treatment for the prevention of recurrent vasovagal syncope. A multicenter, randomized, controlled trial. *Circulation* 2001;104:52–57.
30. Mc Leod KA, Wilson N, Hewit J, et al. Cardiac pacing for severe childhood neurally mediated syncope with reflex anoxic seizures. *Heart* 1999;82:721–725.
31. Johnsrude CL. Current approach to pediatric syncope. *Pediatr Cardiol* 2000;21:522–531.
32. Sokolowski RC. Evaluation and treatment of pediatric patients with neurocardiogenic syncope. *Prog Pediatr Cardiol* 2001;131:117–131.
33. Mc Leod KA, Wilson K, Hewitt J, et al. Cardiac pacing for severe childhood neurally mediated syncope with reflex anoxic seizures. *Heart* 2005;82:721–725.
34. Krediet P, Van Dijk N, Linzer M, et al. Management of vasovagal syncope: Controlling or aborting faints by leg crossing and muscle testing. *Circulation* 2002;106:1684–1689.
35. Brignole M, Croci F, Menozzi C, et al. Isometric arm counter-pressure manoeuvres to abort impending vasovagal syncope. *J Am Coll Cardiol* 2002;40:2054–2060.
36. Shannon JR, Diedrich D, Biaggion I, et al. Water drinking as a treatment for orthostatic syndromes. *Am J Med* 2002;112:355–360.
37. Mtinangi BL, Hainsworth R. Effects of moderate exercise training on plasma volume, baroreceptor sensitivity and orthostatic tolerance in healthy subjects. *Exp Physiol* 1999;84:121–130.
38. Hachul D, Gardenghi G, Rondon MU, et al. The role of physical training in the management of recurrent neurally mediated syncope [abstract]. *Eur Heart J* 2004;25:351.
39. Kosinsky D. Syncope in the athlete. In: Grubb BP, Olshansky B, eds. *Syncope: Mechanisms and Management*. Armonk, NY: Futura Publishing, 1998:317–336.
40. Kapoor W, Peterson J, Wieand HS, et al. Diagnostic and prognostic implications of recurrences in patients with syncope. *Am J Med* 1987;83:700–708.
41. Wieling W, Ganzeboom K, Janousek J. Syncope and other causes of loss of consciousness in children, teenagers and adolescents. In: Benditt DG, Blanc JJ, Brignole M, et al., eds. *The Evaluation and Treatment of Syncope*. New York: Futura Publishing, 2003:163–178.
42. Low PA, ed. *Clinical Autonomic Disorders*. Philadelpia: Lippincott–Raven Publishers, 1997.
43. Robertson D. Assessment of autonomic function. In: Baughman KL, Green BM, eds. *Clinical Diagnosis Manual for the House Officer*. Baltimore: Williams & Wilkins, 1981.

CHAPTER 13 ▪ ELECTROPHYSIOLOGIC STUDIES

JOHN D. KUGLER, MD

Several aspects of electrophysiologic studies—both intracardiac and transesophageal—in infants, children, and adolescents have changed in the past decade. This chapter will emphasize these changes while reviewing the established age-related and disease-related principles (1–4). The expanding therapeutic use of catheter ablation (see Chapter 17) has had a major impact on various aspects of intracardiac electrophysiologic study, including not only objectives and techniques during the study, but also indications for the study. In addition to the influence of ablation, indications for electrophysiologic studies also have changed because of the data from large multicenter studies involving specific arrhythmias and underlying disease processes. Although specific indications for electrophysiologic studies relative to specific underlying disease, symptoms, or arrhythmia are not discussed in this chapter (see Chapter 14), the objectives of electrophysiologic studies are discussed by comparing the intracardiac and transesophageal techniques relative to the advantages and limitations of each technique as viewed in the context of age, risk/benefit, therapy, and especially the clinical questions addressed for the individual patient.

PLANNING THE STUDY

The clinical questions addressed by the electrophysiologic study should be asked in advance, and the procedure should be planned and guided in this manner. The planning should include choice of intracardiac and/or transesophageal technique, needed preprocedure studies (e.g., electrocardiography [ECG], Holter monitoring, exercise testing, imaging studies); preparation or education of the patient and family; choice of sedation or general anesthesia; preparation of the patient in the procedure room or catheterization laboratory; types of equipment (catheters, sheaths); planned recording, pacing, or ablation protocols (with strategies for each); and administration of provocative or antiarrhythmic drugs.

INTRACARDIAC TECHNIQUE

Educational and Emotional Preparation of Patient and Family

The importance of patient and family preparation cannot be overemphasized. The long duration of the study and the use of multiple catheters and protocols necessitate relieving patient and family anxiety, which, in turn, enhances patient cooperation. Age-related patient and family preparation begins with the pediatric electrophysiologist and is continued by pediatric cardiac/congenital heart disease electrophysiology nurses with educational materials.

Sedation

Sedative or general anesthesia is required for virtually all pediatric patients. Sedative anesthesia is generally used for patients who undergo diagnostic electrophysiologic studies and for older, less anxious adolescents and adults who undergo ablations during the studies.

Although sedation is not standardized in electrophysiology laboratories, and multiple regimens are used, chlorpromazine should be avoided because it may have antiarrhythmic action (5). Most sedative regimens include a narcotic (e.g., meperidine, morphine, or fentanyl) and an antiemetic (e.g., Phenergan or droperidol), with benzodiazepines providing effective sedative amnesia (e.g., diazepam or midazolam). Midazolam may be a better choice than diazepam because of its demonstrated lack of electrophysiologic effect (6,7). Continuous intravenous propofol has gained increased acceptance as a deep sedative with low doses and as a general anesthetic with higher doses (8). With propofol's low incidence of postprocedure nausea and vomiting, patients recover faster with less lingering sedation, and because of the decreased vomiting, Valsalva-related catheter site bleeding is minimized (9). However, the electrophysiologic effects of propofol in children are no different from isoflurane-based anesthetics (10).

Preparation of Patient in Catheterization Laboratory

Initial patient preparation involves positioning and then comforting the patient on the table. When a long procedure is planned, securing the arms above the shoulders may promote the undesired complication of brachial plexus injury. Although positioning the arms inferiorly along the thorax interferes with the straight lateral fluoroscopy view, rotating slightly to 10 to 20 degrees right anterior oblique (RAO) with the anterior-posterior tubes and 80 to 70 degrees left anterior oblique (LAO) with the lateral tubes alleviates this problem while still providing acceptable views for catheter manipulation. All limb and chest surface ECG leads are placed initially; this allows for the later choice of displayed leads. Selection of a displayed lead is based on the underlying arrhythmia or conduction disturbance. When an optical disk recording system is used, a full 12-lead ECG is available at any time regardless of the fewer displayed leads.

Many laboratories now use three-dimensional (3-D) mapping systems. Depending on the system used, the initial room setup and preparation of the patient involves steps that are required for proper function of the system (e.g., pads placed/positioned, connections and interfacing as illustrated in Fig. 13.1). Routine use of the disposable (and translucent) defibrillation pad and lead system has improved cardioversion and emergency defibrillation efficiency and has probably improved the safety of the intracardiac study.

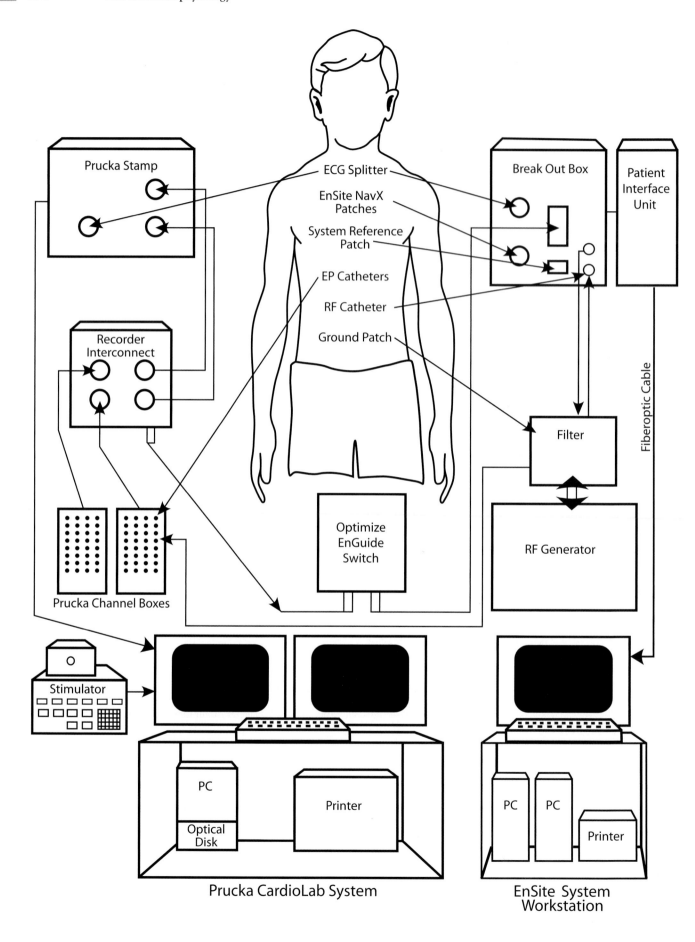

Prucka Stamp

ECG Splitter

EnSite NavX Patches

System Reference Patch

EP Catheters

RF Catheter

Ground Patch

Break Out Box

Patient Interface Unit

Recorder Interconnect

Filter

Fiberoptic Cable

Optimize EnGuide Switch

RF Generator

Prucka Channel Boxes

Stimulator

PC

Optical Disk

Printer

PC

PC

Printer

Prucka CardioLab System

EnSite System Workstation

Sheath and Catheter Placement

In patients undergoing electrophysiologic study, special care is needed when infiltrating skin and subcutaneous areas with lidocaine (1–4). Studies have shown that therapeutic and, therefore, antiarrhythmic serum concentrations have been achieved with routine use of 2% lidocaine (11). One percent or, ideally, 0.5% concentration given in sufficient amounts to achieve local anesthesia, but not in increased volume, is recommended to avoid therapeutic lidocaine serum concentration.

The number, size, and location of the sheaths relates to the age and size of the patient, underlying arrhythmia, and objectives of the study. In most studies, the number of sheaths varies between one and six, with the maximum number consisting of three in the femoral vein, two in the internal jugular vein, and one in the femoral artery. Sheath sizes usually correlate directly with the size of the patient and vary between 4 and 8 French (Fr). The 7 or 8 Fr sheaths are used because when intravenous drug administration is required, a side-arm sheath larger than the catheter within it permits free, unobstructed flow of fluid into the vein. When injecting side arms, it is important to avoid introduction of air emboli.

The ultimate number and location of the sheaths also depends on the success of catheter manipulation and preference of the operator. For example, the coronary sinus catheter can be advanced from the inferior or superior vena caval approach. From the inferior caval approach, a catheter can be manipulated into the coronary sinus from the femoral vein/inferior vena cava by looping the catheter in the right atrium or by directly advancing it from the right atrium (2,3). However, in some particularly obese patients, this is either not successful or not desirable, and a sheath or catheter can be advanced from the superior vena caval approach. This is accomplished from the arm (the median basilic vein in the left arm is preferred), neck (either internal jugular, but right is preferred), or subclavian vein (either right or left) approach (2,3). A limitation to the arm approach is that the arm is extended throughout the procedure, which can be uncomfortable to the patient and can interfere with the lateral fluoroscopy tube positioning. An advantage to the internal jugular vein is that its larger size can more easily accommodate a second sheath if needed (e.g., in a patient such as the one shown in Figure 13.2, in whom a mapping or ablation catheter is manipulated from above to reach a location along the tricuspid annulus not accessible from the femoral approach).

The femoral artery pressure is monitored continuously throughout the procedure for safety reasons (cuff pressure recordings can only be intermittent and may be fraught by challenging mechanical issues, so reliability also can be an issue), regardless of patient size or age or underlying arrhythmia. When a sheath is placed in the femoral artery for retrograde access to the left ventricle, a side-arm sheath one size larger than the catheter permits accurate recordings. Otherwise, a small plastic cannula is used.

The use of anticoagulation to minimize thromboembolic complications varies among laboratories and is difficult to analyze because it is difficult to separate the diagnostic procedure from the various interventional procedures (catheter ablation and the techniques used for ablation). Zhou et al. (12) reviewed the literature to show that heparin use does not eliminate the risk of thromboembolic complications during radiofrequency catheter ablation. Anfinsen et al. (13) in a randomized study in adults showed that heparin administration immediately after sheath placement significantly decreased hemostatic activation. In a separate study, these investigators also showed that the procedure duration prior to heparin administration determined hemostatic activation and fibrinolysis independent of radiofrequency ablation (14). Tse et al. (15) found both platelet and coagulation activation during radiofrequency ablation, but platelet activation was not found during cryoablation. The heparin dose varies among laboratories, but the initial dose is usually 70 to 100 U/kg, to a maximum 5,000 U. Ongoing heparin anticoagulation can be provided by a continuous intravenous infusion (e.g., 15 to 20 U/kg/hr) or by boluses. To follow the degree of optimal anticoagulation during long procedures, the activated clotting time is measured one to three times per hour to achieve a desired value of 200 to 300 seconds except higher values of 300 to 400 seconds when 3-D balloon array mapping systems are used within the left atrium or ventricle.

Electrode Catheters

The catheter sizes vary between 2 and 7 Fr. Formerly, the 4 Fr catheters were used virtually only for infants, whereas the 5 Fr catheters most often were used in young children, and 6 and 7 Fr catheters were used for adolescents and adult-sized patients. Smaller (2 to 3 Fr) catheters are used for intracardiac recordings as well as for epicardial mapping (by advancing the catheters from the coronary sinus into the very small branches throughout the epicardial surface) (16). These small catheters are used in small children to record intracardiac electrograms throughout the conduction system. Although these small catheters may be difficult to manipulate, up to three catheters can be used in the same sheath. Also, 2 Fr active fixation catheters (e.g., Medtronic, Inc.) can be used in patients such as

FIGURE 13.1 Diagram showing the major components of an electrophysiology (EP) cardiac laboratory (lab). An EP lab can be configured using equipment from several companies. In this illustration, the Prucka CardioLab System (General Electric Healthcare, UK) is interfaced with the electronic stimulator. Together, they provide the system by which conventional electrogram recordings are displayed, and pacing protocols are performed and recorded. A three-dimensional mapping system can interface with the conventional system to enhance mapping (see text) and minimize use of fluoroscopy. In this example, the EnSite NavX (St. Jude Medical, St. Paul, MN) provides the ability to view nonfluoroscopic images (see Fig. 13.5) of the catheter positions at the EnSite Workstation also with simultaneous conventional electrogram recordings. As is shown in Figure 13.3 (but not shown here), much greater detailed three-dimensional mapping images can be generated using the intracardiac balloon/electrode array EnSite system. Integration of preprocedure cardiac magnetic resonance images (see Fig. 13.4) or computed tomographic images can be downloaded and interfaced into the EnSite system.

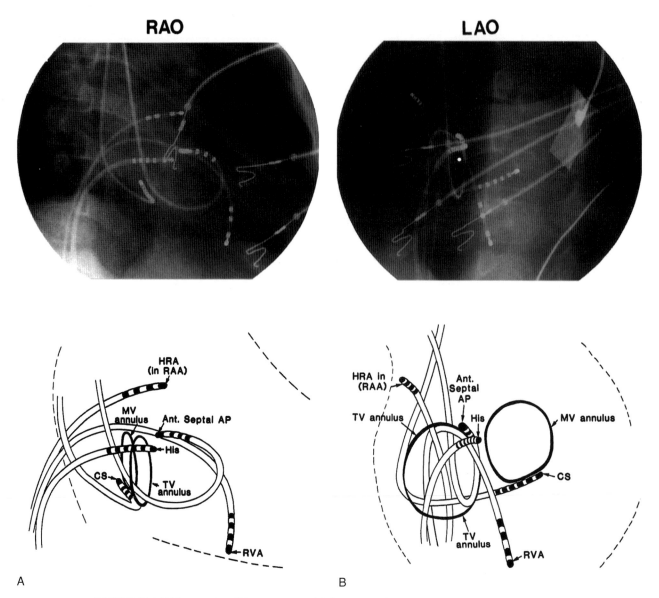

FIGURE 13.2 Right anterior oblique (RAO) and left anterior oblique (LAO) single-frame radiographs **(top)** from biplane cinecardiogram bursts with accompanying diagrammatic illustrations **(bottom)** showing multiple-electrode catheter positions during an intracardiac electrophysiologic study in a 6-year-old boy with Wolff–Parkinson–White's syndrome (right anterior septal accessory atrioventricular pathway). **A:** The RAO view (anterior-posterior tubes rotated 45 degrees) provides the operator with a direct anterior-posterior view (right to left, respectively, as viewed in the radiograph and illustration), with the atrioventricular (AV) valves nearly perpendicular to the operation. **B:** The corresponding LAO biplane view (lateral tubes rotated 45 degrees) provides the operator with a direct left-right view (tricuspid valve annulus on left and mitral valve annulus on right, with septal area between). Note that three 6 Fr catheters were advanced from the femoral veins and positioned in the high right atrium (HRA), right atrial appendage (RAA), right ventricular apex (RVA), and His position. Two 6 Fr catheters were advanced from the right internal jugular vein and positioned in the coronary sinus (CS) posterior to the mitral valve (MV) annulus, and under the tricuspid valve (TV) leaflet anterior (ant. septal) to the His catheter where the accessory atrioventricular pathway (AP) was located. The tricuspid valve annulus and the mitral valve annulus are depicted in positions predicted by the catheter positions to demonstrate approximate locations. The surface electrocardiographic leads and skin electrodes, as well as radiofrequency and defibrillation skin pads, are not labeled. (See Fig. 13.6 for recordings from these electrode catheters in this patient.)

those with pre-excitation/Wolff–Parkinson–White's syndrome who undergo a single-catheter short-duration study to assess risk of rapid A-V conduction of atrial fibrillation. These small catheters can be used in any size patients with the advantage of minimizing the venous puncture site—and therefore skin, muscle, and vein trauma—allowing quick recovery with low groin morbidity.

Catheter electrodes vary in number and interval distance. Most catheters used for recording and pacing are in a quadripolar configuration, whereas catheters used primarily for recording and mapping contain between 6 and 12 electrodes. Short (1 to 2 mm) interelectrode distances are important in attaining the goals of maximum-quality electrograms and precise mapping.

The number of catheters used during a study depends not only on the size of the patient and the underlying problem, but also on whether the electrophysiologist prefers the minimum or maximum possible amount of catheter manipulation during the study. If the least amount of catheter manipulation is desired, a greater number of catheters are positioned initially, and these are left in place for the duration of the procedure. Electrophysiologists who use more catheters prefer the advantage of simultaneous recording from the multiple catheters to optimize data collection. If multiple changes in catheter positions are deemed acceptable, fewer catheters are initially placed. Use of fewer catheters requires moving the catheter from one area to another and perhaps back to the original position during the study. However, it may not be possible without using mapping systems (described later, e.g., the NavX system, shown in Fig. 13.5) to return the catheter to the precise original location, and electrogram consistency may be compromised or the arrhythmia affected by the catheter movement (e.g., arrhythmia may not be inducible thereafter, so optimal gathering and recording of information is lost). Also, with each catheter position change, the otherwise satisfactorily sedated patient may become disturbed.

Manipulation and placement of electrode catheters involves several factors, including patient size and age, underlying arrhythmia, objectives of the individual study, size and type of catheters (e.g., steerable), and underlying cardiac and blood vessel anatomy.

Catheter access to the left atrium or ventricle is desirable for several reasons, usually for the purpose of recording and stimulation of the left atrium and ventricle for evaluation and mapping of supraventricular tachyarrhythmias. With increasing use of catheter ablation, left-sided accessory pathways or ectopic arrhythmia foci require catheter access to the left side. The posterior location of the coronary sinus provides precise mapping of accessory pathways along the mitral valve annulus. For left-sided atrial and ventricular ectopic foci and for ablation catheter manipulation, a lone catheter within the coronary sinus is insufficient. This has prompted use of the retrograde arterial approach or the transatrial septal approach via a patent foramen ovale or the transseptal sheath technique. Limitations are associated with each technique and have been discussed elsewhere (2,17).

Biplane (rather than single-plane) fluoroscopy is virtually essential to minimize the risk of perforation and, moreover, to enhance procedural time efficiency while maximizing the precision of catheter manipulation during mapping. For mapping, especially when it involves the tricuspid annulus, mitral annulus, and posterior septal area, the positioning of the fluoroscopy x-ray tubes in a perpendicular alignment to the long and short cardiac axes optimizes recognition of anatomic relationships (Fig. 13.2). This involves rotation of the anterior-posterior tubes within a 25- to 45-degree RAO position, with

the lateral tubes perpendicular within a 65- to 45-degree LAO position.

Recording and Stimulation Technique

The display and recording of the intracardiac electrograms are undertaken after catheter placement. Most electrograms are displayed and recorded in a bipolar fashion, although unipolar electrograms are easily obtainable (18). Various recordings and stimulation systems are commercially available, and some laboratories customize systems. Most laboratories use an optical disk computer system that maximizes recording and stimulation efficiency by eliminating manual switching of catheter connections, eliminating paper recordings, providing a database/reporting system, and providing on-line measurements with freeze-scope capability (Fig. 13.1). The 3-D mapping systems incorporate the temporal and spatial (anatomic) details and therefore provide much more precise diagnostic data (Figs. 13.3–13.5) (19). Also, many 3-D systems have the capacity to capture single beats for analysis when sustained tachyarrhythmias are not inducible or when the arrhythmia is associated with intolerable hemodynamics. The 3-D mapping systems have added an important diagnostic component to electrophysiologic studies and have also provided increased safety by decreasing radiation exposure because catheter manipulation can be performed without, or by minimizing, fluoroscopy. Regardless of the specific 3-D system used, Packer summarizes the minimal general requirements as follows: (i) Accurately replicate the cardiac anatomy underlying the arrhythmia; (ii) provide a plausible representation of activation of that chamber, as linked to the specific anatomic site of data acquisition; (iii) readily capture and intelligibly display other details of physiology; and (iv) catalogue the site of interventions (19). These features are illustrated in Figures 13.3 to 13.5.

A standard method or order of electrogram display and recording on the optical disk monitor does not exist, but typical examples are illustrated in Figure 13.6. It is advantageous to record at least three or four simultaneous surface ECGs, including two perpendicular limb leads to elicit P or QRS frontal plane axis changes and one or two chest leads to maximize detection of bundle branch changes. A major effort should be undertaken to record a His bundle electrogram (HBE). Virtually all mechanisms of arrhythmias and conduction system disturbances are definitive only when an HBE is recorded. When the usual catheter position (superior or septal tricuspid valve annulus) fails to elicit an HBE, advancing a catheter retrogradely to the noncoronary aortic sinus can allow successful recording. With catheters used for both recording and stimulation, the distal pair of electrodes are best suited for pacing consistency, and all proximal pairs are then used for recording. Because of fast tachycardia rates in children, fast recording capability (200 to 300 mm/s) is essential to differentiate electrograms recorded by the various electrode catheters (Fig. 13.7).

The pacing and recording protocols used are variable, and emphasis should be on flexibility and patient-specific diagnosis and findings. The specific protocols chosen should be adapted to the patient as they relate to the preprocedure diagnosis, but they should also remain flexible during the study, dependent on ongoing elicited findings. It is beyond the scope of this chapter to provide examples of protocols for specific types of arrhythmias and conduction disturbances; these can be found in Chapters 14 and 17 and elsewhere (2–4,17,20–22). However, in Table 13.1, a list of pacing protocols provides examples of options used during intracardiac studies. Also, with the advent

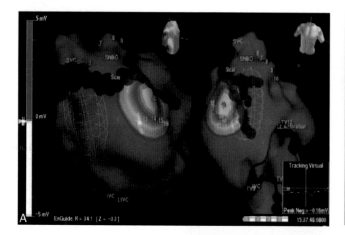
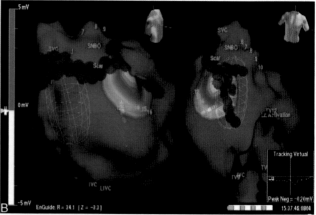
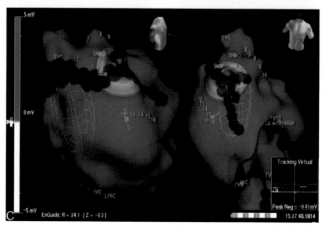

FIGURE 13.3 Three-dimensional (3-D), biplane noncontact (EnSite, St. Jude Medical, St. Paul, MN) map of the right atrium in an adolescent with intra-atrial re-entry tachycardia (IART) owing to postoperative congenital heart disease (Ebstein's anomaly), demonstrating the important features of a 3-D mapping system (see text, reference 19, and Chapter 17 on catheter ablation).

The rotation and view of the images are depicted by the smaller chest views at the upper right of each image. The outline of the 64-electrode mesh, mounted on the outside surface of the 18×40-mm inflated balloon (see Fig. 13.4 for angiographic image in different patient), is shown within each image. The EnSite noncontact mapping system is summarized by Packer (19). By using 5.6-kHz currents driven from the rings on the mesh and on the catheter (displayed here by its green tip, white interelectrode spaces), the catheter is located in 3-D space by sensing the resulting potentials on the mesh electrodes. The images are created by the roving catheter as it is manipulated along the endocardial surface. Nearly 3,300 calculated virtual electrograms, reflecting voltage transients from the endocardial surface, are created using an inverse solution to the Laplace equations. Activation occurring over the course of a cardiac cycle is reflected by unipolar or bipolar activation signals spreading across the right atrium. Both voltage and activation timing maps can be displayed on the system monitor.

In this patient, a series of radiofrequency current ablation applications (each application depicted by a *small circle*) were delivered first in a line from the superior vena cava (SVC), anterior and medial to the atrial septal defect patch because the IART circuit (not shown) was counterclockwise, which involved an area perpendicular to this line. The IART was still inducible (not shown), but the circuit changed to be more horizontal so a second line of ablation applications was placed from the first series inferior, anterior toward the tricuspid annulus. Although the IART was no longer inducible, atrial pacing was performed (shown here) to determine if the lines of block prevented conduction through them. In (**A**), the pacing catheter is shown near the outside (blue/green) edge of the circular activation wave of the right atrium. The atrial activation (center, depicted by *the red asterisk*, then earliest white atrial activation) travels toward the line of scar where in (**B**) 4 ms later, it reaches the ablation line. In (**C**), 10 ms later, it has conducted through the ablation line to the other side. Despite placing additional ablation lesions in this area, the failure to achieve complete block persisted, but IART was not inducible and the patient is off antiarrhythmia drug therapy without IART recurrence 18 months after the procedure.

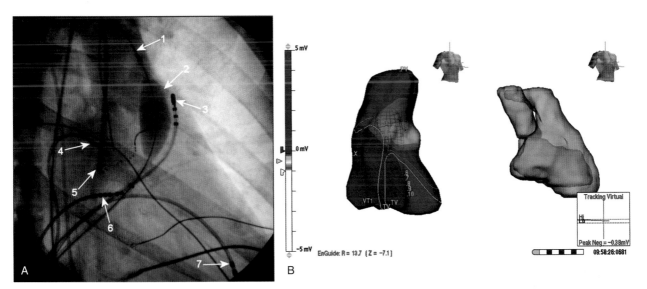

FIGURE 13.4 Two figures show the use of a three-dimensional (3-D) mapping system (EnSite, St. Jude Medical, St. Paul, MN) including the integration of a magnetic resonance image (MRI) in an adolescent with idiopathic adenosine-sensitive ventricular tachycardia that by ECG suggested a left ventricular/aortic sinus location. A cardiac MRI, shown in *right* image in **(B)**, was obtained before the procedure and integrated into the ESI system to optimize the anatomy imaging. The *left* image in **(B)** was derived via the 64-electrode mesh and mapping catheter as explained in Figure 13.3. In **(A)**, the fluoroscopic right anterior oblique image is shown: (1) wire in main pulmonary artery placed to enable advancing the balloon/mesh catheter; (2) 64-electrode mesh inflated balloon in the right ventricular outflow tract (RVOT); (3) mapping/ablation catheter in RVOT; (4) high right atrial catheter; (5) retrograde mapping/ablation catheter in aortic root/sinus; (6) His catheter; (7) RV apex catheter.

Combining fluoroscopic, virtual electrogram-derived, and MRI (or computed tomographic [CT]) images is designed to provide optimal anatomy-based imaging during mapping, especially in patients with complex underlying heart disease and/or arrhythmia substrate.

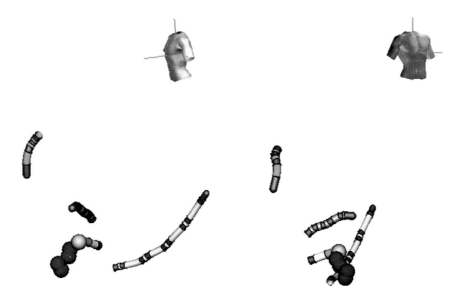

FIGURE 13.5 When imaging of multiple-catheter location is desired without the need for anatomic imaging detail, another simpler mapping system such as the NavX (EnSite, St. Jude Medical, St. Paul, MN) can be used. In this adolescent with atrioventricular nodal re-entry tachycardia (AVNRT) in whom the AVNRT was not easily and reproducibly induced, the NavX system was valuable to demonstrate the line of ablation (4 red, 1 yellow circles) applications along the slow AV nodal slow pathway area (see Chapter 17 on catheter ablation). The image projection is indicated by the small chest images in the upper right of each image. The catheters and location: Green, high right atrium; blue, His; yellow, coronary sinus; white/green, mapping/ablation in the slow AV nodal pathway area.

Although not used in this patient, anatomic details can be added to the catheter location image. Packer summarizes the system (19): Low-level separable currents are injected from three orthogonal electrode pairs positioned on the body surface. The specific catheter position can be established within the chamber based on the three resulting potentials measured in the recording tip with respect to a reference electrode (in this patient, the coronary sinus catheter was used) seen over the distance from each patch set to that recording tip. The chamber image can be created by sequential positioning of a catheter at multiple sites along the endocardial chamber (not shown here). The NavX also provides the ability to reflect real-time motion of catheter positioning, thus minimizing use of fluoroscopy and therefore radiation exposure.

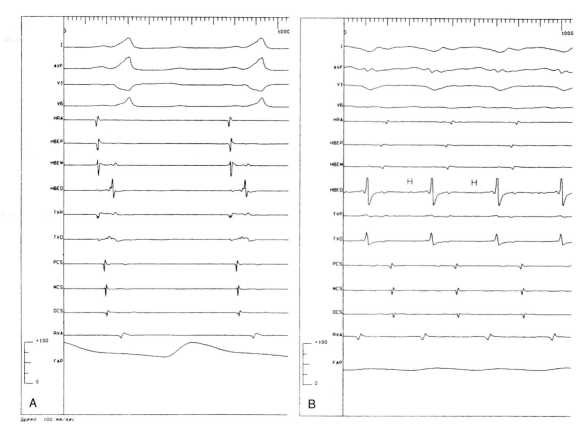

Speed 100 mm/sec

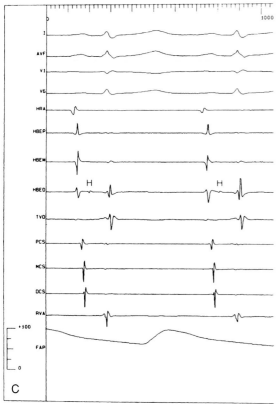

FIGURE 13.6 Three recordings in a 6-year-old boy (same patient as in Fig. 13.2) with pre-excitation owing to a right anterior septal accessory atrioventricular (AV) pathway, showing baseline sinus rhythm (**A**), orthodromic reciprocating AV re-entrant supraventricular tachycardia (SVT) (**B**), and sinus rhythm after successful radiofrequency catheter ablation (**C**). In each plot, the four recordings from surface ECG leads are displayed at the top, followed by intracardiac recordings. The electrograms from the proximal two electrodes on the quadripolar catheter in the high right atrium (HRA) are followed by the proximal (HBEP), middle (HBEM), and distal (HBED) His bundle electrograms from the hexapolar catheter positioned across the anterior septal area of the tricuspid valve. Recordings from this His bundle location elicit activity in the low atrium (best recorded by the HBEP), the His bundle (best recorded by the HBEM or HBED), and the anterior septal inflow area of the right ventricle (best recorded by the HBED). In **A**, note that the presence of pre-excitation from an anterior septal accessory AV pathway eliminated the ability to record an HBE because the septal right ventricular myocardium was activated first by conduction through the accessory AV pathway. The HBE was recorded later, during SVT, when antegrade conduction existed through the His (H) bundle alone (retrograde conduction was via the accessory AV pathway) and after successful ablation (**B** and **C**, respectively) slightly anterior to the His bundle catheter location. This is shown best by the low-amplitude, almost continuous electrogram between the atrial and ventricular electrograms recorded by the distal electrodes (TVD). The electrograms recorded by the proximal, middle, and distal pairs of electrodes on the hexapolar catheter in the coronary sinus are designated PCS, MCS, and DCS, respectively. The next recording was from the proximal pair of electrodes on the quadripolar catheter in the right ventricular apex (RVA). The femoral arterial pressure (FAP) is displayed below.

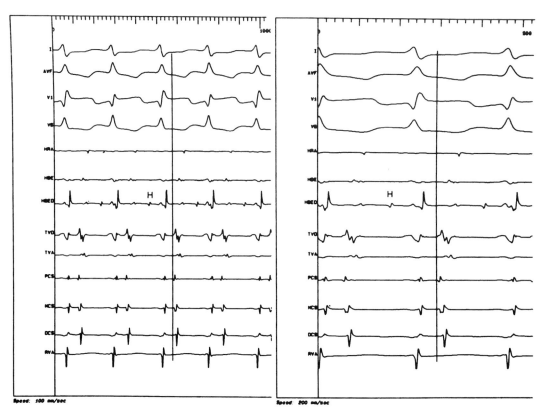

FIGURE 13.7 Two recordings in a 3-year-old boy with incessant, fast (220-ms cycle length; rate 272 beats per minute [bpm]), orthodromic reciprocating atrioventricular (AV) re-entrant supraventricular tachycardia that demonstrate the advantage of fast recording speed. **Left:** Using a recording speed of 100 mm/s, the earliest retrograde (conduction via posterior septal accessory AV pathway) atrial activation was difficult to determine. The atrial activation closest to the vertical line appeared to be either from the distal pair of electrodes on the tricuspid valve annulus mapping catheter (TVD) located at the posterior septal area, or from the proximal pair of electrodes on the coronary sinus (PCS) catheter, located approximately 0.5 cm into the coronary sinus from the os. **Right:** By doubling the recording speed to 200 mm/s, the earliest electrogram not only appeared to be more easily detected by the TVD electrodes, but the low-amplitude earliest electrogram appeared to be from the accessory AV pathway (see also Fig. 13.8). (Other abbreviations are as described in Fig. 13.6.)

of catheter ablation and with the advances in 3-D mapping technology, the techniques and objectives of mapping have assumed a major new role and deserve emphasis (see Chapter 17). The important general mapping concepts include the fluoroscopic image, catheter manipulation techniques, various modes of pacing, nuances of electrogram recordings, and 3-D mapping (Figs. 13.1–13.8).

Administration of Drugs

Intravenous drug administration during an intracardiac study encompasses three general categories: Anesthetic drugs, provocative arrhythmic drugs, and antiarrhythmic drugs. Of the three, anesthetic drugs are the most commonly administered and were discussed earlier in this chapter. The most commonly used provocative arrhythmic drug is isoproterenol. Other less frequently used provocative drugs include epinephrine, caffeine, atropine, procainamide, or flecainide (for Brugada's syndrome) (2,3,26–30). Because of sleep- or sedative-induced vagotonia, one of these provocative drugs may be necessary to induce or sustain tachycardia, which is essential to determine arrhythmia mechanisms and the site of arrhythmia foci or pathways. The doses of isoproterenol and epinephrine continuous-drip infusions are similar and range from 0.01 to 0.1 mg/kg/min. Atropine (0.01 to 0.04 mg/kg) is infrequently used because it cannot be administered as a continuous drip and because of its longer-lasting effects. The caffeine dose is 400 mg during 30 minutes, then 300 mg during 15 minutes.

Before the ablation era, antiarrhythmic drug administration during intracardiac electrophysiologic study was commonly used to assess drug safety and efficiency of planned chronic therapy (31). Although chronic medical therapy still exists as a treatment option (especially for patients with ventricular arrhythmias), its use is declining because of the increased application of ablation treatment and cardioverter-defibrillator device options.

Antiarrhythmic drug administration also is used commonly to achieve acute effects. This is indicated most often during attempts to block atrioventricular (AV) nodal conduction. The AV nodal blocking effects of verapamil, esmolol, propranolol, or adenosine are helpful to elucidate arrhythmia mechanisms and to distinguish the type of AV and ventriculoatrial (VA) conduction, if present (32–34).

TABLE 13.1

PACING PROTOCOLS FOR INTRACARDIAC ELECTROPHYSIOLOGIC STUDY

1. Sinus node function
   a. Sinus node recovery time
   b. Sinoatrial conduction time
2. AV conduction
   a. Continuous atrial decremental pacing
   b. Premature atrial extrastimulus technique (during sinus and/or eight-beat drives of a-paced rhythm)
3. VA conduction
   a. Continuous ventricular decremental pacing
   b. Premature ventricular extrastimulus technique (during sinus and/or eight-beat drives of v-paced rhythm)
4. Atrial muscle conduction and refractory period
   a. Premature atrial extrastimulus technique (during sinus and/or eight-beat drives of a-paced rhythm)
5. Ventricular muscle conduction and refractory period
   a. Premature ventricular extrastimulus technique (during eight-beat drives of v-paced rhythm)
6. Induction of supraventricular tachycardia
   a. One or more of the following: Continuous atrial decremental pacing (or short bursts), premature atrial extrastimulus technique (using one or more drive cycle lengths, one to three extrastimuli, and one or more pacing sites such as HRA, LRA, CS), continuous ventricular decremental pacing, premature ventricular extrastimulus technique (during sinus and/or eight-beat drives of v-paced rhythm)
   b. If unsuccessful, add provocative drug and repeat step 6a
7. Determine SVT mechanism, map location
   a. Results of steps 6a, b
   b. One or more of the following during underlying SVT rhythm with use of recording electrodes in several locations pertinent to type of tachycardia: Premature atrial extrastimulus technique (from one or more pacing sites such as HRA, LRA, CS), premature ventricular extrastimulus technique (from one or more pacing sites such as RV, LV)
8. Induction of ventricular tachyarrhythmia
   a. One or more of the following: Continuous ventricular decremental pacing (or short bursts), premature ventricular extrastimulus technique (using one or more drive cycle lengths, one to four extrastimuli, and one or more pacing sites such as RVA, RVOT, LV), continuous atrial decremental pacing, premature atrial extrastimulus technique (during sinus and/or eight-beat drives of v-paced rhythm)
   b. If unsuccessful, add provocative drug and repeat step 8a
9. Determine VT mechanism, map location
   a. Results of steps 8a, b

AV, atrioventricular; VA, ventriculoatrial; HRA, high right atrium; LRA, lower right atrium; CS, coronary sinus; SVT, supraventricular tachycardia; RV, right ventricle; LV, left ventricle; RVA, right ventricular apex; RVOT, RV outflow tract; VT, ventricular tachycardia.
From references 1–3, 12, 17, 19, and 23–25.)

Complications

Complications have been reported and analyzed for nonelectrophysiologic cardiac catheterizations in children (35–40). Only the 1998 report by Vitiello et al. (39) and the summary in a previous edition of this book by Kugler (17) have separate analyses of electrophysiologic studies. Vitiello et al. conducted an extensive statistical analysis (stepwise multiple logistic regression followed by categorical variable testing of models, which was further tested by Hosmer–Lemeshow's goodness of fit) of 4,952 consecutive cases (3,149 diagnostic, 1,371 interventional, 383 electrophysiologic, 41 ablation) (39). Electrophysiologic procedures had the lowest rate of major complications at 0.7%, similar to the 0.8% of diagnostic procedures, and both were less than the interventional (ablations included in interventional) rate of 2.0%. An electrophysiologic study was not an independent risk factor for complication. However, because ablation was included as an interventional procedure, it was an independent risk factor for complication during electrophysiologic study. It appears that addition of an ablation procedure increases the risk of the procedure to a level similar to that of other interventional catheter procedures (17). For the Pediatric Electrophysiology Society's catheter ablation registry, Schaffer et al. (41) studied the mortality rate and found a mortality rate of 0.89% for all procedures and a correlation of mortality with underlying heart disease, greater number of energy applications, left-sided procedures, and lower body weight. The latter risk factor was also found in the single-center report of Rhodes et al. (40) for patients ≤5 kg, but they included only nonelectrophysiology catheterization procedures.

TRANSESOPHAGEAL TECHNIQUE

Educational and Emotional Preparation of Patient and Family

The preparation of the patient and family for a transesophageal study centers on explaining the technique and addressing expectations and concerns related to placement of

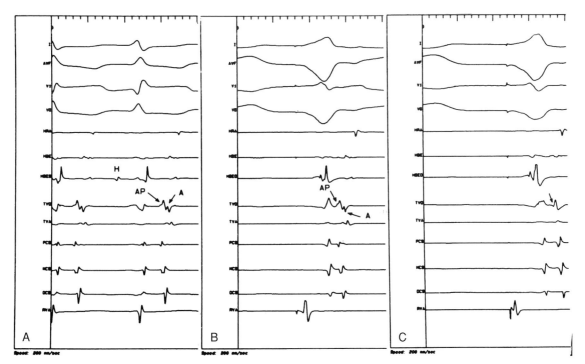

FIGURE 13.8 Three recordings from the same patient as in Fig. 13.7, demonstrating the recording of an electrogram from an accessory atrioventricular (AV) pathway (AP). **A:** During orthodromic reciprocating AV reentrant supraventricular tachycardia (220-ms cycle length, same recording as in Fig. 13.7), an early, low-amplitude electrogram (*arrow*, AP) was recorded before a biphasic electrogram that appeared to be either a fusion with the following atrial (A) electrogram or a biphasic atrial electrogram. H, His bundle. **B:** During ventricular pacing (500-ms cycle length), a virtually identical electrogram was recorded (*arrow*, AP). **C:** During ventricular pacing at the same cycle length after successful radiofrequency catheter ablation, the AP electrogram was eliminated (*arrow*). Also, after the ablation, normal retrograde conduction was verified by several other pacing protocols (not shown). (Other abbreviations are as described in Fig. 13.6.)

the catheter followed by pacing and stimulation. Educational materials backed by an honest but positive and confident approach during the explanation session are important in successfully achieving the goals of a transesophageal study in an older child or adolescent. In infants and small children, the same approach is modified and directed toward the parents.

Sedation

Mild, low levels of sedation usually are sufficient to maximize patient cooperation while relieving discomfort and anxiety. For infants, children, and adolescents, intravenous meperidine (0.5 to 1.0 mg/kg) and midazolam (0.05 to 0.1 mg/kg) is a low-dose, effective analgesic/amnesic sedative combination. Before a peripheral intravenous line is established, oral diazepam (0.2 to 0.4 mg/kg) or intranasal midazolam (0.2 to 0.3 mg/kg) is effective in controlling anxiety and thereby allowing the patient to be more cooperative (42).

Preparation of Patient in the Procedure Room

Whether in an inpatient or outpatient setting, the transesophageal technique is easily adaptable to virtually any type of room or location where the patient can be comfortably supine and where sufficient space exists for equipment and monitoring. After peripheral intravenous access is established,

the surface ECG leads are placed and connected. Although a direct current (DC) defibrillation and cardioversion system should be available, routine placement of chest pads is not necessary. Sedation is administered as needed with appropriate vital sign (heart rate, respiratory rate, and blood pressure) and oximetry monitoring protocols established. In some infants and small children, comfortable extremity restraints are necessary to prevent withdrawal of the catheter by the patient. The success of a transesophageal study depends highly on a positive, encouraging approach during the procedure by the pediatric electrophysiologist, pediatric cardiology nurse, and associated personnel. A soothing, comforting manner is necessary for successful passage of the catheter, as well as for successful recording and stimulation because of the potential mild discomfort encountered during each of these steps.

Catheter Placement

Similar to passage of a nasogastric tube, initial placement of the catheter involves lubrication (water usually is sufficient, but local lidocaine gel can be beneficial). Entry through the nares is followed by firm but gentle advancement through the posterior pharynx into the esophagus. Encouragement of repeated swallowing by the patient facilitates the catheter placement. The distance of catheter advancement required to reach the predicted area best suited for recording and pacing directly correlates with patient height (43) (Fig. 13.9). However, this predicted

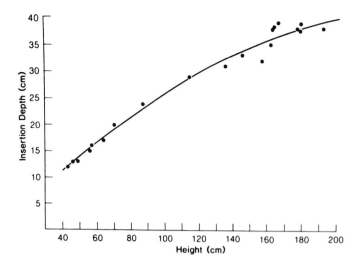

FIGURE 13.9 Graph of depth of transesophageal electrode catheter insertion (measured from distal electrode on catheter) from the nares in pediatric patients of various heights. By plotting the patient's height, in centimeters, the correlating distal electrode depth can be determined. After the distal electrode has been positioned at the predicted depth, small adjustments may be necessary for optimal recording and pacing. (From Benson DW Jr, Sanford M, Dunnigan A, et al. Transesophageal atrial pacing threshold: Role of interelectrode spacing, pulse width and catheter insertion depth. *Am J Cardiol* 1984;53: 1102–1106, with permission.)

depth may not actually be the ideal location, and minor adjustments may be necessary. The optimal catheter electrode position for pacing correlates with the highest atrial electrogram amplitude. Short distances (a few millimeters) of catheter withdrawal and advancement are performed until the maximum atrial electrogram amplitude is found. The catheter is then secured by taping it to the patient's face or nose.

Equipment and Recording/ Stimulation Technique

The three major equipment components are the electrode catheter, the recording apparatus (monitor, strip-chart recorder), and the stimulator (Fig. 13.10). Successful transesophageal recording and stimulation in infants, children, and adolescents have been reported with various types of electrode catheters. Transesophageal electrode catheters differ in size (4 to 12 Fr), interelectrode distance (2 to 30 mm), and number of electrodes (bipolar, quadripolar, hexapolar). Although the adult "pill" electrode can be used in the older child and adolescent, the electrode catheter is better suited for the pediatric patient. Moreover, some transesophageal catheter manufacturers have been receptive to customized catheter design regarding electrode number and interelectrode distance. Benson et al. (43) found that the interelectrode distances (12, 22, and 28 mm) had no significant effect on pacing thresholds regardless of age or size of the patient. Essentially no data are available that compare catheter sizes in pediatric patients; however, intuitively, if electrode contact with the esophageal wall is an important goal, the largest possible catheter size should be used. In normal-sized newborn infants, the nares usually can accommodate catheters in the 7 to 10 Fr range. In older children and adult-sized adolescents, 10 to 12 Fr catheters are most often used. Bipolar electrode configuration limits the technique to either recording or pacing, so quadripolar electrode catheters have been designed to permit simultaneous pacing and recording, with the recording interelectrode distance much shorter (2 mm) than the pacing interelectrode distance (12 to 30 mm).

The recording equipment consists of a strip-chart recorder with or without an ECG monitor. Without a monitor, the strip-chart recorder can run continuously and, therefore, also functions as the monitor. The recording system can be set up in a unipolar or bipolar fashion (Fig. 13.10).

A unipolar recording system is the simplest and involves the lowest investment in equipment because a preamplifier is not required. A three-channel ECG machine can function as both a strip-chart recorder and monitor (Fig. 13.10). A three-channel simultaneous-recording ECG machine uses one channel for a unipolar esophageal lead and the other two channels for two surface ECG leads. For example, the V1 chest lead is connected to one of the electrodes on the transesophageal catheter. The recordings from the V2 and V3 chest leads are then displayed or recorded simultaneously to permit comparison of the QRS and P waves on the surface leads with the electrograms from the unipolar esophageal lead (Figs. 13.10A and 13.11). Alternatively, two simultaneous unipolar esophageal electrograms, each from a separate esophageal electrode, can be displayed or recorded with the recording from one surface ECG lead. Recording during pacing is carried out either without the simultaneous transesophageal electrogram, by reconnecting the V1 chest lead to the V1 skin lead as illustrated in Figure 13.12, or with the simultaneous recording from a transesophageal lead (Figs. 13.10B and 13.13).

A bipolar recording system requires the addition of a preamplifier between the catheter and the monitor/strip-chart recorder (Fig. 13.10A). A bipolar system has certain advantages. More reproducible and reliable atrial electrograms are produced. The baseline wanders less, and the atrial electrograms are more distinct and the ventricular electrograms less prominent, which makes the recordings more distinguishable (Fig. 13.14). However, standard ECG filters are 0.1 to 25 Hz, which are still not ideal for high-quality bipolar electrograms. Optimal recording of bipolar electrograms occurs when the high-pass filter is set at 20 Hz. This requires a preamplifier with the capability for these filter settings (e.g., Arzco Medical Systems, Vernon Hills, IL). The newer quadripolar catheters that use close (2 mm) interelectrode distances for recording an optimally filtered bipolar system permit simultaneous recording of electrograms during pacing with less artifact compared with a unipolar system. In the absence of a quadripolar system, a switch connected from the bipolar catheter to the preamplifier allows a rapid change from pacing to recording when pacing is terminated. Although a bipolar system is better than a unipolar system with regard to artifact, the latter is not eliminated by a bipolar system because the high amplitudes and long pulse widths of bipolar transesophageal pacing present a problem in ECG recording and, therefore, measuring intervals. Benson et al. (44) have reported success using a

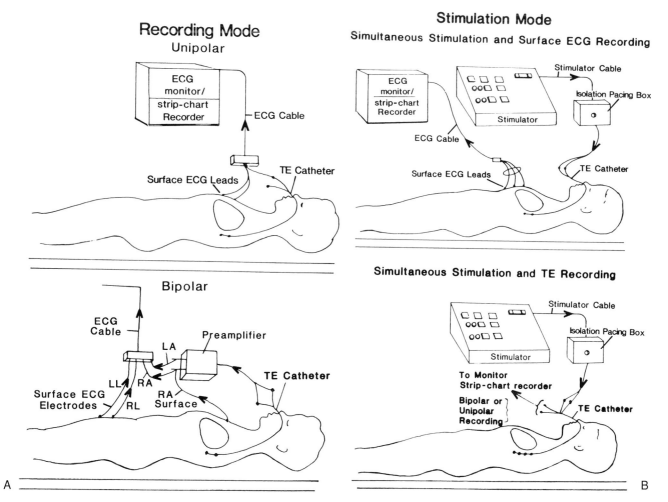

FIGURE 13.10 Diagrammatic illustration showing the recording and stimulation components of the transesophageal (TE) electrophysiologic technique. The recording mode (**A**) can be set up in a simple unipolar system (*top*) by connecting one esophageal electrode terminal to a surface ECG lead (e.g., V1) while recording one or two other simultaneous surface ECG leads (e.g., V2, V3). (See Figs. 13.11 and 13.14A for examples of unipolar recordings.) A bipolar recording system (*bottom*) can be used by adding a preamplifier. (See Fig. 13.14B for an example of a bipolar recording.) The stimulation mode (**B**) can be set up using either a bipolar or a quadripolar transesophageal electrode catheter. The bipolar electrode catheter permits only recording or stimulation, but not both simultaneously. An example of bipolar pacing using a bipolar electrode catheter is shown (*top*) with recording of the surface ECG during pacing. (See Fig. 13.12 for an example of ECG recording during pacing.) Simultaneous esophageal recording during pacing (*bottom*) can be accomplished in a unipolar or bipolar recording mode. (See Fig. 13.13 for an example of unipolar recording during pacing.) LA, left arm; LL, left leg; RA, right arm; RL, right leg.

prototype stimulus artifact suppressor that allowed for much-improved ECG recordings.

The stimulator system requires capability for a long pulse width (10 to 20 ms) and high current (15 to 30 mA) (43,45). Several investigators have shown that pulse widths greater than the standard 2 ms for intracardiac pacing are necessary to overcome high impedance and to penetrate the esophagus to reach the atrial (paraseptal) myocardium. Although reports of pulse width duration for successful transesophageal atrial pacing have included low values of ≤2 ms, atrial pacing is most consistent and reproducible at 6 to 10 ms and current of 10 to 15 mA (30,32). Delivery of stimulus current >15 mA (at a constant pulse width of 10 ms) is associated with patient discomfort (43,45). Moreover, lower stimulus current is needed at higher pulse width settings (e.g., 15 or 22 ms). Therefore, for patients with high thresholds, discomfort can be minimized by increasing the pulse width, limiting the current threshold with a goal of <15 mA.

Transesophageal atrial pacing is most successful and best tolerated when performed at stimulator outputs approximately 50% above threshold. Some investigators use a constant pulse width of 10 ms and vary the stimulus current to obtain a threshold. If, for example, the current threshold is 10 mA at a 10-ms pulse width, then pacing is performed at 15 mA. Others use a constant current and vary the pulse width. If, for example, the pulse width threshold is 8 ms at

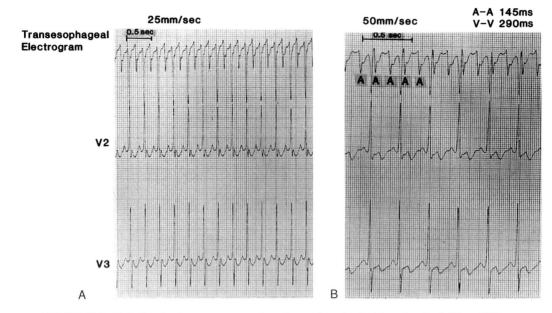

FIGURE 13.11 Unipolar simultaneous transesophageal recordings (*top*) with surface leads V2 and V3 at two recording speeds (**A**: 25 mm/s; **B**: 50 mm/s) from a newborn baby with sustained, regular tachycardia, 206 beats per minute (290-ms cycle length), showing atrial flutter (2:1 atrioventricular block) as the mechanism. The atrial (A-A) cycle length (145 ms) was half of that of the ventricular cycle length (290 ms).

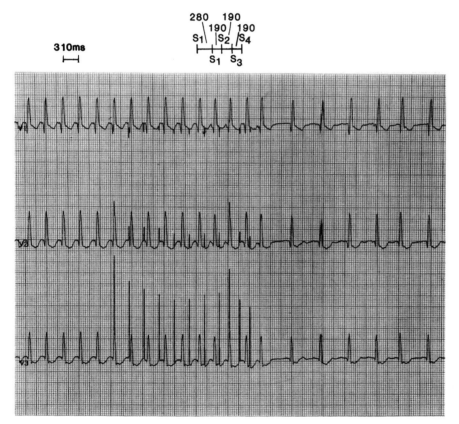

FIGURE 13.12 Recordings (25 mm/s) from simultaneous surface electrocardiographic leads (V1, V2, V3) in a 7-year-old boy with intra-atrial re-entry tachycardia (underlying cardiac diagnosis: Postoperative Fontan's) showing conversion of the atrial tachycardia (310-ms cycle length) by transesophageal atrial pacing using a bipolar electrode catheter. After multiple modes of atrial pacing protocols, successful conversion to sinus was finally accomplished with eight beats of a 280-ms drive cycle length, followed by three extrastimuli (190-ms intervals each).

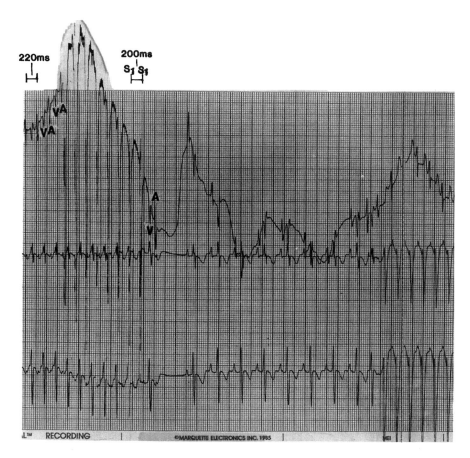

FIGURE 13.13 Unipolar transesophageal simultaneous recordings (*top*) with surface leads V2 and V3 from a 3-year-old boy with incessant normal and wide QRS supraventricular tachycardia (220-ms cycle length), showing simultaneous transesophageal pacing (interelectrode distance 24 mm) and recording (interelectrode distance 2 mm). Using a quadripolar electrode catheter, the esophageal recording (V, ventricular; A, atrial) during tachycardia was interrupted by eight beats of atrial pacing (200-ms cycle length), which converted the tachycardia to several beats of sinus before wide QRS reciprocating atrioventricular re-entrant supraventricular tachycardia recurred. Note the wandering baseline of the unipolar esophageal recording before, during, and after pacing.

10 mA current, then pacing is performed at 12 ms. A third option is to vary both the stimulus current and the pulse width to achieve a combination that results in low amplitude (<15 mA) to avoid patient discomfort.

With either technique, transesophageal atrial pacing can be successfully accomplished in >90% of pediatric patients using presently available transesophageal electrode catheters without discomfort at relatively low stimulator outputs (less than twice threshold) of <10-ms pulse width and 15-mA stimulus current (45–55).

Ventricular transesophageal pacing has been accomplished in adults by stimulating at high outputs currents ranging from 20 to 30 mA with a pulse width of 40 ms and by using a specially designed flexible lead passed into the stomach (56). In a case report of ventricular transesophageal pacing in a 2,400-g premature infant with congenital AV block, high output also was required: 10-ms pulse width with 45-V amplitude (current was not specified) (57). Overall success rates of stable transesophageal ventricular pacing have ranged from 50% to 75% of adult patients; data are not available from a pediatric series.

The pacing protocols for transesophageal pacing are limited on a practical basis to atrial pacing. As with the intracardiac pacing protocols, the specific protocols should be suited

Unipolar

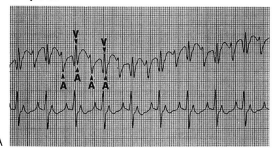

A

Bipolar

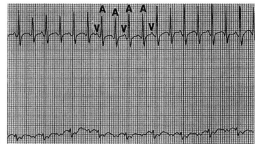

B

FIGURE 13.14 Two transesophageal recordings (50 mm/s) in a 2,250-g newborn with atrial flutter (150 ms atrial cycle length) and 2:1 atrioventricular block, showing a comparison of unipolar (**A**) and bipolar (**B**) recordings. Note that the prominent ventricular electrogram and the wandering baseline in the unipolar recording are eliminated in the bipolar recording. Therefore, the atrial electrogram is better delineated in the bipolar recording.

TABLE 13.2

PACING PROTOCOLS FOR TRANSESOPHAGEAL ELECTROPHYSIOLOGIC STUDY

1. Sinus node function
   a. Sinus node recovery time
2. AV conduction
   a. Continuous atrial decremental pacing
   b. Premature atrial extrastimulation technique (during sinus and/or eight-beat drive of a-paced rhythm)
3. Atrial muscle refractory period
   a. Premature atrial extrastimulation technique (during sinus and/or eight-beat drive of a-paced rhythm)
4. Induction of supraventricular tachycardia
   a. One or more of the following: Short bursts of a-pacing, continuous atrial decremental a-pacing, premature atrial extrastimulation technique (using one or more drive cycle lengths and one to three extrastimuli)
   b. If unsuccessful, add provocative drug and repeat 4a
5. Determine SVT mechanism
   a. Results of 4a, b
   b. Record transesophageal electrogram, determine intervals
6. Determine drug efficacy/safety
   a. Administer drug
   b. For efficacy, repeat provocative a-pacing modes that induced pacing before drug
   c. For safety, repeat steps 1–3
7. Terminate tachycardia
   a. One or more of the following: Short bursts of a-pacing, continuous atrial decremental pacing, premature atrial extrastimulation technique (using one or more drive cycle lengths and one to three extrastimuli)

AV, atrioventricular; SVT, supraventricular tachycardia.
From references 46–58.

to the patient and the preprocedure diagnosis. In Table 13.2, a list of pacing protocols provides examples of several options used during transesophageal electrophysiologic studies.

Administration of Drugs

During transesophageal studies, administration of drugs is similar in scope to that performed during intracardiac studies. Sedative, provocative arrhythmic, and antiarrhythmic drugs are administered intravenously as individually indicated, similar to the intracardiac studies discussed earlier. The major differences relate to the practical application to only supraventricular arrhythmias in transesophageal studies, contrasted with both supraventricular and ventricular arrhythmias in intracardiac studies.

Complications

Complications of transesophageal studies are infrequent and predominantly inconsequential (43–55,58). Mechanical or anatomic problems such as undetected obstructions or mucosal trauma can arise during passage of the catheter through the nares and pharynx. These are usually easily recognized and transient. Using lower stimulation outputs, no esophageal mucosal damage has been documented even after hours of continuous pacing or with the use of excessively high outputs. Although technically not a true complication, transesophageal pacing in rare cases causes intolerable discomfort that is sufficient to disrupt completion of the study. Ventricular arrhythmias may be induced from inadvertent ventricular pacing or from rapidly conducting atrial paced beats (58–60). This rare but serious problem of induced ventricular arrhythmias requires readily accessible DC cardioversion/defibrillation and resuscitative equipment.

OBJECTIVES OF ELECTROPHYSIOLOGIC STUDY AND COMPARISON OF INTRACARDIAC AND TRANSESOPHAGEAL TECHNIQUES

One or more of the objectives listed in Table 13.3 are performed during electrophysiologic studies. The specific objectives performed relate to several factors, including arrhythmia diagnosis, underlying cardiac diagnoses, planned therapy, and which electrophysiologic technique (intracardiac or transesophageal) is used. The following discussion outlines the advantages and limitations of the two techniques relative to the objectives of the electrophysiologic study.

Ample studies of electrophysiologic results for both intracardiac and transesophageal techniques involving the objectives listed in Table 13.3 have been reported. The ability of the two techniques to accomplish the objectives of an electrophysiologic study encompasses multiple factors. It is important to realize the advantages and limitations of the two techniques relative to each objective. In this manner, when presented with an individual patient with a specific diagnostic or therapeutic problem, either the intracardiac or transesophageal technique (or both) can be optimally chosen. It must be emphasized, however, that although the intracardiac technique may be superior in its ability to accomplish virtually all of the specific electrophysiologic objectives, limitations in terms of cost, higher risk, and application in small infants may dominate in specific situations, making the transesophageal technique the best choice for the individual patient.

In Table 13.3, a comparison of the two techniques is graded (by opinion only) on a scale ranging from 0 (−), indicating no ability to accomplish the objective, to 4 (++++), indicating an approximately perfect (or universal) ability to accomplish the objective. Because of the inability of either technique to accomplish any objective in all patients without failure, neither technique received the highest possible grade. The inability to effectively routinely pace the ventricle is the major limitation to the transesophageal technique. Therefore, when the objectives that optimally involve ventricular pacing are analyzed, the transesophageal technique is inferior. Another major limitation of the transesophageal technique involves the fixed site of recording and stimulation, which limits the ability to effectively evaluate mechanisms of supraventricular arrhythmias, sinus node function (increased distance to sinus node), AV conduction, and site of AV block (inability to record HBE). The inability to reach the effective refractory period of the atrium is occasionally overcome by increasing the energy output. This is a potential limitation to the transesophageal technique, especially when attempting to fully evaluate patients with pre-excitation when the accessory

TABLE 13.3

COMPARISON OF INTRACARDIAC AND TRANSESOPHAGEAL TECHNIQUES TO ACCOMPLISH OBJECTIVES OF THE ELECTROPHYSIOLOGIC STUDY

Objective	Intracardiac	Transesophageal
1. Determine cause of unexplained symptoms suggesting arrhythmia	++	+
2. Terminate AV re-entrant SVT, AV nodal SVT, or intra-atrial reentry/atrial flutter	+++	++
3. Determine mechanism of ECG-documented SVT to define treatment options	+++	++
4. Assess efficacy/safety of antiarrhythmic drug therapy for SVT	++	++
5. Assess efficacy/safety of antiarrhythmic therapy for ventricular arrhythmia	++	−
6. Assess sinus node function	++	+
7. Assess AV conduction	+++	+
8. Assess site of AV block	+++	−
9. Evaluate potential risk in patient with:		
a. Pre-excitation	+++	++
b. Ventricular tachycardia	+++	−
10. Determine optimal mode of chronic pacemaker therapy for bradycardia pacing	++	+
11. Determine efficacy/safety and optimal mode of antitachycardia pacemaker therapy	++	+
12. Perform catheter ablation at same setting	+++	−
13. Assess efficacy/safety after catheter ablation	+++	+[a]

AV, atrioventricular; SVT, supraventricular tachycardia.
[a]SVT only.

pathway refractory period is limited by reaching the atrial refractory period first.

Although the major advantages of the intracardiac technique involve its superior ability to accomplish specific objectives, the transesophageal technique is far superior in terms of cost, time commitment, and risk. Therefore, in many situations, limitations of the transesophageal technique are far outweighed by its advantages. Also, it may be better to use one technique for a patient with a specific arrhythmia, but in another patient with an identical arrhythmia it may be better to use the other technique, and in some patients, particularly in unique situations in which catheter access is a problem, the transesophageal technique is used during an intracardiac electrophysiologic procedure to provide additional and/or optional atrial recording/pacing site. By understanding the limitations and advantages of the two techniques in concert with the electrophysiologic objectives, the cardiologist can optimally recommend the appropriate technique for the individual patient.

References

1. Gillette PC, Blair HL. Intracardiac electrophysiology studies. In: Gillette PC, Garson A Jr, eds. *Clinical Pediatric Arrhythmias*. 2nd ed. Philadelphia: WB Saunders, 1999:36–47.
2. Kugler JD. Evaluation of pediatric patients with preexcitation syndromes. In: Benditt DG, Benson DW Jr, eds. *Cardiac Preexcitation Syndromes, Origins, Evaluation and Treatment*. Boston: Martinus Nijhoff, 1986:316–411.
3. Kugler JD. Electrophysiologic studies. In: Allen HD, Gutgessel HP, Clark EB, et al., eds. *Moss and Adams' Heart Disease in Infants, Children, and Adolescents*. 6th ed. Baltimore: Williams & Wilkins, 2001:452–467.
4. Pass RH, Walsh EP. Intracardiac electrophysiologic testing in pediatric patients. In: Walsh EP, Saul JP, Triedman JK, eds. *Cardiac Arrhythmias in Children and Young Adults with Congenital Heart Disease*. Philadelphia: Lippincott Williams & Wilkins, 2001:57–94.
5. Clapp SA, Driscoll DJ, Mitrani I, et al. Comparative effects of age and sedation on sinus node automaticity and AV node conduction. *Dev Pharmacol Ther* 1981;2:180–187.
6. Yip ASB, McGuire MA, Davis L, et al. Lack of effect of midazolam on inducibility of arrhythmias at electrophysiologic study. *Am J Cardiol* 1992;70:593–597.
7. Kumaga K, Yamanouchi Y, Matsuo K, et al. Antiarrhythmic and proarrhythmic properties of diazepam demonstrated by electrophysiological study in humans. *Clin Cardiol* 1991;14:397–401.
8. Lavoie J, Walsh EP, Burrows FA, et al. Effects of propofol or isoflurane anesthesia on cardiac conduction in children undergoing radiofrequency catheter ablation for tachydysrhythmias. *Anesthesiology* 1995;82:884–887.
9. Erb TO, Hall JM, Ing RJ, et al. Postoperative nausea and vomiting in children and adolescents undergoing radiofrequency catheter ablation: A randomized comparison of propofol- and isoflurane-based anesthetics. *Anesth Analg* 2002;95:1577–1581.
10. Erb TO, Kanter RJ, Hall JM, et al. Comparison of electrophysiologic effects of propofol and isoflurane-based anesthetics in children undergoing radiofrequency catheter ablation for supraventricular tachycardia. *Anesthesiology* 2002;96:1386–1394.
11. Buckles CS, Gillette PC, Buckles DS. Subcutaneous lidocaine affects inducibility in programmed electrophysiologic testing of children. *J Cardiovasc Electrophysiol* 1991;2:103–107.
12. Zhou L, Keane D, Reed G, et al. Thromboembolic complications of cardiac radiofrequency catheter ablation: A review of the reported incidence, pathogenesis and current research directions. *J Cardiovasc Electrophysiol* 1999;10:611–620.
13. Anfinsen O-G, Gjesdal K, Aass H, et al. When should heparin preferably be administered during radiofrequency catheter ablation? *Pacing Clin Electrophysiol* 2001;24:5–12.
14. Anfinsen O-G, Gjesdal K, Brosstad F, et al. The activation of platelet function, coagulation, and fibrinolysis during radiofrequency catheter ablation in heparinized patients. *J Cardiovasc Electrophysiol* 1999;10:503–512.
15. Tse H-F, Kwong Y-L, Lau C-P. Transvenous cryoablation reduces platelet activation during pulmonary vein ablation compared with radiofrequency energy in patients with atrial fibrillation. *J Cardiovasc Electrophysiol* 2005;16:1064–1070.
16. Stabile G, De Simone A, Turco P, et al. Feasibility and safety of two French electrode catheters in the performance of electrophysiological studies. *Pacing Clin Electrophysiol* 1998;21(pt 2):2506–2509.
17. Kugler JD. Electrophysiologic studies. In: Emmanouilides GC, Riemenschneider TA, Allen HD, eds. *Moss and Adams' Heart Disease in Infants, Children, and Adolescents*. Baltimore: Williams & Wilkins, 1995:347–366.
18. Stevenson WG, Soejima K. Recording techniques for clinical electrophysiology. *J Cardiovasc Electrophysiol* 2005;16:1017–1022.

19. Packer DL. Three-dimensional mapping in interventional electrophysiology: Techniques and technology. *J Cardiovasc Electrophysiol* 2005;16:1110–1116.

20. Gillette PC, Garson A Jr, eds. *Clinical Pediatric Arrhythmias.* 2nd ed. Philadelphia: WB Saunders, 1999.

21. Deal BJ, Wolff GS, Gelband H, eds. *Current Concepts in Diagnosis and Management of Arrhythmias in Infants and Children.* Armonk, NY: Futura Publishing, 1998.

22. Yabek SM, Gillette PC, Kugler JD, eds. *The Sinus Node in Pediatrics.* New York: Churchill Livingstone, 1984.

23. Kugler JD. Sinus node dysfunction. In: Garson A Jr, Bricker JT, Fisher DJ, et al., eds. *The Science and Practice of Pediatric Cardiology.* Baltimore: Williams & Wilkins, 1998:1995–2031.

24. Hummel JD, Strickberger SA, Daoud E, et al. Arrhythmias/pacing: Results and efficiency of programmed ventricular stimulation with four extrastimuli compared with one, two, and three extrastimuli (clinical investigation and reports). *Circulation* 1994;90:2827–2832.

25. Zipes DP, Jalife J, eds. *Cardiac Electrophysiology from Cell to Bedside.* 4th ed. Philadelphia: WB Saunders, 2004.

26. Przybylski J, Chiale PA, Halpern MS, et al. Unmasking of ventricular pre-excitation by vagal stimulation or isoproterenol administration. *Circulation* 1980;61:1030–1036.

27. Toda I, Kawahara T, Murakawa Y, et al. Electrophysiological study of young patients with exercise related paroxysms of palpitation: Role of atropine and isoprenaline for initiation of supraventricular tachycardia. *Br Heart J* 1989;61:268–273.

28. Huycke EC, Lai WT, Nguyen NX, et al. Role of intravenous isoproterenol in the electrophysiologic induction of atrioventricular node reentrant tachycardia in patients with dual atrioventricular node pathways. *Am J Cardiol* 1989;64:1131–1137.

29. Freedman RA, Swerdlow CD, Echt DS, et al. Facilitation of ventricular tachyarrhythmia induction by isoproterenol. *Am J Cardiol* 1984;54:765–770.

30. Antzelvitch C, Brugada P, Borggrefe M, et al. Brugada syndrome: Report of the Second Consensus Conference. *Heart Rhythm* 2005;2(4):429–440.

31. Kugler JD, Bansal AM, Cheatham JP, et al. Drug-electrophysiology studies in infants, children and adolescents. *Am Heart J* 1985;110:144–154.

32. Milstein S, Dunnigan AN, Buetifkofer J, et al. Usefulness of combined propranolol and verapamil for evaluation of surgical ablation of accessory atrioventricular connections in patients without structural heart disease. *Am J Cardiol* 1990;66:1216–1221.

33. Dorostkar PC, Dick M II, Serwer GA, et al. Effect of adenosine on atrioventricular conduction in children and young patients with supraventricular tachycardia. *Cardiol Young* 1996;6:308–314.

34. Belhassen B. Adenosine triphosphate in cardiac arrhythmias: From therapeutic to diagnostic use. *Pacing Clin Electrophysiol* 2002;25:98–102.

35. Stanger P, Heymann MA, Tarnoff H, et al. Complications of cardiac catheterization of neonates, infants, and children. *Circulation* 1974;50:595–608.

36. Cohn HE, Freed MD, Hellenbrand WF, et al. Complications and mortality associated with cardiac catheterization in infants under one year: A prospective study. *Pediatr Cardiol* 1985;6:123–131.

37. Mullins CE, Latson LA, Neches WH, et al. Balloon dilation of miscellaneous lesions: Results of valvuloplasty and angioplasty of congenital anomalies registry. *Am J Cardiol* 1990;65:802–803.

38. Cassidy SC, Schmidt KG, Van Hare GF, et al. Complications of pediatric catheterization: A 3-year study. *J Am Coll Cardiol* 1992;19:1285–1293.

39. Vitiello R, McCrindle BW, Nykanen D, et al. Complications associated with pediatric cardiac catheterization. *J Am Coll Cardiol* 1998;32:1433–1440.

40. Rhodes JF, Asnes JD, Blaufox AD, et al. Impact of low body weight on frequency of pediatric cardiac catheterization complications. *Am J Cardiol* 2000;86:1275–1278.

41. Schaffer MS, Gow RM, Moak JP, et al. Mortality following radiofrequency catheter ablation (from the Pediatric Radiofrequency Ablation Registry). *Am J Cardiol* 2000;86:639–643.

42. Latson LA, Cheatham JP, Gumbiner CH, et al. Midazolam nose drops for outpatient echocardiography sedation in infants. *Am Heart J* 1991;121:209–210.

43. Benson DW Jr, Sanford M, Dunnigan A, et al. Transesophageal atrial pacing threshold: Role of interelectrode spacing, pulse width and catheter insertion depth. *Am J Cardiol* 1984;53:1102–1110.

44. Benson DW Jr, Jadvar H, Strasburger JF. Utility of a stimulus artifact suppressor for transesophageal pacing. *Am J Cardiol* 1990;65:393–394.

45. Dick M II, Campbell RM, Jenkins JM. Thresholds for transesophageal atrial pacing. *Cathet Cardiovasc Diagn* 1984;10:507–513.

46. Dick M II, Scott WA, Serwer GS, et al. Acute termination of supraventricular tachyarrhythmias in children by transesophageal atrial pacing. *Am J Cardiol* 1988;61:925–927.

47. Campbell RM, Dick M, Jenkins JM, et al. Atrial overdrive pacing in conversion of atrial flutter in children. *Pediatrics* 1985;75:730–740.

48. Butto F, Dunnigan A, Overholt ED, et al. Transesophageal study of recurrent atrial tachycardia after atrial baffle procedures for complete transposition of the great arteries. *Am J Cardiol* 1986;57:1356–1362.

49. Drago F, Turchetta A, Calzolari A, et al. Detection of atrial vulnerability by transesophageal atrial pacing and the relation of symptoms in children with Wolff–Parkinson–White syndrome and in a symptomatic control group. *Am J Cardiol* 1994;74:400–401.

50. Samson RA, Deal BJ, Strasburger JF, et al. Comparison of transesophageal and intracardiac electrophysiologic studies in characterization of supraventricular tachycardia in pediatric patients. *J Am Coll Cardiol* 1995;26:159–163.

51. Fenici R, Ruggieri MP, di Lillo M, et al. Reproducibility of transesophageal pacing in patients with Wolff–Parkinson–White syndrome. *Pacing Clin Electrophysiol* 1996;19:1951–1957.

52. Blomstrom-Lundqvist C, Edvardsson N. Transesophageal versus intracardiac atrial stimulation in assessing electrophysiologic parameters of the sinus and AV nodes and of the atrial myocardium. *Pacing Clin Electrophysiol* 1987;10:1081–1095.

53. Alboni P, Paparella N, Cappato R, et al. Reliability of transesophageal pacing in the assessment of sinus node function in patients with sick sinus syndrome. *Pacing Clin Electrophysiol* 1989;12:294–300.

54. Weindling SN, Saul JP, Walsh EP. Efficacy and risks of medical therapy for supraventricular tachycardia in neonates and infants. *Am Heart J* 1996;131:66–72.

55. Lemler MS, Schaffer MS. Neonatal supraventricular tachycardia: Predictors of successful treatment withdrawal. *Am Heart J* 1997;133:130–131.

56. McEneaney DJ, Escalona O, Anderson JA, et al. A gastroesophageal electrode for electrophysiological studies. *Pacing Clin Electrophysiol* 1999;22:487–499.

57. Serwer GA, Eckerd JM, Kelly EE, et al. Emergency ventricular pacing from the esophagus in infancy. *Am J Cardiol* 1986;58:1105–1106.

58. Benson DW Jr. Transesophageal electrocardiography and cardiac pacing: State of the art. *Circulation* 1987;75(suppl 3):86–90.

59. Kugler JD, Danford DA, Gumbiner CH. Ventricular fibrillation during transesophageal atrial pacing in an infant with Wolff–Parkinson–White syndrome. *Pediatr Cardiol* 1991;12:36–38.

60. Sanatani S, Saul JP, Walsh EP, et al. Spontaneously terminating apparent ventricular fibrillation during transesophageal electrophysiological testing in infants with Wolff-Parkinson-White syndrome. *Pacing Clin Electrophysiol* 2001;24:1816–1818.

CHAPTER 14 ■ DISORDERS OF CARDIAC RHYTHM AND CONDUCTION

PRINCE J. KANNANKERIL, MD, MSCI, AND FRANK A. FISH, MD

Disorders of cardiac rhythm range from benign to life-threatening. Arrhythmias may be classified according to various schemes. While no single one addresses all pertinent issues, an expanded classification based primarily on electrophysiologic and functional mechanisms will be used in this chapter (Table 14.1). Arrhythmias can be attributed to various and often combined *abnormalities in impulse formation*, such as automaticity or triggered depolarizations; *abnormalities in impulse propagation*, such as conduction block or delay, functional or fixed re-entry circuits; and *abnormalities in autonomic influence*.

TABLE 14.1

FUNCTIONAL CLASSIFICATION OF ARRHYTHMIAS AND CONDUCTION ABNORMALITIES

I. Extrasystoles: supraventricular, ventricular, junctional
II. Conduction abnormalities
  a. Right and left bundle branch block
  b. Left anterior and posterior hemiblock
  c. Bifascicular block
  d. First-degree atrioventricular (AV) block
  e. Rate-related bundle branch block
  f. Pre-excitation syndromes: Wolff–Parkinson–White's syndrome (WPW), Mahaim's fibers
III. Bradycardias
  a. Sinoatrial (SA) node dysfunction
  b. Second-degree AV block
  c. Complete AV block
IV. Tachycardias with normal QRS (supraventricular tachycardias)
  a. AV re-entry (orthodromic reciprocating tachycardia)
  b. AV node re-entry: typical and atypical forms
  c. Primary atrial tachycardias
    1. Ectopic atrial
    2. Atrial flutter, intra-atrial re-entry
    3. Atrial fibrillation
    4. Chaotic atrial tachycardia
  d. Junctional (ectopic) tachycardia
V. Tachycardias with wide QRS
  a. Supraventricular tachycardias (SVTs) with aberrant conduction
  b. Pre-excited tachycardias
    1. Antidromic tachycardias
    2. Bystander accessory pathway
  c. Ventricular tachycardias (VT)
    1. Monomorphic: re-entrant, triggered, automatic
    2. Polymorphic: including torsades de pointes, bidirectional VT
  d. Ventricular fibrillation

For bradycardias, the most important distinction is the differentiation of transient, functional abnormalities related to factors such as autonomic tone from those caused by underlying disease of the conduction system. In the case of tachycardias, the initial distinction drawn is often between supraventricular and ventricular mechanisms. However, it may prove just as important to differentiate arrhythmias owing to re-entry from those owing to triggered depolarizations or abnormal automaticity.

PRESENTATION AND EVALUATION

Some arrhythmias produce only mild, nonspecific symptoms such as decreased appetite, lethargy, nausea, chest pain (discomfort), and light-headedness; these may be particularly subtle in infancy. Chronic, incessant arrhythmias, in particular, often produce few, if any, immediate symptoms but may have significant long-term consequences on cardiac performance by producing progressive ventricular dysfunction, so-called tachycardia-induced cardiomyopathy. Paroxysmal arrhythmias often produce overt acute symptoms including palpitations, hypotension, syncope, or cardiac arrest.

Specific electrocardiographic (ECG) documentation correlated with reported symptoms is critical in establishing a diagnosis. If ECG documentation cannot be obtained, then provocative testing may be useful to establish the cause of severe or even life-threatening symptoms (Fig. 14.1).

Symptoms Owing to Bradycardias

In pediatric patients, symptoms owing to primary bradycardias are relatively uncommon. Most symptoms associated with true sinus node dysfunction are caused by inadequate chronotropic response to stress or exertion. Overt symptoms are relatively uncommon in patients with first- and second-degree atrioventricular (AV) block, except when there is limited ability to increase the ventricular rate during stress or exercise. Syncope and sudden death owing to complete AV block may result from bradycardia-dependent polymorphic ventricular tachycardia with degeneration to ventricular fibrillation. The fetus and infant with congenitally complete AV block and no associated heart disease usually are asymptomatic. However, if the escape rate is inadequate, symptoms may range from subtle growth failure to overt congestive heart failure, including fetal hydrops. Older patients with congenital AV block may manifest varying degrees of exercise limitation or syncope. Sudden death is uncommon during the first decade but increases thereafter. Both syncope and sudden

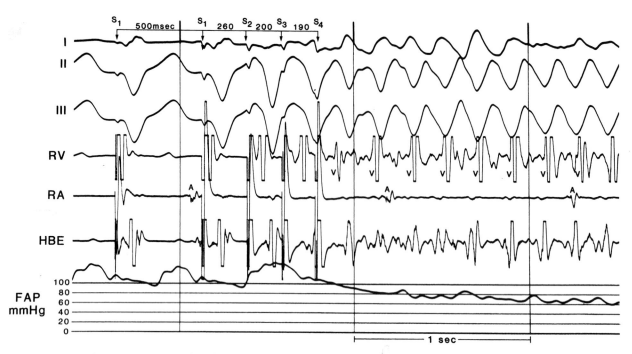

FIGURE 14.1 Intracardiac electrograms from a patient who experienced syncope after intracardiac surgery for tetralogy of Fallot. Ventricular tachycardia was induced with three extrastimuli (S$_2$, S$_3$, S$_4$) delivered at a drive train of 500 ms. Arterial pressure tracing demonstrates no pulse during tachycardia. FAP, femoral arterial pressure; HBE, His-bundle electrogram; RA, right atrium; RV, right ventricle.

death may be due to bradycardia-dependent ventricular tachycardia (torsades de pointes) rather than to the bradycardia itself.

Symptoms Owing to Tachycardia

Patients with incessant tachycardia at relatively slow rates may have few overt symptoms until congestive heart failure develops after weeks or months of ongoing tachycardia. On the other hand, patients with paroxysmal tachycardia may have hemodynamic collapse soon after tachycardia begins. Sustained tachycardia in the fetus may result in congestive heart failure or *hydrops fetalis*. Whereas in the neonate, rapid tachycardia of 12 to 24 hours' duration typically results in heart failure, in the fetus, intermittent tachycardia, at relatively slow rates, may produce heart failure only over days to weeks. Usually, tachycardia is recognized only during routine prenatal testing or during evaluation of suspected fetal distress (Fig. 14.2). Fetal tachycardia should be suspected if there is nonimmune fetal hydrops, even when tachycardia has not been documented.

Symptoms associated with tachycardia usually are nonspecific in infants and neonates. Consequently, tachycardia may go unrecognized for many hours and significant hemodynamic compromise may result. Palpitations are the usual presenting symptom in older children or adolescents with paroxysmal tachycardia, but other nonspecific symptoms such as lightheadedness, chest pain, dyspnea, pallor, or nausea may occur. Syncope is uncommon with tachycardia.

In contrast to paroxysmal tachycardia, incessant tachycardia may produce negligible symptoms and may go unrecognized by the patient until symptoms related to cardiac dysfunction develop.

Arrhythmias Presenting in the Asymptomatic Newborn

The spectrum of abnormalities that are detected in normal infants can include transient bradycardia, including sinus bradycardia, sinus pauses, and junctional escape beats, all of which can occur in 20% to 90% of infants (1). Such rhythms may be detected in utero. Transient bradycardias and mild QT-c prolongation (≤470 ms) may occur following stressful

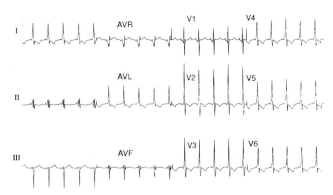

FIGURE 14.2 Standard ECG from neonate with large cardiac rhabdomyomas detected prenatally. Both mother and infant were diagnosed with tuberous sclerosis. Ventricular pre-excitation (Wolff–Parkinson–White syndrome [WPW]) may result from a tumor traversing the arteriovenous (AV) groove. Tachycardias with both normal QRS and wide QRS occurred after birth. Both orthodromic reciprocating tachycardia and ventricular tachycardia were induced at electrophysiology study.

labor or delivery but usually resolve within 48 to 72 hours. Premature atrial contractions (PACs) are quite common. Atrial bigeminy may occur in association with AV block, mimicking sinus bradycardia when the blocked P wave is superimposed on the T wave. When detected in utero, frequent premature beats carry approximately 1% risk of associated supraventricular tachycardia (SVT), and postnatally, that risk may be even lower.

Premature ventricular contractions (PVCs) are less common than PACs (1,2). The distinction between PVCs and PACs may be difficult for various reasons. Modest QRS prolongation in a neonate may be less evident, particularly if only a single ECG lead is examined. Also, aberrantly conducted PACs are common. Ventricular tachycardia is rare, even among otherwise well infants with PVCs.

Accelerated ventricular rhythm is a relatively uncommon, benign entity and is characterized by a regular, wide QRS rhythm with sustained or nonsustained rates exceeding the concurrent sinus rate by no more than 20% (3). This rhythm tends to resolve with time and should not be associated with acute or progressive hemodynamic compromise.

In general, none of the above rhythm abnormalities warrant specific therapy. The signs or symptoms likely to result from sustained tachycardia should be reviewed with parents. Continuous home monitoring usually is not warranted. Follow-up monitoring for PACs can usually be minimal, but more careful attention is warranted for PVCs.

Evaluation of Palpitations

Palpitations are more commonly due to SVT in the adolescent compared with the younger child (4). Precipitating circumstances such as fever, exercise, or emotional stress are common but variable. Abrupt onset and termination usually are apparent to older patients with paroxysmal tachycardias, but are less commonly described by patients with sinus tachycardia, incessant tachycardia at relatively slow rates, or ectopic beats. When symptom severity warrants or when standard monitoring attempts prove unsuccessful in capturing ECG during symptoms, provocative EP testing may be indicated.

Recently, newer monitoring modalities have become available, including continuous outpatient telemetry monitoring or implantable loop recorders (ILR). The latter are implanted subcutaneously (5). They have a slightly longer recording time per event than loop recorders, can be worn during swimming or other vigorous exercises, and can provide monitoring capabilities for >1 year.

Genetic/Familial Basis of Arrhythmias

Familial or genetic disorders of cardiac rhythm or conduction can be classified by their patterns of inheritance as autosomal dominant, autosomal recessive, X-linked, or matrilinear. For the electrophysiologist, understanding the mode of inheritance is essential for identifying individuals at risk of developing these disorders.

Identification of genes causing arrhythmias promises to lead to improved understanding of the pathophysiologic basis and natural history of arrhythmias. Establishing the genotype of individuals with arrhythmia phenotypes will provide an unambiguous way to identify siblings, offspring, and other genotype-positive family members at risk for developing arrhythmias.

GENERAL PRINCIPLES OF TREATMENT

Autonomic Interventions

Symptomatic bradycardias caused by AV block or severe sinus node dysfunction often are responsive to atropine, epinephrine, or isoproterenol until temporary pacing is available. The utility of other stimulants such as caffeine and theophylline is less clearly established. Autonomic modulation through vagal stimulation may also be useful in terminating certain supraventricular and occasionally ventricular tachycardias. This can be achieved in older children with the Valsalva maneuver or carotid sinus massage, and in younger children by applying ice to the face to elicit a dive reflex (Fig. 14.3). These maneuvers usually produce transient AV node block sufficient to terminate most reciprocating tachycardias or alter the AV relationship, allowing diagnostic recognition of other supraventricular or ventricular tachycardias. Continuous ECG recording during these interventions is essential. Beta-blockade can be useful for acute tachycardia termination or suppression. Conversely, beta-stimulation with isoproterenol, by increasing the heart rate and enhancing repolarization, is useful in the acute management of drug-induced torsades de pointes.

Antiarrhythmic Agents

Antiarrhythmic drugs are usually grouped using the modified Vaughan-Williams classification.

Class I: Sodium Channel Blocking Drugs

Class I antiarrhythmic agents block sodium channels. The resulting decrease in depolarizing current (dv/dt) slows conduction

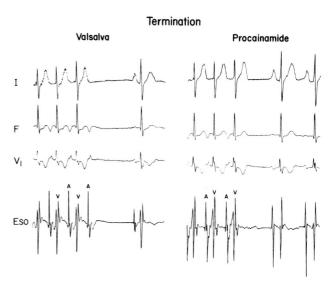

FIGURE 14.3 Termination of supraventricular tachycardia (SVT) (orthodromic reciprocating tachycardia) during esophageal ECG (*Eso*) recording. **Left:** Termination with antegrade block in the AV node following Valsalva maneuver. **Right:** Termination owing to retrograde block in the accessory connection following intravenous procainamide.

velocity within the myocardium. They are further subdivided into class IA, IB, and IC according to time course of recovery from block. This, in turn, determines the extent and rate-dependence of QRS prolongation and influences relative regional effects on atrial versus ventricular myocardium and diseased versus healthy tissue (6).

The class IA agents, quinidine, procainamide, and disopyramide, are characterized by intermediate recovery of block such that the QRS is prolonged slightly at normal rates and more markedly at faster rates. In addition to blocking sodium channels, these agents also produce anticholinergic effects and prolong the Q-T interval. The latter effect, now referred to as class III action (see below), is due to potassium channel blockade and may contribute substantially to their antiarrhythmic and proarrhythmic actions.

Class IB agents, lidocaine, phenytoin, and mexiletine, are characterized by rapid recovery of sodium channel block such that QRS prolongation is evident only at rapid rates. Q-T intervals may be slightly shortened. Typically Class IB agents affect ventricular tissue to a greater degree than atrial tissue.

Class IC agents, flecainide, propafenone, Ethmozine, and encainide (no longer marketed), are characterized by slower recovery of sodium channel blockade, such that tonic block and notable QRS prolongation occurs, even at normal heart rates.

Class IA and IC agents may be useful for various supraventricular and ventricular arrhythmias; class IB agents are generally useful only for ventricular arrhythmias. This tissue specificity is attributed to tissue-specific action potential characteristics, which may also vary during development. Class IC agents may be particularly potent for various arrhythmias, but may also be more prone to produce certain proarrhythmic effects. These include slow, incessant wide QRS tachycardia responsive to high-dose sodium bicarbonate, AV block, and an apparent risk of ventricular fibrillation and sudden death in certain populations. Class IA agents may aggravate SA node dysfunction and produce torsades de pointes owing to their associated QT prolonging (class III) effects. Class IA and IC agents may also depress ventricular function and thus aggravate congestive heart failure. A large body of evidence now indicates that class I agents do not reduce and may increase long-term mortality in patients with various ventricular arrhythmias in the setting of ischemic heart disease and congestive heart failure, even when apparent short-term efficacy is demonstrated. The degree to which these findings can be extrapolated to the pediatric setting remains incompletely established.

Class II: Beta-Blocking Drugs

Beta-adrenergic blocking agents may be useful for various tachycardias, used alone or in combinations with other agents. Antiarrhythmic effects include, but are not limited to, inhibition of sinus node and AV node conduction, resulting in decreased resting and peak heart rate, and P-R prolongation. Protective effects in relation to ischemia or surges in sympathetic tone may be particularly important in various ventricular arrhythmias. Propranolol is the prototype, but this group includes various agents characterized by very brief action (esmolol) or longer action and specificity for cardiac β-receptors (atenolol, nadolol, metoprolol).

β-blocking agents are often effective in treating reciprocating tachycardias using the AV node. They are also indicated for long Q-T syndrome and sometimes suppress various automatic tachycardias and reperfusion-related arrhythmias. Other antiarrhythmic agents possessing significant β-blocking

properties include the class III agents sotalol and amiodarone and the class IC agent propafenone.

For chronic treatment of congenital long QT syndromes (LQTS), nonselective agents with long duration of action such as Inderal LA™ or nadolol are now generally favored over selective β_1 blockers. In other situations, selective beta-blockers may be more preferable. Use of β-blocking agents may be limited by depression of ventricular function, bradycardia, AV block, exacerbation of bronchospasm, and their potential to exacerbate insulin-induced hypoglycemia. Nonspecific complaints such as irritability, depression, fatigue, and constipation often are reported.

Class III: Potassium Channel Blocking Drugs

The principal effect of class III antiarrhythmic agents is to produce Q-T prolongation and prolong cardiac action potential duration. Q-T prolongation appears to result from block of one or more potassium channels and reflects delay in myocardial repolarization with prolonged refractoriness. Amiodarone, sotalol, and dofetilide are available for oral administration.

Amiodarone may be the single most potent antiarrhythmic agent available for various supraventricular and ventricular arrhythmias. However, in addition to blocking potassium channels, it also blocks, to some degree, sodium channels, calcium channels, and β-adrenergic receptors. Its use is complicated by its very slow tissue uptake, delayed onset of action, and delayed clearance, as well as an unusually high incidence of adverse effects. Most of the other currently available agents with class III action are also "impure," exhibiting various other antiarrhythmic properties, such as sodium channel blockade (class IA agents), β-blocking properties (racemic sotalol), or α-adrenergic stimulation (disopyramide, bretylium). Several agents with more "pure" class III effects have been developed, such as dofetilide and d-sotalol (the non–β-blocking enantiomer), but their future role in clinical practice remains uncertain.

Class III agents have the theoretical advantage of decreasing the excitable gap of re-entrant arrhythmias without aggravating (and possibly improving) ventricular dysfunction. Amiodarone and d,l-sotalol also slow AV nodal conduction in contrast with the anticholinergic action of Class IA drugs. The chief concern during treatment with all drugs displaying Class III action is the potential for excessive Q-T prolongation, particularly in the presence of hypokalemia and hypomagnesemia, which may lead to torsades de pointes, a potentially lethal proarrhythmic effect. Recent reports have attributed some cases of excessive QT prolongation owing to subclinical forms of LQTS that become manifest only in the presence of a QT-prolonging drug. As a result, class IA and class III agents are contraindicated in patients with known or suspected long Q-T syndrome, and should be used with extreme caution in their unaffected family members or in patients with any previous history of drug-induced torsades de pointes. They should generally be instituted only during inpatient monitoring with frequent serial ECGs.

Class IV: Calcium Channel Blocking Drugs

Calcium channel blocking agents such as verapamil and diltiazem depress sinus and AV node depolarization, prolonging the P-R interval and slowing the sinus rate. They are particularly useful in controlling reciprocating supraventricular tachycardias by inhibiting AV node conduction. They also may be useful for slowing the ventricular response during primary atrial tachycardias by inhibiting AV node conduction, but they should not be used for this purpose in the presence of ventricular pre-excitation (Wolff–Parkinson–White syndrome [WPW]). Though not generally used for ventricular tachycardias, they may be quite effective in two specific idiopathic ventricular tachycardias: Left ventricular fascicular tachycardias and ventricular outflow tract tachycardias.

Calcium channel blocking drugs can depress ventricular function, lower blood pressure, slow heart rate, and increase AV block, all of which may limit their use in some patients. Infants are particularly prone to these effects, although oral therapy may be tolerated. Calcium channel blockers are not recommended in WPW patients, since enhanced antegrade accessory connection conduction has been described during atrial fibrillation.

Digoxin

Because it impairs AV conduction and has positive inotropic action, digoxin, alone or in combination with other drugs, has traditionally been regarded as first-line therapy for various supraventricular arrhythmias, especially in infants. However, its efficacy has not been subjected to the same critical study as most other agents. Although its use remains prevalent, some data suggest that much of its apparent efficacy may be attributable to the natural history of the arrhythmia rather than to any actual therapeutic effect of the drug (7,8). Digoxin may enhance antegrade accessory connection conduction during atrial fibrillation in WPW patients, and its use in infants with WPW may contribute to early mortality described in this population.

When used in conjunction with other therapies, digoxin dosage must often be reduced owing to altered binding or clearance by quinidine, amiodarone, flecainide, propafenone, and verapamil, whereas its efficacy may be offset by phenytoin. Caution should be exercised when instituting any combination of antiarrhythmic regimens, and the apparent benefits of combination therapies versus single agent therapy should always be carefully considered.

Adenosine

When administered as a rapid intravenous bolus, adenosine should produce transient AV node block, terminating tachycardias using the AV node (Fig. 14.4) (9). These effects on the AV node and SA node will be brief, allowing normal sinus

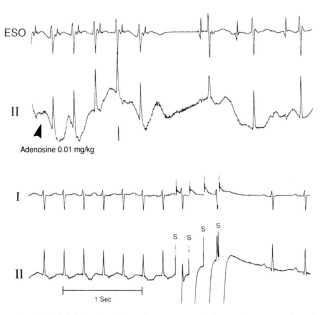

FIGURE 14.4 Termination of supraventricular tachycardia (SVT) (orthodromic reciprocating tachycardia). **Upper panel:** Termination with block in the AV node (antegrade) following intravenous adenosine. **Lower panel:** Termination with transesophageal pacing.

rhythm to resume. Even if AV node block fails to terminate tachycardia, the resultant alteration in the AV relationship provides important diagnostic information (Fig. 14.5). Primary atrial tachycardias or ventricular tachycardias occasionally may terminate with adenosine. Adenosine should be used cautiously in patients with known sinus node dysfunction or with severe reactive airway disease because of the risk of bronchospasm.

Temporary Pacing

Temporary pacing may be superior to acute pharmacologic therapy for both bradycardias and many tachycardias. Ventricular pacing generally is preferred over atrial pacing for

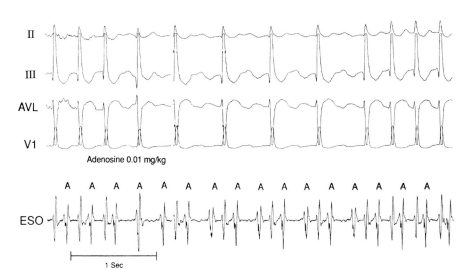

FIGURE 14.5 ECG recording during atrial tachycardia (atrial flutter) in a child with sick sinus syndrome following congenital heart surgery. P waves are not evident on the surface ECG. Transesophageal ECG (*ESO*) demonstrates 1:1 AV conduction. Adenosine produces transient AV block without terminating tachycardia, confirming the diagnosis of a primary atrial tachycardia.

most bradycardias, since AV node conduction may be tenuous. Transcutaneous pacing is tolerable for short periods and has been used for tachycardia conversion or for bradycardia treatment prior to insertion of a transvenous pacing catheter.

Whenever temporary pacing is necessary, careful and frequent determination of the pacing and sensing thresholds is necessary to ensure appropriate function of the pacing system. The pacing device should be set to at least twice the pacing threshold and half the sensing threshold whenever possible. Bipolar catheters with inflatable balloon tips and distal electrode placement well suited for pediatric use are available in 3 Fr and 5 Fr calibers and are superior to standard pacing catheters. Careful assessment and readjustment of temporary pacing modes may be necessary during acute pacing to accommodate changes in the patient's underlying rhythm. Demand pacing modes (AAI, DDD, and VVI, described later) usually are preferred over asynchronous pacing to avoid inadvertent pace induction of a tachycardia or fibrillation. However, when sensing characteristics are marginal, asynchronous pacing at rates just above the spontaneous heart rate may be an acceptable alternative.

Temporary pacing also is an extremely effective means of terminating various supraventricular and ventricular tachycardias (Fig. 14.6). The most frequent application is for terminating intra-atrial re-entrant tachycardias and atrial flutter. Pace termination should be considered when pharmacologic termination is ineffective, when frequent recurrences require repeated terminations, and as an alternative to DC cardioversion in non–life-threatening ventricular tachycardias.

Pace termination of tachycardias always carries the risk of accelerating or destabilizing re-entrant tachycardias and should be used only with appropriate equipment and personnel for emergency resuscitation and defibrillation. Though the terms overdrive pacing and burst suppression are often applied, termination of the tachycardia usually is achieved when one or more appropriately timed stimuli enters the re-entrant circuit during the excitable gap and advances the depolarization wavefront sufficiently that tissue still refractory from the preceding cycle is encountered. Ideally, a successful antitachycardia algorithm would methodically scan the tachycardia cycle to ensure stimulation during the excitable gap, minimize the potential for reinitiation or acceleration, and minimize discomfort to the patient. In the acute setting, rapid, short pacing bursts are most likely to terminate tachycardia without accelerating or reinitiating the arrhythmia. Often, termination is preceded by oscillations owing to destabilization of the circuit or when transient atrial fibrillation results. Even greater precautions in terms of the number of extrastimuli delivered to prevent ventricular fibrillation and preparedness for defibrillation are required when ventricular tachycardias are pace terminated.

Pace termination of tachycardias similarly can be accomplished at the bedside, during cardiac catheterization (usually in the context of an invasive electrophysiology study), or using an implanted pacing device. Most contemporary single-chamber and dual-chamber pacemakers and implantable cardioverter defibrillator (ICDs) may be reprogrammed temporarily for terminating tachycardias by pacing the appropriate chamber, or automatic antitachycardia therapies may be used when available. Temporary antibradycardia pacing may also help suppress reinitiation of bradycardia-dependent tachycardias such as torsades de pointes and possibly atrial fibrillation. Despite the feasibility of pace termination, cardioversion should never be deferred for hemodynamically unstable tachycardia.

Cardioversion and Defibrillation

For life-threatening symptoms due to tachycardia, DC cardioversion or defibrillation should be performed without delay, regardless of the suspected mechanism. In the unconscious patient, cardiopulmonary resuscitation (CPR) should be instituted until delivery of DC current (1 to 2 joules/kg). An amnestic sedative should be administered immediately afterward to the semiconscious patient. Semielective DC cardioversion should be performed with short-acting general anesthesia. The dose used for atrial tachycardias may be significantly lower, particularly with devices using biphasic waveforms (0.25 to 0.5 J/kg). Under no circumstances should an awake patient undergo transthoracic cardioversion.

When feasible, transesophageal echocardiography should be performed to exclude atrial thrombus prior to elective conversion of atrial fibrillation or atrial flutter of more than 24 to 48 hours, or when the duration is unknown. If thrombus is evident, cardioversion should be deferred 3 to 4 weeks while

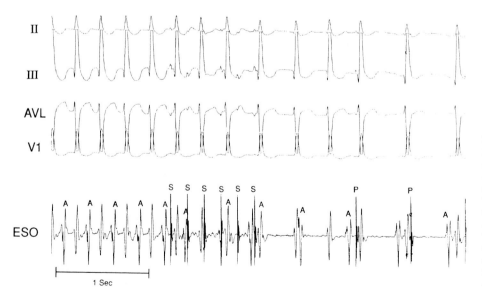

FIGURE 14.6 Pace termination of primary atrial tachycardia by a permanent antitachycardia pacemaker functioning in AAIT mode (see Table 14.2). Six extrastimuli (*S*) delivered at 80% of the tachycardia cycle length terminate tachycardia. Note that termination does not represent "overdrive pacing," but rather the fourth and sixth stimuli appear to enter the re-entrant circuit, rendering a critical portion refractory. The pacemaker temporarily reverts to AOO mode after delivering the burst.

anticoagulation therapy is instituted. The ventricular rate usually can be controlled with antiarrhythmic drugs such as diltiazem until cardioversion can be performed.

For organized tachycardias, countershock should be synchronized with the QRS to avoid inadvertent ventricular fibrillation due to the R-on-T phenomenon. For ventricular fibrillation or polymorphic tachycardias, unsynchronized delivery is necessary (otherwise the DC shock will be indefinitely delayed while attempting to track a consistent QRS). An ECG strip should be recorded continuously prior to delivery of the shock and should be continued for several seconds afterward to detect the recovery rhythm or possible tachycardia reinitiation.

As with other termination measures, it is important to distinguish unsuccessful cardioversion (or defibrillation) from termination followed by prompt reinitiation of the arrhythmia. In the case of failed conversion, technical errors, such as inadequate energy or improper electrode placement, should be distinguished from diagnostic errors. For reinitiation, measures to prevent reinitiation (such as antiarrhythmic therapy or temporary pacing) are warranted. It should be noted that both amiodarone and lidocaine, although often used for ventricular tachycardia or fibrillation refractory to DC shock, may actually increase the energy requirements for successful defibrillation. In contrast, class III agents actually lower defibrillation energy requirements in animal models and may also favorably inhibit fibrillation. However, if DC cardioversion, administered appropriately, continually fails to interrupt a tachycardia, an automatic or triggered mechanism should be considered and subsequent measures modified accordingly. Intracardiac defibrillation for atrial fibrillation occasionally is useful when transthoracic conversion has failed, but again, an alternative mechanism such as chaotic atrial tachycardia should be considered.

The growing proliferation of automatic external defibrillators in the community has vastly improved the potential for successful resuscitation in the out-of-hospital setting. Initially, appropriate concerns were raised regarding accuracy in arrhythmia recognition and appropriateness for use in pediatric patients. Now, early use of the AED is stipulated in the most recent pediatric advanced life support (PALS) guidelines, even in younger patients with out-of-hospital arrest.

Implantable Pacemakers and Defibrillators

Historically, simple ventricular demand pacemakers prevented the ventricular rate from dropping below a selected value. Progressive advances in pacing technologies enabled establishment of AV synchrony, rate-response, and antitachycardia therapies. More recently new algorithms have been developed to minimize adverse effects of chronic ventricular pacing by minimizing unnecessary ventricular pacing or allowing biventricular pacing. Furthermore, advances in electronic and lead design allow an ever-expanding array of complex functions to be housed in devices ever more suitable for use in smaller patients. These devices allow a number of physiologic goals to be met, and the reader is referred to recent reviews for detailed discussion of device selection (10).

Common pacing modes are listed in Table 14.2. Pacing modes are characterized by three- or four-letter codes wherein the first letter refers to the chamber paced, the second letter refers to the chamber sensed, the third letter refers to the response to sensed events, and the fourth refers to special functions. In general, DDD, VDD, or DVI modes allow AV synchrony to be maintained in the presence of AV block. When AV conduction is present, AAI mode permits synchro-

---

TABLE 14.2

COMMON PACING MODES

Single chamber	
AAI, AAIR	Atrial demand modes
VVI, VVIR	Ventricular demand modes
ADI, ADIR	Atrial demand with additional ventricular sensing
AOO, VOO	Asynchronous atrial, ventricular pacing
AAT, VVT	Atrial and ventricular triggered modes (e.g., track external pacemaker, stimulator)
VDD	Ventricular pacing, atrial and ventricular sensing with tracking (atrial sensing, but no pacing)
Dual chamber	
DDD, DDDR	Standard dual chamber pacing
DDI, DDIR	Dual-chamber pacing without atrial tracking
DVI, DVIR	Dual-chamber pacing, ventricular sensing only
DOO	Asynchronous dual chamber

---

nized AV conduction. VVIR, AAIR, and DDDR modes use an internal sensor to monitor vibration, motion, chest wall impedance, mixed venous saturation, or other physiologic parameters, and to adjust the pacing rate according to exercise or metabolic demands. VDD pacing systems using a single transvenous lead have been employed in patients with intact SA node function and complete AV block; their use in patients with congenital heart disease may not be appropriate owing to the significant potential for eventual atrial arrhythmias for which atrial pacing (in addition to sensing) would be warranted. Table 14-3 lists pediatric indications for a permanent pacemaker.

Simple antitachycardia functions are available in most pacemakers using temporary programming functions. Many newer generators have programmed stimulation capabilities, allowing limited noninvasive electrophysiologic evaluation. Alternatively, this capability can be mimicked using triggered modes (AAT or VVT) to track a cutaneously applied external programmed stimulator. In addition to the precautions discussed above for other pace terminations, it should be noted that antibradycardia pacing may be temporarily suspended during such maneuvers with certain devices. Therefore, familiarity with the specific features of a given device is necessary to ensure patient safety during use in this context.

Antitachycardia pacemakers, specifically designed to pace for bradycardia and automatically detect and respond to tachycardias, also are available (11). These devices use adjustable algorithms to promptly detect and terminate each tachycardia episode by automatically delivering preselected rapid pacing sequences (Fig. 14.6). Because of the risk of inducing ventricular fibrillation with the high-rate burst, these are used only for atrial tachycardias, although identical algorithms are available for pace termination of ventricular tachycardia in implantable defibrillators. Pharmacologic depression of AV node conduction often is necessary to prevent a rapid ventricular response during these episodes and the consequent pacing bursts. Newer dual-chamber defibrillators able to pace-terminate atrial arrhythmias as well as perform atrial or ventricular fibrillation are also available and are often preferable over simple antitachycardia pacemakers.

Implantable cardiac defibrillators (ICDs) have emerged as the treatment of choice in preventing sudden cardiac death in

TABLE 14.3

PEDIATRIC INDICATIONS FOR PERMANENT PACEMAKER

Class I: General agreement of indication
  Advanced second- or third-degree AV block with symptoms
    or ventricular dysfunction
  Sinus node dysfunction with symptoms
  Postop advanced second- or third-degree AV block, not
    expected to resolve or persistent >7 days
  Complete AV block with wide QRS escape, ventricular
    ectopy, or ventricular dysfunction
  Congenital third-degree AV block in infancy with
    HR <50–55 bpm
    HR <70 bpm with congenital heart disease

Class IIa: No consensus
  Bradycardia–tachycardia syndrome with need for
    longer-term antiarrhythmic therapy
  Congenital third degree AV block beyond infancy with
    Average HR <50 bpm
    Abrupt pauses in HR more than two to three times basic
      cycle length
    Symptoms associated with chronotropic incompetence
  Long QT syndrome with 2:1 or third-degree AV block
  Asymptomatic sinus bradycardia in child with CHD and
    Resting HR <40 bpm
    Pauses in ventricular rate >3 s
    Impaired hemodynamics owing to sinus bradycardia or
      loss of AV synchrony

Class IIb
  Congenital third-degree AV block with acceptable rate,
    narrow QRS, and normal LV function
  Asymptomatic sinus bradycardia with resting HR <40 or
    pauses >3 s
  Neuromuscular diseases with any degree of AV block
    (including first-degree AV block)

Class III: Not indicated
  Postsurgical AV block with return of normal conduction

AV, atrioventricular; bpm, beats per minute; CHD, congenital heart disease; HR, heart rate.
Adapted from Gregoratos G, Abrams J, Epstein AE, et al. ACC/AHA/NASPE 2002 guideline update for implantation of cardiac pacemakers and antiarrhythmia devices: summary article: a report of the American College of Cardiology/American Heart Association Task Force on Practice Guidelines (ACC/AHA/NASPE Committee to Update the 1998 Pacemaker Guidelines). *Circulation* 2002;106: 2145–2161, with permission.

TABLE 14.4

INDICATIONS FOR IMPLANTABLE DEFIBRILLATOR

Class I: General agreement of indication
  – Spontaneous sustained VT in association with structural
    heart disease
  – Nonsustained VT in patients with
    a. Prior MI
    b. LV dysfunction and inducible VT or VF
  – Spontaneous sustained VT in patients without structural
    heart disease that is not amenable to other forms of therapy

Class II: No consensus
  – Cardiac arrest presumed to be due to VF
  – Severe symptoms attributable to ventricular arrhythmias
    in patient awaiting cardiac transplantation
  – Inherited conditions with high risk of life-threatening ven-
    tricular arrhythmias
  – Recurrent syncope of undetermined origin with ventricular
    dysfunction and inducible ventricular arrhythmias at EPS
  – Syncope in advanced structural heart disease with no
    other identifiable cause

Class III
  – Syncope of undetermined cause and without structural
    heart disease and no inducible arrhythmias
  – Incessant VT or VF
  – VF or VT resulting from arrhythmias amenable to surgical
    or catheter ablation
  – Ventricular arrhythmias associated with reversible disorder
  – Psychiatric illness that is likely to be aggravated by ICD
  – Terminal illness, life expectancy <6 months

Class IV
  – CHF patients who are not candidates for transplant

CHF, congestive heart failure; EPS, electrophysiologic stimulation; ICD, implantable cardioverter defibrillator; LV, left ventricular; MI, myocardial infarction; VF, ventricular fibrillation; VT, ventricular tachycardia.
Adapted from Gregoratos G, Abrams J, Epstein AE, et al. ACC/AHA/ NASPE 2002 guideline update for implantation of cardiac pacemakers and antiarrhythmia devices: summary article: a report of the American College of Cardiology/American Heart Association Task Force on Practice Guidelines (ACC/AHA/NASPE Committee to Update the 1998 Pacemaker Guidelines). *Circulation* 2002;106:2145–2161, with permission.

most clinical situations. ICDs may be used in patients with prior life-threatening events (secondary therapy), or in certain conditions where the risk of sudden death is deemed sufficient to warrant ICD placement in the absence of a prior event (primary therapy). Table 14.4 presents ICD indications. These indications include patients with sustained ventricular tachycardia and underlying heart disease, ventricular fibrillation, or patients with hypertrophic cardiomyopathy, LQTS, or arrhythmogenic right ventricular cardiomyopathy who are at high risk of sudden death. An ICD is the treatment of choice for idiopathic ventricular fibrillation, though risk stratification algorithms are discussed later in this chapter (12).

In large studies of adult patients with ventricular tachycardias, ICD therapy consistently has proven superior to antiar-

rhythmic drug therapy in preventing sudden death, and these findings are presumed to be applicable to young patients at risk of sudden death. The role of ICDs in patients with dilated cardiomyopathies is less clear, although they may be useful adjuncts in some patients awaiting cardiac transplantation.

As with pacemakers, smaller-diameter transvenous lead systems and small generators suitable for most children and adolescents are now available. Current systems allow tiered therapies including pacing bursts, low-energy shocks, or high-energy shocks to be selected for use in a given patient, according to the rate and regularity of the arrhythmia. They also provide emergency antibradycardia ventricular pacing. Algorithms for discriminating atrial and ventricular arrhythmias are continually being refined in both single-chamber and dual-chamber devices.

For patients with complex anatomy, ICD implantation often requires novel approaches to both pace-sensing lead placement (e.g., epicardial) (Fig. 14.7), and to the placement of the high-voltage (HV) defibrillation lead. Increasingly,

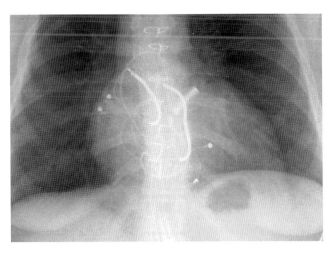

FIGURE 14.7 Posteroanterior (PA) chest radiograph of epicardial ICD system in teenager with prior Fontan repair who experienced cardiac arrest with documented ventricular tachycardia. A transvenous dual-coil ICD lead was draped over the anterior epicardial surface of the heart. The patient has experienced successful pace-termination atrial tachycardia and ICD discharge for ventricular tachycardia since implantation.

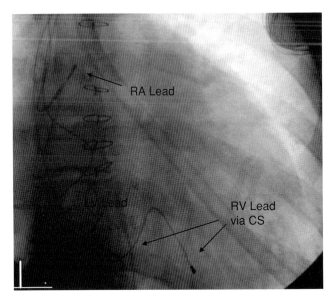

FIGURE 14.8 Posteroanterior (PA) chest radiograph of biventricular pacemaker in teenager with congenitally corrected transposition of the great arteries, complete AV block, and mechanical tricuspid valve prosthesis who developed progressive exercise intolerance associated with severe right ventricular (RV) dyssynchrony during chronic (right-sided) left ventricular (LV) pacing. Implantation of coronary sinus (CS) lead was complicated by unusually acute angulation of coronary sinus and posterior coronary vein used for left-sided lead. RA, right atrial.

when transvenous (HV) leads are not feasible, subcutaneous or epicardial coils are being used in lieu of traditional epicardial patches whenever possible (13).

Antitachycardia pacing or implantable defibrillators require careful patient selection, often including electrophysiologic study. Assessment of lead sensing and pacing characteristics are tested at implant and may need to be reassessed during follow-up, particularly when there has been a significant change in medical therapy, significant somatic growth, or other changes in clinical status. Concomitant antiarrhythmic therapy may be useful in facilitating tachycardia termination or limiting recurrences but also may alter sensing, pacing, or defibrillation thresholds. Stored electrograms should be reviewed promptly following automatic discharge to assess the relative appropriateness of the treatment delivered.

Biventricular Pacing

In recent years, a link between asynchronous electrical depolarization within the ventricles, regional myocardial wall motion abnormalities, and overall ventricular performance increasingly has become recognized. In adult patients with prolonged QRS duration and congestive heart failure, simultaneous pacing of the right and left ventricles to restore synchronous contraction has the potential to improve ventricular performance and lessen symptoms of congestive heart failure (Fig. 14.8). Usually, biventricular pacing is combined with defibrillation capabilities (biventricular ICD), given the potential for sudden death in the congestive heart failure (CHF) population. Typically, when vascular access allows, biventricular pacing is accomplished by pacing a bipolar pacing lead in the right ventricular apex and a second specially designed unipolar lead via the coronary sinus into a lateral coronary vein on the lateral surface of the left ventricle (with a third bipolar lead in the atrium).

Despite anecdotal reports of sometimes remarkable benefits with biventricular pacing in pediatric patients, the overall indications and utility of this modality remain largely undefined in this population. Preliminary data suggest particularly limited benefit among patients with univentricular hearts (14).

In addition to biventricular pacing, the role of ventricular resynchronization has fueled resurgence of interest in pacing from alternate sites, such as the right ventricular (RV) septum or left ventricular (LV) epicardium to achieve similar goals. It is hoped that advances in assessing appropriate indications for biventricular pacing and for optimizing timing parameters to maximize its utility will allow improved application of this new pacing modality.

Ablative or Surgical Procedures

Radiofrequency (RF) catheter ablation was developed in the late 1980s and applied to pediatric patients in the early 1990s. Ablation of accessory AV connections and modification of the AV node quickly proved to be highly effective with a low incidence of associated morbidity. More complex arrhythmias proved amenable to catheter ablation, including idiopathic ventricular tachycardias from the right or left ventricle; Mahaim fibers; the permanent form of junctional reciprocating tachycardias; and even junctional ectopic tachycardias. The detailed mapping and opportunity to immediately test therapy at putative targeted tissues has improved the mechanistic understanding of many complex arrhythmias.

Catheter ablation techniques continue to evolve, allowing application of the technique to increasingly complex arrhythmias. Ablation catheters allowing creation of larger lesions are now available, including those with larger tips. Saline irrigation of catheter tips allows conductive cooling of the catheter tip so that more RF energy can be applied to the tissue. The ability to create large lesions may be particularly important in the ablation of ventricular tachycardias and intra-atrial reentrant tachycardias. Conversely, cryoablation is now available as an alternative to radiofrequency catheter ablation.

In certain situations, smaller or more discrete lesions are desired. Cryoablation offers an advantage for ablation near the normal conduction system because lesions take longer to deliver, allowing the opportunity to recognize development of unwanted effects on normal conduction. Abortion of cryolesions typically allows recovery of conduction, virtually eliminating the complication of inadvertent AV block. This increased safety is somewhat offset by a greater potential for late recurrence of the tachycardia.

Advances in mapping techniques also are responsible for increasing success of ablation for complex atrial and ventricular tachycardias. Various specialized mapping modalities allow true three-dimensional electroanatomic mapping to recreate the activation pattern of a particular arrhythmia in the context of the patient's anatomy. The anatomy is typically created by positioning the mapping catheter along throughout the surface of the chamber of interest. However, importation of high-definition images created by MRI or CT scan should allow a more true representation of anatomic details and characterizing their relationship to the arrhythmia substrate.

As experience accumulates, ablation therapy now is offered earlier as a treatment option for various arrhythmias, often in lieu of any prior medical therapy. The relative indications for ablation versus medical treatments should be individualized for each patient, and ablation recommended only after careful consideration and explanation of the risk/benefit for each mode of treatment. Recommendations should always consider the age and size of the patient, impact of associated cardiac and noncardiac conditions on risk or treatments, and receptiveness of parents and patient to a given therapy.

Certain patients may be candidates for surgical procedures directed at both structural abnormalities and associated arrhythmias. Examples include incorporating the atrial Maze with left-sided AV valve surgery; atrial cryoablation during surgical revision of previous Fontan procedure; right-sided accessory connection division at the time of tricuspid valve surgery in the setting of Ebstein anomaly of the tricuspid valve; or surgical ablation of ventricular tachycardia during RV outflow tract reconstruction in tetralogy of Fallot.

On the other hand, preemptive RF catheter ablation of known arrhythmias should be performed prior to operations for congenital heart disease whenever feasible. Elimination of these pre-existing arrhythmias should decrease the operative and postoperative risk associated with perioperative arrhythmia recurrence. The choice of preoperative RF ablation or intraoperative ablation must be considered carefully, relative to the experience and success rates of each technique at the institution.

BRADYCARDIAS, CONDUCTION ABNORMALITIES, AND PREMATURE BEATS

Abnormalities of impulse propagation and/or inhibitory neural influence in the AV conduction system may result in abnormalities including intra-atrial block, block within the AV node, block within the His, or aberrant ventricular conduction owing to block within one of the specialized intraventricular fascicles. When block occurs within the specialized AV conduction system, depolarization of the affected region of myocardium may occur in an aberrant fashion, a slower subsidiary pacemaker may emerge, or distal structures may fail to depolarize altogether. When aberrant conduction occurs within the ventricles, depolarization spreads through ventricular myocardium less efficiently than through the specialized Purkinje cells, resulting in regional delays in depolarization and a prolonged QRS duration. Aberrant conduction with QRS prolongation also can occur if an abnormal impulse arises distal to the His bundle (such as a ventricular premature depolarization) or if an accessory connection bypasses the normal conduction system as in WPW.

SINUS NODE DYSFUNCTION

Electrocardiographic Features

Any inappropriately slow sinus mechanism for a given clinical situation can be considered sinus node dysfunction. The diagnosis is subjective and requires an evaluation of rate and rhythm over a period of observation. ECG features may include low resting heart rate; low mean heart rate; decreased variability (insensitivity to autonomic input); decreased peak heart rate (chronotropic incompetence); and prolonged sinus pauses, sinus arrest, or sinus node exit block with junctional rhythm may be present. The expressions tachycardia–bradycardia syndrome and sick sinus syndrome typically are used to characterize the frequent association of sinus node dysfunction with atrial tachycardias.

Etiology

Rarely, congenital sinus node dysfunction may be observed in unoperated patients with or without underlying structural heart disease. More commonly sick sinus syndrome develops following operations for congenital heart disease, particularly those involving atrial surgery such as the Mustard, Senning, and Fontan operations and ASD closure. Both direct injury to the sinoatrial (SA) node and intra-atrial conduction abnormalities with intra-atrial block have been shown to underlie the frequent bradycardias in these patients. Fibrosis and hypertrophy, both before and after, likely contribute. Long-term follow-up studies reveal a steady loss of predominant sinus rhythm following these operations.

The increasing prevalence of frequent pauses may contribute to abnormal triggered activity, which, coupled with abnormalities of atrial activation and repolarization, forms the basis for the concomitant appearance of atrial tachycardias. The potential role of damage to local neural inputs has not been completely evaluated, but they likely contribute more to loss of heart rate variability and altered chronotropic response.

Various other causes for transient bradycardia and long sinus pauses are often observed. These include neurocardiogenic syncope, apnea of prematurity, breathholding spells, and sleep apnea. These events are typically episodic, but may be profound and symptomatic. However, when seen in otherwise healthy patients with normal rate, rhythm, and chronotropic response to normal daily stresses and exercise, they are unlikely to be life threatening. A potential role for pacing his been proposed for many such indications (15). However, the response to pacing in alleviating symptoms may vary greatly from patient to patient, such that the potential limitations should be discussed thoroughly before recommending pacing.

Management

Treatment for sinus node dysfunction depends on symptoms, which may include syncope, exercise intolerance, and/or cardiac dysfunction aggravated by loss of AV synchrony, all of which are treated with pacing. Therapy should be directed toward both the tachycardia and bradycardia. To date, the prevention of sudden death has been the most difficult aspect of patient management. ECG documentation during cardiac arrest or sudden death rarely has been accomplished, and prophylactic pacing has not been shown to lessen the risk of sudden death. Nevertheless, atrial rate support may sometimes be a useful adjunct to antiarrhythmic therapy for suppressing tachycardia recurrences and may help maintain AV synchrony, both of which may ultimately improve prognosis. Prophylactic pacemaker implantation for asymptomatic patients with sinus node dysfunction is controversial. Likewise, presyncope or syncope associated with profound sinus pauses often is due to neurally mediated cardioinhibitory syncope rather than sinus node dysfunction and can often be prevented without pacing.

Prognosis

Current pacing systems provide reliable, physiologic, rate-responsive pacing with preservation of AV conduction in virtually all patients. For the survivor of congenital heart disease surgery, the prevention of sudden death remains a challenge, and the extent to which early pacing improves the risk is uncertain, at best. The modes of sudden death among these patients remain poorly characterized, and neither pacing nor antiarrhythmic regimens completely prevent this complication.

ATRIOVENTRICULAR BLOCK

AV block refers to any abnormality in which conduction of sinus or atrial impulses to the ventricle is delayed or interrupted. It may vary in the extent of block as well as in the anatomic level at which block occurs and may represent normal physiologic behavior, a transient functional abnormality, or a fixed anatomic interruption of the normal conduction system (Fig. 14.9). These and other factors affect the clinical significance of the varied manifestations of AV block.

Electrocardiographic Features

AV block can be characterized by the anatomic site of block (atrial, AV nodal, or infranodal), the degree of block (first, second, and third degree), and by the ratio of atrial to ventricular impulses (e.g., 1:1, 2:1, 4:3). The surface ECG provides a convenient way to classify AV block, but there are problems with this approach. For example, first-degree AV block is present when the P-R interval is prolonged. The P-R interval can be subdivided into subintervals relating to conduction through specific areas: P-A interval (sinus node to low septal atrium), A-H interval (low septal atrium to His bundle depolarization), and H-V interval (His bundle depolarization to onset of ventricular depolarization). Thus, first-degree block may be due to delay in any of these regions, yet the site of block or conduction delay may have important implications with regard to prognosis and natural history.

First-degree AV block is defined as prolongation of the P-R interval, according to normative values for age and heart rate. Usually this occurs at the level of the AV node (A-H interval), but it may also occur in the atrium (P-A interval) or in the distal conduction system (H-V interval). Perturbations from

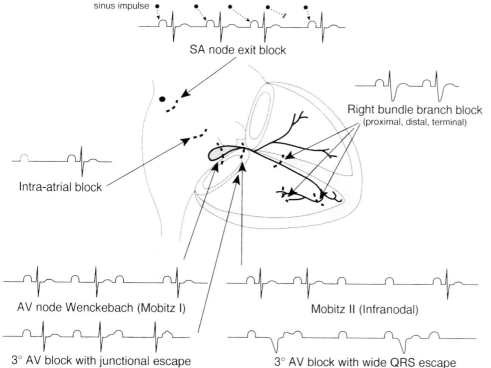

FIGURE 14.9 Diagram of different levels of conduction block. Sinoatrial (SA) node exit block, intra-atrial block, Mobitz I and II atrioventricular block, and three levels of right bundle branch block are illustrated.

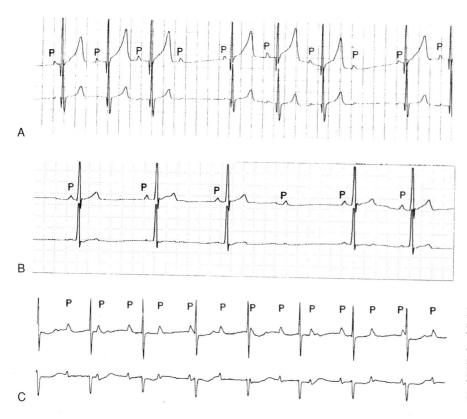

FIGURE 14.10 Rhythm strips during second- and third-degree atrioventricular (AV) block. The top tracing (**A**) shows Wenckebach's periodicity of the P-R interval (Mobitz I). The middle tracing (**B**) shows abrupt conduction loss without P-R interval change (Mobitz II). The bottom tracing (**C**) shows complete AV block.

normal resting conditions such as increased vagal tone, PR-prolonging medications, or a nonsinus atrial rhythm may result in appropriate deviations in the P-R interval from the normal range for age and rate without implying intrinsic conduction system disease.

Second-degree AV block traditionally is characterized as either type I or type II (Fig. 14.10). Type I AV block, also referred to as Wenckebach periodicity, is characterized by progressive P-R prolongation, usually owing to changes in the A-H interval (reflecting AV node delay), with successive cycles prior to a single blocked atrial impulse, and the subsequently conducted atrial impulse is followed by a shortened PR interval. In contrast, type II AV block refers to abrupt failure of AV conduction of one or more atrial impulses without prior PR prolongation. Type II block usually occurs below the AV node (H-V interval block). In addition to the absence of progressive P-R prolongation prior to block, type II block may abruptly progress to third-degree block with an inadequate escape rhythm (16).

During second-degree AV block, multiple atrial impulses may be blocked for each impulse conducted. Conduction may occur in a regular or irregularly recurring pattern. When regular, block can be characterized by the conduction ratio as 2:1, 4:1, and so on. High-grade AV block (3:1 or greater) during sinus rhythm usually involves infranodal block, alone or in combination with AV nodal block. Variation in the R-R interval or regular R-R intervals that are integer multiples of the atrial cycle length distinguish high-grade second-degree block from third-degree AV block.

In third-degree or complete AV block, no atrial impulses conduct to the ventricles. Congenital AV block is usually characterized by a somewhat variable heart rate in response to varying physiologic conditions, whereas in surgical block there may be a relatively fixed ventricular rate. Irregular variation in R-R intervals suggests intermittent AV conduction

and second-degree AV block. Third-degree AV block should not be confused with AV dissociation, which results from a sinus or atrial bradycardia and has a faster, dissociated escape rhythm. In the latter, appropriately timed atrial impulses should conduct to the ventricles, shortening the R-R interval and advancing the escape rhythm. If block occurs within the AV node and the escape rhythm has a normal QRS, intracardiac recording should demonstrate a His bundle potential preceding each ventricular electrogram. Block below the His bundle recording site will result in appropriately related atrial and His depolarizations that are completely dissociated from ventricular depolarizations. Often, the escape rhythm will have a prolonged QRS duration.

Etiology

First- and second-degree AV block may represent a variant of normal in neonates, in adolescents and young adults, and particularly in athletes. In this context, the block is thought to be due to changes in heart rate or autonomic tone. Conduction abnormalities may be a nonspecific finding in various pathologic conditions including congenital heart disease, infectious or inflammatory conditions, or surgical injury to the AV node or His–Purkinje system. High-grade second-degree block at normal sinus rates or sustained third-degree block should always be regarded as abnormal.

The causes of high-grade atrioventricular block are diverse (Table 14.5). AV block has been associated with certain forms of congenital heart disease, particularly AV septal defects and those involving abnormalities in the bulboventricular looping such as l-transposition of the great arteries or left atrial isomerism. In this setting, AV block may occur either as the result of fibrous disruption between the atrium and the AV node or

TABLE 14.5

CONDITIONS ASSOCIATED WITH HIGH-GRADE ATRIOVENTRICULAR BLOCK

Infectious	Viral myocarditis
	Lyme disease
	Chagas disease
	Diptheria
	Typhoid
	Valvular endocarditis
Inflammatory	Rheumatoid arthritis
	Reiter syndrome
	Guillain–Barré syndrome
Neurodegenerative and muscular dystrophies	Myotonic dystrophy
	Emery–Dreyfus muscular dystrophy
	Facioscapulohumeral muscular dystrophy
	Myotonic dystrophy
	Kearns–Sayre syndrome
Infiltrative	Tuberous sclerosis
	Lymphoma
	Amyloidosis
	Sarcoidosis
Trauma	Cardiac surgery
	Blunt chest trauma
	Penetrating chest trauma
	Radiation therapy
Functional	Resting vagal tone (athlete's heart)
	Head trauma, cerebral edema
	Neurally mediated reflex
	Bezold–Jarisch
	Carotid sinus hypersensitivity
Pharmacologic	Tricyclic antidepressants
	Antiarrythmic drugs
	Digoxin
	Clonidine

because of absence of the penetrating bundles of the AV node (17). On the other hand, some patients affected with Holt–Oram syndrome, characterized by deformity of the upper extremity and congenital heart defects and caused by mutations in *TBX5*, a cardiac transcription factor, have associated abnormalities of AV conduction (18,19). Mutations in another cardiac transcription factor, *Nkx2.5*, result in autosomal dominant inheritance of AV node conduction abnormality associated with congenital heart defects (20).

Congenital AV block occurs in association with maternal antibodies in 1/15,000 to 1/20,000 live births. Specific antibodies (Anti-Ro and Anti-La) directed against ribonuclear proteins are transmitted across the placenta, often in the absence of prior maternal symptoms. These antibodies presumably cross-react with fetal cardiac tissue at a critical stage of development, disrupting the normal conduction system. Varying degrees of myocardial dysfunction are occasionally observed in isolated congenital AV block (21). Occasionally, infants with congenital LQTS will present with bradycardia owing to second-degree AV block. In these infants, 2:1 functional AV block occurs as a consequence of prolonged ventricular repolarization, such that every other atrial impulse finds ventricular myocardium or His–Purkinje tissue. It is refractory and unable to propagate to the ventricles (22,23).

Most cases of acquired AV block in children are the result of direct or indirect trauma to the AV nodal or infranodal conduction system at the time of intracardiac surgery. Transient block may represent damage adjacent to the specialized conduction system with edema or hemorrhage resolving within 7 to 8 days postoperatively, although a risk of late recurrence of AV block may persist. AV block persisting beyond 8 days is usually permanent and reflects obliteration of or fibrous infiltration of the conducting tissue.

AV block has been described following surgical treatment of atrial or ventricular septal defects, tetralogy of Fallot, total anomalous pulmonary venous connections to the coronary sinus, mitral valve replacement, relief of ventricular outflow obstruction in hypertrophic cardiomyopathy, single ventricle with a subaortic outflow chamber, or Konno procedure for relief of aortic or subaortic stenosis. Membranous ventricular septum or atrial septum in the regions of Koch's triangle can be involved. Displacement of the AV node and His bundle in endocardial cushion defects and congenitally corrected transposition of the great arteries place the conduction system at particular risk. The incidence of postoperative AV block has been reduced to <5% for most lesions as the predictable anatomic variations in the course of the conduction system are well known. Nevertheless, temporary epicardial pacing wires should be placed during cardiac operations that have a known risk of producing AV block.

A more recent iatrogenic cause of acquired AV block is inadvertent injury to the conduction system during RF ablation. Effects on the conduction system can be monitored closely during RF administration, such that permanent injury can usually be avoided. The risk of AV block is higher in young patients, at centers with decreased procedural experience, and typically occurs during ablation in the septal region of the tricuspid annulus and Koch's triangle for such arrhythmias as AV node re-entry, AV re-entry or WPW using midseptal accessory connections, the permanent form of junctional reciprocating tachycardias, and junctional ectopic tachycardias. Familiarity with specific anatomic variations found in patients with congenital heart disease is essential in minimizing the risk of inadvertent postsurgical AV block.

AV block of varying severity may be an acute or chronic manifestation of other genetically acquired diseases, including muscular dystrophies, myotonic dystrophy, and cardiomyopathy (24,25). Kearns–Sayre syndrome, characterized by progressive external ophthalmoplegia, retinal pigmentation, and severe cardiac conduction abnormality early in life, is due to partial deletions of mitochondrial DNA (mtDNA) (26–28). Genetic causes for isolated AV block have also been described (29,30). Various infectious processes involving the heart may also produce AV block, notably acute rheumatic fever, diphtheria, Rocky Mountain spotted fever, and infection with *Yersinia enterocolitica*. Bacterial endocarditis and viral myocarditis can also produce AV block, including persistent third-degree AV block (31). The potential for recovery of conduction in such patients and the potential for ongoing bacteremia warrant a period of antimicrobial treatment and temporary pacing when necessary, prior to permanent pacing in the latter group. Untreated infection with the spirochete *Borrelia burgdorferi* (Lyme disease) may produce carditis with AV block as a stage II manifestation in ≤8% of patients (32). Nearly half of these patients present with acute, high-grade AV block, which may be the only manifestation of this infection. Block is usually within the AV node and shows a corresponding response to atropine and isoproterenol, despite sometimes dangerously slow escape rhythms. AV conduction usually recovers following antimicrobial therapy.

Management

Effective, immediate treatments of symptomatic complete AV block include infusion of atropine and/or adrenergic agonists or even chest compressions until pacing can be implemented.

Temporary pacing can be accomplished by transcutaneous or transvenous (endocardial) pacing. Transcutaneous pacing may be most useful as a temporary measure until a transvenous catheter is successfully placed for extended pacing. With any temporary pacing modality, pacing thresholds should be evaluated regularly to ensure a safe pacing margin and radiographic confirmation of appropriate lead placement should be regularly repeated as long as pacing is required. Active-fixation (screw-in) temporary pacing leads are now available, but must be positioned under fluoroscopy whereas balloon-tipped (floating) leads can often be positioned at the bedside from an internal jugular or subclavian vein.

The mainstay of management for symptomatic AV block is cardiac pacing. The relative indications for treatment are based on either the presence or absence of symptoms. Guidelines for permanent pacing in pediatric patients were revised in 2002 (Table 14.3) (12). Nevertheless, determining the relative need for chronic pacing is often a more difficult consideration than choosing the most appropriate type of device, once the decision has been made to implant the pacemaker. It can be anticipated that as more is learned about the etiologic factors of AV conduction including genetic causes, the indications will evolve to include more prophylactic use of pacing.

In general, any patient who is symptomatic as the result of AV block should receive permanent pacing. Kearns–Sayre syndrome and persistent postoperative AV block are two situations that pose a sufficient long-term risk to warrant prophylactic pacemaker implantation prior to development of symptoms (24–26). It is also generally accepted that pacemaker implantation should be performed for complete AV block with a wide QRS (i.e., infranodal) escape rhythm.

Prognosis

The two important aspects to consider regarding prognosis are the reversibility of the block and the extent of underlying heart disease. Congenital AV block almost uniformly is irreversible (33). In contrast, acquired AV block associated with myocarditis, with Lyme carditis, and cardiac surgery often is transient. In general, patients with permanent AV block and normal cardiac structure and function have a better prognosis than patients with associated heart disease.

Congenital AV block often is detected first by fetal echocardiography, which also can provide useful details of cardiac anatomy. Fetal magnetocardiograms are also feasible in assessing fetal rhythm, particularly when echo-based rhythm is ambiguous (34). Symptoms can occur prenatally, and *hydrops fetalis* in the presence or absence of structural heart disease requires prompt intervention, if any hope of survival can be expected. On the other hand, the fetus with complete AV block, an adequate escape rate, and no evidence of congestive heart failure usually can be followed to term with serial ultrasound examinations to monitor for signs indicating fetal distress. The prognosis for the fetus with complete AV block, associated structural heart disease, and hydrops fetalis is poor, with a high rate of fetal demise. This increased risk appears even worse when considering total perinatal mortality, which approaches 100%, despite pacing postpartum. Attempts to perform intrauterine pacing have not resulted in fetal salvage.

Postoperative AV block can be characterized as either transient or persistent, with spontaneous recovery of AV conduction occurring in 40% to 56% of patients. Older studies suggested recovery of conduction ≤10 to 14 days postoperatively, but more recent reports indicated recovery of conduction ≥7 to 8 days is uncommon. As more suitable pacing systems for young children are available, earlier implantation in persistent postsurgical AV block is now advocated. With appropriate pacemaker therapy, the long-term prognosis appears good, or at least comparable to patients without postoperative AV block and similar anatomic residua.

Despite the frequent need for temporary pacing owing to inadequate escape rates or even asystole, permanent pacing usually is not required for acute rheumatic fever or Lyme carditis. Antibiotic therapy (ceftriaxone, intravenous penicillin, erythromycin, tetracycline) for 10 to 20 days is recommended, sometimes in combination with salicylates or corticosteroids, both to eradicate symptoms and to prevent stage III (rheumatologic and neurologic) manifestations. However, the effect of anti-inflammatory therapy on the carditis has not been clearly established.

BUNDLE BRANCH BLOCK AND FASCICULAR BLOCK

Electrocardiographic Features

Nearly synchronous depolarization of the left and right ventricles is accomplished by rapid conduction through the specialized ventricular conduction system. As a consequence, ventricular depolarization proceeds rapidly and the QRS complex is of relatively short duration. When activation is delayed or blocked in the conduction system, the QRS duration is prolonged. Common patterns include a large superior terminal deflection in lead V_1 (right bundle branch block) or lead V_6 (left bundle branch block) with QRS prolonged for age (usually >80 to 100 ms). The term incomplete right bundle branch block is used to describe an rSR′ pattern in lead V_1 without QRS prolongation. This term is probably a misnomer since the ECG pattern may be due to variation in the right ventricular free wall thickness rather than a conduction system abnormality.

Etiology

The proximal aspect of the conduction network is the transition from the distal portion of the AV node to the penetrating bundle, distinguished by its encasement in fibrous annulus tissue. The penetrating bundle traverses the AV ring and travels beneath the central fibrous body and between the membranous RV septum and the muscular septum, which it then traverses. Beneath the right coronary and noncoronary leaflets, the penetrating bundle branches into the right bundle and the sheetlike left bundle. The penetrating bundle continues intramyocardially as the right bundle inferiorly to the right ventricular apex and then turns anteriorly and is continuous within the moderator band to the outflow tract (35,36). The left bundle quickly divides into two or three sheetlike fascicles that fan out over the left ventricular subendocardial surface and interconnect distally. The proximal portions supply the muscular septum, which depolarizes left to right and corresponds with the initial electrocardiographic QRS deflection. The right ventricle depolarizes only after subendocardial fibers arise from the right bundle at the apex, and both right and left ventricles depolarize from their subendocardial to epicardial surfaces.

As with AV block, abnormalities in intraventricular conduction may be congenital or acquired. Congenital right bundle branch block may be hereditary or it may occur in association with Ebstein's anomaly of the tricuspid valve. More commonly, right bundle branch block is acquired following cardiac surgery, and may occur in the proximal, distal, or terminal branches of the conduction system (Fig. 14.9).

Several systemic diseases predisposing to acquired AV block can initially manifest bundle branch block (Table 14.4); the potential for abrupt progression to complete AV block in Kearns–Sayre syndrome or myotonic dystrophy must be recognized. Right bundle branch block also frequently is seen following cardiac transplantation, but progression to complete AV block is uncommon. Bundle branch block may also occur as a physiologic response to fast or, less commonly, slow heart rates.

Management

Children with isolated right bundle branch block or even bifascicular block generally do not require invasive evaluation unless symptoms suggesting higher-grade AV block are reported. The occurrence of the latter constitutes a class I pacing indication. Kearns–Sayre syndrome constitutes a class I indication for permanent ventricular pacing to prevent complete AV block and sudden death. Patients with residual bifascicular block following transient postsurgical AV block may not need pacing acutely, but should be followed longitudinally because of an increased risk for late AV block. This constitutes a class II pacing indication (12) (Table 14.3). Patients presenting with syncope or cardiac arrest with right bundle branch block require particularly careful attention, since symptoms may not be the result of transient AV block, but rather, owing to ventricular arrhythmias.

Right bundle branch block in a patient with syncope or cardiac arrest without apparent heart disease may indicate arrhythmogenic right ventricular cardiomyopathy or the Brugada syndrome. Similarly, patients with dilated cardiomyopathy and associated bundle branch block may develop various ventricular tachycardias, including bundle branch re-entry. Each of these situations would generally warrant an implantable defibrillator, and in the case of bundle branch re-entry, adjunctive RF ablation may also be considered.

Prognosis

The prognosis for bifascicular block or right or left bundle branch block depends on the cause. Residual bundle branch block following transient complete postsurgical AV block, myocarditis, or cardiomyopathies may have a risk of progression to late complete AV block. Measurement of the HV interval may be helpful in risk assessment of these patients.

EXTRASYSTOLES

Atrial and ventricular extrasystoles have been described in healthy fetuses, infants, and older children. Most studies suggest that these premature beats are more common among fetuses and decline during infancy and childhood through the first 10 years.

Supraventricular Extrasystoles

Supraventricular premature beats (SVPBs, supraventricular extrasystoles) usually arise from the atria, though junctional extrasystoles are occasionally seen. They may conduct with normal or aberrant QRS, or may block in the AV node, resulting in an apparent pause. When the premature atrial impulse resets the sinus node, the ensuing sinus complex will follow a conducted SVPB by less than a full compensatory pause. However, entrance block may prevent resetting of the sinus node such that the SVPB is instead followed by a full compensatory pause. Frequent, blocked SVPBs may mimic bradycardia, and aberrantly conducted extrasystoles may be difficult to distinguish from VPBs, particularly junctional extrasystoles.

In neonates, atrial extrasystoles may be quite frequent, yet tend to decline within the first few weeks of age and usually do not predispose to symptomatic arrhythmias. Atrial bigeminy with associated block is an occasional but benign cause of neonatal bradycardia. Therapy is indicated only in the occasional neonate in whom atrial extrasystoles serve as initiating events for recurrent episodes of supraventricular tachycardia. In older children, frequent SVPBs may herald the development of sinus node dysfunction, particularly following surgery for congenital heart disease or in association with cardiomyopathies. Even in these situations, treatment of SVPBs is not warranted.

Ventricular Extrasystoles

Ventricular extrasystoles (VPBs) are characterized by an aberrant and premature QRS that is not preceded by an atrial depolarization. In young patients, the QRS duration may be only modestly prolonged since QRS duration is age dependent. Though typically followed by a full compensatory pause, VPBs conducting in a retrograde manner over the AV node may reset the sinus node and be followed by a less than full compensatory pause in a manner similar to atrial extrasystoles. Regularly recurring VPBs alternating with every two or three sinus beats are referred to as ventricular bigeminy or trigeminy. They may not affect the underlying rhythm (interpolated VPBs), or may be only slightly premature so that the extrasystole merges with a normally conducted impulse. The resulting fusion complexes are intermediate between the normal and aberrant QRS morphology, and are usually preceded by a P wave with a shortened P-R interval. Fusion complexes owing to late VPBs should be differentiated from those owing to intermittent pre-excitation. A pair of VPBs often is referred to as a couplet, whereas three or more consecutive VPBs define nonsustained ventricular tachycardia. When coupling intervals vary in their relationship to sinus impulses, but are related to each other by a fixed interval between ectopic beats, ventricular *parasystole* may be diagnosed.

Ventricular extrasystoles commonly are regarded as markers for significant underlying heart disease, and patient evaluation is usually directed to this question. However, their incidence at certain ages may be sufficiently frequent to be considered a variation of normal rhythm (37). Like atrial extrasystoles, isolated VPBs can occur in otherwise healthy neonates, after which the incidence falls off rapidly until adolescence.

In adolescents, isolated VPBs become even more commonplace and usually display characteristic features. These so-called benign VPBs of adolescence usually have left bundle branch block QRS morphology with inferior axis, indicating an origin in the right ventricular outflow tract. They typically predominate at slow heart rates, are often suppressed with exercise, and only occasionally occur in pairs or three to four brief salvos at relatively slow rates. Although often a source of considerable angst, isolated VPBs and even nonsustained VT in an otherwise asymptomatic individual without underlying heart disease have a generally benign course (38). However, the likelihood of associated heart disease increases with frequent and more complex arrhythmias (39,40). In certain conditions, including hypertrophic and dilated cardiomyopathies, nonsustained ventricular tachycardia imparts an increased risk of sudden death (41,42). The significance of ventricular arrhythmias among survivors of congenital heart disease surgery remains to be determined, but programmed electrical stimulation may help delineate the prognosis and risk of future events (43).

At present, there is no indication for treating asymptomatic patients with isolated VPBs. Indeed, this practice may be hazardous owing to the potential for proarrhythmia, even when the presence of frequent VPBs suggests an increased risk of sudden death (44). In symptomatic patients, the cause of the symptoms should be defined, and then management should be directed toward the prevention of symptoms. Asymptomatic patients with underlying heart disease require management on an individual basis. In most cases, the prognosis of SVPBs is excellent, whereas the prognosis of VPBs largely depends on the underlying heart disease.

ATRIOVENTRICULAR NODAL RE-ENTRY, ATRIOVENTRICULAR TACHYCARDIAS, AND PRE-EXCITATION SYNDROMES

Atrioventricular Re-entrant Tachycardias

The tachycardias collectively referred to as supraventricular tachycardia (SVT) and paroxysmal atrial tachycardia (PAT) represent the most common tachycardias encountered in pediatric patients. The characteristic features include abrupt onset and termination, fixed cycle length, normal QRS complexes, and usually an absence of clearly discernible P waves or flutter waves. The terms SVT and PAT are imprecise, and diverse electrophysiologic mechanisms may produce this phenotype.

In pediatric patients, two tachycardia mechanisms, atrioventricular re-entry tachycardia (AVRT) and AV nodal re-entry tachycardia (AVNRT), predominate in an age-dependent manner (45). Despite fundamental differences in substrate, both are reciprocating tachycardias in that they use two functionally and anatomically discrete antegrade and retrograde limbs in the re-entry circuit. Even among these two mechanisms, electrocardiographically distinct variants occur. As they share a number of clinical, electrocardiographic, and therapeutic similarities, they will be discussed together in this section. For clarity, SVT will be used to refer to these tachycardias collectively, whereas AVRT or AVNRT will refer to each individually. Other forms of supraventricular tachycardias, including various primary atrial tachycardias and junctional ectopic tachycardias, will be discussed separately.

Electrocardiographic Features

Both AVRT and AVNRT most commonly manifest as regular tachycardias with normal QRS duration. When P waves are evident, they typically follow the QRS and there is usually a 1:1 AV relationship with a regular rate, although beat-to-beat oscillation in the cycle length may occur. Variations in AV and VA conduction may occur in AVNRT; 2:1 AV block occasionally is observed, and intermittent retrograde block or VA dissociation occur rarely during ongoing AVNRT. However, they more typically display a 1:1 AV relationship, allowing these tachycardias to be distinguished from other tachycardia mechanisms such as primary atrial tachycardias, junctional ectopic tachycardia, and ventricular tachycardias, all of which may at times manifest a variable AV relationship. It is important to note that any tachycardia mechanism may have a 1:1 AV relationship depending on antegrade or retrograde conduction properties, but only the various forms of AVRT and AVNRT tend to terminate when this relationship is interrupted.

Depending on the particulars of antegrade and retrograde conduction in the re-entry circuit, AVNRT and AVRT may display both typical and atypical electrophysiologic patterns as displayed on the surface ECG. These tachycardias usually occur episodically and abruptly (paroxysmal) since they are initiated by a specific event such as a premature extrasystole or a junctional escape complex following a sinus pause to initiate the re-entry. Less commonly, sinus acceleration may serve as the initiating event in infants with AVRT and in the permanent form of junctional reciprocating tachycardia (PJRT), an incessant variant of AVRT. PJRT usually perpetuates continuously with only brief interruptions that often last for no more than a few sinus beats. Other forms of AV re-entry may behave incessantly, particularly in response to adrenergic stimulation or certain antiarrhythmic medications. The ECG pattern of a normal P-R interval (long R-P interval) and inverted P waves in the inferior ECG leads (II, III, aVF) is characteristic of both PJRT and atypical AVNRT, which is electrocardiographically identical to PJRT but usually more paroxysmal in occurrence (Fig. 14.11).

Usually, QRS duration is normal (Fig. 14.12), but a wide QRS may occur in some situations (Fig. 14.13). QRS prolongation owing to transient, rate-related bundle branch block occurs commonly with AVRT, particularly in the presence of antiarrhythmic medications that slow intraventricular conduction. Marked QRS prolongation can also occur in pre-excitation syndromes when the tachycardia uses the accessory connection as the antegrade rather than retrograde limb of the circuit, resulting in pre-excited or antidromic tachycardia. Other pre-excited tachycardias are discussed below. Patients

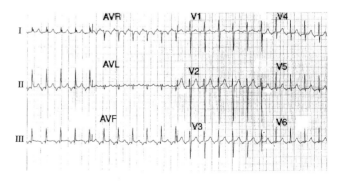

FIGURE 14.11 Electrocardiogram during the permanent form of junctional reciprocating tachycardia. The characteristic inverted P-wave axis in inferior leads indicates retrograde conduction with a long RP interval. Radiofrequency catheter ablation adjacent to the coronary sinus successfully eliminated the tachycardia.

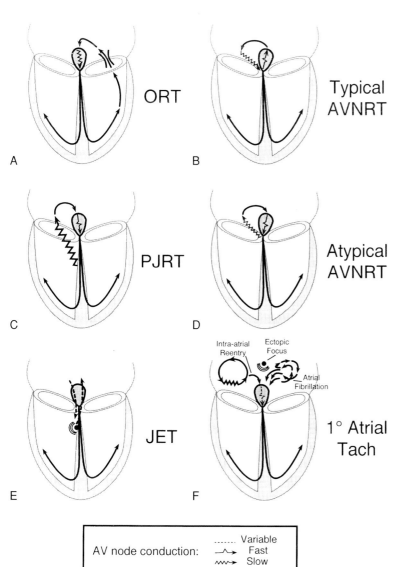

FIGURE 14.12 Diagrammatic representation of tachycardias with normal QRS. **A:** Orthodromic reciprocating tachycardia (ORT). **B:** Typical atrioventricular nodal re-entry tachycardia (AVNRT). **C:** Permanent form of junctional reciprocating tachycardia (PJRT). **D:** Atypical AVNRT. **E:** Junctional ectopic tachycardia (JET). **F:** Primary atrial tachycardias owing to re-entrant, automatic, or possibly triggered mechanisms.

with underlying conduction system disease will also manifest QRS prolongation during tachycardia.

Etiology

As the names suggest, the AV node is an important part of the re-entrant circuit. These tachycardias are subdivided into those where the re-entry involves the peri-AV nodal region (AVNRT) and those using an accessory AV connection (AVRT). AVRT uses an accessory connection and represents one of the best-understood paradigms for re-entrant tachycardias. The accessory connection can functionally link atrial tissue and ventricular tissue at virtually any site along either AV valve ring except where the mitral and aortic valves are in fibrous continuity. These connections may lie in a subendocardial, endocardial, or epicardial location, and may vary considerably in their ability to conduct in either antegrade or retrograde directions.

AVRT can be subdivided further according to the direction of conduction in the accessory AV connection during tachycardia. In the most common situation, orthodromic reciprocating tachycardia, the accessory connection serves as the retrograde limb of tachycardia with antegrade conduction over the AV node. Antegrade conduction (pre-excitation) over the accessory connection during sinus rhythm is characteristic of patients with the Wolff–Parkinson–White (WPW) syndrome, but many accessory connections conduct exclusively retrogradely and thus do not exhibit pre-excitation during sinus rhythm. Orthodromic reciprocating tachycardia results in a normal QRS unless rate-related bundle branch block is present. Less commonly, the accessory connection serves as the antegrade limb with the AV node or a second accessory connection serving as the retrograde limb. This antidromic reciprocating tachycardia is maximally pre-excited with prolonged QRS duration (Fig. 14.13) and may be electrocardiographically indistinguishable from ventricular tachycardia surface ECG. Two other distinct forms of AVRT exist, each using a slowly conducting accessory connection with decremental (AV node–like) conduction properties. PJRT, the incessant form of AVRT, uses retrograde conduction over a slowly conducting accessory connection that usually inserts into the atrial septum. Most tachycardias attributed to Mahaim fibers (see below) represent a variant of antidromic reciprocating tachycardia in which the accessory connection, referred to as an

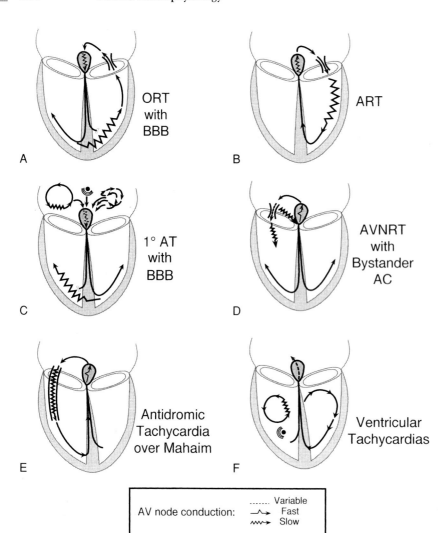

FIGURE 14.13 Diagrammatic representation of tachycardias with prolonged (wide) QRS. Such tachycardias may be due to (A) orthodromic reciprocating tachycardia (ORT) with bundle branch block (BBB), (B) antidromic tachycardia using an accessory AV connection (ART), (C) primary atrial tachycardia with BBB, (D) atrioventricular nodal reentry tachycardia (AVNRT) with a bystander accessory connection (AC), (E) tachycardia using a Mahaim fiber, or (F) ventricular tachycardia. Despite the diversity of mechanisms, ventricular tachycardia should be assumed until or unless additional data to the contrary are available.

atriofascicular connection, originates from the right atrial free wall and inserts into the right ventricular His–Purkinje system (atriofascicular connection or tract). This produces a characteristically prolonged QRS with RBBB pattern on ECG during tachycardia.

In AVNRT, antegrade and retrograde conduction occurs over two functionally and anatomically discrete regions of atrial inputs that display differential conduction properties. Classically, the "slow" connection refers to posterior and inferior inputs into the AV node and is characterized by slow conduction and a short refractory period. The "fast" pathway usually represents anterior and superior inputs that propagate conduction more rapidly but block at longer coupling intervals because of a longer refractory period. This situation permits the development of unidirectional block (usually in the fast limb) with conduction propagating over the other (slow) limb with sufficient delay to allow subsequent recovery in the fast limb and resultant re-entry.

Two distinct types of AVNRT are also described. In the common typical AV node re-entry, the fast pathway serves as the retrograde limb and the slow pathway serves as the antegrade limb. Because of the very rapid retrograde conduction to the atrium over the fast pathway, local atrial activation occurs almost immediately after the onset of ventricular activation, and the surface P wave is usually obscured in the QRS.

This corresponds to a short V-A interval (<70 ms) during intracardiac or transesophageal recordings. Less commonly, the slow pathway conducts retrograde with a long V-A interval, and antegrade conduction over the fast pathway results in a short P-R interval during atypical AV node re-entry. This tachycardia has electrocardiographic features similar to PJRT.

Considerable controversy previously surrounded the notion of functionally versus anatomically separate AV node pathways and whether a portion of atrial tissue is required to complete the proximal circuit between two anatomically separate pathways during AVNRT. Results of radiofrequency ablation have provided compelling evidence that selective ablation of either the fast or slow pathway eliminates tachycardia while preserving antegrade AV node conduction (46). Typically, the fast pathway is located in the anteroseptal right AV ring in the region of an otherwise normal AV node. The slow pathway typically is found posterior to the compact AV node in the posteroseptal to midseptal region of the tricuspid annulus. These pathways likely represent functionally and regionally distinct inputs with differential conduction into the AV node rather than anatomically distinct tracts in the manner of an accessory pathway. Nonetheless, the areas necessary to successfully target this arrhythmia with ablation are often quite local, and distinct electrogram characteristics can sometimes be identified on local recordings at these sites.

Management

Management strategies are dictated by the clinical setting, including the age of the patient, the severity and duration of symptoms, the duration of tachycardia, the presence of underlying heart disease, and prior diagnostic information. In general, management can be divided into two strategies: termination of established tachycardia and prevention of recurrences.

In patients with established tachycardia and severe symptoms, DC cardioversion should be performed. In hemodynamically stable patients, the participation of the AV node can be used for both diagnostic and therapeutic benefit. Transient block in the AV node with vagal maneuvers or adenosine will consistently result in prompt termination of both AVRT and AVNRT. Failure to terminate tachycardia suggests that either the AV node is not integral to the tachycardia circuit, or the maneuver was ineffective in producing AV block. Failure to terminate also must be differentiated from termination followed by immediate reinitiation. If repeated reinitiation results, options include transesophageal pacing for termination and intravenous procainamide, esmolol, verapamil (beyond infancy), or amiodarone to help suppress acute reinitiation until maintenance treatment can be established.

Following termination of an acute episode of tachycardia, an ECG should be obtained in sinus rhythm to assess for ventricular pre-excitation, other conduction abnormalities, or clues to underlying heart disease. Although the role of echocardiography in defining structural or functional heart disease has not been agreed on, occult abnormalities such as nonobstructive hypertrophic cardiomyopathy, tachycardia-induced myopathy, Ebstein's anomaly, or myocardial tumors may have important prognostic and therapeutic implications. In contrast, the utility of laboratory studies sometimes recommended such as thyroid function, serum electrolytes, and possibly bacterial cultures, is usually limited for AVRT or AVNRT.

The decision of whether or not to initiate therapy following a single episode of SVT rests on several factors, including patient age, severity of symptoms, propensity for spontaneous termination, and presence of other cardiac or noncardiac diseases. Socioeconomic, parental, and geographic issues impacting on the prompt recognition of recurrences and access to prompt medical treatment must also be considered. The decision to begin medical treatment must take into account the need for daily treatment to prevent an unpredictable pattern of recurrence, a scenario that may be unacceptable to some patients, particularly adolescents and teenagers. In these older patients, catheter ablation represents a viable, generally safe, and effective alternative to long-term medical therapy. However, the decision to offer ablation as an alternative to initial medical therapy requires carefully individualized consideration and involvement of the family and patient in the decision-making process. In many cases, it may be preferable to initiate short-term medical therapy until the patient and family are ready to discuss ablation therapy.

In the absence of pre-excitation, medical therapy usually can be initiated without regard to the underlying mechanism (i.e., AVRT vs. AVNRT). This is usually accomplished with beta-blocking agents or verapamil (in patients beyond infancy). Digoxin, although still commonly used, is less effective. In the presence of pre-excitation, both verapamil and digoxin are contraindicated.

In older patients, treatment efficacy may be regarded as the elimination of symptomatic recurrences. However, in young patients, prolonged observation may be necessary to ensure efficacy. Infants undergoing frequent, repeated recurrences over short periods of time can usually be monitored for suppression of SVT as a measure of efficacy. However, the simple suppression of triggering events may underestimate the overall potential for later recurrences. Transesophageal pacing can, therefore, be used as an alternative means of evaluating treatment. Complete elimination of inducible tachycardia may be an overly stringent end point of therapy, but adequate therapy may render tachycardia less easily inducible or more likely to terminate spontaneously following initiation. In addition to thoughtful selection and evaluation of therapy, careful parental education is essential to ensure prompt recognition of tachycardia following discharge in infants and younger children who have been diagnosed with SVT.

Virtually all other antiarrhythmic classes (with the exception of class IB antiarrhythmics such as phenytoin and mexiletine) have been used successfully as treatment for both AVNRT and AVRT. Class IC medications such as flecainide and propafenone appear to be highly effective for both AVNRT and AVRT, whereas class IA drugs such as quinidine or disopyramide are less useful for AVNRT and may even potentiate tachycardia because of anticholinergic effects. PJRT, because of its incessant nature and the relative properties of antegrade and retrograde conduction, may be particularly refractory to pharmacologic therapy. Tachycardias refractory to other drugs may be suppressed adequately with sotalol, amiodarone, or drug combinations. However, such combinations are now generally reserved only for very young patients in whom RF ablation may carry a higher risk of complications.

Prognosis

The long-term outcomes of AVRT and AVNRT are dependent primarily on the age of presentation and presence or absence of associated structural heart disease. The most concerning risks are confined to hemodynamic instability in the face of serious structural heart disease, cardiovascular collapse in infants with unrecognized tachycardia of many hours duration, and the risks inherent to atrial fibrillation associated with pre-excitation, which will be discussed in the following section.

Tachycardia presenting in the fetus or early infancy is most commonly due to an accessory connection. Symptoms may be severe and most likely are related to tachycardia duration. However, following initial diagnosis, the prognosis of infants is particularly good, with tachycardia recurrences abating by 6 to 12 months of age in 60% to 90% of infants, regardless of the severity or frequency of initial symptoms. This abatement may be due to age-related changes in the conduction over the accessory connection or the AV node, or it may be due to changes in initiating events.

Spontaneous regression of accessory connection function has been demonstrated in at least one third of infants undergoing serial transesophageal electrophysiology study between the time of initial diagnosis and follow-up evaluation at a mean age of 12 months (8). A second large group of patients in whom conduction over the accessory connection persists nevertheless have shown dramatic cessation of tachycardia recurrences during their early childhood years. Although most of these patients likely will experience tachycardia by adolescence, symptomfree intervals of several years' duration are likely, allowing successful discontinuation of therapy in most. A comparatively small proportion of patients have ongoing recurrences during and beyond the first year despite ongoing therapy. This group often proves difficult to control medically and may benefit from ablation during early childhood. However, aggressive short-term antiarrhythmic strategies including combination regimens should be exhausted before resorting to ablation in infancy.

A relatively large group of patients presents with their first apparent episodes in later childhood or adolescence. Despite the relatively frequent phenomenon of accessory connection regression in infants diagnosed with AVRT, the same phenomenon does not appear to hold in patients experiencing tachycardia beyond infancy. Most of these patients will experience tachycardia recurrences of varying frequency throughout their lifetime such that eventual curative treatment is usually sought. However, most can be controlled successfully with acceptable medical regimens with low risk.

Syncope can occur in association with supraventricular tachycardia and may warrant more aggressive evaluation and treatment. At least three possibilities can account for this symptom. In the presence of pre-excitation, syncope may occur as a consequence of rapid conduction during atrial fibrillation and represent a hazardous situation. Indeed, rapid antegrade accessory connection conduction was demonstrated in one series of young patients with WPW experiencing syncope (47). However, the second possibility of an exaggerated drop in blood pressure during tachycardia onset has also been demonstrated in patients with SVT owing to WPW who experience syncope with no relation to accessory connection conduction characteristics (48). Finally, the high prevalence of simple neurocardiogenic syncope in the adolescent population makes a chance association inevitable in a proportion of patients who are also susceptible to SVT. Although it may be difficult to substantiate a causative relationship between WPW and syncope in many cases, ablation increasingly is being recommended in this setting. The potential for ongoing susceptibility to neurocardiogenic syncope despite successful ablation should be acknowledged beforehand to limit anxiety in the event of subsequent symptoms.

Pre-excitation Syndromes

The pre-excitation syndromes represent a group of electrocardiographic and electrophysiologic abnormalities in which atrial impulses are conducted partly or completely prematurely to the ventricles via a mechanism other than the normal AV node. Collectively, they are associated with a wide array of tachycardias with both normal QRS and prolonged QRS duration.

The nomenclature for pre-excitation syndromes in many cases predated characterization of the electroanatomic bases for these disorders (49). The European Study Group for Pre-excitation suggested the term tract be used to describe accessory conduction tissue that inserts into the specialized conduction and the term connection for accessory conduction inserting into myocardium. There have been several classification schemes for the various pre-excitation syndromes. Historically, the goal has been to relate functional disturbances (electrophysiology) with cardiac morphologic abnormalities. Our discussion will focus on the most common situations where both morphologic and functional features have been defined (Fig. 14.14).

Wolff–Parkinson–White Syndrome

Wolff–Parkinson–White syndrome (WPW) is the most commonly form of cardiac pre-excitation syndrome. Although most commonly seen in structurally normal hearts, there is an

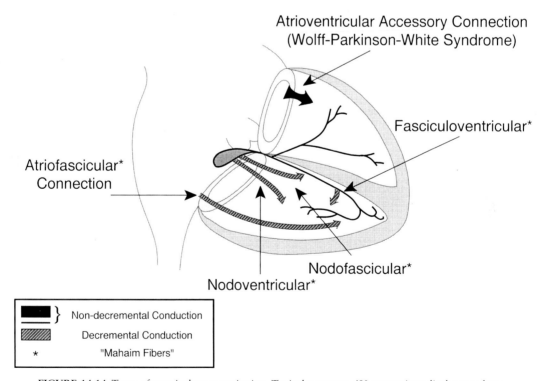

FIGURE 14.14 Types of ventricular pre-excitation. Typical accessory AV connections display nondecremental (all-or-none) conduction. Various patterns of pre-excitation with decremental antegrade conduction have been included under the designation Mahaim fibers. Catheter and surgical ablation results have indicated atriofascicular connections.

increased prevalence among patients with congenital heart disease, hypertrophic cardiomyopathy, and cardiac rhabdomyomas (50). The overall prevalence of WPW is estimated at 0.1% to 0.3% among the general population, although the incidence of newly diagnosed cases reported by Munger et al. (51) was only 4 per 100,000 patient-years, varying considerably with age. The prevalence is slightly higher among patients with congenital heart disease (0.27% to 0.86%). Among the variety of associated lesions, Ebstein's anomaly predominates, representing between 10% and 29% of pediatric patients with congenital heart disease and WPW syndrome (52). Estimates of multiple accessory AV connections have varied in structurally normal hearts, but probably occur in 10% to 15% of cases. The prevalence of multiple accessory connections is increased in the presence of congenital heart disease, particularly Ebstein's anomaly where abnormal development of the valve annulus is fundamental to both the electrical and anatomic anomalies.

Most cases of WPW appear to be sporadic, but about 3% of probands have an affected first-degree relative. An autosomal dominant mode of transmission has been described in familial WPW-associated hypertrophic cardiomyopathy and AV block owing to a defect in PRKAG2, the gamma-2–regulatory subunit of AMP-activated protein kinase (53). Although several candidate genes have been proposed, a genetic basis for WPW in the absence of structural heart disease has remained elusive.

In WPW, fusion of early anomalous depolarization via an accessory AV connection with simultaneous depolarization over the AV node results in the shortened P-R interval, QRS prolongation, and characteristic early slurring in the QRS complex referred to as a delta wave. The accessory connection also may serve as one limb of a re-entrant circuit during tachycardia. The association of the electrocardiographic abnormality with a muscular connection traversing the AV groove was first described in the 1940s. Over 20 years later, Burchell demonstrated that the site of earliest ventricular depolarization during sinus rhythm was just across the AV ring from the earliest site of atrial depolarization during tachycardia in a patient undergoing surgery for atrial septal defect. The report of the first surgical division of an accessory AV connection followed in 1968 (49). These observations have been confirmed and expanded by countless additional morphologic, surgical, and electrophysiologic studies.

Several lines of reasoning suggest that defects in the fibrous annulus may occur during normal cardiac development as the atria and ventricles become electrically isolated and the normal conduction system develops (54). Although these connections normally regress during development, their persistence may provide the basis for some forms of pre-excitation. Not only are accessory AV connections more common early in development, but their increased occurrence in certain congenital cardiac lesions such as Ebstein's anomaly and congenitally corrected transposition of the great arteries reinforces the developmental basis for this disorder. Furthermore, these connections may be derived from either normal ventricular myocardium or from specialized conduction tissue, possibly contributing to some of the variations described for accessory connection location (right vs. left, subendocardial vs. epicardial) or function (bidirectional vs. unidirectional conduction, decremental vs. nondecremental conduction).

As previously noted, WPW may be associated with both orthodromic and, less commonly, antidromic reciprocating tachycardias (Figs. 14.12 and 14.13). Arrhythmias not directly attributable to the accessory connection, including atrial flutter, atrial fibrillation, and AVNRT, also are common in patients with WPW and may greatly impact the clinical course and prognosis (55). Loss of pre-excitation in some infants indicates complete loss of accessory connection function, whereas in others tachycardia recurs later in childhood (8,56). The long-term outcome of patients with accessory connections beyond childhood is variable. Klein et al. (57) found that 9% of asymptomatic adults with WPW lost evidence of pre-excitation during a 36- to 79-month follow-up. However, it is also clear that when symptomatic WPW persists beyond infancy, many individuals will experience recurrent tachycardia (56).

A few patients with WPW experience life-threatening events such as cardiac arrest and sudden death. These potentially lethal events usually are attributed to a rapid ventricular response over the accessory connection during atrial fibrillation. The mechanism for the association of atrial fibrillation with orthodromic reciprocating tachycardia has been well described (58). Digoxin, and possibly verapamil, may further potentiate this phenomenon in patients with pre-excitation by enhancing antegrade conduction over the accessory connection (59).

The exact incidence of sudden death among patients with WPW is uncertain but has been estimated at approximately 1 to 2 per 1,000 patient-years (51). Although electrophysiologic study (EPS)–derived criteria may help identify a subgroup at increased risk, prospective EPS (and intervention) to prevent sudden death remains controversial in asymptomatic patients. It has been presumed that sudden death occurs less commonly among children with WPW, owing to decreased frequency of atrial fibrillation in the young. However, sudden death has been well documented among otherwise healthy young patients with WPW, including infants (60). A recent study prospectively evaluated young patients with asymptomatic WPW undergoing risk stratification for sudden death (61). A small subgroup of 27 at-risk patients was followed conservatively for a median of 19 months, and 3 of these patients suffered ventricular fibrillation, cardiac arrest, or sudden death.

The cumulative risk over time must be considered against the otherwise expected longevity of these young patients with WPW. Although recent guidelines reserve EPS for selected asymptomatic patients at particular risk owing to vocation or sports participation, the option of pursuing such evaluation is left open in any patient for whom the potential of sudden death risk is unacceptable (62). It may be helpful to consider in such patients that the procedural risk of fatal complications during RF ablation is estimated to be between 0.2% and 0.02%. In contrast, the approximately 20% of patients with the potential for rapid accessory connection conduction may have an annual risk of 1 in 200 patient-years, or a cumulative risk of 5% over a period of 10 years. Given the low risk of EPS, and the availability of a low-risk and effective intervention, a proactive approach to asymptomatic WPW in childhood warrants consideration.

NODOVENTRICULAR, NODOFASCICULAR, FASCICULOVENTRICULAR, AND ATRIOFASCICULAR CONNECTIONS

Nodofascicular, nodoventricular, fasciculoventricular, and atriofascicular connections are collectively referred to as Mahaim fibers. Mahaim described connections between the His bundle and the interventricular septum in 1938, although a correlation of electrophysiologic and anatomic findings has been described in only a single patient with a Mahaim fiber. Although often seen in the absence of structural heart disease, there is an association with Ebstein's anomaly (52).

Subsequent electrophysiologic characterization of Mahaim fibers led to the conclusion that these fibers arose from either the distal aspect of the AV node or infranodally from the His bundle and inserted into the right ventricular myocardium (nodoventricular fiber) or right ventricular Purkinje network (nodofascicular fiber). This characterization has been extended by subsequent epicardial mapping studies and experience with radiofrequency catheter ablation (55). Most pre-excited tachycardias fulfilling the electrophysiologic features of Mahaim fibers do not originate from classic nodoventricular or nodofascicular connections. Instead, atriofascicular connections, typically located along the lateral aspect of the tricuspid ring, appear to predominate. These connections have antegrade conduction properties similar to the AV node and connect into the right ventricular Purkinje network. Careful mapping typically reveals an electrogram similar to a typical His bundle potential on the free wall of the tricuspid annulus, and successful ablation can be accomplished at the site of this electrogram recording. The concept of an accessory AV node has been proposed, and indeed, ablation of such connections typically produces a transient pre-excited rhythm analogous to accelerated junctional rhythm during RF ablation of the AV node. Classic nodoventricular and nodofascicular fibers still are occasionally identified, but appear to be quite uncommon relative to atriofascicular fibers.

In most patients with Mahaim fibers, the ECG appears normal during sinus rhythm, or may reveal very subtle suggestion of a small delta wave. However, with increasing atrial rates (particularly with right atrial pacing), delay over the AV node allows preferential conduction to occur over the accessory connection. The resulting P-R prolongation and the appearance of a prolonged QRS with a left bundle branch block and left-axis deviation morphology are most readily demonstrated by pacing from the lateral right atrial wall close to the tricuspid annulus and thus close to the atrial insertion of the connection. Retrograde conduction over the atriofascicular connection can sometimes also be demonstrated. However, tachycardia uses the atriofascicular connection as the antegrade limb and the AV node (or a second accessory connection) as the retrograde limb. Thus, this tachycardia represents a variant of antidromic AV re-entry and could be considered the antidromic counterpart to permanent junctional reciprocating tachycardia (PJRT).

Fasciculoventricular connections have been less commonly observed. They are thought to arise from the His bundle or bundle branches. Since they arise below the level of the AV node, the extent of pre-excitation remains relatively fixed at all rates. They usually are associated with enhanced AV node conduction, and specific tachycardias owing to the existence of these fibers appear to be rare or nonexistent. Occasionally, fascicular ventricular fibers coexist with other tachycardia substrates, in which case a mildly pre-excited tachycardia with QRS morphology identical to sinus is expected. Ablation is directed at the underlying tachycardia substrate, and specific mapping and ablation of the fascicular connection is not warranted.

OTHER SUPRAVENTRICULAR TACHYCARDIAS

This large group of tachycardias affects relatively few patients and accounts for only 14% of supraventricular tachycardias in pediatric patients without other heart disease (45). Among pediatric patients with associated heart disease, tachycardias in this group are common. In contrast to AV reciprocating and AV node re-entrant tachycardias, which with rare exceptions occur with a 1:1 AV relationship, tachycardias discussed in this section are often identified by the lack of interdependence of the atria and ventricles for the continuation of tachycardia. Although these tachycardias may at times manifest the ECG features ascribed to PSVT or PAT, it is important that they be distinguished from the AV reciprocating tachycardias (AVNRT and AVRT) for both acute and long-term management.

ATRIAL FLUTTER AND INTRA-ATRIAL RE-ENTRY

Electrocardiographic Features

Atrial flutter, atrial fibrillation, and intra-atrial re-entry share many clinical and electrocardiographic features, making their distinction sometimes obscure and somewhat arbitrary. Furthermore, spontaneous transitions between these rhythms are common. For example, the observation that an organized and regular atrial flutter may degenerate to a more irregular fibrillation has led to the hybrid term atrial fib-flutter. In this and the following sections we will make specific distinctions between atrial flutter and atrial fibrillation.

Atrial flutter specifically refers to a regular, rapid atrial tachycardia with visible saw-toothed flutter waves that are usually best appreciated in certain leads (typically II, III, and aVF). During atrial flutter, AV block is usually present and regular RR intervals are usually integer multiples of the atrial cycle length. However, continually varying R-R intervals may occur, and the resulting variations in RR may lead to an erroneous diagnosis of atrial fibrillation. This is especially likely when viewing only a single-lead ECG. As with all tachycardias, multiple ECG leads should be examined to correctly ascertain the atrial rhythm. See Figure 14.15 for different patterns of intra-atrial re-entrant tachycardia (IART).

The distinction between atrial flutter and IART can be even less clear (63). In atrial flutter, the atrial rate is typically 240 to 360 beats per minute (bpm), and there is typically continuous atrial activation on the surface ECG. In IART, the tendency is for a slower atrial rate, and usually a clear isoelectric segment separates discrete P waves, which may assume various morphologies, depending on the pattern of atrial activation. Furthermore, the slower atrial rate and generally robust AV node conduction seen in many congenital heart disease (CHD) patients often favors 1:1 AV conduction, and depending on the P wave morphology, may closely resemble sinus tachycardia.

The term IART is reserved for patients who have undergone previous cardiac surgery for congenital or acquired heart disease. However, the electrophysiologic substrates of atrial flutter and IART have many similarities, and a significant proportion of atrial tachycardia in repaired congenital heart disease could be characterized as bona fide atrial flutter. Thus, clinically, the distinction may at times seem more semantic than substantive. To further confuse the issue, two forms of atrial flutter are usually described. Typical, common, or type I atrial flutter has saw-tooth flutter waves with an inverted P-wave axis in the inferior frontal leads. In patients without structural heart disease, this electrocardiographic appearance correlates with a very reproducible re-entry circuit as described below. Atypical, uncommon, or type II atrial flutter usually refers to a similar arrhythmia with less dramatic saw-toothed appearance and with an upright P-wave axis in the

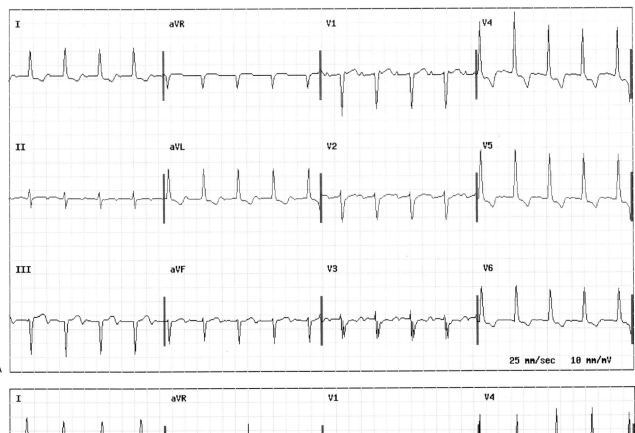

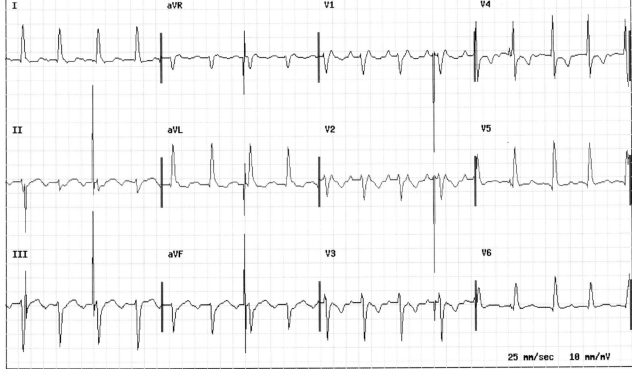

FIGURE 14.15 Various electrocardiographic patterns associated with IART. **A:** Slow intra-atrial re-entry tachycardia (IART) with 1:1 conduction in adult post-Fontan. **B;** 2:1 AV conduction in a different adult post-Fontan (second P wave obscured by QRS). **C:** ECG simulating typical (type I) atrial flutter in adult post-Senning. Although the so-called flutter isthmus was used by this circuit, successful radiofrequency (RF) ablation required ablation in pulmonary venous atrium (accessed via retrograde approach from aorta and right ventricle). **D:** IART in a different adult post-Senning that was initially misdiagnosed with atrial fibrillation owing to the highly irregular ventricular response; hemodynamic compromise ensued soon after presentation, requiring emergency transesophageal echo and DC cardioversion.

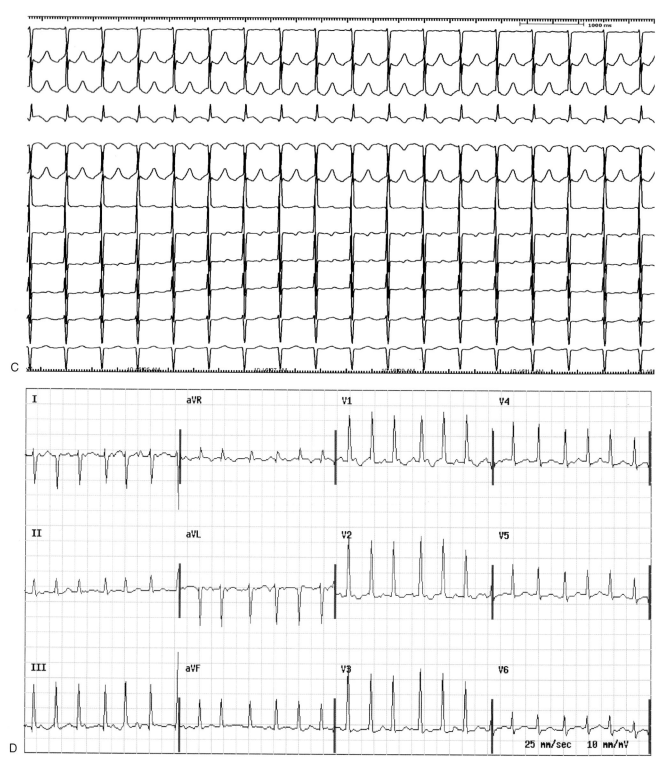

FIGURE 14.15 (*Continued*)

frontal ECG leads. Unfortunately, the term atypical atrial flutter has sometimes been used interchangeably with intra-atrial re-entrant tachycardia (IART), and this should generally be discouraged. The precise tachycardia circuit in any CHD patient cannot be presumed from the P-wave morphology alone, but only with carefully intracardiac mapping. It there-fore remains most appropriate to refer to all paroxysmal atrial tachycardias in CHD patients as IART.

A key feature of IART and atrial flutter is the regularity of the P-P intervals, and this may be difficult to ascertain in the presence of variable AV conduction. For therapeutic purposes, it is important to distinguish IART and atrial flutter from atrial fibrillation and chaotic atrial tachycardia, both of which are characterized by irregularly irregular or intermittently varying atrial activation. It may be feasible to unmask atrial activation with adenosine or obtain a direct atrial recording via transesophageal, epicardial, or transvenous atrial lead to make this distinction.

Other forms of intra-atrial re-entry are described, including left-sided atrial flutter (often observed in patients with prior mitral valve surgery), as well as the entity often referred to as sinus node re-entry. This arrhythmia is characterized by atrial rates generally <200 bpm and P waves that appear identical to sinus P waves. It can be initiated and terminated with atrial pacing, and may also be terminated with adenosine or vagal maneuvers. Often, this arrhythmia is regarded as an artifact of programmed atrial stimulation, although occasional patients experience symptomatic tachycardia on this basis. Whether a given tachycardia represents microre-entry in the region of the sinus node or macrore-entry with an exit site of the circuit close to the sinus node can only be determined in the electrophysiology (EP) laboratory. However, SA node re-entry generally is more apt to terminate with vagal maneuvers or adenosine than IART with a similar morphology. Again, this distinction may be somewhat arbitrary and imprecise, since a continuum may exist between IART and SA node re-entry in some cases.

Etiology

The underlying basis for both IART and atrial flutter is a stable macrore-entry circuit within atrial muscle. Both assume a fixed, stable activation pattern. Activation mapping in both animal models and in patients demonstrate that re-entry during IART and atrial flutter may use either fixed anatomic boundaries or areas of functional conduction block. Normal cardiac structures such as the tricuspid valve annulus, the pulmonary veins, and the junction of the cavae with the heart contribute to the boundaries of conduction delay or block necessary for these arrhythmias. Additional conduction abnormalities may result from postsurgical scars and less discrete changes in the intercellular matrix owing to atrial dilation, hypertrophy, fibrosis, and even prior ablation procedures.

In typical atrial flutter, re-entry uses a predictable and critical zone of slow conduction as the tachycardia propagates in a counterclockwise fashion from the atrial free wall through the isthmus of myocardium between the inferior vena cava and tricuspid annulus toward the septum (64–66). Activation is inferior to superior along the atrial septum and returns inferiorly along the right atrial free wall along the crista terminalis, which serves as an additional inner boundary to the circuit. In congenital heart disease patients, IART often uses this same isthmus, but additional conduction anomalies owing to anatomic defects or postoperative scars may further contribute to many re-entrant conduction patterns. Indeed, such patients often have multiple, stable re-entrant circuits identified during electrophysiology study, complicating efforts to treat this arrhythmia with ablation techniques.

Among young patients beyond infancy, these tachycardias occur predominantly in association with underlying heart disease (Fig. 14.15), most often following operations for congenital heart disease (67). In contrast, among infants, atrial flutter usually occurs in the absence of apparent heart disease (Fig. 14.16); instead, there it is frequently associated with the presence of an atrioventricular accessory connection, with or without pre-excitation (68).

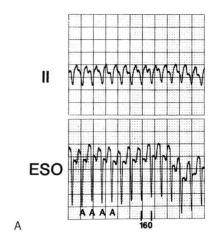

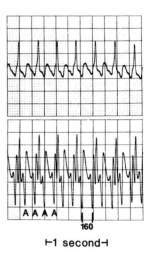

FIGURE 14.16 Electrocardiographic rhythm strip of atrial flutter in an infant. The atrial cycle length is very short (160 ms) characteristic of this tachycardia. **A:** 1:1 conduction with aberrant QRS is present, simulating ventricular tachycardia or SVT with aberrancy. **B:** The QRS becomes normal during 2:1 AV conduction.

Management

Management strategies for IART focus on four goals: (i) controlling symptoms during recurrences, (ii) terminating tachycardia, (iii) re-establishing sinus rhythm, and (iv) preventing recurrences. Symptoms during IART are largely, but not completely, a function of the ventricular rate. Ongoing atrial arrhythmias may be associated with rapid AV conduction leading to hemodynamic compromise, exertional symptoms owing to rapid ventricular rates, or progressive ventricular dysfunction. The potential for rapid hemodynamic deterioration cannot be understated in CHD patients. Thrombus formation may lead to cerebral embolic events, or in the case of the Fontan circulation, pulmonary emboli. Management may be complicated by coexisting bradycardia as seen in sick sinus or tachycardia–bradycardia syndromes. DC cardioversion remains the treatment of choice in the acute setting when severe hemodynamic compromise is evident. However, in hemodynamically stable patients, acute therapy requires a more considered approach.

Like atrial fibrillation, the more organized atrial tachycardias, IART and atrial flutter, usually are amenable to DC cardioversion, but may also be terminated with temporary transvenous or transesophageal pacing. Pacing may transiently convert atrial tachycardia to atrial fibrillation, which often spontaneously terminates. In the case of rare episodes, particularly in a patient with an implanted pacemaker, pace termination may be used very effectively to terminate otherwise well-tolerated atrial tachycardia in lieu of any chronic medical therapy. In such circumstances, it may be useful to treat patients with a medication able to slow the ventricular response to minimize the impact during such recurrences. Finally, acute pharmacologic conversion of IART can often be achieved. Ibutilide appears to be more effective for this purpose than procainamide but at increased risk of proarrhythmia. Occasionally, adenosine, administered for diagnostic purposes in IART or atrial flutter, results in tachycardia termination of this arrhythmia.

The potential for acute cerebral embolic events is well recognized with long-standing (24 to 48 hour) atrial fibrillation. Atrial thrombi have been demonstrated by transesophageal echo in patients with IART, but there have been few reports of embolic events even when tachycardia is long-standing. Nevertheless, for atrial fibrillation, echocardiography (preferably transesophageal) should be performed in patients presenting with flutter (IART) of uncertain duration to screen for intracardiac thrombi prior to acute termination. Alternatively, cardioversion can be delayed for 3 to 4 weeks while instituting anticoagulation. However, careful reassessment during this period of rate control is advisable to ensure ongoing toleration of the arrhythmia. Calcium channel blockers and beta-blockers generally are more reliable at control of the ventricular response than digoxin.

In the acute setting, calcium channel blockers generally are preferred as the treatment of choice for acute control of rapid ventricular rate. Diltiazem can be administered as an intravenous bolus or continuous infusion, as measures to screen for thrombi or perform cardioversion ensue. Digoxin and verapamil should be avoided in patients with atrial fibrillation associated with WPW because of the risk of enhancing antegrade conduction over the accessory connection (59,69).

The primary objective of long-term therapy is to maintain sinus rhythm. Improvement in cardiac function has been demonstrated following conversion of atrial tachycardia; thus maintenance of sinus rhythm is favored over simply controlling the ventricular rate. Medications that seem to be most effective for suppressing recurrences include class I and class III drugs. Class IA medications also have anticholinergic effects that potentiate antegrade conduction over the AV node during atrial flutter or fibrillation and should be administered with a medication that offsets this effect, such as diltiazem, digoxin, or a beta-blocker. The efficacy of class IC drugs such as propafenone and flecainide may be slightly better, but patients with atrial flutter and fibrillation may be at increased risk for serious proarrhythmia during treatment with these agents (70). Furthermore, the degree to which atrial conduction velocity is slowed with class IC drugs relative to the degree of AV node block may actually potentiate 1:1 AV conduction such that the ventricular rate increases despite a substantially slowed atrial rate, worsening symptoms during recurrences. Class III drugs appear to be equally effective and tend to reduce symptoms experienced with recurrences, possibly by slowing atrial conduction more so than the atrial rate, favoring a slower ventricular rate.

Unfortunately, none of these medical regimens is uniformly effective, and many patients seems to be refractory to all medications. Nonmedical therapies therefore often are necessary. The choices include antitachycardia pacing, catheter ablation, surgical revision, or a combination thereof. The role of antibradycardia pacing remains uncertain. Some studies suggest that atrial pacing may help limit recurrences of atrial fibrillation. Pacing also may be warranted owing to aggravation of bradycardia related to antiarrhythmic drug therapy and may lessen the risk of proarrhythmia. If pacing is necessary for SA node dysfunction associated with IART or atrial fibrillation, either an atrial pacemaker with rate response (AAIR) or dual-chamber pacemaker (DDDR) with both rate response and mode switching are preferred. These also provide the opportunity for temporarily programmed pacing algorithms for terminating recurrences (Fig. 14.6) (11).

Initial reports of catheter ablation of IART were somewhat encouraging, although acute success rates lagged behind the success rates for most other tachycardia mechanisms. Furthermore, recurrences following seemingly successful ablation have been problematic. Because of the complex atrial anatomy, identifying ablation sites that lead to successful prevention of IART has been a challenge. Variability in placement of suture lines and orientation of atriotomy incisions, distinguishing early activation within the circuit from concurrent late activation peripheral to the circuit, and the frequent occurrence of multiple tachycardia circuits in individual patients combine to make this a challenging undertaking. Additionally, successful ablation requires creation of an uninterrupted line of complete conduction block extending completely across a corridor or isthmus of conduction participating within the circuit. Newer ablation devices and mapping techniques are being developed and applied to this problem, notably multielectrode basket catheters allowing simultaneous recordings in multiple sites and various systems to create three-dimensional (3-D) electroanatomic models correlating chamber anatomy with electrical activation. Those tachycardias using the flutter isthmus are likely most amenable to successful ablation, whereas other sites can be more challenging. Even so, recent results have proven more encouraging with acute success rates of >90% now feasible (71). The issue of recurrence remains, often with new re-entry circuits encountered when repeat mapping and ablation are undertaken. This may be a consequence of incomplete lines of block created by noncontiguous ablation lesions, ongoing progression of the underlying myocardial disease processes contributing to IART, or even a proarrhythmic effect of the scars left behind by previous ablation procedures.

Because of the limitations of catheter ablation, alternative surgical techniques have been advocated for treating IART, most notably in patients with prior Fontan operation for single ventricle (72). Surgical conversion from more traditional Fontan's connections to either streamlined lateral tunnel or extracardiac connection has been combined with intraoperative cryoablation along regions likely to participate in IART. In doing so, more laminar and presumably hemodynamically favorable flow characteristics are created, and lines of conduction block intended to truncate all anticipated re-entry circuits are created. Even when not completely successful in eliminating IART, improved response to antiarrhythmic and/or antitachycardia pacing therapy has often been achieved with this approach.

Despite present limitations, nonpharmacologic therapies for IART continue to occupy an increasing role in management. Ongoing improvements in mapping techniques and ablation devices allowing more precise anatomic correlation through the use of MRI-generated images and methods to create more complete transmural and linear lesions continue.

Implantable devices allowing pace termination of IART with backup defibrillation capabilities and intracardiac atrial defibrillators are also available, although certain requirements, including bipolar pacing leads on both atrium and ventricle, along with the requirement that the atrial rate exceeds the ventricular rate to enable therapy, can prove problematic when applied to the CHD population with IART.

Prognosis

Prognosis of IART is dependent, in large measure, on the extent of underlying disease. Atrial flutter in infants without other heart disease is generally a self-limited process, and most patients do not require therapy beyond initial conversion. Late recurrences have been reported, but the relationship to earlier arrhythmias remains uncertain (68).

Management is most complicated for postoperative congenital heart disease with bradycardia and atrial tachycardia. A consensus has evolved that intra-atrial re-entrant tachycardia carries a substantial morbidity and mortality in patients with underlying congenital heart disease, and aggressive treatment is therefore advocated. The appropriate selection among potential treatments available is less clear, and longitudinal data comparing various treatment strategies is lacking. The degree to which coexisting abnormalities such as ventricular dysfunction, valvular disease, residual intracardiac shunts, and coexisting ventricular arrhythmias contribute to sudden death in this population is poorly understood. Symptomatic bradycardia warrants pacemaker implantation, and it has also been suggested that patients with tachycardia requiring antiarrhythmic therapy other than digoxin also be paced. However, this has recently been deemed a class II indication for pacing, and adverse events during pharmacologic treatment of atrial flutter and fibrillation are not necessarily prevented by pacemaker implantation.

The risk of cerebral thromboembolic phenomena contributes to the morbidity of chronic atrial arrhythmias, particularly in patients with chronic rheumatic heart disease. Chronic anticoagulation is recommended in all patients with chronic or frequently recurrent atrial flutter. Although embolic events may be less frequent with atrial flutter, patients with congenital heart disease and atrial flutter often have additional risk factors for thromboembolic complications. Increasingly, anticoagulation is being offered to these patients.

ATRIAL FIBRILLATION

Electrocardiographic Features

Atrial fibrillation is best distinguished from atrial flutter by the marked irregularity in the R-R intervals and the inconsistent pattern of atrial depolarizations. Because of the consequent irregular arrival of impulses into the AV node, the ventricular response is best characterized as irregularly irregular. It sometimes may be difficult to distinguish atrial fibrillation from atrial flutter with variable AV conduction on a short rhythm strip. Careful comparison of atrial cycle lengths is best made by measuring a group of four to five atrial cycles rather than a single cycle. Deviations in the apparent atrial P-wave morphology, axis, and cycle length are clues against atrial flutter, even when a saw-toothed appearance is perceived, and this may be best appreciated during longer tracings with multiple simultaneous ECG leads. Transesophageal or transvenous atrial electrogram recordings also are useful in making the distinction between atrial flutter and fibrillation. Atrial flutter, atrial fibrillation, and IART all are based on re-entry within atrial tissue.

Etiology

Although the mechanism underlying atrial fibrillation is well understood, the underlying causes among pediatric patients is largely speculative. This largely accounts for its infrequent occurrence among otherwise healthy young patients (73,74).

Atrial fibrillation generally is attributed to a disorganized re-entrant process involving multiple wavelets that perpetuate throughout the atria with varying degrees of organization and repetitiveness. As a result, periods more closely resembling atrial flutter may occur, and it can closely resemble chaotic atrial tachycardia. Indeed, the latter may often be mistaken for atrial fibrillation, prompting inappropriate treatment. In atrial fibrillation, the substrate for re-entry is largely dependent on functional rather than anatomic conduction abnormalities, such that fixed, consistent re-entrant circuits are lacking (75). Focal origins of atrial fibrillation can originate from the ostia of the pulmonary veins (Fig. 14.17).

The phenomenon of atrial remodeling refers to the occurrence of time-dependent alterations in atrial action potential configuration; this feature of atrial fibrillation favors the perpetuation of this arrhythmia. These changes likely have both electrical and mechanical implications and contribute to the delayed recovery of atrial contractile function following successful conversion to sinus rhythm (69).

Older children and adolescents with WPW also are susceptible to atrial fibrillation. As noted above, this tendency poses a risk of sudden death when atrial fibrillation is conducted rapidly over the accessory connection (Fig. 14.18). Ablation of the accessory connection eliminates this risk of rapid conduction and appears to decrease overall susceptibility to subsequent atrial fibrillation. Occasionally, atrial fibrillation may be the initial manifestation of hyperthyroidism, myocarditis, or digoxin toxicity (69).

A genetic basis for atrial fibrillation was suspected since the initial report of familial atrial fibrillation in 1943. Subsequently, genetic loci were identified using linkage studies in large kindreds with familial atrial fibrillation, and recently, the first genes for atrial fibrillation have been reported: *KCNQ1* and *KCNE2* (76). Electrophysiologic analysis of identified mutations shows gain of function of the currents generated by KCNQ1/KCNE1 and KCNQ1/KCNE2. These studies establish the role of potassium ion channels in the pathogenesis of some cases of atrial fibrillation. Monogenic familial atrial fibrillation likely is rare, although genetic susceptibility to atrial fibrillation may be more prevalent than previously suspected. Young patients with atrial fibrillation in the absence of other hemodynamic or electrophysiologic abnormalities may have a greater likelihood of a genetic basis for atrial fibrillation.

Management

The basic principles described above for acute IART management generally apply to atrial fibrillation as well. Ascertaining the time since atrial fibrillation onset is key in determining whether transesophageal echo is necessary. Pharmacologic measures to slow AV node conduction to the ventricles may be somewhat more feasible in atrial fibrillation compared with IART. In contrast, the thromboembolic risk is probably

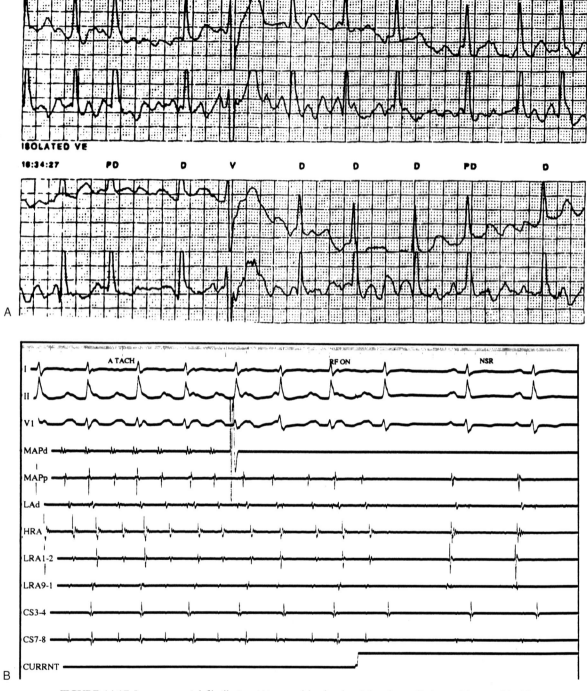

FIGURE 14.17 Incessant atrial fibrillation (**A**) caused by focal atrial tachycardia in an 11-year-old girl without structural heart disease. Periods of regular, narrow QRS tachycardia and atrial flutter were also observed. Radiofrequency ablation of the focus adjacent to the left upper pulmonary vein eliminated the arrhythmia (**B**).

greater for atrial fibrillation. Patients awaiting cardioversion for longer than very brief periods should receive intravenous anticoagulation and a rate-controlling medication. The capability for temporary pacing must be available, since there may be significant bradycardia prior to emergence of a stable spontaneous escape rhythm. In contrast to IART, there is little role for pace-termination attempts with atrial fibrillation.

The choice of chronic antiarrhythmic medications mirrors that for IART. Often the goal is to decrease both the frequency and duration of episodes. Patients with brief, self-limited episodes of atrial fibrillation without a rapid ventricular response may even be observed conservatively.

One of the earliest nonpharmacologic interventions for atrial fibrillation was ablation of the AV node with implantation of a

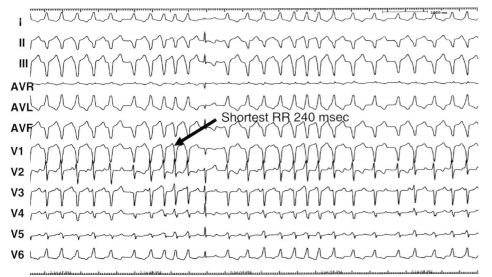

FIGURE 14.18 Rapid antegrade conduction over a right posterior accessory connection in 12-year-old athlete with Wolff–Parkinson–White syndrome and frequent palpitations with exertion. Although induced at electrophysiologic stimulation (EPS) prior to radiofrequency (RF) ablation, sustained and nonsustained atrial fibrillation were repeatedly provoked with single extrastimuli while the patient received propofol anesthesia.

ventricular pacemaker. The permanent loss of AV synchrony, lifelong dependence on a ventricular pacemaker, and the ongoing need for anticoagulation may be offset by the restoration of both a controlled ventricular rate, more appropriate rate response to activity, and elimination of the irregular ventricular rate. This approach should be reserved for patients in whom multiple medical regimens have proven ineffective.

Focal atrial fibrillation results from a rapidly firing tachycardia focus propagating from one of the pulmonary veins into the left atrium. These rapidly discharged impulses encounter varying degrees of local refractoriness such that the beat to beat pattern of atrial depolarization appears highly variable and disorganized. It is important to recognize this entity, since it has proven highly amenable to ablation (73). In adults, a few patients with atrial fibrillation have tachycardia of this type. More commonly atrial fibrillation is a diffuse process involving a myriad of variable and functional macrore-entrant circuits. Whether specific focal targets within one or more pulmonary veins can be isolated or targeted varies greatly. The risk of iatrogenic pulmonary vein stenosis should be noted and discussed with patients prior to ablation.

Efforts are ongoing to develop a clinically feasible and effective catheter-based treatment of atrial fibrillation. The model for such an effort is the Maze operation, which essentially partitions regions of atrial tissue while maintaining routes of electrical activation (77). The basis for this approach was the hypothesis that atrial fibrillation could perpetuate only if sufficiently large segments of tissue to complete a re-entrant "rotor" were available. In selected centers performing this procedure in sufficiently large numbers, excellent results have been reported.

Because of the infrequency of atrial fibrillation among the young, the potential for discrete pulmonary vein foci, and the frequent association with other SVT mechanisms, it would seem prudent to recommend comprehensive EPS in young patients presenting with this arrhythmia. However, the potential morbidity associated with focal pulmonary vein ablation and more generalized pulmonary vein isolation procedures need to be weighed carefully before attempting ablation, especially with initial or infrequently recurring episodes.

Prognosis

As with IART, prognosis is largely a function of the underlying cardiac disease. Certainly, recurrence is the rule for late repair of atrial septal defects, postoperative cardiac lesions with associated AV valve regurgitation, dilated cardiomyopathy, hypertrophic cardiomyopathy, chronic rheumatic mitral valve disease, and Emery-Dreyfus muscular dystrophy. Once established, surgical interventions (short of a surgical Maze) are unlikely to alter the relentless recurrence of the associated arrhythmia.

In contrast, atrial fibrillation associated with hyperthyroidism typically resolves after re-establishment of a euthyroid state. Otherwise healthy adolescents and teens presenting with atrial fibrillation typically have very infrequent recurrences, at least prior to the third decade of life. Whether these individuals will eventually develop early onset of frequent paroxysmal atrial fibrillation or chronic atrial fibrillation has not been ascertained.

Perhaps the greatest overall risk of atrial fibrillation is among those patients who fail to recognize atrial fibrillation because of an absence of palpitations. These patients may remain in unrecognized atrial fibrillation for prolonged periods of time before eventually developing deteriorating hemodynamic function or experiencing a cerebral embolic event. Patients with chronic atrial fibrillation or repeated recurrences that fail to be perceived at the time of onset require chronic anticoagulation with their own inherent risks. For this reason, an aggressive stance in trying to maintain a stable spontaneous or paced atrial rhythm appears warranted, whenever possible. However, except for focal ablation of pulmonary vein foci, the long-term efficacy of catheter ablation procedures remains generally unknown.

ECTOPIC ATRIAL TACHYCARDIAS

Electrocardiographic Features

Ectopic atrial tachycardias (EAT) (Fig. 14.19) are primary atrial tachycardias that appear to result from localized automatic foci

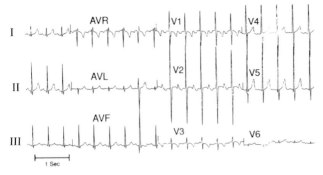

FIGURE 14.19 ECG during atrial automatic tachycardia originating at the base of the right atrial appendage. P waves with unusual bifid morphology in leads II and V1 were distinct from sinus P waves. An automatic mechanism and origin was ultimately confirmed at successful radiofrequency catheter ablation.

within the atrium rather than from re-entry. Tachycardia is usually chronic and often incessant. Associated cardiac dysfunction may be severe, and the tachycardia may be mistaken as an appropriate sinus tachycardia in response to heart failure. Analysis of P-wave morphology precludes ready distinction of EAT from sinus tachycardia. Because of the insidious nature of the problem and the subtle heart rate changes, patients rarely perceive palpitations. A high index of suspicion and careful inspection of multiple ECG recordings is therefore essential to the diagnosis.

Typically, tachycardia rates are moderately elevated and often are within the normal range for age. However, resting heart rates tend to be inappropriately elevated, and an exaggerated response to exercise may occur. Although heart rates may fluctuate considerably over sustained periods of time, there is little short-term or beat-to-beat variation in heart rate, and prolonged recordings appear quite monotonous. Although typically incessant, interruptions of tachycardia often occur (particularly during sleep), revealing discrete but often subtle changes in P-wave morphology between the ectopic and sinus rhythms. Characteristic acceleration (warm-up) occurs with tachycardia onset, and converse slowing (cool-down) may precede termination (78). Additionally, first- or second-degree AV block during apparent sinus tachycardia may be an important diagnostic clue.

Etiology

The basis for abnormal atrial automaticity in otherwise normal pediatric patients is not known, and the tendency for spontaneous cessation in some patients is mystifying. Some attempts have been made to subdivide microre-entrant foci from tachycardia foci owing to abnormal automaticity. Features suggestive of automatic foci include warm-up, or tachycardia acceleration at onset; failure to initiate or terminate with extrastimulus testing; and demonstration of reset phenomena during atrial extrastimuli delivered during tachycardia. However, these features do not definitively exclude microre-entrant circuits.

Mapping studies have identified two regional clusterings of ectopic foci, either near the right atrial appendage or near the pulmonary venous connections with the left atrium (79). The anatomic and developmental significance of these sites and the nature of the tissues involved remain uncertain. The notion of anatomically isolated nests of embryologic sinus node tissue

that are not subject to normal parasympathetic influence would be compatible with the clinical behavior of this tachycardia. However, appearance of ectopic atrial tachycardia after previously documented normal ECGs and heart rates argues against a simple developmental basis for this entity. Likewise, gross and histologic inspection of surgically resected foci have identified various abnormalities.

Management

Often, the most critical step is to establish a correct diagnosis. In addition to recognizing an inappropriate tachycardia, the ineffectiveness of pace termination, DC cardioversion, vagal maneuvers and adenosine in restoring sinus rhythm are further clues to the diagnosis of EAT. The typical sensitivity of EAT to adrenergic stimulation also should be recognized during acute management (78). Even in the face of overt congestive heart failure, adrenergic stimulation should be avoided, and beta-blockade may be an important component of therapy.

Various antiarrhythmic regimens have been used with varying success for EAT. These have included class IA, IC, β-blocking drugs, and class III agents, alone or in combination, with amiodarone appearing most effective (78–80). In contrast, digoxin seems to be particularly ineffective, except as a component of treatment for secondary congestive heart failure. Complete cessation of tachycardia, normalization of mean heart rate, slowing of the fastest tachycardia rates, and normalization of associated ventricular dysfunction may all represent appropriate end points of therapy. Careful monitoring is warranted during initiation of therapy in these patients, particularly if ventricular dysfunction coexists.

Surgical mapping and resection of the automatic foci are feasible and potentially allow a cure in drug-refractory cases. Radiofrequency (RF) ablation is equally successful in this arrhythmia and has supplanted the surgical approach. Although recurrences occur, repeat ablation usually can be successful.

With curative therapy available, the role of initial medical therapy prior to attempting RF ablation has been debated. Spontaneous resolution has been common in some series and less frequently observed in others (79,80). However, even severe ventricular dysfunction typically resolves with successful heart rate control such that initial medical therapy usually is warranted. Thus, younger patients and those with ventricular dysfunction at the time of diagnosis may be particularly likely to benefit from a period of medical suppression (80).

Prognosis

Several factors influence the long-term outcome of EAT, including the number or size of automatic foci, the tendency for spontaneous regression over time, and the possibility of late sequelae owing to the tachycardia or its treatment. Ventricular dysfunction improves and resolves in most cases. The potential for spontaneous regression favors at least short-term medical therapy in most patients. On the other hand, the relative resistance of this tachycardia to antiarrhythmic therapy makes ablation increasingly attractive. Thus, the potential risks of catheter ablation must be weighed against the likelihood of long-term cure and the potential risks of the aggressive antiarrhythmic regimens sometimes necessary to achieve long-term tachycardia control.

CHAOTIC ATRIAL TACHYCARDIA

Electrocardiographic Features

Chaotic atrial tachycardia (or chaotic atrial rhythm) is an unusual atrial tachycardia characterized by ECG evidence of multiple (three or more) distinct P-wave morphologies during tachycardia with an isoelectric baseline, distinguishing it from atrial flutter or fibrillation. Tachycardia with identical features is typically seen in adults with advanced pulmonary disease and is referred to as multifocal atrial tachycardia. Chaotic atrial tachycardia is described in young children and infants with otherwise normal hearts (81). Tachycardia rates vary considerably, with irregular P-P intervals despite discrete P waves. This tachycardia sometimes is difficult to distinguish from atrial fibrillation, and periods of apparent atrial fibrillation may be associated.

The anatomic or functional substrates responsible for chaotic atrial tachycardia remain poorly defined. Whether the rhythm is related to multiple competing automatic foci, multiple re-entrant circuits, or triggered mechanisms is uncertain, although in adults a relationship between stress and adrenergic tone has been implicated. Although most infants with chaotic atrial tachycardia have no major structural heart disease, various cardiac and noncardiac conditions were present among two thirds of patients reviewed by Yeager et al. (82). In several series, associated respiratory illnesses, particularly bronchiolitis with respiratory syncytial virus occurred (81,83). Nevertheless, the presence of severe and occasionally lethal bradycardias may belie a more fundamental cardiac or autonomic abnormality in some patients.

Chaotic atrial tachycardia is refractory to pace termination, DC cardioversion, and adenosine. Therefore, treatment strategies are similar to those outlined for EAT. Because of the age of the patient, symptoms may be fairly subjective, although ventricular dysfunction can result. Drugs such as verapamil or propranolol that slow the ventricular response during tachycardia alone may be sufficient in alleviating symptoms, whereas complete suppression of the tachycardia usually requires treatment with class IA, IC, and class III agents. Propafenone and amiodarone are particularly effective.

Like EAT, this tachycardia frequently regresses within days to months. However, sudden death occurred in 17% of the young patients reviewed by Yeager et al. (82), including two witnessed deaths attributed to severe bradycardia. As with other deaths during antiarrhythmic therapy, it is difficult to distinguish those resulting from therapy from those resulting from the tachycardia. Nevertheless, close inpatient monitoring is essential during initiation of therapy along with careful follow-up evaluation.

JUNCTIONAL ECTOPIC TACHYCARDIA

Electrocardiographic Features

Junctional ectopic tachycardia (JET) is an uncommon automatic tachycardia in pediatric patients. It generally is observed in two clinical settings. The most frequent presentation is in the early postoperative period following cardiopulmonary bypass in infants and toddlers with congenital heart disease. In this setting, the tachycardia may have acute and catastrophic hemodynamic consequences but it is a transient problem (84).

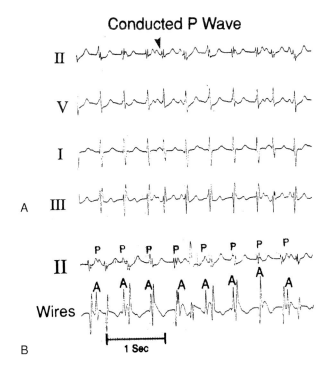

FIGURE 14.20 Junctional ectopic tachycardia with AV dissociation and typical cycle length changes. **A:** Surface leads demonstrate regular tachycardia with normal QRS and AV dissociation. P waves identify slower atrial rate. Tachycardia cycle length is irregular when P waves conduct to the ventricles and advance the tachycardia. **B:** Single surface lead and unipolar recording from atrial epicardial wire (*Wires*) delineated the atrial and ventricular electrograms.

Less frequently, a congenital form occurs in nonoperated patients.

The hallmark electrocardiographic appearance is a tachycardia with normal QRS duration at a rate of 180 to 240 bpm with AV dissociation and a slower atrial rate. Often, appropriately timed atrial beats conduct through the AV node with a recurring periodicity, resulting in periodic shortening of the R-R interval (Fig. 14.20). The resultant grouped beating often is an important initial clue to the diagnosis. However, the ventricular rate may be regular if VA conduction is present (1:1 AV association) or in the presence of complete antegrade AV block. In the former case, tachycardia appears identical to paroxysmal forms of SVT but is refractory to measures such as atrial pacing, DC cardioversion, or adenosine. The possibility of complete AV block should be suspected when the R-R intervals are unvarying (despite AV dissociation) and eventual heart rate slowing fails to yield to appropriate sinus rhythm. An ECG from atrial epicardial wires or transesophageal electrode facilitates making the diagnosis of this rhythm.

Congenital JET usually is recognized prenatally or within the first month of life and has an extremely high familial incidence (85); recessive inheritance has been suggested. Heart rates are variable but rates up to 370 bpm have been reported. Patients usually present with varying degrees of congestive heart failure, although acute cardiovascular collapse may also occur.

In postoperative patients, JET may occur in association with prolonged QRS duration and be indistinguishable from ventricular tachycardia. Invasive electrophysiologic recordings during this tachycardia should reveal His depolarizations preceding each ventricular depolarization, confirming the diagnosis of JET. Unlike His bundle re-entry, atrial or ventricular pacing may entrain the rhythm but fail to terminate the tachycardia.

Etiology

Both forms of JET are attributed to enhanced automaticity of tissues in or near the AV node. The exact cause of this automaticity remains poorly characterized. Presumably, surgical trauma to these tissues could result in an irritable automatic focus, an impression supported by the transient nature of this arrhythmia. Conceivably, other undetermined factors may be involved, including an abnormal cellular response to reperfusion injury or anesthetic agents. Temperature elevation and use of pancuronium bromide frequently are associated, although no link with malignant hyperthermia has been established.

The cause of the congenital form of JET remains even more obscure. An association with late-onset AV block has been postulated, and histologic degeneration of the His bundle has been demonstrated in patients who died suddenly of JET (85). The familial association may indicate an intrauterine insult analogous to congenital AV block owing to maternal connective tissue disease. The arrhythmia has also been associated with a Purkinje cell tumor in one instance (86).

Management

The hemodynamic consequences of JET warrant aggressive therapy to slow the rate, or when possible, to restore sinus rhythm. Yet, almost invariably, both the postoperative and the congenital forms of JET have proven unusually resistant to most standard antiarrhythmic therapy. Amiodarone appears to be the single most effective agent used for the congenital form of JET, yielding control or partial control in 80% of cases (85). Ablation of the His conduction system surgically or with radiofrequency catheter ablation may be a reasonable alternative in persistent cases, particularly when amiodarone fails to successfully control the rhythm. However, selective ablation of the ectopic junctional focus with preservation of AV conduction is often feasible (87).

Because of its transient course, treatment of postoperative JET usually is limited to temporizing measures. Discontinuation of inotropic agents and modest cooling remain the most easily instituted measures to ameliorate postoperative JET. Historically, various other measures have been used with varying success. R-wave synchronized atrial pacing has been performed to achieve AV synchrony, but is associated with a risk of induced atrial tachycardia owing to asynchronous atrial pacing (88). Intravenous agents used effectively include flecainide and amiodarone (89,90). Digoxin, beta-blockers, and calcium channel blockers are generally ineffective for JET, and response to various class IA and class IC drugs has been highly variable. The goal of treatment should be either restoration of sinus rhythm or slowing the junctional rate sufficiently to allow atrial pacing at a slightly faster rate, improving hemodynamics. When medical measures are ineffective, extracorporeal membrane oxygenation (ECMO) and emergency AV node ablation have been used.

Prognosis

In the multicenter study of Villain et al. (85), congenital JET was associated with an extremely high incidence of congestive heart failure at presentation and with high mortality. Deaths occurred <13 months of life, sometimes as a consequence of attempted treatment, but also suddenly in patients thought to be under good medical control. Late AV block has been postulated as a cause for death in some patients, and a possible role for backup ventricular pacing has been proposed. Amiodarone was the most effective therapy and was successfully withdrawn in nearly half of all survivors at a mean age of 3.6 years. Thus, ablation should probably be reserved for medically refractory or persistent tachycardias.

Postoperative JET, despite its deleterious acute effects, is transient. Slowing of the tachycardia to rates allowing return of normal sinus rhythm usually occurs within 24 to 72 hours regardless of the temporizing therapy used. The potential for late sequelae such as AV block following postoperative JET has not been systematically examined. However, the apparent link between congenital and postoperative JET and disease of the AV node or His conduction system appears sufficient to warrant long-term follow-up of all patients who have recovered from JET.

GENERAL ASPECTS OF VENTRICULAR TACHYCARDIAS

The differential diagnosis of tachycardias with a prolonged QRS includes ventricular tachycardias, pre-excited supraventricular tachycardias and any other tachycardia conducted aberrantly owing to fixed, functional, or rate-related bundle branch block. Additionally, pacemaker-mediated tachycardia (a wide complex tachycardia with paced QRS morphology) should be considered in patients with implanted pacemakers. Since ventricular tachycardias (VT) are less common than the various forms of SVT among young patients, tachycardias with prolonged QRS duration sometimes inappropriately are presumed to represent SVT with aberrant intraventricular conduction. Even when patients appear hemodynamically stable, the hazards of such an assumption may be substantial, especially in patients with underlying heart disease. Initial treatment based on a presumed diagnosis of ventricular tachycardia is rarely deleterious, even when the mechanism subsequently proves to be supraventricular. Tachycardias with prolonged QRS duration should be considered ventricular tachycardia and treated as such until a more definitive diagnosis can be established. Electrophysiology study may be necessary to establish the diagnosis and guide therapy accordingly.

Electrocardiographic Features

The hallmark electrocardiographic features of ventricular tachycardia are prolonged QRS duration and dissociation of the P waves from QRS during tachycardia (with a slower atrial rate). However, in infants and children with ventricular tachycardia, one or both of these features may not be evident. Since the normal QRS duration is age and rate dependent, the QRS may be significantly prolonged for age but still appear to be within the normal range (Fig. 14.21). Conversely, many patients with congenital heart disease may display a prolonged QRS during sinus rhythm. In such patients, ventricular tachycardia may result in a change in QRS morphology rather than further prolongation of the QRS duration. Comparison with a previous ECG obtained during sinus rhythm is helpful in this determination. Young patients also may maintain retrograde

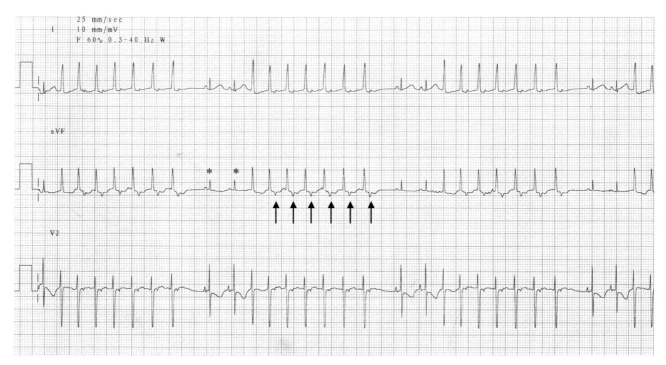

FIGURE 14.21 Nonsustained ventricular tachycardia in a neonate. After two beats of sinus rhythm (*asterisks*), there are seven beats of tachycardia; the last six beats are followed by inverted P waves (*arrows*), consistent with retrograde activation of the atria. The first beat is dissociated from the atrium, excluding a supraventricular origin. The QRS duration during tachycardia is <80 ms but significantly prolonged compared to sinus rhythm.

conduction over the specialized conduction system at high rates, resulting in a 1:1 VA relationship during ventricular tachycardia, eliminating the second major electrocardiographic feature of ventricular tachycardia.

A transesophageal ECG recording during tachycardia may be helpful to delineate the atrial-ventricular relationship. If either VA dissociation (with slower atrial rate) or variations in retrograde conduction are demonstrated during ongoing tachycardia, particularly following vagal maneuvers or intravenous adenosine administration, ventricular tachycardia is confirmed. However, 1:1 VA conduction does not exclude the diagnosis, unless antegrade or retrograde block consistently terminates tachycardia. Variations in the R-R interval owing to sinus capture beats may also be helpful when VA dissociation is present; intermittent fusion complexes distinguish ventricular tachycardia from SVT with variable AV conduction. Additional electrocardiographic features favoring ventricular tachycardia over other tachycardias with a prolonged QRS have been reviewed (91), but these features, including the absence of an RS complex in the precordial leads and QRS duration >100 ms, have not been systematically evaluated in pediatric patients.

Symptoms caused by ventricular tachycardia vary widely, and the clinical presentation itself is of little benefit in distinguishing these tachycardias from SVT with aberrant conduction. Patients may present with modest symptoms comparable to those experienced during various supraventricular tachycardias or may experience cardiac arrest and sudden death. Likewise, successful termination using interventions such as vagal maneuvers, adenosine, atrial pacing, or verapamil should not be construed as evidence of a supraventricular mechanism, since these also may terminate certain types

of ventricular tachycardias. Prior knowledge of certain conditions predisposing individual patients to supraventricular arrhythmias (such as WPW) may be helpful, particularly in recognizing antidromic reciprocating tachycardia or atrial fibrillation in association with ventricular pre-excitation. However, many cardiac diseases may predispose to both atrial and ventricular tachycardias, and ECG features alone may not permit a precise electrophysiologic diagnosis. Again, the prognostic and therapeutic implications are such that tachycardia with a prolonged QRS usually warrants electrophysiologic evaluation to define the tachycardia mechanism.

Nomenclature such as nonsustained (defined as ≥3 but <30 consecutive ventricular depolarizations) versus sustained or self-limited, and spontaneous versus induced (such as with programmed stimulation) are used. Ventricular tachycardias may also be characterized as monomorphic or polymorphic, depending on the constancy or variation of QRS complexes during tachycardia.

Two specific types of polymorphic ventricular tachycardia are torsades de pointes and bidirectional ventricular tachycardia (Fig. 14.22). The former, by definition, is associated with prolongation of the QT interval, as occurs in congenital and acquired long QT syndromes, and the QRS complexes appear to undulate or twist about the isoelectric line as the QRS morphology gradually changes shape and axis. Bidirectional ventricular tachycardia is described in association with digitalis toxicity, Andersen-Tawil syndrome, or catecholaminergic polymorphic ventricular tachycardia (CPVT). As the name suggests, beat-to-beat alternation in the QRS axis occurs during ongoing tachycardia, a phenomenon that easily can be mistaken for ventricular bigeminy (Fig. 14.23).

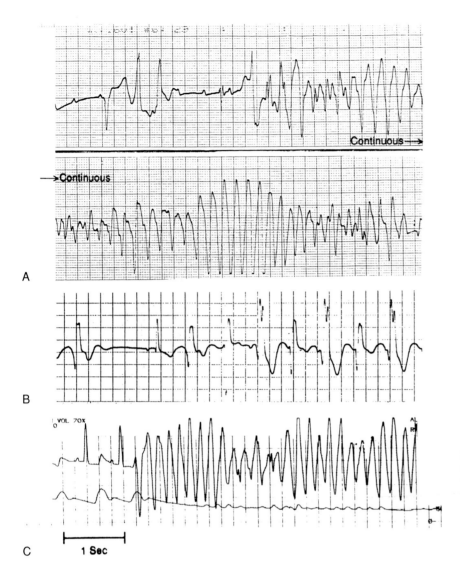

FIGURE 14.22 Polymorphic ventricular tachycardias. **A:** Torsades de pointes in a patient with complete AV block and a history of syncope. QRS morphology continually twists about the isoelectric line. **B:** Bidirectional ventricular tachycardia with alternating QRS morphologies during tachycardia. **C:** Ventricular fibrillation with erratic disorganized activity and no discernible QRS.

Etiology

Many of the prevailing views about ventricular arrhythmias have been derived from experience in older patients. While certain similarities exist, extrapolating this huge body of experience to pediatric patients is tenuous. There are clear distinctions of the underlying substrate and disease processes. In adults, prior myocardial infarction with a healed scar, intermittent ischemia, or changes associated with dilated cardiomyopathies prevail.

Although many pediatric patients with ventricular tachycardia appear to have no obvious underlying heart disease, on close scrutiny an underlying basis for ventricular tachycardia often is identifiable. These may include myocarditis or subtle forms of cardiomyopathy (39). In other young patients, a history of surgery for congenital heart disease or reversible myocardial derangements owing to some metabolic abnormality, such as electrolyte disturbances or drug toxicity, may provide a clue as to the basis. A partial listing of diagnoses associated with ventricular tachycardia is shown in Table 14.6.

Emphasis sometimes is placed on classifying ventricular tachycardias according to whether they result from a re-entrant mechanism, a triggered mechanism, or abnormal automaticity. Criteria favoring each of these may be established by electrophysiologic study. Re-entry may occur around a scar or around an area of electrically abnormal myocardium. Automaticity may arise from a myocardial tumor. Considerable evidence has been presented for triggered activity as the basis for both digoxin-mediated tachycardia (delayed afterdepolarizations), torsades de pointes (early afterdepolarizations), and reperfusion-related arrhythmias (early and/or late afterdepolarizations). Other classification schemes have emphasized response to programmed stimulation (atrial versus ventricular) or response to various pharmacologic agents (isoproterenol, verapamil, adenosine, or vagal maneuvers). These observations support the idea that ventricular tachycardias have many diverse causes or mechanisms, which may overlap in some instances.

Management

For sustained ventricular tachycardia with hemodynamic compromise, synchronized DC cardioversion is the acute treatment of choice. In rare instances, careful pharmacologic termination with intravenous lidocaine or procainamide may be attempted, although DC cardioversion should performed at

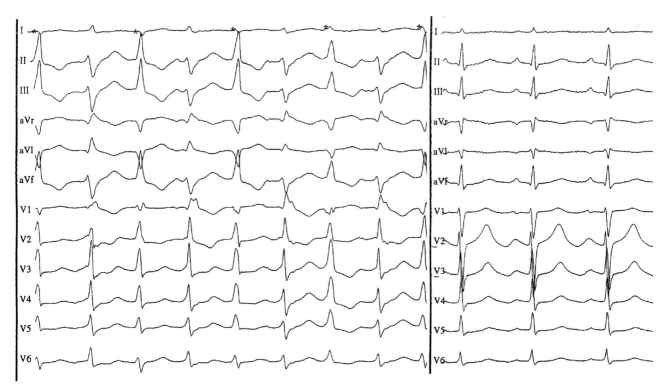

FIGURE 14.23 Bidirectional ventricular tachycardia. **Left:** Sustained bidirectional ventricular in a patient with Andersen-Tawil syndrome. The relatively slow rate and deceptively normal appearance of QRS complexes in some leads may result in misdiagnosis of sinus rhythm with premature ventricular beats in a bigeminal pattern. All QRS complexes, however, are prolonged compared with the QRS complexes in sinus rhythm (**right**).

the first suggestion of compromise during such infusions. More often, drugs are initiated following cardioversion in an attempt to suppress reinitiation. Transvenous pace termination should be reserved for the electrophysiology laboratory, again with immediate DC cardioversion or defibrillation available. Intravenous amiodarone now is used in otherwise drug-refractory ventricular tachycardias. Rarely, if clinical features suggest idiopathic tachycardia from the right ventricular outflow region or left fascicular tachycardia, verapamil may be cautiously infused, providing important diagnostic (and indirectly, prognostic) information if tachycardia terminates.

Unlike SVT, where careful follow-up alone may be sufficient, chronic therapy of sustained ventricular tachycardias is almost always mandatory. The only possible exceptions are patients for whom the cause of the tachycardias can be eliminated or for asymptomatic patients without structural heart disease. Virtually all classes of antiarrhythmic agents have been used for ventricular tachycardias, including all class I and class III drugs. The appropriate selection of the best drug remains problematic. Treatment also may include implantable cardioverter defibrillators and catheter ablation.

In the past, serial electrophysiology study to assess inducibility before and after treatment was considered a standard strategy. However, prospective data from adults with ischemic heart disease demonstrated unacceptably high tachycardia recurrence using either this approach or simple suppression of ectopy as determined by Holter monitoring. Furthermore, in some settings, treatment was associated with increased mortality (44). For this reason, implantable cardioverter defibrillators have become the established standard for treating many,

if not most, forms of ventricular tachycardia. Antiarrhythmic therapy and catheter ablation often are useful adjuncts to ICD therapy, particularly to limit recurrent discharges. Amiodarone is sometimes used for patients considered poor candidates for defibrillator therapy.

It can be assumed that most patients with prior cardiac arrest and documented ventricular tachycardia or fibrillation should receive an ICD. Likewise, those with sustained monomorphic ventricular tachycardias associated with heart disease generally are at sufficient risk of sudden death to warrant ICD implantation (12). Incessant ventricular tachycardias may be amenable to surgical or catheter ablation and even may regress spontaneously following a period of medical therapy. Exercise-induced tachycardia arising in the right (or left) ventricular outflow tract and those owing to fascicular re-entry are particularly amenable to drugs or catheter ablation.

The life-threatening nature of most ventricular tachycardias requires more reliable therapy than most SVTs since even occasional treatment failures may have disastrous consequences. Neither reduction in the frequency of ventricular extrasystoles nor the suppression of previously inducible tachycardia with serial electrophysiologic testing are sufficiently specific to ensure complete freedom from further arrhythmias. With the ongoing improvements in ICD design, this modality has emerged as the primary therapy for potentially lethal arrhythmias. Electrophysiologic assessment remains useful in the assessment of ventricular tachycardias for risk stratification, selection of specific devices and associated medical regimens, and to guide therapy of any associated supraventricular arrhythmias.

TABLE 14.6

ETIOLOGIC FACTORS UNDERLYING VENTRICULAR TACHYCARDIAS

Functional
Dilated cardiomyopathy
Pulmonary hypertension
Inherited arrhythmia syndromes
Myocardial ischemia
Myocarditis

Idiopathic
Posterior fascicular re-entry
LV outflow tract VT
RV outflow tract VT

Structural heart disease
Tetralogy of Fallot and double-outlet RV
Univentricular heart disease (Fontan)
Hypertrophic cardiomyopathy
Eisenmenger syndrome
Aortic stenosis
Myocardial tumors

Metabolic and pharmacologic
Hypoxia, acidosis
Hypomagnesemia
Hyperkalemia, hypokalemia
Digoxin and catecholamine toxicity
Cocaine, methamphetamine
Psychotropic agents (phenothiazines, antidepressants)
Severe hypothermia
Antiarrhythmic drugs (class Ia, IC, III)

LV, left ventricular; RV, right ventricle/ventricular; VT, ventricular tachycardia.

Prognosis

The prognosis of patients with ventricular tachycardias depends largely on the specific arrhythmia and associated heart disease or genetic factors. Risk factors have been identified only partially. Risk factors for developing ventricular arrhythmias after surgery for congenital heart disease include older age at surgery, prolonged cardiopulmonary bypass time, residual hemodynamic abnormalities (including elevated ventricular pressure and severe semilunar valve regurgitation), prolonged QRS duration during sinus rhythm, and the presence of frequent ventricular premature beats (VPBs) (92). None of these factors sufficiently discriminates between patients at low and high risk. The clustering of multiple risk factors may help identify some of the most likely at-risk patients. Interventions, such as revising the repair of a congenital heart defect, may be offered in the hope that ventricular tachycardias may be averted. The role of programmed stimulation for risk stratification has not been well established in young patients with brief, asymptomatic ventricular arrhythmias.

The risk of ventricular tachycardia also is clearly related to the specific type of tachycardia. Torsades de pointes and other polymorphic ventricular tachycardias pose an extremely high risk of death because of the profound hemodynamic consequences of these tachycardias and their propensity to quickly degenerate to ventricular fibrillation. In contrast, certain exercise-induced ventricular tachycardias that are generally not associated with underlying heart disease may have a prognosis similar to that for SVT.

SPECIFIC VENTRICULAR TACHYCARDIAS

Incessant tachycardias are characterized as persisting >10% of the time. A QRS pattern resembling right bundle branch block is most common among these patients, but there are no pathognomonic ECG features other than the incessant behavior.

Incessant ventricular tachycardias usually are encountered in infancy and early childhood. Most are due to a hamartoma or Purkinje cell tumor, and less commonly, rhabdomyoma or focal myocarditis (93). Ventricular function may be depressed, and this usually is the result rather than the cause of the sustained tachycardia. The tachycardia usually is well tolerated, and symptoms correspond to the degree of ventricular dysfunction. However, cardiac arrest has also been described, attesting to the need for aggressive therapy.

Because of the incessant nature of the tachycardia, the usual absence of acute symptoms, and probable automatic or triggered mechanism, acute measures such as DC cardioversion or pace termination are generally ineffective. These tachycardias may prove difficult to treat with standard antiarrhythmic regimens, leading to the recommendation of resection or ablation of the focus. However, reports have demonstrated that if satisfactory medical suppression of the tachycardia is achieved, many patients ultimately experience spontaneous regression of the tachycardia within 12 months (94).

In the absence of effective tachycardia suppression, the long-term prognosis is likely to be poor. However, with effective treatment, ventricular function typically recovers, and long-term prognosis appears to be favorable. Thus, the approach to long-term therapy depends on the success of medical suppression versus surgical resection. The success of ablation depends on the location and size of the focus. These factors must be weighed against the apparent response to aggressive antiarrhythmic drug therapy. Purkinje cell tumors are too diffuse to be amenable to RF ablation, though there is little published experience with this entity.

Genetic Arrhythmia Syndromes

Long QT Syndrome

Long QT syndrome is characterized by abnormal QT interval prolongation (rate-corrected QT or QTc) and susceptibility for cardiac arrest and sudden death owing to a specific type of polymorphic ventricular tachycardia, torsades de pointes. A long QT interval and torsades de pointes have been associated with both the congenital and acquired long QT syndromes.

Electrocardiographic Features. In addition to prolongation of the QT interval, bradycardia, torsades de pointes, AV block, and abnormal T-wave morphology may be electrocardiographic manifestations of long QT syndrome. The diagnosis may become manifest in the neonatal period, when it may be associated with second-degree AV block. The diagnosis more often is made during the course of evaluating children and adolescents with syncope or seizures, or occasionally in association with neurosensory deafness. Asymptomatic individuals may be identified after the diagnosis in a family member. Occasionally, the diagnosis can be made retrospectively after a patient experiences drug-induced torsades de pointes, followed by persistent QTc prolongation despite withdrawal of the offending agent.

Borderline QTc prolongation without other clinical, historical, or electrocardiographic features suggesting the long QT syndrome may merely represent the upper range of the normal population. Other electrocardiographic features, such as bizarrely shaped T waves, exaggerated U waves, and T-wave alternans are helpful when considering this diagnosis (95). In some patients, the QTc prolongation may be only modest on a resting ECG, becoming more exaggerated only at increased heart rates as the QT interval fails to shorten. In others, the QTc prolongation may be most evident at slow heart rates. Evaluation of the QT interval during exercise, or with epinephrine infusion, can aid in diagnosis (96,97). A thorough family history and careful scrutiny of family members' electrocardiograms is paramount in the evaluation of any patient in whom this diagnosis is suspected.

The hallmark rhythm disturbance associated with long QT syndrome (LQTS) is torsades de pointes. Often, repeated bursts or salvos of tachycardia are self-limited and associated with mild symptoms of palpitations or presyncope. Longer episodes lead to cardiac arrest or death as the tachycardia degenerates to ventricular fibrillation. The subsequent postpause escape complex is associated with markedly prolonged repolarization, which, in turn, gives rise to a premature ventricular depolarization that may then go on to initiate the tachycardia (Fig. 14.22A). In congenital LQTS, syncope may occur with specific triggers such as physical or emotional stress, a sudden startle, loud auditory stimuli, or at rest or sleep when relatively bradycardic (98).

Etiology. Since the initial description of congenital deafness, prolongation of the QT interval, and sudden death by Jervell and Lange-Nielsen in 1957 (99), our understanding of the genetic basis of LQTS has progressed significantly. Shortly after the autosomal recessive Jervell–Lange-Nielsen syndrome was described, Romano et al. (100) and Ward (101) each independently described an autosomal dominant form without congenital deafness. The findings that the QT interval could be prolonged by right stellectomy, and the successful treatment of a medically refractory young patient with LQTS by left stellectomy, led to the hypothesis that the disease was primarily a disorder of cardiac sympathetic innervation (102). Although we now know that this is not the primary cause of LQTS, the importance of these early observations is evident in that autonomic modulation is a vital therapeutic approach in LQTS patients.

The subsequent theory that the underlying cause of LQTS was an alteration of one of the repolarizing potassium currents was proposed nearly 10 years prior to the identification of the first LQTS genes in 1995 (103–106). Indeed, four forms of LQTS, and the two most common forms (LQT1 and LQT2), are caused by mutations in genes that encode proteins that form repolarizing potassium channels. In the late 1990s the first five LQTS genes were identified (Table 14.7), all of which encoded proteins that form ion channels that underlie the cardiac action potential. The most commonly identified genes, KCNQ1 and KCNH2, encode proteins that form the α-subunits of two major repolarizing potassium currents, IKs and IKr. Two other LQTS genes encode for the corresponding β-subunits (KCNE1 and KCNE2). The other major LQTS gene, SCN5A, encodes the α-subunit of the cardiac sodium channel. Either loss-of-function mutations in potassium channel genes, or gain-of-function mutations in the cardiac sodium or calcium channels leads to prolongation of ventricular repolarization, and therefore, a prolonged QT interval. Furthermore, we now know that the Jervell–Lange-Nielsen syndrome is simply a more severe form of LQTS, as

patients with Romano–Ward syndrome carry a single mutation, while it is now accepted that homozygous mutations of KCNQ1 or KCNE1 cause Jervell–Lange-Nielsen syndrome (107). Congenital deafness requires the presence of two mutant alleles and results from lack of functioning IKs in the inner ear (108). These first five forms of LQTS represent classic LQTS, in that single mutations in ion channel genes resulted in action potential prolongation and prolonged QT intervals, with an increased risk for torsades de pointes and sudden death, with no significant extracardiac manifestations.

With the finding of ANK2 mutations underlying LQT4 (109), the spectrum of LQTS genes is not limited to genes that encode ion channel proteins. ANK2 encodes ankyrin-B, one isoform of a ubiquitously expressed family of proteins originally identified in the erythrocyte as a link between membrane proteins. Cardiomyocytes heterozygous for a null mutation in ankyrin B display reduced expression and abnormal localization of the Na/Ca exchanger, Na/K ATPase, and InsP3 receptor but normal expression and localization of other cardiac proteins, including the L-type Ca^{2+} channel and the cardiac Na^{+} channel (110). Action potential duration is normal, but myocytes display abnormalities in calcium homeostasis leading to early and delayed afterdepolarizations. Further clinical characterization of patients with ANK2 mutations show that they, while at risk for sudden death, do not uniformly display prolonged QT intervals, suggesting that ankyrin-B diseases are distinct from LQTS (111). Andersen-Tawil syndrome (ATS), termed by some as LQT7 (112), is due to mutations in KCNJ2 and is associated with significant extracardiac findings, including periodic paralysis, hypertelorism, and clinodactyly (113,114). Although at risk for torsades de pointes, the predominant arrhythmia observed in ATS is bidirectional VT (115). As many patients with ATS have mild or no prolongation of the QT interval, and the clinical manifestations, ECG characteristics, and outcomes are quite different from LQTS, it seems that ATS is not a subtype of the long QT syndrome. It has been recommended that the annotation of KCNJ2-positive ATS individuals should be ATS1 rather than LQT7 (116). Recently, mutations in the gene encoding the L-type calcium channel have been found to underlie Timothy's syndrome, a rare multisystem disorder characterized by QT prolongation as well as syndactyly, autism, and immune deficiencies (117). This has been termed LQT8 (118), and does cause a gain of function of ICa owing to slowed inactivation, which directly prolongs the QT interval, similar to the other forms of LQTS. However, the first described case of Timothy's syndrome differs from classic forms of LQTS in that it is associated with significant extracardiac manifestations. More recently, other Ca^{2+} channel gene (CACNA1C) mutations have been identified that increase the QT interval but result in less severe extracardiac manifestations (119).

Even when limited to classic forms of LQTS, important clinical differences among affected patients depending on the specific gene (and in some cases the specific mutation) have been observed. As most (>90%) genotyped LQTS patients have LQT1, LQT2, or LQT3 (120), most of the differences are observed among these genotypes. Important differences among LQTS types 1–3 include different ECG T-wave patterns, clinical course, triggers of cardiac events, response to sympathetic stimulation, and effectiveness and limitations of β-blocker therapy (121). In some cases, it also appears that disease "hot spots" may confer enhanced proarrhythmic risk. For example, among patients with LQT2, increased risk has been associated with mutations located in the pore region of the protein compared with mutations in other locations (122). In patients with LQT1, transmembrane domain mutations

TABLE 14.7

GENETIC ARRHYTHMIA SYNDROMES ASSOCIATED WITH SUDDEN DEATH

Syndrome	Inheritance	Locus	Ion current/protein	Gene
Long QT syndrome (RW)				
LQT1	AD	11p15	IKs	*KCNQ1*
LQT2		7q35	IKr	*KCNH2*
LQT3		3p21	INa	*SCN5A*
LQT4		4q25	Ankyrin B	*ANK2*
LQT5		21q22	IKs	*KCNE1*
LQT6		21q22	IKr	*KCNE2*
LQT7		17q23	IK1	*KCNJ2*
LQT8		12p13.3	ICa–L	*CACNA1C*
Long QT syndrome (JLN)	AR	11p15	IKs	*KCNQ1*
		21q22	IKr	*KCNE1*
Catecholaminergic polymorphic VT	AD	1q42		*RYR2*
	AR	1p13-p11		*CASQ2*
Brugada syndrome	AD	3p21	INa	*SCN5A*
		3p22-25		
Short QT syndrome	AD	21q22	IKr	*KCNH2*
		21q22	IKs	*KCNQ1*
		17q23	IK1	*KCNJ2*
Arrhythmogenic right ventricular cardiomyopathy				
ARVC1	AD	14q23-24		
ARVC2	AD	1q42	Ryanodine receptor 2	*RYR2*
ARVC3	AD	14q11-q12		
ARVC4	AD	2q32		
ARVC5	AD	3p23		
ARVC6	AD	10p12-p14		
ARVC7	AD	10q22		
ARVC8	AD	6p28	Desmoplakin	*DSP*
ARVC9	AD	12p11	Plakophilin 2	*PKP2*
Naxos disease	AR	17q21	Plakoglobin	*JUP*
Hypertrophic cardiomyopathy	AD	14q12	β-Myosin heavy chain	*MYH7*
	AD	11p11.2	Myosin binding protein-C	*MYBPC3*
	AD	1q32	Cardiac troponin T	*TNNT2*
	AD	19p13.2	Cardiac troponin I	*TNN13*
	AD	15q22.1	α-Tropomyosin	*TPM1*
	AD	3p21.3	Essential myosin light chain	*MYL3*
	AD	12q23-24.3	Regulatory myosin light chain	*MYL2*
	AD	15q11	Cardiac α-actin	*ACTC*
	AD	2q24.1	Titin	*TTN*
	AD	14q1	α-Myosin heavy chain	*MYH6*
	AD	3p21.3-3p14.3	Cardiac troponin C	*TNNC1*

AD, autosomal dominant; AR, autosomal recessive; JLN, Jervell–Lange-Nielsen; RW, Romano–Ward; VT, ventricular tachycardia.

were associated with more frequent events, as well as longer QTc and longer peak to end of QT interval, than those with C-terminal mutations (123). Despite these findings and the hope for genotype-guided therapy, there is tremendous clinical variability even within families with a single specific mutation, with variable penetrance and expression (124,125), likely owing to modifier genes that alter the phenotype. Multiple genes may influence cardiac repolarization and alter the phenotype in patients with the same LQTS mutation. One example is the finding of additional gene variants in LQTS patients resistant to β-blocker therapy (126).

Management. The major goals of therapy are to prevent torsades de pointes or to prevent sudden death by terminating torsades de pointes. Acutely, asynchronous cardioversion usually is effective in terminating torsades de pointes, though immediate reinitiation may ensue, requiring further preventative interventions. These include ventricular pacing to prevent bradycardia or long pauses that might potentiate initiation and correction of hypokalemia. Magnesium, which suppresses early afterdepolarizations (EADs) in vitro, may be particularly useful in suppressing reinitiation of torsades de pointes and may be beneficial regardless of the serum magnesium level

(127). Responses to beta-blockers or isoproterenol infusion are variable and may depend on the underlying cause. Experimental data suggest that calcium channel blockers also may be of some acute benefit (128).

Long-term therapy to prevent recurrences of torsades de pointes generally has used a stepped approach. Beta-blockers have remained the mainstay for chronic therapy of long QT syndrome and appear to be particularly effective in previously asymptomatic individuals (129). The dosage of beta-blocker should be titrated to sufficiently blunt the maximal heart rate on exercise testing. In patients with syncope or torsades de pointes despite adequate beta-blockade, implantation of an ICD is warranted. ICD implantation is sometimes recommended as initial therapy in patients at particularly high risk. Left cardiac sympathetic denervation can be useful in patients in whom beta-blockers are ineffective or contraindicated (130). Extreme vigilance in avoiding any medications with the potential of further prolonging the QT interval is necessary. The list of medications is ever-expanding, and an excellent web site that maintains such a list can be found at www.qtdrugs.org.

The improved understanding of the molecular mechanisms underlying the various forms of LQTS has allowed a framework for developing some genotype specific therapies (121). Since beta-adrenergically mediated increases in IKs are the predominant mechanism of QT shortening with adrenergic stimulation (131), patients with defective IKs (LQT1 and LQT5) are most sensitive to autonomic influences, and beta-blockers and left cardiac sympathetic denervation seem most effective for these LQTS types. Increased extracellular potassium paradoxically increases IKr (132), therefore supplemental potassium seems most appropriate for patients with defective IKr (LQT2 and LQT6) and has been shown to shorten the QT interval in patients with LQT2, both acutely and chronically (133,134). Patients with augmented INa, (LQT3) would be expected to improve with sodium channel blockers, and the QT interval has shortened with mexiletine (135). LQT3 patients also have bradycardia and shorten their QT interval with increases in heart rate, leading to the recommendation for treatment with pacemakers. Despite genotype-specific mechanisms, many therapies have beneficial effects on patients with any form of LQTS. Beta-blockers are recommended for all patients with LQTS, and mexiletine may have beneficial effects in LQT1 and LQT2 (136,137). This is consistent with the concept of reduced repolarization reserve (138). Multiple redundant mechanisms contribute to normal repolarization, and when an alteration in one or more of these causes a net increase in inward current during repolarization, it manifests as QT prolongation with increased risk for torsades de pointes. A specific therapy may target the underlying defect as when a sodium channel blocker normalizes the QT interval in a LQT3 patient. Alternatively, a therapy may enhance a normal mechanism and thereby offset the diseased one. For example, a patient with LQT1 with reduced IKs may benefit from supplemental potassium, which augments normal IKr and thereby helps restore the balance of repolarization.

Patients with long QT syndrome should be restricted from vigorous exercise, competitive sports, and high-risk occupations such as flying. Immediate family members should be screened with 12-lead ECG, and if other family members appear to be affected or if there is a history of sudden death, the extended family also should be screened for risk factors. At this point, it seems unwarranted to treat patients with a normal QT interval. In the absence of a clearly established family history or genetic confirmation of the diagnosis, serial exercise testing, epinephrine challenge, or Holter monitoring may be useful in screening minimally symptomatic patients with borderline QTc prolongation and no family history. If no additional features suggesting long QT syndrome are discovered, conservative follow-up probably is sufficient.

Genetic testing is now commercially available. It must be noted that nearly one third of patients with unambiguous LQTS have no identifiable mutations in the known LQTS genes. The failure to identify mutations may be attributed to mutations in noncoding regions, novel genes, or relatively large genomic alterations not detected by standard techniques (139).

Prognosis. Mortality of untreated, symptomatic patients may exceed 20% annually after the first syncopal episode and may approach 50% in 10 years. However, with adrenergic blocking drugs and/or stellate gangliectomy, 5-year mortality has been reduced to 3% to 5% (140). During childhood and early adulthood, untreated symptomatic long QT syndrome carries a cumulative mortality of 71%, the greatest risk being within the first year after appearance of symptoms. Adolescence may be a time of particularly high risk. Cardiac events can be reduced substantially with beta-blockers, although not entirely eliminated in patients with LQT2 or LQT3 (141). The extent of QT prolongation alone does not correlate closely with a patient's risk to develop torsades de pointes, and not all interventions that reduce risk shorten the QTc. Other electrocardiographic features, including QT dispersion on 12-lead ECG, may be more predictive than the QTc alone. The interval from the peak to the end of the T wave has been correlated with transmural dispersion of refractoriness and risk for torsades de pointes in left ventricular wedge preparations (142). Clinical studies have demonstrated increased transmural dispersion of repolarization, as measured by the peak to end of the T wave, in patients with congenital LQTS (143). This marker may be a more specific marker of risk than QT prolongation alone.

Acquired LQTS may be secondary to AV block, myocardial infarction, central nervous system injury, electrolyte abnormalities, or starvation, but is most commonly caused by drugs (144). Many commonly used drugs block IKr, resulting in exaggerated QT prolongation in certain patients. In contrast to congenital long QT syndrome, these patients have normal QT intervals when not taking the drug. Risk factors for acquired long QT syndrome include female gender, hypokalemia, hypomagnesemia, and bradycardia. A few patients with acquired LQTS have mutations or polymorphisms in LQTS genes (145). The possibility of other genes contributing to susceptibility to acquired LQTS is suggested by increased risk in family members of those with acquired LQTS (146). In accordance with the concept of reduced repolarization reserve (138), it seems that genetically susceptible individuals appear normal until subjected to the additional stressor of a drug that blocks IKr, at which point they manifest LQTS. Therapy consists of removal of the offending agent and avoidance of drugs known to prolong the QT interval.

Short QT syndrome

Just as patients with prolonged QT intervals (whether congenital or acquired) have an increased risk of sudden death, it has been recognized since the 1990s that excessively short QT intervals also are associated with increased mortality (147). In 2000, the possibility of a new genetic arrhythmia syndrome was raised when persistently short QT intervals were noted in a family with atrial fibrillation and in an unrelated patient with sudden death (148). Subsequently, two other families with short QT intervals, short atrial and ventricular effective refractory periods, and inducible VF at electrophysiology study were reported, and the term short QT syndrome was coined (149).

Electrocardiographic Features. The ECG in short QT syndrome reveals a short QT interval, and an absence of the ST segment with abnormally high amplitude T waves. Importantly, the QT interval remains short at slow heart rates. Atrial fibrillation commonly is observed, and patients are at risk for ventricular fibrillation. As with any new syndrome, the initially recognized cases tend to be the most severe. The reported cases of short QT syndrome have corrected QT intervals between 250 and 320 ms (150). The high incidence of sudden death in this cohort is, therefore, not surprising.

Etiology. Identification of mutations in *KCNH2*, *KCNQ1*, and *KCNJ2* in short QT syndrome patients followed only 4 to 5 years after the initial description of the syndrome (151–153). In each case, the mutations result in a gain of function of the respective potassium currents, causing short QT intervals. Loss-of-function mutations in *KCNQ1*, *KCNH2*, and *KCNJ2* underlie LQT1, LQT2, and Andersen-Tawil syndrome, respectively. Interestingly, the family with short QT syndrome owing to the *KCNJ2* mutation was reported not to have any extracardiac phenotype. The risk for ventricular fibrillation in short QT syndrome also may stem from an increased transmural dispersion of repolarization (154).

Management. Defibrillator therapy has been recommended for these high-risk patients but is complicated by the potential for frequent inappropriate shocks owing to oversensing of the high-amplitude T waves in this disorder (155). As more patients with short QT syndrome are identified, clinical heterogeneity likely will be uncovered, and risk stratification may become possible. Multiple drugs, including flecainide, sotalol, ibutilide, and quinidine, have been tested in a few patients with short QT syndrome (156). Quinidine significantly prolonged the QT interval and ventricular refractory period, and prevented inducibility of ventricular fibrillation. Importantly, drug testing has been reported in only a few patients, all with *KCNH2* mutations. This limited experience leaves the role of pharmacologic therapy uncertain at this time.

Catecholaminergic Polymorphic Ventricular Tachycardia

Leenhardt et al. (157) described the clinical course and prognosis of 21 cases of catecholaminergic polymorphic ventricular tachycardia (CPVT). This entity may lead to syncope or sudden death in young children with normal hearts.

Electrocardiographic Features

In contrast to LQTS, the baseline ECG reveals a normal QT interval and exercise induces a characteristic bidirectional ventricular tachycardia (VT). The bidirectional VT may be asymptomatic. However, polymorphic VT and ventricular fibrillation also may occur (158). Electrophysiology study with programmed ventricular stimulation usually does not provoke any arrhythmias, but the characteristic bidirectional VT is seen with exercise or catecholamine infusion (159). The familial transmission, risk from physical or emotional stress, and benefits of beta-blocker therapy were recognized since the first reports. Recently, swimming-triggered events, previously

thought to be specific for LQT1, have been associated with CPVT (160). Furthermore, a relative sinus bradycardia prior to beta-blocker therapy has been recognized in patients with CPVT (161).

Etiology

Linkage of CPVT to chromosome 1q42-q43 was described in two unrelated families in 1999 (162), followed by identification of mutations in the cardiac ryanodine receptor (RYR2) in 2001 (163). The ryanodine receptor resides on the membrane of sarcoplasmic reticulum (SR) and releases calcium from the SR in response to calcium influx from the L-type calcium channels (calcium-induced calcium release) (164). Functional assessment of mutant RYR2 showed increased calcium release from mutant RYR2 under adrenergic stimulation (165). Mutations in calsequestrin 2 (CASQ2) have also been identified in an autosomal recessive form of CPVT (166). Functional assessment in a CASQ2 mutant confirms abnormal calcium release from the SR underlying CPVT mutations (167). Experimental studies simulating adrenergic stimulation in the setting of abnormal calcium release reveal epicardial origin of ectopic beats increasing transmural dispersion of repolarization, providing the substrate for catecholaminergic VT. Furthermore, bidirectional VT results as a consequence of alternation in the origin of ectopic activity between endocardial and epicardial regions (168).

Management

Beta-blockers, often in high doses, and restriction from vigorous exercise and competitive sports should be recommended for all patients with CPVT. Immediate family members should be screened with 12-lead ECG and exercise testing. The efficacy of beta-blockers to prevent sudden death in CPVT has been variable, suggesting that a defibrillator may be required in ≤30% who are resistant to beta-blocker therapy (157,158). Calcium channel blockers in combination with beta-blockers have demonstrated partial efficacy in a few cases, whereas sodium channel blockers may contribute to mortality (159).

Brugada Syndrome

The syndrome of ST elevation in the right precordial leads associated with a risk of ventricular arrhythmias and sudden death, now termed Brugada syndrome, is attributed to Brugada and Brugada from their description in 1992 (169). The characteristic ECG was published in 1953 by Osher and Wolff (170) and associated with a risk for sudden death by Martini et al. in 1989 (171). With improved recognition of the syndrome, it is now apparent that some sudden infant death syndrome (SIDS) cases are due to Brugada syndrome (172,173).

Electrocardiographic Features

The typical electrocardiographic findings in Brugada syndrome consist of J-point elevation and downsloping ST-segment elevation in the right precordial leads (Fig. 14.24). Atypical cases with repolarization abnormalities evident in the inferior and lateral leads have been reported (172,174). The ECG findings are dynamic and may be concealed, but can be unmasked by sodium channel blocking drugs such as flecainide, ajmaline, or procainamide (175). Superior placement of the right precordial leads may increase the sensitivity of the ECG in detecting the Brugada pattern (176). In contrast to most forms of LQTS and CPVT, cardiac events in Brugada syndrome occur during rest or sleep, similar to LQT3.

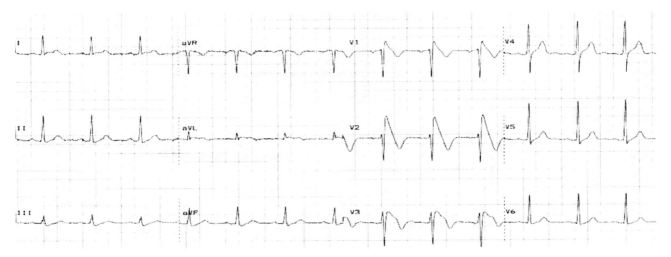

FIGURE 14.24 Brugada's syndrome. This ECG from a 10-year-old boy with Brugada syndrome shows the typical downsloping ST-segment elevation in the right precordial leads.

Etiology

To date, only one Brugada syndrome gene has been identified, *SCN5A*, the same gene underlying LQT3 (177), but most patients with Brugada syndrome do not have identified *SCN5A* mutations, suggesting that other genes are also important. Brugada syndrome *SCN5A* mutations result in reduced sodium current, as opposed to augmented late sodium current in LQT3. Experimental studies have revealed loss of sodium current leaves the transient outward current (Ito) unopposed, resulting in the characteristic ECG as well as an increased risk for ventricular tachycardia and fibrillation (178). Interestingly, fever has been reported to unmask the ECG findings and elicit storms of ventricular tachycardia in Brugada syndrome (179). Correspondingly, some mutations have temperature-dependent functional consequences (180).

Management

Although quinidine, likely by blocking Ito, has some protective effects (181), the only proven effective therapy for Brugada syndrome is an ICD (182). Patients with Brugada syndrome and a history of syncope or aborted cardiac arrest warrant ICD implantation. Patients who are asymptomatic, and who require drug challenge to elicit the ECG abnormalities, are felt to be at sufficiently low risk. Those with no symptoms but a spontaneously abnormal ECG are at intermediate risk. The use of electrophysiology study with programmed stimulation to assess the inducibility of ventricular fibrillation is controversial but endorsed by some for those at intermediate risk (183). Patients who receive an ICD should undergo electrophysiology study to assess for supraventricular tachycardias, as these are commonly associated with Brugada syndrome. Restriction from exercise does not seem warranted, as the risk for cardiac events is highest during rest or sleep.

Arrhythmogenic Right Ventricular Dysplasia/Cardiomyopathy

Arrhythmogenic right ventricular dysplasia/cardiomyopathy (ARVD/C) is a genetic cardiomyopathy characterized by ventricular arrhythmias and structural abnormalities of the right ventricle, resulting from progressive fibrofatty infiltration of the right ventricular myocardium (184). It may be a relatively common cause of ventricular tachycardia in young patients with previously unrecognized heart disease, and accounts for up to 10% of unexpected sudden death (185), although its prevalence may vary by geographic location (186). The diagnosis of ARVD/C is based on clinical criteria including structural abnormalities, tissue characterization, abnormalities in depolarization or repolarization, arrhythmias, and family history (187). These criteria are often subjective and may be too stringent, especially for family members of patients with known ARVD/C (188).

Electrocardiographic Features

Because the tachycardia arises in the right ventricle, a left bundle branch block QRS pattern is most common during tachycardia. However, most patients have multiple QRS morphologies during tachycardia induced at electrophysiology study. Some patients experience exercise-induced tachycardia or incessant tachycardia similar to idiopathic RV outflow tachycardia. T-wave inversion over the right precordial leads during sinus rhythm is present in 87% of patients with ARVD/C but only 3% of healthy subjects aged 19 to 45 years (189). This criterion is less helpful among pediatric patients in whom such a finding is normal. Undulations in the ST segment, the so-called epsilon waves, are postexcitation low-amplitude potentials that constitute a major criterion for diagnosis (Fig. 14.25). Other ECG abnormalities include localized widening of the QRS complex in the right precordial leads and prolonged S-wave upstroke in V_1 through V_3, which is seen in 95% of patients and correlates with disease severity (190).

Etiology

Familial occurrence of ARVD/C is well recognized, most commonly with autosomal dominant inheritance. Genetic heterogeneity has been firmly established, and linkage analysis has been used to define nine distinct genetic loci. To date, three genes have been identified in autosomal dominant ARVD/C: the cardiac ryanodine receptor (*RYR2*) in ARVD/C2 (191), desmoplakin (*DSP*) in ARVD/C8 (192), and plakophilin-2

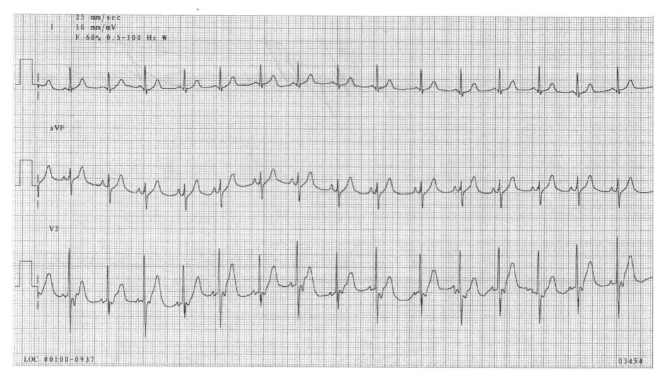

FIGURE 14.25 Epsilon waves in arrhythmogenic right ventricular cardiomyopathy. This rhythm strip was taken from an 8-year-old boy with chest pain and palpitations. High-frequency potentials are observed after the QRS complex in the ST segment in lead V2, consistent with delayed depolarization of myocytes in the right ventricle.

(*PKP2*) in ARVD/C9 (193). ARVD/C2 is a rare and atypical form, with only mild structural abnormalities and a characteristic bidirectional VT very similar to CPVT. It is still unclear whether such patients fulfil the diagnostic criteria for ARVD/C. Plakophilin-2 mutations are likely the major cause of familial ARVD/C. One form of ARVD/C, inherited in an autosomal recessive fashion, is associated with wooly hair and palmoplantar keratoderma (Naxos disease) and caused by mutations in plakoglobin (JUP) (194). Three of the four identified genes encode key components of the desmosome protein complexes that provide structural and functional integrity to adjacent cells, suggesting that ARVD/C is a disease of the desmosome.

Management

Management is problematic in patients with ARVD/C. Patients simultaneously may be at risk for lethal arrhythmias, yet experience frequent, short episodes of minimally symptomatic arrhythmias. Patients with ARVD/C who have a history of aborted sudden cardiac death or sustained ventricular tachycardia warrant placement of an ICD. Otherwise, there currently is little information available to help guide which patients merit placement of a prophylactic ICD. In the absence of firm guidelines, several clinical features have been proposed as markers of an increased risk of sudden death, including disease severity, history of syncope, family history of sudden death, and inducible ventricular tachycardia on electrophysiologic testing. In the United States, most patients who meet Task Force criteria for diagnosis undergo placement of an ICD. Adjunctive medical or attempted ablation therapy often is necessary to limit the frequency of discharges, especially for minimally symptomatic

arrhythmias. Although response to beta-blockers is variable, they generally are recommended as first-line therapy (184). Among other antiarrhythmic agents, sotalol has appeared particularly promising. Among nonmedical therapies, surgical ablation may be only temporarily effective. Likewise, catheter ablation techniques, despite promising early results, remain unproven as long-term therapy in this condition. Complete electrical disarticulation of the right ventricle has been described for patients with diffuse right ventricular involvement (195). However, recurrences occur frequently, particularly when disease extends beyond the right ventricular free wall.

Hypertrophic Cardiomyopathy

Hypertrophic cardiomyopathy (HCM) represents a genetically diverse group of disorders associated with various cardiac arrhythmias. It is an important cause of sudden death in children and adolescents. Indeed, the reported incidence of sudden death among this age group is 2% to 4% per year, compared with 1% in adults with HCM. It is a leading cause of sudden death in young athletes (196). This condition is discussed in detail in Chapter 56.

Electrocardiographic Features

ECG findings include repolarization abnormalities, left atrial enlargement, or pathologic Q waves. Giant negative T waves in the midprecordial leads occur in the apical variant of HCM, with hypertrophy confined to the distal left ventricle, a common variant in Japan. Both accelerated AV conduction and AV block may be observed. Wolff–Parkinson–White syndrome may be observed, but a short PR interval and slurred QRS upstroke also may occur as the result of accelerated AV node conduction with associated incomplete left bundle branch block. Mutations in PRKAG2 underlie a specific phenotype consisting of hypertrophic cardiomyopathy, Wolff–Parkinson–White syndrome (WPW), premature conduction disease, and the presence of glycogen vacuoles in myocytes (53). Supraventricular tachycardias including atrial fibrillation and flutter, ventricular tachycardia, and ventricular fibrillation are observed. Nonsustained VT is infrequent in children, but is a an important risk factor for sudden death in young patients with HCM (42).

Management

It is important to recognize that treatment strategies for relief of left ventricular outflow obstruction and associated symptoms such as exercise and chest pain are completely independent of arrhythmia management in HCM. Patients with symptoms suggestive of arrhythmias such as palpitations, syncope, or presenting with sustained supraventricular arrhythmias should have comprehensive invasive electrophysiology testing, as should patients with associated WPW. Survivors of cardiac arrest should have implantation of an ICD (197). The details of arrhythmia management in HCM are beyond the scope of this chapter and have been reviewed elsewhere (198).

Hypertrophic cardiomyopathy also represents one of the few pediatric indications for ICD implantation as primary prevention in minimally symptomatic individuals. Aside from previous cardiac arrest, the highest risk factors include a history of syncope, family history of sudden death owing to HCM, abnormal blood pressure response to exercise, nonsustained ventricular tachycardia (NSVT) during Holter monitoring, and septal thickness >3 cm. Intracardiac electrophysiology study does not appear to provide additional prognostic information in addition to these risk factors (199). Asymptomatic patients with no risk factors are at low risk, whereas those with two or more risk factors carry a 3% per year risk of sudden death and warrant ICD implantation. Those with one risk factor are at intermediate risk, and decisions regarding ICD implantation should be individualized. There are important differences between children and adults with HCM that alter the above scheme for risk stratification (200). A history of unexplained syncope is an independent predictor of risk in all ages, particularly in children, in whom other potential causes for syncope (atrial fibrillation) are less prevalent. Furthermore, 20% of adults with HCM have NSVT on Holter monitoring, and the absence of NSVT is particularly reassuring, with a negative-predictive value of 97%. In children and adolescents with HCM, NSVT is infrequent, limiting its utility and providing little reassurance with its absence. If detected, however, it is a particularly ominous finding, with an eightfold increase in risk. It has been recommended, therefore, that the finding of NSVT alone in children or adolescents with HCM is sufficient to warrant therapy with an ICD. As most sudden deaths in HCM occur during or shortly after exertion, patients should be restricted from vigorous exercise and competitive sports.

Ventricular Tachycardia Associated with Congenital Heart Disease

Since the initial association of ventricular arrhythmias and cardiac arrest in survivors of congenital heart disease surgery, there has been considerable interest in these rhythm disturbances in postoperative patients. The risk of sudden death following CHD surgery is greatest in double-outlet right ventricle/ tetralogy of Fallot, complete transposition of the great arteries palliated with Mustard or Senning repairs, and left-sided obstructive lesions (201). However, patients with tetralogy of Fallot seem to be particularly prone to develop sustained, monomorphic ventricular tachycardia and make up a large portion of the population with repaired congenital heart disease, thus serving as the prototype for ventricular tachycardia following surgery for congenital heart disease. Some of the features are analogous to those following healed myocardial infarction.

Electrocardiographic Features

Patients with congenital heart disease may present with various ventricular rhythm disturbances. Some of these may be detected during routine evaluation, whereas others come to attention during evaluation for palpitations, presyncope, or syncope. Occasionally, tachycardias may be induced at electrophysiology study in an effort to explain possible arrhythmia-related symptoms or as part of an investigational protocol being used to evaluate these patients (Fig. 14.1). Sustained spontaneous tachycardia is relatively uncommon among these patients, but when present, it usually originates from the right ventricle and produces a left bundle branch block QRS configuration. This helps distinguish the ventricular tachycardia from a supraventricular tachycardia with aberrant conduction, which usually produces a right bundle branch block QRS configuration in this population with perioperative injury damage to right ventricular conduction.

Etiology

Most ventricular tachycardias in postoperative tetralogy of Fallot patients are monomorphic and macrore-entrant, often in the areas of surgical scar in the right ventricular outflow tract or conal septum. There is also evidence that chronic volume or pressure overload, sometimes associated with previous cyanosis, lead to areas of myocardial fibrosis that may serve as a substrate for ventricular tachycardias. Although ventricular arrhythmias appear to be the most likely precursor to sudden death, the terminal arrhythmia is usually undetermined in sudden death victims. Thus, whether these individuals experience primarily ventricular fibrillation, polymorphic ventricular tachycardia, rapid monomorphic ventricular tachycardia that impairs cardiac output, a supraventricular arrhythmia that degenerates to ventricular fibrillation, or, possibly in some cases, a lethal bradycardia cannot be ascertained except when an event is captured and stored in an ICD.

Management

Acute treatment of sustained ventricular tachycardias is determined in part by the patient's clinical status and the type of tachycardia recognized (i.e., polymorphic vs. monomorphic). Because of the frequent misdiagnosis as supraventricular tachycardia with aberrant conduction, appropriate recognition is essential. When possible, a 12-lead ECG prior to treatment is useful for determining QRS duration, morphology, and axis. If possible, the VA relationship should be ascertained, often by transesophageal recording, which may facilitate its determination. However, if the patient is compromised, immediate DC cardioversion is indicated whether a supraventricular or ventricular mechanism seems more likely. Occasionally, if the clinical situation and available expertise permit, temporary ventricular pacing may be used to acutely terminate the rhythm. Likewise, loading with intravenous lidocaine, amiodarone, or procainamide may be cautiously attempted with careful monitoring, but only in the most stable patients.

The choices of chronic therapy for ventricular tachycardia include antiarrhythmic drug therapy, ICD implantation, further operative intervention to improve hemodynamics, or ablation of the arrhythmia. Each approach has its relative shortcomings, which include potential for arrhythmia recurrence despite antiarrhythmic drug or ablation therapies and the associated risk of surgical revision. Catheter ablation for monomorphic, hemodynamically stable VT in postoperative patients can be performed with good acute results (Fig. 14.26), but the risk of recurrent tachycardia is unknown (202). Technological

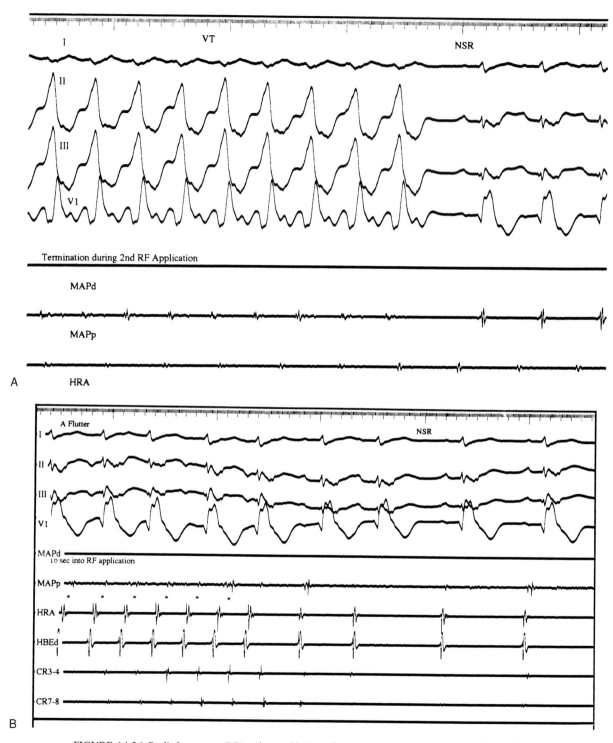

FIGURE 14.26 Radiofrequency (RF) catheter ablation of macrore-entrant ventricular tachycardia in a 34-year-old man with previously repaired tetralogy of Fallot (**A**). The patient presented with syncope owing to sustained ventricular tachycardia. He had also experienced previous atrial flutter, and type I atrial flutter was induced and ablated at the same session (**B**). VT, ventricular tachycardia; NSR, normal sinus rhythm; MAPd, distal mapping catheter; MAPp, proximal mapping catheter; HRA, high right atrium; HBEd, distal His-bundle electrogram; CR3-4, distal crista catheter; CR7-8, proximal crista catheter.

advances such as electroanatomic mapping systems to aid in localizing target sites, as well as irrigated-tip catheters to produce deep, transmural lesions may improve the success of catheter ablation for VT.

The ability to adequately risk stratify patients with repaired congenital heart disease has remained elusive. Many factors have been associated with increased risk for sudden death, such as older age of repair and QRS duration as a measure of ventricular enlargement, but there are few quantitative factors with adequate predictive value (203). Even a history of syncope may not be as predictive as one might imagine, since neurocardiogenic syncope has clearly been observed in this population, and supraventricular tachycardias are more prevalent than ventricular tachycardias (204). Electrophysiology study with programmed ventricular stimulation has been shown to provide prognostic information, and the finding of inducible polymorphic VT, often interpreted as a nonspecific finding, has also been correlated with future VT and sudden death (43).

Prognosis

The prognosis of sustained ventricular tachycardia or prior cardiac arrest may depend on the underlying diagnosis. In otherwise well-palliated congenital heart disease, substantially increased survival may be expected with appropriate therapy (ICD implantation). In patients with certain cardiomyopathies (dilated and hypertrophic), sudden death mortality can be decreased with ICD implantation, but overall survival may not be affected because of increased mortality from nonsudden cardiac events. The cumulative risk, in tetralogy of Fallot and in congenital heart disease collectively, may be lower than previously assumed. Still, the inability to prospectively identify patients at risk remains an issue of frustration and concern.

Miscellaneous Ventricular Tachycardia in Ostensibly Normal Patients

Despite the prevalence of underlying heart disease among patients with ventricular tachycardias, rarely, patients without any identifiable heart disease present with fairly well-tolerated ventricular tachycardias. Two distinct forms have been described that are differentiated by clinical and ECG features: Fascicular ventricular tachycardia and right ventricular outflow tract tachycardia.

Electrocardiographic Features

Recurrent sustained ventricular tachycardia with right bundle branch block pattern and left-axis deviation, commonly referred to as fascicular ventricular tachycardia or verapamil-sensitive ventricular tachycardia, was recognized in 1979 by Zipes et al. (205), who described the characteristic diagnostic triad: Induction with atrial pacing, right bundle branch block (RBBB) and left-axis deviation, and manifestation in patients without structural heart disease. In 1981, Belhassen et al. (206) demonstrated the fourth feature: Verapamil sensitivity of the tachycardia. This tachycardia frequently is misdiagnosed as SVT with aberrancy because of its paroxysmal nature, characteristically mild symptoms, relatively narrow QRS, and termination with intravenous verapamil. Although VA dissociation may not be readily evident from the surface ECG, the diagnosis must be suspected when QRS morphology of right bundle branch block with left-axis deviation is present during tachycardia in a seemingly normal individual (Fig. 14.27). In addition to the commonly observed left posterior fascicular VT, with its characteristic RBBB/LAD pattern, two

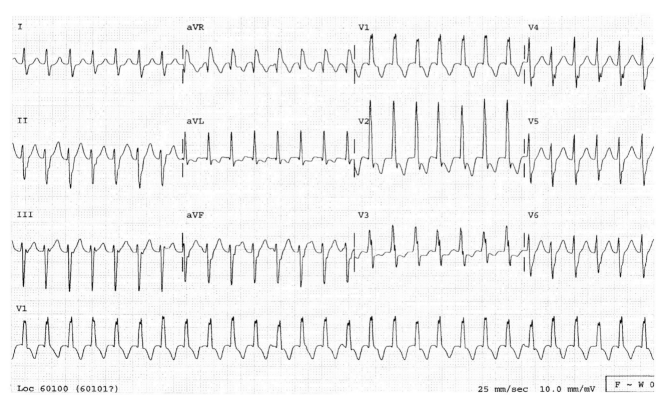

FIGURE 14.27 Idiopathic ventricular tachycardia with characteristic right bundle branch block and left-axis deviation in a 12-year-old girl with syncope and palpitations. Tachycardia was mapped and ablated at the site of pre-systolic fascicular potentials in the left posterior fascicular region of the left ventricular septum.

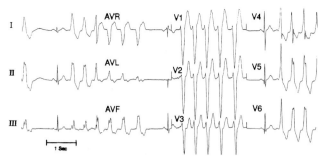

FIGURE 14.28 Idiopathic right ventricular outflow tract tachycardia (also referred to as repetitive monomorphic ventricular tachycardia). Tachycardia is characterized by an inferior QRS axis, incessant behavior, an absence of other causes (myocarditis, arrhythmogenic right ventricular cardiomyopathy [ARVC]), and suppression with verapamil and beta-blocker therapy. Intracardiac mapping confirmed that the origin was in the RV outflow tract.

uncommon forms have been observed: Left anterior fascicular VT with a RBBB/RAD pattern and the rare left upper septal fascicular VT with a narrow QRS and normal axis (207).

Tachycardia originating from the right ventricular outflow tract (RVOT VT) has ECG resemblance to tachycardia seen in ARVC/D. However, unlike the latter, it tends to occur in a repetitive, self-limited fashion with only a single morphology (Fig. 14.28). Episodes are typically interrupted by relatively brief periods of sinus rhythm, in contrast to tachycardia with ARVC/D, which is more frequently sustained and is likely to require DC cardioversion. The electrocardiographic and clinical features of right ventricular outflow tachycardia (also referred to as repetitive monomorphic ventricular tachycardia) have been well characterized. Unlike monomorphic ventricular tachycardias owing to re-entry, RVOT VT is usually not inducible with programmed extrastimuli but can be induced with long sustained burst pacing, often in combination with adrenergic stimulation. Likewise, it can often be provoked during exercise testing.

Etiology

These tachycardias may be suspected from the clinical features, but electrophysiology study is often necessary to confirm their diagnoses and to demonstrate the characteristic features of each. Although sometimes mistaken for SVT, fascicular tachycardia usually can be induced and terminated with pacing from either the atrium or the ventricle, it is not associated with pre-excitation, and early retrograde His deflections during tachycardia may be evident during tachycardia in the presence of VA conduction. The mechanism of this tachycardia appears to be re-entry using portions of the left posterior fascicle. The presence of a false tendon or fibromuscular band from the posteroinferior left ventricle to the septum in many patients with fascicular VT has suggested its role in the pathogenesis of this arrhythmia (208). However, false tendons and muscular bands in the left ventricle are not specific to patients with fascicular VT (209). This tachycardia only occasionally is observed in the first decade, then becomes increasingly prevalent in teenagers and young adults. Whether this tachycardia results from a congenital anomaly of the conduction system or occurs during postnatal development is not known.

As the name implies, the cause of idiopathic RV outflow tachycardia also remains uncertain, although embryologic migration of cells with pacemaker properties is touted as a potential cause. Somatic point mutations in the cAMP signaling cascade localized to the myocardium from the outflow tract have also been suggested (210). Variants of this arrhythmia with origins from the LV outflow tract and the RV free wall have been increasingly recognized. Anatomically, these foci lie adjacent to the most common RVOT origins, and they appear to represent a single clinical entity. The lack of reproducible induction with pacing and the catecholamine-responsive nature of RVOT suggests an automatic or triggered mechanism rather than re-entry.

Management

Fascicular tachycardia and right ventricular outflow tract tachycardia usually are well tolerated compared with other ventricular tachycardias and characteristically responsive to medical therapy. The therapeutic approach can usually be adjusted accordingly, with suppression of symptomatic or sustained recurrences (as in the patient with SVTs) as representing an adequate end point. Fascicular tachycardia generally is sensitive to verapamil, and RVOT VT is sensitive to beta-blockers and calcium channel blockers. Both are also amenable to catheter ablation, reflecting the localized nature of the underlying tissue substrate. Fascicular potentials frequently are recorded at the successful ablation site of fascicular VT. Neither of these tachycardias appear to be related to significant underlying heart disease, and the prognosis appears to be generally good.

References

1. Southall DP, Richards J, Mitchell P, et al. Study of cardiac rhythm in healthy newborn infants. *Br Heart J* 1980;43:14–20.
2. Nagashima M, Matsushima M, Ogawa A, et al. Cardiac arrhythmias in healthy children revealed by 24-hour ambulatory ECG monitoring. *Pediatr Cardiol* 1987;8:103–108.
3. Scagliotti D, Kumar SP, Williamson GD. Ventricular rhythm with intermediate rate in the neonate without heart disease. *Clin Perinatol* 1988;15:609–618.
4. Pongiglione G, Saul JP, Dunnigan A, et al. Role of transesophageal pacing in evaluation of palpitations in children and adolescents. *Am J Cardiol* 1988;62:566–570.
5. Kannankeril PJ, Bibeau DA, Fish FA. Feasibility of the inframammary location for insertable loop recorders in young women and girls. *Pacing Clin Electrophysiol* 2004;27:492–494.
6. Stanton M. Class I antiarrhythmic drugs: Quinidine, procainamide, disopyramide, lidocaine, mexiletine, tocainide, phenytoin, moricizine, flecainide, propafenone. In: Zipes D, Jalife J, eds. *Cardiac Electrophysiology: From Cell to Bedside.* Philadelphia: WB Saunders, 2000:890–901.
7. Benson DW Jr, Dunnigan A, Benditt DG, et al. Prediction of digoxin treatment failure in infants with supraventricular tachycardia: Role of transesophageal pacing. *Pediatrics* 1985;75:288–293.
8. Benson DW Jr, Dunnigan A, Benditt DG. Follow-up evaluation of infant paroxysmal atrial tachycardia: Transesophageal study. *Circulation* 1987;75:542–549.
9. Camm AJ, Garratt CJ. Adenosine and supraventricular tachycardia. *N Engl J Med* 1991;325:1621–1629.
10. Sliz NB Jr, Johns JA. Cardiac pacing in infants and children. *Cardiol Rev* 2000;8:223–239.
11. Stephenson EA, Casavant D, Tuzi J, et al. Efficacy of atrial antitachycardia pacing using the Medtronic AT500 pacemaker in patients with congenital heart disease. *Am J Cardiol* 2003;92:871–876.
12. Gregoratos G, Abrams J, Epstein AE, et al. ACC/AHA/NASPE 2002 guideline update for implantation of cardiac pacemakers and antiarrhythmia devices: Summary article: A report of the American College of Cardiology/American Heart Association Task Force on Practice Guidelines (ACC/AHA/NASPE Committee to Update the 1998 Pacemaker Guidelines). *Circulation* 2002;106:2145–2161.

13. Stephenson EA, Batra AS, Knilans TK, et al. A multicenter experience with novel implantable cardioverter defibrillator configurations in the pediatric and congenital heart disease population. *J Cardiovasc Electrophysiol* 2006;17:41–46.

14. Dubin AM, Janousek J, Rhee E, et al. Resynchronization therapy in pediatric and congenital heart disease patients: An international multicenter study. *J Am Coll Cardiol* 2005;46:2277–2283.

15. Villain E, Lucet V, Do Nqoc ND, et al. Cardiac pacing in children with breath-holding spells [in French]. *Arch Mal Coeur Vaiss* 2000;93:547–552.

16. Rosen KM, Mehta A, Rahimtoola SH, et al. Sites of congenital and surgical AV block as defined by His bundle electrocardiography. *Circulation* 1971;44:833–841.

17. Lev M. Pathogenesis of congenital atrioventricular block. *Prog Cardiovasc Dis* 1972;15:145–157.

18. Basson CT, Bachinsky DR, Lin RC, et al. Mutations in human TBX5 [corrected] cause limb and cardiac malformation in Holt-Oram syndrome. *Nat Genet* 1997;15:30–35.

19. Li QY, Newbury-Ecob RA, Terrett JA, et al. Holt-Oram syndrome is caused by mutations in TBX5, a member of the Brachyury (T) gene family. *Nat Genet* 1997;15:21–29.

20. Schott JJ, Benson DW, Basson CT, et al. Congenital heart disease caused by mutations in the transcription factor NKX2-5. *Science* 1998;281:108–111.

21. Buyon JP, Hiebert R, Copel J, et al. Autoimmune-associated congenital AV block: Demographics, mortality, morbidity and recurrence rates obtained from a national neonatal lupus registry. *J Am Coll Cardiol* 1998;31: 1658–1666.

22. Scott WA, Dick M. Two:one atrioventricular block in infants with congenital long QT syndrome. *Am J Cardiol* 1987;60:1409–1410.

23. Van Hare GF, Franz MR, Roge C, et al. Persistent functional atrioventricular block in two patients with prolonged QT intervals: Elucidation of the mechanism of block. *Pacing Clin Electrophysiol* 1990;13:608–618.

24. Dickey RP, Ziter FA, Smith RA. Emery-Dreifuss muscular dystrophy. *J Pediatr* 1984;104:555–559.

25. Gallastegui J, Hariman RJ, Handler B, et al. Cardiac involvement in the Kearns-Sayre syndrome. *Am J Cardiol* 1987;60:385–388.

26. Stevenson WG, Perloff JK, Weiss JN, et al. Facioscapulohumeral muscular dystrophy: Evidence for selective, genetic electrophysiologic cardiac involvement. *J Am Coll Cardiol* 1990;15:292–299.

27. Anan R, Nakagawa M, Miyata M, et al. Cardiac involvement in mitochondrial diseases. A study on 17 patients with documented mitochondrial DNA defects. *Circulation* 1995;91:955–961.

28. Kerr DS. Protean manifestations of mitochondrial diseases: A minireview. *J Pediatr Hematol Oncol* 1997;19:279–286.

29. Kass S, MacRae C, Graber HL, et al. A gene defect that causes conduction system disease and dilated cardiomyopathy maps to chromosome 1p1-1q1. *Nat Genet* 1994;7:546–551.

30. Brink PA, Ferreira A, Moolman JC, et al. Gene for progressive familial AV block type I maps to chromosome 19q13. *Circulation* 1995;91:1633–1640.

31. DiNubile MJ, Calderwood SB, Steinhaus DM, et al. Cardiac conduction abnormalities complicating native valve active infective endocarditis. *Am J Cardiol* 1986;58:1213–1217.

32. Pinto DS. Cardiac manifestations of Lyme disease. *Med Clin North Am* 2002;86:285–296.

33. Michaelsson M, Riesenfeld T, Jonzon A. Natural history of congenital complete atrioventricular block. *Pacing Clin Electrophysiol* 1997;20: 2098–2101.

34. Li Z, Strasburger JF, Cuneo BF, et al. Giant fetal magnetocardiogram P waves in congenital atrioventricular block: A marker of cardiovascular compensation? *Circulation* 2004;110:2097–2101.

35. Ho SY, Anderson RH. Embryology and anatomy of the conduction system. In: Gilette PC, Garson A Jr, eds. *Pediatric Arrhythmias: Pacing and Electrophysiology*. Philadelphia: WB Saunders, 1990:2–27.

36. Bharati S, Lev M, Kirklin J. The anatomy of the normal human conduction system: Cardiac surgery and the conduction system. 2 ed. Mt. Kisco, NY: Futura Publishing, 1992.

37. Yabek SM. Ventricular arrhythmias in children with an apparently normal heart. *J Pediatr* 1991;119:1–11.

38. Kennedy HL, Whitlock JA, Sprague MK, et al. Long-term follow-up of asymptomatic healthy subjects with frequent and complex ventricular ectopy. *N Engl J Med* 1985;312:193–197.

39. Wiles HB, Gillette PC, Harley RA, et al. Cardiomyopathy and myocarditis in children with ventricular ectopic rhythm. *J Am Coll Cardiol* 1992;20:359–362.

40. Paul T, Marchal C, Garson A Jr. Ventricular couplets in the young: Prognosis related to underlying substrate. *Am Heart J* 1990;119:577–582.

41. Muller G, Ulmer HE, Hagel KJ, et al. Cardiac dysrhythmias in children with idiopathic dilated or hypertrophic cardiomyopathy. *Pediatr Cardiol* 1995;16:56–60.

42. Monserrat L, Elliott PM, Gimeno JR, et al. Non-sustained ventricular tachycardia in hypertrophic cardiomyopathy: An independent marker of sudden death risk in young patients. *J Am Coll Cardiol* 2003;42: 873–879.

43. Khairy P, Landzberg MJ, Gatzoulis MA, et al. Value of programmed ventricular stimulation after tetralogy of Fallot repair: A multicenter study. *Circulation* 2004;109:1994–2000.

44. Echt DS, Liebson PR, Mitchell LB, et al. Mortality and morbidity in patients receiving encainide, flecainide, or placebo. The Cardiac Arrhythmia Suppression Trial. *N Engl J Med* 1991;324:781–788.

45. Ko JK, Deal BJ, Strasburger JF, et al. Supraventricular tachycardia mechanisms and their age distribution in pediatric patients. *Am J Cardiol* 1992;69:1028–1032.

46. Kwaku KF, Josephson ME. Typical AVNRT-an update on mechanisms and therapy. *Card Electrophysiol Rev.* 2002;6:414–421.

47. Paul T, Guccione P, Garson A Jr. Relation of syncope in young patients with Wolff-Parkinson-White syndrome to rapid ventricular response during atrial fibrillation. *Am J Cardiol* 1990;65:318–321.

48. Leitch JW, Klein GJ, Yee R, et al. Syncope associated with supraventricular tachycardia. An expression of tachycardia rate or vasomotor response? *Circulation* 1992;85:1064–1071.

49. Burchell H. Introduction. In: Benditt DG, Benson DW, eds. *Cardiac Preexcitation Syndromes: Origins, Evaluation and Treatment*. Hingham, MA: Martinus Nijhoff, 1986:3–19.

50. Van Hare GF, Phoon CK, Munkenbeck F, et al. Electrophysiologic study and radiofrequency ablation in patients with intracardiac tumors and accessory pathways: Is the tumor the pathway? *J Cardiovasc Electrophysiol* 1996;7:1204–1210.

51. Munger TM, Packer DL, Hammill SC, et al. A population study of the natural history of Wolff-Parkinson-White syndrome in Olmsted County, Minnesota, 1953–1989. *Circulation* 1993;87:866–873.

52. Porter CJ, Holmes DR. Preexcitation syndromes associated with congenital heart disease. In: Benditt DG, Benson DW Jr, eds. *Cardiac Preexcitation Syndromes: Origins, Evaluation and Treatment*. Hingham, MA: Martinus Nijhoff, 1986:289–302.

53. Gollob MH, Green MS, Tang AS, et al. Identification of a gene responsible for familial Wolff-Parkinson-White syndrome. *N Engl J Med* 2001;344: 1823–1831.

54. Dunnigan A. Developmental aspects and natural history of preexcitation syndromes. In: Benditt DG, Benson DW, eds. *Cardiac Preexcitation Syndromes: Origins, Evaluation and Treatment*. Hingham, MA: Martinus Nijhoff, 1986:21–29.

55. Yee R, Klein GJ, Prystowski E. The Wolff-Parkinson-White Syndrome and related variants. In: Zipes D, Jalife J, eds. *Cardiac Electrophysiology: From Cell to Bedside*. Philadelphia: WB Saunders, 2000:845–861.

56. Perry JC, Garson A Jr. Supraventricular tachycardia due to Wolff-Parkinson-White syndrome in children: Early disappearance and late recurrence. *J Am Coll Cardiol* 1990;16:1215–1220.

57. Klein GJ, Yee R, Sharma AD. Longitudinal electrophysiological assessment of asymptomatic patients with the Wolff-Parkinson-White electrocardiographic pattern. *N Engl J Med* 1989;320:1229–1233.

58. Roark SF, McCarthy EA, Lee KL, et al. Observations on the occurrence of atrial fibrillation in paroxysmal supraventricular tachycardia. *Am J Cardiol* 1986;57:571–575.

59. Gulamhusein S, Ko P, Carruthers SG, et al. Acceleration of the ventricular response during atrial fibrillation in the Wolff-Parkinson-White syndrome after verapamil. *Circulation* 1982;65:348–354.

60. Deal BJ, Keane JF, Gillette PC, et al. Wolff-Parkinson-White syndrome and supraventricular tachycardia during infancy: Management and follow-up. *J Am Coll Cardiol* 1985;5:130–135.

61. Pappone C, Manguso F, Santinelli R, et al. Radiofrequency ablation in children with asymptomatic Wolff-Parkinson-White syndrome. *N Engl J Med* 2004;351:1197–1205.

62. Blomstrom-Lundqvist C, Scheinman MM, Aliot EM, et al. ACC/AHA/ESC guidelines for the management of patients with supraventricular arrhythmias—executive summary: A report of the American College of Cardiology/American Heart Association Task Force on Practice Guidelines and the European Society of Cardiology Committee for Practice Guidelines (Writing Committee to Develop Guidelines for the Management of Patients With Supraventricular Arrhythmias). *Circulation* 2003;108:1871–1909.

63. Saoudi N, Cosio F, Waldo A, et al. Classification of atrial flutter and regular atrial tachycardia according to electrophysiologic mechanism and anatomic bases: A statement from a joint expert group from the Working Group of Arrhythmias of the European Society of Cardiology and the North American Society of Pacing and Electrophysiology. *J Cardiovasc Electrophysiol* 2001;12:852–866.

64. Klein GJ, Guiraudon GM, Sharma AD, et al. Demonstration of macroreentry and feasibility of operative therapy in the common type of atrial flutter. *Am J Cardiol* 1986;57:587–591.

65. Olshansky B, Okumura K, Hess PG, et al. Demonstration of an area of slow conduction in human atrial flutter. *J Am Coll Cardiol* 1990; 16:1639–1648.

66. Feld GK, Fleck RP, Chen PS, et al. Radiofrequency catheter ablation for the treatment of human type 1 atrial flutter. Identification of a critical zone in the reentrant circuit by endocardial mapping techniques. *Circulation* 1992;86:1233–1240.

67. Muller GI, Deal BJ, Strasburger JF, et al. Electrocardiographic features of atrial tachycardias after operation for congenital heart disease. *Am J Cardiol* 1993;71:122–124.

68. Dunnigan A, Benson W Jr, Benditt DG. Atrial flutter in infancy: Diagnosis, clinical features, and treatment. *Pediatrics* 1985;75:725–729.

69. Prystowsky EN, Benson DW Jr, Fuster V, et al. Management of patients with atrial fibrillation. A statement for healthcare professionals. From the Subcommittee on Electrocardiography and Electrophysiology, American Heart Association. *Circulation* 1996;93:1262–1277.

70. Kanter RJ, Garson A Jr. Atrial arrhythmias during chronic follow-up of surgery for complex congenital heart disease. *Pacing Clin Electrophysiol* 1997;20:502–511.

71. Kannankeril PJ, Anderson ME, Rottman JN, et al. Frequency of late recurrence of intra-atrial reentry tachycardia after radiofrequency catheter ablation in patients with congenital heart disease. *Am J Cardiol* 2003;92:879–881.

72. Deal BJ, Mavroudis C, Backer CL, et al. Comparison of anatomic isthmus block with the modified right atrial maze procedure for late atrial tachycardia in Fontan patients. *Circulation* 2002;106:575–579.

73. Nanthakumar K, Lau YR, Plumb VJ, et al. Electrophysiological findings in adolescents with atrial fibrillation who have structurally normal hearts. *Circulation* 2004;110:117–123.

74. Frustaci A, Chimenti C, Bellocci F, et al. Histological substrate of atrial biopsies in patients with lone atrial fibrillation. *Circulation* 1997;96:1180–1184.

75. Janse MJ. Mechanisms of atrial fibrillation. In: Zipes D, Jalife J, eds. *Cardiac Electrophysiology: From Cell to Bedside.* Philadelphia: WB Saunders, 2000:476–481.

76. Wiesfeld AC, Hemels ME, Van Tintelen JP, et al. Genetic aspects of atrial fibrillation. *Cardiovasc Res* 2005;67:414–418.

77. Cox JL. Surgical treatment of atrial fibrillation: A review. *Europace* 2004;5(suppl 1):S20–S29.

78. Mehta AV, Sanchez GR, Sacks EJ, et al. Ectopic automatic atrial tachycardia in children: Clinical characteristics, management and follow-up. *J Am Coll Cardiol* 1988;11:379–385.

79. Walsh EP, Saul JP, Hulse JE, et al. Transcatheter ablation of ectopic atrial tachycardia in young patients using radiofrequency current. *Circulation* 1992;86:1138–1146.

80. Naheed ZJ, Strasburger JF, Benson DW Jr, et al. Natural history and management strategies of automatic atrial tachycardia in children. *Am J Cardiol* 1995;75:405–407.

81. Fish FA, Mehta AV, Johns JA. Characteristics and management of chaotic atrial tachycardia of infancy. *Am J Cardiol* 1996;78:1052–1055.

82. Yeager SB, Hougen TJ, Levy AM. Sudden death in infants with chaotic atrial rhythm. *Am J Dis Child* 1984;138:689–692.

83. Bradley DJ, Fischbach PS, Law IH, et al. The clinical course of multifocal atrial tachycardia in infants and children. *J Am Coll Cardiol* 2001;38:401–408.

84. Grant JW, Serwer GA, Armstrong BE, et al. Junctional tachycardia in infants and children after open heart surgery for congenital heart disease. *Am J Cardiol* 1987;59:1216–1218.

85. Villain E, Vetter VL, Garcia JM, et al. Evolving concepts in the management of congenital junctional ectopic tachycardia. A multicenter study. *Circulation* 1990;81:1544–1549.

86. Rossi L, Piffer R, Turolla E, et al. Multifocal Purkinje-like tumor of the heart. Occurrence with other anatomic abnormalities in the atrioventricular junction of an infant with junctional tachycardia, Lown-Ganong-Levine syndrome, and sudden death. *Chest* 1985;87:340–345.

87. Van Hare GF, Velvis H, Langberg JJ. Successful transcatheter ablation of congenital junctional ectopic tachycardia in a ten-month-old infant using radiofrequency energy. *Pacing Clin Electrophysiol* 1990;13:730–735.

88. Janousek J, Vojtovic P, Gebauer RA. Use of a modified, commercially available temporary pacemaker for R wave synchronized atrial pacing in postoperative junctional ectopic tachycardia. *Pacing Clin Electrophysiol* 2003;26:579–586.

89. Laird WP, Snyder CS, Kertesz NJ, et al. Use of intravenous amiodarone for postoperative junctional ectopic tachycardia in children. *Pediatr Cardiol* 2003;24:133–137.

90. Bronzetti G, Formigari R, Giardini A, et al. Intravenous flecainide for the treatment of junctional ectopic tachycardia after surgery for congenital heart disease. *Ann Thorac Surg* 2003;76:148–151.

91. Brugada P, Brugada J, Mont L, et al. A new approach to the differential diagnosis of a regular tachycardia with a wide QRS complex. *Circulation* 1991;83:1649–1659.

92. Kannankeril PJ, Fish FA. Management of common arrhythmias and conduction abnormalities. *Prog Pediatr Cardiol* 2003;17:41–52.

93. Garson A Jr, Smith RT Jr, Moak JP, et al. Incessant ventricular tachycardia in infants: Myocardial hamartomas and surgical cure. *J Am Coll Cardiol* 1987;10:619–626.

94. Bostan OM, Celiker A, Ozme S. Spontaneous resolution of ventricular tachycardia with right bundle branch block morphology: A case report. *Turk J Pediatr* 2003;45:170–173.

95. Moss AJ, Zareba W, Benhorin J, et al. ECG T-wave patterns in genetically distinct forms of the hereditary long QT syndrome. *Circulation* 1995;92:2929–2934.

96. Ackerman MJ, Khositseth A, Tester DJ, et al. Epinephrine-induced QT interval prolongation: A gene-specific paradoxical response in congenital long QT syndrome. *Mayo Clin Proc* 2002;77:413–421.

97. Walker BD, Krahn AD, Klein GJ, et al. Burst bicycle exercise facilitates diagnosis of latent long QT syndrome. *Am Heart J* 2005;150:1059–1063.

98. Schwartz PJ, Priori SG, Spazzolini C, et al. Genotype-phenotype correlation in the long-QT syndrome: Gene-specific triggers for life-threatening arrhythmias. *Circulation* 2001;103:89–95.

99. Jervell A, Lange-Nielsen F. Congenital deaf-mutism, functional heart disease with prolongation of the Q-T interval and sudden death. *Am Heart J* 1957;54:59–68.

100. Romano C, Gemme G, Pongiglione R. Rare cardiac arrhythmias of the pediatric age. II. Syncopal attacks due to paroxysmal ventricular fibrillation [in Italian]. (Presentation of 1st case in Italian pediatric literature.). *Clin Pediatr (Bologna)* 1963;45:656–683.

101. Ward OC. A new familial cardiac syndrome in children. *J Ir Med Assoc* 1964;54:103–106.

102. Schwartz PJ, Periti M, Malliani A. The long Q-T syndrome. *Am Heart J* 1975;89:378–390.

103. Moss AJ. Prolonged QT-interval syndromes. *JAMA* 1986;256:2985–2987.

104. Wang Q, Shen J, Splawski I, et al. SCN5A mutations associated with an inherited cardiac arrhythmia, long QT syndrome. *Cell* 1995;80:805–811.

105. Curran ME, Splawski I, Timothy KW, et al. A molecular basis for cardiac arrhythmia: HERG mutations cause long QT syndrome. *Cell* 1995;80:795–803.

106. Wang Q, Curran ME, Splawski I, et al. Positional cloning of a novel potassium channel gene: KVLQT1 mutations cause cardiac arrhythmias. *Nat Genet* 1996;12:17–23.

107. Tyson J, Tranebjaerg L, Bellman S, et al. IsK and KvLQT1: Mutation in either of the two subunits of the slow component of the delayed rectifier potassium channel can cause Jervell and Lange-Nielsen syndrome. *Hum Mol Genet* 1997;6:2179–2185.

108. Neyroud N, Tesson F, Denjoy I, et al. A novel mutation in the potassium channel gene KVLQT1 causes the Jervell and Lange-Nielsen cardioauditory syndrome. *Nat Genet* 1997;15:186–189.

109. Mohler PJ, Schott JJ, Gramolini AO, et al. Ankyrin-B mutation causes type 4 long-QT cardiac arrhythmia and sudden cardiac death. *Nature* 2003;421:634–639.

110. Mohler PJ, Splawski I, Napolitano C, et al. A cardiac arrhythmia syndrome caused by loss of ankyrin-B function. *Proc Natl Acad Sci USA* 2004;101:9137–9142.

111. Mohler PJ, Bennett V. Ankyrin-based cardiac arrhythmias: A new class of channelopathies due to loss of cellular targeting. *Curr Opin Cardiol* 2005;20:189–193.

112. Tristani-Firouzi M, Jensen JL, Donaldson MR, et al. Functional and clinical characterization of KCNJ2 mutations associated with LQT7 (Andersen syndrome). *J Clin Invest* 2002;110:381–388.

113. Plaster NM, Tawil R, Tristani-Firouzi M, et al. Mutations in Kir2.1 cause the developmental and episodic electrical phenotypes of Andersen's syndrome. *Cell* 2001;105:511–519.

114. Smith A, Fish FA, Kannankeril PJ. Andersen-Tawil Syndrome. *Indian Pacing Electrophysiol J* 2006;6:32–43.

115. Kannankeril PJ, Roden DM, Fish FA. Suppression of bidirectional ventricular tachycardia and unmasking of prolonged QT interval with verapamil in Andersen's syndrome. *J Cardiovasc Electrophysiol* 2004;15:119.

116. Zhang L, Benson DW, Tristani-Firouzi M, et al. Electrocardiographic features in Andersen-Tawil syndrome patients with KCNJ2 mutations: Characteristic T-U-wave patterns predict the KCNJ2 genotype. *Circulation* 2005;111:2720–2726.

117. Splawski I, Timothy KW, Sharpe LM, et al. Ca(V)1.2 calcium channel dysfunction causes a multisystem disorder including arrhythmia and autism. *Cell* 2004;119:19–31.

118. Priori SG, Cerrone M. Genetic arrhythmias. *Ital Heart J* 2005;6:241–248.

119. Splawski I, Timothy KW, Decher N, et al. Severe arrhythmia disorder caused by cardiac L-type calcium channel mutations. *Proc Natl Acad Sci USA* 2005;102:8089–8096.

120. Splawski I, Shen J, Timothy KW, et al. Spectrum of mutations in long-QT syndrome genes. KVLQT1, HERG, SCN5A, KCNE1, and KCNE2. *Circulation* 2000;102:1178–1185.

121. Shimizu W. The long QT syndrome: Therapeutic implications of a genetic diagnosis. *Cardiovasc Res* 2005;67:347–356.

122. Moss AJ, Zareba W, Kaufman ES, et al. Increased risk of arrhythmic events in long-QT syndrome with mutations in the pore region of the human ether-a-go-go-related gene potassium channel. *Circulation* 2002;105:794–799.

123. Shimizu W, Horie M, Ohno S, et al. Mutation site-specific differences in arrhythmic risk and sensitivity to sympathetic stimulation in the LQT1 form of congenital long QT syndrome: multicenter study in Japan. *J Am Coll Cardiol* 2004;44:117–125.

124. Priori SG, Napolitano C, Schwartz PJ. Low penetrance in the long-QT syndrome: Clinical impact. *Circulation* 1999;99:529–533.

125. Benhorin J, Moss AJ, Bak M, et al. Variable expression of long QT syndrome among gene carriers from families with five different HERG mutations. *Ann Noninvasive Electrocardiol* 2002;7:40–46.

126. Kobori A, Sarai N, Shimizu W, et al. Additional gene variants reduce effectiveness of beta-blockers in the LQT1 form of long QT syndrome. *J Cardiovasc Electrophysiol* 2004;15:190–199.

127. Tzivoni D, Banai S, Schuger C, et al. Treatment of torsade de pointes with magnesium sulfate. *Circulation* 1988;77:392–397.

128. Milberg P, Reinsch N, Osada N, et al. Verapamil prevents torsade de pointes by reduction of transmural dispersion of repolarization and suppression of early afterdepolarizations in an intact heart model of LQT3. *Basic Res Cardiol* 2005;100:365–371.

129. Moss AJ, Zareba W, Hall WJ, et al. Effectiveness and limitations of beta-blocker therapy in congenital long-QT syndrome. *Circulation* 2000;101:616–623.

130. Schwartz PJ, Priori SG, Cerrone M, et al. Left cardiac sympathetic denervation in the management of high-risk patients affected by the long-QT syndrome. *Circulation* 2004;109:1826–1833.

131. Kass RS, Wang W. Regulatory and molecular properties of delayed potassium channels in the heart: Relationship to human disease. In: Zipes DP, Jalife J, eds. *Cardiac Electrophysiology: From Cell to Bedside.* Philadelphia: WB Saunders, 2000:104–112.

132. Sanguinetti MC, Jurkiewicz NK. Role of external Ca2+ and K+ in gating of cardiac delayed rectifier K+ currents. *Pflugers Arch* 1992;420:180–186.

133. Compton SJ, Lux RL, Ramsey MR, et al. Genetically defined therapy of inherited long-QT syndrome. Correction of abnormal repolarization by potassium. *Circulation* 1996;94:1018–1022.

134. Etheridge SP, Compton SJ, Tristani-Firouzi M, et al. A new oral therapy for long QT syndrome: Long-term oral potassium improves repolarization in patients with HERG mutations. *J Am Coll Cardiol* 2003;42:1777–1782.

135. Schwartz PJ, Priori SG, Locati EH, et al. Long QT syndrome patients with mutations of the SCN5A and HERG genes have differential responses to Na+ channel blockade and to increases in heart rate. Implications for gene-specific therapy. *Circulation* 1995;92:3381–3386.

136. Shimizu W, Antzelevitch C. Sodium channel block with mexiletine is effective in reducing dispersion of repolarization and preventing torsade des pointes in LQT2 and LQT3 models of the long-QT syndrome. *Circulation* 1997;96:2038–2047.

137. Shimizu W, Antzelevitch C. Cellular basis for the ECG features of the LQT1 form of the long-QT syndrome: Effects of beta-adrenergic agonists and antagonists and sodium channel blockers on transmural dispersion of repolarization and torsade de pointes. *Circulation* 1998;98:2314–2322.

138. Roden DM. Taking the "idio" out of "idiosyncratic": Predicting torsades de pointes. *Pacing Clin Electrophysiol* 1998;21:1029–1034.

139. Darbar D. Screening for genomic alterations in congenital long QT syndrome. *Heart Rhythm* 2006;3:56–57.

140. Chiang CE. Congenital and acquired long QT syndrome. Current concepts and management. *Cardiol Rev* 2004;12:222–234.

141. Priori SG, Napolitano C, Schwartz PJ, et al. Association of long QT syndrome loci and cardiac events among patients treated with beta-blockers. *JAMA* 2004;292:1341–1344.

142. Antzelevitch C. T peak-Tend interval as an index of transmural dispersion of repolarization. *Eur J Clin Invest* 2001;31:555–557.

143. Lubinski A, Lewicka-Nowak E, Kempa M, et al. New insight into repolarization abnormalities in patients with congenital long QT syndrome: The increased transmural dispersion of repolarization. *Pacing Clin Electrophysiol* 1998;21:172–175.

144. Roden DM. Long QT syndrome: Reduced repolarization reserve and the genetic link. *J Intern Med* 2006;259:59–69.

145. Yang P, Kanki H, Drolet B, et al. Allelic variants in long-QT disease genes in patients with drug-associated torsades de pointes. *Circulation* 2002;105:1943–1948.

146. Kannankeril PJ, Roden DM, Norris KJ, et al. Genetic susceptibility to acquired long QT syndrome: Pharmacologic challenge in first-degree relatives. *Heart Rhythm* 2005;2:134–140.

147. Algra A, Tijssen JG, Roelandt JR, et al. QT interval variables from 24 hour electrocardiography and the two year risk of sudden death. *Br Heart J* 1993;70:43–48.

148. Gussak I, Brugada P, Brugada J, et al. Idiopathic short QT interval: A new clinical syndrome? *Cardiology* 2000;94:99–102.

149. Gaita F, Giustetto C, Bianchi F, et al. Short QT syndrome: A familial cause of sudden death. *Circulation* 2003;108:965–970.

150. Schimpf R, Wolpert C, Gaita F, et al. Short QT syndrome. *Cardiovasc Res* 2005;67:357–366.

151. Brugada R, Hong K, Dumaine R, et al. Sudden death associated with short-QT syndrome linked to mutations in HERG. *Circulation* 2004;109:30–35.

152. Bellocq C, van Ginneken AC, Bezzina CR, et al. Mutation in the KCNQ1 gene leading to the short QT-interval syndrome. *Circulation* 2004;109:2394–2397.

153. Priori SG, Pandit SV, Rivolta I, et al. A novel form of short QT syndrome (SQT3) is caused by a mutation in the KCNJ2 gene. *Circ Res* 2005;96:800–807.

154. Extramiana F, Antzelevitch C. Amplified transmural dispersion of repolarization as the basis for arrhythmogenesis in a canine ventricular-wedge model of short-QT syndrome. *Circulation* 2004;110:3661–3666.

155. Schimpf R, Wolpert C, Bianchi F, et al. Congenital short QT syndrome and implantable cardioverter defibrillator treatment: Inherent risk for inappropriate shock delivery. *J Cardiovasc Electrophysiol* 2003;14:1273–1277.

156. Gaita F, Giustetto C, Bianchi F, et al. Short QT syndrome: Pharmacological treatment. *J Am Coll Cardiol* 2004;43:1494–1499.

157. Leenhardt A, Lucet V, Denjoy I, et al. Catecholaminergic polymorphic ventricular tachycardia in children. A 7-year follow-up of 21 patients. *Circulation* 1995;91:1512–1519.

158. Priori SG, Napolitano C, Memmi M, et al. Clinical and molecular characterization of patients with catecholaminergic polymorphic ventricular tachycardia. *Circulation* 2002;106:69–74.

159. Sumitomo N, Harada K, Nagashima M, et al. Catecholaminergic polymorphic ventricular tachycardia: electrocardiographic characteristics and optimal therapeutic strategies to prevent sudden death. *Heart* 2003;89:66–70.

160. Choi G, Kopplin LJ, Tester DJ, et al. Spectrum and frequency of cardiac channel defects in swimming-triggered arrhythmia syndromes. *Circulation* 2004;110:2119–2124.

161. Postma AV, Denjoy I, Kamblock J, et al. Catecholaminergic polymorphic ventricular tachycardia: RYR2 mutations, bradycardia, and follow up of the patients. *J Med Genet* 2005;42:863–870.

162. Swan H, Piippo K, Viitasalo M, et al. Arrhythmic disorder mapped to chromosome 1q42-q43 causes malignant polymorphic ventricular tachycardia in structurally normal hearts. *J Am Coll Cardiol* 1999;34:2035–2042.

163. Priori SG, Napolitano C, Tiso N, et al. Mutations in the cardiac ryanodine receptor gene (hRyR2) underlie catecholaminergic polymorphic ventricular tachycardia. *Circulation* 2001;103:196–200.

164. Fabiato A, Fabiato F. Contractions induced by a calcium-triggered release of calcium from the sarcoplasmic reticulum of single skinned cardiac cells. *J Physiol* 1975;249:469–495.

165. George CH, Higgs GV, Lai FA. Ryanodine receptor mutations associated with stress-induced ventricular tachycardia mediate increased calcium release in stimulated cardiomyocytes. *Circ Res* 2003;93:531–540.

166. Lahat H, Pras E, Olender T, et al. A missense mutation in a highly conserved region of CASQ2 is associated with autosomal recessive catecholamine-induced polymorphic ventricular tachycardia in Bedouin families from Israel. *Am J Hum Genet* 2001;69:1378–1384.

167. Viatchenko-Karpinski S, Terentyev D, Gyorke I, et al. Abnormal calcium signaling and sudden cardiac death associated with mutation of calsequestrin. *Circ Res* 2004;94:471–477.

168. Nam GB, Burashnikov A, Antzelevitch C. Cellular mechanisms underlying the development of catecholaminergic ventricular tachycardia. *Circulation* 2005;111:2727–2733.

169. Brugada P, Brugada J. Right bundle branch block, persistent ST segment elevation and sudden cardiac death: A distinct clinical and electrocardiographic syndrome. A multicenter report. *J Am Coll Cardiol* 1992;20:1391–1396.

170. Osher HL, Wolff L. Electrocardiographic pattern simulating acute myocardial injury. *Am J Med Sci* 1953;226:541–545.

171. Martini B, Nava A, Thiene G, et al. Ventricular fibrillation without apparent heart disease: Description of six cases. *Am Heart J* 1989;118:1203–1209.

172. Todd SJ, Campbell MJ, Roden DM, et al. Novel Brugada SCN5A mutation causing sudden death in children. *Heart Rhythm* 2005;2:540–543.

173. Priori SG, Napolitano C, Giordano U, et al. Brugada syndrome and sudden cardiac death in children. *Lancet* 2000;355:808–809.

174. Potet F, Mabo P, Le Coq G, et al. Novel Brugada SCN5A mutation leading to ST segment elevation in the inferior or the right precordial leads. *J Cardiovasc Electrophysiol* 2003;14:200–203.

175. Brugada R, Brugada J, Antzelevitch C, et al. Sodium channel blockers identify risk for sudden death in patients with ST-segment elevation and right bundle branch block but structurally normal hearts. *Circulation* 2000;101:510–515.

176. Sangwatanaroj S, Prechawat S, Sunsaneewitayakul B, et al. New electrocardiographic leads and the procainamide test for the detection of the Brugada sign in sudden unexplained death syndrome survivors and their relatives. *Eur Heart J* 2001;22:2290–2296.

177. Chen Q, Kirsch GE, Zhang D, et al. Genetic basis and molecular mechanism for idiopathic ventricular fibrillation. *Nature* 1998;392:293–296.

178. Yan GX, Antzelevitch C. Cellular basis for the Brugada syndrome and other mechanisms of arrhythmogenesis associated with ST-segment elevation. *Circulation* 1999;100:1660–1666.

179. Dinckal MH, Davutoglu V, Akdemir I, et al. Incessant monomorphic ventricular tachycardia during febrile illness in a patient with Brugada syndrome: Fatal electrical storm. *Europace* 2003;5:257–261.

180. Dumaine R, Towbin JA, Brugada P, et al. Ionic mechanisms responsible for the electrocardiographic phenotype of the Brugada syndrome are temperature dependent. *Circ Res* 1999;85:803–809.

181. Hermida JS, Denjoy I, Clerc J, et al. Hydroquinidine therapy in Brugada syndrome. *J Am Coll Cardiol* 2004;43:1853–1860.
182. Nademanee K, Veerakul G, Mower M, et al. Defibrillator versus beta-blockers for unexplained death in Thailand (DEBUT): A randomized clinical trial. *Circulation* 2003;107:2221–2226.
183. Antzelevitch C, Brugada P, Borggrefe M, et al. Brugada syndrome: Report of the second consensus conference: Endorsed by the Heart Rhythm Society and the European Heart Rhythm Association. *Circulation* 2005;111:659–670.
184. Calkins H. Arrhythmogenic right-ventricular dysplasia/cardiomyopathy. *Curr Opin Cardiol* 2006;21:55–63.
185. Tabib A, Loire R, Chalabreysse L, et al. Circumstances of death and gross and microscopic observations in a series of 200 cases of sudden death associated with arrhythmogenic right ventricular cardiomyopathy and/or dysplasia. *Circulation* 2003;108:3000–3005.
186. Corrado D, Basso C, Thiene G. Sudden cardiac death in young people with apparently normal heart. *Cardiovasc Res* 2001;50:399–408.
187. McKenna WJ, Thiene G, Nava A, et al. Diagnosis of arrhythmogenic right ventricular dysplasia/cardiomyopathy. Task Force of the Working Group Myocardial and Pericardial Disease of the European Society of Cardiology and of the Scientific Council on Cardiomyopathies of the International Society and Federation of Cardiology. *Br Heart J* 1994;71:215–218.
188. Hamid MS, Norman M, Quraishi A, et al. Prospective evaluation of relatives for familial arrhythmogenic right ventricular cardiomyopathy/dysplasia reveals a need to broaden diagnostic criteria. *J Am Coll Cardiol* 2002;40:1445–1450.
189. Marcus FI. Prevalence of T-wave inversion beyond V1 in young normal individuals and usefulness for the diagnosis of arrhythmogenic right ventricular cardiomyopathy/dysplasia. *Am J Cardiol* 2005;95:1070–1071.
190. Nasir K, Bomma C, Tandri H, et al. Electrocardiographic features of arrhythmogenic right ventricular dysplasia/cardiomyopathy according to disease severity: A need to broaden diagnostic criteria. *Circulation* 2004;110:1527–1534.
191. Tiso N, Stephan DA, Nava A, et al. Identification of mutations in the cardiac ryanodine receptor gene in families affected with arrhythmogenic right ventricular cardiomyopathy type 2 (ARVD2). *Hum Mol Genet* 2001;10:189–194.
192. Rampazzo A, Nava A, Malacrida S, et al. Mutation in human desmoplakin domain binding to plakoglobin causes a dominant form of arrhythmogenic right ventricular cardiomyopathy. *Am J Hum Genet* 2002;71:1200–1206.
193. Gerull B, Heuser A, Wichter T, et al. Mutations in the desmosomal protein plakophilin-2 are common in arrhythmogenic right ventricular cardiomyopathy. *Nat Genet* 2004;36:1162–1164.
194. McKoy G, Protonotarios N, Crosby A, et al. Identification of a deletion in plakoglobin in arrhythmogenic right ventricular cardiomyopathy with palmoplantar keratoderma and woolly hair (Naxos disease). *Lancet* 2000;355:2119–2124.
195. Zacharias J, Forty J, Doig JC, et al. Right ventricular disarticulation. An 18-year single centre experience. *Eur J Cardiothorac Surg* 2005;27:1000–1004.
196. Maron BJ, Shirani J, Poliac LC, et al. Sudden death in young competitive athletes. Clinical, demographic, and pathological profiles. *JAMA* 1996;276:199–204.
197. Maron BJ, Shen WK, Link MS, et al. Efficacy of implantable cardioverter-defibrillators for the prevention of sudden death in patients with hypertrophic cardiomyopathy. *N Engl J Med* 2000;342:365–373.
198. Elliott P, McKenna WJ. Hypertrophic cardiomyopathy. *Lancet* 2004;363:1881–1891.
199. Behr ER, Elliott P, McKenna WJ. Role of invasive EP testing in the evaluation and management of hypertrophic cardiomyopathy. *Card Electrophysiol Rev* 2002;6:482–486.
200. McKenna WJ, Behr ER. Hypertrophic cardiomyopathy: Management, risk stratification, and prevention of sudden death. *Heart* 2002;87:169–176.
201. Gatzoulis K, Frogoudaki A, Brili S, et al. Implantable defibrillators: From the adult cardiac to the grown up congenital heart disease patient. *Int J Cardiol* 2004;97(suppl 1):117–122.
202. Gonska BD, Cao K, Raab J, et al. Radiofrequency catheter ablation of right ventricular tachycardia late after repair of congenital heart defects. *Circulation* 1996;94:1902–1908.
203. Gatzoulis MA, Till JA, Somerville J, et al. Mechanoelectrical interaction in tetralogy of Fallot. QRS prolongation relates to right ventricular size and predicts malignant ventricular arrhythmias and sudden death. *Circulation* 1995;92:231–237.
204. Harrison DA, Siu SC, Hussain F, et al. Sustained atrial arrhythmias in adults late after repair of tetralogy of Fallot. *Am J Cardiol* 2001;87:584–588.
205. Zipes DP, Foster PR, Troup PJ, et al. Atrial induction of ventricular tachycardia: Reentry versus triggered automaticity. *Am J Cardiol* 1979;44:1–8.
206. Belhassen B, Rotmensch HH, Laniado S. Response of recurrent sustained ventricular tachycardia to verapamil. *Br Heart J* 1981;46:679–682.
207. Nogami A. Idiopathic left ventricular tachycardia: Assessment and treatment. *Card Electrophysiol Rev* 2002;6:448–457.
208. Thakur RK, Klein GJ, Sivaram CA, et al. Anatomic substrate for idiopathic left ventricular tachycardia. *Circulation* 1996;93:497–501.
209. Lin FC, Wen MS, Wang CC, et al. Left ventricular fibromuscular band is not a specific substrate for idiopathic left ventricular tachycardia. *Circulation* 1996;93:525–528.
210. Farzaneh-Far A, Lerman BB. Idiopathic ventricular outflow tract tachycardia. *Heart* 2005;91:136–138.

CHAPTER 15 ■ SUDDEN CARDIAC DEATH

MICHAEL J. SILKA, MD, AND YANIV BAR-COHEN, MD

Sudden cardiac death (SCD) is defined as death that is abrupt, unexpected, and due to a cardiovascular cause, occurring in the absence of other potentially fatal conditions (1). The term *sudden* has been used to describe various intervals, but usually refers to a time <1 hour from the onset of symptoms to death or irreversible neurologic injury. In distinction, *sudden death* is defined by the World Health Organization as "a natural death within 24 hours of the onset of symptoms" irrespective of the cause. However, if the interval between the onset of symptoms and biologic death is limited to <2 hours, a cardiovascular cause of death is identified in 88% of all cases (2).

In spite of recent advances in medical therapy, SCD remains a significant national health problem, accounting for >350,000 deaths annually in the United States (3). Although primarily associated with coronary artery disease and consequences of myocardial ischemia, infarction, and dysfunction, SCD is increasingly recognized in diverse groups of young patients, such as athletes, individuals who have undergone prior repair of congenital heart defects, and some victims of sudden infant death syndrome (SIDS). The identification of young individuals at risk for SCD remains a major health challenge. The probability of survival to hospital discharge with minimal disability following an out-of-hospital cardiac arrest in the United States ranges between 2% and 17%, depending on the initial cardiac rhythm (4).

The continuing advances in electrophysiology and genetic testing, antiarrhythmic drugs, and implantable cardioverter defibrillators (ICDs) have stimulated efforts to define individuals who are at risk of SCD prior to a first event as well as to improve the prognosis of survivors of cardiac arrest. However, because of the very low incidence of SCD among young patients, criteria for prospective identification and risk stratification remain elusive.

PHASES AND MECHANISMS OF SUDDEN CARDIAC DEATH

Although SCD is by definition an abrupt event, several phases in the sequence of SCD are recognized (5). Prodrome (phase 1) refers to premonitory symptoms such as palpitations, weakness, or chest pain. Onset (phase 2) refers to the development of sustained pathophysiologic disturbances, such as ischemia or arrhythmia, which result in cardiac arrest. Cardiac arrest (phase 3) is defined by the abrupt loss of consciousness owing to impaired cerebral perfusion. The interval between cardiac arrest and biologic death (phase 4) is variable, depending on whether interventions are performed. Resuscitative efforts may restore spontaneous circulation, resulting in *aborted sudden cardiac death*. Biologic death is defined as an irreversible event with failure of resuscitative efforts and cessation of electrical and mechanical cardiac activity. In the absence of effective resuscitative efforts, irreversible neurologic injury and biologic death generally follow cardiac arrest within minutes.

There are diverse mechanisms of sudden death, which may be classified as (a) arrhythmic (proven or presumptive); (b) circulatory (congestive heart failure or thromboembolic events); and (c) noncardiac (Table 15.1) (6,7). Arrhythmic deaths are defined by the abrupt loss of consciousness and pulse in the absence of other medical conditions likely to cause death. Circulatory or nonarrhythmic sudden deaths are defined by the collapse of circulation before the disappearance of an organized cardiac rhythm, such as cardiac tamponade or pulmonary or systemic embolism. Noncardiac causes of sudden death are diverse and include trauma, respiratory failure, and neurologic events. This chapter will be limited to discussion of sudden deaths due to proven or probable cardiovascular causes. There is limited precision even within this classification as, first,

TABLE 15.1

MECHANISMS OF SUDDEN CARDIAC DEATH

Arrhythmic death
Proven
Presumptive
Nonarrhythmic cardiac deaths
Circulatory (cardiac: congestive heart failure)
(vascular: embolic, aneurysm)
Noncardiac

Adapted from Hinkle LE, Thaler HT. Clinical classification of cardiac deaths. *Circulation* 1982;65:457–464; and Greene HL, Richardson DW, Barker AH, et al. Classification of deaths after myocardial infarction as arrhythmic or nonarrhythmic. *Am J Cardiol* 1989;63:1–6, with permission.

noncardiac causes of death identified at autopsy may clinically simulate SCD and, second, terminal arrhythmias or ICD discharges may occur as secondary and incidental responses to the primary pathophysiologic process leading to death (8).

PATHOPHYSIOLOGY OF ARRHYTHMIC SUDDEN CARDIAC DEATH

Prior to the use of ICDs, there were few cases of unexpected out-of-hospital SCD in children when electrocardiographic documentation of the terminal arrhythmias had been recorded. Those reports demonstrated either an atrial or ventricular tachycardia (VT) resulting in ventricular fibrillation (VF) (Fig. 15.1) (9).

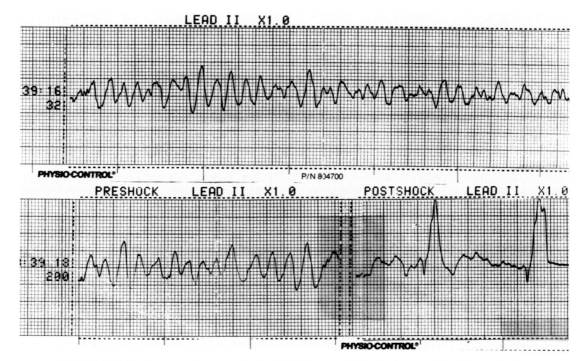

FIGURE 15.1 Cardiac arrest due to ventricular fibrillation recorded during the out-of-hospital resuscitation of a 12-year-old with prior surgical valvotomy for aortic stenosis. These recordings demonstrate ventricular fibrillation that was terminated by an asynchronous 100-J countershock, followed by an idioventricular rhythm (with subsequent return of sinus rhythm). An apical left ventricular aneurysm was identified by angiography in this patient, and sustained ventricular tachycardia was inducible at electrophysiologic testing.

Several recent studies of young patients with cardiovascular disease and ICDs have confirmed that pulseless VT or VF is often the cause of out-of-hospital SCD (10,11). This is in contrast to death in chronically ill children, in whom profound bradycardia progressing to asystole has been observed most commonly (12).

The development of VF may be an age-dependent variable, with VF reported at the time of initial attempted resuscitation in only 6% of patients younger than 18 years of age, compared with 31% in those 19 to 35 years old and 48% in those 36 years of age or older (13). It has been suggested that although the capability to fibrillate is inherent to the human myocardium, a critical mass of disorganized, depolarized cells may be required to sustain VF (14). Thus, it is hypothesized that the small heart of a young child may not be able to sustain VF, which may account for the relative infrequency of this rhythm in pediatric patients.

Definition of the arrhythmic causes of SCD may be complicated by the fact that extreme bradycardia, such as pacemaker failure in a patient with complete heart block, may result in asystole, followed by polymorphic VT degenerating into VF. In such a case, the triggering event is bradycardia, even though the terminal arrhythmia may be VF. Conversely, estimates of the incidence of VF are limited by the time-limited nature of this arrhythmia, with asystole the final arrhythmia regardless of antecedent events. This has clinical relevance as survival and neurologic outcome of patients, irrespective of age, is consistently better for those whose resuscitation begins in VF as compared with asystole (4).

EPIDEMIOLOGY OF SCD IN CHILDREN AND ADOLESCENTS

Population-based studies of the incidence of sudden death in pediatric patients have reported a rate between 1.3 and 4 per 100,000 patient years (Table 15.2) (15–19). In comparison, the incidence of SCD in adult males >35 years of age is 1 to 2 per 1,000 patient years (20). Two points are worth noting regarding these studies. First, most studies of SCD in pediatric patients have excluded SIDS victims, the validity of which may be questioned (21). Second, between 1989 and 1998, age-adjusted SCD rates in the United States declined 11.7% in males and 5.8% in females, primarily attributed to prevention and improved therapy for coronary artery disease (22).

Several groups of pediatric and young adult patients who are at increased risk of SCD compared with the general population have been identified. These include patients with congenital heart disease, cardiomyopathies, and primary arrhythmic diagnoses such as the long QT syndromes and Wolff–Parkinson–White syndrome.

SUDDEN CARDIAC DEATH IN PATIENTS WITH CONGENITAL HEART DISEASE

Sudden cardiac death has been reported in patients with both unoperated and unrecognized forms of congenital heart disease, as well as following surgical or catheter interventional treatment for these defects. Because of differences in both the mechanisms and relative risks of SCD, these patient groups will be discussed separately. The pathophysiology that is the basis for the risk of SCD is discussed in the specific chapters for each type of congenital heart defect.

Unoperated Congenital Heart Disease

Aortic Stenosis

Most young patients with aortic stenosis are clinically asymptomatic, although some patients may be reluctant to report cardiac symptoms. In a study of the long-term outcome of patients with congenital heart defects, the Natural History Study-II reported six sudden deaths (2.8%) among 217 children medically managed for valvar aortic stenosis (23). Virtually all cases of SCD were associated with moderate to severe left ventricular obstruction. Clinical symptoms of syncope, exertional dyspnea, or chest pain, as well as findings of severe left ventricular obstruction, hypertrophy, and strain on the ECG were identified as risk factors for SCD.

Surgical or balloon valvuloplasty treatment of aortic valve obstruction may reduce but not eliminate the risk of SCD. The development of myocardial ischemia is thought to be the initiating factor for the terminal ventricular arrhythmias in patients with severe aortic stenosis who experience SCD. Persistent pulmonary hypertension is also a recognized consequence of neonatal aortic stenosis, with the failure of normalization of pulmonary vascular resistance attributed to chronic elevation of left atrial and left ventricular end-diastolic pressures (24).

Coronary Artery Anomalies

Sudden cardiac death may be the presenting symptom of congenital coronary artery anomalies as well as acquired forms of coronary artery disease (25). Patients with either form of

TABLE 15.2

POPULATION-BASED STUDIES OF SUDDEN CARDIAC DEATH IN CHILDREN AND ADOLESCENTS

Author	Dates	Total population (N)	Sudden deaths (N)	Cardiac disease (N)
Molander (15)	1974–1979	1,800,000	43	7
Driscoll and Edwards (16)	1950–1982	NA	12	4
Niiruma and Maki (17)	1975–1986	15,000,000	18	4
Wren et al. (18)	1985–1992	3,800,000	226	42
Young et al. (19)	1994–1997	3,000,000	600	48

coronary disease are at increased risk for SCD, especially during exertion. These anomalies may be first recognized on postmortem examination, after years or decades of relatively symptom-free status (26).

The most common congenital coronary anomaly associated with SCD is origin of the left main coronary artery from the right sinus of Valsalva (see Chapter 34). In this anomaly, the left coronary artery courses between the aorta and the pulmonary artery. It is hypothesized that during exercise, expansion of the pulmonary artery and aorta results in compression of the left main coronary artery, resulting in acute myocardial ischemia and ventricular arrhythmias. Clinical recognition may be difficult, since only one third of patients with this anomaly who died suddenly reported prior symptoms of angina or exertional syncope (27). Patients with anomalous origin of the right coronary artery from the left sinus are at a similar risk for SCD. In general, surgical revascularization is indicated on diagnosis. Other reported causes of acute myocardial ischemia resulting in SCD owing to congenital coronary artery anomalies include acute angle origin of a coronary artery, left main coronary artery atresia, an intramural coronary artery, or a single right coronary artery (28). Anomalous origin of the left coronary artery from the pulmonary artery usually presents with severe congestive heart failure during infancy; however, it may be unrecognized in 5% to 10% of cases and present during childhood or adolescence as SCD, often during exertion.

Acquired Coronary Artery Anomalies

In the initial reports, SCD was reported early in the course of Kawasaki's disease in 2% of patients, with late development of coronary artery aneurysms or thrombosis in 10% to 20% of patients. However, with the introduction of gamma globulin and aspirin therapy, there has been a marked reduction in the development of late coronary artery disease (29). Some patients may still die suddenly during the acute phase of Kawasaki's disease from rupture of a coronary aneurysm, acute myocarditis, or later owing to consequences of myocardial ischemia and infarction (30). In the current era, late sudden death is reported to be most common in patients with persistent bilateral giant aneurysms. The cause of late SCD appears to be sustained VT, which develops at the site of a prior myocardial infarction (31).

An accelerated form of coronary vasculopathy may occur in pediatric patients after cardiac transplantation (32). The pathogenesis consists of marked intimal hyperplasia and small vessel coronary artery stenosis. These may result in myocardial ischemia and dysfunction, resulting in a significant risk of SCD.

Atherosclerotic heart disease has been identified as the cause of death in 23% of men who died suddenly between the ages of 18 and 35 years (33). In general, these patients did not have prior symptoms of angina or exertional syncope, and nearly all had single vessel disease, involving the left main or proximal left anterior descending coronary artery.

Pulmonary Hypertension

Sudden cardiac death is often the mode of death in patients with pulmonary hypertension, either as a primary disorder or when associated with congenital heart disease (Eisenmenger syndrome). In early studies of SCD in pediatric patients, 11% occurred in patients with pulmonary hypertension associated with congenital heart disease with an additional 4% in patients with primary pulmonary hypertension (34,35). The risk of SCD appears to be related to severity of the pulmonary

vascular disease, advancing age, and presence of syncope. Such patients are at increased risk for SCD during pregnancy and delivery, during noncardiac surgery, at altitudes >5,000 feet, and during strenuous physical activities. The pathophysiology of SCD in patients with intracardiac shunts and severe pulmonary hypertension appears to be related to an acute decrease in systemic vascular resistance or an increase in pulmonary vascular resistance, which increases the right-to-left shunting and decreases pulmonary blood flow. This results in profound arterial desaturation and acidosis, which further increase peripheral vasodilation and pulmonary vasoconstriction. This may result in either a lethal ventricular arrhythmia or profound bradycardia.

Other Cardiac Diseases

SCD may occur in patients with Ebstein anomaly of the tricuspid valve and in patients with congenitally corrected transposition of the great arteries. Both defects are associated with a high incidence of accessory AV connections and, in the presence of severe AV valve dysfunction, supraventricular arrhythmias may result in marked compromise of cardiac output (36). The development of spontaneous AV block is an additional risk factor for patients with congenitally corrected transposition of the great arteries (37). Adolescents or adults with either of these defects may also develop atrial flutter or fibrillation owing to atrial dilation associated with chronic AV valve insufficiency. SCD has also been reported in infants with pulmonary atresia with intact ventricular septum and unoperated cyanotic congenital heart disease, most notably tetralogy of Fallot and tricuspid atresia due to hypercyanotic spells (38).

Sudden Cardiac Death following Surgery for Congenital Heart Disease

Sudden cardiac death has been recognized as a late complication following surgical treatment of congenital heart disease for many decades. Although relatively infrequent, the absolute number of patients who are survivors of surgery for congenital heart disease makes this issue a major concern (39). Clinical criteria to define patients at increased risk for SCD remain undefined because most studies have been retrospective, single-center studies with limited statistical power and inconsistent conclusions. Further confounding factors are the diverse spectrum of postoperative congenital heart defects, evolving surgical treatments and defect-specific risk factors. This has resulted in considerable controversy regarding the indications for evaluation and need for treatment of postoperative congenital heart disease patients.

An initial issue to address is the incidence of SCD following surgery for congenital heart defects. Morris et al. (40) reported findings on 4,208 patients who were followed for 2 to 40 years after surgery for common congenital heart defects. During the study, there was a total of 196 deaths (4.7%). This overall mortality rate was three times the anticipated death rate for an age-matched control population. The causes of death were noncardiac in 61 patients (31%) and cardiac in the other 135 patients. The principle cardiac causes of death were sudden ($n = 44$), reoperation ($n = 28$), pulmonary hypertension ($n = 26$), and heart failure ($n = 24$). Thus, 22% of all deaths in this population were due to sudden cardiac causes (Fig. 15.2).

Silka et al. (41) further studied the risk of late SCD in the same cohort of patients. This study was composed of 3,589

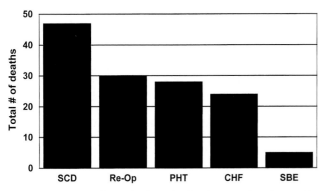

FIGURE 15.2 This figure displays the distribution of cardiovascular causes of death following surgery for common congenital heart defects. Of 133 deaths, sudden cardiovascular death was most common, occurring in 46 of 133 patients. SCD, sudden cardiac death; Re-op, reoperation for congenital heart disease; PHT, pulmonary hypertension; CHF, congestive heart failure; SBE, subacute bacterial endocarditis. (Adapted from Morris CD, Silka MJ, Reller MD. Comparative causes of late mortality after surgery for 14 congenital heart defects: Sudden, non-sudden cardiac, and non-cardiac [abstract]. *Circulation* 1998;98:1–619, with permission.)

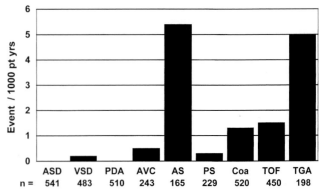

FIGURE 15.3 The prevalence of sudden cardiac death (SCD) among patients following surgery for various forms of congenital heart disease. The SCD rate for aortic stenosis (AS) and d-transposition of the great arteries (TGA) was significantly greater than for all other defects. The incidence of SCD was also increased for tetralogy of Fallot (TOF) and coarctation of the aorta (Coa). ASD, atrial septal defect; VSD, ventricular septal defect; PDA, patent ductus arteriosus; AVC, atrioventricular canal; PS, pulmonic stenosis; *n*, number of patients with the specific defect for whom follow-up was available. (Adapted from Silka MJ, Hardy BG, Menashe VD, et al. A population-based prospective evaluation of risk of sudden cardiac death after operation for common congenital heart defects. *J Am Coll Cardiol* 1998;32: 245–251, with permission.).

patients and limited to forms of congenital heart disease with at least 20 years of follow-up and at least 150 patients with each type of congenital heart defect. This study identified a total of 41 late sudden deaths during 45,857 total years of patient follow-up, for a calculated overall risk of 1 late SCD per 1,118 patient years of follow-up for the entire cohort of patients.

Subgroup analysis identified late SCD as a concern primarily for patients with four types of congenital heart disease: Tetralogy of Fallot, transposition of the great arteries, aortic stenosis, and coarctation of the aorta. The overall risk for SCD among these four defects was one event per 454 years of follow-up; in contrast, the risk for late SCD among atrial, ventricular or atrioventricular septal defects, patent ductus arteriosus, and pulmonic stenosis was one event per 7,154 years of follow-up. Defect-specific analysis of the SCD rates demonstrated an observed incidence of late SCD of 5 per 1,000 patient years of follow-up for postoperative transposition of the great arteries and aortic stenosis. In comparison, the observed rates of late sudden death following surgery for coarctation and tetralogy were 1.3 and 1.5 per 1,000 patient years, respectively (Fig. 15.3). The relative risk of late SCD for patients with these forms of congenital heart disease was nonlinear, increasing with longer duration of follow-up with the exception of transposition of the great arteries. This suggests that the risk of SCD may be a time-dependent factor, as the observed rates of SCD increased primarily after 20 years of follow-up. One other finding of this study was that most, but not all, SCDs were owing to an arrhythmia. Of the 41 total sudden deaths, the causes were either a documented or presumed arrhythmia in 30, circulatory in 7 (embolic in 5 and rupture of an aneurysm in 2), and acute ventricular failure in 4. These data provide a compelling argument for the continued long-term evaluation of postoperative congenital heart disease patients.

Specific Defects and Sudden Cardiac Death

Tetralogy of Fallot. Based on comprehensive review of the medical literature, Garson (42) performed a meta-analysis of 39 studies regarding 4,627 patients who had undergone surgical treatment for tetralogy of Fallot. In this study, SCD was

reported in 57 patients (1.2%) during an average of 8.4 years of follow-up (an incidence of 1.5 events per 1,000 patient years of follow-up). Analysis of the risk factors associated with SCD identified the combination of ventricular arrhythmias on Holter monitor and abnormal hemodynamics as present in 80% of SCD victims, but in only 8% of 4,570 survivors (Table 15.3). Prior symptoms (syncope, sustained palpitations) were not predictive of SCD and were identified in only 18% of SCD victims. Based on this analysis, a mathematical decision model proposed that further investigation or treatment was indicated in patients with both abnormal hemodynamics and complex ventricular ectopy following repair of tetralogy of Fallot.

Over the past years, at least 20 factors have been proposed as associated with an increased risk for SCD following repair of tetralogy of Fallot (43). These may be classified as conduction disturbances, atrial or ventricular arrhythmias, residual hemodynamic abnormalities, surgical era, or technique and duration of follow-up. Most SCDs in this population have been attributed to ventricular arrhythmias that originate at the ventriculotomy incision or are related to intrinsic abnormalities of the right ventricular outflow tract (44).

The indications and optimal methods for risk evaluation in postoperative tetralogy of Fallot patients remain debated topics. In an early multicenter study of 359 patients, Chandar et al. (45) reported that the response to programmed ventricular stimulation (induction of VT) was not predictive of subsequent syncope or SCD. This study was limited by significant variability in the stimulation protocol used. Subsequently, Khairy et al. (46) reported the positive prognostic value of programmed stimulation in the risk stratification of these patients. Of the 252 patients in this series, 87 had inducible sustained VT, with 48 (55%) of these patients experiencing subsequent clinical VT or SCD. In contrast, of the remaining 165 patients with no inducible sustained arrhythmia, only 14 experienced subsequent VT or SCD (8.5%).

Gatzoulis et al. (47) have reported that a markedly prolonged QRS complex (>180 ms) identifies tetralogy of Fallot

TABLE 15.3

FACTORS ASSOCIATED WITH SCD FOLLOWING SURGERY FOR TETRALOGY OF
FALLOT (*n* = 4,627)

	Sudden death (%)[a]	Alive (%)[b]
Symptoms	18	—
Ventricular arrhythmia on		
ECG	61	8
Exercise test	50	18
Holter	93	46
EPS	38	17
Abnormal RVSP	77	20
Abnormal RVEDP	85	20
Ventricular arrhythmia on Holter and abnormal hemodynamics	80	8

ECG, electrocardiogram; EPS, electrophysiologic stimulation; RVSP, right ventricular systolic pressure;
RVEDP, RV end-diastolic pressure.
[a] *n* = 57.
[b] *n* = 4,570.
Adapted from Garson (42), with permission.

patients at risk for sustained VT and SCD (Fig. 15.4). However, QRS prolongation may be a surrogate marker for either
impaired ventricular function or slow intraventricular conduction, both of which may favor the development of re-entrant
sustained VT. Although QRS duration >180 ms was more
likely in patients with inducible sustained VT in the Khairy

study, it was not an independent risk factor for subsequent
events by multivariate analysis.

An appreciation of the relationship between abnormal
hemodynamics and arrhythmias has more recently focused
attention on right ventricular volume overload associated with
pulmonary regurgitation following repair of tetralogy of Fallot.

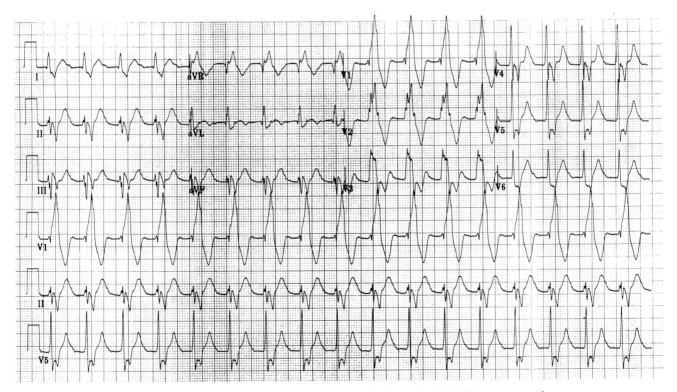

FIGURE 15.4 This electrocardiogram demonstrates two risk factors for SCD following surgery for congenital heart disease. The first is prolonged duration of the QRS complex (210 ms), which may identify
patients at risk for syncope, ventricular tachycardia, or sudden death following surgery for tetralogy of
Fallot. The second risk factor is that the cardiac rhythm is atrial flutter (intra-atrial reentrant tachycardia), which is an independent risk factor following surgery for several forms of congenital heart disease.

In a multicenter study, Gatzoulis et al. (48) reported that pulmonary regurgitation was the primary hemodynamic lesion associated with SCD in tetralogy of Fallot patients. This finding is supported by animal work demonstrating that chronic right ventricular volume load, as opposed to chronic pressure load, increases the incidence of inducible ventricular arrhythmias (49). In addition, moderate to severe left ventricular dysfunction had been observed to be more common in adult tetralogy of Fallot patients who were victims of SCD (50).

Postoperative patients with tetralogy of Fallot who experience syncope, sustained tachycardia, or aborted SCD may benefit from surgical repair of significant residual hemodynamic abnormalities or lesions, whether an intracardiac shunt, valvar insufficiency, or stenosis or right ventricular outflow tract aneurysm. This repair is ideally performed in conjunction with electrophysiologic mapping and ablation or surgical resection of arrhythmogenic foci. In the absence of definitive therapy, implantation of an ICD is indicated (Fig. 15.5) (51).

Evaluation of asymptomatic or minimally symptomatic patients years or decades following repair of tetralogy of Fallot requires consideration of both hemodynamics and electrophysiology. In the absence of a definitive prospective randomized clinical trial, identification of patients at risk for SCD will continue to be based on individual judgment and experience.

Transposition of the Great Arteries. Late postoperative complications are common in patients who have undergone either the Mustard or the Senning operation for transposition of the great arteries. These include atrial arrhythmias, venous pathway obstruction, and impaired ventricular function. Each of the factors may result in an increased risk of SCD. Although the arterial switch operation has replaced the atrial switch procedures, many patients had undergone either the Mustard or Senning procedure and remain at risk for late SCD. Table 15.4 summarizes the largest series of postoperative Mustard and/or Senning patients (52–57). The cumulative incidence of late SCD among these studies was 6 per 1,000 patient years of follow-up.

The mechanism(s) of SCD in these patients remains uncertain. However, in a retrospective study of SCD in 47 post–atrial switch patients, either VT or VF was recorded during attempted resuscitation in all 18 patients in whom ECG documentation was available (58). The statistically significant risk factors for SCD in this study were symptoms owing to either atrial flutter/fibrillation or heart failure. Previously, it had been proposed that atrial flutter (intra-atrial re-entrant tachycardia) with 1:1 AV conduction may result in hypotension and myocardial ischemia with subsequent ventricular arrhythmias as the mechanism of SCD (59). Although profound bradycardia may result in low cardiac output and dispersion of refractoriness, it has not been consistently identified as a risk factor for an increased risk of SCD.

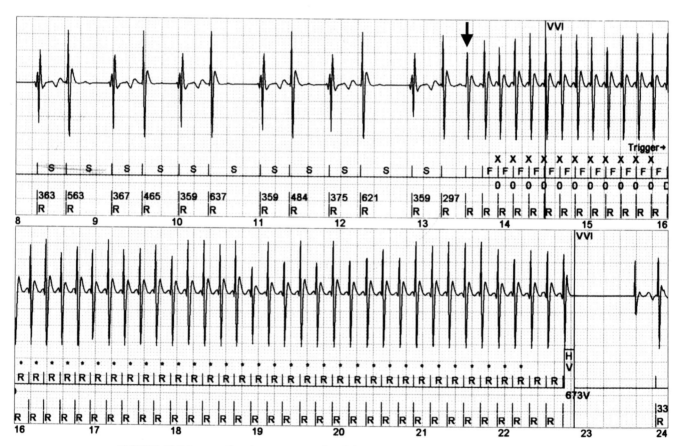

FIGURE 15.5 Intracardiac electrograms retrieved from an implantable cardioverter defibrillator following a brief syncopal event in a patient with prior repair of tetralogy of Fallot. Immediately prior to collapse, the patient had noted frequent palpitations, with the first 12 beats of this recording demonstrating a bigeminal rhythm. The thirteenth ventricular electrogram (*arrow*) initiates a sustained ventricular tachycardia at a cycle length of 190 ms (rate, 316/minute). A 20-J shock (labeled HV) results in termination of tachycardia and return to sinus rhythm.

TABLE 15.4

INCIDENCE OF SCD FOLLOWING THE MUSTARD OR SENNING PROCEDURE FOR d-TGA

Author	Date	Patients (n)	Follow-up years (total)	SCD (n)
Flinn et al. (52)	1984	372	1,674	9
Turina et al. (53)	1988	220	2,266	8
Gewillig et al. (54)	1991	226	2,644	37
Gelatt et al. (55)	1997	478	5,544	31
Silka et al. (41)	1998	172	1,413	7
Moons et al. (56)	2004	257	4,369	10
Dos et al. (57)	2005	137	767	3
TOTAL		1,862	18,677	105

Long-term follow-up of patients who have undergone the arterial switch repair of TGA will also be required to confirm the superiority of this operation in reducing the risk of late SCD. The primary concern for these patients appears to be coronary artery insufficiency, related to stenosis at the site of coronary ostial reimplantation or lack of vasodilatory reserve resulting in exertionally related subendocardial ischemia (60).

Left Heart Obstructive Lesions. Few studies have specifically evaluated the risk of late SCD following surgery or balloon valvuloplasty for aortic stenosis (23,41,61). The Natural History Study II reported 19 unexpected SCDs among 240 postoperative patients (7.9%) with aortic stenosis (23). Ventricular arrhythmias were present in 45% of patients with aortic stenosis and were correlated with an increased left ventricular end diastolic pressure, aortic regurgitation, functional class, and aortic valve replacement. Reported mechanisms of SCD include arrhythmias (possibly related to ischemia), cerebral or coronary embolism, and acute ventricular failure.

Late SCD may occur decades following surgical treatment of coarctation of the aorta (62). Causes of late SCD may include coronary artery disease or the rupture of an aortic aneurysm, either native or related to patch aortoplasty. Advanced left ventricular dysfunction following previous hypertrophy of the left ventricle has been noted in the two series reporting SCD following coarctation repair (41,61). In these series, given the absence of any autopsy-defined abnormality, the cause of death was presumed to be arrhythmic.

Complex Congenital Heart Disease. Long-term survival is increasingly observed in the current era following staged surgical treatment of various forms of complex CHD. Most of these repairs involve defects with only one functional ventricle, and often incorporate the Norwood procedure followed by serial superior (Glenn) and inferior cavopulmonary (Fontan) connections.

Unexplained sudden death has been reported in 4% to 15% of patients following the initial Norwood procedure and preceding the second-stage superior cavopulmonary connection (63,64). Potential causes of unexpected SCD include aortopulmonary shunt occlusion, arrhythmias, coronary hypoperfusion, and residual anatomic lesions (65). Whether SCD in this group of patients will be reduced with the Sano modification (right ventricular to pulmonary artery conduit) is a topic of ongoing clinical study.

Postoperative complications after the Fontan procedure include frequent atrial arrhythmias, ventricular dysfunction, and chronic low output owing to elevated pulmonary vascular resistance (66,67). Unexpected late SCD has been reported in these patients and has been attributed to atrial and ventricular arrhythmias, ischemia, thromboembolism, or heart failure.

Other Risk Factors for Late SCD following Surgery for Congenital Heart Disease

Postoperative Complete Heart Block. Prior to the development of reliable and commercially available permanent pacemakers, the observed 12-month incidence of SCD for nonpaced patients with postoperative complete heart block was 80% (68). Because of this, permanent pacemaker implantation is a class I indication for all patients with postoperative persistent complete heart block (69). A controversial population of patients, who may be at risk for late postoperative SCD, are those with transient postoperative complete heart block, who have persistent late bifascicular or trifascicular block. These patients may be at risk for SCD, potentially because of either late recurrence of complete heart block or ventricular arrhythmias (70).

Antiarrhythmic Drug Therapy. Owing to concern regarding ventricular arrhythmias as a cause of late SCD following surgery for congenital heart disease, antiarrhythmic drugs were often recommended for the suppression of ventricular ectopy. However, subsequent clinical studies identified several adverse effects of these drugs, primarily class I and class III antiarrhythmic agents. These include an increased incidence of SCD compared with nontreated patients, impairment of ventricular function, and loss of pacemaker function owing to change in stimulation threshold (71,72). One mechanism of SCD appears to be prolongation of the QT interval and development of polymorphic ventricular tachycardia in genetically susceptible individuals (73).

Postoperative Valvular Disease. SCD may occur in patients with prosthetic aortic, mitral, or tricuspid valves. The causes of death include mechanical failure, thrombosis or endocarditis of the valve, or development of late postoperative complete heart block (74). Patients with prior valve replacement require lifelong follow-up for assessment of hemodynamics and arrhythmias as well as for monitoring of anticoagulation. Acute thrombosis of the low-flow mitral and tricuspid valves has been reported in infants and young children as a complication of hypovolemia and dehydration.

CARDIOMYOPATHIES

Sudden cardiac death is a significant risk for young patients with hypertrophic, dilated, or restrictive cardiomyopathies.

TABLE 15.5

HYPERTROPHIC CARDIOMYOPATHY IN THE YOUNG: INCIDENCE OF SCD OR CARDIAC ARREST

Author	n	Mean age (y) at diagnosis	Follow-up years (total)	SCD/Arrest (n)
Maron et al. (75)	20	<1	3.3	2 (10%)
McKenna et al. (76)	53	15.3	3	7 (15%)
Hordof et al. (77)	135	7.7	15	17 (13%)
Romeo et al. (78)	37	7.0	9.2	9 (24%)
Yetman et al. (79)	99	5.0	4.8	18 (18%)
Nugent et al. (80)	80	0.5	5.2	1 (1%)
Ostman-Smith et al. (81)	128	8.5	10.8	16 (13%)
TOTAL	552	7.9[a]	9.1[a]	70

[a]Weighted average based on sample size.

In many instances, SCD may be the initial manifestation of a cardiomyopathy during childhood.

Hypertrophic Cardiomyopathy

The annual risk of SCD for young patients with hypertrophic cardiomyopathy (HCM) is approximately 2% per year (Table 15.5) (75–81) and is among the most common causes for unexpected SCD in adolescents and young athletes (82). Among patients with hypertrophic cardiomyopathy, factors associated with an increased risk for SCD include a family history of sudden death, syncope, an abnormal blood pressure response to exercise, nonsustained VT, septal thickness >30 mm, and impaired ventricular function (83). The exact significance of these risk factors continues to be debated.

Many young patients with hypertrophic cardiomyopathy who experience SCD do not have significant outflow tract gradients at rest. The mechanism(s) of SCD may involve either the dynamic development of left ventricular obstruction during exercise or be related to myocardial ischemia, possibly owing to an intramural course of a coronary artery (myocardial bridge) (84). Patients with hypertrophic obstructive cardiomyopathy also may experience SCD owing to supraventricular arrhythmias, which may result in myocardial ischemia or hemodynamic collapse resulting in VF.

All patients with HCM should undergo risk stratification for SCD, with a decision regarding treatment based on the number and relative risk of the factors present. The long-term benefit of empiric therapy with beta-blockade, calcium channel blockade, or amiodarone is a matter of debate. Similarly, other therapies including dual chamber pacing or surgical relief of left ventricular obstruction have not been demonstrated to eliminate the risk of SCD. The treatment of high-risk young patients with a hypertrophic cardiomyopathy with an implantable cardioverter defibrillator (ICD) has been reported to improve survival, provided there is not severe impairment of ventricular function (85,86). In the future, clarification of the genotype–phenotype correlation in HCM may further assist the decision regarding need for and type of treatment.

Dilated Cardiomyopathies

Compared with SCD in adults, SCD is relatively uncommon in young patients with dilated cardiomyopathies. Diverse causes of SCD have been reported in patients with dilated cardiomyopathies, including progressive bradycardia, electromechanical dissociation, massive pulmonary embolism, and ventricular arrhythmias (87–89). A high incidence of appropriate ICD therapies has been reported in young patients with both advanced ventricular dysfunction and ventricular arrhythmias who are listed for heart transplantation (90). However, most young patients with advanced forms of dilated cardiomyopathy do not have complex ventricular arrhythmias, and isolated ventricular dysfunction is not an indication for ICD implantation.

Arrhythmogenic Right Ventricular Dysplasia

Arrhythmogenic right ventricular dysplasia (ARVD) is a specific cardiomyopathy that is associated with a high prevalence of ventricular arrhythmias and SCD in young patients. Although this diagnosis may not be suspected until postmortem examination, it should be considered in individuals with exercise-induced arrhythmias or syncope, one or multiple left bundle branch QRS morphology tachycardias, or unexplained right ventricular enlargement on the echocardiogram (91,92). The primary pathology is fibro-fatty replacement of myocytes, resulting in patchy areas of fibrosis and ventricular enlargement. Endomyocardial biopsy and magnetic resonance imaging are of limited reliability in establishing a diagnosis of ARVD. Although ventricular arrhythmias are cited as the primary cause of unexpected SCD, profound sinus node dysfunction and progressive heart failure also have been observed in young patients with ARVD. It is unclear whether antiarrhythmic therapy, catheter ablation or surgical disarticulation of the right ventricular free wall will reduce the risk of SCD in these patients. Studies of ICDs in these patients suggest a high rate of appropriate therapies, with prior VT/VF and a younger age at diagnosis independent predictors of subsequent ICD discharge (93).

Isolated Left Ventricular Noncompaction

Isolated left ventricular noncompaction is a cardiomyopathy characterized by prominent trabeculations and deep intratrabecular recesses in the left ventricular myocardium. Two distinct myocardial layers may be demonstrated by echocardiography, with a thin epicardial layer and a thicker noncompacted endocardial layer resulting in a trabecular meshwork with deep endomyocardial spaces (94). Proposed criteria for an echocardiographic diagnosis include a maximal end systolic ratio of noncompacted to compacted layers of >2, although a cutoff of >1.4 has been suggested for children (95). Initially thought to be a rare disorder, noncompaction may account for 9% of childhood cardiomyopathies (96).

The etiologic factors of sudden cardiac death in noncompaction have not been defined. Evidence of coronary microcirculatory dysfunction suggests that ischemia may have a role in the development of both impaired systolic function and ventricular arrhythmias (97). On the other hand, ventricular arrhythmias have been seen in those without systolic dysfunction, suggesting the possibility of an intrinsic electrophysiologic disorder. Noncompaction has also been associated with Wolff–Parkinson–White syndrome, sinus bradycardia, and AV block (98).

Restrictive Cardiomyopathies

Restrictive cardiomyopathies are uncommon but associated with a very high incidence of SCD, which may be the presenting symptom of this disorder (99). Although sporadic cases may occur, familial clustering of restrictive cardiomyopathy suggest a genetic basis. Myocardial ischemia and intrinsic arrhythmic substrate have both been suggested as the causes of SCD in these patients. Because of the absence of any effective medical therapy and the unpredictable occurrence of events, ICD implantation has been suggested when this diagnosis has been made, with heart transplantation reserved for patients with global impairment of function (100).

Myocarditis

Both acute and chronic myocarditis have been reported as pathologic findings in 42% of young patients who experience SCD (28). Clinical findings prior to SCD may vary considerably, from overt congestive heart failure with cardiomegaly and exercise intolerance to subtle findings such as persistently elevated heart rate or low-grade ventricular ectopy (101). In the absence of unexplained acute-onset ventricular dysfunction, a diagnosis of myocarditis may be difficult to establish. Among patients with SCD, pathologic studies have shown lymphocyte infiltration, necrosis of myocardial fibers, and multifocal scars. Myocarditis may cause transient complete AV block, which in combination with ventricular dysfunction, may result in low cardiac output and ventricular arrhythmias. Temporary pacing is indicated as AV block usually resolves within 7 days (102).

PRIMARY CARDIAC ARRHYTHMIAS

Although most cases of SCD occur in young patients with structural heart disease, primary cardiac arrhythmias (i.e., those not associated with structural heart disease) may cause SCD. In pediatric patients, SCD may occur with the Wolff–Parkinson–White syndrome, congenital complete AV block, supraventricular and ventricular tachycardias, and genetic channelopathies such as the long QT syndromes.

Wolff–Parkinson–White Syndrome

The proposed mechanism of SCD in patients with the Wolff–Parkinson–White syndrome (WPW) is rapid antegrade conduction of atrial impulses over an accessory AV connection during atrial flutter or atrial fibrillation, resulting in the development of VF (Fig. 15.6). Although the Wolff–Parkinson–White syndrome is common among pediatric-age patients, with an estimated incidence of 1:1,500, documented SCD is a rare event.

The largest series to date consisted of 42 pediatric patients (mean age 11.0 ± 7.6 years of age) with Wolff–Parkinson–White syndrome who experienced cardiac arrest (103). Fifteen of these patients died, and 9 of 27 survivors sustained severe neurologic injury. The notable characteristics of these patients included cardiac arrest as the initial arrhythmia in 20 patients, structural heart disease in 13 of the other 22 patients, and multiple accessory AV connections in 6 of the 28 patients in whom electrophysiologic studies were performed. One conclusion of this study was that the absence of symptoms did not provide a reliable basis for classification of a patient with Wolff–Parkinson–White syndrome as having a low risk for SCD.

Risk stratification for the asymptomatic patient with Wolff–Parkinson–White syndrome remains difficult owing to the infrequency of SCD. Historically, the incidence of SCD in the asymptomatic patient with WPW has been estimated at 1 per 1,000 patient years (104), with an increased risk of SCD reported in patients with multiple pathways, syncope, structural heart disease, or a family history of Wolff–Parkinson–White syndrome. However, in a prospective study, Pappone et al. (105) reported that 3 of 27 untreated patients with asymptomatic WPW and a "high risk for arrhythmia" experienced either ventricular fibrillation ($n = 2$) or SCD ($n = 1$) during a median follow-up of 19 months. Of note, high risk was defined as inducibility of AV reciprocating tachycardia or atrial fibrillation, whereas others have defined high risk in the Wolff–Parkinson–White syndrome by antegrade accessory connection conduction properties (106). Additional prospective studies will be necessary to more clearly define the risk of SCD in the Wolff–Parkinson–White syndrome, which is especially vital in guiding treatment decisions for asymptomatic patients. In the current era, radiofrequency catheter ablation of the accessory AV connection is the preferred mode of therapy for patients who are at risk for SCD, intolerant or not responsive to drug therapy, or have a strong preference for definitive cure (107).

Congenital Complete Atrioventricular Block

Congenital complete AV block (CCAVB) in the absence of congenital heart disease occurs in an estimated 1 of 20,000 infants. There is a definite association between the finding of CCAVB and maternal autoimmune disorders (108). In the absence of congenital heart disease, the risk of death in infants with CCAVB is highest when the average heart rate is <55 beats per minute. However, beyond infancy, SCD has not correlated specifically with either heart rate or prior symptoms. In two series of patients with isolated CCAVB, there were 10 sudden deaths among 145 patients, with SCD as the initial symptom in 8 of the 10 deaths (109,110). Severe mitral insufficiency and ventricular failure may develop in the second or third decade of life in previously asymptomatic patients with CCAVB (110). Because of the lack of reliable methods of risk stratification and the significant risk of late SCD, elective cardiac pacing has now been classified as a class II b indication for asymptomatic CCAVB patients with an acceptable rate (69).

Another population at risk for unexpected SCD is infants with the long QT syndrome and 2:1 atrioventricular block or complete AV block. Sustained VT resulting in hemodynamic

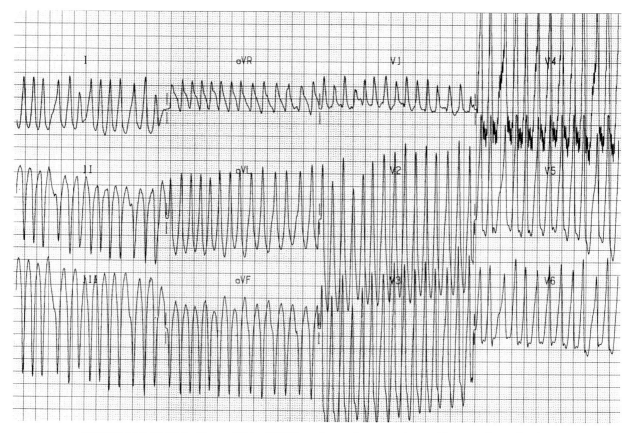

FIGURE 15.6 Wolff–Parkinson–White (WPW) syndrome demonstrating rapid antegrade conduction over an accessory pathway during atrial fibrillation. This electrocardiogram was recorded from a 14-year-old who had collapsed after several hours of palpitations. Prior to this event, neither supraventricular tachycardia nor WPW had been recognized in this patient. Catheter ablation of a posteroseptal accessory pathway associated with a coronary sinus diverticulum was performed, resulting in elimination of pre-excitation and inducible tachycardia.

collapse may be the cause of SCD. However, the benefit of pacemaker or pharmacologic therapy remains limited, with a significant percentage of these infants failing to survive the first year of life (111).

Tachycardias

Supraventricular and ventricular tachycardias in the absence of structural heart disease have been reported as the cause of SCD in pediatric patients, most commonly in infants. Cardiovascular collapse may occur in infants following a prolonged, unrecognized episode of sustained supraventricular tachycardia. SCD in this setting is attributed to low cardiac output and progressive acidosis as a consequence of impaired ventricular function (112). Sustained VT may also occur in infants or children at extremely rapid rates resulting in cardiovascular collapse. VT in infants is associated with discrete myocardial tumors (113). It is critical to correctly diagnose VT, as the administration of digoxin for presumed supraventricular tachycardia may result in ventricular fibrillation. Surgical excision of the involved area(s) may result in cure of tachycardia and an improved long-term prognosis.

The evaluation and potential risk of SCD for children and adolescents with complex ventricular ectopy in the absence of symptoms and with no identifiable structural heart disease

remains a matter of debate. Paul et al. (114) reported that children with couplets in the absence of structural heart disease had no inducibility of sustained ventricular arrhythmias and no death during follow-up. Patients with documented complex ventricular ectopy require a thorough evaluation to exclude heart disease, including Holter monitoring, exercise testing, and echocardiography. Idiopathic forms of VT originating at the right ventricular outflow tract or septal aspect of the left ventricle have characteristic electrocardiographic patterns and are associated with a very low risk of SCD. Conversely, patients with exercise-induced VT may have a cardiomyopathy or genetic channelopathy and are at an increased risk for SCD.

Genetic Channelopathies

Over the past decade, considerable progress has been made in understanding the molecular basis of arrhythmias and SCD in patients with no identifiable structural heart disease. It is now well established that certain individuals have a genetic basis for the development of lethal cardiac arrhythmias, involving either cardiac depolarization or repolarization or both, and that specific physiologic or pharmacologic triggers may be required to initiate these arrhythmias (115). Although the long QT syndromes have been the most extensively studied of the channelopathies, a genetic basis for the Brugada syndrome, catecholaminergic VT, and short QT syndrome has also been defined.

Long QT Syndromes

The long QT syndromes refer to a group of disorders with the common features of prolongation of the QT interval (corrected for heart rate) on the surface electrocardiogram and associated syncope, polymorphic VT, or familial SCD (116). This is a heterogeneous disorder, usually involving genetic disorders of either sodium or potassium ion channels, and may be either congenital or acquired. An autosomal dominant pattern of transmission occurs in 50% of patients with the congenital form of this disorder.

The mechanism of SCD in the long QT syndrome is a characteristic form of polymorphic VT (torsade de pointes), which may degenerate into VF. It is proposed that mutations in ion channel subunits result in reduction of repolarization currents, which in turn result in prolongation of the action potential duration, electrocardiographic prolongation of the QT interval, after depolarizations, and an increased dispersion of refractoriness. These consequences of altered repolarization result in a proarrhythmic substrate and the basis to initiate and sustain polymorphic VT.

The diagnosis of a prolonged QT interval on the surface electrocardiogram may be problematic in children. This is because of the presence of sinus arrhythmia, uncertainty regarding inclusion of U waves, and the transient prolongation of the QT interval frequently observed in newborn infants (117). Owing to the imprecision inherent in measurement of the ECG and diverse clinical presentations, clinical criteria have been proposed for diagnosis of the long QT syndrome (118). Patients with four or more points are categorized as a high probability, 2 to 3 points as intermediate and one or less as low probability of having the long QT syndrome (Table 15.6).

In a collaborative series of 287 children (mean age 6.8 years) with the long QT syndrome (119), the initial presentation included cardiac arrest in 9%, syncope in 26%, and seizures in 10%. During 5 ± 4 years of follow-up, 5% of the patients experienced cardiac arrest, 4% had syncope, and 1% seizures. SCD occurred in 8% of the patients, with a corrected QT interval >0.60 seconds and noncompliance with medication (β-blockade) the multivariate predictors of SCD. Because cardiac arrest was the initial presentation of the long QT syndrome in 9% of the patients, pharmacologic treatment of asymptomatic patients with QT prolongation and a positive family history was advised.

There is continuing debate regarding whether some cases of the sudden infant death syndrome may be due to the presence of an unrecognized long QT syndrome. Renewed interest in this possibility developed when Schwartz et al. (21) reported that a large proportion of victims of sudden infant death syndrome displayed a prolonged QT (<440 ms) in the first week of life. Others have suggested that some cases of SIDS may be specifically related to mutations in the HERG gene, which is a known cause of long QT syndrome (120). This issue remains a topic of debate but does not appear to explain most deaths from SIDS (121).

The initial treatment of minimally symptomatic patients with the congenital long QT syndromes most often is beta-blockade, with the possible exception of those with long QT3 owing to SCN5A mutations. Combined treatment with pacing and pharmacologic therapy has not proven to provide adequate prophylaxis against SCD in symptomatic patients (122). Therefore, patients with prolonged QT who are SCD survivors or experience recurrent syncope on medication generally require implantation of an ICD.

Prolongation of the QT interval may also be acquired secondary to electrolyte abnormalities, hypothermia, central nervous system injury, liquid protein diets, and starvation. A number of antiarrhythmic medications, nonsedating antihistamines, and macrolide antibiotics have been associated with QT interval prolongation (123). There is increasing evidence that some individuals are genetically predisposed to QT prolongation and that these drugs may unmask this disorder.

Short QT Syndrome

The short QT syndrome is a recently described primary electrical disease of the heart. It is defined by an abnormally short QTc interval (<300 ms) and a propensity for atrial fibrillation and sudden cardiac death (SCD) (124). The short QT syndrome has been linked to mutations in several genes, each encoding a different potassium ion channel involved in repolarization. It is proposed that shortening of the effective refractory period combined with increased dispersion of repolarization is the substrate for re-entry and life-threatening arrhythmias. Diagnosis in children may be difficult because the short QT interval may become apparent only at heart rates <80 per minute. Therapies have not been defined, although quinidine may lengthen ventricular refractoriness and reduce vulnerability to VF (125).

Brugada Syndrome

Brugada syndrome is defined by VF in the absence of structural heart disease but associated with right precordial electrocardiographic abnormalities. The syndrome originally was described in 1992 in eight patients with right bundle branch block, ST elevation in the right precordial leads, and sudden cardiac death (126).

The disorder exhibits a pattern of autosomal dominant inheritance with variable penetrance and is believed to be caused by mutations in the cardiac sodium channel. Mutations in the SCN5A gene have been found in 20% of patients with

TABLE 15.6

CLINICAL CRITERIA FOR DIAGNOSIS OF PROLONGED QT SYNDROMES

	Points
ECG findings:	
QTc duration	
≥480 ms	3
460–470 ms	2
≥450 ms (if male)	1
Torsade de pointes	2
T-wave alternans	1
Notched T wave in three leads	1
Low heart rate for age (<2nd percentile)	0.5
Clinical history:	
Syncope[a]	
With stress	2
Without stress	1
Congenital deafness	0.5
Family history:	
Family members with definite LQTS	1
Unexplained sudden cardiac death <30 years of age among immediate family members	0.5

Adapted from Schwartz et al. (118), with permission.
[a]Mutually exclusive.

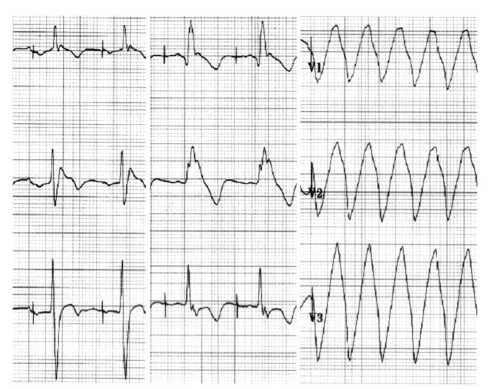

FIGURE 15.7 Procainamide infusion in an 11-year-old with recurrent syncope, sinus bradycardia, and both atrial and ventricular tachyarrhythmias. The **left panel** shows the preinfusion electrocardiogram, leads V1 to V3, with equivocal findings for the Brugada syndrome. The **center panel**, after procainamide infusion, demonstrates marked elevation of the ST-T segments consistent with Brugada's syndrome. In the **right panel**, the patient develops a wide QRS complex (ventricular) tachycardia, which was terminated using overdrive pacing from a previously implanted pacemaker. Following this testing, the pacemaker was removed and replaced with an implantable cardioverter defibrillator.

Brugada syndrome and result in a loss of function of the sodium channel alpha-subunit (127). This loss of function can be exacerbated by sodium channel blocking agents (class I antiarrhythmic medications), and these medications may be used to unmask the diagnostic ECG findings in this syndrome, specifically the coved ST segment followed by a negative T-wave (Fig. 15.7) (128). Brugada syndrome also has been associated with other arrhythmias including sinus node dysfunction, supraventricular and ventricular arrhythmias, and AV node conduction delay.

Although the syndrome typically presents in adulthood with a mean age of SCD of 41 years, Brugada syndrome has been diagnosed in children, generally older than 5 years of age (129). Diagnosis in children is difficult owing to the dynamic ECG findings, variations in prevalence in different populations, and the fact that electrocardiographic features that are similar to those characteristic of the Brugada syndrome may occur in healthy young children (130).

Risk stratification and management of Brugada syndrome continue to be defined at this time. Spontaneous ST-segment elevation in leads V1 through V3 (as opposed to diagnostic ECG findings only after sodium channel blocker challenge) and a history of syncope are associated with a greater risk of an arrhythmic event. However, the induction of VT or VF by programmed electrical stimulation has not been a consistent risk factor for SCD.

Antiarrhythmic agents have been ineffective in the treatment of Brugada syndrome, although quinidine has been shown to normalize ST-segment elevation. The Consensus Statement on Brugada Syndrome offers some recommendations to guide management (131). In general, symptomatic patients with diagnostic ECG findings who present with aborted sudden cardiac death (or syncope or seizure) should undergo ICD implantation. Asymptomatic patients with diagnostic findings (either spontaneous or drug induced) should undergo programmed electrical stimulation if a family history of SCD exists. If no family history of SCD exists but a spontaneous diagnostic ECG is seen, then programmed electrical stimulation is justified. If no family history of SCD is present and the diagnostic ECG findings are only seen with drug challenge, the patient is considered to be at low risk and observation is sufficient. For patients undergoing programmed electrical stimulation, the finding of inducible VT/VF warrants ICD implantation.

Catecholaminergic Ventricular Tachycardia

Catecholaminergic VT is a malignant disorder that presents in childhood or adolescence as syncope, polymorphic VT, or SCD preceded by exertion or stress (132). Several ventricular arrhythmias have been described in this disorder, including bidirectional VT, polymorphic VT, and VF (Fig. 15.8). The disease is genetically heterogeneous, involving mutations in the cardiac ryanodine and calsequestrin receptors (133). In spite of diverse mutations, the arrhythmias occur as a functional result of hypersensitivity to inward calcium currents and abnormal release of calcium ions from the sarcoplasmic reticulum. The calcium overload results in delayed cardiac after-depolarizations, which trigger the sustained ventricular arrhythmias. Adrenergic stimulation owing to emotional stress or physical activity can lead to calcium overload and precipitate tachyarrhythmias in this disease; however, programmed stimulation usually does not induce the arrhythmias (134). Leenhardt et al. (135) reported 21 children (mean age 9.9 years) with stress- or emotion-related syncope secondary to polymorphic ventricular tachycardia. Treatment with β-blockade was effective in reducing, but not completely eliminating, the risk of SCD.

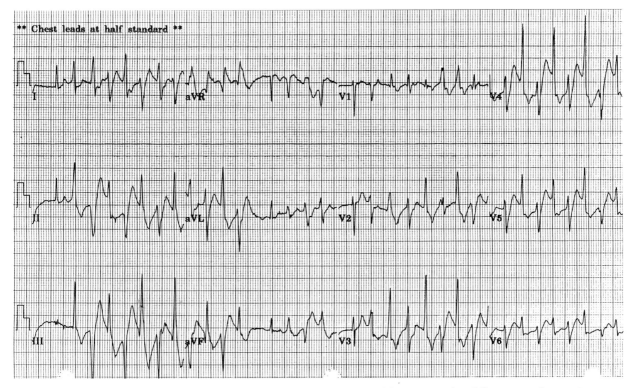

FIGURE 15.8 Bidirectional ventricular tachycardia (VT) recorded from a young boy following anesthesia and the use of epinephrine for local vasoconstriction. Alternating polarity of the QRS complexes is present, most evident in the lateral precordial leads. Degeneration to ventricular fibrillation on several occasions occurred, requiring defibrillation to restore an organized ventricular rhythm.

SUDDEN CARDIAC DEATH IN ATHLETES

It is estimated that 70% of nontraumatic sudden deaths in young individuals occur during moderate to strenuous physical exertion (17,18,136). The vast majority of sudden deaths during sports occur in males, with the incidence increasing with age as coronary artery disease becomes more prevalent.

In the United States, the most common type of heart disease associated with SCD during sports is hypertrophic cardiomyopathy (36%) (82). Less commonly, SCD during sports is related to congenital coronary artery anomalies (19%) and dilated cardiomyopathies or myocarditis (9%). Although the mechanism of death is most commonly a cardiac arrhythmia, traumatic causes such as aortic rupture owing to Marfan syndrome may also occur. Primary cardiac arrhythmias are only rarely cited in pathology studies as the cause of SCD during athletics.

Although SCD during sports is extremely rare, the impact is enormous. The familial and social ramifications of an apparently healthy adolescent dying suddenly are monumental. Controversy therefore centers on the need for and type of preparticipation screening to reduce the risk of SCD in competitive athletes. In 1996, the American Heart Association published a consensus statement on cardiovascular preparticipation screening of competitive athletes (137). An initial health assessment including a comprehensive personal and family history as well as physical examination was recommended for all competitive athletes, regardless of age. In 1998, an additional statement advised serial screening every 2 years in high school athletes. For collegiate athletics, an initial screening at entrance to the institution followed by an interim history and blood pressure in each of the subsequent years was recommended (138). The most recent 2005 Guidelines continued the above recommendations, with an electrocardiogram, echocardiogram, or other testing recommended only when there was a suspicion of cardiovascular disease based on screening (139). This decision was based on the large number of competitive athletes in the United States (10 to 12 million), the low prevalence of the cardiovascular diseases that potentially could cause SCD, and recognition that it was impossible to eliminate all risks associated with competitive sports. Furthermore, the high number of anticipated false-positive results was expected to create undue problems for the athletes and their families, as well as unjustified exclusion from life insurance coverage and athletic competition.

In contrast, a European task force in 2005 recommended a screening electrocardiogram for all young athletes (140). This proposal was based on the report of a significant decline in athletic deaths in Italy following institution of a mandatory national preparticipation screening program that included a routine electrocardiogram (141). In this study of 33,735 screened athletes, 3,016 (8.9%) were referred for echocardiographic evaluation and 22 were found to have hypertrophic cardiomyopathy and were disqualified from sports. Only 5 of the 22 disqualified athletes (23%) had a positive family history and/or cardiac murmur, suggesting a 77% greater power for detecting hypertrophic cardiomyopathy with inclusion of an electrocardiogram.

In assessing the differences between these recommendations, it is important to consider differences in the population bases for these two guidelines. The higher mortality previously reported in the Italian studies may reflect the greater mean age of their athletes and a local clustering of deaths owing to arrhythmogenic right ventricular dysplasia (142). The current American Heart Association guidelines continue to recommend only history and physical examination as initial screening for athletic participation.

Commotio Cordis

Commotio cordis is defined as sudden death resulting from nonpenetrating trauma to the chest wall, occurring in the absence of obvious injury to the precordium, thoracic cavity, or heart. This phenomenon primarily affects children and adolescents from 5 to 15 years of age and usually occurs during sports, most notably baseball, hockey, and lacrosse (143,144). Although first described in 1856, the etiology of SCD following chest trauma remained elusive until recent years. In the few cases of commotio cordis with a recorded cardiac rhythm, VF was most common, although complete heart block and an idioventricular rhythm were reported. In 1998, a swine model of commotio cordis was developed to help define the cause of SCD. This study demonstrated that chest impact (a baseball striking the sternum) occurring 15 to 30 ms before the peak of the T wave consistently induced VF, whereas VF did not occur with the same impact at any other time during the cardiac cycle (145). Of note, impact during the QRS complex often resulted in transient complete heart block.

Commotio cordis generally is fatal, with survival in only 15% of cases (146). When survival occurs, usually it is associated with the rapid initiation of resuscitation and occasionally a precordial thump. Preventive guidelines have focused on the use of safer equipment (such as softer "safety" baseballs), but the universal use of commercial chest protectors has not been advised due to insufficient evidence regarding their benefit. Public and policy efforts to provide automated external defibrillators at sports events may improve the chance for meaningful survival after commotio cordis. For patients who survive commotio cordis, neither invasive testing nor ICD implantation are generally indicated, although noninvasive testing with 12-lead ECG, Holter monitoring, and echocardiography is advised.

EVALUATION AND TREATMENT OF THE PATIENT RESUSCITATED FROM CARDIAC ARREST

As discussed earlier in this chapter, the meaningful survival rate for pediatric patients who experience cardiac arrest remains <20%, with a much poorer outcome for those found in bradycardia or asystole compared with VT or VF. However, with improved emergency medical response systems, the increased availability of automated external defibrillators, and advances in neurologic and cardiovascular resuscitation, it is reasonable to anticipate an increased number of survivors of aborted SCD in the future.

To date, there have been limited data regarding the prognosis in pediatric patients resuscitated from SCD. Benson et al. (147) reported 11 young patients (mean age 18 years) with ostensibly normal hearts who were evaluated following resuscitation from ventricular fibrillation ($n = 10$) or tachycardia ($n = 1$). No patient had a congenital heart defect, pro-longed QT, or cardiomyopathy. However, sustained tachyarrhythmias were identified in 8 of 11 patients by programmed stimulation. Silka et al. (148) reported a series of 15 patients (mean age 11.2 years) who were evaluated following resuscitation from cardiac arrest. In this series there were six patients with primary cardiac arrhythmias, five with prior surgery for congenital heart disease, and four with a cardiomyopathy. Ventricular arrhythmias were identified in eight patients, an accessory pathway with rapid conduction in three patients, atrial flutter in two patients with congenital heart disease, and no arrhythmias in two patients. During 33 ± 17 months of follow-up, two patients died suddenly and three others experienced recurrent cardiac arrest. Recurrent events were limited to patients with persistent inducibility of tachycardia or an undefined arrhythmia. More recently, provocative testing with adrenaline and procainamide has been reported as diagnostic of a genetic or primary electrical disease in 67% of patients with unexplained cardiac arrest (128).

These studies, consistent with several large studies in adult populations, suggest that, first, there is a limited role for antiarrhythmic drug therapy, and second, there is a significant risk of recurrence of SCD following an initial event. Thus, one focus of therapy for patients at risk for SCD is the attempted reversal or inhibition of the substrate for electrical instability, which often is related to abnormal structural remodeling of the myocardium. This includes correction of residual hemodynamic defects resulting in pressure or volume overload, such as severe pulmonary insufficiency following surgery for tetralogy of Fallot, or coronary artery reimplantation for anomalous origin of the left coronary artery. Additionally, the role of beta-blockade and angiotensin-converting enzyme inhibition in the reduction of SCD is established in adults but is undefined in pediatrics.

Reversible causes will be identified in only a small proportion of young cardiac arrest survivors. In most cases, the physician will need to confront the issue that SCD is a complex and unpredictable pathophysiologic process with many cofactors resulting in a common arrhythmic endpoint—VF. Because of uncertainties of causation and a high risk of recurrence, the ICD is the recommended therapy for survivors of arrhythmic SCD. The ACC/AHA/HRS Guidelines for pacemakers and antitachycardia devices has classified "cardiac arrest due to VT or VF, not due to a reversible cause" as a class 1 indication for ICD implantation (69). Individuals with high risk familial or inherited conditions such as hypertrophic cardiomyopathy or long QT syndrome are classified as having a class IIb indication for ICD implantation.

The long-term prognosis for young SCD survivors who have received ICDs appears improved, unless there is severe impairment of ventricular function (87). With continued decrease in device size and improvements in design, the use of these devices in young patients is becoming increasingly accepted. At the same time, the primary objective must remain risk identification to allow prevention of SCD, rather than attempted resuscitation and subsequent ICD implantation.

A final issue is the evaluation of family members of a young relative with unexplained sudden death. Extensive clinical and genetic testing of family members may identify an inherited cause in ≤40% of such cases (149). Asymptomatic family members who are affected by the same mutation may thus be identified, although the most appropriate therapy and limitations for these individuals is an unresolved issue.

References

1. Zipes DP, Wellens HJJ. Sudden cardiac death. *Circulation* 1998;98: 2334–2351.
2. Kuller L, Lilienfeld A, Fisher R. An epidemiological study of sudden and unexpected deaths in adults. *Medicine* 1967;46:341–361.
3. Rubart M, Zipes DP. Mechanisms of sudden cardiac death. *J Clin Invest* 2005;115:2305–2315.
4. Mogayzel C, Quan L, Graves JB, et al. Out-of-hospital ventricular fibrillation in children and adolescents: Causes and outcomes. *Ann Emerg Med* 1995;4:484–491.
5. Myerburg RJ. Epidemiology of ventricular tachycardia/ventricular fibrillation and sudden cardiac death. *Pacing Clin Electrophysiol* 1986;9:1334–1338.
6. Hinkle LE, Thaler HT. Clinical classification of cardiac deaths. *Circulation* 1982;65:457–464.
7. Greene HL, Richardson DW, Barker AH, et al. Classification of deaths after myocardial infarction as arrhythmic or nonarrhythmic. *Am J Cardiol* 1989;63:1–6.
8. Pratt CM, Greenway PS, Schoenfeld MH, et al. Exploration of the precision of classifying sudden cardiac death: Implications for the interpretation of clinical trials. *Circulation* 1996;93:519–524.
9. Silka M, Kron J, McAnulty J. Supraventricular tachyarrhythmias, congenital heart disease, and sudden cardiac death. *Pediatr Cardiol* 1992;13: 116–118.
10. Alexander ME, Cecchin F, Walsh EP, et al. Implications of implantable cardioverter defibrillator therapy in congenital heart disease and pediatrics. *J Cardiovasc Electrophysiol* 2004;15:72–76.
11. Korte T, Koditz H, Neihaus M, et al. High incidence of appropriate and inappropriate ICD therapies in children and adolescents with implantable cardioverter defibrillator. *Pacing Clin Electrophysiol* 2004;27:924–932.
12. Walsh CK, Krongrad E. Terminal cardiac electrical activity in pediatric patients. *Am J Cardiol* 1983;51:557–561.
13. Safranek DJ, Eisenberg MS, Larsen MP. The epidemiology of cardiac arrest in young adults. *Ann Emer Med* 1992;21:1102–1106.
14. Zipes DP. Electrophysiological mechanisms involved in ventricular fibrillation. *Circulation* 1975;51(suppl):III120–130.
15. Molander N. Sudden natural death in later childhood and adolescence. *Arch Dis Child* 1982;57:572–576.
16. Driscoll DJ, Edwards WD. Sudden unexpected death in children and adolescents. *J Am Coll Cardiol* 1985;5:118B–121B.
17. Niimura I, Maki T. Sudden cardiac death in childhood. *Jpn Circ J* 1989;53:1571–1580.
18. Wren C, O'Sullivan JJ, Wright C. Sudden death in children and adolescents. *Heart* 2000;83:410–413.
19. Young KD, Gausche-Hill M, McClung CD, et al. A prospective, population-based study of the epidemiology and outcome of out-of-hospital pediatric cardiopulmonary arrest. *Pediatrics* 2004;114:157–164.
20. Myerburg RJ, Interian A Jr, Mitrani RM, et al. Frequency of sudden cardiac death and profiles of risk. *Am J Cardiol* 1997;80:10F–19F.
21. Schwartz PJ, Stramba-Badiale M, Segantini A, et al. Prolongation of the QT interval and the sudden infant death syndrome. *N Engl J Med* 1998;338:1709–1714.
22. Zheng ZJ, Croft JB, Giles WH, et al. Sudden cardiac death in the United States, 1989–1998. *Circulation* 2001;104:2158–2163.
23. Keane JF, Driscoll DJ, Gersony WM, et al. Second natural history study of congenital heart defects. Results of treatment of patients with aortic valvar stenosis. *Circulation* 1993;87:I16–I27.
24. Burch M, Kaufmann L, Archer N, et al. Persistent pulmonary hypertension late after neonatal aortic valvotomy: A consequence of an expanded surgical cohort. *Heart* 2004;90:918–920.
25. Taylor AJ, Rogan KM, Virmani R. Sudden cardiac death associated with isolated congenital coronary artery anomalies. *J Am Coll Cardiol* 1992; 20;640–647.
26. Choi JH, Kornblum RN. Pete Maravich's incredible heart. *J Forensic Sci* 1990;35:981–986.
27. Liberthson RR, Dinsmore RE, Fallon JT. Aberrant coronary artery origin from the aorta: Report of 18 patients, review of literature and delineation of natural history and management. *Circulation* 1979;59:748–754.
28. Liberthson RR. Sudden death from cardiac causes in children and young adults. *N Eng J Med* 1996;334:1039–1044.
29. Newburger JW, Takahashi M, Burns JC, et al. The treatment of Kawasaki syndrome with intravenous gamma globulin. *N Engl J Med* 1986;315: 341–347.
30. Johnsrude CL, Towbin JA, Cecchin F, et al. Postinfarction ventricular arrhythmias in children. *Am Heart J* 1995;129:1171–1177.
31. Tsuda E, Arakaka Y, Shimizu T, et al. Changes in causes of sudden deaths by decade in patients with coronary arterial lesions due to Kawasaki disease. *Cardiol Young* 2005;15:481–488.
32. Addonizio LJ, Hsu DT, Smith CR, et al. Late complications in pediatric cardiac transplant recipients. *Circulation* 1990;82:IV295–301.
33. Corrado D, Basso C, Poletti A, et al. Sudden death in the young. Is acute coronary thrombosis the major precipitating factor? *Circulation* 1994;90: 2315–2323.
34. Lambert EC, Menon VA, Wagner HR, et al. Sudden unexpected death from cardiovascular disease in children. *Am J Cardiol* 1974;34:89–96.
35. Garson A Jr, McNamara DG. Sudden death in a pediatric cardiology population, 1958 to 1983: Relation to prior arrhythmias. *J Am Coll Cardiol* 1985;5:134B–137B.
36. Ross L, Thiene G. Mild Ebstein's anomaly associated with supraventricular tachycardia and sudden death: Clinicomorphologic features in 3 patients. *Am J Cardiol* 1984;53:332–334.
37. Presbitero P, Somerville J, Rabajoli F, et al. Corrected transposition of the great arteries without associated defects in adult patients: Clinical profile and follow up. *Br Heart J* 1995;74:57–59.
38. Leonard H, Derrick G, O'Sullivan J, et al. Natural and unnatural history of pulmonary atresia. *Heart* 2000;84:499–503.
39. Perloff JK, Warnes CA. Challenges posed by adults with repaired congenital heart disease. *Circulation* 2001;103:2637–2643.
40. Morris CD, Silka MJ, Reller MD. Comparative causes of late mortality after surgery for 14 congenital heart defects: Sudden, non-sudden cardiac, and non-cardiac [abstract]. *Circulation* 1998;98;1–619.
41. Silka MJ, Hardy BG, Menashe VD, et al. A population-based prospective evaluation of risk of sudden cardiac death after operation for common congenital heart defects. *J Am Coll Cardiol* 1998;32:245–251.
42. Garson A Jr. Ventricular arrhythmias after repair of congenital heart disease: Who needs treatment? *Cardiol Young* 1991;1:177–181.
43. Bricker JT. Sudden death and tetralogy of Fallot: Risks, markers, and causes. *Circulation* 1995;92:158–159.
44. Harrison DA, Harris L, Siu SC, et al. Sustained ventricular tachycardia in adult patients late after repair of tetralogy of Fallot. *J Am Coll Cardiol* 1997;30:1368–1373.
45. Chandar JS, Wolff GS, Garson A, et al. Ventricular arrhythmias in postoperative tetralogy of Fallot. *Am J Cardiol* 1990;65:655–661.
46. Khairy P, Landzberg MJ, Gatzoulis MA, et al. Value of programmed ventricular stimulation after tetralogy of Fallot repair: A multicenter study. *Circulation* 2004;109:1994–2000.
47. Gatzoulis MA, Till JA, Somerville J, et al. Mechanoelectrical interaction in tetralogy of Fallot: QRS prolongation relates to right ventricular size and predicts malignant ventricular arrhythmias and sudden death. *Circulation* 1995;92:231–237.
48. Gatzoulis MA, Balaji S, Webber SA, et al. Risk factors for arrhythmia and sudden cardiac death late after repair of tetralogy of Fallot: A multicentre study. *Lancet* 2000;356:975–981.
49. Zeltser I, Gaynor JW, Petko M, et al. The roles of chronic pressure and volume overload states in induction of arrhythmias: An animal model of physiologic sequelae after repair of tetralogy of Fallot. *J Thorac Cardiovasc Surg* 2005;130:1542–1548.
50. Ghai A, Silversides C, Harris L, et al. Left ventricular dysfunction is a risk factor for sudden cardiac death in adults late after repair of tetralogy of Fallot. *J Am Coll Cardiol* 2002;40:1675–1680.
51. Walsh EP. Arrhythmias in patients with congenital heart disease. *Card Electrophysiol Rev* 2002;6:422–430.
52. Flinn CJ, Wolff GS, Dick M, et al. Cardiac rhythm after the Mustard operation for complete transposition of the great arteries. *N Eng J Med* 1984;310:1635–1638.
53. Turina M, Siebenmann R, Nussbaumer P, et al. Long-term outlook after atrial correction of transposition of the great arteries. *J Thorac Cardiovasc Surg* 1988;95:828–835.
54. Gewillig M, Cullen S, Merten B, et al. Risk factors for arrhythmia and death after Mustard operation for simple transposition of the great arteries. *Circulation* 1991;84:III187–192.
55. Gelatt M, Hamilton RM, McCrindle BW, et al. Arrhythmia and mortality after the Mustard procedure: A 30-year single-center experience. *J Am Coll Cardiol* 1997;29:194–201.
56. Moons P, Gewillig M, Sluysmans T, et al. Long term outcome up to 30 years after the Mustard or Senning operation: A nationwide multicentre study in Belgium. *Heart* 2004;90:307–313.
57. Dos L, Ferriera IJ, Rodriguez-Larrea J, et al. Late outcome of Senning and Mustard procedures of correction of transposition of the great arteries. *Heart* 2005;91:652–656.
58. Kammeraad JAE, van Deurzen CHM, Sreeram N, et al. Predictors of sudden cardiac death after Mustard or Senning repair for transposition of the great arteries. *J Am Coll Cardiol* 2004;44:1095–1102.
59. Rhodes LA, Walsh EP, Gamble WJ, et al. Benefits and potential risks of atrial antitachycardia pacing after repair of congenital heart disease. *Pacing Clin Electrophysiol* 1995;18:1005–1016.

60. Bonhoeffer P, Bonnet D, Piéchaud JF, et al. Coronary artery obstruction after the arterial switch operation for transposition of the great arteries in newborns. *J Am Coll Cardiol* 1997;29:202–206.

61. Oeschslin EN, Harrison DA, Connelly MS, et al. Mode of death in adults with congenital heart disease. *Am J Cardiol* 2000;86:1111–1116.

62. Forfang K, Rostad H, Sörland S, et al. Late sudden death after surgical correction of coarctation of the aorta. *Acta Med Scand* 1979;206:375–379.

63. Azakie T, Merklinger SL, McCrindle BW, et al. Evolving strategies and improving outcomes of the modified Norwood procedure: A 10-year single-institution experience. *Ann Thorac Surg* 2001;72:1349–1353.

64. Mahle WT, Spray TL, Gaynor JW, et al. Unexpected death after reconstructive surgery for hypoplastic left heart syndrome. *Ann Thorac Surg* 2001;71:61–65.

65. Mahle WT, Spray TL, Gaynor JW, et al. Causes of death after the modified Norwood procedure: A study of 122 postmortem cases. *Ann Thorac Surg* 1997;64:1795–1802.

66. Cetta F, Feldt RH, O'Leary PW, et al. Improved early morbidity and mortality after Fontan operation: The Mayo Clinic experience. *J Am Coll Cardiol* 1996;28:480–486.

67. Abrams D, Schilling R. Mechanism and mapping of atrial arrhythmia in the modified Fontan circulation. *Heart Rhythm* 2005;2:1138–1144

68. Lillehei CW, Seller RD, Bonnabeau RC, et al. Chronic postsurgical complete heart block. *J Thorac Cardiovasc Surg* 1963;46:436–456.

69. Gregoratos G, Abrams J, Epstein AE, et al. ACC/AHA/NASPE 2002 guideline update for implantation of cardiac pacemakers and antiarrhythmia devices—summary article: A report of the American College of Cardiology/American Heart Association Task Force on Practice Guidelines. *J Am Coll Cardiol* 2002;40:1703–1719.

70. Hokanson JS, Moller JS. Significance of early transient complete heart block as a predictor of sudden death late after operative correction of tetralogy of Fallot. *Am J Cardiol* 2001;87:1271–1277.

71. The Cardiac Arrhythmia Suppression Trial (CAST) Investigators. Preliminary report: Effect of encainide and flecainide in a randomized trial of arrhythmia suppression after myocardial infarction. *N Engl J Med* 1989;321:406–412.

72. Fish FA, Gillette PC, Benson DW. Proarrhythmia, cardiac arrest and death in young patients receiving encainide and flecainide. *J Am Coll Cardiol* 1991;18:156–165.

73. Heist EK, Ruskin JN. Drug-induced proarrhythmia and use of QTc prolonging agents: Clues for clinicians. *Heart Rhythm* 2005;2:S1–S8.

74. Raghuveer G, Caldarone CA, Hills CB, et al. Predictors of prosthesis survival, growth, and functional status following mechanical mitral valve replacement in children aged <5 years, a multi-institutional study. *Circulation* 2003;108(suppl 1):II174–179.

75. Maron BJ, Tajik AJ, Ruttenberg HD, et al. Hypertrophic cardiomyopathy in infants: Clinical features and natural history. *Circulation* 1982;65:7–17.

76. McKenna WJ, Franklin RC, Nihoyannopoulos P, et al. Arrhythmia and prognosis in infants, children and adolescents with hypertrophic cardiomyopathy. *J Am Coll Cardiol* 1988;11:147–153.

77. Hordof A, Kuehl K, Vetter V. Risk factors for sudden death in patients with hypertrophic obstructive cardiomyopathy [abstract]. *Circulation* 1988;78:II595.

78. Romeo F, Cianfrocca C, Pelliccia F, et al. Long-term prognosis in children with hypertrophic cardiomyopathy: An analysis of 37 patients aged less than or equal to 14 years at diagnosis. *Clin Cardiol* 1990;13:101–107.

79. Yetman AT, Hamilton RM, Benson LN, et al. Long-term outcome and prognostic determinants in children with hypertrophic cardiomyopathy. *J Am Coll Cardiol* 1998;32:1943–1950.

80. Nugent AW, Daubeney PEF, Chondros P, et al. Clinical features and outcomes of childhood hypertrophic cardiomyopathy. *Circulation* 2005;112:1332–1338.

81. Ostman-Smith I, Wettrell G, Keeton B, et al. Echocardiographic and electrocardiographic identification of those children with hypertrophic cardiomyopathy who should be considered at high-risk of dying suddenly. *Cardiol Young* 2005;15:632–642.

82. Maron BJ, Shirani J, Poliac LC, et al. Sudden death in young competitive athletes: Clinical, demographic, and pathological profiles. *JAMA* 1996;276:199–204.

83. McKenna WJ, Behr ER. Hypertrophic cardiomyopathy: Management, risk stratification, and prevention of sudden death. *Heart* 2002;87:169–176.

84. Yetman AT, MacDonald C, McCrindle BW, et al. Myocardial bridging with coronary compression in children with hypertrophic cardiomyopathy: A risk factor for sudden death. *N Engl J Med* 1998;339:1201–1209.

85. Maron BJ, Shen WK, Link MS, et al. Efficacy of implantable cardioverter-defibrillators for the prevention of sudden death in patients with hypertrophic cardiomyopathy. *N Engl J Med* 2000;342:365–373.

86. Biagini E, Coccolo F, Ferlito M, et al. Dilated-hypokinetic evolution of hypertrophic cardiomyopathy: Prevalence, incidence, risk factors and prognostic implications in pediatric and adult patients *J Am Coll Cardiol* 2005;46:1543–1550.

87. Silka MJ, Kron J, Dunnigan A, et al. Sudden cardiac death and the use of implantable cardioverter-defibrillators in pediatric patients. *Circulation* 1993;87:800–807.

88. Luu M, Stevenson WG, Stevenson LW, et al. Diverse mechanisms of unexpected cardiac arrest in advanced heart failure. *Circulation* 1989;80:1675–1680.

89. Hsu DT, Addonizio LJ, Hordof AJ, et al. Acute pulmonary embolism in pediatric patients awaiting heart transplantation. *J Am Coll Cardiol* 1991;17:1621–1625.

90. Dubin AM, Berul CI, Bevilacqua LM, et al. The use of implantable cardioverter-defibrillators in pediatric patients awaiting heart transplantation. *J Card Fail* 2003;9:375–379.

91. Marcus FI, Fontaine GH, Guiraudon G, et al. Right ventricular dysplasia: A report of 24 adult cases. *Circulation* 1982;65:384–398.

92. Thiene G, Nava A, Corrado D, et al. Right ventricular cardiomyopathy and sudden death in young people. *N Engl J Med* 1988;318:129–133.

93. Corrado D, Leoni L, Link MS, et al. Implantable cardioverter-defibrillator therapy for prevention of sudden death in patients with arrhythmogenic right ventricular cardiomyopathy/dysplasia. *Circulation.* 2003;108:3084–3091.

94. Jenni R, Oechslin E, Schneider J, et al. Echocardiographic and pathoanatomical characteristics of isolated left ventricular non-compaction: A step towards classification as a distinct cardiomyopathy. *Heart* 2001;86:666–671.

95. Pignatelli RH, McMahon CJ, Dreyer WJ, et al. Clinical characterization of left ventricular noncompaction in children: A relatively common form of cardiomyopathy. *Circulation.* 2003;108:2672–2678.

96. Nugent AW, Daubeney PE, Chondros P, et al. National Australian Childhood Cardiomyopathy Study. The epidemiology of childhood cardiomyopathy in Australia. *N Engl J Med* 2003;348:1639–1646.

97. Jenni R, Wyss CA, Oechslin EN, et al. Isolated ventricular noncompaction is associated with coronary microcirculatory dysfunction. *J Am Coll Cardiol* 2002;39:450–454.

98. Celiker A, Ozkutlu S, Dilber E, et al. Rhythm abnormalities in children with isolated ventricular noncompaction. *Pacing Clin Electrophysiol* 2005;28:1198–1202.

99. Denfield SW. Sudden death in children with restrictive cardiomyopathy. *Card Electrophysiol Rev* 2002;6:163–167.

100. Rivenes SM, Kearney DL, Smith EO, et al. Sudden death and cardiovascular collapse in children with restrictive cardiomyopathy. *Circulation* 2000;102:876–882.

101. Friedman RA, Kearney DL, Moak JP, et al. Persistence of ventricular arrhythmia after resolution of occult myocarditis in children and young adults. *J Am Coll Cardiol* 1994;24:780–783.

102. Batra AS, Epstein D, Silka MJ. The clinical course of acquired complete heart block in children with acute myocarditis. *Pediatr Cardiol* 2003;24:495–497.

103. Deal BJ, MacDonald D, Beerman L, et al. Cardiac arrest in young patients with Wolff-Parkinson-White syndrome [Abstract]. *Pacing Clin Electrophysiol* 1995;18:815.

104. Klein GJ, Yee R, Sharma AD. Longitudinal electrophysiologic assessment of asymptomatic patients with the Wolff-Parkinson-White electrocardiographic pattern. *N Engl J Med* 1989;320:1229–1233.

105. Pappone C, Manguso F, Santinelli R, et al. Radiofrequency ablation in children with asymptomatic Wolff-Parkinson-White syndrome. *N Engl J Med* 2004;351:1197–1205.

106. Bromberg BI, Lindsay BD, Cain ME, et al. Impact of clinical history and electrophysiologic characterization of accessory pathways on management strategies to reduce sudden death among children with Wolff-Parkinson-White syndrome. *J Am Coll Cardiol* 1996;27:690–695.

107. Kugler JD, Danford DA, Deal B, et al. Radiofrequency catheter ablation in children and adolescents: Early results in 572 patients from 24 centers. *N Engl J Med* 1994;330:1481–1487.

108. Buyon JP, Biebert R, Copel J, et al. Autoimmune-associated congenital heart block: Demographics, mortality, morbidity and recurrence rates obtained from a national neonatal lupus registry. *J Am Coll Cardiol* 1998;31:1658–1666.

109. Sholler GF, Walsh EP. Congenital complete heart block in patients without anatomic cardiac defects. *Am Heart J* 1989;118:1193–1198.

110. Michaelson M, Jonzon A, Riesenfeld T. Isolated congenital complete atrioventricular block in adult life: A prospective study. *Circulation* 1995;92:442–449.

111. Trippel DL, Parsons MK, Gillette PC. Infants with long-QT syndrome and 2:1 atrioventricular block. *Am Heart J* 1995;130:1130–1134.

112. Gikonyo BM, Dunnigan A, Benson DW Jr. Cardiovascular collapse in infants: Association with paroxysmal atrial tachycardia. *Pediatrics* 1985;76:922–926.

113. Garson A Jr, Smith RT Jr, Moak JP, et al. Incessant ventricular tachycardia in infants: Myocardial hamartomas and surgical cure. *J Am Coll Cardiol* 1987;10:619–626.

114. Paul T, Marchal C, Garson A Jr. Ventricular couplets in the young: Prognosis related to underlying substrate. *Am Heart J* 1990;119:577–582.

115. Shah M, Akar FG, Tomaselli GF. Molecular basis of arrhythmias. *Circulation* 2005;112:2517–2529.

116. Priori SG, Schwartz PJ, Napolitano C, et al. Risk stratification in the long-QT syndrome. *N Engl J Med* 2003;348:1866–1874.

117. Villain E, Levy M, Kachaner J, et al. Prolonged QT interval in neonates: benign, transient, or prolonged risk of sudden death. *Am Heart J* 1992;124:194–197.

118. Schwartz PJ, Moss AJ, Vincent GM, et al. Diagnostic criteria for the long QT syndrome: An update. *Circulation* 1993;88:782–784.

119. Garson A Jr, Dick M 2d, Fournier A, et al. The long QT syndrome in children: An international study of 287 patients. *Circulation* 1993;87:1866–1872.

120. Christiansen M, Tonder N, Larsen LA, et al. Mutations in the HERG K+-ion channel: A novel link between long QT syndrome and sudden infant death syndrome. *Am J Cardiol* 2005;95:433–434.

121. Task Force on Sudden Infant Death Syndrome. The changing concept of sudden infant death syndrome: Diagnostic coding shifts, controversies regarding the sleeping environment, and new variables to consider in reducing risk. *Pediatrics* 2005;116:1245–1255.

122. Dorostkar PC, Eldar M, Belhassen B, et al. Long-term follow-up of patients with long-QT syndrome treated with beta-blockers and continuous pacing. *Circulation* 1999;100:2431–2436.

123. Roden DM, Viswanathan PC. Genetics of acquired long QT syndrome. *J Clin Invest* 2005;115:2025–2035.

124. Bjerregaard P, Gussak I. Short QT syndrome. *Ann Noninvasive Electrocardiol* 2005;10:436–440.

125. Gaita F, Guisetto C, Bianchi F, et al. Short QT syndrome: Pharmacological treatment. *J Am Coll Cardiol* 2004;43:1494–1499.

126. Brugada P, Brugada J. Right bundle branch block, persistent ST segment elevation and sudden cardiac death: A distinct clinical and electrocardiographic syndrome. *J Am Coll Cardiol* 1992;20:1391–1396.

127. Chen Q, Kirsch GE, Zhang D, et al. Genetic basis and molecular mechanism for idiopathic ventricular fibrillation. *Nature* 1998;392:293–296.

128. Krahn AD, Gollob M, Yee R, et al. Diagnosis of unexplained cardiac arrest: Role of adrenaline and procainamide infusion. *Circulation* 2005;112:2228–2234.

129. Beaufort-Krol GC, van den Berg MP, Wilde AA, et al. Developmental aspects of long QT syndrome type 3 and Brugada syndrome on the basis of a single SCN5A mutation in childhood. *J Am Coll Cardiol* 2005;46:331–337.

130. Yoshinaga M, Anan R, Nomura Y, et al. Prevalence and time of appearance of Brugada electrocardiographic pattern in young male adolescents from a three-year follow-up study. *Am J Cardiol* 2004;94:1186–1189.

131. Antzelevitch C, Brugada P, Borggrefe M, et al. Brugada syndrome: Report of the second consensus conference. *Heart Rhythm* 2005;2:429–440.

132. Priori SG, Napolitano C, Memmi M, et al. Clinical and molecular characterization of patients with catecholaminergic polymorphic ventricular tachycardia. *Circulation* 2002;106:69–74.

133. Postma AV, Denjoy I, Hoorntje TM, et al. Absence of calsequestrin 2 causes severe forms of catecholaminergic polymorphic ventricular tachycardia. *Circ Res* 2002;91:e21–e26.

134. Sumitomo N, Harada K, Nagashima M, et al. Catecholaminergic polymorphic ventricular tachycardia: Electrocardiographic characteristics and optimal therapeutic strategies to prevent sudden death. *Heart* 2003;89:66–70.

135. Leenhardt A, Lucet V, Denjoy I, et al. Catecholaminergic polymorphic ventricular tachycardia in children: A 7-year follow-up of 21 patients. *Circulation* 1995;91:1512–1519.

136. Scoville SL, Gardner JW, Magill AJ, et al. Nontraumatic deaths during U.S. Armed Forces basic training. *Am J Prev Med* 2004;26:205–212.

137. Maron BJ, Thompson PD, Puffer JC, et al. Cardiovascular preparticipation screening of competitive athletes. A statement for health professionals from the Sudden Death Committee (clinical cardiology) and Congenital Cardiac Defects Committee (cardiovascular disease in the young), American Heart Association. *Circulation* 1996;94:850–856.

138. Maron BJ, Thompson PD, Puffer JC, et al. Cardiovascular preparticipation screening of competitive athletes: addendum: An addendum to a statement for health professionals from the Sudden Death Committee (Council on Clinical Cardiology) and the Congenital Cardiac Defects Committee (Council on Cardiovascular Disease in the Young), American Heart Association. *Circulation* 1998;97:2294.

139. Maron BJ, Douglas PS, Graham TP, et al. 36th Bethesda conference: Eligibility recommendations for competitive athletes with cardiovascular abnormalities. Task force 1: Preparticipation screening and diagnosis of cardiovascular disease. *J Am Coll Cardiol* 2005;45:1322–1326.

140. Corrado D, Pelliccia A, Bjornstad HH, et al. Study Group of Sport Cardiology of the Working Group of Cardiac Rehabilitation and Exercise Physiology and the Working Group of Myocardial and Pericardial Diseases of the European Society of Cardiology. Cardiovascular pre-participation screening of young competitive athletes for prevention of sudden death: Proposal for a common European protocol. Consensus Statement of the Study Group of Sport Cardiology of the Working Group of Cardiac Rehabilitation and Exercise Physiology and the Working Group of Myocardial and Pericardial Diseases of the European Society of Cardiology. *Eur Heart J* 2005;26:516–524.

141. Corrado D, Basso C, Schiavon M, et al. Screening for hypertrophic cardiomyopathy in young athletes. *N Engl J Med* 1998;339:364–369.

142. Corrado D, Thiene G, Nava A, et al. Sudden death in young competitive athletes: Clinicopathologic correlations in 22 cases. *Am J Med* 1990;89:588–596.

143. Maron BJ, Poliac LC, Kaplan JA, et al. Blunt impact to the chest leading to sudden death from cardiac arrest during sports activities. *N Engl J Med* 1995;333:337–342.

144. Zangwill SD, Strasburger JF. Commotio cordis. *Pediatr Clin North Am* 2004;51:1347–1354.

145. Link MS, Wang PJ, Pandian NG, et al. An experimental model of sudden death due to low-energy chest-wall impact (commotio cordis). *N Engl J Med* 1998;338:1805–1811.

146. Maron BJ, Estes NA 3rd, Link MS. 36th Bethesda Conference. Eligibility recommendations for competitive athletes with cardiovascular abnormalities. Task Force 11: Commotio cordis. *J Am Coll Cardiol* 2005;45:1371–1373.

147. Benson DW, Benditt DG, Anderson RW, et al. Cardiac arrest in young, ostensibly healthy patients: Clinical, hemodynamic, and electrophysiologic findings. *Am J Cardiol* 1983;52:65–69.

148. Silka MJ, Kron J, Walance CG, et al. Assessment and follow-up of pediatric survivors of sudden cardiac death. *Circulation* 1990;82:341–349.

149. Tan HL, Hofman N, van Langen IM, et al. Sudden unexplained death: Heritability and diagnostic yield of cardiological and genetic examination in surviving relatives. *Circulation* 2005;112:207–213.

PART IV   THERAPEUTIC METHODS

CHAPTER 16 ■ THERAPEUTIC CARDIAC CATHETERIZATION

RALF J. HOLZER, MD, MSc, AND JOHN P. CHEATHAM, MD

Catheter-based techniques, whether palliative or corrective, are now the accepted therapy for many congenital cardiac defects. Interventional, or better-termed therapeutic, catheterizations were initiated by Dotter and Judkins (1), who first reported the treatment of peripheral vascular lesions during a catheterization in 1964, when they dilated a stenotic peripheral vessel through a cutdown on the vessel. The next major innovative accomplishment and the first intracardiac therapeutic catheterization procedure for pediatric congenital heart disease was the balloon atrial septostomy done by Rashkind and Miller in 1966 (2). That procedure really set the stage for all therapeutic catheterization procedures used today. In 1967, Porstmann et al. (3) reported the first nonsurgical corrective procedure in the catheterization laboratory with their description of a technique for closure of a patent ductus. Vascular occlusion coils were introduced by Wallace et al. in 1975 (4), and in 1976 King et al. (5) were the first to describe the closure of atrial septal defects in the catheterization laboratory. Even though their device has not found widespread use, it set the stage for future development of transcatheter devices. One of the largest contributions to interventional cardiology has probably been made by Gruentzig, a Swiss native who in 1976 reported on dilation of peripheral vessels with noncompliant balloons. This initiated a rapid innovative spurt within the congenital cardiac community during which narrowed lesions at various locations were treated with balloon angioplasty, frequently initially in a noncontrolled fashion. In 1982, Dr. Jean Kan et al. (6) reported the first successful transcatheter static balloon pulmonary valvuloplasty, and Dr. James Lock et al. (7) in 1987 reported use of the clamshell device to occlude a ventricular septal defect (VSD) using a percutaneous approach. Dr. Charles Mullins introduced endovascular stents into the management of patients with congenital cardiac lesions (8), and the long list of innovations reached another milestone when Dr. Phillip Bonhoeffer, a German cardiologist working in France in 2000, performed the first transcatheter pulmonary valve replacement in a human (9).

In this section, the most important therapeutic catheterization procedures performed as of this writing are discussed. This chapter is not intended as a complete and exhaustive textbook of interventional techniques, but instead should give the reader a general overview of therapeutic catheterization. It should be emphasized that not every pediatric cardiologist, or, for that matter, every center, should offer every therapeutic catheterization procedure. For any procedures to be performed at any particular institution, minimal specific skills are involved, special techniques must be mastered and maintained, and a large inventory of specialized and expensive catheters and devices must be stocked to offer the patient an optimal procedure. Absence of appropriate qualifications and equipment can result in unnecessary risk to the patient without a reasonable chance of the therapeutic catheterization procedure being successfully accomplished. In fact, even if the patient is not acutely harmed by the attempt, it is important to be aware of the fact that the next procedure in a more appropriate setting might be compromised by a previously unsuccessful attempt.

We have used and expanded on this chapter published in other editions of this textbook and therefore acknowledge the previous contributions made by Drs. Nancy Bridges, Martin O'Laughlin, Charles Mullins, and Michael Freed.

THE INTERVENTIONAL ARMAMENTARIUM

General Considerations

The spectrum of transcatheter procedures available for the treatment of children and adults with congenital heart disease has rapidly increased over the last three decades. Although the technical skills of the operator combined with a sound anatomic and hemodynamic understanding of a patient's condition remain without a doubt the most important ingredients for successful outcome of an interventional catheter procedure, the choice of the appropriate equipment is almost equally as important for a successful outcome. With rapid progress that is being made in the development of new and more refined equipment, the operator has an inherent responsibility to keep up-to-date with these development efforts and to avoid procedural failures in situations where the use of a different type of equipment may lead to a very different outcome. Even though most interventional meetings center on new device developments, the choice of appropriate balloon, catheters, sheaths, and wires is in many situations even more important for a successful outcome. It is beyond the scope of this discussion to describe all available balloon catheters, but the operator has to make a well-informed decision on which balloon to use based on profile, rated maximum pressure, available lengths, and degree of compliance and adjust his or her choice to suit specifically the therapeutic intervention that is intended. For example, balloon-in-balloon (BIB) catheters (NuMED, Hopkinton, NY) are specifically suited for stent deployment, whereas the family of high-pressure Mullins balloons (NuMED, Hopkinton, NY) aids exquisitely when high-pressure balloon angioplasty or stent re-expansion to a larger diameter is required.

The following discussion focuses mainly on transcatheter devices and has been taken to a large extent from an article on this topic that was recently published in *Expert Review of Medical Devices* (10).

Even though transcatheter devices have long been available for the management of congenital cardiac lesions, the greatest progress has been made through introduction of a large variety of newer devices that were specifically developed for individual congenital cardiac lesions over the last 10 years. This progress has enabled many procedures to be safely performed in a much wider range of clinical centers.

The following discussion is centered on transcatheter devices that are presently approved or investigated within the United States and includes a discussion of devices available for the occlusion of septal defects as well as occlusion of vascular structures. Additionally, a very brief discussion is centered on the off-label use of endovascular stents in the management of congenital heart disease. The spectrum of devices that are discussed below is not intended to be complete, but rather, represents subjective choices of the authors.

Devices for Occlusion of Septal Defects

The development of transcatheter devices for the occlusion of septal defects has been progressing at a rapidly accelerating pace, ever since King et al. (5) first described a percutaneous technique to close atrial septal defects (ASD). Various devices are presently approved by the Federal Drug Administration (FDA), either for regular use or under a humanitarian device exemption (HDE), whereas others are presently being evaluated in phase I and II clinical trials. Even though devices are usually developed to address a specific type of septal defect, it is not uncommon that they are also used for occlusion of other types of defects on an off-label basis, once regular premarket approval (PMA) has been obtained.

The Amplatzer septal occluder gained FDA approval in December 2001 for occlusion of secundum atrial septal defects as well as fenestrations after surgical completion of a Fontan-type circulation. It is presently the most frequently used transcatheter device for occlusion of septal defects within the United States and worldwide. Modifications of the principle device design have since been developed to accommodate the specific requirements of patent foramen ovale (Amplatzer PFO occluder), multifenestrated ASD (Amplatzer cribriform septal occluder), muscular VSD (Amplatzer muscular VSD occluder), perimembranous VSD (Amplatzer membranous VSD occluder), as well as post–myocardial infarction VSD (Amplatzer muscular VSD [post–myocardial infarction] occluder), most of which are presently undergoing or have just completed phase 1 or phase 2 FDA-sponsored clinical trials. The Amplatzer muscular VSD occluder is presently available for investigational use (investigational device exemption [IDE]) in high-risk muscular VSD and is pending PMA approval by the FDA as of this writing. Figure 16.1 shows the family of Amplatzer devices. (All of these devices are manufactured by AGA Medical Corporation, Golden Valley, MN.)

The CardioSEAL ASD occlusion device (Nitinol Medical Technologies, Boston, MA) was developed as a successor to the Clamshell device. At the same time as the Amplatzer septal

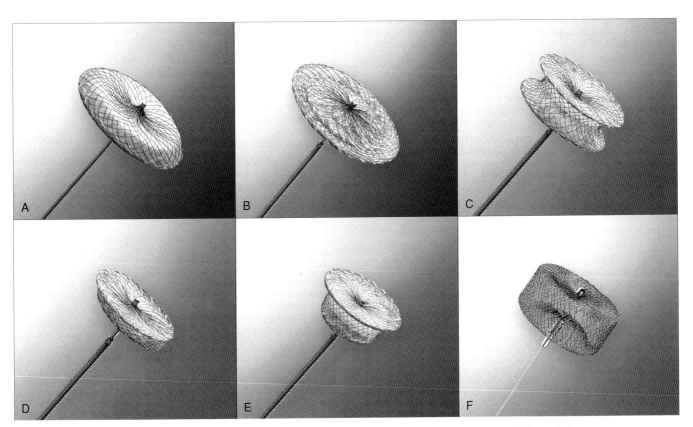

FIGURE 16.1 Amplatzer devices. **A:** Amplatzer septal occluder. **B:** Amplatzer PFO occluder. **C:** Amplatzer muscular VSD occluder. **D:** Amplatzer membranous VSD occluder. **E:** Amplatzer duct occluder. **F:** Amplatzer vascular plug. (The images were provided by AGA Medical Corporation [AGA Medical, Golden Valley, MN].)

occluder was approved, the CardioSEAL device gained regular use approval by the FDA for occlusion of high-risk muscular ventricular septal defects, under a registry requirement. Furthermore, it gained HDE approval for occlusion of patent foramen ovale (PFO) with associated recurrent stroke in patients who were taking therapeutic warfarin. A self-centering modification of the CardioSEAL device, the STARFlex occluder is presently under IDE study for the treatment of PFO and stroke, as well as for migraine headaches considered to be associated with PFO (11).

Another device that has recently acquired FDA premarket approval for the occlusion of ASD is the HELEX septal occluder (W.L. Gore & Associates, Flagstaff, AZ) (12). Devices that have been used outside the United States but have not gained FDA approval include the Sideris buttoned device (Pediatric Cardiology Custom Medical Devices, Athens, Greece) (13,14), the Das-Angel Wings (Microvena Corporation, White Bear Lake, MN, U.S.A.) (15), the PFO-STAR, as well as the ASDOS (Osypka, GmbH; Grenzach-Wyhlen, Germany) (16).

Amplatzer Septal Occluder

The Amplatzer septal occluder (ASO) is a double-disc device formed of 0.005-inch nitinol mesh, which was first described in 1997 (17,18). It consists of two discs that are linked to each other through a central connecting waist. Dacron fabric is incorporated into each disc as well as the connecting waist to enhance thrombosis. The device size is defined by the diameter of the connecting waist and is available from 4 to 38 mm. A 40-mm device is available outside the United States; it has completed tests under an investigational device exemption (IDE) and is currently awaiting FDA approval. The connecting waist has a length between 3 and 4 mm with the diameter of the left atrial disc exceeding the connecting waist by 12 to 16 mm, whereas the diameter of the right atrial disc exceeds the connecting waist by 8 to 10 mm.

The ease of use of this device combined with high closure rates and a low rate of device- or procedure-related complications has allowed transcatheter closure of atrial septal defects to be performed at a much wider range of institutions (19,20). Electrophysiologic abnormalities are frequently seen during the first 24 hours after device implantation but usually do not require any treatment (21). These abnormalities usually resolve quickly, with rhythm or conduction abnormalities 1 year after device occlusion being extremely rare (22). A release of nickel from the device with a peak at 1 month postimplantation has been described (23). However, its clinical significance is questionable, and reports of clinically significant allergic reactions to nickel after device implantation are rare (24). A rare but serious complication is erosion of the device through the anterior atrial wall and into the aortic root. Its incidence is estimated at approximately 0.1%, and most of the described cases have occurred in older female patients. Even though oversizing of the device has been implicated as a potential causal factor, it could not be documented in all affected patients, and therefore, the exact cause and disposition of this very serious complication remains unclear (25).

Amplatzer PFO Occluder

The design of the Amplatzer patent foramen ovale (PFO) occluder, albeit similar to the Amplatzer septal occluder, accommodates very specific morphologic characteristics of the PFO. Similar to the ASO, the PFO occluder is a double-disc device formed of 0.005 inch (18- and 25-mm device) or 0.006 inch (35-mm device) nitinol wire mesh. However, it is non–self-centering and consists of two discs that are linked to each other

through a central connecting waist, with Dacron fabric being incorporated into each disc. The connecting waist is thin with a length of 3 mm, thereby accommodating the tunnel-type morphology of a PFO without distorting the atrial septal anatomy. In contrast to the ASO, the right atrial disc is equal to or larger in size than the left atrial disc. The device is available in three size configurations of right and left atrial disc: 18/18 mm (18-mm device) (26), 25/18 mm (25-mm device) and 35/25 mm (35-mm device). The relatively large size of the discs in relation to the connecting waist makes this device particularly useful to flatten any coexisting atrial septal aneurysm. Its clinical use was first described in 2000 by Waight et al. (27).

Similar to the ASO, the PFO occluder has a low risk of procedure- or device-related complications (28). However, the rare but serious complication of device erosion into the aortic root has also been observed with the PFO occluder (29), with its exact cause and disposition remaining unclear. Thrombus formation on implanted Amplatzer devices can occur (30) but is significantly less common when compared with other devices that are used for occlusion of PFO or ASD, where the incidence averages 2.5% (31). It usually can be expected to resolve under anticoagulation therapy, with postprocedural atrial fibrillation as well as persistent atrial septal aneurysms having been identified as significant predictors for thrombus formation (31). The effectiveness of PFO device closure in reducing the risk of recurrent neurologic events compared with established treatment modalities is currently being evaluated in the RESPECT trial. Braun et al. (32) reported an annual risk of recurrence of transient ischemic attack (TIA) of 0.6% after PFO closure, whereas the rate of complete closure as determined by echocardiogram with bubble-contrast evaluation has been reported to be about 94% at a mean follow-up of 16.5 months (28).

Amplatzer Muscular VSD Occluder

The Amplatzer muscular VSD occluder was added to the interventional armamentarium in 1999 (33,34). Similar to most Amplatzer devices, it is a double-disc device made of 0.0005-inch nitinol mesh wire. Both discs are equal in size and exceed the diameter of the central connecting waist by 8 mm. Dacron fabric is incorporated into both discs as well as the central connecting waist, which has a length of 7 mm to accommodate the increased septal thickness of muscular VSD. This determines the size of the device, which is available from 4 to 18 mm.

An early multicenter U.S.A. experience of 75 patients was reported by Holzer et al. in 2004 (35). Procedure- and device-related complications occurred in ≤39% of patients, almost a quarter of which were classified as major. The mortality in this early multicenter trial was 2.6%. Weight <10 kg has been identified as a significant risk factor for adverse events. Closure rates were 40% immediately after device deployment and increased further to 92% at 12-month followup (35). In 2005, Thanopoulos and Rigby (36) reported one case of subsequent development of complete heart block 1 year after device implantation in a series of 30 patients with a median follow-up of 2.2 years. Closure rates as high as 93% were described. Reports suggest that the relatively high rate of procedure-related complications in infants may be reduced through a perventricular approach through the beating heart without need for cardiopulmonary bypass (37,38). It has been suggested that when the advantages and disadvantages of the surgical approach to muscular ventricular defects are weighed against the risks and difficulties of the catheterization technique, the transcatheter route may be an effective alternative in selected patients with a decreased morbidity.

Amplatzer Muscular VSD (Post–Myocardial Infarction) Occluder

The Amplatzer muscular VSD (post–myocardial infarction) occluder was first described in 2003 in a small series by Goldstein et al. (39). It was developed as a modification of the Amplatzer muscular VSD occluder to take account of the increased septal thickness in adults. It is a double-disc device made of 0.0005-inch nitinol mesh wire. The discs are symmetrical, slightly larger than those of the muscular VSD device, and exceed the connecting waist by 10 mm. The length of the central connecting waist is 10 mm, which is longer than the waist of the muscular VSD occluder. The device is available in sizes from 16 to 24 mm. Similar to the muscular VSD device, Dacron fabric is incorporated into both discs as well as the central connecting waist.

The largest series to date has been reported by Holzer et al. (40) in 2004, including 18 patients in whom occlusion of a postinfarct VSD was attempted using the Amplatzer muscular VSD (post–myocardial infarction) occluder. A device was successfully placed in 89% of procedures, with early 30-day mortality being about 28%. On follow-up, two patients required re-catheterization to close residual VSD. At a median follow-up of 332 days, 20% of patients had complete closure, 60% a small residual shunt, and a further 20% a moderate residual shunt (40). Even though results of device closure of post–myocardial infarction VSD are poor, they have to be interpreted on the background of an early surgical mortality of as high as 27% to 46%, with the mortality in untreated patients >90% (41–43).

Unfortunately, so far the device design for postinfarction VSD remains suboptimal, both in sizes available as well as device configuration. Residual shunts are not uncommon. It is possible that the addition of further Dacron fabric to the device may help. From our own experience, we have found that the maximum available device size of 24 mm is frequently insufficient to occlude larger postinfarct VSDs. Whether a perventricular approach may aid in reducing the perioperative mortality has not been evaluated.

Amplatzer Membranous VSD Occluder

The inherent morphologic and anatomic characteristics of perimembranous VSD have in the past resulted in suboptimal outcomes of attempts at percutaneous device closure (44). The Amplatzer membranous VSD occluder is the first device that has been specifically designed for occlusion of these defects. It was first described in a natural swine model in 2000 (45) with Hijazi et al. (46) reporting the first clinical experience in 2002.

In contrast to other Amplatzer devices, the membranous VSD occluder is an asymmetrical double-disc device made of 0.004-inch nitinol wire mesh. The asymmetrical left ventricular (LV) disc exceeds the central connecting waist at the superior, aortic end by just 0.5 mm and at the inferior, apical end by about 5.5 mm. A platinum marker is incorporated into the apical end of the LV disc to aid device positioning. In contrast, the right ventricular (RV) disc is symmetrical in relation to the connecting waist and exceeds its diameter by a total of 4 mm. The connecting waist has a length of just 1.5 mm, and the device is available with the diameter of the connecting waist ranging from 4 to 18 mm.

A serious and worrisome complication after implantation of the Amplatzer membranous VSD occluder is the development of complete heart block. Its incidence in reported studies ranged from 2% to 3% (47,48). However, more recent reports of even higher incidences of complete heart block, ≤4% to 5%, have appeared in several international registries. Even though heart block may develop during the procedure itself (49), it has been reported to occur at any time from within a few days to within a few months after an otherwise uncomplicated procedure (47,50). So far, no specific factors have been identified that would allow prediction of these serious events. However, device modifications that would allow a reduction in external forces exposed onto the conduction system are presently being evaluated. The general outcome after transcatheter occlusion of perimembranous VSD has otherwise been encouraging, with closure rates being as high as 84% to 96% at 6-month follow-up (47,48). Complications are observed in as many as 29% of procedures, mostly minor and self-resolving (47). New or increased aortic or tricuspid regurgitation is observed in as many as 9% of patients, most of which resolves by 6 months follow-up or is described as trivial or mild in degree (51,52). Similar to muscular VSD, a weight of <10 kg has been identified as a significant risk factor for device- or procedure-related adverse events (47). The feasibility of perventricular device deployment has been evaluated in an animal model with encouraging results (53).

HELEX Septal Occluder

The HELEX septal occluder was first described by Zahn et al. in 2001 (12). Its frame is made of a long nitinol wire, with a strip of polytetrafluoroethylene (PTFE) fabric attached alongside. Three eyelets are embedded along the device to facilitate accurate positioning, one at each end and one in central position between both discs. In its deployed status, the device forms two circular discs that are composed of the spiraling nitinol wire with its attached PTFE membrane. The device is available in sizes from 15 to 35 mm (diameter of discs) in 5-mm increments with a device-to-defect ratio of 1.7 to 2:1 being recommended. When compared with the Amplatzer septal occluder, the device has a lower profile and a more atraumatic contour. It is delivered through a 9 Fr catheter, rather than relying on a long sheath. It also creates less distortion of the atrial septum prior to its release.

Vincent et al. (54) reported on the results of 14 patients who were enrolled in an FDA phase II multicenter trial. Devices were successfully placed and released in 13 of 14 (93%) patients, without procedure- or device-related complications. Closure rates at 6 months were 85%, with residual shunts in the remaining patients being classified as hemodynamically insignificant. One patient required removal of the device owing to nickel allergy. Outside the United States, the HELEX septal occluder has also been used to occlude PFO. Sievert et al. (55) reported their experience of 33 patients and identified residual shunts at 6-month follow-up in 5.5% of patients without any procedure- or device-related complications. No recurrent neurologic event was observed in these patients during a mean follow-up of 12 months (55). Serious complications, such as erosions into the aortic root that have been described with the Amplatzer devices, have not been observed with the HELEX septal occluder thus far. The HELEX septal occluder has recently gained FDA premarket approval, and with its low-profile design characteristics, it may provide a suitable alternative for occlusion of smaller ASDs and PFOs.

CardioSEAL and STARFlex Septal Occlusion System

The CardioSEAL and STARFlex septal occlusion devices represent second- and third-generation modifications of the original Clamshell device, which was ultimately withdrawn because of the occurrence of stress fractures in some of the device arms (56–60). Both devices are classic double-umbrella devices with the umbrella frame being composed of four arms made of 0.009-inch MP35n, a cobalt-based alloy that is more flexible and less corrosive than stainless steel. Each arm contains two hinges, with the umbrella material itself being woven Dacron fabric. The two umbrellas are attached to each other at the center, and the devices are available in sizes of 17, 23, 28, and 33 mm, which represents the maximum diagonal diameter of the expanded umbrella (61). The STARFlex device, introduced in 1999 (11), differs from the CardioSEAL device through four central nitinol springs that facilitate a device self-centering mechanism. The main disadvantage of this group of devices is related to the implantation process, which does not allow repositioning of the device. Device retrieval is cumbersome and often impossible.

In 2000, Carminati et al. (62) reported on the European multicenter experience of using the CardioSEAL and STARFlex double-umbrella devices to close intra-atrial communications in 334 patients with a mean age of 12 years. Implantation was achieved in 97% of patients, with early device embolization being seen in 4% of procedures, most of which required surgical removal of the device. Residual shunting has been observed more frequently when compared with the Amplatzer septal occluder. Immediately after the procedure, 41% of patients had a detectable residual shunt, which decreased gradually to 21% at 12-month follow-up. However, when excluding trivial leaks, the rate of complete closure was as high as 93% at 1-year follow-up. Two patients required late explantation of the device, one owing to malposition and one owing to late embolization. Fractures of the device arms were seen in 6% of patients, not associated with clinically significant adverse events. Device erosions into adjacent structures were not observed, and no patient died as a result of the device implantation. Unfortunately, only defects ≤20 mm can be reliably closed using these devices, a significant limitation for patients with larger defects.

Other Devices and Device Modifications

Of those devices that are less frequently used, the Amplatzer cribriform septal occluder has very specific characteristics that make it an excellent choice for closing multifenestrated ASDs. The device was introduced in 2003 and has recently gained FDA premarket approval after completing phase II clinical U.S. trials (63). Its design resembles the Amplatzer PFO occluder, with the notable exception of both discs being equally sized. It is available in sizes of 18, 25, and 35 mm diameter. The thin central connecting waist allows a much larger area of the device to be available to cover the atrial septum when compared with the ASO, while at the same time avoiding any septal distortion through the central connecting waist. This not only makes it an excellent choice for multifenestrated atrial septal defects, but it also allows stabilization of an associated aneurysmal atrial septum. However, placement of the device through the most central defect is important, and therefore, high-quality transesophageal echocardiography (TEE) or intracardiac echocardiography (ICE) guidance is imperative to achieve the desired result.

The Sideris "buttoned device" was first introduced in the late 1980s and is a single umbrella of a thin foam square of polyurethane mounted on crossing arms of spring guidewire (13). This umbrella is held on the septum by a single strand of spring guidewire on the opposite side of the ASD, which is "buttoned" against the crossed wires of the main umbrella. This device has been used extensively in many centers throughout the world, even though it has not gained FDA approval in the United States. In the process, it has undergone a series of modifications and corrections of deficiencies (14),

currently resulting in the use of fifth-generation devices. Even though the buttoned device can be retrieved fairly easily, its lack of a self-centering mechanism and square shape remain significant disadvantages that often require significant oversizing to achieve adequate closure.

Devices for Occlusion of Vascular Structures

Porstmann et al. (3) introduced a technique of transcatheter closure of the ductus arteriosus in 1967. The procedure was complicated and required a large arterial cannulation, and as a result, this technique never found widespread use.

Rashkind and Cuaso (64), while still working on the septostomy balloon, also developed a device for closure of the patent ductus. This device was a small umbrella that attached to the ductus by tiny hooks at the ends of the umbrella arms. The first successful use of this early device was reported in 1979. It was modified into a double umbrella, which was fixed in the ductus by a spring mechanism of the arms expanding against the vessel walls. Even though the device had undergone extensive trials, resulting in >700 prospectively monitored PDA occlusion procedures performed in the United States, it never quite made it to regular use approval (65,66). However, the extensive experience gained in this process formed the basis on which virtually all subsequent devices have been developed.

A large variety of devices has been developed to facilitate occlusion of vascular structures. Embolization coils have been used by general interventional radiologists for almost three decades (4). However, it was not until the 1980s that these were introduced into the interventional armamentarium of the pediatric cardiologist, initially for occlusion of abnormal collateral vessels (67) and subsequently in 1992 for the occlusion of the patent arterial duct in children (68). Gianturco coils are available in various sizes, but their lack of a controlled-release mechanism ultimately stimulated the development of the Jackson coils, which are presently available only outside the United States (69), and its U.S. counterpart, the Flipper coil (Cook, Bloomington, IN). Even though coils were and still are used off-label for the occlusion of the patent arterial duct, it was not until 2003 that a custom-made device designed specifically for the occlusion of the PDA gained FDA premarket approval (70). The Amplatzer duct occluder (AGA Medical Corporation, Golden Valley, MN), which was first introduced into clinical use in 1997, has since remained the only device approved specifically for this indication (70). However, the Nit-Occlud PDA occlusion device (pfm AG, Cologne, Germany), a modification of the Duct-Occlud device, has since undergone phase II clinical trials with promising results (71,72). An additional coil modification, the Gianturco–Grifka vascular occlusion device (Cook, Bloomington, IN), has gained FDA approval, even though its cumbersome delivery technique has prevented its widespread use. A large variety of additional coils is available for regular use, such as Target coils (Target therapeutics, Fremont, CA), Tornado coils (Cook, Bloomington, IN) as well as Nester coils (Cook, Bloomington, IN). However, these are seldom used in congenital cardiac interventions and therefore will not be further discussed in this review. The most recent addition to the interventional armamentarium, the Amplatzer vascular plug, first described in 2003, has since acquired regular use approval for peripheral arterial and venous embolizations (73).

Amplatzer Duct Occluder

The Amplatzer duct occluder (ADO) was introduced into clinical use in 1997 (70). It is, at present, the most commonly used device to close medium- or larger-sized PDA. The device is mushroom shaped and made of 0.005-inch nitinol wire mesh. The central skirt of the device is cone shaped with the pulmonary end being about 1 to 2 mm smaller than the aortic end. A microscrew for attachment of the delivery cable is recessed into the pulmonary end of the device. The device is further expanded at the aortic end through a symmetrical retention disc, the diameter of which exceeds the size of the aortic end of the skirt by about 4 to 6 mm. Dacron fabric is incorporated into the retention disc as well as the skirt. The size of the device, defined by a combination of the diameters at aortic and pulmonary end of the skirt, is available from 5/4 mm to 16/14 mm. The total length of the device ranges from 5 to 8 mm.

Pass et al. (74) reported the results of a multicenter U.S. trial that enrolled 484 patients with a median age of 1.8 years between 1999 and 2002. The Amplatzer duct occluder was successfully implanted in 99% of suitable patients. Occlusion rates increased from 76% immediately at the end of the procedure to 89% at day one postprocedure and further to 99.7% at 1-year follow-up. Major complications were reported in 2.3% of patients whereas the incidence of minor adverse events was about 4.8%. Partial occlusion of the left pulmonary artery was seen in two patients. However, no case of significant aortic obstruction was identified. Device embolization occurred in two patients, requiring surgical retrieval in one. Vascular complications or blood loss requiring transfusion was reported in 18 patients, and one patient died 5 months after the procedure of overwhelming sepsis. Embolized Amplatzer duct occluders are more difficult to retrieve compared with other Amplatzer devices, as a result of the recess of the microscrew into the device, and therefore devices are usually retrieved using at least a 4 Fr larger delivery sheath to be able to collapse a device that has been snared circumferentially. Ducts of atypical (non–type A) morphology are technically more challenging and may require variations in the type and positioning of devices used.

Amplatzer Vascular Plug

The use of the Amplatzer vascular plug in transcatheter therapy of congenital cardiac lesions was first reported in 2003 (73). The device is cylindrical and formed of 0.0015- to 0.003-inch 144 nitinol wire mesh. It is available in diameters from 4 to 16 mm in 2-mm increments, with a device length of 7 to 8 mm. In contrast to other Amplatzer devices, Dacron fabric is not incorporated into the device.

Hill et al. (75) reported on a multicenter experience of 52 patients in whom 84 vessels were occluded using 89 Amplatzer vascular plugs. The most commonly occluded vessels included 45 aortopulmonary or venovenous collaterals, 28 pulmonary arteriovenous malformations (AVMs), 7 transhepatic tracts, and 4 shunts. Complete occlusion of the vascular structure was accomplished within 10 minutes in 94% of implanted devices. More than one vascular plug was required for five vascular structures. Two vascular plugs were electively removed because of residual shunts. Even though the device has been used to occlude persistent arterial ducts (73,76), caution has to be applied for this indication, because the lack of Dacron fabric in these devices may prevent complete occlusion in moderate-sized high-flow PDA, as was demonstrated in a patient with a type C PDA (75,77).

Embolization Coils

Stainless steel coils for embolization of vascular structures were introduced in the early 1970s (4) and have since undergone few modifications. At present, Gianturco embolization coils (Cook, Bloomington, IN) are made of stainless steel spring wire (0.004 to 0.008 inches) with synthetic Dacron fibers being added for increased thrombogenicity. Each extended spring coil has a stiffening core wire that facilitates the forming of a coil of variable length and diameter, once the extending forces are removed. The coils are delivered in their extended length, requiring delivery catheters of 0.025, 0.035, 0.038, or 0.052 inches, depending on the size of the spring coil. The coils are available in diameters between 2 and 15 mm and a length that allows formation of between 1.1 to 5.3 loops. Even though the 0.035- and 0.038-inch varieties are most frequently used, 0.025- and 0.052-inch coils have maintained their usefulness for very specific occasions. The detachable Flipper coil (Cook, Bloomington, IN) is a variation of the standard 0.035-inch Gianturco coil and includes a controlled-release mechanism. It became available in the United States in 2001. However, early versions of this coil lacked thrombogenic Dacron fibers, and the 0.035-coil remains less robust than the 0.038-inch standard Gianturco coil (61).

As early as 1989, Perry et al. (67) reported on their experience of occluding 77 vessels in 54 patients using Gianturco coils. The rates of total or subtotal occlusion immediately during the procedure were as high as 95%. Complications included six cases of inadvertent embolization into the pulmonary or systemic circulation, half of which were retrieved using transcatheter techniques and half of which were left without symptoms. This, however, represents early results. Current practice is to continue to place multiple coils until complete or near complete occlusion of a vessel is confirmed angiographically, and detachable Flipper coils are usually preferred for any attempted occlusion that may be associated with a slightly higher risk of inadvertent coil embolization.

In 1999, Patel et al. (78) reported their experience of PDA coil occlusion in 149 patients. Out of 146 patients who had coils implanted, the rate of immediate complete closure was 97%. In three of four patients with a residual shunt, complete occlusion was achieved during a second transcatheter procedure, whereas the residual shunt spontaneously resolved in another. The study documented zero mortality and very low morbidity. Coil migration during the procedure was seen in six patients (4%), four of which were successfully retrieved. Recanalization or delayed coil migration was not observed during a median follow-up period of 3 years. The risk of inadvertent coil embolization when attempting to close large PDA with a PA diameter >4 mm has been documented to be as high as 16% (79). However, most published data about PDA coil occlusion preceded the introduction of the controlled-release Flipper coil as well as the introduction of the Amplatzer duct occluder, which is now available for moderate- or large-sized PDA. Therefore, the rate of inadvertent embolization can today be expected to be <1% if full use is made of all available devices and techniques.

Nit-Occlud

The Nit-Occlud PDA occlusion system, developed as a successor to the Duct-Occlud device, was introduced in 2001. The device is made up of wound 0.01-inch nitinol wire, which forms a secondary helix-type loop, thereby conforming to a double opposing cone shape (Fig. 16.2) (61,71,72). The device has reinforced distal windings at the aortic end that prevent it from pulling through the PDA, while tighter and softer central windings allow the device to conform to the narrow portions of the PDA at the pulmonary end, thereby allowing more efficient occlusion of the duct. No fabric is attached to the device, with occlusion being facilitated through the metal

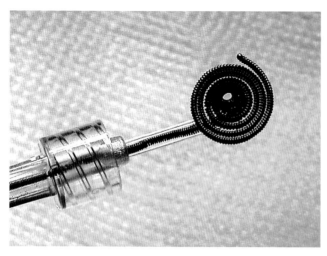

FIGURE 16.2 Nit-Occlud patent ductus arteriosus (PDA) occlusion system. The image shows the aortic spiral disc with the device still attached to the delivery system.

windings alone. The device is available in three principal versions, the Nit-Occlud Flex, the Nit-Occlud Medium, and the Nit-Occlud Stiff, which differ from each other through an increasing stiffness. The devices are available in various dimensions, with the distal (aortic) diameter ranging from 4 to 14 mm, whereas the proximal pulmonary winding diameter ranges from 4 to 6 mm.

A phase II clinical trial has been completed in the United States, and results are expected soon. In 2003, Chisolm et al. (71) reported on 19 patients in whom a Nit-Occlud was implanted as part of the phase II U.S. clinical trial. Devices used were either Nit-Occlud Flex or Nit-Occlud Medium of various sizes. At 24 hours 17 of 19 (89%) had no residual flow, whereas there was trivial residual flow in one and a small degree of residual flow in another patient. Procedural complications or device embolizations were not observed. In 2005, Celiker et al. (72) reported a closure rate ≥93% at 6-month follow-up.

Other Devices and Device Modifications

In 1995, Grifka et al. (80) reported on the evaluation of a new vascular occlusion device in a canine model. The Gianturco–Grifka vascular occlusion device (GGVOD) is essentially an oblong nylon bag that is filled with a long, stainless steel spring guidewire. The length of the wire determines the size of the device, which is available in diameters of 3, 5, 7 and 9 mm. A radiopaque marker is attached to the proximal end of the bag. The GGVOD has been used to occlude various tubular structures, including shunts and pulmonary AVMs, but its design and cumbersome delivery technique make it less suitable for occlusion of the standard type A PDA (61,81,82).

In addition to the aforementioned, a wide variety of devices has been used off-label to occlude the patent arterial duct and other vascular communications, including the Amplatzer muscular VSD occluder (83), the Amplatzer septal occluder (84), the buttoned device (85), and the Amplatzer vascular plug (73).

Endovascular Stents

Charles E. Mullins, MD, pioneered the introduction of endovascular stents into the armamentarium of the congenital

cardiac interventionalist in the late 1980s and early 1990s (8,86). The most common indications for stent placement include rehabilitation of branch pulmonary artery stenosis as well as treatment of primary and recurrent coarctation of the aorta or aortic arch obstruction. However, stents are also used to rehabilitate stenotic lesions in systemic and pulmonary veins and to maintain patency of structures that would otherwise close, such as the arterial duct or a foramen ovale. Endovascular stents are particularly helpful in locations that are either inaccessible to surgical techniques, or where the scarring resulting from surgical intervention is unlikely to achieve an improvement of the lesion, which applies to thin-walled vessels such as distal pulmonary arteries or pulmonary veins.

Virtually all approved stents that are used in the United States in transcatheter therapy of congenital cardiovascular lesions have not been designed specifically for these indications, and are therefore used on an off-label basis. The choice of which stent to use for a particular lesion depends not only on the age and size of the patient, but also on the expected adult dimensions of the vascular structure that is being treated, the morphology of the specific lesion, expected future surgical procedures, as well as previous surgical and transcatheter procedures and their outcomes.

An ideal stent would combine various characteristics, which are often exclusive to each other and may require opposing design goals:

- Low profile that allows introduction through small delivery sheaths
- Easy crimp ability or availability as premounted stents
- Possibility for re-expansion with maximum achievable diameter being sufficient to accommodate the growth of a vessel to adult size
- High degree of flexibility for placement around curved structures
- Allowance for rehabilitation of vessels that are overlapped by the placed stent through the stent meshwork/cells (e.g., open-cell design)
- High radial force to accommodate very tight and scarred lesions
- Rounded atraumatic edges that avoid damage to the vessel and the balloon on which it is mounted
- Nonexisting or low degree of stent-shortening during expansion
- Stent material that is magnetic resonance imaging (MRI)–compliant, noncorrosive, and does not lead to increased blood levels of metal
- Low risk of neointimal proliferation, possibly through internal coating
- Possibility of biodegradable material with a platform to sustain drug coating to minimize tissue reaction

Unfortunately, an ideal stent does not exist; therefore, a careful decision has to be made on which to use. Dr. Charles Mullins always emphasized that the interventional cardiologist should not create a later surgical stenosis by failure of the stent to be able to be dilated to the adult-sized diameter of the vessel. However, it is important to note that the use of premounted and smaller-diameter stents as a palliative procedure to relieve critical vascular narrowings in small infants and children who will have later surgery as a staged repair or conduit change is now a very important treatment option. When judging the suitability of stent implantation, one always has to remember that suboptimal balloon angioplasty may result in impaired interval growth of the pulmonary arterial tree.

Table 16.1 summarizes the most important characteristics of those stents that are presently most frequently used in

TABLE 16.1

STENTS

Name (manufacturer)	Material	Max diameter (mm)	Available length (mm)	Profile	Radial force	Flex	Short	Nontraumatic edges	Crimp	Cells
Genesis XD (Cordis)	Stainless steel	18	19, 25, 29, 39, 59	+	+	−	−	−	++	Closed
Premounted Genesis (Cordis)	Stainless steel	10	12, 15, 18, 24	++	0	0	0	0	NA	Closed
Mega LD (EV3)	Stainless steel	18	16, 26, 36	+	+	++	++	+	0	Open
Max LD (EV3)	Stainless steel	25	16, 26, 36	−	++	+	++	+	−	Open
Cheatham-Platinum 8z (NuMED)	Platinum/ iridium + Gold	25	22–45	−	++	0	−	++	+	Closed

Characteristics of the most commonly used endovascular stents in congenital heart disease (US). Manufacturers listed are Cordis (Warren, NJ), EV3 (Plymouth, MN), and NuMED (Hopkinton, NY). Stent characteristics range from −− (poor stent characteristic) to ++ (excellent stent characteristic). Max, maximum; Flex, flexibility; Short, stent shortening; Crimp, crimp ability; Cells, open or closed cell design.

congenital heart disease in the United States. The Cheatham-Platinum stent (NuMED, Hopkinton, NY), as well as its covered variety, is available in the United States for compassionate use only but is approved outside the United States as the only stent specifically approved for the treatment of congenital heart disease, and has favorable design characteristics for use in native and recurrent coarctation. Covered stents are especially useful for the treatment of ruptured vessels, including aortic aneurysms. Even though the early versions of the Palmaz stent (P108, P188, P308) (Johnson & Johnson, Warren, NJ), as well as the ITI Double Strut and Double Strut LD stent (Intra Therapeutics Inc., St Paul, NM), are still available, they have largely been replaced by the Genesis XD stents (Cordis, Warren, NJ), as well as the EV3 Mega LD and Max LD stents (EV3, Plymouth, MN), and are therefore not listed in this summary. Other stents that are occasionally used in the congenital pediatric population include self-expandable nitinol stents as well as various coronary stents.

The use of intravascular stents has provided a definitive solution to the problem of overdilation that is frequently required when performing standard balloon angioplasty. There has been extensive favorable experience and ≤15 years' follow-up in patients with pulmonary artery branch stenosis and systemic vein stenosis. In the single-center series of Charles E. Mullins et al. at Texas Children's Hospital, >655 stents were implanted in 340 patients with pulmonary artery and systemic vein stenoses. The largest group of patients in this series had lesions involving the central pulmonary arteries in postoperative patients and postoperative central systemic vein or systemic venous baffle stenosis. Many of these stenotic veins had a totally occluded initial lumen; some of the venous channels were purposely perforated with a wire or long needle. The mean vessel diameter increased from 5 to 12 mm, and there was lasting success, with <0.5% showing restenosis during the follow-up period. The number of complications from the procedure or the stents themselves was minimal.

HOW TO CREATE, ENLARGE, AND MAINTAIN INTRA-ATRIAL COMMUNICATIONS

Balloon Atrial Septostomy

Balloon atrial septostomy (BAS), introduced by Rashkind and Miller (2) in 1966, is a lifesaving procedure and one of the few remaining indications for an emergency catheterization in infants. BAS should be available in every institution that cares for infants with congenital heart disease. Because of septal thickening with age, BAS is consistently effective only in infants younger than 1 month of age. The BAS procedure is indicated in all infants with simple transposition of the great arteries (TGA) who are younger than 1 month of age with a restrictive intra-atrial communication and not otherwise scheduled for immediate surgical correction. Emergency BAS is imperative in any infant with simple TGA who exhibits evidence of acidosis as a result of an inadequate intra-atrial communication. This procedure also may be indicated for palliation in other congenital heart lesions in equally young infants, in whom all systemic, pulmonary, or mixed venous blood must traverse through a restrictive intra-atrial communication to return to the active circulation. These lesions include those complex single-ventricle defects associated with hypoplastic right or left ventricles and some instances of total anomalous pulmonary venous connection. Balloon atrial septostomy is rarely indicated in cases of pulmonary valve atresia and intact ventricular septum. It can be extremely hazardous in left-sided heart hypoplasia if the left atrium is diminutive, as there is a heightened risk of perforation or avulsion of atrial appendage or pulmonary vein. In such cases, static balloon dilation of the atrial septum may be preferable.

The preferable approach for performing a BAS is percutaneously through the femoral vein. In addition, balloon atrial septostomy can be accomplished successfully using an umbilical venous approach. For acute, temporary palliation, many of these procedures can performed under echocardiographic guidance in the neonatal intensive care unit, but whenever possible, the availability of fluoroscopy in the cardiac catheterization laboratory adds an additional safety margin to the procedure. BAS catheters are available from various manufacturers and in different designs. The classic Miller–Edwards balloon septostomy catheter (Edwards Lifescience, Irvine, CA), is a single-lumen catheter with a fairly compliant latex balloon at the end that is rated ≤4 mL capacity but can be inflated with larger quantities if required. It requires the use of a 7 French sheath and is still in widespread use, even though newer catheter varieties offer more favorable balloon characteristics. Because of the single lumen it cannot be tracked over a wire, and the fairly high compliance often requires large balloon inflations to successfully perform a septostomy, which is a considerable disadvantage especially in smaller infants <3 kg. Other catheter varieties include the USCI Rashkind balloon catheter (USCI, Glens Falls, NY) which has a 6 French shaft, as well as the newer NuMED Z5 atrioseptostomy catheters (NuMED, Hopkinton, NY) that are available on a 4 or 5 French shaft and can be passed through a 5 or 6 French introducer. These balloons have the advantage of being noncompliant at inflation volumes of 1 mL or 2 mL, which is very important when attempting to tear, rather then stretch, the atrial septum. The balloons also have the additional benefit of being able to be passed over a wire.

Once the deflated balloon catheter is introduced into the venous system and while it is observed on fluoroscopy or by echocardiography, it is advanced through the right atrium and through the foramen ovale or small ASD into the left atrium. While continually observed on fluoroscopy and/or two-dimensional echocardiography, the balloon is inflated with dilute contrast to the maximum diameter of the balloon or, in the smaller atrium, to the maximum diameter tolerated within the particular left atrium. It is essential to determine that the balloon is completely free within the left atrium before initiating the jerk across the septum. Failure to do so can result in laceration or even separation of the left atrium from the pulmonary veins. The balloon is pulled rapidly or, better stated, jerked across the atrial septum into the right atrium (RA) using as forceful and rapid, but at the same time, as short and controlled a pull as possible. Especially when using the fairly noncompliant NuMED atrioseptostomy catheters, it is important to avoid pulling the balloons into the inferior vena cava (IVC), as the rapid jerk can easily create a laceration or disruption of the IVC-RA junction. The entire procedure should be performed one to four times or until no resistance to withdrawal of the fully inflated balloon is encountered or until enlargement of the defect and looseness or flipping of the septum primum tissue are documented by echocardiography. Following a successful septostomy, there should be an immediate equalization or near equalization of pressures across the atrial septum. Performed carefully with precise attention to details, the procedure carries only a small risk, yet it has the potential for a dramatic improvement in the infant's hemodynamic and symptomatic status.

Blade Atrial Septostomy and Cutting Balloon Atrial Septostomy

In infants older than 1 month of age, and certainly for older children who might require an atrial septostomy for palliation of their cardiac defect, the atrial septum usually is too tough or thick for a simple BAS to tear the septum. In 1975, Park et al.

introduced the Park Blade Septostomy Catheter (Cook, Inc., Bloomington, IN) and the blade atrial septostomy procedure to obviate this difficulty. A collaborative study from 1978 to 1982 (87) demonstrated the safety and effectiveness of the blade procedure. The indications for blade atrial septostomy are the same as considered for a balloon septostomy or for surgical atrial septostomy that otherwise would be needed in the older infant.

Blade catheters are available with three blade lengths: 1.0, 1.34, and 2.0 cm. The two smaller blades (the PBS 100 and 200) are available on a 6 French catheter, and the 2.0 cm blade (the PBS 300) is on an 8 French catheter. Both blade catheter sizes require a sheath one size larger than the catheter shaft for smooth introduction.

The most consistent method of delivering the blade into the left atrium is to pass a long Mullins sheath over a catheter or dilator from the femoral vein through the right atrium, through the septum (either through the patent foramen ovale or through a transseptal puncture), and into the left atrium. The blade catheter is advanced through this sheath, and the sheath is withdrawn well into the inferior vena cava. The blade is opened carefully in the left atrium while it is continuously observed on fluoroscopy. Transesophageal echocardiographic guidance can add an additional safety margin to this procedure. The tip is directed anteriorly and to either the patient's right or left side. In contrast to the balloon septostomy, the blade catheter is withdrawn slowly in a controlled but, at the same time, forceful maneuver until the blade snaps through the septum. The blading is repeated four to eight times while changing the angle of extension of the blade as necessary and changing the blade direction from side to side until there is no further resistance to the withdrawal of the fully opened blade catheter.

The blade septostomy is followed by a balloon septostomy. In most patients, this can be accomplished using the Rashkind balloon technique; however, in larger or older patients, when the septum is tough or resistant to tearing, the blade incision can be extended by the use of static dilation balloons placed in the defect and inflated. Alternatively, balloon dilation alone after transseptal placement of a guidewire can be effective in creating or enlarging an atrial septal defect. The resultant defect will be somewhat smaller than the balloon or balloons used for dilation, so the balloon catheters must be oversized relative to the final defect diameter desired. As a result of the combined blade and ballooning, equalization of pressures between the two atria as well as a measurable increase in the mixing of the systemic and pulmonary venous blood should occur. In most cases, an adequate and permanent atrial septal defect is created, palliating the patient indefinitely or until a more permanent correction is possible. Stenting of the atrial septum has been performed in a few cases to ensure a lasting opening. The blade atrial septostomy can be accomplished in patients of any age or any size. Prior to the introduction of the transhepatic approach, congenital absence or acquired blockage of the inferior vena cava had been the only absolute prohibition to a blade atrial septostomy.

With the availability of larger cutting balloons of ≤8 mm in diameter (Boston Scientific, Boston, MA), the combination of static cutting balloon septoplasty, followed by the use of larger diameter static balloons or standard balloon atrial septostomy, has become an important alternative to blade atrial septostomy in patients with a thickened atrial septum. The smaller the pre-existing septal defect, the higher the likelihood that the use of a cutting balloon will achieve an adequate result (Fig. 16.3). This is especially important if the patient size is rather small or prohibitive to use of even a small PBS

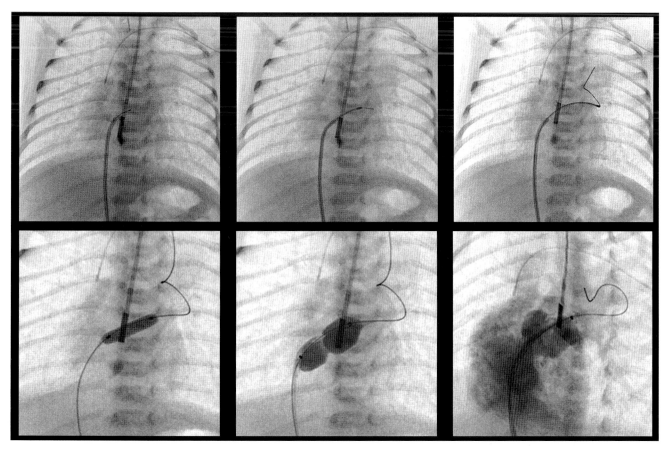

FIGURE 16.3 Radiofrequency (RF) perforation of the atrial septum followed by cutting and standard atrial balloon septoplasty in a 7-day-old infant with hypoplastic left heart syndrome, intact atrial septum, and a restrictive decompressing vein. Images (from **left** to **right** and **top** to **bottom**) demonstrate the RF wire across the atrial septum, the coaxial catheter advanced over the RF wire into the left atrium (LA), wire position through the coaxial catheter into the decompressing vein, and cutting balloon septoplasty followed by standard balloon atrial septoplasty and final left atrial angiogram demonstrating the newly created intra-atrial communication. An intracardiac echocardiographic probe is used in the trans-esophageal echocardiography (TEE) position.

100 blade catheter. If the existing intra-atrial communication is stretched, cutting balloon septoplasty may not be feasible, and it may be more beneficial to perform a transseptal puncture to start with a fresh diminutive opening to facilitate a better result of cutting balloon atrial septoplasty.

Transseptal Puncture

Access to left heart structures is required at times to obtain accurate left atrial pressure recordings, or to facilitate interventional procedures such as the creation or closure of an intra-atrial communication or balloon mitral valvuloplasty. In addition, access to left heart structures from a venous approach avoids the use of larger sheaths in the femoral artery, which can be especially beneficial in small children and infants. Most catheterization laboratories use the standard Brockenbrough transseptal needle, although the use of radiofrequency energy has recently added a more controlled technique specifically for infants with small left atria (88).

The Brockenbrough needle is available in sizes of 62 cm and 72 cm of usable length and is usually used in conjunction with a transseptal Mullins introducer set (Cook, Bloomington, IN).

A fairly stiff exchange-length wire is placed in the SVC or preferably innominate vein, and the Mullins sheath and dilator are advanced to a position within the SVC. The wire is withdrawn, and the transseptal needle is advanced through the sheath to a position just 1 to 2 mm below the tip of the dilator. Occasionally, difficulty can be encountered when introducing the transseptal needle through the hub or dilator and sheath, at which point the two components should be separated temporarily by 1 to 2 cm to allow passage of the needle through the hub. Once the needle has been positioned appropriately, the whole system needs to be flushed and the needle connected to a pressure-monitoring system. There is usually a 1- to 2-cm separation between the needle and the hub of the dilator, and care has to be taken to maintain this distance throughout the procedure. Needle, sheath, and dilator are then removed carefully as one unit with the system being gently pointed toward the patient's left scapula (and posterior) when withdrawing from the SVC and sliding along the atrial septum. Any harsh movement or torque should be avoided at this stage as it can create injury to adjacent vessel or chamber walls. Once the unit has passed about two thirds of the atrial septal length inferiorly, one often notices the tip of the dilator suddenly moving slightly to the left while advancing into the fossa ovalis. At this stage, sheath dilator and needle are withdrawn inferiorly for a few millimeters farther just below the limbus of the ovale fossa. At this point, sheath and dilator are fixed while the needle is advanced slightly out of the tip of the dilator until it fully engages the dilator. At this point the whole unit is advanced while the operator not only carefully observes the recorded pressure tracing but also maintains a left and posterior direction. The operator usually feels a slight pop when the needle traverses the atrial septum, and this should be followed by the emergence of a left atrial pressure tracing. If any untoward resistance or inappropriate pressure tracings appear, the operator should stop any advances of needle, sheath, and dilator. If a position is unclear, a small amount of contrast can be instilled through the needle. If a left atrial pressure tracing is obtained, the entire system is advanced slightly farther toward the patient's left to allow at least the proximal portion of the dilator to pass through the atrial septum. This is performed in very diminutive steps while maintaining careful observation for left atrial pressure tracings. At this point, the needle is withdrawn just inside the dilator to add additional stiffness to the system, and the Mullins sheath is advanced over the dilator and needle across the atrial septum into the left atrium. If at any stage during the procedure doubt about the accurate position occurs, then the system is either withdrawn in very small steps until appropriate pressure recording reoccurs, or a small amount of contrast is injected to confirm the sheath's location.

An alternative to the use of the classic Brockenbrough needle is the use of radiofrequency energy. At the present time, two techniques of radiofrequency (RF) perforation of the atrial septum are available, depending on patient and left atrial size. In larger patients, the Toronto transseptal catheter can be used in combination with the 8 Fr TorFlex transseptal sheath and dilator (Both: Baylis Medical Corporation, Montreal, Quebec, Canada). The Toronto transseptal catheter is curved at the end by about 210 degrees to avoid continued perforation of adjacent structures once the atrial septum is traversed. It also has a slightly increased stiffness when compared with the Nykanen RF perforation wire (Baylis Medical Corporation, Montreal, Quebec, Canada) that is specifically suited to allow tracking of the transseptal sheath across the perforated atrial septum. Initial positioning of the transseptal sheath is very similar to the Brockenbrough transseptal technique. However, instead of using a stiff and forceful needle to traverse the atrial septum, low power and high-intensity electrical current is used to allow the transseptal catheter to advance through the atrial septum, usually with minimal force and a much lower risk of injuring adjacent structures.

In small infants, especially in neonates with a small left atrium, the curve of the Toronto transseptal catheter is too large to fit snugly into the small left atrium. Therefore in these patients, a 4 or 5 French Judkins right (JR) catheter is used to obtain an appropriate position along the atrial septum to facilitate radiofrequency puncture (Fig. 16.3). A 180-cm 0.035-inch outer diameter coaxial injectable catheter (Baylis Medical Corporation, Montreal, Quebec, Canada) is loaded over a 260-cm 0.024-inch Nykanen RF perforation wire, and the RF wire is advanced to the tip of the positioned JR catheter. The use of TEE-guided perforation of the atrial septum has greatly improved the safety and success of this challenging procedure. In infants <3.0 kg, placing the 8 Fr ICE catheter (Acuson-Siemens Co., Mountain View, CA) transesophageally has been suggested by Hill et al [89]. Once an accurate position is confirmed with hand injections of contrast through the side port of a Tuohy Borst adapter, RF energy is applied while the operator also exerts a gentle push on the RF wire. Once perforation has occurred, an orientating injection of contrast can be performed through the Tuohy Borst adapter before the operator advances the coaxial catheter over the RF wire across the perforated lesion. The RF wire is then exchanged to an appropriate exchange-length wire that can be preshaped according to the size of the left atrium. This positioned wire then facilitates cutting balloon septoplasty, possibly followed by balloon atrial septostomy, depending on the size of the intra-atrial communication that is required.

BALLOON AORTIC VALVULOPLASTY

The possibility of creating significant aortic regurgitation has always been the main concern when considering balloon dilation of congenitally stenotic aortic valves, especially in infants and small children. In 1984, Lababidi et al. (30a) reported for the first time on a series of 23 patients with congenital aortic valve stenosis, in whom the procedure was documented to be safe and effective [31]. Despite this report, general acceptance of the technique was relatively slow. One of the fundamental problems of the procedure remains the risk of creating significant aortic insufficiency, which then may accelerate the need for any surgical aortic valve procedure. Although this is less of a concern in the adolescent, where all other treatment options are available in such a situation, the problems are more significant in the infant who has a moderate degree of aortic valve stenosis, where severe aortic regurgitation may require a surgical procedure to be performed at an age where one would have otherwise preferably waited a little longer for the patient to grow.

Several other centers have demonstrated that the results of balloon aortic valve dilation approximated the results of surgical valvotomy but with less risk and much less morbidity. However, the disease has very wide morphologic variations, ranging from the critically ill neonate with borderline LV and left ventricular outflow tract (LVOT) size and a very dysplastic aortic valve, to the young adult with isolated valvar stenosis and well-formed aortic valve.

Guidelines for the treatment of congenital aortic valve stenosis in children are derived from the adult population, where a peak-to-peak gradient >60 mm Hg in asymptomatic patients is considered an indication for transcatheter intervention. However, in a symptomatic patient, or with the presence of ischemic or repolarization changes on ECG, a gradient of 50 mm Hg should be used. However, peak systolic gradients are only meaningful if left ventricular function is normal. Documented aortic valve stenosis in the critically ill neonate with a dilated left ventricle and poor left ventricular function would be considered a candidate for transcatheter intervention irrespective of any obtained transvalvar gradient.

Balloon aortic valvuloplasty is now considered a standard technique performed in virtually any center that offers interventional treatment for congenial cardiac lesions (Fig. 16.4). In contrast to balloon pulmonary valvuloplasty, where the vast majority of patients can be expected not to require any further transcatheter or surgical intervention, aortic valvuloplasty is usually palliative and not infrequently aimed at delaying an inevitable surgical procedure, be it valve replacement or a Ross procedure, until a time when the child has reached close-to-adult size.

In general, aortic valve dilation is performed retrogradely with a catheter introduced into the femoral artery. Although an antegrade approach with transseptal puncture offers a

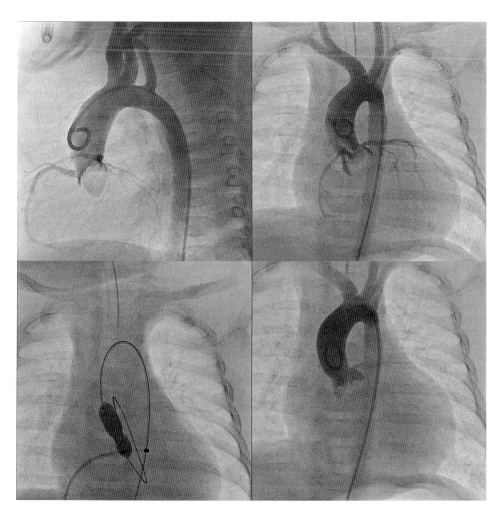

FIGURE 16.4 Balloon aortic valvuloplasty in a 3-month-old infant with congenital aortic stenosis (gradient: pre: 92 mm Hg, post 25 mm Hg). **Top left and right:** Aortogram in lateral and AP projection profiling the doming aortic valve annulus. **Bottom left:** Balloon inflation centered across the aortic valve with concomitant rapid right ventricle (RV) pacing for cardiac output control. **Bottom right:** Aortogram after balloon valvuloplasty documenting absence of aortic insufficiency.

slight advantage in maintaining a centered balloon position across the aortic valve during balloon inflation, the technique is more cumbersome and is associated with risk of injuring the mitral valve apparatus with resulting mitral insufficiency, and is therefore not routinely used. An end-hole catheter is passed from the femoral artery across the aortic valve to a stable position in the left ventricle. A double-balloon technique with the introduction procedure repeated from both femoral arteries may offer advantages for the aortic valve dilation in selected older patients, even though today, the spectrum of available high-pressure balloons usually allows the successful use of a single-balloon technique.

The catheter/wire passage retrogradely across the stenotic aortic orifice is the most difficult maneuver in the entire procedure and therefore should ideally be performed only once during the procedure. Before crossing the aortic valve, an aortogram with 25 degrees left anterior oblique (LAO)/cranial angulation of the AP and straight lateral projection should initially be performed to exactly delineate the size of the aortic valve annulus, while at the same time demonstrating any angiographic evidence of pre-existing aortic valve insufficiency. The exact technique for passing the wire or catheter into the left ventricle varies from operator to operator. A Judkins right coronary catheter curve or multipurpose catheter was initially used with success in crossing the aortic valve from this approach. However, the Judkins left coronary catheter may offer advantages in many patients, as the curvature is automatically

directed to the leftward and posterior opening of the congenitally stenotic aortic valve. Once the end-hole catheter is in place within the ventricle, it is replaced with an extra-stiff exchange-length wire with a long floppy tip, which is looped within the ventricle to protect the ventricular apex from perforation by the catheter tip and to minimize ventricular ectopy. A left ventricular angiogram is optional. In neonates and infants, a floppy-tipped coronary wire with a relatively stiff body may be advanced across the valve and allowed to loop in the left ventricle. Care has to be taken to prevent the wire from being ejected from the left ventricle, and therefore, once positioned, wire control should be maintained throughout the procedure. By using a floppy-tipped, high-torque guidewire, the wire does not need to be changed, and the first catheter to cross the valve can be the dilation balloon (thus minimizing the period of potential low output). The use of stiffer exchange wires and longer-dilation balloons may aid in maintaining an exact position of the balloon across the valve during inflation and, in turn, eliminate the shear trauma to the valve from balloon movement during inflation. With the wire secured within the left ventricle, the deflated balloon is manipulated through arterial sheaths and passed retrogradely over the wire. We do not believe that direct introduction of the balloon through the skin should have any role to play, as the profile of balloons has considerably decreased, thereby allowing the appropriately sized balloon to be introduced through fairly small sheaths. In addition, it is quite conceivable that the pulling of a deflated balloon directly through the femoral and iliac arteries may cause more harm to the vessel than using the appropriately sized sheath. Once the balloon is positioned across the stenotic valve, the balloon is rapidly inflated to the recommended maximal pressure and then rapidly deflated.

One difficulty of the procedure is to keep the balloon positioned across the aortic valve during inflation. Once it is inflated, a balloon tends naturally to move toward the ascending aorta because of the ejecting forces created by the left ventricle. It is generally difficult to push against these forces (unless using an antegrade approach), but a longer balloon length aids this process. Adenosine has been used to achieve a temporary cardiac standstill, but its timing in relation to balloon inflation is often difficult to predict. A more controllable method of reducing the cardiac output is through rapid right ventricular pacing (90). The rate of pacing can be adjusted prior to balloon inflation to achieve a drop in blood pressure by at least 50%, and these settings are then available to be used during the inflation process. An inflation device that can be operated using a single hand is preferential, as this allows the operator to use the other hand to maintain control of the balloon catheter, making very fine adjustments as the balloon is inflated. The balloon is then immediately and rapidly deflated, with the entire process taking no more than 5 to 10 seconds. Arterial pressures should be monitored throughout the procedure. The inflation should be repeated until the operator is assured that (a) the balloon remained properly positioned in the valve, (b) the balloon was of adequate size, and (c) the waist disappeared early and at low pressures during subsequent inflations. Regardless of the technique, a marked drop in systemic pressure, a rise in left ventricular pressure, and resultant bradycardia may transiently result. The double-balloon technique using two balloons placed side by side across the valve may minimize this problem, but more important, one has to avoid prolonged inflations with any technique when performing aortic balloon dilations. With successful valve dilation, after the balloon is deflated, both the blood pressure and heart rate should return spontaneously to normal.

For a single-balloon technique, the balloon is chosen with a diameter of about 80% of the measured aortic annulus diameter. After each set of inflations, the hemodynamic result and the degree of aortic insufficiency are evaluated. If no or only minimal change in the degree of aortic insufficiency has been observed with still a significant residual gradient (>40 mm Hg), repeat dilation valvuloplasty is done with a balloon sized just 1 to 2 mm greater than the one previously used. When using the double-balloon technique, the combined diameters of the two balloons should approximate 1.2 times the measured diameter of the aortic annulus. Because of the extensive manipulation in the left side of the heart and arteries, all these patients are systemically anticoagulated with heparin at the beginning of the procedure.

In the past, the most common complication of aortic balloon dilation was damage to the femoral arteries by the large balloon-dilation catheters. That problem has been minimized by newer lower-profile balloon designs, use of the double-balloon technique where required, and diligent monitoring of activated clotting time (ACT) levels throughout the procedure. When arterial damage does occur, it usually can be managed medically or rarely, surgically. In small infants, because of the increased risk of femoral artery injury from the introduction of the dilating balloon catheters into the vessels, several other approaches to aortic valve dilation have been introduced. The prograde approach, first passing a catheter, then a wire, and finally the balloon from the femoral vein to the right atrium, foramen ovale, left atrium, left ventricle, and prograde across

the aortic valve is chosen by some. Although frequently successful, this approach has a high incidence of failure in delivering the balloons and, even more disturbing, a significant incidence of damage to the mitral valve apparatus. Another approach that is gaining popularity is through a controlled cutdown on the carotid artery. As a result of extensive experience with extracorporeal membrane oxygenation (ECMO) and the safe introduction of cannulae into the carotid arteries, several centers, with the help of pediatric or vascular surgeons, began dilating aortic valves in infants with this approach. The approach is direct to the aortic valve and requires less catheter manipulation and less overall time, and has resulted in no reported complications related to the technique. The ideal procedure for the small infant is still to be determined.

With a conservative dilation of the aortic valve, the gradient should be reduced by 60% to 70% or to a gradient ≤30 to 40 mm of Hg. This usually can be accomplished without inducing significant aortic insufficiency, no more than that seen after surgical valvotomy. The long-term results, like surgical valvotomy, will be palliative; however, the catheter balloon dilation procedure is accomplished without a sternotomy or cardiopulmonary bypass with their inherent risks and morbidity. Balloon dilation of congenital aortic valve stenosis in pediatric patients and young adults is now the standard initial procedure for this lesion in most centers.

BALLOON PULMONARY VALVULOPLASTY

With the development of the special larger-dilation balloons, a transcatheter technique for balloon pulmonary valve dilation was first introduced by Kan et al. in 1982 (6). The technique performed acutely was successful and, at the same time, carried little risk beyond the basic risk of a catheterization. By December 1986, 28 centers, voluntarily reporting to a collaborative registry (Valvuloplasty and Angioplasty of Congenital Anomalies [VACA]), demonstrated the successful and safe application of the technique in >680 cases of pulmonary valve stenosis (91). With these data and many subsequent reports of successful use (92,93), balloon dilation has been accepted as the standard therapeutic procedure for pulmonary valvar stenosis. It is applicable to patients of all ages from the newborn period throughout adult life. With its excellent results and low rate of procedure-related complications, maximum instantaneous systolic echo gradients of as little as 35 mm Hg, when combined with evidence of right ventricular hypertrophy, should be considered an indication for balloon pulmonary valvuloplasty (94).

The degree of pulmonary valve stenosis is documented by accurate hemodynamic measurements in the catheterization laboratory. However, if the pulmonary valve is not easily crossed, then right ventricular angiography should be obtained prior to further attempts at crossing the valve.

The valve anatomy, size, and exact location are visualized angiographically, with standard anteroposterior (AP) (with some cranial angulation) and lateral being the most appropriate projections. Accurate determination of the valve annulus diameter is obtained using appropriate calibration techniques. With this information available, a long exchange guidewire is passed through an end-hole catheter into a distal pulmonary artery. The left pulmonary artery is preferable for this position because of the straighter course from the valve and main pulmonary artery to the left. However, in neonates with a patent arterial duct, the wire may be passed through the duct into the descending aorta. The chosen wire should be fairly stiff to allow the balloon to track over the wire and across the stenosed pulmonary valve. In infants and smaller children, a stiff 0.018-inch wire with a floppy tip is frequently appropriate for this purpose. However, infants with critical pulmonary stenosis and a closed arterial duct may poorly tolerate placement of a wire or catheter across the valve; therefore, the valve should be crossed only when all equipment has been prepared to immediately proceed with balloon pulmonary valvuloplasty.

McCrindle (95) documented that the optimum balloon diameter should be between 1.2 and 1.3 times the size of the pulmonary valve annulus for a single-balloon dilation. Lower balloon-to-valve annulus ratios are associated with an increased risk of recurrent or residual pulmonary valve stenosis, whereas ratios in excess of 1.4 are associated with an increased risk of clinically significant pulmonary insufficiency (95).

The choice of balloon catheters that can be used for this procedure is wide and depends to a degree on the individual valve morphology. In general, inflation pressures of more than six atmospheres are rarely necessary in patients with typical valve morphology, and therefore, low-pressure balloons, such as Tyshak II (NuMED, Hopkinton, NY) with a lower profile are the preferred initial balloon types to be used. However, the maximum rated inflation pressures decline sharply when using the larger varieties of these balloons. Therefore, high-pressure balloons, such as ZMed II (NuMED, Hopkinton, NY) or the double-balloon technique should be considered in these situations as the primary approach to balloon valvuloplasty (Fig. 16.5). High-pressure balloons may also be more beneficial when dealing with very dysplastic, thickened pulmonary valves in the older patient, or if there is associated supravalvar narrowing. In neonates with critical pulmonary valve stenosis and a closed arterial duct, a low-profile balloon with fairly rapid deflation characteristics such as the Tyshak II balloon should be used. Very low profile balloons, such as the mini Tyshak balloons (NuMED, Hopkinton, NY), may cross the valve more readily, but their very slow deflation characteristics make these balloons an inappropriate choice in patients who

have critical pulmonary stenosis without a patent arterial duct. If the valve cannot be crossed with the appropriate-sized balloon, smaller coronary balloons can facilitate predilating the valve to allow the larger balloon to be subsequently passed.

With the wire fixed in place in the distal pulmonary artery, the end-hole catheter is removed and the catheter with its deflated balloon is passed over this wire until the center of the balloon length is positioned exactly at the area of the stenotic valve. The balloon is then rapidly inflated to the pressure recommended by the manufacturer and is observed for the appearance of a circumferential indentation or waist in the balloon. Full inflation results in disappearance of the waist. An inflation device that can be operated using a single hand is preferential, as this allows the operator to use the other hand to maintain control of the balloon catheter, making very fine adjustments as the balloon is inflated. The balloon is then immediately and rapidly deflated, with the entire process taking no more than 5 to 10 seconds. Arterial pressures should be monitored throughout the procedure. The inflation should be repeated until the operator is assured that (a) the balloon remained properly positioned in the valve; (b) the balloon was of adequate size; and (c) the waist disappeared early and at low pressures during subsequent inflations. When a single balloon is used, there is a significant drop in both systemic blood pressure and heart rate during inflation. With successful valve dilation, after the balloon is deflated, both the blood pressure and heart rate should return spontaneously to normal.

To avoid the marked drop in systemic blood pressure and to reduce the trauma to the peripheral introductory veins, a double-balloon technique was introduced (96). This technique also allows the use of higher inflation pressures in patients with a large pulmonary valve annulus, where a single balloon would provide an inadequate rated burst pressure. The double-balloon technique uses two separate balloon catheters, each on a smaller shaft and with a smaller balloon profile. Each is introduced into a separate vein. With this technique, a second exchange wire is introduced from the opposite femoral vein and positioned across the pulmonary valve into a distal pulmonary artery, possibly next to the first wire. Two smaller-diameter balloon-dilation catheters are advanced over the separate wires and centered in the valve orifice, and the two balloons are simultaneously inflated. Various formulae have been used to estimate the equivalence of double-balloon to single-balloon technique (94), ultimately resulting in comparison charts that allow choice of sizes of the two smaller balloons, depending on the size that would have been chosen if a single-balloon technique would have been used.

With pure valve stenosis and a closed PDA, regardless of the initial gradient, one should expect to reduce the pressure gradient across the nondysplastic pulmonary valve to <10 mm Hg by balloon valvuloplasty, with an equivalent reduction in the RV-to-systemic pressure ratio. If the initial results are suboptimal, the balloon size should be increased ≤130% to 140% of the pulmonary valve annulus, and high-pressure balloons should be used, after obtaining an intermittent angiographic evaluation, using, for example, a Multi-Track catheter that is positioned over the *in situ* guidewire in the right ventricular outflow tract. However, it is important to recognize that relief of the valvar stenosis may unmask a dynamic infundibular obstruction, in some cases resulting in a persistent residual right ventricular outflow gradient. This secondary area of obstruction can be documented by pressure recording during careful catheter withdrawal from the pulmonary artery to the right ventricular outflow tract or with simultaneous pressure recordings from a double-lumen catheter or from separate catheters in each of the two areas.

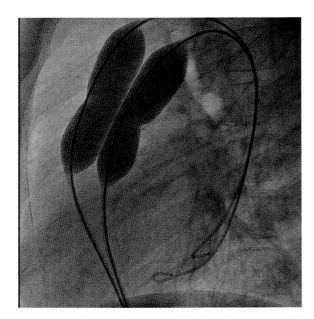

FIGURE 16.5 Balloon pulmonary valvuloplasty in a 5-year-old boy with valvar and supravalvar pulmonary stenosis, using the double-balloon technique to facilitate the use of higher inflation pressures.

Experience has shown that the infundibular obstruction is dynamic and that it will regress with time. In <10% of patients, a dysplastic pulmonary valve is encountered, with thickened, redundant leaflets resembling a cauliflower; frequently supravalve stenosis may coexist. This condition is more common in some genetic conditions, such as Noonan's syndrome. A higher-pressure balloon is usually required with a gradient reduction frequently less than what would be expected with nondysplastic valves.

The long-term effects of the procedure have not yet been determined. However, studies so far have documented rates of restenosis of between 5% and 11% within 10 years after the procedure (92,93). The risk of recurrence or restenosis may be greater in patients who present in infancy or with very dysplastic pulmonary valves, as well as those in whom an undersized balloon was used in the initial procedure. So far, reports have not provided evidence to suggest an increased risk of patients requiring pulmonary valve replacement because of pulmonary insufficiency, secondary to balloon pulmonary valvuloplasty. Dr. Charles Mullins pointed out that, in the presence of otherwise normal heart and lungs, the regurgitant fraction is usually small and at low diastolic pressure, owing to 80% to 85% of the ejection fraction having "diffused completely into the distal pulmonary capillary bed by the end of systole." However, we have also learned that progressive right ventricular dilation secondary to pulmonary insufficiency should be considered a potential indication for pulmonary valve replacement.

PERFORATION OF THE ATRETIC PULMONARY VALVE

The diagnosis of pulmonary atresia with intact ventricular septum (PA/IVS) is usually made within the neonatal period. Pulmonary blood flow after birth is maintained through a patent arterial duct until a more definitive source of pulmonary blood supply can be established. An intra-atrial communication allows the systemic venous return to pass into the systemic circulation. The long-term prognosis of patients with PA/IVS can be extremely poor, especially when a diminutive right ventricle is combined with an RV-dependent coronary circulation with multiple coronary abnormalities. In this situation, patients may require cardiac transplantation early in life. However, although patients with the diagnosis of PA/IVS and a single-ventricle pathway usually have a very poor long-term outcome, the outlook for those patients with a biventricular or a "one-and-a-half ventricle" circulation is much better.

Perforation of the atretic pulmonary valve plate has an important role to play within the available treatment modalities for these patients (88). Achieving antegrade pulmonary flow not only acutely decompresses the right ventricle, but more important, serves as an incentive to facilitate further growth of an initially hypoplastic right ventricle. Although various sharp instruments as well as laser-guided techniques have been used to perforate the atretic pulmonary valve, these techniques are often poorly controlled and associated with a variably high risk of creating inadvertent injury to surrounding structures, often with disastrous results. Consequently, the use of RF energy was introduced into therapeutic cardiac catheterization in the early 1990s as an alternative to laser-guided perforation of the pulmonary valve plate (97).

The equipment presently used most frequently to achieve perforation of the atretic pulmonary valve with RF energy is the Nykanen RF perforation wire and the Baylis radiofrequency puncture generator (Both: Baylis Medical Corpora-

tion, Montreal, Quebec, Canada). Suitability for transcatheter RF perforation of the pulmonary valve plate is ascertained by two-dimensional echocardiography with minimal criteria in most cases being the presence of a tripartite right ventricle as well as a membranous atretic pulmonary valve with a well formed infundibulum (98). Vascular access is routinely obtained via right femoral venous cannulation. A femoral arterial pressure-monitoring line is placed. Initial hemodynamic evaluation includes measurement of right ventricular and systemic arterial pressures, followed by right ventricular angiography with 20-degree cranial angulation of the frontal tubes and standard lateral projection. This allows measurement of the pulmonary valve plate diameter and exclusion of RV-dependent coronary circulation. Further angiography is obtained in the left ventricle in the same projection. The combination of these two ventriculograms allows documentation of the relationship between the blind-ending right ventricular infundibulum and main pulmonary artery. A 4 or 5 Fr Judkins 2.5 right coronary artery catheter is placed below the pulmonary valve plate within the right ventricular outflow tract using a Tuohy Borst adapter to allow passage of the RF wire and simultaneous contrast injections. Once the RF wire and coaxial catheter are loaded, and accurate positioning is confirmed, RF energy is applied while the operator maintains a gentle push on the RF wire toward the valve membrane. In most patients a power setting of 5 W/s should be sufficient to perforate the pulmonary valve plate, and it is important for the operator to be particularly suspicious of creating a false track if high-power settings are required. RF energy is discontinued once the wire has advanced through the valve plate. Appropriate positioning is confirmed using contrast injection through the Tuohy Borst adapter. The coaxial catheter is then advanced over the RF wire into the main pulmonary artery, and the RF wire is exchanged to a 0.014-inch or 0.018-inch coronary wire, which can be directed either to a position in a distal branch pulmonary artery or preferably through the PDA into the descending aorta. Even though a wire position in the distal pulmonary arteries or preferably across the PDA needs to be established, this should not be attempted with the Nykanen RF wire, as it can easily cause perforation of the main pulmonary artery (88). Once the valve plate is crossed, the coaxial catheter should be advanced into the main pulmonary artery (MPA) and then the RF wire exchanged to a 0.018-inch or 0.014-inch wire with a softer tip that can be more readily maneuvered across the PDA or into the distal pulmonary arteries. This presence of a coaxial catheter is a significant advantage when comparing the Baylis with the Osypka RF system that is still in widespread use elsewhere. A low-profile balloon valvuloplasty catheter, such as the Mini-Tyshak (NuMED, Hopkinton, NY), with a diameter of about 130% of the valve plate annulus is then advanced over the coronary wire and balloon dilation performed (Fig. 16.6). In cases where the balloon catheter cannot be advanced across the valve, sequential dilation can be performed starting with a lower-profile 2.5-mm coronary balloon. Trackability can also be improved through arterial fixation or snaring of the coronary wire (99). Balloon valvuloplasty is followed by assessment of the pressure gradient across the pulmonary valve as well as the RV-to-systemic pressure ratio, and a final RV angiogram is performed to document the result of the procedure.

Studies on the outcome of RF perforation of the pulmonary valve have been reported, and results have been summarized by Benson et al. (100–106). Most series are very small and include fewer than five patients. The overall procedural mortality is about 8% with incidence of procedural complications being about 15%.

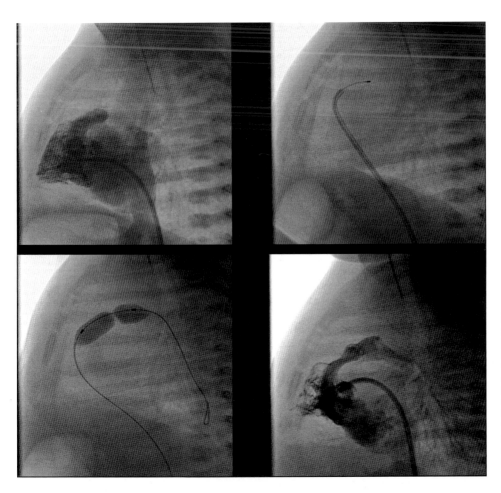

FIGURE 16.6 Radiofrequency (RF) perforation of the pulmonary valve plate in a neonate with pulmonary atresia with intact ventricular septum (PA/IVS). **Top left:** RV angiogram delineating the right ventricular outflow tract (RVOT). **Top right:** RF wire across the pulmonary valve plate. **Bottom left:** Balloon valvuloplasty with a wire positioned in distal right pulmonary artery. **Bottom right:** RV angiogram demonstrating the newly created continuity between right ventricle and main pulmonary artery.

It has been advocated that the combination of ductal stenting with RF perforation in one single procedure may reduce the number of transcatheter interventions and prevent prolonged postprocedural care. Approximately 50% of all neonates undergoing successful perforation and balloon valvuloplasty required additional pulmonary blood flow (107), even though it remains difficult to predict this for each individual patient. Some authors have suggested the use of the tricuspid valve z-score (108), but this has not consistently been identified as being predictive of the need for pulmonary blood flow augmentation. Regardless, after failing to wean from prostaglandin E (PGE) infusion after 7 to 10 days, one should proceed with either PDA stenting or surgical aortopulmonary shunt placement. If performed appropriately, the technique allows ≤75% of suitable patients to ultimately sustain a biventricular or one-and-a-half ventricle circulation (88).

TRANSCATHETER TREATMENT OF STENOTIC ATRIOVENTRICULAR VALVES

Mitral Valve Dilation

When discussing balloon dilation of stenotic atrioventricular (AV) valves, it is very important to distinguish between congenitally stenotic AV valves and acquired AV valve stenosis as a result of rheumatic fever. In many countries outside the United States, rheumatic mitral valve stenosis is still a common lesion in children. These acquired valve lesions with commissural fusion lend themselves naturally to a dilation procedure, which has been demonstrated to be effective in children. In contrast, the anatomy of congenital mitral stenosis is quite variable and is generally less favorable for balloon dilation, although the procedure has occasionally been effective for this lesion. The decision to proceed with balloon valvuloplasty of congenital mitral stenosis should be based on a complete echocardiographic assessment of mitral valve anatomy.

The mitral valve is approached from the femoral veins using a transseptal approach into the left heart. Various techniques have been described, which include predilating the atrial septum to allow passing a single large mitral dilation balloon, the passing of two balloons through two large transseptal sheaths, the passing of two balloons over separate guidewires without long sheaths and without the need for specific dilation of the septum, as well as a double-balloon technique using a MultiTrack system over a single guidewire (NuMED, Hopkinton, NY) (109). The Inoue balloon (Toray Industries, Houston, TX) is a custom-made hourglass-shaped balloon that is available as a complete set, including sheath, guidewire, and mandrill. It specifically facilitates balloon valvuloplasty using a single-balloon technique without the use of a guidewire in the left ventricle (Fig. 16.7). The Inoue balloon is available in three sizes, allowing balloon dilation diameters between 22 and 30 mm. Its use has demonstrated success in treating rheumatic mitral valve stenosis (110). When using a double-balloon technique, the left atrium is entered and one or two separate transseptal punctures are made. Exchange wires are manipulated from the

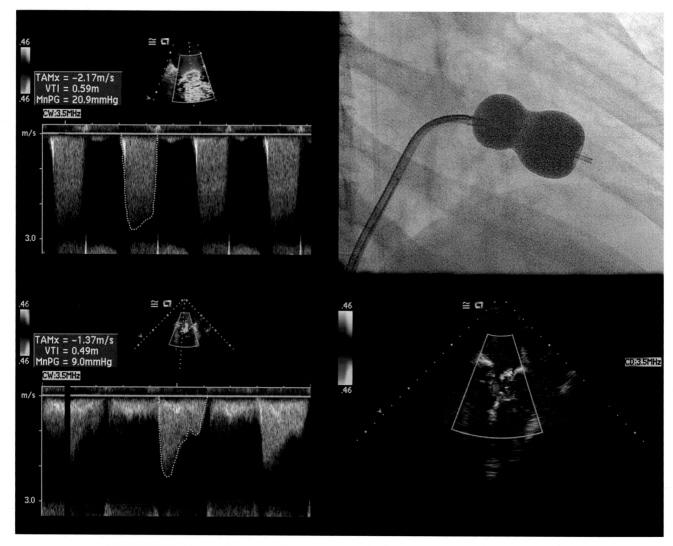

FIGURE 16.7 A 38-year-old woman with rheumatic mitral valve stenosis. Inoue balloon mitral valvuloplasty reduced the mean gradient from 21 mm Hg to 9 mm Hg with mitral regurgitation increasing from trivial to mild. **Top left:** A 28-mm Hg mean Doppler gradient across mitral valve prior to balloon valvuloplasty. **Bottom left:** A 9-mm Hg mean Doppler gradient across mitral valve post balloon valvuloplasty. **Top right:** Inoue balloon inflated across mitral valve. **Bottom right:** Mild mitral insufficiency by color Doppler after balloon valvuloplasty.

right atrium through previously positioned catheters or long sheaths across the septum, across the mitral valve, and into the left ventricle with the transition and floppy portions of the wires looped in the ventricle. It is important to remember that if a guidewire is to be used for balloon dilation, a balloon-tipped end-hole catheter should be initially directed from the left atrium across the mitral valve to lessen the chance of crossing between cordal attachments. Once the wires are in place, either the two long sheath/dilator sets or the two separate uncovered balloons are passed over the wires into the left atrium. The balloons are advanced and positioned across the mitral valve. The sheaths are withdrawn from the balloons, and the balloons are simultaneously inflated. Again, longer balloons (5 to 6 cm in older children and adolescents) help to stabilize during inflation. The sum of the two balloon diameters equals the measured or estimated maximal normal mitral valve diameter for a patient of that particular body size. The two balloons allow an adequate total balloon diameter for the much larger mitral annulus without coincident destruction of

the entry veins or the atrial septum during balloon passage. As with any interventional catheterization, these patients undergo anticoagulation with heparin.

The initial success of transcatheter balloon dilation of congenital mitral valve stenosis appears equal to that of surgical commissurotomy, depending on the mitral valve apparatus. However, the total experience is limited, and the duration of the relief of the obstruction is unpredictable. McElhinney et al. (111) recently described a series of 108 patients with congenital mitral stenosis who underwent balloon mitral valvuloplasty (BMVP) or surgical intervention at a median age of 18 months. BMVP was effective in creating a reduction of the mean gradient by 38%, although significant mitral regurgitation was identified as a result in 28% of procedures. Overall 5-year survival was 69% whereas patients at the later stages of the institutional experience had a 5-year survival of 87%. The early mortality was similar for balloon valvuloplasty and surgical mitral valvuloplasty, whereas the need for initial mitral valve replacement was a significant predictor of worse acute and long-term outcomes. The 5-year survival free from failure of biventricular repair after balloon valvuloplasty was 75%. Although the authors suggest that the initial procedure for congenital mitral stenosis (MS) in patients with either typical congenital MS or double-orifice mitral valve (MV) should be balloon valvuloplasty, they concede that the surgical approach is more appropriate in patients with supravalve mitral ring and parachute mitral valve.

Although in general a parachute MV is not a contraindication to balloon valvuloplasty, the procedure is probably less likely to be effective when there is a single papillary muscle or severe shortening or virtual absence of the chordal apparatus (the arcade-type mitral valve). Ultimately, it is difficult to predict which intervention is the more appropriate for congenital mitral stenosis, and most series report institutional preferences. Therefore, comparisons between surgical and percutaneous approaches are biased at best.

Tricuspid Valve Dilation

Congenital tricuspid stenosis, as well as rheumatic, carcinoid, and rare other types of acquired tricuspid valve stenosis, occur less frequently than mitral stenosis but, as with mitral stenosis, may be amenable to balloon valve dilation. Congenital forms of tricuspid valve stenosis are usually associated with other cardiac lesions and, similar to mitral valve stenosis, are less amenable to balloon valvuloplasty than rheumatic tricuspid valve stenosis. The diagnosis of tricuspid stenosis is confirmed hemodynamically. As much information as possible about the valve anatomy and the exact location of the obstruction is obtained by echocardiography, then angiography. The tricuspid valve is approached by passing one or two guidewires across the valve, either into the pulmonary artery or to the right ventricular apex. With the use of the calculated or estimated maximum tricuspid valve annulus diameter according to the patient's body surface area, the balloon diameter or combined balloon diameters are chosen to equal this measurement (except in cases of annular hypoplasia). The dilation balloons are introduced through standard venous sheaths and over the wires. When the balloons are positioned across the stenotic valve, they are inflated simultaneously. Disappearance of the indentations or waists in the balloons at maximal inflation is sought. As with mitral valve dilation, the use of the longer balloons facilitates appropriate positioning and maintaining positioning across the valve during dilation. A successful dilation should eliminate any transvalvar gradient. Experience with tricuspid valve dilation is limited, but, on the basis of even limited experience and minimal risk, this procedure is offered to the appropriate patients before considering surgery for tricuspid stenosis.

TRANSCATHETER MANAGEMENT OF COARCTATION, RECOARCTATION, AND AORTIC ARCH OBSTRUCTIONS

Dilation of peripheral arteries was the first therapeutic catheterization procedure and represents yet another area in which the vascular radiologist introduced the techniques. Dotter and Judkins (112) reported on the dilation of atherosclerotic peripheral arteries at the same time that Rashkind et al. (2) were working on the atrial septostomy catheter.

The technique for dilation of vessel stenosis uses small, cylindrical, fixed maximal-diameter dilating balloons passed over a spring guidewire, positioned across the area of stenosis, and inflated with relatively high pressures. This stretches or tears the area of stenosis up to the predetermined diameter of the balloon. This balloon technique is not only used to treat recurrent or native coarctation of the aorta, but similarly is used for branch pulmonary artery stenoses as well as central and peripheral venous stenoses. As many vessel dilation procedures are associated with immediate recoil and subsequent restenosis, the addition of balloon-expandable stents has further improved on the available therapeutic interventional armamentarium and is frequently the treatment of choice in adult patients.

In 1979, Sos et al. (113) first experimented with balloon angioplasty of native coarctation in postmortem specimens, and this was followed by some fundamental work by Dr. James Lock et al. (114,115) in the early 1980s. He performed balloon angioplasty on excised human coarctations as well as experimentally induced coarctations in lambs. He showed that balloon angioplasty achieved its therapeutic result by creating microscopic or macroscopic intimal and medial tears over a variable distance in the vessel. These intimal injuries appeared to have healed completely on late pathologic examination, leaving the ballooned segment with a normal-looking intima. The studies also documented that a balloon diameter of less than twice the size of the coarctation segment was unlikely to achieve a successful dilation, whereas diameters greater than three times appeared to carry a higher risk of deep and extensive tears.

Dr. Ronald Grifka and Dr. Charles E. Mullins et al., a group from Texas Children's Hospital surroundings, set the stage for early evaluation of endovascular stent therapy to treat coarctation (Fig. 16.8) (116). In animal experiments,

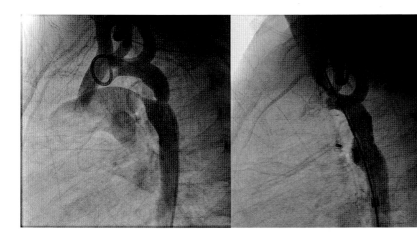

FIGURE 16.8 Coarctation and patent ductus arteriosus (PDA). A 14-month-old child who was referred for elective PDA closure. Coarctation with 30-mm Hg peak systolic gradient incidentally found during procedure. PDA closed with 6/4-mm Amplatzer duct occluder (ADO), followed by placement of a 19-mm Genesis XD in the descending aorta (DAO), completely abolishing the gradient. **Left:** PDA and coarctation prior to intervention. **Right:** After intervention.

they implanted Palmaz P308, 188, and 108 stents in the abdominal aorta and documented that stents can be safely redilated after initial stent implantation. Dr. Andrew Redington et al. added to this in 1993 by implanting a self-expandable stent into a 10-week-old girl who had previously had palliative surgery for hypoplastic left heart syndrome (117). Although one should generally avoid endovascular stent therapy in small infants, in some circumstances the implantation of a low-profile stent in very sick infants may be justifiable, even though one has to accept that these low-profile stents are not expandable to adult size and therefore will eventually require surgical removal. In 1995, Suarez de Lezo reported the first large series of stent implantation to treat native and recurrent coarctation in humans using the Palmaz stent (118) and in 1999 Cheatham first reported on a new stent design, the Cheatham-Platinum (CP) stent, which is also available in a PTFe-covered variety (119). Chisolm et al. (120) at Columbus Children's Hospital, recently reported a larger experience of stent therapy for complex aortic arch lesions, which further expanded the indications for transcatheter stent therapy with excellent results (Fig. 16.9).

One of the major difficulties when comparing the various treatment modalities for native or recurrent coarctation of the aorta, such as surgery, balloon angioplasty, and endovascular stenting, is the fundamental lack of prospective, evidence-based data. Therefore, one has to rely on institutional series, the results of which are necessarily influenced by not only the skill of the individual interventional cardiologist and cardiac surgeon in the respective institution, but also by the common institutional policy and experience in treating these lesions.

Similar to the comparison of surgical and interventional approaches to coarctation, the decision between balloon angioplasty and primary stenting is often dependant on the individual institutional policy, rather than being guided by evidence-based data. Although both balloon angioplasty and endovascular stenting have an important role to play in the primary management of aortic coarctation, several valid reasons make primary stenting the more suitable treatment modality, if the size of the patient permits this procedure. First, the results of balloon angioplasty are limited owing to elastic recoil of the coarcted segment, and the rigidity of an endovascular stent obviously overcomes this problem. Second, the degree of trauma to the aortic vessel wall plays an important role in the potential development of complications such as aneurysm formation. Whereas balloon angioplasty often requires a degree of overexpansion of the coarctation and adjacent vessel wall to achieve a maintainable result, endovas-

cular stenting allows having a successful result while dilating the vessel wall only to the desired diameter—overexpansion is not required. Last, a subgroup of longer-segment coarctation or arch hypoplasia typically has a poorer outcome after balloon angioplasty alone. Even though primary endovascular stenting offers significant benefits, it is usually avoided in small children and infants because of the potential for injury to the arterial vessels and access sites as well as the higher likelihood of developing in-stent stenosis when stents are expanded only to fairly small diameters. As with any other aspect of interventional therapy, the catheterization laboratory has to be equipped to allow the operator to deal with potential complications that are specific to the procedure performed (Fig. 16.10).

The goal of the procedure is to achieve reduction in the gradient to <10 mm Hg or a ≥90% relief of the obstruction angiographically. In an observational study, Zabal et al. (121) analyzed a cohort of 54 consecutive adult patients who underwent transcatheter treatment for coarctation with the primary end point being a composite index of failure, made up of heart-related death, a gradient on follow-up of >20 mm Hg, and the need for reintervention or complications such as aneurysm formation. They identified that a residual gradient of >10 mm Hg was associated with a significantly higher failure index. Although this is not a prospective or randomized study, it does fit with the results of other observational series and appears to be a good guideline when delivering interventional therapy to these patients. With the present techniques and equipment, dilation and/or stent implantation for native or recurrent coarctation appears to be successful in achieving immediate relief of the obstruction in >90% of cases. However, balloon angioplasty alone for native coarctation in smaller children and infants has lower long-term success rates, and the results are frequently not well maintained, with ≤66% recoarctation rate. An additional concern when discussing transcatheter interventions for native coarctation is the concern that there may be a greater incidence of aortic aneurysm formation in the area of the coarctation dilation. Aneurysms have occurred both immediately and late after the coarctation dilation. Catastrophic events as a direct result of these aneurysms are rare. However, the long-term follow-up is relatively short, and the long-term outcome is uncertain at best. From several surgically removed segments and from intravascular ultrasound of the area, it appears that both the aortic intima and media are often disrupted, with only the adventitial layer constraining the aortic pressure. Another concern with these aneurysms, particularly following an otherwise successful dilation, is that if subsequent surgery is necessary, it could be more

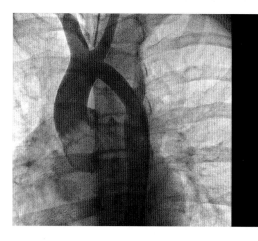
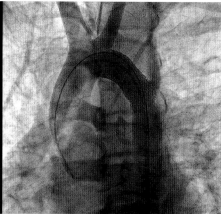

FIGURE 16.9 Complex arch stenting. A 15-year-old with h/o coarctation repair (end-to-end) during infancy, Shone complex with transverse arch hypoplasia. Placement of a 36-mm Max LD stent in the transverse arch led to a gradient reduction from 22 mm Hg peak systolic to 2 mm Hg peak systolic. **Left:** Aortogram before stent placement. **Right:** Aortogram after stent placement.

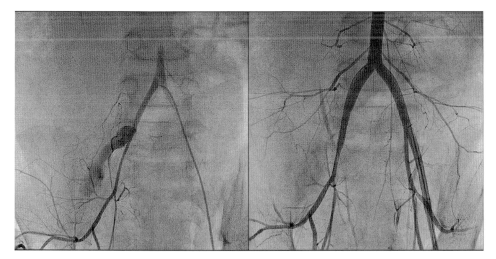

FIGURE 16.10 Iliac rupture. A 9-year-old boy with localized coarctation undergoing placement of a Max LD stent with complete abolishment of the gradient. On sheath removal, injury occurred to right iliac artery, which was treated through implantation of a covered Atrium Cast stent. **Left:** Injured iliac artery with significant extravasation of contrast. **Right:** Same vessel after placement of the covered stent.

hazardous because of the disappearance of collaterals following a hemodynamically successful dilation. As more follow-up information is gathered regarding dilation of native coarctation, this technique appears more reasonable for discrete lesions in patients >7 to 12 months of age (122). Continued long-term follow-up is still recommended. In the larger child, primary stent therapy for native coarctation is a suitable treatment alternative to balloon angioplasty, even though aneurysms can occur with these stent implants. It has been suggested that gradual conservative expansion of these stents be performed over two or three procedures to reduce the incidence of dissection or aneurysm formation.

The technique itself is relatively straightforward. The coarctation and adjacent aorta are visualized by quantitative angiography, usually using lateral as well as left anterior oblique projections. Intravascular ultrasound can further assist the preinterventional assessment of coarctation and may be specifically useful in the postoperative group of patients (123–125). If balloon angioplasty alone is performed, a balloon of the same diameter as the narrowest aortic diameter adjacent to the coarctation is prepared. A 'J' or curved-tip stiff guidewire is positioned retrogradely through the coarctation, around the aortic arch, and into the aortic root or occasionally into the right innominate artery. The dilation balloon catheter is passed over the wire and across the area of coarctation. When the balloon is centered in the coarctation, it is inflated to the manufacturer's listed maximum pressure. The inflation may be repeated several times until the waist in the balloon or the gradient disappears. In smaller children and infants, cutting balloon angioplasty frequently adds an additional treatment alternative in patients where endovascular stent placement should be avoided.

In the slightly larger patient, when the results of the dilation are not satisfactory and where larger sheaths can be introduced into the arteries, intravascular stents can be used to support the dilated segment of aorta. When stents are used, it is imperative that only stents that eventually can be dilated to the full diameter of the adult descending aorta are used. In smaller patients with an expected diameter below average adult size, the Genesis XD or the Mega LD stents with a maximum expandable diameter of ≤18 mm would be perfectly appropriate. If larger maximum diameters are required, the Max LD, the Cheatham-Platinum, or older Palmaz XL (Cordis, Warren, NJ) stents with maximum expandable diameters >25 mm are available, even though the NuMED CP stent is not approved for use within

the United States. If aortic arch vessels must be crossed, the Mega or Max LD stents offer additional advantages because of their open-cell design, whereas the ePTFE-covered variety of the Cheatham-Platinum stent is specifically useful for very tight coarctation where an increased risk of injury to the aortic wall is expected as well as in the adult population, where catastrophic aortic rupture has been reported (126–128). Stents implanted in children can gradually be expanded to adult size in subsequent transcatheter procedures to accommodate a child's growth. It is hoped that the prospective enrollment of patients undergoing balloon angioplasty, stent therapy, or surgical treatment in the Congenital Cardiovascular Interventional Study Consortium (CCISC), organized by Dr. Thomas Forbes in Detroit with participating centers worldwide, helps shed light on this subject.

REHABILITATION OF (BRANCH) PULMONARY ARTERY STENOSES

Transcatheter therapy of all varieties of branch pulmonary artery stenoses is a widely accepted standard procedure, in large part because most of these lesions are not amenable to surgical repair. However, rehabilitation of branch pulmonary artery stenoses can be one of the most challenging tasks in congenital pediatric patients. Transcatheter therapy has to strive to achieve the optimum possible outcome, which sometimes requires repeated and staged procedures to achieve some improvement for an individual complex patient. The treatment modalities available include the use of cutting balloons, standard balloon angioplasty, or the placement of endovascular stents.

The individual success of treating these lesions is sometimes difficult to assess, but in patients with a biventricular circulation, a reduction in the right ventricular-to-systemic pressure ratio is a good indicator for a successful outcome. Individual pressure gradients to branch pulmonary arteries may be less meaningful, and in fact angiographically significant branch pulmonary artery stenoses can be associated with surprisingly low pressure gradients, especially in the presence of significant pulmonary insufficiency. However, when assessing these gradients across individual stenoses, it is important to avoid a catheter-induced damping; therefore, the use of the RADI PressureWire (Radi Medical Systems, Wilmington, MA) may aid in accurately assessing the hemodynamic data. The angiographic appearance of the vessel before and after transcatheter intervention is equally important, and while one should strive to aim to achieve a "normal" vessel diameter, frequently the percentage of improvement in the anatomic measured stenosis is a good outcome parameter.

Although standard balloon angioplasty can be performed using a normal balloon-over-the-wire technique, it is frequently helpful to place long sheaths toward the area of intended interventional therapy to facilitate simultaneous therapies of adjacent lesions, balloon exchanges, and subsequent placement of stents if required. In many patients, especially in adults, placements of long sheaths from a femoral venous approach may be difficult. Therefore alternative approaches should be considered. Internal jugular venous or transhepatic approaches offer the advantages of eliminating some of the double-S curves that have to be traversed from a femoral venous approach, while also requiring a shorter sheath length and allowing improved "pushability" of the catheter.

Standard balloon angioplasty alone rarely achieves a sustainable long-term improvement to an individual stenosis and therefore is usually performed only in situations where other forms of transcatheter treatment are not available or where the size of the patient or vessel prevents the use of endovascular stents that can be expanded to adult size. No absolute rules exist for determining the correct balloon size; however, it appears that the balloon should preferably be larger then two times the diameter of the stenotic segment while avoiding exceeding a diameter of three times the actual narrowing. However, when using standard balloon angioplasty, overdilation of a vessel is frequently required to achieve an adequate outcome. In very resistant stenoses, high-pressure balloons should be used, rather than exceeding the size of the dilation balloons. Cutting balloon angioplasty is available for maximum diameters of ≤8 mm and is a suitable alternative to endovascular stenting, especially in small distal pulmonary arteries. It is frequently beneficial to open up very tight stenoses and can be followed either by standard balloon angioplasty or endovascular stent placement if required.

Standard balloon angioplasty of pulmonary branch stenosis has not been highly successful at correcting the lesions, and many of the vessels that initially are dilated satisfactorily reconstrict immediately (recoil) with the deflation of the balloon or, if not immediately, a short time later. Few of these dilated vessels are maintained at a normal diameter. The true success rate at achieving a vessel of normal diameter with no gradient is <20%; at the same time, there is a definite morbidity and even mortality for the procedure. It is not possible to determine in advance which case will be successful, so the procedure is often performed as a therapeutic trial.

The clinical use of intravascular stents in patients with congenital heart lesions was introduced in 1988 by Mullins et al. (86) with the use of large Johnson and Johnson Interventional System (JJIS; Sommerville, NJ) iliac stents in branch pulmonary artery and central systemic vein stenoses. The experience with stents in these lesions has significantly changed the approach to branch pulmonary stenosis. Results in eliminating any gradients and opening the vessels to their normal diameters have been excellent (8). The implant dilation does not require overdilation of the vessel to achieve a normal end diameter. The initial results have been sustained over years. In addition, it has been demonstrated that if the appropriate stents are implanted initially, these stents can be dilated further in the future up to the adult diameter of the vessel. In the 15 years since their introduction for this use, intravascular stents have become the primary mode of therapy for branch pulmonary artery stenoses in most large institutions that care for congenital heart patients. Implanting stents that may not be expandable to adult size (such as premounted stents) may be indicated in certain infants and small children requiring a palliative procedure. Holzer et al. (129) recently presented a series of pulmonary arterial stent implantation in children weighing <15 kg and documented that stent implantation may prevent or defer the need for subsequent surgical intervention to a time when this can be performed with a lower risk. The authors documented that the *in situ* stents may not necessarily present a major difficulty for the surgeons and can be excised or patched where required. Although this may be challenging, it may present the preferred treatment alternative for selected patients.

The delivery and implant of intravascular stents in the branch pulmonary arteries are performed through the use of long sheaths, and these procedures are usually a fairly complex undertaking. An end-hole catheter is advanced well beyond the lesion to be treated and is replaced with a stiff exchange wire. Appropriate and diligent guidewire positioning is a key to successful stent therapy. A long sheath/dilator large enough in diameter to accommodate the stent mounted on the appropriate delivery balloon is passed over the wire beyond the area of stenosis. This is usually one of the most challenging parts of the procedure and may require changing the approach from femoral venous to internal jugular or transhepatic in selected patients. The chosen long sheath should be kink resistant and reinforced if possible, such as the Super ArrowFlex sheath (Arrow, Reading, PA), but these suitable sheaths are presently not available in all sizes that would accommodate larger-sized balloon–stent combinations, as required in many adult patients. The dilator is then removed over the wire, leaving the sheath and wire in place. The balloon with the mounted stent is advanced over the wire and through the long sheath to the area of stenosis. The sheath is withdrawn from the balloon/stent; when the stent is verified to be in the exact position, the balloon is inflated, expanding the stent into the lesion, and with deflation of the balloon, fixes the vessel at the dilated diameter (Fig. 16.11). During stent positioning, angiography can be obtained either through the sidearm of the long hemostatic sheath or by using an additional angiographic catheter advanced from a separate venous entry site. To achieve precise delivery and positioning of the stent, specialized balloon-delivery catheters are often helpful. The balloon-in-balloon (BIB) balloon catheter allows adjustment of the partially deployed stent after inflation of the inner balloon alone, before full deployment using the outer balloon. When expanding the stent to a diameter greater or equal to 12 mm, the BIB catheter is chosen. The addition of rapid RV pacing also reduces systolic stent movement during deployment.

TRANSCATHETER MANAGEMENT OF PULMONARY VEIN STENOSES

Surgical as well as transcatheter interventions for pulmonary vein stenoses have a uniformly bad long-term outcome (130,131). Pulmonary vein stenoses are frequently not isolated. Transcatheter interventions, whether (cutting) balloon angioplasty or endovascular stenting, are often performed as a last resort in patients in whom no other treatment alternatives are available before considering heart–lung transplantation. These procedures are technically challenging and have a higher-than-average associated procedural risk. The procedures are often

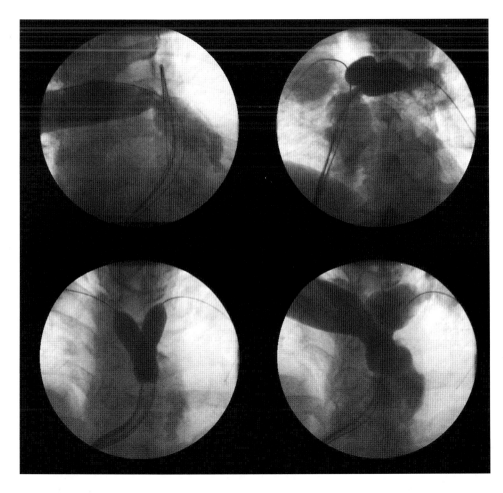

FIGURE 16.11 Bilateral branch pulmonary artery stenosis (PAS) after repair of tetralogy of Fallot. Implantation of "kissing" stents to the PAS abolished 25-mm Hg gradients to the branch PAS and reduced the right ventricular (RV)/systemic pressure ratio from 60% to 35%. **Top left:** RPA origin stenosis. **Top right:** LPA origin stenosis. **Bottom left:** Simultaneous expansion of kissing stents (Genesis XD as well as Max LD). **Bottom right:** Angiographic result after stent deployment.

acutely successful, but restenosis is observed in most cases. Attempted dilation of these lesions may be recommended in an infant or child who is severely symptomatic. The experience with intravascular stents in pulmonary vein stenosis to date has had no better medium- or long-term results than (cutting) balloon angioplasty alone, but has been associated with a high percentage of complications, including systemic stent embolization. However, in selected patients, short-term results of endovascular stenting may be superior to cutting balloon angioplasty and, therefore, may serve as a temporizing measure in critically ill children (Fig. 16.12). Stents have been surgically placed into pulmonary veins under direct vision as well as during brief ECMO support as hybrid procedures. The ultimate prognosis of these lesions remains poor.

TRANSCATHETER MANAGEMENT OF SYSTEMIC VEIN STENOSES

Dilation of stenosed systemic veins, particularly those narrowed after surgical or other interventions, often is acutely successful and carries little risk. Zahn et al. (132) recently demonstrated the feasibility of transcatheter interventions even in freshly operated lesions. The surgical alternative for these lesions is poor to nonexistent. As for pulmonary branch stenosis, the results are not uniform or predictable. As with balloon dilation of other vessels, there is immediate hemody-

namic, anatomic, and symptomatic improvement; however, stenosis recurs in most cases. The technique for dilation of systemic veins, as with the other vascular balloon dilation procedures, involves crossing the stenosed lesion with a catheter and exchanging the catheter for a wire over which the dilation balloon (or balloons) can be advanced across the lesion. The balloon size is chosen so as to vary between two and three times the diameter of the stenosed segment. The balloons are inflated in the lesion to the pressure recommended for the particular balloons. Balloon angioplasty is frequently the preferred intervention when fairly fresh thrombotic material is responsible for the stenosis, as placement of endovascular stents often does not offer additional advantages because of protrusion of thrombotic material through the struts of the placed stent (unless covered stents are used).

Similar to results seen in pulmonary artery branch stenoses, the incidence of restenosis is high. Therefore, primary therapy for the more long-standing venous lesions has become the implantation of intravascular stents. In many patients, the use of radiofrequency energy combined with the subsequent placement of covered stents may allow the recanalization of even completely obstructed venous structures (Fig. 16.13) (88). As with any other lesion, stents are chosen to be expandable to adult size, and therefore usually include the Genesis XD or the Max/Mega LD stents, or the covered Cheatham-Platinum stent, if available. The venous stent delivery procedure is similar to other intravascular stent deliveries in congenital heart lesions with the stents delivered over a stiff wire and through a long sheath. For stent delivery, a single balloon

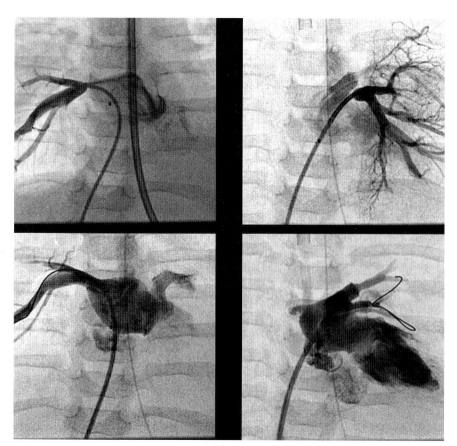

FIGURE 16.12 Stenting of pulmonary vein stenosis. A 13-month-old infant with Adams-Oliver syndrome, primary pulmonary hypertension, as well as pulmonary vein stenoses (procedure performed on extracorporeal membrane oxygenation [ECMO] support). **Top left:** Right lower pulmonary vein stenosis. **Bottom left:** Right lower pulmonary vein after stent implantation. **Top right:** Left lower pulmonary vein stenosis with drainage partially via stented left upper pulmonary vein. **Bottom right:** Left pulmonary veins after stent placement in upper as well as lower pulmonary vein.

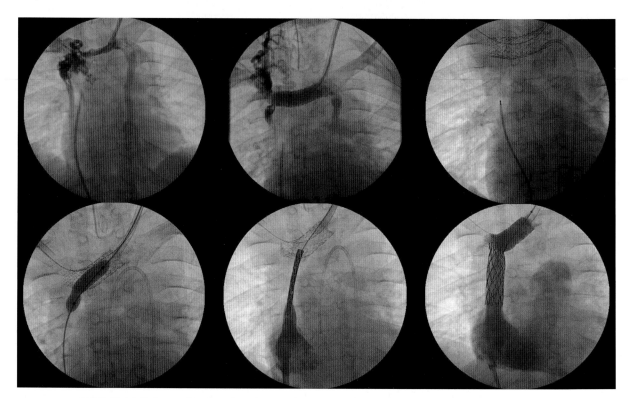

FIGURE 16.13 Recanalization of an obstructed superior vena cava (SVC) and stenotic innominate vein in a 16-year-old boy. **Top left:** Occluded SVC and stenotic innominate vein with collateral formation. **Top middle:** Innominate vein appearance after placement of a Mega LD stent. **Top right:** RF wire positioning from right atrium to innominate vein. **Bottom left:** Balloon angioplasty of the open cell Mega LD stent (over wire loop). **Bottom middle:** Final positioning of a covered NuMED CP stent in SVC. **Bottom right:** Final result with significantly improved drainage from innominate vein via SVC to right atrium.

of a diameter not less than that of the adjacent nearest normal vein is used. Results of central venous stent implantations have been excellent. No adverse reactions or long-term complications of the stents have occurred. Some venous restenoses have occurred when stents were dilated to a diameter significantly larger than the adjacent vessel at the time of implant. In these instances, the lumen within the stent remodels with neointima to the size of the normal adjacent vessel.

DEVICE CLOSURE OF SEPTAL DEFECTS

Transcatheter Closure of Atrial Septal Defects

Presently, the Amplatzer septal occluder is by far the most commonly used device to close intra-atrial communications worldwide as well as in the United States, ranking superior with regard to closure rates, rates of complications, and ease of use. However, clinical trials that compare these devices in a controlled and randomized fashion have not been conducted.

Technique

Transcatheter closure of atrial septal defects is usually performed under general anesthesia using transesophageal echocardiography (TEE) as guidance for device deployment and delivery. However, studies have documented that intracardiac echocardiography (ICE) is equally suitable for echocardiographic guidance, thereby allowing these procedures to be performed under conscious or deep sedation in older children and adults (19,133).

Every study requires a full echocardiographic evaluation of the atrial septal defect. This should include assessment of the defect size in different planes (four-chamber view, short-axis view, and superior vena cava [SVC] view), confirmation of normal pulmonary venous drainage, as well as evaluation of the atrioventricular (AV) valves for the presence of pre-existing AV valve regurgitation. It is extremely important to evaluate all septal rims, including the superior rim with distance to pulmonary vein insertion and SVC, the inferior rim toward the AV valves, the anterior retroaortic rim, as well as the posterior-inferior rim that is in continuity with the inferior vena cava. With TEE it can at times be difficult to achieve a clear definition of the posterior-inferior rim toward the IVC, in which case ICE has a clear advantage. Although studies have documented that closure of atrial septal defects even with multiple septal rim deficiency is feasible, this clearly increases demands of the operator's technical skills (20,134).

Vascular access is usually obtained in the right femoral vein, placing an additional arterial monitoring cannula in the right femoral artery. Additional venous access from the right or left femoral veins may be required for intracardiac echocardiography. In patients with bilateral occluded femoral veins, device deployment and delivery should usually be performed using transhepatic access, which may even provide for better alignment of the device to the atrial septum (135). Internal jugular venous access is the least preferable access route and is unsuitable for device delivery in most patients. Heparin at a dose of 100 IU/kg is administered to maintain an activated clotting time of >200 seconds. A standard hemodynamic left and right heart catheter evaluation should be performed prior to device closure. This should include evaluation of pulmonary artery pressures, pulmonary vascular resistance, and estimation of the atrial level shunt. Angiographic evaluation

of the atrial septal defect through an injection in the right upper pulmonary vein is not uniformly required, but may aid as a road map for device orientation, especially when larger defects are being closed in smaller children. Angiography is usually performed in 35-degree left anterior oblique (LAO) and cranial angulation. However, as the ASD's position varies between patients, so does the best view to *en face* profile the atrial septum. Therefore, tube angulations may have to be adjusted after initial angiography to achieve a better profile of the atrial septum. This view is then used throughout the device delivery and deployment process. In general, biplane views are not necessary to aid ASD device closure, and in fact may hinder accessibility to the patient for the echocardiographer.

The left upper or lower pulmonary vein is entered using either a wedge, multipurpose, or Judkins right coronary catheter, and a preshaped exchange length, extra stiff, j-tipped wire is advanced. Most operators would at this stage perform static Doppler stop-flow balloon sizing under echocardiographic guidance, using either a 24-mm or 34-mm AGA sizing balloon (AGA Medical Corporation, Golden Valley, MN) or a NuMED sizing balloon (NuMED, Hopkinton, NY). It is extremely important to expand the balloon until the atrial level shunt is just abolished. The dimensions are then recorded on echocardiography as well as on cine recording. However, unless a mild waist is visible, cine recordings can be misleading at times, as the angle of the atrial septum in relation to the sizing balloon may vary. One should clearly avoid any oversizing in an attempt to achieve a clear waist on the balloon, as oversizing of the device has been linked to the rare but serious complication of device erosion into the aortic root that has been described after ASD closure using the ASO (25). Many centers now completely avoid balloon sizing, especially in small children, and instead use an averaged maximum diameter taken from the three standard views to determine the appropriate device size. One would then add 25% to this diameter to determine the appropriate device size, which is often very similar to the atrial septal defect size determined when using color flow mapping. In patients with a deficient retroaortic rim where the two discs are expected to hug the aortic root on either side, the device size should be increased by a further 1 to 2 mm. In very large defects, the maximum septal length is determined using echocardiography as well as the initial angiographic recording. By subtracting 12 to 14 mm (depending on the device size), one can then estimate the maximum left atrial (LA) disc size that is suitable to close the defect without exceeding the septal length. Where balloon sizing is performed, the AGA sizing balloon may be advanced directly through the skin without the use of a hemostatic sheath, whereas the NuMED sizing balloon (NuMED, Hopkinton, USA) can pass through an 8 Fr sheath.

Once the device size has been determined, the appropriate delivery sheath is placed over the guidewire into the mouth of the left upper pulmonary vein. In addition to the standard AGA 45-degree delivery sheath, other long hemostatic sheaths can be used. The dilator and wire are gently removed, and extreme care has to be taken to avoid any inadvertent air entry into the sheath and left atrium at this stage. The device is then prepared for delivery, attaching either a Tuohy-Borst adapter or the standard bleedback valve that is supplied with the AGA delivery system to the loader. The delivery cable is passed through the assembly, and the device, after being carefully inspected, is screwed onto the cable, avoiding any force on the screwing mechanism. The device is then loaded under water seal and the whole assembly flushed with hand-warm saline. Once the loader is screwed onto the delivery sheath, the device is pushed forward under fluoroscopic guidance until the tip of the sheath is reached. The deployment is conducted under simultaneous echocardiographic and fluoroscopic guidance. The whole assembly is pulled back until the tip of the delivery sheath exits the mouth of the pulmonary vein, at which stage the delivery sheath is pulled back while fixing the delivery cable to deploy the left atrial disc. Once the LA disc has been deployed, the position and orientation of the device is further evaluated on echocardiography, and while the operator gently pulls toward the atrial septum, he or she evaluates the alignment of device and septum. At this stage, gentle rotation of the sheath may aid a better alignment. Once alignment appears suitable, the central connecting waist is deployed allowing self-centering, and the whole assembly is pulled back against the atrial septum. In quick succession this is followed by deployment of the right atrial disc once the connecting waist stents the defect itself. If the device pulls through the septum, the device is recaptured, the delivery sheath repositioned, and the deployment process started again. Various techniques have been used to achieve better alignment of the device, such as the use of specialized s-curved delivery sheaths (Hausdorf sheath, Cook, Bloomington, IN), deployment of the left atrial disc into the left or right upper pulmonary vein, use of a dilator advanced through additional venous access to prevent the device from pulling through the defect, and use of Judkins right coronary guide catheters for smaller devices (20,136,137). Before release, the device must be carefully evaluated by echocardiography. This should include assessment for residual shunts around the device, obstruction of adjacent structures, as well as possible interference with the AV valves. The tension of

the delivery cable will frequently distort device orientation and allow a moderate shunt between the separated discs. A careful push/pull action of the delivery cable should clearly demonstrate that the two discs are separate in all echocardiographic views as well as on fluoroscopy, and the device should not easily be displaced through this very gentle push/pull maneuver. Sometimes right atrial angiography through the delivery sheath may be helpful to unmask inappropriate device position. Once the operator and the echocardiographer are satisfied with the device position, the device is released through counterclockwise rotation of the delivery cable using the supplied pin vise. The device usually reorients itself into a more appropriate position, and therefore a final echocardiographic assessment is performed after release of the device.

Results

Procedure- or device-related complications after ASD device closure are extremely rare. Even though the risk of device embolization is low, about 0.5%, it can occur, especially during attempts to close very large defects with deficient rims (138). Therefore it is mandatory that any physician attempting to close atrial septal defects should be sufficiently trained and skilled in device retrieval, using for example a gooseneck snare (Microvena Corporation, White Bear Lake, MN). Early electrophysiologic abnormalities are common within the first 24 hours after ASD device closure (21), but most of these resolve quickly, and persistent rhythm or conductance disturbances 1 year after device closure are extremely rare (22). One of the most serious

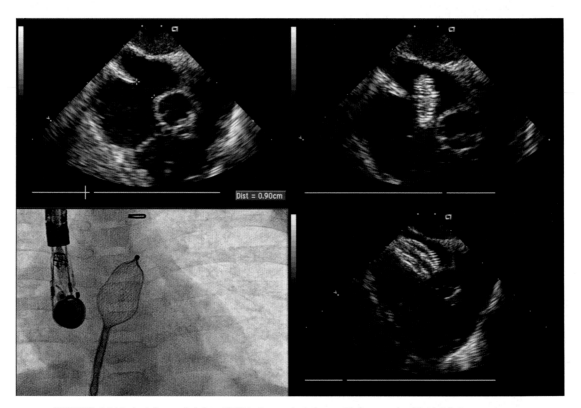

FIGURE 16.14 Atrial septal defect (ASD) closure in infancy. Eight-month-old (6.5 kg) expremature ventilator-dependent infant with bronchopulmonary dysplasia and a moderate (9 mm, unstretched) secundum atrial septal defect with deficient retroaortic rim (**top left**). **Top right:** Standard deployment technique was unsuccessful in aligning the device with the atrial septum. **Bottom left:** Left upper pulmonary venous deployment technique. **Bottom right:** Device alignment and position after release (11-mm Amplatzer septal occluder [ASO]). Patient was subsequently weaned off the ventilator.

complications after ASD closure is erosion of the device into the aortic root, observed at an incidence of 0.1%, which may be related to the oversizing of devices and deficiency of the retroaortic rim (25). Closure rates are excellent with residual shunts being <5% at 1 year follow-up (18,20,139,140). The right ventricular diastolic diameter tends to decrease after ASD closure, suggesting some degree of remodeling when the exposure to volume loading is eliminated (141).

ASD closure in small children is particularly challenging owing to the small left atrial size and the relationship between device size and limited septal length in these patients (Fig. 16.14). Holzer et al. (141a) recently reported on 26 patients with a weight <10 kg (2.4 kg to 10 kg) in whom ASD closure was attempted. Rim deficiencies were present in 31% of patients, and the overall procedural success was 95%. One unsuccessful procedure was related to a deficiency of the inferior rim. In small children, especially when the weight is <3 kg, the ICE catheter can be used as echocardiographic guidance in the TEE position. Because of the reduced left atrial size, it is often necessary to pull up the TEE probe prior to device deployment to avoid the device being tilted into an unfavorable position owing to impingement of the TEE probe

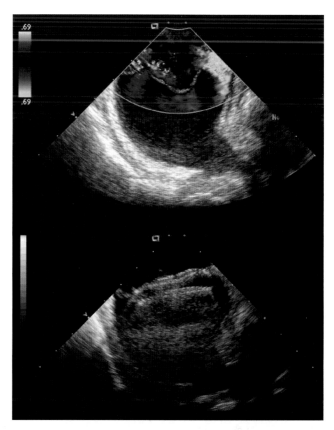

FIGURE 16.16 Closure of multifenestrated atrial septum defect (ASD). Multifenestrated atrial septum with at least three separate shunts on echo color flow mapping. **Top:** Multifenestrated septum before device placement associated with atrial septal aneurysm. **Bottom:** Atrial septum after device placement—note the flat appearance of the device and septum without a significant central waist.

posteriorly (which frequently would let a device pull through at the anterior retroaortic rim). Figure 16.15 demonstrates closure of multiple ASDs using two Amplatzer septal occluders, whereas Figure 16.16 demonstrates closure of a multifenestrated atrial septum using the Amplatzer cribriform septal occluder.

Transcatheter Closure of Fontan Fenestrations

Transcatheter closure of fenestrations created surgically during the completion of a Fontan is usually being considered in patients who have transcutaneous oxygen saturations ≤90% after Fontan completion. Although the CardioSEAL ASD occlusion device has standard use approval under the FDA for occlusion of these defects, many other approved devices have been used on an off-label basis, and the most commonly used devices for this indication are presently the smaller varieties of the Amplatzer septal occluder (Fig. 16.17) (142,143). Although in general these defects are closed in a similar fashion to secundum atrial septal defects, there are a few important considerations. Balloon test-occlusion of the fenestration should be undertaken for 10 to 15 minutes, allowing for careful evaluation of right atrial pressures, systemic pressure, oxygen saturations, and cardiac index. If test-occlusion is well tolerated, the defect can be closed using various approaches.

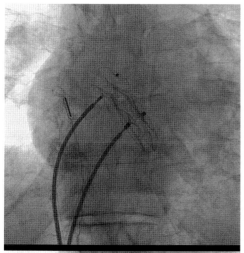
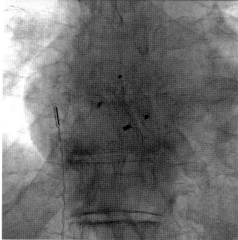

FIGURE 16.15 Closure of two secundum atrial septal defects in a 59-year-old man using a 20-mm and a 13-mm Amplatzer septal occluder. **Top:** Two devices deployed but not released with the larger device being sandwiched within the smaller device. **Bottom:** Both devices after release.

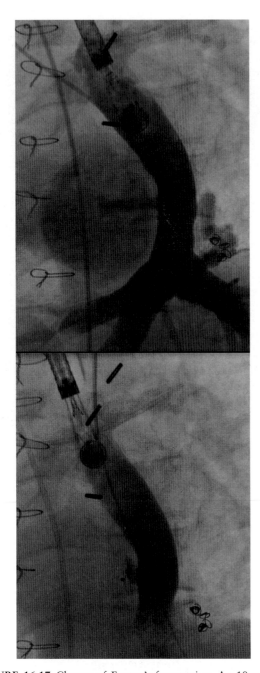

FIGURE 16.17 Closure of Fontan's fenestration. An 18-year-old woman with heterotaxia and an extracardiac Fontan's (hepatic confluence to left pulmonary artery [LPA]). Fenestration occluded using 5-mm Amplatzer septal occluder. **Top:** Before occlusion. **Bottom:** After occlusion.

Even though the jugular venous approach is unsuitable for occlusion of atrial septal defects, small surgically created fenestrations are usually more amenable to this approach, as the small size of the defect allows a much harder pulling force to be exerted, which overcomes the disadvantages otherwise encountered through inappropriate alignment. The location of surgical fenestrations may be close to the tricuspid valve, and therefore careful echocardiographic assessment is necessary to avoid the device dropping into the tricuspid apparatus. Ideally, the left atrial disc should be deployed close to the fenestration.

In many cases, the smallest device size of an Amplatzer septal occluder (4 mm) is sufficient for occlusion. In patients with extracardiac Fontan's circulation and a short tubular connection to the atrial mass, the Amplatzer duct occluder may be more suitable to close this fenestration (144).

Transcatheter Closure of Ventricular Septal Defects

Background and History

Transcatheter closure of muscular ventricular septal defects (VSDs) was first attempted on a compassionate basis using the larger Rashkind patent ductus arteriosus (PDA) occluding device (7). In 1988, Lock et al. reported on a series of six patients in whom muscular VSDs—including postinfarct VSDs—were closed using the Rashkind device (7). Although the device and technique were successful in some cases, the device frequently was too small and resulted in significant residual leaks or actual embolization of the device. Some shortcomings of the PDA device were overcome by the design and by the larger sizes of the Clamshell ASD device, making this a useful technique for some otherwise difficult-to-treat VSDs (145). Its successor, the CardioSEAL, has since been used to close various muscular ventricular septal defects (146) and is presently the only device that has regular use FDA approval for this indication.

Other devices have been used off-label to close muscular as well as perimembranous (44) ventricular septal defects, including the buttoned device (147), detachable coils (148–150), and the Amplatzer septal occluder (151). However, theses devices, as well as the approved CardioSEAL device, were designed for different indications and as such are not generally adapted to suit the very different anatomic and morphologic parameters (such as septal thickness) that are encountered with muscular ventricular septal defects.

In 1999, Thanopoulos first reported on the use of a custom-made device for closure of muscular ventricular septal defects (34). Early results of the Amplatzer muscular VSD occluder are promising, but in the United States the device can presently be used only under a high-risk IDE protocol, with PMA approval expected in the near future. In contrast to muscular ventricular septal defects, perimembranous defects pose much higher demands on device design because of their proximity to the aortic valve, and early trials with off-label use of the Rashkind double-umbrella were quickly abandoned (44). In 2002, Hijazi et al. (46) first reported on the use of a custom-designed device to close perimembranous ventricular septal defects. Phase I trials investigating the Amplatzer membranous VSD occluder have been conducted in the United States (48), but at present the device does not have FDA approval, even though the device is used outside the United States (48).

Technique

The principle approach to device closure of muscular as well as perimembranous ventricular septal defects (Fig. 16.18) is similar, with the device usually being deployed from an antegrade approach. For apical and midmuscular locations of the defects, the device delivery usually is from the superior vena cava; defects in the anterior muscular septum as well as perimembranous defects generally are approached from the inferior vena cava. This combination of circumstances results in a complex delivery technique requiring an arterial-venous guidewire "rail" passing from the arterial approach to the left ventricle, through

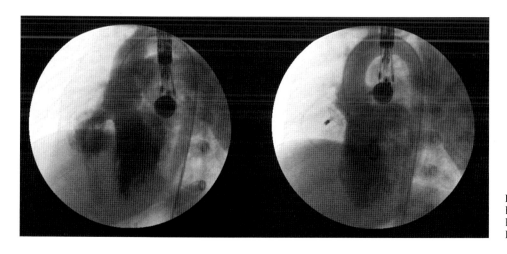

FIGURE 16.18 Closure of perimembranous VSD. Closure of a perimembranous ventricular septal defect. **Left:** Before closure. **Right:** After closure.

the defect into the right ventricle, and ultimately being exteriorized either via femoral or internal jugular vein.

The procedure is performed using continuous transesophageal echocardiography. After an initial hemodynamic evaluation and left ventricular angiography, the VSD is usually crossed from the LV using a Judkins right coronary catheter as well as a 0.035-inch exchange-length angled glidewire. In case of perimembranous ventricular septal defects, the wire is then exchanged to a 0.035-inch, soft, j-tipped exchange-length wire. The wire is snared using an Amplatz gooseneck snare (Microvena Corporation, White Bear Lake, MN) either in SVC or pulmonary arteries and exteriorized via femoral vein or internal jugular vein, thereby establishing a rail that can then be used to advance the appropriate-diameter long-delivery sheath through the defect and into the left ventricle. Device delivery is similar to that of the Amplatzer septal occluder for ASD closure; especially, the closure of posterior-inferior defects is frequently complicated by kinking of the delivery sheath. Perimembranous defects require a special technique to position the delivery sheath in the left ventricular apex, and the delivery system has significant differences from the system being used to deliver the standard muscular VSD occluder. Because of the complexity of the procedure, transcatheter muscular and membranous VSD closure should be limited to a few centers that have the necessary interventional expertise. For general results of this technique, refer to the device-specific section in this chapter.

TRANSCATHETER OCCLUSION OF PERSISTENT DUCTUS ARTERIOSUS

At present the most commonly used device to close medium- or larger-sized arterial ducts is the Amplatzer duct occluder (ADO), which was introduced in the late 1990's (70), and which presently is the only device that has been FDA approved specifically for closure of the patent arterial duct. However, many small PDAs are still being occluded using various coils.

Technique

Coil occlusion of the arterial duct can be performed using either an antegrade or retrograde approach. For very small PDAs, a retrograde arterial approach is usually sufficient. Before crossing the patent arterial duct an aortogram is performed just at the origin of the PDA using standard lateral projection as well as 30-degree right anterior oblique (RAO) projection of the AP tube. Measurements are obtained at the pulmonary arterial end and the aortic end, as well as the total length of the arterial duct. According to a classification by Krichenko et al. (152), the arterial duct can be described angiographically as classically cone shaped (type A), short with a narrow aortic end (type B), tubular (type C), having multiple constrictions (type D), or elongated conical with a distant constriction (type E). Hemodynamic evaluation is performed prior to angiography, including assessment for any pressure gradient across the aortic arch, as well as a full right heart catheterization in cases where an antegrade ductal closure is anticipated. Care should be taken to avoid inadvertently entering the duct before angiographic evaluation can be completed, as that may trigger ductal spasm that may make it impossible to obtain accurate measurements and could in the worst case lead to the patient having to be rescheduled for a repeat procedure. The antegrade approach has the advantage of allowing angiographic evaluation before the coil is completely deployed, but both techniques are equally used and suitable.

A coil usually twice the size of the pulmonary end of the duct is chosen, and coils are deployed in a way to usually allow about one loop being placed distal to the pulmonary arterial end, while the remainder of the loops are placed in the ductal ampulla. The length of the coil is usually three to five loops and depends on the length of the aortic ampulla. Delivery of Flipper or Jackson coils is technically fairly easy, and the controlled-release mechanism allows an extra safety margin to prevent inadvertent coil embolization. If the coil position appears suboptimal, the coil can be recaptured and redeployed into a more appropriate position. However, Flipper coils with their reduced amount of filament are not always suitable to close medium-sized PDAs in particular. Therefore, techniques have been developed that allow delivery of the standard Gianturco coils in a more controlled fashion, such as the use of a snare (153) or bioptome (154) to hold onto the coil, the use of a tightened catheter tip (155), or the use of a balloon (156) to tamp the coil within the ductus during deployment. Even without these aids, closure of many arterial ducts is feasible using just the standard Gianturco coils, as has been demonstrated through many successful procedures, performed before any other devices became available. If a residual shunt is present after placement of a coil, attempts should be made to place an additional coil. Residual shunts not only fail to abolish the risk of bacterial endocarditis, but in addition are associated with an increased risk of intravascular hemolysis (157). Sufficient time (10 to 15 minutes) should be given to allow clotting to occur before attempting to place an additional coil, which is usually placed using a retrograde approach. The duct is carefully crossed using a 0.018-inch V18 wire. A soft 4 Fr catheter, such as an angled glide catheter, should then be tracked over the wire and advanced carefully across the PDA before placing an additional coil that is usually of smaller diameter than the one that was originally placed. Before introduction of the Amplatzer duct occluder, many moderate- to large-sized PDAs were occluded using multiple coils in this fashion (79).

The technique of closing the arterial duct using the Amplatzer duct occluder has been described in detail by Masura et al. (70). After hemodynamic and angiographic evaluation, the PDA is crossed antegradely and a 0.035-inch exchange-length wire is advanced into the descending aorta. The appropriate delivery sheath is advanced over the wire with the tip being positioned in the lower descending aorta. The wire is removed and the device loaded in a way similar to the Amplatzer septal occluder. The device size is chosen so that the pulmonary end of the skirt is about 2 mm larger than

the size of the narrowest PA portion of the arterial duct. In a typical type A PDA with a 3- to 4-mm pulmonary arterial end, one would therefore choose an 8/6 mm Amplatzer duct occluder. However, in very small patients, the device size is chosen to be frequently on the smaller side. The device is advanced until it reaches the tip of the delivery sheath. At this point the whole assembly is gradually withdrawn in small increments. One should begin to deploy the retention disc when a position just in midportion of the descending aorta opposite to the PDA insertion is reached. It is important to have the angiographic recordings as a road map when deploying the device, using specifically the anterior end of the trachea and its relation to the PDA as a reference point. Once the retention disc is deployed, the whole assembly is withdrawn into the mouth of the aortic ductal ampulla, at which point the skirt is then deployed while the operator fixes the delivery cable and retracts the sheath. In type E PDA, tubular type C PDA, or elongated arterial ducts with a typical cone shape, it may be necessary to withdraw (or begin to deploy) the retention disc inside the PDA. Once the device is deployed, a pigtail catheter is advanced and positioned opposite the PDA in the descending aorta and aortography is performed, carefully evaluating for the presence of any residual shunt around the device. One can repeat the aortogram after 10 to 15 minutes to allow clotting to occur if required. Without any residual shunt, the device can be released, and its position should again be evaluated through a final angiogram (Fig. 16.19). Pressure recordings before and after device deployment in the ascending and descending aorta should be obtained. Even though the device is recommended only for use in infants >5 kg, it is our experience that the ease with which the device can be recaptured if the position is not satisfactory should allow an attempt at PDA occlusion in any duct beyond the neonatal period, even if the patient's weight is <5 kg. The key to successful deployment in small patients is not necessarily the size of the PDA, but more so its length.

Results of PDA closure using the various available devices have been described in the device-specific section of this chapter.

CLOSURE OF OTHER PERSISTENT OR ABNORMAL VASCULAR COMMUNICATIONS

Embolization of abnormal or persistent arterial or arteriovenous vascular structures has been available for >30 years. Embolization techniques were developed and perfected primarily by the vascular radiologists working in the abdominal viscera, gastrointestinal areas, and central nervous system, particularly in end artery vessels. Many materials and devices, including the patient's own clotted blood, Gelfoam, colloidal plugs, "glues," detachable balloons, and coil occlusion devices, have been used for these peripheral occlusions.

Gianturco (Cook, Inc.) coils are the most commonly used of all occlusion devices for patients with congenital cardiac defects. These coils are made of spring wire with polyester fibers enmeshed in the coils and are available in several sizes and multiple diameters and lengths. The coil is introduced into the delivery catheter through a straight metal loader as a straight wire. When it is delivered by extrusion out of the distal end of the catheter, it coils like a small pigtail. Once delivery with this particular coil has been started, there is no way of withdrawing the coil back into the wire. The Gianturco coil occludes the vessel by the creation of a mass of fabric and wire in which a thrombus is formed. The coil occlusion device usually

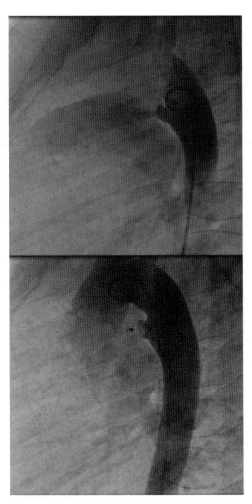

FIGURE 16.19 A 9-year-old girl with a medium-sized patent ductus arteriosus (PDA) who underwent PDA occlusion using an Amplatzer duct occluder. **Top:** Before closure. **Bottom:** After closure.

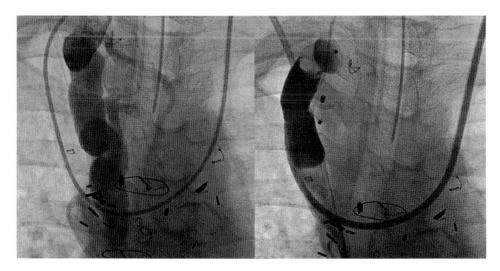

FIGURE 16.20 Closure of venovenous collaterals. A 10-year-old girl with hypoplastic left heart syndrome (HLHS) and status post-Norwood's procedure and bidirectional Glenn's shunt, with low transcutaneous saturations. A large venovenous collateral was occluded using two 16-mm Amplatzer vascular plugs. **Left:** Collateral before occlusion. **Right:** Collateral after occlusion.

is delivered into a vessel with a discrete distal narrowing, where it will fix in place and not migrate farther through the vessel. Often, several coils are placed in a single vessel to achieve complete occlusion. In the absence of a distal narrowing or some other type of device for fixation, coils are generally usable only in tubular structures with a distended diameter ≤7 to 8 mm. For larger vessels or vessels without an area of discrete stenosis, coils can be used in conjunction with other intravascular occlusion devices to complete the occlusion of the vessel. Other devices that are available to occlude slightly larger vascular structures include the Amplatzer vascular plug (Fig. 16.20), the Amplatzer duct occluder, as well as the Gianturco–Grifka vascular occlusion device.

Many abnormal collateral vessels or persistent surgically created systemic-to-pulmonary artery shunts are associated with the more complex lesions. These vessels should be occluded when systemic flow competes with normal pulmonary flow, particularly after the major defect is corrected. These communications traditionally required surgical division during the corrective procedure or as a separate procedure. Other lesions in which these devices may be useful are AV fistulae, including systemic, coronary-cameral, and peripheral as well as pulmonary AV fistulae. In these lesions, it is critical to identify the stenotic or end vessel into which the device can be fixed to reduce the dangers of migration to a vital structure. Various other persistent and abnormal vascular communications can be occluded with the available devices and include a left superior vena cava to the left atrium, systemic-to-pulmonary artery shunts in postoperative tetralogy of Fallot or pulmonary atresia patients, persistent systemic venous-to-right atrial connections after the Fontan or Glenn procedures and others.

RETRIEVAL OF FOREIGN BODIES

With the proliferation of various types of chronic parenteral therapy, central line monitoring, chronic indwelling intravenous chemotherapeutic devices, and now the catheter-delivered therapeutic devices, the nonsurgical removal of embolized foreign bodies from the heart or great vessels has become a more frequent challenge for the interventional cardiologist. The pediatric interventional cardiologist, who is more familiar with complex intracardiac anatomy and with the routine use of biplane fluoroscopy, is generally best qualified to perform these procedures, regardless of the patient's age. Fortunately, and

thanks mostly to urologists, various catheter devices are available for the grabbing, snaring, looping, or lassoing of any type of debris that works its way into the vascular system and must be available in any interventional catheterization laboratory.

Most embolized materials end up in the pulmonary artery branches. Retrieval involves the delivery of a large sheath (8 to 15 French) into the specific branch pulmonary artery just proximal to the foreign body. The specific type of retrieval catheter used is determined by the size of the patient, the type of foreign body, and exactly how and where the foreign body is situated within the vascular system. Then, either directly through the sheath or through a catheter delivered through the sheath, the particular retrieval device is advanced to the foreign body and manipulated to grasp it. Once firmly grasped, the foreign material is withdrawn into the large sheath and out of the body through the sheath. With the use of the large, long sheaths with these retrieval devices, it is usually no longer necessary to perform a venous cutdown even for the final removal of the foreign body from the vessel or skin entry site.

MANAGEMENT OF PERIPROSTHETIC LEAKS

Periprosthetic leaks are notoriously difficult to treat. Various devices have been used successfully in selected patients, using either an antegrade or a retrograde approach (158–161). However, the crescent-shaped form of many of these defects combined with the biophysical characteristics of the adjacent prosthetic valves do not lend themselves to the use of any of the currently available transcatheter devices. Development efforts are presently underway to design a custom-made device specifically designed for the closure of periprosthetic leaks, which, it is hoped, will improve on the currently available devices that have been used for these indications.

TRANSCATHETER VALVE THERAPY

The groundbreaking work by Dr. Phillip Bonhoeffer has initiated one of the most exiting developments in transcatheter therapy of recent years. Patients with significant pulmonary insufficiency and right ventricular dilation have so far required surgical (re)placement of a valved conduit between the right ventricle and pulmonary arteries. The longevity of these conduits has been limited, requiring further conduit replacements every 5 to 15 years for recurrent conduit stenosis or new or recurrent valve insufficiency. The prospect of frequent open-heart procedures is very undesirable in this group of patients, who usually already have undergone a series of cardiac surgical procedures, each adding further potential insults to global left and right ventricular function. Because of scarring, these operations are potentially very difficult to perform. Therefore, a less-invasive procedure that would further extend the need for surgical conduit replacement has been most desirable. In 2000, Bonhoeffer et al. (9) reported on the first human implantation of a stent-mounted valve into an RV-PA conduit in a 12-year old boy. The technique has been modified since and until now >100 patients have received a transcatheter-stented valve in the pulmonary position (Fig. 16.21) (162). The Bonhoeffer-Medtronic valve uses a bovine jugular venous valve that is preserved in glutaraldehyde and mounted within a 34-mm-long Cheatham-Platinum (CP) stent. The valve is ideally implanted into a pre-existing RV-PA conduit, preferably with a degree of associated stenosis, and expanded up to a maximum of 22 mm in diameter. At the present time, the valve is not suitable for use in patients with a dilated right ventricular outflow tract. Difficulties of adequately positioning a valved stent in pulmonary position, owing to an unusual location of the right ventricular outflow tract, could potentially be overcome using a hybrid approach with direct perventricular placement of the balloon expandable valve. This approach has been successfully adopted in an animal experiment in six adult pigs (163). Additional advantages of this approach include the fact that cardiopulmonary bypass would be readily available to convert to a classic surgical valve insertion if required.

In addition to the Bonhoeffer–Medtronic valve, the Cribier–Edwards valve has recently been percutaneously implanted in the pulmonary position in the first patient within the United States (164). The valve has been derived from Cribier's original experiments of percutaneous valve implantation in the aortic position. Cribier et al. (165) were the first to report a successful percutaneous placement of an aortic valve stent using an antegrade transseptal technique through a size 24 Fr sheath in a 57-year-old patient with calcific aortic stenosis. No impairment to coronary blood flow was observed, and immediate function of the prosthesis 48 hours postprocedure was excellent. The Cribier–Edwards valve has achieved investigational device exemption (IDE) approval for aortic implantation within the

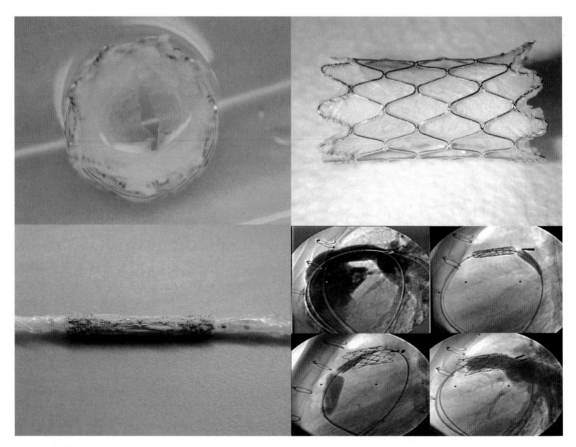

FIGURE 16.21 Transcatheter pulmonary valve implantation. **Top left:** En face view of a bovine jugular venous valve mounted on a Cheatham-Platinum (CP) stent. **Top right:** Side view of the transcatheter bovine jugular venous valve mounted on a CP stent. **Bottom left:** Transcatheter pulmonary valve mounted on a balloon-in-balloon (BIB) catheter. **Bottom right:** Sequential steps of transcatheter pulmonary valve implantation with documentation of free pulmonary insufficiency (PI) before valve implantation (**top left**) and no residual PI after implantation (**bottom right**).

United States. Modifications in the delivery sheath as well as the delivery approach have since occurred, changing from the original antegrade delivery technique to a retrograde approach.

Parallel to the percutaneous valve techniques, development efforts have been made to facilitate percutaneous mitral valve repair. The two primary techniques include either annuloplasty, which is usually facilitated through implantation of a device into the coronary sinus (coronary sinus technique), or the direct edge-to-edge clip or suture techniques, which adhere opposing mitral valve leaflets using a technique similar to the Alfieri stitch. However, these are primarily adult-based techniques and, therefore, are not discussed in greater detail.

HYBRID PROCEDURES

For many years the relationship between the cardiothoracic surgeon and cardiac interventionalist was marked by competition and occasional "turf wars" between both groups, especially in adult acquired heart disease. However, one of the most valuable lessons learned over the last decade is the need to embrace a collaborative approach between the congenital interventionalist and cardiac surgeon. Today, it should be commonplace to find a cardiac surgeon giving advice in the cardiac catheterization laboratory, whereas an interventionalist may aid his/her surgical colleague in the operating room by providing specific interventional techniques in selected patients. It should be routine and standard to involve the surgical team in any patient who is expected to undergo further surgical procedures prior to engaging in any transcatheter intervention. These discussions have to be open and directed toward the specific patient who is being considered for interventional and/or surgical treatment. For example, in a patient undergoing transcatheter evaluation in preparation for conduit replacement, it may well be justified to place a stent for a more distal pulmonary artery stenosis, while proximal branch stenosis is not addressed because it is felt that this lesion could easily be treated during subsequent conduit replacement. The knowledge of the combined treatment capabilities allows the development of new and complex treatment strategies. One of the most notable examples of this cooperation has been in the fenestrated Fontan patients, in whom the immediate surgical morbidity is dramatically reduced by a purposeful conduit fenestration, which can subsequently be closed in the catheterization laboratory once the patient has recovered from the initial procedure. Another dramatic example of this type of collaboration is in patients with pulmonary valve atresia and ventricular septal defect, in whom the surgical creation of a right ventricle-to-pulmonary artery connection early in the course of management provides the cardiologist access to the pulmonary vessels for dilation and intrapulmonary stenting in preparation for eventual definitive repair. This type of cooperation with inclusion of the adjunct procedures of the cardiologist in the staging of the surgery will contribute to a better outcome for many patients with extremely complex lesions.

In addition to the aforementioned collaboration between cardiac surgeon and cardiac interventionalist, a selection of new therapeutic hybrid catheterization and surgical procedures has been added to the spectrum of therapeutic interventions in complex congenital heart disease. These include the staged hybrid approach to the management of hypoplastic left heart syndrome (166–168), perventricular closure of ventricular septal defects (37,38), as well as intraoperative stent placements (169).

Hypoplastic Left Heart Syndrome

Hypoplastic left heart syndrome carries a grave short- and long-term prognosis despite improvements made in the traditional staged surgical approach. Even though the surgical management has evolved over time, the basic concept has remained the same, and any possible improvements are capped by the limitations of this basic surgical approach. Using the conventional palliative surgical approach, the 5-year survival has been documented in multicenter experiences to be as low as 54% (170). The stage I palliation in the neonate appears to carry the greatest risk, contributing to the high morbidity and mortality in these patients. This is not surprising given the many physiologic changes that occur in the neonatal period, which significantly influence the overall balance of this very fragile circulation. Combining this with an additional insult of a major open-heart procedure results in quite variable results among institutions, with mortality ranging from just under 10% to >50%. This has led to the development of alternative treatment strategies that are based on smaller off-pump interventions in the early neonatal period that can be performed with minimal morbidity and mortality, thereby deferring the need for major cardiac surgical procedures and allowing the necessary time for improved growth and development of the patient and cardiac structures. This sets the stage for a subsequent comprehensive surgical procedure that combines the classic bidirectional Glenn shunt with a Norwood-type palliation as well as potential setup for subsequent transcatheter completion of the Fontan-type circulation. This staged approach requires a close collaboration between the cardiac surgeon, interventional cardiologist, and Heart Center staff. As is the case with many new innovative techniques, modifications have evolved over time as a result of the associated learning curve.

In 2002, Akintuerk et al. (171) reported on their experience with 11 patients who underwent transcatheter stenting of the arterial duct using balloon-expandable Jo stents, followed by bilateral pulmonary arterial banding 1 to 3 days after the transcatheter procedure. Balloon atrial septoplasty or balloon atrial septostomy was performed if required on an as-needed basis. This early palliation was then followed by a bidirectional Glenn procedure as well as a Damus–Kaye–Stansel procedure and arch reconstruction between the ages of 3.5 and 6 months. Two deaths were encountered in this smaller series. In 2003, Michel-Behnke et al. (166) of the same group published an updated experience of 20 patients with very similar results.

The technique has further been modified by Galantowicz and Cheatham (167). Initial attempts at a sole transcatheter technique with implantation of the Amplatzer pulmonary artery (PA) flow restrictor (AGA Medical, Golden Valley, MN) and PDA stents had a suboptimal outcome with significant hemodynamic compromise owing to the combination of the stiffness of the delivery cable as well as the need for placing a long sheath through tricuspid and pulmonary valves into the branch PAs, resulting in significant regurgitation. The approach was thus modified to a true hybrid technique, in which the cardiac surgeon initially performs bilateral pulmonary arterial banding, followed by transpulmonary placement of a stent to maintain patency of the arterial duct during the same procedure. This technique is performed preferably in a specially designed hybrid cardiac catheterization or operative suite that facilitates the specific needs of the cardiac surgeon as well as the interventional cardiologist (Fig. 16.22). The first suite dedicated to hybrid therapies in complex

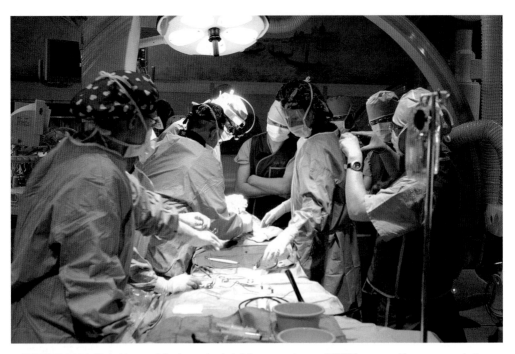

FIGURE 16.22 Hybrid stage I for hypoplastic left heart syndrome (HLHS)—setup. Team approach during a hybrid stage I palliation in the specifically designed hybrid catheterization suites.

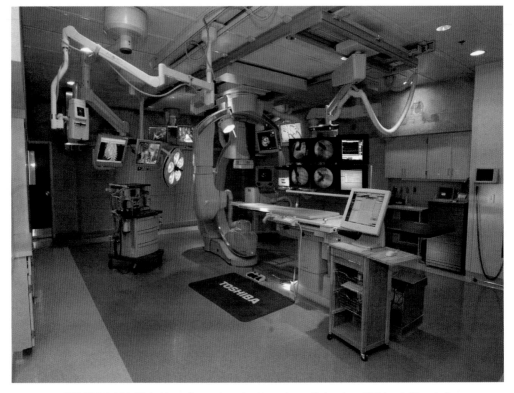

FIGURE 16.23 Hybrid cardiac catheterization suite at Columbus Children's Hospital.

congenital heart disease opened in June 2004 at Columbus Children's Hospital (Fig. 16.23).

After LPA and RPA bands are placed, using a 3.5-mm or 3.0-mm Gore-Tex tube, and cut into 1- to 2-mm-wide strips, the PDA stent is then delivered through a short delivery sheath placed transpulmonary directly through a purse-string suture secured by snares. The initial choice of stents included balloon-expandable premounted Genesis (Cordis, Warren, NJ) or Formula 418 stents (Cook, Bloomington, IN), but more recently, self-expandable Protégé (EV3, Plymouth, MN) stents have been implanted and are felt to be more beneficial owing to the increased flexibility when compared with the balloon-expandable varieties. Additionally, being able to drag the partially deployed stent backward if required during the delivery process is useful. The use of these stents has become even more appropriate since the length of the delivery sheath has been decreased from 135 to 80 cm.

The hybrid stage I procedure is feasible for most patients with hypoplastic left heart syndrome (Fig. 16.24), an exception being those patients with stenosis of the retrograde aortic arch with accelerated flow noted on screening Doppler echocardiography. In these patients, a classic Norwood-type procedure remains the preferred treatment choice. Size has not been an issue, with hybrid stage I palliation being successfully performed in preterm neonates as small as 1.1 kg. After the hybrid stage I procedure, patients are usually evaluated prior to discharge for the presence of any significant atrial-level restriction, and balloon atrial septostomy or atrial septoplasty is performed when the mean gradient across the intra-atrial communication is ≥8 mm Hg. Patients are closely monitored during the follow-up period not only for the development of recurrent atrial-level restriction, but also for the presence of any obstruction at the level of the retrograde aortic arch or the PDA stent, as well as for assessing the flow to both branch PAs. Ideally, a single catheterization procedure is performed prior to the comprehensive stage II procedure. This includes assessment of the distal pulmonary artery pressures using the RADI PressureWire (Radi Medical Systems, Uppsala, Sweden) (88), as well as assessment for any residual or recurrent stenosis across the PDA stent or retrograde arch. Again, a septostomy at this stage usually allows the use of a larger septostomy balloon and is performed if any significant atrial-level restriction is identified.

The comprehensive stage II procedure is purely surgical. It combines a bidirectional Glenn's shunt with debanding of the pulmonary arteries and patch augmentation, if required. A Damus–Kaye–Stansel anastomosis is performed with arch reconstruction. The PDA stent is removed and atrial septectomy is performed. During the same procedure, radiopaque bands are placed across the IVC and a blind-ending pouch of SVC below the pulmonary arteries is created. Another radiopaque marker facilitates subsequent transcatheter completion of a Fontan-type circulation. The transcatheter completion

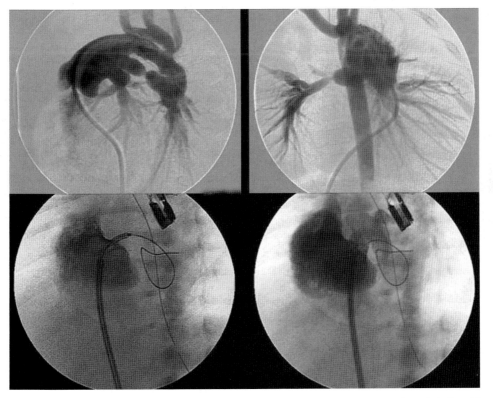

FIGURE 16.24 Hybrid stage I for hypoplastic left heart syndrome (HLHS)—procedure. A 2-day-old infant with hypoplastic left heart syndrome undergoing stage I palliation. **Top left and right:** Main pulmonary artery (MPA) angiography after placement of bilateral pulmonary artery (PA) bands as well as a patent ductus arteriosus (PDA) stent. **Bottom left:** Placement of a stent across a restrictive intra-atrial communication. **Bottom right:** Angiography after placement of a stent across the restrictive intra-atrial communication.

of the Fontan-type circulation requires the availability of a covered balloon-expandable stent, which can be implanted between the IVC and SVC pouch using a transcatheter technique. A catheter-based approach was first described by Hausdorf et al. (172), but it was only recently that this approach was modified by Galantowicz and Cheatham (168). However, its practical use has been limited in the United States because of the lack of FDA approval of the covered stent. Outside the United States, the covered varieties of the NuMED CP stent are more widely available, and this has resulted in further development of this technique being presently pursued by larger Canadian centers (173).

The hybrid approach has been documented to achieve acceptable short- and mid-term outcome in patients with hypoplastic left heart syndrome. This technique is still evolving with an expected learning curve. With refinements in patient selection, improved morbidity and mortality should be realized.

Perventricular Closure of Ventricular Septal Defects

Device closure of muscular ventricular septal defects using the Amplatzer muscular VSD occluder has been shown to be safe and effective. However, even though the transcatheter approach can be safely and effectively performed in most patients, patient weight <10 kg has been associated with a significantly higher risk of procedure- or device-related complications, as well as a higher risk of procedural failure (35,52). This is mainly related to the need for establishing an arteriovenous wire loop and the use of a long and relatively stiff delivery system, which in infants frequently not only stents open the tricuspid and aortic valves, but also creates a significant amount of tension that may result in bradycardia and/or temporary heart block. As a result, a perventricular approach has been adopted whereby the heart is exposed through a midline sternotomy off cardiopulmonary bypass. Under TEE and/or epicardial echo guidance, the appropriate entry site in relation to the VSD is identified and secured by placing a purse-string suture around its location at the RV free wall. Subsequently a direct puncture is performed with the needle directed toward the VSD. A 0.035-inch angled glide wire is used to cross the VSD. An appropriately sized short hemostatic sheath can then be advanced across the VSD under echo guidance, keeping an appropriate distance from the LV free wall and the mitral valve apparatus. The correctly sized Amplatzer muscular VSD occluder is then loaded and advanced across the sheath and deployed under echo guidance,

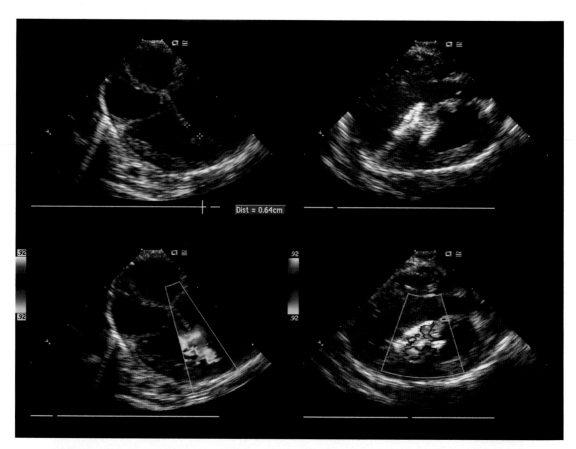

FIGURE 16.25 Closure of a moderate-sized muscular ventricular septal defect (VSD) in a 3-month-old infant using a perventricular hybrid approach. **Top left:** Four-chamber view demonstrating large VSD. **Bottom left:** Four-chamber view with color flow mapping demonstrating VSD. **Top right:** Long-axis view documenting excellent device position after VSD closure. **Bottom right:** Long-axis view demonstrating only minimal foaming through the device after relapse on color flow mapping.

with the operator again being especially careful to establish some distance to the mitral valve apparatus before deploying the LV disc. Once deployed across the VSD, the device position is evaluated for any evidence of residual shunts or interference with adjacent structures that could create, for example, mitral or tricuspid regurgitation. Once a satisfactory device position has been confirmed, the device is released, followed by a final echo evaluation (Fig. 16.25). The earliest experience describing this technique was reported by Bacha et al. in 2003 (38). In 2005, a multicenter experience documented successful application of this technique in 12 of 13 patients without mortality (37). At follow-up, residual shunts were present in two patients, without evidence of volume overload, congestive heart failure, or pulmonary hypertension. Modifications of this perventricular approach to facilitate closure of perimembranous ventricular septal defects have recently been evaluated in animal experiments by Amin et al. (53).

The perventricular technique of VSD closure is specifically suitable for small infants with high-risk muscular ventricular septal defects. It combines the safety of the hybrid surgical approach, avoidance of cardiopulmonary bypass, and relatively short procedure time. Its safety and efficacy are presently evaluated in a formal FDA-sponsored clinical trial under a high-risk protocol. Whether perventricular closure of perimembranous ventricular septal defects will ultimately gain acceptance as an alternative to surgical closure in infants is uncertain and will to a large extent depend on whether device modifications will significantly reduce the incidence of complete heart block that has so far been associated with the use of this device.

Other Hybrid Procedures

The cooperation between cardiac surgeon and interventional cardiologist is not limited to the management of infants with HLHS or perventricular VSD closure, but instead the hybrid approach can and has been adapted to various lesions and indications, such as the stent placement in various locations (Fig. 16.26) on and off cardiopulmonary bypass, vascular access in preterm neonates requiring interventional therapy (such as carotid cutdown or direct puncture via sternotomy), as well as intraoperative balloon occlusion of aortopulmonary collaterals or shunts. The ability of the surgeon to provide safe access to a vascular structure not amenable to conventional transcatheter therapy and the ability of the interventionalist to use less invasive techniques and materials creates a unique "marriage" benefiting patients with complex congenital heart disease (Fig. 16.27). The essential ingredients to achieve a successful outcome of these procedures are the close cooperation between surgeon and interventionalist as well as their flexibility to adapt nonstandard approaches that are specifically tailored toward each individual patient. Intraoperative stent placement is aided by the direct visualization in the operative field and can be further enhanced through the use of endoscopic equipment that facilitates a more detailed view of the stenosed or compressed area. In addition, it is essential to have a high-resolution, digital, mobile C-arm readily available to obtain intraoperative angiograms whenever necessary. Future hybrid cardiothoracic operative suites with integrated permanent imaging

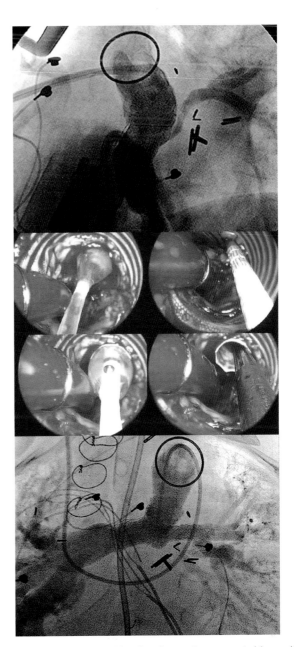

FIGURE 16.26 A 7-year-old girl with complex congenital heart disease (CHD) who underwent intraoperative left pulmonary artery (LPA) stent placement during a Mustard procedure. **Top:** PA angiography demonstrating a severely hypoplastic LPA. **Middle:** Intraoperative PA rehabilitation monitored endoscopically, from **left** to **right** and **top** to **bottom**, cutting balloon angioplasty, (covered) stent positioning followed by expansion, stent appearance after expansion. **Bottom:** PA angiography demonstrating significantly improved LPA appearance.

equipment will allow even more complex CHD to be treated using innovative management strategies. It is expected that the hybrid approach will establish a new dimension in the treatment of neonates, children, and adults with CHD, regardless of patient size or lesion complexity.

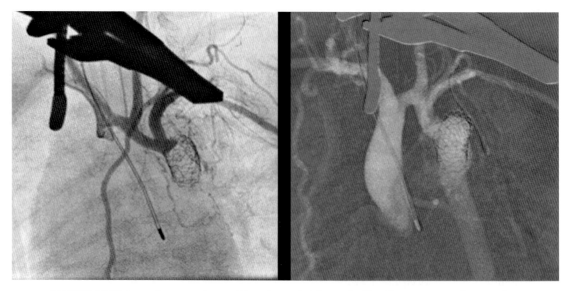

FIGURE 16.27 Stent placement via carotid cutdown. A 2.5-month-old male premature infant (2.1 kg), who initially underwent hybrid stage 1 palliation for complex congenital heart disease. He developed a significant recoarctation distal to the left subclavian artery (LSA) and therefore underwent hybrid placement of a premounted stent using a surgical carotid cutdown. **Left:** Almost complete interruption distal to LSA before stent placement. **Right:** Aortogram after stent placement demonstrating significantly improved flow through the descending aorta (DAO).

SUMMARY

The therapeutic cardiac catheterization procedures discussed in this chapter represent significant advances in the care of patients with congenital heart disease. The procedures are ordinarily performed without an incision, cardiopulmonary bypass, or chest tubes. Some of the therapeutic procedures are possible only in the catheterization laboratory, and the subsequent surgery is possible only after preparation in the catheterization laboratory.

Even with the additional expense of the specialized catheters and devices and the added cost of the more extensive catheterization procedures, the direct costs of the therapeutic procedure in the catheterization laboratory are significantly lower than those for the comparable surgical procedure. The indirect savings for a patient or the patient's family may be even greater. The patient and family are away from home and work for only 1 or 2 days for the entire hospital stay. Following the catheterization procedure, the patient is able to return home and immediately return to full activity of either school or work. These advantages of therapeutic catheterization procedures have led to their wide acceptance.

However, therapeutic catheterization has advanced beyond the confines of the cardiac catheterization laboratory. Many cutting-edge procedures can be facilitated only through the unique cooperation between cardiac surgeon and interventional cardiologist, and therefore patient care is advanced through this combined expertise. With further developments and improvements in catheter and surgical techniques, it is to be expected that additional nonsurgical or hybrid corrections will become standard within the next several years.

References

1. Dotter CT, Judkins MP. Transluminal treatment of arteriosclerotic obstruction. Description of a new technic and a preliminary report of its application. *Circulation* 1964;30:654–670.
2. Rashkind WJ, Miller WW. Creation of an atrial septal defect without thoracotomy. A palliative approach to complete transposition of the great arteries. *JAMA* 1966;196:991–992.
3. Porstmann W, Wierny L, Warnke H. Closure of ductus arteriosus persistens without thoracotomy [in German]. 2. *Fortschr Geb Rontgenstr Nuklearmed* 1968;109:133–148.
4. Wallace S, Gianturco C, Anderson JH, et al. Therapeutic vascular occlusion utilizing steel coil technique: Clinical applications. *AJR Am J Roentgenol* 1976;127:381–387.
5. King TD, Thompson SL, Steiner C, et al. Secundum atrial septal defect. Nonoperative closure during cardiac catheterization. *JAMA* 1976;235:2506–2509.
6. Kan JS, White RI Jr, Mitchell SE, et al. Percutaneous balloon valvuloplasty: A new method for treating congenital pulmonary-valve stenosis. *N Engl J Med* 1982;307:540–542.
7. Lock JE, Block PC, McKay RG, et al. Transcatheter closure of ventricular septal defects. *Circulation* 1988;78:361–368.
8. O'Laughlin MP, Perry SB, Lock JE, et al. Use of endovascular stents in congenital heart disease. *Circulation* 1991;83:1923–1939.
9. Bonhoeffer P, Boudjemline Y, Saliba Z, et al. Percutaneous replacement of pulmonary valve in a right-ventricle to pulmonary-artery prosthetic conduit with valve dysfunction. *Lancet* 2000;356:1403–1405.
10. Holzer R, Chisolm J, Hill SL, et al. Transcatheter devices used in the management of patients with congenital heart disease. *Expert Rev Med Devices* 2006;2:603–615.
11. Hausdorf G, Kaulitz R, Paul T, et al. Transcatheter closure of atrial septal defect with a new flexible, self-centering device (the STARFlex Occluder). *Am J Cardiol* 1999;84:1113–1116, A10.
12. Zahn EM, Wilson N, Cutright W, et al. Development and testing of the Helex septal occluder, a new expanded polytetrafluoroethylene atrial septal defect occlusion system. *Circulation* 2001;104:711–716.
13. Sideris EB, Sideris SE, Thanopoulos BD, et al. Transvenous atrial septal defect occlusion by the buttoned device. *Am J Cardiol* 1990;66:1524–1526.
14. Rao PS, Berger F, Rey C, et al. Results of transvenous occlusion of secundum atrial septal defects with the fourth generation buttoned device: Comparison with first, second and third generation devices. International Buttoned Device Trial Group. *J Am Coll Cardiol* 2000;36:583–592.

15. O'Laughlin MP. Microvena atrial septal defect occlusion device—update 2000. *J Interv Cardiol* 2001;14(1):77–80.

16. Hausdorf G, Schneider M, Franzbach B, et al. Transcatheter closure of secundum atrial septal defects with the atrial septal defect occlusion system (ASDOS): Initial experience in children. *Heart* 1996;75:83–88.

17. Sharafuddin MJ, Gu X, Titus JL, et al. Transvenous closure of secundum atrial septal defects: Preliminary results with a new self-expanding Nitinol prosthesis in a swine model. *Circulation* 1997;95:2162–2168. Erratum in: *Circulation* 1998;97:413.

18. Masura J, Gavora P, Formanek A, et al. Transcatheter closure of secundum atrial septal defects using the new self-centering Amplatzer septal occluder: Initial human experience. [See comment.] *Cathet Cardiovasc Diagn* 1997;42:388–393.

19. Zanchetta M, Rigatelli G, Pedon L, et al. Transcatheter atrial septal defect closure assisted by intracardiac echocardiography: 3-year follow-up. *J Interv Cardiol* 2004;17:95–98.

20. Varma C, Benson LN, Silversides C, et al. Outcomes and alternative techniques for device closure of the large secundum atrial septal defect. *Cathet Cardiovasc Interv* 2004;61:131–139.

21. Hill SL, Berul CI, Patel HT, et al. Early ECG abnormalities associated with transcatheter closure of atrial septal defects using the Amplatzer septal occluder. *J Interv Card Electrophysiol* 2000;4:469–474.

22. Hessling G, Hyca S, Brockmeier K, et al. Cardiac dysrhythmias in pediatric patients before and 1 year after transcatheter closure of atrial septal defects using the Amplatzer septal occluder. *Pediatr Cardiol* 2003;24:259–262.

23. Ries MW, Kampmann C, Rupprecht HJ, et al. Nickel release after implantation of the Amplatzer occluder. *Am Heart J* 2003;145:737–741.

24. Lai DW, Saver JL, Araujo JA, et al. Pericarditis associated with nickel hypersensitivity to the Amplatzer occluder device: A case report. *Cathet Cardiovasc Interv* 2005;66:424–426.

25. Amin Z, Hijazi ZM., Bass JL, et al. Erosion of Amplatzer septal occluder device after closure of secundum atrial septal defects: Review of registry of complications and recommendations to minimize future risk. *Cathet Cardiovasc Interv* 2004;63:496–502.

26. Ewert P, Kretschmar O, Peters B, et al. Preliminary experience with a new 18 mm Amplatzer PFO occluder for small persistent foramen ovale. *Cathet Cardiovasc Interv* 2003;59:518–521.

27. Waight DJ, Cao QL, Hijazi ZM. Closure of patent foramen ovale in patients with orthodeoxia-platypnea using the Amplatzer devices. [See comment.] *Cathet Cardiovasc Interv* 2000;50:195–198.

28. Hong TE, Thaler D, Brorson J, et al. Amplatzer PFO, I. Transcatheter closure of patent foramen ovale associated with paradoxical embolism using the Amplatzer PFO occluder: Initial and intermediate-term results of the U.S. multicenter clinical trial. *Cathet Cardiovasc Interv* 2003;60:524–528.

29. Trepels T, Zeplin H, Sievert H, et al. Cardiac perforation following transcatheter PFO closure. *Cathet Cardiovasc Interv* 2003;58:111–113.

30. Schrader R. Incidence and clinical course of thrombus formation on atrial septal defect and patent foramen ovale closure devices [comment]. *J Am Coll Cardiol* 2004;44:1714; author reply 1714–1716.

30a. Lababidi Z, Wu JR, Walls JT. Percutaneous balloon aortic valvuloplasty: Results in 23 patients. *Am J Cardiol* 1984;53(1):194–197.

31. Krumsdorf U, Ostermayer S, Billinger K, et al. Incidence and clinical course of thrombus formation on atrial septal defect and patient foramen ovale closure devices in 1,000 consecutive patients. [See comment.] *J Am Coll Cardiol* 2004;43:302–309.

32. Braun M, Gliech V, Boscheri A, et al. Transcatheter closure of patent foramen ovale (PFO) in patients with paradoxical embolism. Periprocedural safety and mid-term follow-up results of three different device occluder systems. [See comment.] *Eur Heart J* 2004;25:424–430.

33. Amin Z, Gu X, Berry JM, et al. New device for closure of muscular ventricular septal defects in a canine model. *Circulation* 1999;100:320–328.

34. Thanopoulos BD, Tsaousis GS, Konstadopoulou GN, et al. Transcatheter closure of muscular ventricular septal defects with the Amplatzer ventricular septal defect occluder: Initial clinical applications in children. *J Am Coll Cardiol* 1999;33:1395–1399.

35. Holzer R, Balzer D, Cao QL, et al., Amplatzer Muscular Ventricular Septal Defect Investigators. Device closure of muscular ventricular septal defects using the Amplatzer muscular ventricular septal defect occluder: Immediate and mid-term results of a U.S. registry. *J Am Coll Cardiol* 2004;43:1257–1263.

36. Thanopoulos BD, Rigby ML. Outcome of transcatheter closure of muscular ventricular septal defects with the Amplatzer ventricular septal defect occluder. *Heart* 2005;91:513–516.

37. Bacha EA, Cao QL, Galantowicz ME, et al. Multicenter experience with perventricular device closure of muscular ventricular septal defects. *Pediatr Cardiol* 2005;26:169–175.

38. Bacha EA, Cao QL, Starr JP, et al. Perventricular device closure of muscular ventricular septal defects on the beating heart: Technique and results. *J Thorac Cardiovasc Surg* 2003;126:1718–1723.

39. Goldstein JA, Casserly IP, Balzer DT, et al. Transcatheter closure of recurrent postmyocardial infarction ventricular septal defects utilizing the Amplatzer postinfarction VSD device: A case series. *Cathet Cardiovasc Interv* 2003;59:238–243.

40. Holzer R, Balzer D, Amin Z, et al. Transcatheter closure of postinfarction ventricular septal defects using the new Amplatzer muscular VSD occluder: Results of a U.S. Registry. *Cathet Cardiovasc Interv* 2004;61:196–201.

41. Crenshaw BS, Granger CB, Birnbaum Y, et al. Risk factors, angiographic patterns, and outcomes in patients with ventricular septal defect complicating acute myocardial infarction. GUSTO-I (Global Utilization of Streptokinase and TPA for Occluded Coronary Arteries) Trial Investigators. *Circulation* 2000;101:27–32.

42. Cooley DA. Postinfarction ventricular septal rupture. *Semin Thorac Cardiovasc Surg* 1998;10:100–104.

43. Dalrymple-Hay MJ, Monro JL, Livesey SA, et al. Postinfarction ventricular septal rupture: The Wessex experience. *Semin Thorac Cardiovasc Surg* 1998;10:111–116.

44. Rigby ML, Redington AN. Primary transcatheter umbrella closure of perimembranous ventricular septal defect. *Br Heart J* 1994;72:368–371.

45. Gu X, Han YM, Titus JL, et al. Transcatheter closure of membranous ventricular septal defects with a new Nitinol prosthesis in a natural swine model. *Cathet Cardiovasc Interv* 2000;50:502–509.

46. Hijazi ZM, Hakim F, Haweleh AA, et al. Catheter closure of perimembranous ventricular septal defects using the new Amplatzer membranous VSD occluder: Initial clinical experience. *Cathe Cardiovasc Interv* 2002;56:508–515.

47. Holzer R, De Giovanni JV, Walsh KP, et al. Transcatheter closure of perimembranous ventricular septal defects using the Amplatzer membranous VSD occluder: Immediate and midterm results of an international registry. *Cathet Cardiovasc Interv* 2006;68:620–628.

48. Fu YC, Bass J, Amin Z, et al. Transcatheter closure of perimembranous ventricular septal defects using the new Amplatzer membranous VSD occluder: Results of the U.S. Phase I Trial. *J Am Coll Cardiol* 2006;47:319–325.

49. Masura J, Gao W, Gavora P, et al. Percutaneous closure of perimembranous ventricular septal defects with the eccentric Amplatzer device: Multicenter follow-up study. *Pediatr Cardiol* 2005;26:216–219.

50. Yip WC, Zimmerman F, Hijazi ZM. Heart block and empirical therapy after transcatheter closure of perimembranous ventricular septal defect. *Cathet Cardiovasc Interv* 2005;66:436–441.

51. Boutin C, Musewe NN, Smallhorn JF, et al. Echocardiographic follow-up of atrial septal defect after catheter closure by double-umbrella device. *Circulation* 1993;88:621–627.

52. Holzer R, de Giovanni J, Walsh KP, et al. Transcatheter closure of perimembranous ventricular septal defects using the Amplatzer membranous VSD occluder: Immediate and midterm results of an international registry. *Cathet Cardiovasc Interv* 2006;68:620–628.

53. Amin Z, Danford DA, Lof J, et al. Intraoperative device closure of perimembranous ventricular septal defects without cardiopulmonary bypass: Preliminary results with the perventricular technique. *J Thorac Cardiovasc Surg* 2004;127:234–241.

54. Vincent RN, Raviele AA, Diehl HJ. Single-center experience with the HELEX septal occluder for closure of atrial septal defects in children. *J Interv Cardiol* 2003;16:79–82.

55. Sievert H, Horvath K, Zadan E, et al. Patent foramen ovale closure in patients with transient ischemia attack/stroke. *J Interv Cardiol* 2001;14:261–266.

56. Lock JE, Rome JJ, Davis R, et al. Transcatheter closure of atrial septal defects. Experimental studies. *Circulation* 1989;79:1091–1099.

57. Latson LA, Benson LN, Hellenbrand WF, et al. Transcatheter closure of ASD—early results of multi-center trial of the Bard clamshell septal occluder. *Circulation* 1991;84(suppl II):544.

58. Bridges ND, Perry SB, Parness I, et al. Transcatheter closure of a large patent ductus arteriosus with the clamshell septal umbrella. *J Am Coll Cardiol* 1991;18:1297–1302.

59. Schlesinger AE, Folz SJ, Beekman RH. Transcatheter atrial septal defect occlusion devices: Normal radiographic appearances and complications. *J Vascul Interv Radiol* 1992;3:527–533.

60. Latson LA. The CardioSEAL device: History, techniques, results. *J Interv Cardiol* 1998;11:501–505.

61. Mullins CE. *Cardiac Catheterization in Congenital Heart Disease.* Malden, MA: Blackwell, 2006.

62. Carminati M, Giusti S, Hausdorf G, et al. A European multicentric experience using the CardioSEAL and Starflex double umbrella devices to close interatrial communications holes within the oval fossa. *Cardiol Young* 2000;10:519–526.

63. Cheatham JP, Hill SL, Chisolm JL. Initial results using the new cribriforme Amplatzer septal occluder for transcatheter closure of multifenestrated atrial septal defects with septal aneurysm [abstract]. *Cathet Cardiovasc Interv* 2003;60:126.

64. Rashkind WJ, Cuaso CC. Transcatheter closure of patent ductus arteriosus; successful use in a 3.5 kilogram infant. *Pediatr Cardiol* 1979;1:3–7.

65. Rashkind WJ, Mullins CE, Hellenbrand WE, et al. Nonsurgical closure of patent ductus arteriosus: Clinical application of the Rashkind PDA Occluder System. *Circulation* 1987;75:583–592.

66. Rashkind WJ. Therapeutic interventional procedures in congenital heart disease. *Radiol Diagn* 1987;28:449–460.

67. Perry SB, Radtke W, Fellows KE, et al. Coil embolization to occlude aortopulmonary collateral vessels and shunts in patients with congenital heart disease. *J Am Coll Cardiol* 1989;13:100–108.

68. Cambier PA, Kirby WC, Wortham DC, et al. Percutaneous closure of the small (less than 2.5 mm) patent ductus arteriosus using coil embolization. *Am J Cardiol* 1992;69:815–816.

69. Uzun O, Hancock S, Parsons JM, et al. Transcatheter occlusion of the arterial duct with Cook detachable coils: Early experience. *Heart* 1996;76:269–273.

70. Masura J, Walsh KP, Thanopoulous B, et al. Catheter closure of moderate-to large-sized patent ductus arteriosus using the new Amplatzer duct occluder: Immediate and short-term results. *J Am Coll Cardiol* 1998;31:878–882.

71. Chisolm JL, Hill SL, Hardin J, et al. Initial experience with the Nit-Occlud PDA occlusion system for closure of patent ductus arteriosus [abstract]. *Cathet Cardiovasc Interv* 2003;60:123.

72. Celiker A, Aypar E, Karagoz T, et al. Transcatheter closure of patent ductus arteriosus with Nit-Occlud coils. *Cathet Cardiovasc Interv* 2005;65:569–576.

73. Holzer R, Cao QL, Sandhu S, et al. The Amplatzer vascular plug—an addition to our interventional armantarium. *Pediatr Cardiol Today* 2004;2(6):6–8.

74. Pass RH, Hijazi Z, Hsu DT, et al. Multicenter USA Amplatzer patent ductus arteriosus occlusion device trial: Initial and one-year results. *J Am Coll Cardiol* 2004;44:513–519.

75. Hill SL, Hijazi ZM, Hellenbrand WE, et al. Evaluation of the Amplatzer vascular plug for embolization of peripheral vascular malformations associated with congenital heart disease. *Cathet Cardiovasc Interv* 2006;67:113–119.

76. Hoyer MH. Novel use of the Amplatzer plug for closure of a patent ductus arteriosus. [See comment.] *Cathet Cardiovasc Interv* 2005;65:577–580.

77. Cheatham JP. Not so fast with that Novel use: Does AVP = PDA? [comment]. *Cathet Cardiovasc Interv* 2005;65:581–583.

78. Patel HT, Cao QL, Rhodes J, et al. Long-term outcome of transcatheter coil closure of small to large patent ductus arteriosus. *Cathet Cardiovasc Interv* 1999;47:457–461.

79. Hijazi ZM, Geggel RL. Transcatheter closure of large patent ductus arteriosus (> or = 4 mm) with multiple Gianturco coils: Immediate and mid-term results. *Heart* 1996;76:536–540.

80. Grifka RG, Mullins CE, Gianturco C, et al. New Gianturco-Grifka vascular occlusion device. Initial studies in a canine model. *Circulation* 1995;91:1840–1846.

81. Hoyer MH, Leon RA, Fricker FJ. Transcatheter closure of modified Blalock-Taussig shunt with Gianturco-Grifka Vascular Occlusion Device. [See comment.] *Cathet Cardiovasc Interv* 1999;48:365–367.

82. Ebeid MR, Gaymes CH, Smith JC, et al. Gianturco-Grifka vascular occlusion device for closure of patent ductus arteriosus. *Am J Cardiol* 2001;87:657–660.

83. Demkow M, Ruzyllo W, Siudalska H, et al. Transcatheter closure of a 16 mm hypertensive patent ductus arteriosus with the Amplatzer muscular VSD occluder. *Cathet Cardiovasc Interv* 2001;52:359–362.

84. Pedra CA, Sanches SA, Fontes VF. Percutaneous occlusion of the patent ductus arteriosus with the Amplatzer device for atrial septal defects. *J Invasive Cardiol* 2003;15:413–417.

85. Rao PS, Sideris EB, Haddad J, et al. Transcatheter occlusion of patent ductus arteriosus with adjustable buttoned device. Initial clinical experience. *Circulation* 1993;88:1119–1126.

86. Mullins CE, O'Laughlin MP, Vick GW III, et al. Implantation of balloon-expandable intravascular grafts by catheterization in pulmonary arteries and systemic veins. *Circulation* 1988;77:188–199.

87. Park SC, Neches WH, Mullins CE, et al. Blade atrial septostomy: Collaborative study. *Circulation* 1982;66:258–266.

88. Holzer RJ, Hardin J, Hill SL, et al. Radiofrequency energy—a multifaceted tool for the congenital interventionist. *Congenital Cardiol Today* 2006;4:1–8.

89. Hill SL, Mizelle KM, Vellucci SM, et al. Radiofrequency perforation and cutting balloon septoplasty of intact atrial septum in a newborn with hypoplastic left heart syndrome using transesophageal ICE probe guidance. *Cathet Cardiovasc Interv* 2005;64:214–217.

90. Daehnert I, Rotzsch C, Wiener M, et al. Rapid right ventricular pacing is an alternative to adenosine in catheter interventional procedures for congenital heart disease. *Heart* 2004;90:1047–1050.

91. Stanger P, Cassidy SC, Girod DA, et al. Balloon pulmonary valvuloplasty: Results of the Valvuloplasty and Angioplasty of Congenital Anomalies Registry. *Am J Cardiol* 1990;65:775–783.

92. Jarrar M, Betbout F, Farhat MB, et al. Long-term invasive and noninvasive results of percutaneous balloon pulmonary valvuloplasty in children, adolescents, and adults. *Am Heart J* 1199;138(pt 1):950–954.

93. Rao PS, Galal O, Patnana M, et al. Results of three to 10 year follow up of balloon dilatation of the pulmonary valve. *Heart* 1998;80:591–595.

94. Mullins CE. Pulmonary valve balloon dilation. In: Mullins CE, ed. *Cardiac Catheterization in Congenital Heart Disease*. Malden, MA: Blackwell, 2006:430–440.

95. McCrindle BW. Independent predictors of long-term results after balloon pulmonary valvuloplasty. Valvuloplasty and Angioplasty of Congenital Anomalies (VACA) Registry Investigators. *Circulation* 1994;89:1751–1759.

96. Mullins CE, Nihill MR, Vick GW III, et al. Double balloon technique for dilation of valvular or vessel stenosis in congenital and acquired heart disease. *J Am Coll Cardiol* 1987;10:107–114.

97. Redington AN, Cullen S, Rigby ML. Laser or radiofrequency pulmonary valvotomy in neonates with pulmonary atresia and intact ventricular septum—description of a new method avoiding arterial catheterization. *Cardiol Young* 1992;2:387–390.

98. Cheatham JP. To perforate or not to perforate—that's the question ... or is it? Just ask Richard! *Cathet Cardiovasc Diagn* 1997;42:403–404.

99. Latson L, Cheatham J, Froemming S, et al. Transductal guidewire "rail" for balloon valvuloplasty in neonates with isolated critical pulmonary valve stenosis or atresia. *Am J Cardiol* 1994;73:713–714.

100. Benson LN, Nykanen D, Collison A. Radiofrequency perforation in the treatment of congenital heart disease. *Cathet Cardiovasc Interv* 2002;56:72–82.

101. Gournay V, Piechaud JF, Delogu A, et al. Balloon valvotomy for critical stenosis or atresia of pulmonary valve in newborns. *J Am Coll Cardiol* 1995;26:1725–1731.

102. Walsh KP, Abdulhamed JM, Tometzki JP. Importance of right ventricular outflow tract angiography in distinguishing critical pulmonary stenosis from pulmonary atresia. *Heart* 1997;77:456–460.

103. Wang JK, Wu MH, Chang CI, et al. Outcomes of transcatheter valvotomy in patients with pulmonary atresia and intact ventricular septum. *Am J Cardiol* 1999;84:1055–1060.

104. Alwi M, Geetha K, Bilkis AA, et al. Pulmonary atresia with intact ventricular septum percutaneous radiofrequency-assisted valvotomy and balloon dilation versus surgical valvotomy and Blalock Taussig shunt. *J Am Coll Cardiol* 2000;35:468–476.

105. Agnoletti G, Piechaud JF, Bonhoeffer P, et al. Perforation of the atretic pulmonary valve. Long-term follow-up. *J Am Coll Cardiol* 2003;41:1399–1403.

106. Justo RN, Nykanen DG, Williams WG, et al. Transcatheter perforation of the right ventricular outflow tract as initial therapy for pulmonary valve atresia and intact ventricular septum in the newborn. [See comment.] *Cathet Cardiovasc Diagn* 1997;40:408–413.

107. Cheatham JP. The transcatheter management of the neonate and infant with pulmonary atresia and intact ventricular septum. *J Interven Cardiology* 1998;11:363–387.

108. Alwi M, Kandavello G, Choo KK, et al. Risk factors for augmentation of the flow of blood to the lungs in pulmonary atresia with intact ventricular septum after radiofrequency valvotomy. *Cardiol Young* 2005;15:141–147.

109. Bonhoeffer P, Piechaud JF, Sidi D, et al. Mitral dilatation with the Multi-Track system: An alternative approach. *Cathet Cardiovasc Diagn* 1995;36:189–193.

110. Inoue K, Owaki T, Nakamura T, et al. Clinical application of transvenous mitral commissurotomy by a new balloon catheter. *J Thorac Cardiovasc Surg* 1984;87:394–402.

111. McElhinney DB, Sherwood MC, Keane JF, et al. Current management of severe congenital mitral stenosis: Outcomes of transcatheter and surgical therapy in 108 infants and children. *Circulation* 2005;112:707–714.

112. Dotter CT, Judkins MP. Transluminal treatment of arteriosclerotic obstruction. Description of a new technic and a preliminary report of its application. 1964. *Radiology* 1989;172(pt 2):904–920.

113. Sos T, Sniderman KW, Rettek-Sos B, et al. Percutaneous transluminal dilatation of coarctation of thoracic aorta post mortem. *Lancet* 1979;2:970–971.

114. Lock JE, Niemi T, Burke BA, et al. Transcutaneous angioplasty of experimental aortic coarctation. *Circulation* 1982;66:1280–1286.

115. Lock JE, Castaneda-Zuniga WR, Bass JL, et al. Balloon dilatation of excised aortic coarctations. *Radiology* 1982;143:689–691.

116. Grifka RG, Vick GW III, O'Laughlin MP, et al. Balloon expandable intravascular stents: Aortic implantation and late further dilation in growing minipigs. *Am Heart J* 1993;126:979–984.

117. Redington AN, Hayes AM, Ho SY. Transcatheter stent implantation to treat aortic coarctation in infancy. *Br Heart J* 1993;69(1):80–82.

118. Suarez de Lezo J, Pan M, Romero M, et al. Percutaneous interventions on severe coarctation of the aorta: A 21-year experience. *Pediatr Cardiol* 2005;26(2):176–189.

119. Cheatham JP. Stenting of coarctation of the aorta. *Cathet Cardiovasc Interv* 2001;54:112–125.

120. Chisolm JL, Hill SL, Holzer RJ, et al. Stenting complex aortic arch obstruction—a challenge, not a taboo [abstract]. *Cathet Cardiovasc Interv* 2006;68:461–462.

121. Zabal C, Attie F, Rosas M, et al. The adult patient with native coarctation of the aorta: Balloon angioplasty or primary stenting? [See comment.] *Heart* 2003;89:77–83.

122. Fletcher SE, Nihill MR, Grifka RG, et al. Balloon angioplasty of native coarctation of the aorta: midterm follow-up and prognostic factors. *J Am Coll Cardiol* 1995;25:730–734.
123. DeGroff CG, Rice MJ, Reller MD, et al. Intravascular ultrasound can assist angiographic assessment of coarctation of the aorta. *Am Heart J* 1994;128:836–839.
124. Tong AD, Rothman A, Atkinson RL, et al. Intravascular ultrasound imaging of coarctation of the aorta: Animal and human studies. *Am J Card Imaging* 1995;9:250–256.
125. Xu J, Shiota T, Omoto R, et al. Intravascular ultrasound assessment of regional aortic wall stiffness, distensibility, and compliance in patients with coarctation of the aorta. *Am Heart J* 1997;134:93–98.
126. Tan JL, Mullen M. Emergency stent graft deployment for acute aortic rupture following primary stenting for aortic coarctation. *Cathet Cardiovasc Interv* 2005;65:306–309.
127. Hijazi ZM. Catheter intervention for adult aortic coarctation: Be very careful! [comment]. *Cathet Cardiovasc Interv* 2003;59:536–537.
128. Varma C, Benson LN, Butany J, et al. Aortic dissection after stent dilatation for coarctation of the aorta: A case report and literature review. [See comment.] *Cathet Cardiovasc Interv* 2003;59:528–535.
129. Holzer RJ, Chisolm JL, Hill S, et al. PA Rehabilitation using endovascular stents in children with a weight below 15 kg: Stents are for kids too [abstract]. *Cathet Cardiovasc Interv* 2006;67:836.
130. Seale AN, Daubeney PE, Magee AG, et al. Pulmonary vein stenosis: Initial experience with cutting balloon angioplasty. *Heart* 2006;92:815–820.
131. Devaney EJ, Chang AC, Ohye RG, et al. Management of congenital and acquired pulmonary vein stenosis. *Ann Thorac Surg* 2006;81:992–995; discussion 995–996.
132. Zahn EM, Dobrolet NC, Nykanen DG, et al. Interventional catheterization performed in the early postoperative period after congenital heart surgery in children. *J Am Coll Cardiol* 2004;43:1264–1269.
133. Koenig P, Cao QL, Heitschmidt M, et al. Role of intracardiac echocardiographic guidance in transcatheter closure of atrial septal defects and patent foramen ovale using the Amplatzer device. *J Interv Cardiol* 2003;16:51–62.
134. Du ZD, Koenig P, Cao QL, et al. Comparison of transcatheter closure of secundum atrial septal defect using the Amplatzer septal occluder associated with deficient versus sufficient rims. *Am J Cardiol* 2002;90:865–869.
135. Holzer RJ, Chisolm J, Hill S, et al. Transhepatic cardiac catheterization in complex congenital heart disease: Where there is a will there is a way. *Congenital Cardiol Today* 2005;3:1–7.
136. Wahab HA, Bairam AR, Cao QL, et al. Novel technique to prevent prolapse of the Amplatzer septal occluder through large atrial septal defect. *Cathet Cardiovasc Interv* 2003;60:543–545.
137. Berger F, Ewert P, Abdul-Khaliq H, et al. Percutaneous closure of large atrial septal defects with the Amplatzer Septal Occluder: Technical overkill or recommendable alternative treatment? *J Interv Cardiol* 2001;14:63–67.
138. Levi DS, Moore JW. Embolization and retrieval of the Amplatzer septal occluder. *Cathet Cardiovasc Interv* 2004;61:543–547.
139. Masura J, Gavora P, Podnar T. Long-term outcome of transcatheter secundum-type atrial septal defect closure using Amplatzer septal occluders. *J Am Coll Cardiol* 2005;45:505–507.
140. Fischer G, Stieh J, Uebing A, et al. Experience with transcatheter closure of secundum atrial septal defects using the Amplatzer septal occluder: A single centre study in 236 consecutive patients. *Heart* 2003;89:199–204.
141. Veldtman GR, Razack V, Siu S, et al. Right ventricular form and function after percutaneous atrial septal defect device closure. *J Am Coll Cardiol* 2001;37:2108–2113.
141a.Holzer RJ, Chisolm JL, Hill SL, et al. ASD closure in small children. *Cath Cardio Inter* 2006;68(3):485.
142. Tofeig M, Walsh KP, Chan C, et al. Occlusion of Fontan fenestrations using the Amplatzer septal occluder. *Heart* 1998;79(4):368–370.
143. Cowley CG, Badran S, Gaffney D, et al. Transcatheter closure of Fontan fenestrations using the Amplatzer septal occluder: Initial experience and follow-up. [See comment.] *Cathet Cardiovasc Interv* 2000;51:301–304.
144. Rueda F, Squitieri C, Ballerini L. Closure of the fenestration in the extracardiac Fontan with the Amplatzer duct occluder device. [See comment.] *Cathet Cardiovasc Interv* 2001;54:88–92.
145. Bridges ND, Perry SB, Keane JF, et al. Preoperative transcatheter closure of congenital muscular ventricular septal defects. *N Engl J Med* 1991;324:1312–1317.
146. Pienvichit P, Piemonte TC. Percutaneous closure of postmyocardial infarction ventricular septal defect with the CardioSEAL septal occluder implant. [See comment.] *Cathet Cardiovasc Interv* 2001;54:490–494.

147. Sideris EB, Walsh KP, Haddad JL, et al. Occlusion of congenital ventricular septal defects by the buttoned device. "Buttoned device" Clinical Trials International Register. *Heart* 1997;77:276–279.
148. Chaudhari M, Chessa M, Stumper O, et al. Transcatheter coil closure of muscular ventricular septal defects. *J Interv Cardiol* 2001;14:165–168.
149. Kalra GS, Verma PK, Singh S, et al. Transcatheter closure of ventricular septal defect using detachable steel coil. *Heart* 1999;82:395–396.
150. Latiff HA, Alwi M, Kandhavel G, et al. Transcatheter closure of multiple muscular ventricular septal defects using Gianturco coils. *Ann Thorac Surg* 1999;68:1400–1401.
151. Lee EM, Roberts DH, Walsh KP. Transcatheter closure of a residual postmyocardial infarction ventricular septal defect with the Amplatzer septal occluder. *Heart* 1998;80:522–524.
152. Krichenko A, Benson LN, Burrows P, et al. Angiographic classification of the isolated, persistently patent ductus arteriosus and implications for percutaneous catheter occlusion. *Am J Cardiol* 1989;63:877–880.
153. Sommer RJ, Gutierrez A, Lai WW, et al. Use of preformed Nitinol snare to improve transcatheter coil delivery in occlusion of patent ductus arteriosus. *Am J Cardiol* 1994;74:836–839.
154. Hays MD, Hoyer MH, Glasow PF. New forceps delivery technique for coil occlusion of patent ductus arteriosus. *Am J Cardiol* 1996;77:209–211.
155. Kuhn MA, Latson LA. Transcatheter embolization coil closure of patent ductus arteriosus—modified delivery for enhanced control during coil positioning. *Cathet Cardiovasc Diagn* 1995;36:288–290.
156. Dalvi B, Goyal V, Narula D, et al. New technique using temporary balloon occlusion for transcatheter closure of patent ductus arteriosus with Gianturco coils. *Cathet Cardiovasc Diagn* 1997;41:62–70.
157. Henry G, Danilowicz D, Verma R. Severe hemolysis following partial coil-occlusion of patent ductus arteriosus. [See comment.] *Cathet Cardiovasc Diagn* 1996;39:410–412.
158. Hourihan M, Perry SB, Mandell VS, et al. Transcatheter umbrella closure of valvular and paravalvular leaks. *J Am Coll Cardiol* 1992;20;1371–1377.
159. Moore JD, Lashus AG, Prieto LR, et al. Transcatheter coil occlusion of perivalvular mitral leaks associated with severe hemolysis. *Cathet Cardiovasc Interv* 2000;49:64–67.
160. Boudjemline Y, Abdel-Massih T, Bonhoeffer P, et al. Percutaneous closure of a paravalvular mitral regurgitation with Amplatzer and coil prostheses [in French]. *Arch Mal Coeur Vaiss* 2002;95:483–486.
161. Piechaud JF. Percutaneous closure of mitral paravalvular leak. *J Interv Cardiol* 2003;16:153–155.
162. Khambadkone S, Coats L, Taylor A, et al. Percutaneous pulmonary valve implantation in humans: Results in 59 consecutive patients. *Circulation* 2005;112:1189–1197.
163. Zhou JQ, Corno AF, Huber CH, et al. Self-expandable valved stent of large size: Off-bypass implantation in pulmonary position. *Eur J Cardiothorac Surg* 2003;24(2):212–216.
164. Garay F, Webb J, Hijazi ZM. Percutaneous replacement of pulmonary valve using the Edwards-Cribier percutaneous heart valve: First report in a human patient. *Cathet Cardiovasc Interv* 2006;67:659–662.
165. Cribier A, Eltchaninoff H, Bash A, et al. Percutaneous transcatheter implantation of an aortic valve prosthesis for calcific aortic stenosis: First human case description. [See comment.] *Circulation* 2002;106:3006–3008.
166. Michel-Behnke I, Akintuerk H, Marquardt I, et al. Stenting of the ductus arteriosus and banding of the pulmonary arteries: Basis for various surgical strategies in newborns with multiple left heart obstructive lesions. *Heart* 2003;89:645–650.
167. Galantowicz M, Cheatham JP. Lessons learned from the development of a new hybrid strategy for the management of hypoplastic left heart syndrome. *Pediatr Cardiol* 2005;26:190–199.
168. Galantowicz M, Cheatham JP. Fontan completion without surgery. *Semin Thora Cardiovasc Surg Pediatr Card Surg Annu* 2004;7:48–55.
169. Hjortdal VE, Redington AN, de Leval MR, et al. Hybrid approaches to complex congenital cardiac surgery. *Eur J Cardiothorac Surg* 2002;22:885–890.
170. Ashburn DA, McCrindle BW, Tchervenkov CI, et al. Outcomes after the Norwood operation in neonates with critical aortic stenosis or aortic valve atresia. *J Thorac Cardiovasc Surg* 2003;125:1070–1082.
171. Akintuerk H, Michel-Behnke I, Valeske K, et al. Stenting of the arterial duct and banding of the pulmonary arteries: Basis for combined Norwood stage I and II repair in hypoplastic left heart. *Circulation* 2002;105:1099–1103.
172. Hausdorf G, Schneider M, Konertz W. Surgical preconditioning and completion of total cavopulmonary connection by interventional cardiac catheterisation: A new concept. *Heart* 1996;75:403–409.
173. Crystal M, Yoo S, Van Arsdell GS, et al. Catheter-based completion of the Fontan: A non-surgical approach [abstract]. *Cathet Cardiovasc Interv* 2006;68:460.

CHAPTER 17 ■ ELECTROPHYSIOLOGIC THERAPEUTIC CATHETERIZATION

J. PHILIP SAUL, MD

In 1932, based on surface electrocardiographic data alone, Wolferth and Wood (1) correctly hypothesized that the structural abnormality underlying Wolff–Parkinson–White (WPW) syndrome (2) was an accessory atrioventricular (AV) connection or accessory pathway. However, it was not until Sealy et al. (3) surgically cured a patient with WPW syndrome and a right-sided accessory pathway that the anatomic basis of the disease proposed so long before was confirmed. This milestone also heralded the beginning of a prolonged debate concerning the optimal management of symptomatic and asymptomatic WPW syndrome: medical, surgical, or none. That debate has now changed from which to one of when, as definitive catheter therapy for elimination of accessory pathways has progressed from application of uncontrolled mini-explosions generated by high-energy defibrillator shocks delivered through the tip of a catheter, to precise localization of the atrial or ventricular accessory pathway insertion sites followed by temperature-controlled heating or freezing of a small volume of myocardium with various energy forms (4). However, despite these changes, various questions regarding the early and late implications of catheter therapy in small children whose myocardial development is still underway remain unanswered (5,6).

This introduction has used the treatment of accessory pathway–mediated tachyarrhythmias as a focal point for discussion; however, catheter therapy has now been applied to the cure or modification of most pediatric arrhythmias, including AV node re-entry tachycardia (7), ectopic atrial tachycardia (EAT), atrial re-entry/flutter, congenital junctional ectopic tachycardia (JET), and some forms of ventricular tachycardia (VT) (8). This chapter will include a review of the techniques available, proposed or conceivable for catheter therapy of arrhythmias, as well as both the current and potential applications of this important therapeutic modality.

THE DECISION TO ABLATE: SAFETY VERSUS EFFICACY

One overriding theme in the management of arrhythmias in children compared with adults is an emphasis on *safety* over *efficacy*. Although there are few cases at any age where safety is not an important concern, the relatively benign course of many arrhythmia conditions in childhood, the potential disruption even therapies such as permanent pacing cause for a child, and the fact that parents are usually the decision-making surrogate for the child, often lead to a different decision tree for children than for adults. Furthermore, for some situations and technologies, e.g., the potential for coronary damage with radiofrequency (RF) energy application at the AV groove, size (of the patient and the heart) may really matter.

Ablation in patients with WPW is an excellent example of how decision making may be highly age dependent (9). In this chapter, the term WPW will be used to describe the condition of pre-excitation on the surface ECG, with or without coexisting tachycardia. Because of various concerns, even the most symptomatic infant with WPW and paroxysmal supraventricular tachycardia (SVT) is only rarely a candidate for ablation (10–12). Myocardial (6) and potentially severe coronary injury (13–16) are more likely with ablation in this age group. Furthermore, about 40% of accessory pathways APs in infants spontaneously stop functioning in the first year of life (17,18), and an additional third of patients are unlikely to have symptoms between infancy and early childhood (19). In children older than 4 years of age with symptomatic arrhythmias, the balance between risks and benefits clearly shifts toward ablation therapy, but generally only if the ablation can be performed safely (9). In contrast to the situation in infants, even asymptomatic WPW patients between the ages of 10 and 18 years may be managed more aggressively than in adults. Unlike asymptomatic adults older than 28 years of age, who are unlikely to ever have symptoms (20,21), the older child with a high-risk pathway is exactly the type of patient who may present with sudden arrhythmic death as the initial symptom, leading to the recommendation that such patients undergo risk stratification and those who are *high risk* be offered catheter ablation as a therapeutic option (22). Furthermore, the guidelines for sports participation in patients with WPW recommend risk stratification prior to approval for this age group (23). Other age-dependent differences in management decisions will be addressed when discussing individual arrhythmias below.

ENERGY SOURCES

Various energy sources have been used for ablation of myocardial tissue. Although many of the techniques rely on the generation of heat to destroy tissue, alternate mechanisms include chemically induced cell death, application of high current densities to disrupt intracellular membranes, and cooling to first reversibly silence cells followed by freezing to burst them. A brief review follows.

Direct Current

In 1979, Vedel et al. (24) reported the first use of a direct current (DC) shock through a catheter to produce complete AV block (inadvertently, in that case). His findings soon led to the use of DC catheter ablation for intentional production of complete heart block in a limited number of patients with drug-refractory supraventricular arrhythmias (25). Although the method was moderately successful in producing clinically effective AV block (approximately 90% of 127 patients in one large series), complications were sometimes severe, including production of new arrhythmias, cardiac tamponade, and sudden death (26). With the possible exception of one series (27), similar results were obtained when DC ablation techniques were applied to the elimination of accessory AV connections or VT; moderate success was attained with infrequent but serious complications (28). Based on the results in adults, appropriate skepticism concerning the use of DC ablation in small hearts led to limited use of the technique in pediatric patients. Although success was possible, a high incidence of complications has resulted in there being no current circumstances in which DC ablation is recommended for the treatment of arrhythmias in children (29,30). The so-called low-energy DC ablation technique (2 to 40 joules) introduced in 1986 (31) was significantly safer than standard DC ablation, even within the coronary sinus, but its introduction was nearly simultaneous with the much more controllable RF techniques described below.

Radiofrequency

The theoretical advantages of controlled lesion formation using RF current to heat tissue combined with an existing neurosurgical experience using RF current (32) led Huang et al. (33) to attempt closed-chest ablation of the AV node with catheter-delivered RF energy. Their use of relatively low power (<50 W) appeared to provide adequate tissue heating to induce permanent AV block without significant complications, such as perforation or proarrhythmia, and with a lesion that was histologically well demarcated. The appeal of this technique was noted immediately by several investigators, such that by 1987, reports of the use of this technique in humans for both AV node and accessory pathway ablation were appearing (34).

Since 1987, a number of studies, both *in vitro* and *in vivo*, in adult animals have confirmed that the cause of tissue destruction with RF ablation is tissue heating to a temperature greater than approximately 50°C (4). Tissue heating to >90°C to 100°C usually is associated with coagulum formation on the tip of the catheter, an increase in impedance, and a decrease in delivered current (35). Cell death appears to occur almost immediately, suggesting that cell death is the result of both protein denaturation and dehydration. The histologic changes have been described as coagulation necrosis (33). Haines and Watson (4) demonstrated that the lesion size grows exponentially with time, with a half-time of about 18 seconds. The temperature decreases hyperbolically with distance away from the electrode tip (inversely proportional to the radial distance) so that the lesion dimensions are directly proportional to the temperature measured at the tip–tissue interface. We have demonstrated similar findings for RF lesions made in immature myocardium (Fig. 17.1) (6). Thus, theoretically, it is possible to accurately control lesion size by controlling the RF power output such that a particular preset temperature is achieved at the tip–tissue interface.

Current commercial systems supply RF energy at 500 KHz using either a generator that can supply unmodulated voltage/power or control the temperature of the catheter tip through power modulation between 0 and 50, 60, or 100 W, depending on the manufacturer and catheter used (36). Energy is delivered in a unipolar fashion from the catheter tip to a large skin reference electrode, positioned either on the

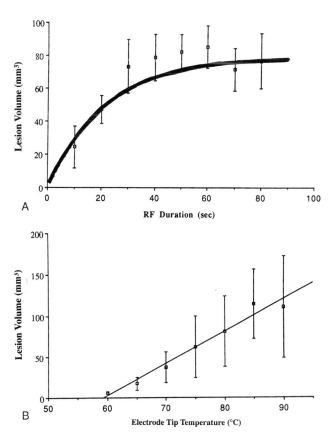

FIGURE 17.1 Lesion volume as a function of the duration of radiofrequency application (**A**) and the electrode tip temperature (**B**). Volume increases exponentially as a function of lesion duration. For (**A**), the tip temperature was held constant at 80°C. The time constant (time required to reach 63% of the ultimate asymptotic lesion size of 79 mm³) was 22 seconds. Ninety percent of the maximum lesion was reached by 45 seconds. Lesion volume appeared to grow linearly as a function of electrode tip temperature. Previous data in adult animals had shown linear increase in width and depth with tip temperature.

patient's chest, buttocks, or leg. During each RF application, voltage, power, current, impedance, and temperature are available and can be continuously monitored. Appropriate filters are available in most recording systems so that intracardiac electrograms and surface ECG leads can be monitored during RF delivery (Fig. 17.2). Control of catheter tip temperature during power application has not necessarily improved the success rate of ablation procedures, but has (a) almost completely eliminated overheating, impedance increase, and coagulum formation; (b) helped determine whether inadequate heating rather than incorrect catheter location is responsible for lack of success at a particular site; and (c) allowed for low-temperature heat mapping by intentionally producing low-temperature (45°C to 50°C) applications, which cause reversible electrical changes in the tissue (Fig. 17.2) (37).

As noted elsewhere, chronic lesions in adult dogs appear to be well demarcated histologically and are approximately the same size as the acute lesions (33); however, in 1994 we reported that chronic atrial and ventricular lesions produced in immature (approximately 1-month-old) sheep may increase in size during the subsequent 6 to 8 months of normal development (6). This finding may have important implications for the use of RF ablation in very small children.

50° C Test

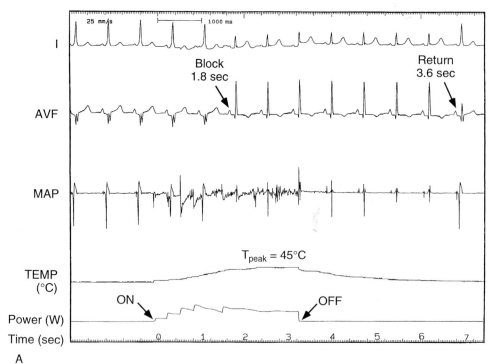

A

70°C Application

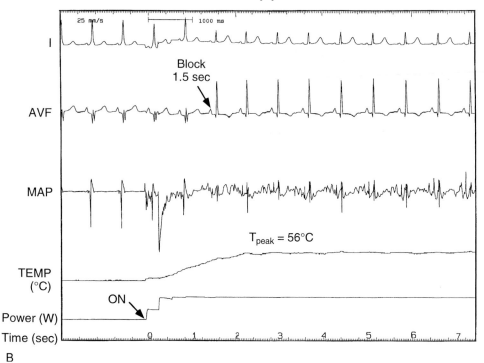

B

FIGURE 17.2 A: Test application with radiofrequency (RF) generator set to 50°C. Maximum temperature achieved is 45°C. Accessory pathway (AP) block occurs after 1.8 seconds, and power is turned off after 3.1 seconds. Accessory pathway conduction returns 3.6 seconds after turning off the power. **B:** After return of AP conduction, a full application is delivered with the RF generator set to 70°C. Peak temperature achieved is 56°C, and AP conduction block occurs at 1.5 seconds.

Cooled-Tip Radiofrequency

As noted, one of the limitations in creating larger RF lesions is that high temperatures at the tip–tissue interface lead to boiling, coagulum formation, and impedance increase, preventing further delivery of RF energy to the tissue. Over the past few years, it has become apparent that tip cooling can decrease the tip–tissue interface temperature, allowing the delivery of more RF power, pushing the peak temperature farther into the tissue, and increasing lesion size by as much as a factor of two (38). Tip cooling can be accomplished passively with a more thermally massive tip (e.g., 8 mm long, gold, etc.) (39), or actively using various methodologies (e.g., shower head, internal flow, porous metal, sheath flow) (38,40), achieving lesion widths and depths of 10 to 15 mm. Although this technique already has been critically useful for treatment of several arrhythmias, there are two important caveats. First, lesions can be too large, creating unintentional damage to structures, such as coronary arteries; second, cooling will reduce lesion size when maximum power is already being delivered with a noncooled ablation tip.

Microwave

In contrast to RF heating, which is primarily resistive, microwaves heat with a propagating magnetic field that has the potential to heat tissue at a distance from the origin of the field. *In vitro* studies with microwave antennas have shown that the volume of heating is probably somewhat larger than that seen with RF, but is more dependent than RF on antenna construction characteristics, electromagnetic frequency, and geometry of the antenna in relation to the tissue (41). Although there are no commercial microwave systems available now, microwave ablation may someday have a much greater bearing on the treatment of VT or atrial flutter, where larger lesions may be necessary, than for common forms of SVT, where RF techniques have been adequate.

Cryotherapy

Catheter-based cryotherapy has been introduced recently for ablation of various cardiac arrhythmias (42–47), but only limited reports involving children are available (44,48,49). Cryoablation has several potential advantages over RF ablation, including (a) reversible cryomapping prior to the production of a permanent lesion (46,50,51), (b) adherence of the catheter tip to the endocardium on freezing, (c) a well-defined edge of the cryolesion (50), (d) minimal effects on adjacent coronary arteries (52,53), and (e) a lower incidence of thrombus (54). The first four of these issues are particularly relevant to small children because of the close proximity of various critical cardiac structures to the ablation target and the reported potential for RF lesion growth in immature myocardium (6). In fact, the most common major complication during RF ablation in pediatric patients is AV block (12,55,56), and there appears to be a higher potential for coronary artery injury in this patient group (14–16,57,58), even during slow pathway modification (16).

Cryotherapy is performed with a system that cools the tip of a catheter by expanding a liquid gas within the tip and removing heat from the surrounding blood and tissue. Typically, the systems allow for both ice *mapping* at a tip temperature of $-25°C$ to $-35°C$ in which the catheter adheres and nearby tissue loses electrical activity but few cells are killed, and *ablation* at a tip temperature of $<-65°C$ in which a lesion will be formed. Once cells freeze, they expand and burst. After 4 minutes at the ablation temperature, a typical lesion size is 3 to 6 mm in diameter, smaller than those seen for RF. One of the contrasting features of cryoablation compared with RF is that there is a much larger zone of reversibility as the lesion expands because tissue cooling above the freezing point will lead to loss of electrical activation well before the loss of viability. This feature has dramatically enhanced the safety profile in clinical trials to date. In fact, despite frequent use of the technology for septal tachycardia substrates, there are no reports of AV block with cryoablation (42–47), even in children as small as 20 kg, in the presence of a His potential (Fig. 17.3) (49).

The primary disadvantage of cryoablation is that, inherent in its high level of safety, is a smaller lesion size than for RF ablation. For ablation of septal tachycardia substrates (AV node modification, anterior and posterior septal pathways), cryoablation success rates have been statistically similar to those for RF techniques (42–47). However, most operators are less aggressive with RF in septal areas and have had to be highly aggressive with cryotherapy to achieve success. Furthermore, even aggressive application of cryoenergy has not yielded similar success rates to RF for ablation of nonseptal accessory pathways. Although the data are limited in very small children and infants, anecdotal evidence suggests that cryoablation may be effective for all accessory pathway locations in these unique patient groups. Given the above considerations, as discussed below for individual arrhythmia substrates, the use of cryoablation is most important for septal substrates, small children, and patients with abnormal anatomy where the precise location of the AV conduction system is not known.

Other

Any energy source that creates tissue heat has the potential to ablate myocardium in a similar manner to RF and microwave. Laser energy has been used to successfully ablate ventricular myocardium in both normal animals and humans with VT (59–61). The use of high-power ultrasound delivered through a catheter also has been reported as a means of heat ablation. One potential advantage might be the simultaneous use of diagnostic ultrasound to monitor lesion production (62). Finally, chemical ablation achieved by delivering a toxic agent such as alcohol into the coronary artery or vein supplying the myocardium responsible for an arrhythmia has been used in both animals and humans; however, technical problems with selective delivery will probably prevent this technique from ever reaching widespread use.

Summary—Energy Sources

Several energy types are available currently for use in catheter ablation procedures. However, currently, for procedures in children, cryotherapy and RF energy with or without tip cooling appear to have the best safety and efficacy profile. Both energy sources can reproducibly control lesion characteristics through assessment of tip temperature and application time. In general, RF ablation is more effective, but for the reasons discussed above, cryoablation is safer. At this time, the balance between which source is used for which procedure depends on the arrhythmia substrate, the location of the target, including the proximity of the AV node and coronary arteries, and the preference of the center and operator.

PROCEDURE—GENERAL

Sedation and Anesthesia

The pain and discomfort of an ablation procedure does not appear to be very much higher than that for a typical diagnostic catheterization, even accounting for some patients feeling pain during the application of RF energy. Thus, general anesthesia is by no means necessary. However, we began

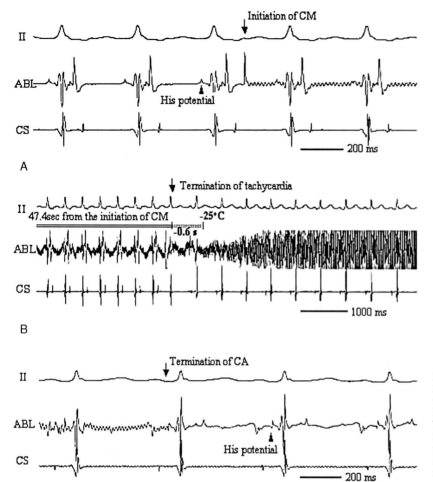

FIGURE 17.3 Successful cryoablation of a right anterior septal accessory pathway. **A:** ECG at the initiation of cryomapping (CM) during tachycardia. A His potential can be seen on the ablation catheter. **B:** Termination of tachycardia during cryomapping. Supraventricular tachycardia (SVT) terminates with ventriculoatrial (VA) block just 0.6 seconds before reaching −25°C and 47.4 seconds from the initiation of cryomapping. **C:** ECG at the termination of cryoablation shows sinus rhythm and a His potential still on the ablation catheter. CS, coronary sinus.

using general or near general anesthesia for most patients early in our experience for two reasons. First and foremost, uncontrolled patient movement that dislodges the catheter may inadvertently occur at a critical point in the procedure, particularly if the RF application produces pain. In fact, our only case of complete heart block in the first decade of performing ablations occurred in part from untimely movement of an uncooperative patient during ablation of a midseptal accessory pathway, leading us to replace heavy, often disorienting sedation with general anesthesia for most younger patients. Second, after beginning the use of general anesthesia, we found that even older cooperative children and young adults find a long procedure much more tolerable under anesthesia and are more willing to return for follow-up procedures, when needed. For these reasons, the vast majority of pediatric centers use general anesthesia for ablation procedures when available.

Preablation

Prior to the ablation procedure, standard electrophysiologic techniques should be used to identify the tachycardia mechanism, and, if appropriate, the location of the arrhythmia substrate. Differences from the standard study are related primarily to the actual mapping and ablation. Although not

absolutely necessary, biplane fluoroscopy is very useful for precise two-dimensional localization of catheter tip positions. For most accessory pathways and AV node modifications, cameras are placed in the 30-degree right anterior oblique and 60-degree left anterior oblique positions, with 15-degree caudal projections (Fig. 17.4). In addition to camera angles, the development of deflectable tipped catheters with closely spaced electrode configurations, which are now available from a number of manufacturers, has greatly facilitated accurate mapping and ablation in all parts of the heart.

Three-Dimensional Electroanatomic Mapping

Over the past 10 years, a few novel methods have been introduced to simultaneously present three-dimensional (3-D), detailed electrical and anatomic information, facilitating mapping and reducing fluoroscopy exposure. One, termed *nonfluoroscopic*, uses a technology similar to a global positioning system to identify the precise catheter tip position and orientation (Fig. 17.5) (CARTO, Biosense–Webster, Baldwin Park, CA). Another, termed *noncontact*, uses the electrical signals in the blood pool of a cardiac chamber to derive an inverse solution for the signals on the endocardial surface (Fig. 17.6) (EnSite, Endocardial Solutions, St. Paul, MN). Other systems provide simpler 3-D localizations of the catheter electrodes,

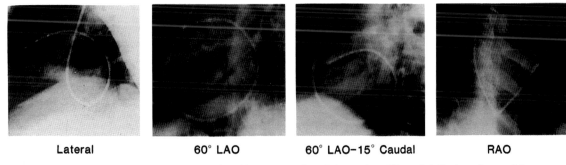

| Lateral | 60° LAO | 60° LAO-15° Caudal | RAO |

FIGURE 17.4 Catheter projections for ablation. Note how left anterior oblique (LAO) view plus caudal angulation maximally elongates the mitral annulus. (From Saul JP, Hulse JE, De W, et al. Catheter ablation of accessory atrioventricular pathways in young patients: Use of long vascular sheaths, the transseptal approach and a retrograde left posterior parallel approach. *J Am Coll Cardiol* 1993;21:571–583, with permission.)

using either impedance (NavX, Endocardial Solutions, St. Paul, MN; and Loca-Lisa, Medtronic, Minneapolis, MN) or ultrasound localization (RPM, Cardiac Pathways, Sunnyvale, CA), and can catalogue catheter locations and timing signals during either mapping or ablation. This location tracking and cataloguing feature is an important component of all 3-D systems, enabling the operator to be aware of where critical cardiac structures are, where applications have been made, and their outcome. Although all of these systems have their limitations, including high cost for the CARTO catheter and EnSite balloon catheter, it already is clear that they can contribute significantly to our understanding of arrhythmias and their mechanisms, and probably enhance success for complex cases (63–68). Some of the uses of these systems will be addressed below in the discussion of specific arrhythmias.

PROCEDURE—SUBSTRATE SPECIFIC

Accessory Pathways

Mapping

Jackman et al. (69) and others have described important electrogram characteristics that help identify the precise location of antegrade- and retrograde-conducting accessory pathways. Electrograms should be examined for the presence of probable accessory pathway potentials (Fig. 17.7), as well as the shortest AV time in pre-excited sinus rhythm or atrial-paced rhythm, and the shortest ventriculoatrial (VA) time during orthodromic reciprocating tachycardia or ventricular-paced rhythm (69). To help localize left free wall and left posteroseptal accessory pathways, a multielectrode catheter may be used in the coronary sinus (Fig. 17.8), but is probably not always necessary because it is the electrogram from the tip of the ablation catheter that ultimately determines the final ablation site. Typically, a deflectable-tip mapping/ablation catheter is used to localize right-sided accessory pathways on the tricuspid annulus either from the right femoral vein or the left subclavian vein. These techniques have been well described elsewhere (69,70). Some of the 3-D mapping techniques described above may be particularly useful for septal accessory pathways, to better understand the local anatomy, identify the location of critical structures, and identify prior ablation locations.

Ablation Catheter Manipulation—General

After initial localization, additional mapping and RF ablation are performed with introduction of a large-tipped (4 to 10 mm) steerable electrode catheter. These catheters are now available from several manufacturers in multiple sizes (5, 6, and 7 French [Fr]) and with various deflecting curve options. For technical reasons, cryoablation catheters are not available in <7 Fr. The following standard approaches to accessory pathway ablation have been reported (69,70).

Left Free Wall Pathways. Left free wall accessory pathways can be approached using a deflectable-tip catheter advanced retrograde from the aorta into the left ventricle (69,70) or transseptal (70). For the retrograde approach, an attempt is made to place the catheter tip under and perpendicular to the mitral leaflet (aorta [Ao]–left ventricle [LV]) (Fig. 17.8) or through the mitral valve and above the mitral leaflet (LV–LV) (Fig. 17.9).

For the transseptal approach, the area of the foramen ovale is first probed with the mapping/ablation catheter for patency. If not patent, a standard transseptal puncture is performed using any of various techniques and sheaths. The mapping/ablation catheter then is placed through the transseptal sheath into the left atrium. Generally, the tip of the ablation catheter is maneuvered so that fluoroscopically it appears to be near the AV groove, confirming such location by the electrical recording from the distal pair of electrodes. Then the catheter tip is manipulated through deflection, rotation, and longitudinal movement to map the left AV groove. In many cases, catheter stabilization for mapping and ablation can be enhanced by deflecting the catheter and pulling it back into the sheath until only the four electrodes protrude, giving the appearance of a hockey stick (Fig. 17.9). Then the sheath and catheter are moved along their long axis as a single unit from septum to lateral free wall and the catheter torqued either clockwise (posterior groove) or counterclockwise (anterior groove) within the sheath. Access to left lateral pathways in larger patients sometimes requires exchange of the typical Mullins-type transseptal sheath for one of various specialized sheaths that are now available.

Most operators today prefer the transseptal approach for left free wall pathways in both adults and children because it is generally more consistent, cannot damage the aortic valve or the left or right coronary artery orifices, and theoretically is less likely to damage ventricular myocardium. However, the overall results and complications from the transseptal and retrograde techniques do not differ significantly.

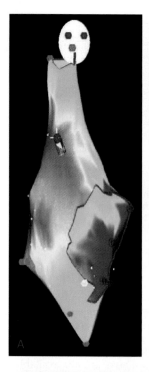

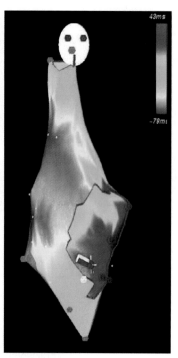

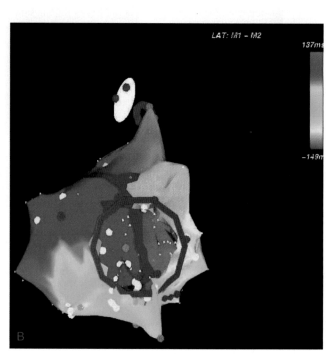

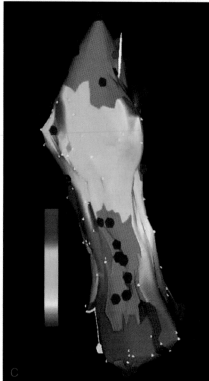

FIGURE 17.5 Three-dimensional mapping using the CARTO, Biosense nonfluoroscopic system. Color scales go from red-orange (the earliest activation) to blue-purple (the latest) (see *scale bar* in images). Gray represents an area of low voltage determined to be scar tissue. Each white dot represents one point where the catheter was placed and activation times determined. The "face" at the top of each image shows the direction of the image. **A:** Sinus rhythm— right anterior oblique (RAO) projection (see face) of the right atrium (RA) in an adult patient with prior repair of a ventricular septal defect (VSD) as a child. As expected with sinus rhythm, activation spreads from the anterolateral RA down toward the tricuspid valve. Activation lasts 122 ms, from 79 ms before to 43 ms after the fiducial point (*bar at upper left*). The two images show the mapping catheter tip in two locations acquiring mapping data: High lateral RA on the left and low septal RA just behind the tricuspid valve on the right. **B:** Atrial re-entry/flutter—left anterior oblique (LAO) caudal image (see face) of the RA from **A**. Tricuspid valve is now seen en face. Activation proceeds from high anterior (red) down the septum, under the tricuspid valve, and up the lateral RA wall. Activation lasts 286 ms from 149 ms before to 137 ms after the fiducial point (*bar at left*), encompassing the entire cardiac cycle. This could be considered typical atrial flutter circling the tricuspid valve, but in a clockwise direction. **C:** Atypical intra-atrial re-entry tachycardia (IART). Straight left lateral view of the septal surface of the RA (see edge of face with eyes forward). This 27-year-old patient with tricuspid atresia began to have IART soon after an atriopulmonary Fontan's. After failing multiple medications and catheter ablation procedures, he underwent a right atriectomy and conversion to a lateral tunnel, but continued to have IART. After many subsequent years of failed medical therapy, he underwent mapping with the CARTO system demonstrating extensive atrial scarring, and a single IART circuit was identified encircling a large septal scar or atrial septal defect (ASD) patch. Note counterclockwise procession from red to yellow to green to blue to purple in this left septal view. Ablation was successful with an actively cooled tip system to block conduction in the inferior segment of the circuit (around the purple color). The patient has been asymptomatic since.

Right Free Wall Pathways. Right posterior and right posterior paraseptal pathways almost always can be approached from the right femoral vein with a deflectable-tip catheter placed above the tricuspid valve (inferior vena cava [IVC]–right atrium [RA]). Right lateral and right anterior pathways can be approached either from the right femoral vein and IVC or from the right internal jugular vein and superior vena cava (SVC).

For right lateral pathways, most operators find the use of a long vascular sheath (see below) very important to enhance catheter stability and improve access. Right anterior pathways also can be ablated on the ventricular side of the tricuspid leaflet (SVC–right ventricle [RV]), using an approach from the superior vena cava and placing the catheter tip through the tricuspid valve orifice, as previously described (70).

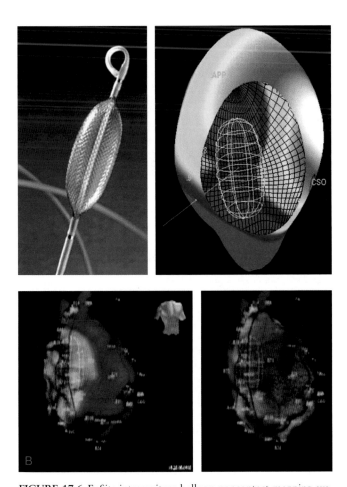

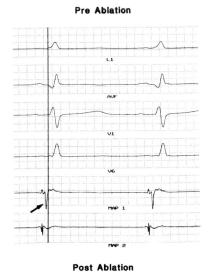

Pre Ablation

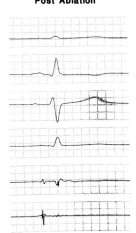

Post Ablation

FIGURE 17.6 EnSite intracavitary balloon noncontact mapping system. Endocardial voltages are represented by the colors on the chamber surfaces. Purple is zero volts, representing inactivated or previously activated tissue. White is peak voltage, representing the area of current activation. Red, yellow, and white are progressively smaller voltages, representing prior or impending activation. **A:** Picture of mapping balloon shows a grid of wires crisscrossing the surface of the balloon, creating 64 individual electrodes. The image on the right is a computer reconstruction of the right atrium (CSO, coronary sinus os; APP, appendage) showing the endocavitary location of the balloon and voltages on the endocardial surface at a single point in time. Activation is currently septal, shown by the white color above the CSO. **B:** Right atrium (RA) during intra-atrial re-entry tachycardia (IART) in a 14-year-old boy after an atriopulmonary Fontan operation. The torso shows this is a slight right anterior oblique (RAO) projection. The atrium is large and bulbous. Although a little fuzzy, an area of presumed block secondary to a right lateral atrial scar is shown by a dark line along the anterolateral RA. When played as a movie, the tachycardia proceeded around the scar inferior to superior on the anterior surface and superior to anterior on the posterolateral. The two images show posterior activation on the left and lateral activation on the right. The image of the balloon can be seen within the chamber.

Posterior Septal Pathways. Left and right posterior septal pathways can be approached in various ways. For left-sided pathways, the retrograde aortic technique can be used with an attempt to deflect the catheter tip under the mitral valve near the aortic annulus. Alternatively, a transseptal approach can be used by extending the catheter all the way around the mitral annulus to the area of the septum. However, many of these pathways are intimately related to the coronary sinus (CS) (71–80) and can be ablated only within or around the CS

FIGURE 17.7 Accessory pathway potentials. The first four signals are surface ECG leads. The second two come from the mapping/ablation catheter. Note that there is minimal pre-excitation in the surface leads preablation; however, a very large potential is seen in the distal electrode pair of the mapping catheter (*arrow*) preceding the surface QRS. This probable accessory pathway potential is no longer present after the ablation. (From Saul JP, Hulse JE, De W, et al. Catheter ablation of accessory atrioventricular pathways in young patients: Use of long vascular sheaths, the transseptal approach and a retrograde left posterior parallel approach. *J Am Coll Cardiol* 1993;21:571–583, with permission.)

(70,70). The CS and the region around the CS os can be approached from the right atrium, using the right femoral vein/inferior vena cava or the subclavian vein/superior vena cava. (IVC-CS and SVC-CS). Regardless of approach, one must be aware of the small size and close proximity of the coronary arteries in this region. In fact, over the last few years there has been a realization that the coronary arteries in the posterior septal region may be at a higher than previously realized risk for collateral damage during application of RF energy in this region (15,16,57,58,81). Consequently, a number of operators now perform preablation coronary angiograms for any pathway near the posterior septum to evaluate the proximity of the ablation site to a small coronary artery. Pathway locations near a small coronary artery are either not ablated or are ablated using cryotherapy, for the reasons stated above in the description of cryotherapy and below in the discussion of

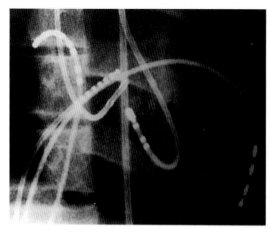 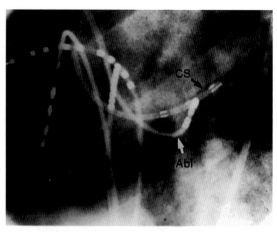

30° RAO   **60° LAO, 15° Caudal**

FIGURE 17.8 Standard retrograde approach from the aorta. The point of successful ablation is along the posterior AV groove at the sight of the large catheter tip. Note: Overlapping of coronary sinus catheter in the left anterior oblique (LAO) view, but catheter position well below the coronary sinus catheter in right anterior oblique (RAO) view, indicating that the tip of the catheter is in the left ventricle.

safety. This issue is particularly important for small children and infants, who have smaller coronary arteries and shorter distances from the ablation sites to the coronary artery.

Right Anterior Septal Pathways. These pathways are perhaps the most difficult to ablate safely because of the close proximity

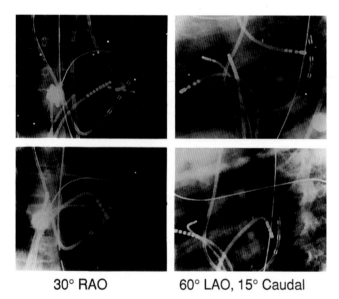

30° RAO   **60° LAO, 15° Caudal**

FIGURE 17.9 Transseptal approach. The **top** two cine frames show a failed attempt to place the catheter retrograde through the mitral valve on top of the mitral anulus. The transseptal approach (**bottom** two frames) was successful with the catheter in position very close to, but slightly different from, the retrograde mitral approach. Note the hockey stick appearance of the catheter tip (*arrow*) using the transseptal approach. As with Figure 17.8, a Jackman orthogonal catheter is in the coronary sinus, an octapolar catheter is at the His bundle, and a quadripolar catheter is at the right ventricular apex. The deflectable ablation catheter has a large tip. (From Saul JP, Hulse JE, De W, et al. Catheter ablation of accessory atrioventricular pathways in young patients: Use of long vascular sheaths, the transseptal approach and a retrograde left posterior parallel approach. *J Am Coll Cardiol* 1993;21:571–583, with permission.).

to the AV conduction system. As with other anterior right-sided pathways, they can be approached from below via the IVC or above via the SVC. It is not uncommon that the best location for accessory pathway ablation also has a relatively large His potential on the ablation catheter, raising concern about unintended damage to the normal AV conduction system (Fig. 17.4). In fact, permanent complete AV block has been reported during RF ablation in as many as 10% of patients with right anterior septal pathways (56,82,83). Although rapid junctional acceleration during application of RF energy in such locations may predict impending permanent AV conduction system damage, AV block can be quite sudden in onset and permanent. Several techniques can be used to help avoid AV block. We have found that approaching the AV groove from above via the SVC allows for somewhat easier separation of the ablation location from the bundle by deflecting the catheter superiorly away from the His bundle. If the ablation catheter is seen lateral to the His catheter in the LAO caudal view, theoretically the His bundle should be at least a few millimeters from the ablation location. However, the most important advance we have found for these pathways is the use of cryoablation (43,49,84–87). Cryo systems allow for (a) observation of the effects without junctional acceleration when close to the normal AV conduction system, (b) reversibility during mapping at higher temperatures around −30°C, (c) catheter adhesion, and (d) the ability to electrically test AV conduction continuously during ablation. Furthermore, even if cryoablation is unsuccessful because of early recurrence, it often is possible to identify a safe location for the application of RF energy to permanently ablate the pathway. As with coronary injury for posterior septal pathways, AV conduction system damage may be an even more important issue in children than in adults because of the close proximity of all cardiac structures in the smaller heart and the larger impact of needing permanent AV pacing in a child. Thus, cryoablation is probably the therapy of choice for septal pathways in the pediatric patient.

Use of Long Vascular Sheaths

The approach to left and right free wall pathways in particular can often be improved by use of one of various long sheaths, including 6, 7, and 8 Fr straight and specially designed sheaths. The presence of the sheath provides catheter stability, markedly improves torque transmission from the catheter handle to the tip of the catheter, and allows for coaxial steering of the catheter tip (70). These characteristics may be critical for the atrial approach on either the right or left side, even when a patent foramen ovale is present. The set of sheaths that have gained the widest appeal are designed to facilitate an approach to the left and right AV groove in which the catheter tip ends up parallel to the plane of the groove (Swartz Left SL1-4 and Right SR0-4, Daig Corp., Minnetonka, MN); however, any sheath that helps deliver the catheter to the correct location will facilitate stability and enhance efficacy. These sheaths seem to be most helpful for right free wall pathways but are designed for use in every right- and left-sided location.

Ablation

Ablation can be performed in either sinus rhythm or orthodromic reciprocating tachycardia; however, if performed in tachycardia, the catheter is likely to move when the accessory pathway blocks and the tachycardia terminates. Thus, catheter stability during ablation of retrograde conduction can be improved by performing the ablation during right ventricular pacing and observing for loss of retrograde VA conduction during the ablation (Fig. 17.10).

When RF energy is being used and permanent ablation is desired, the initial catheter tip setpoint is usually 70°C. However, as noted above, a particular site can be tested for success by setting the desired temperature to 50°C and stopping RF application at 5 to 10 seconds if success is not achieved, reducing myocardial damage to an absolute minimum (Fig 17.2) (37). Based on the observation that permanent success is highly associated with early disappearance of accessory pathway conduction (69,88), lesions should be made for only 5 to 10 seconds unless the delta wave disappears, tachycardia terminates, or there is a noted change in VA conduction. If any of these three conditions is met, the temperature should be set at 70°C and the RF application continued for 30 to 60 seconds. Without temperature monitoring, the delivered power is likely to be too high or too low. Thus, with temperature monitoring, the delivered power varies dramatically in an individual patient between individual applications, depending on catheter tip location and stability.

When cryoablation is used, the system may be used in either the mapping or ablation mode, as described above. In either case, as with RF energy, the earlier the effect, the more likely conduction block will be permanent. Accessory pathway block prior to 15 seconds after a tip temperature of $-25°C$ is reached is desirable. Once accessory pathway block is observed, cryoablation is performed at the lowest possible temperature ($-70°C$ to $-80°C$) for 4 minutes. There is evidence that repeating the application for 4 minutes in the same location will significantly increase the lesion size and reduce the risk of recurrence, which may be higher with cryoablation than with RF ablation (43,49,84). However, as experience is gained with cryotherapy, initial and long-term results have improved.

Following creation of a successful lesion, patients usually are observed in the electrophysiology laboratory for 30 to 60 minutes, after which repeat electrophysiologic testing is performed, usually with and without an infusion of isoproterenol. A bolus of adenosine also may be used to unmask residual accessory pathway function by briefly reducing or eliminating AV node function. Most patients can be discharged the day of the procedure or the morning after.

Results

Regardless of pathway location, the presence of multiple pathways, catheter approach, or patient age, it appears that initial success rates for elimination of accessory pathways can be as high as 98% (8,70,89,90) and typically range between 85% and 95% (8,36,70,89–91). The most reliable outcome data in children probably come from the Prospective Assessment after Pediatric Catheter Ablation (PAPCA) (90,92,93) in which 2,761 ablation patients from a wide variety of U.S. centers were enrolled prospectively and 481 of them followed for a period of 2 years. Overall initial success rates for accessory pathway ablation were about 94%, with results varying significantly by locations (left free wall 98%, right free wall 90%, left septal 88%, right septal 89%). Fluoroscopy times can be long compared to other pediatric catheter procedures but have generally come down over time (94,95). High variance in the difficulty of individual procedures, combined with the variability of observations between investigators, probably attest to a large number of poorly defined factors that affect each procedure. However, the overall high success rates, sometimes requiring a second procedure, also indicate that these factors can be overcome.

From the 481 PAPCA patients followed prospectively, 12.3% of the 361 with an accessory pathway substrate had a recurrence within 12 months of the procedure (92). As with initial success, recurrence also varied by pathway location, varying from 4.8% for left free wall pathways to 24.6% for right septal pathways. Left septal had the lowest rate at 4.8%, and right free wall was intermediate at 15.8%. Although these rates may be higher than in other reports from single centers or uncontrolled registries, they are the only data from a prospectively controlled trial in children, and the subjects have the broadest center representation of any prospective ablation trial. Thus, these recurrence rates may be the most accurate representation of what can be expected in the average pediatric ablation center.

Complications will be discussed together for all substrates below.

Permanent Form of Junctional Reciprocating Tachycardia

The permanent form of junctional reciprocating tachycardia (PJRT) is not strictly a pediatric disease; however, it occurs primarily in young patients, causing a nearly incessant tachycardia that is frequently refractory to medical therapy and often leads to ventricular dysfunction (96). Despite the name, PJRT is caused by a concealed (retrograde only) accessory pathway with decremental conduction properties that has classically been described as having a posterior septal location (96). Recently, the results of RF ablation studies that can confirm a precise accessory pathway location have demonstrated that, first, most (>95%) of these pathways can be ablated, and second, their location may be in almost any position around the AV groove (Fig. 17.11) (97). The high safety and efficacy of RF ablation for PJRT, combined with the fact that pharmacologic therapy is often ineffective, suggest that catheter ablation is probably appropriate as first-line therapy for this syndrome, particularly if ventricular dysfunction is present (98).

As with any other accessory pathway, the methodology for ablation of PJRT pathways is dependent on location. Because many of the pathways are posteroseptal, ablation within the mouth or veins of the coronary sinus often is necessary. For such cases, coronary angiography should be performed prior to ablation. If a small coronary artery is within 2 to 3 mm of the

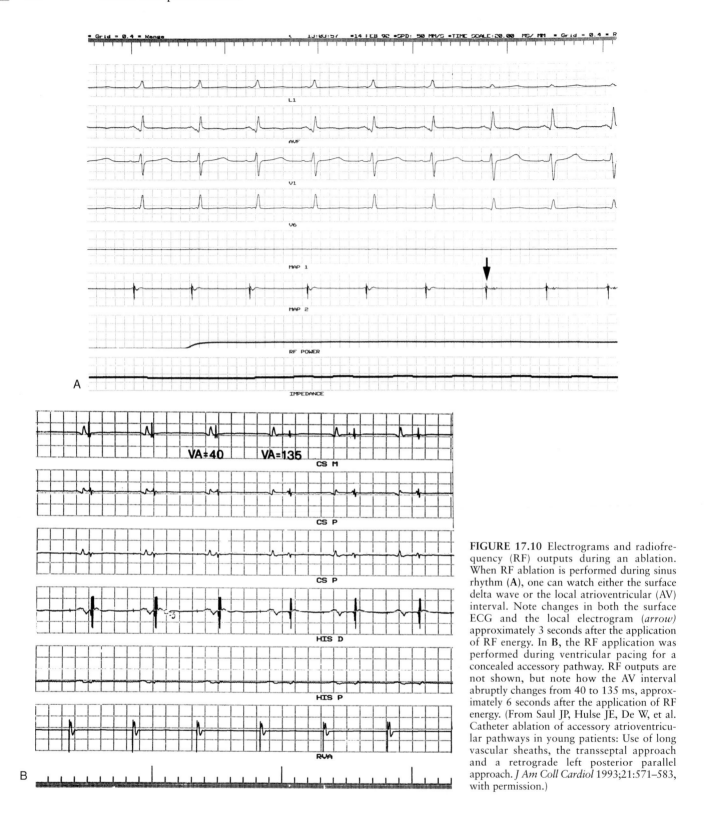

FIGURE 17.10 Electrograms and radiofrequency (RF) outputs during an ablation. When RF ablation is performed during sinus rhythm (**A**), one can watch either the surface delta wave or the local atrioventricular (AV) interval. Note changes in both the surface ECG and the local electrogram (*arrow*) approximately 3 seconds after the application of RF energy. In **B**, the RF application was performed during ventricular pacing for a concealed accessory pathway. RF outputs are not shown, but note how the AV interval abruptly changes from 40 to 135 ms, approximately 6 seconds after the application of RF energy. (From Saul JP, Hulse JE, De W, et al. Catheter ablation of accessory atrioventricular pathways in young patients: Use of long vascular sheaths, the transseptal approach and a retrograde left posterior parallel approach. *J Am Coll Cardiol* 1993;21:571–583, with permission.)

expected ablation site, cryoablation should be strongly considered in place of RF energy. If cryotherapy is either unavailable or ineffective, RF energy application should be minimized by reducing catheter size, temperature setpoint, maximum power, and/or duration. High-energy RF application with active or passive cooled-tip technology should be entirely avoided within the coronary sinus or used with extreme caution.

Mapping virtually always should be performed during tachycardia. The VA interval during tachycardia is generally long with a long isoelectric segment between the ventricular

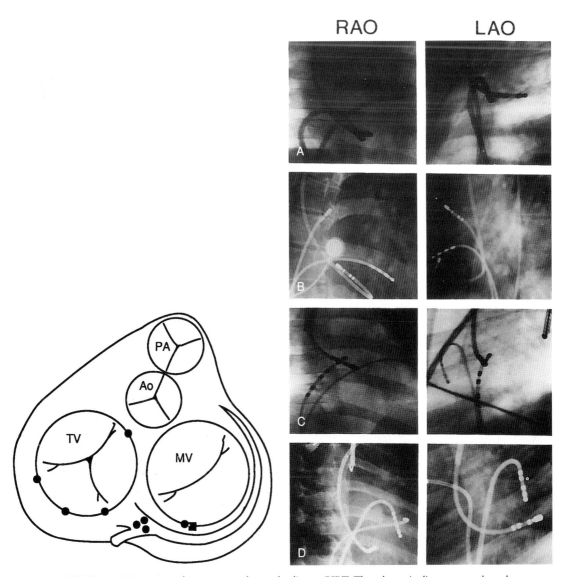

FIGURE 17.11 Location of accessory pathways leading to PJRT. The schematic diagram reveals pathway locations as identified by successful radiofrequency ablation site. *Circles* represent pathways causing permanent junctional reciprocating tachycardia (PJRT) whereas the *square* represents a typical concealed pathway found as a second pathway in one patient. Note that four pathways were located outside of the typical posteroseptal location. Ao, aorta; MV, mitral valve; PA, pulmonary artery; TV, tricuspid valve. **A** through **D** show representative angiograms of catheter electrode positions in four locations. **A:** The large-tipped ablation catheter approaches from the inferior vena cava. Its final position is in the mouth of the coronary sinus, near the ostium of the middle coronary vein (posteroseptal pathway). **B:** The ablation catheter approaches from the superior vena cava and loops on itself in the right anterior oblique (RAO) view; together with the left anterior oblique (LAO) view, the findings demonstrate a right lateral position. **C:** The ablation tip is positioned via the superior vena cava and overlies the distal His electrode, indicating a right anterior pathway. **D:** The large-tip catheter positioned in the coronary sinus was used for mapping only. A deflectable-tip catheter with a dumbbell-shaped electrode was used for ablation and was positioned transseptally from the inferior vena cava to the posterior mitral anulus (left posterior pathway). (From Ticho BS, Saul JP, Hulse JE, et al. Variable location of accessory pathways associated with the permanent form of junctional reciprocating tachycardia and confirmation with radiofrequency ablation. *Am J Cardiol* 1992;70:1559–1564, with permission.)

and atrial signals, and an accessory pathway potential may be present in as many as 75% of cases (99). Recurrence rates are higher than for typical APs, and some patients may require more than one procedure for initial success (89,92,97,99–102). Of note, despite the proximity to the AV node, AV block has not been reported in the larger series of patients with PJRT who have undergone RF ablation (97,99–101).

Atrioventricular Node Modification

Dual AV nodal physiology is the substrate for AV node re-entry tachycardia. Regardless of whether this physiology is the result of anatomic or functional dissociation of AV nodal conduction, it now seems clear that either the fast or slow AV nodal pathways can be modified to eliminate AV node re-entry. Most early reports using either DC or RF energy to modify the AV node concentrated on eliminating conduction over the fast AV nodal pathway by delivering energy to an area just proximal to the His bundle, where a relatively large atrial and relatively small or absent His potential were recorded (103,104). When successful (80% to 95% of cases), this so-called fast pathway ablation usually results in significant prolongation of the AH and PR intervals, and, unfortunately, regardless of the energy form used, most investigators have inadvertently produced complete AV block in 2% to 10% of patients (103). Although these characteristics make the technique undesirable for most children and adolescents, a few successful fast pathway ablations were reported in pediatric patients without significant complications (7,8). However, since around 1994, most AV node modifications have been directed at the slow pathway by positioning the catheter inferior and posterior to the AV node (105).

The advantages of the slow pathway technique are that normal AV node function can be preserved in the fast pathway, and the risk of complete AV block is lower than with a fast pathway ablation (8,89,105). Importantly, even this small risk of AV block has been virtually eliminated by the use of cryoenergy in place of RF energy for slow pathway ablation. In fact, as of December 2005, no cases of unintended permanent AV block have been reported using cryoablation for the treatment of AV node reentry (43,46,48,49,84,106). However, initial recurrence rates in these early reports have been somewhat higher with cryoablation than RF ablation of the slow pathway.

When mapping the slow pathway, some investigators have found that the presence of a small electrical potential from a presumably discrete slow pathway potential is a highly sensitive indicator of an appropriate catheter position (105), whereas others have found this slow pathway potential to have very poor specificity (107). Thus, many ablation techniques have been developed, including a purely anatomic approach to the inferior aspects of the AV node (107) and the use of slow junctional acceleration as an indicator of slow pathway node proximity. This latter observation is not useful for cryoablation because cooling of the slow pathway does not lead to junctional acceleration as does heating. Consequently, the technique with cryoablation focuses more on elimination of slow pathway conduction with only transient changes to fast pathway conduction as procedural end points (48,49).

Using RF energy to modify the slow AV nodal pathway, the PAPCA study reported that between 97% and 99% of AV node re-entry tachycardia can be eliminated in children <17 years of age, but with a 2.1% incidence of AV block (90). Similar success rates can be obtained with cryoablation, but as noted above, most if not all of the AV block can be avoided (43,46,48,49,84,106). Cryoablation may be particularly important in smaller children, in whom the close proximity of both the fast and slow pathways to each other and the bundle of His provides a much higher theoretical risk of inadvertent AV conduction system damage. This potential for AV block with the subsequent need for long-term electronic pacing has led to a formal guideline recommendation that RF ablation for well-controlled SVT be delayed until age 5 years (9).

In addition to the risk of AV block, we reported coronary damage in a child undergoing slow pathway modification for AV node re-entry resistant to drug therapy (16). After transient ST changes were observed, selective coronary angiography revealed a dominant right coronary artery giving off a posterior left ventricular branch artery that had an 80% stenosis (Fig. 17.12). The vessel course was within 2 to 3 mm of where the catheter tip was placed during the last RF application ablation. Acute management was conservative, and after 2 days, repeat angiography revealed some improvement with an approximately 50% stenosis. Repeat selective right coronary angiography 2 months later revealed complete resolution of the narrowing (Fig. 17.12). Although this is the first case of coronary injury reported for AV node modification, coronary damage has been reported in many other posterior locations during accessory pathway animals (13–15,81,108–110). Furthermore, this case highlights several important issues regarding the potential for coronary artery injury during RF ablation in children.

First, coronary artery injury may occur with slow pathway ablation for atrioventricular nodal re-entry tachycardia (AVNRT). Second, acute coronary artery injury has the potential to be missed and is likely an underreported phenomenon. Third, infants and young children may be at particular risk. The inflammatory component of tissue injury caused by RF energy has been shown to invade layers of the right coronary artery, leading to acute narrowing when RF energy is applied to the atrial side of the lateral tricuspid annulus in pigs (13). Further maturation of this injury can result in significant late coronary stenosis (57). Thus, with RF energy application, coronary stenosis may occur acutely or be delayed. Our patient's injury was nearly missed because ST-segment changes did not occur until 100 seconds after the last RF application and resolved spontaneously within minutes despite a significant persistent

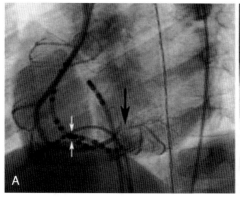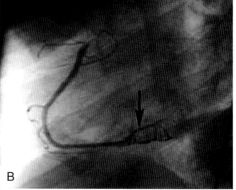

FIGURE 17.12 A: Left anterior oblique (LAO) projection of right coronary angiogram a few minutes after the ST-segment changes in Figure 17.2 had spontaneously normalized. An approximately 80% stenosis (*arrow*) is seen in a posterior left ventricular branch off a dominant right coronary. The ablation catheter was moved away from the septum at the time of angiogram, but had been immediately adjacent to the stenosis during the radiofrequency (RF) application. **B:** Similar LAO projection of right coronary angiogram 2 months following ablation. *Arrow* marks are of prior stenosis, which is now resolved.

stenosis of the involved artery. Other instances of coronary artery injury following radiofrequency ablation (RFA) have also been nearly missed because of this delay (15,110).

To absolutely minimize the chance of coronary injury in children, the following is recommended for patients <40 kg undergoing slow pathway modification for AVNRT: (i) cryotherapy is the preferred ablation methodology; (ii) in all patients in whom RF energy is used, selective coronary angiography of the artery supplying the posterior septum should be performed prior to ablation; (iii) if a small coronary artery is within 2 to 3 mm of the expected ablation location, RF energy should not be delivered; and (iv) if any RF energy is delivered, acute follow-up angiography should be performed postablation. Furthermore, it may be prudent to perform preablation and postablation angiography in all patients <20 kg regardless of the ablation technology used.

Ectopic Atrial Tachycardia

Ectopic atrial tachycardia (EAT) is an uncommon form of chronic SVT seen primarily in pediatric patients that often leads to cardiomyopathy and can be difficult to control medically (111). EAT in children is typically caused by automaticity in a single nonsinus focus, which may occur almost anywhere in the left or right atria but tends to occur more frequently in the locations shown in Fig. 17.13. Left-sided foci near the pulmonary veins are more common in children (112–114), as opposed to right atrial foci in adults (115). Although EAT has been reported to resolve spontaneously in a few cases, the sometimes devastating effects of the arrhythmia on cardiac function, combined with the hypothesis that the arrhythmia arises from a single nonsinus atrial focus and some reports of successful surgical excision of the focus (111), led to relatively early attempts at eliminating EAT with DC catheter ablation techniques (116). These attempts were promising, but the technique never gained wide acceptance because of the risks of acute damage and the fears of chronic myocardial damage associated with the DC technique. In addition, there was considerable speculation that elimination of one EAT focus was inadequate owing to the later appearance of others, particularly for right-sided foci (111).

EAT Focus Location

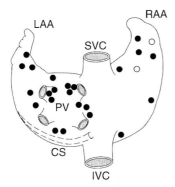

FIGURE 17.13 Location of ectopic atrial tachycardia (EAT) foci in the first 25 patients ablated at Children's Hospital in whom detailed mapping was possible. Closed circles (*n* = 23) indicate sites of successful ablation, and open circles (*n* = 2) indicate foci that could not be eliminated, in one case because of a broad area of fibrous dysplasia that was resected at surgery, and another patient because of multiple atrial foci of which this was only one. CS, coronary sinus; IVC, inferior vena cava; LAA, left atrial appendage; PV, pulmonary vein; RAA, right atrial appendage; SVC, superior vena cava.

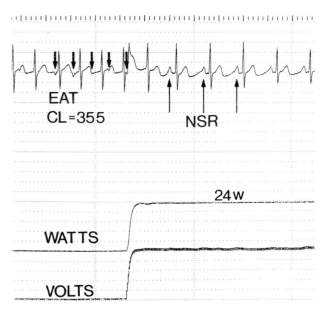

FIGURE 17.14 Ectopic atrial tachycardia ablation (EAT). Note how ectopic P waves terminate immediately at the onset of application of radiofrequency (RF) energy. CL, cycle length; NSR, normal sinus rhythm. (From Walsh EP, Saul JP, Hulse JE, et al. Transcatheter ablation of ectopic atrial tachycardia in young patients using radiofrequency current. *Circulation* 1992;86:1138–1146, with permission.)

Impressively, the use of RF catheter ablation for EAT has revolutionized its treatment. The first reported experience in a group of 12 patients who all presented with cardiomyopathy and drug-resistant EAT demonstrated that in all but 1 patient with diffuse atrial dysplasia, RF catheter ablation could successfully and safely eliminate the arrhythmia without long-term recurrence up to a median of what is currently approximately 2 years (112,114). Furthermore, the data have demonstrated that the arrhythmia focus is anatomically very small, because tachycardia termination took place in a median of 2.0 seconds after application of RF energy (Fig. 17.14). These results have now been confirmed in larger series in which ≤96% of EAT foci in children have been successfully eliminated with RF ablation (8,89,90). Because of these high success rates using ablation and the morbidity of drug therapy, the question of drug therapy generally has been reduced to one of whether it should be attempted at all in patients with ventricular dysfunction, and if so, how long should one wait for reversion to sinus rhythm before proceeding to ablation.

Initial procedure failure and late recurrence tend to be associated with the presence of multiple foci or intermittent EAT during the procedure. Multiple foci portend poorly for long-term success (111), both because of the increased difficulty in differentiating the foci during mapping and because more than one focus seems to be indicative of other foci emerging after the ablation procedure. Fortunately, in the pediatric population, most EAT is caused by a single nonsinus focus.

Overall, EAT ablation seems to be extremely low risk. Pulmonary vein stenosis is the only unique complication and can occur when the EAT focus is near or within a pulmonary vein (Fig. 17.13), eliciting concerns over stenosis. Clinically significant stenosis has not been reported for a pediatric case but is quite common in adults undergoing atrial fibrillation ablation procedures in similar locations (117–119). There is also a potential for damage to the sinus node or the right phrenic nerve for foci that occur along the crista terminalis, but injury is less likely in a patient who has never had heart surgery because the phrenic nerve continuously slides over the epicardial surface of the heart. Most other EAT foci are not near vital structures, such as the AV node or a coronary artery (Fig. 17.13).

Atrial Flutter or Fibrillation in the Absence of Other Heart Disease

In the pediatric patient, atrial re-entry tachycardias are relatively rare in the absence of either structural or functional heart disease. The term *lone atrial flutter* or *fibrillation* has been applied here, referring to the isolated nature of the arrhythmia findings. However, both of these tachyarrhythmias are occasionally observed in pediatric patients. There are two age ranges for presentation. Perhaps the most common is during third-trimester fetal life when atrial flutter accounts for up to a third of fetal tachycardias (120), often lasting through delivery and leading to ventricular dysfunction. Neonatal atrial flutter almost universally resolves without recurrence if the baby can be managed successfully during fetal and early neonatal life (121). Consequently, ablation therapy for such infants should not be necessary and has never been reported.

A second presentation peak occurs during adolescence when both atrial flutter and fibrillation may present in the absence of any identifiable structural, hormonal, or chemical cause. Although initial management should be conservative, in contrast to that with infants, the arrhythmia typically recurs multiple times in this age group despite medical therapy, creating a need for ablation therapy similar to the scenario in adults. The use of catheter ablation has been reported for both flutter and fibrillation in young patients. Success rates have been >90% for the flutter subgroup in a relatively large series of patients in the Pediatric Ablation Registry (55). Interestingly, acute success also recently was reported in seven of eight pediatric patients with paroxysmal atrial fibrillation who underwent ablation of either a single ectopic atrial focus or pulmonary vein electrical isolation (122). Furthermore, one of the cases we included in a series of EAT ablations in 1992 (112) was a 12-year-old boy who presented with recurrent atrial fibrillation, which was permanently eliminated after ablation of a single left pulmonary vein ectopic focus.

Specific technical details for ablation of either atrial flutter or fibrillation in the larger child are not particularly different from those in adults (123–125), so they will not be reviewed here. However, the decision of when to ablate can be quite different, particularly for fibrillation. After conversion from a first episode of one of these arrhythmias, either no therapy or a drug to block the AV node response is adequate. After recurrences, the threshold for ablation of atrial flutter can be similar to that in adults. The use of ablation therapy for the rare cases of atrial fibrillation in pediatric patients is also appealing, but the high emphasis on safety over efficacy noted above for all children necessitates that a decision to use RF ablation in this age group be considered only after failure of multiple anti-arrhythmic agents. Furthermore, the technique chosen should be the most conservative in terms of safety, since complications such as pulmonary vein stenosis and stroke may be devastating in a child.

Intra-atrial Re-entry Tachycardia in the Presence of Congenital Heart Disease

Commonly known as atrial flutter, intra-atrial re-entry tachycardia (IART) is uncommon in children with structurally and functionally normal hearts, but quite common after surgery for congenital heart disease. Although the prevalence is highest after either an atrial repair of transposition of the great arteries (Mustard or Senning techniques) (126) or after the Fontan repair (127), IART may occur after any repair that includes an atrial scar (atrial septal defect, tetralogy of Fallot, etc.) (128). IART generally is easy to convert to sinus rhythm with DC cardioversion or atrial pacing via either an esophageal lead, an intracardiac lead, or an implantable antitachycardia device (129). However, prevention is critically important in some patients because IART can be life threatening (126,129) and increases the likelihood of atrial thrombus formation. Unfortunately, prevention of IART is much more difficult than cardioversion, with drugs of all classes being generally ineffective and, even worse, often unsafe (130). Consequently, RF catheter ablation to either prevent IART (130,131) or to eliminate AV conduction and institute ventricular rate responsive pacing has recently gained prominence as a therapeutic option. IART in postoperative congenital heart patients may have multiple circuits in the same patient and be much more complex to ablate than typical atrial flutter, which is generally easily treated by electrically dividing the tricuspid annulus–inferior vena cava isthmus (130) (Fig. 17.15). Despite these complexities and a relatively high recurrence rate (132,133), acute success rates were initially reported at about 75%, and more recently, we and others have approached a rate of 95% (63,130,132–134). The use of 3-D mapping techniques is probably most important in this patient group (Figs. 17.5 and

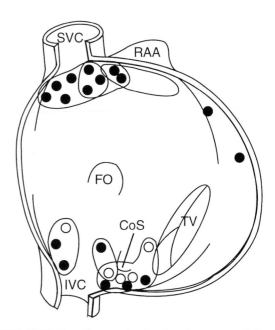

FIGURE 17.15 Sites of mapped exit points from zones of slow conduction at which ablation was attempted. In this schematic drawing of the right atrium, *filled circles* represent 17 sites of successful termination of atrial re-entry, and *open circles* represent the presumed exit point of the circuit from the zone of slow conduction for five circuits not successfully ablated. A right atriotomy would normally be performed along the lateral reflected wall of the atrium in this view and may extend across the reflected opening to the base of the right atrial appendage; it is not possible to define with precision the sites of right atriotomy in individual cases. The crista terminalis would be expected to run along the line in which the right atrium has been opened in this view. CS, coronary sinus; FO, fossa ovalis; IVC, inferior vena cava; RAA, right atrial appendage; SVC, superior vena cava; TV, tricuspid valve. (From American Heart Association. *Circulation* 1995;91: 707–714, with permission.)

17.6). Recurrence remains a problem, probably secondary to inadequate lesion development, but it is likely that technologies, such as the tip cooling described above, will improve even late outcome (63).

Junctional Ectopic Tachycardia

In the pediatric population, unlike in adults, junctional ectopic tachycardia (JET) is seen in two relatively distinct settings: Postoperative and congenital (135,136). The electrophysiologic characteristics of both varieties are similar to those of EAT (136), suggesting they are also due to abnormal automaticity, in this case arising from either low in the AV node or high in the His-Purkinje system. However, direct intracellular recordings have not been obtained.

The postoperative and congenital forms of JET differ primarily in their duration and response to therapy (137–140). Postoperative JET is typically transient after ventricular septal defect repair, either alone or at the time of repair of more complex anomalies (141). It responds to cooling and a variety of antiarrhythmic agents (138–140). In contrast, congenital JET is typically chronic and incessant but may resolve spontaneously over a period of years (136). Both JET types may result in severe hemodynamic compromise and appear to be exacerbated by both endogenous and exogenous adrenergic stimulation (136,140), and both arrhythmias seem to respond well to amiodarone (142).

The propensity for JET to eventually resolve spontaneously and the high theoretical risk of AV block from either catheter (29) or surgical (136) ablation of the JET focus in the AV junction suggest that JET may initially be best treated medically by minimizing adrenergic stimulation and beginning either intravenous or oral amiodarone (136,142,143), particularly in infants. However, there are now anecdotal data from a few reports (144–149) that have demonstrated that with ablation, it may be possible to eliminate JET while preserving AV conduction. Thus, when JET is resistant to medical therapy, persistent after a prolonged period of control, or producing intractable hemodynamic compromise, RF or cryoablation should probably be attempted. Because of anecdotal reports of sudden death and one case of AV block with JET, some investigators have recommended ventricular demand pacing in all patients with congenital JET (136), but this recommendation has remained controversial.

The specific details from the small number of reported cases of successful JET ablation provide few overarching recommendations to use when approaching these patients. Although in most cases the region of interest has ended up in the anterior septum near the bundle of His, successful ablation in at least one case was reported in the posteroseptal region below the coronary sinus os, with the site identified using retrograde atrial activation as a guide (145). This region corresponds to the site used for slow pathway modification and should be associated with a low incidence of permanent AV block. However, the data presented in the manuscript may be most consistent with frequent paroxysms of AV node re-entry tachycardia triggered by junctional escape beats, and other reports have not found mapping of earliest retrograde activation to be useful (147–150). Nonetheless, because this area is generally safe, initial attempts at ablation may be applied in the posterior septal region. If unsuccessful, mapping should focus on identifying the site of the earliest His potential during JET. Prior to ablation, the catheter should be moved very slightly posterior to that site, attempting to increase the atrial electrogram size and minimize the His activation from the distal ablation tip, similar to the methodology used in the past for fast pathway ablation. Most prior reports of successful elimination of JET without causing AV block have used this technique with brief, lower-power applications of RF energy. However, there is clearly a high risk of AV block in children using this technique. Recently, we had the opportunity to use cryotherapy for ablation of JET in a 10-year-old with intermittently incessant tachycardia. Earliest His activation during tachycardia was actually found with retrograde mapping just under the aortic valve (Fig. 17.16). The high degree of safety of this methodology around the AV conduction system made it ideal for both cryomapping and cryoablation, with successful elimination of the JET and preservation of the AV node, despite a catheter signal and location suggesting very close proximity to the His bundle. Although this case is a single anecdote, its outcome combined with the demonstrated reversibility of cryomap applications suggests that cryotherapy should be the treatment of first choice for ablation of JET.

Ventricular Tachycardia

High success rates for both DC and RF ablation have been reported for two forms of ventricular tachycardia (VT) in pediatric patients. In 1990, Morady et al. (150) first reported successful elimination of idiopathic right-sided VT in ten relatively young patients without structural heart disease using catheter-delivered DC energy. Other reports soon followed. In all of these series, pace mapping, as well as the site of earliest endocardial activation, were used as guides to the appropriate ablation site, but neither method was clearly superior. The youngest patient in any of these series was 18 years old, but a number of

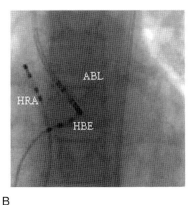

FIGURE 17.16 Successful cryoablation at location with His potential in a patient with junctional ectopic tachycardia (JET). **A:** Identical His potentials are clearly seen from the ablation catheter (retrograde approach through the aortic valve) and from the His catheter (in a usual position) just prior to initiation of cryomapping (CM). **B:** Fluoroscopic images in the anteroposterior (AP) view shows the cryoablation catheter overlapping the image of the His position catheter. ABL, ablation; HBE, His bundle electrogram.

younger patients have now been reported (8,89,90). Both DC and RF energy also have been used to eliminate bundle branch re-entry VT and idiopathic left VT by ablation of the right bundle branch or a left posterior Purkinje fiber (151,152). More recently, an entrainment technique that can identify sites most likely to ablate re-entrant VT after myocardial infarction (153) has been used to successfully ablate re-entrant VT in patients with tetralogy of Fallot and its variants (152,154–158).

COMPLICATIONS AND FOLLOW-UP

In most larger series in children, acute major complications appear to occur in 1% to 2% of cases and include complete AV block when ablating septal pathways (8,56,69,89,90), inadvertent coronary damage or coronary vein perforation (14–16,69,81), and vascular and embolic injury (7). Other minor complications have included Doppler-detectable increases in valvular regurgitation, minor vascular injury, and minor skin burns at the reference electrode skin site (8,70).

Follow-up studies have revealed no evidence of new coronary abnormalities by traditional angiography at 1 to 6 months postablation (69,70) and no significant increase in ventricular arrhythmias as late as 2 to 3 years. Importantly, however, acute coronary injury may not resolve postablation, and animal studies have revealed coronary intimal thickening in arteries near the ablation site (15,57). Currently no data exist that assess the long-term effects of RF lesions on coronary function or arrhythmogenicity in developing infants and children.

The PAPCA study did not report any deaths in its 2,761 patients; however, in prior reports death has been a rare complication of RF ablation procedures in children. Kugler et al. (8) reported a total of 4 procedure-related deaths in 4,135 children (0.097%) from 1991 to 1996, whereas Schaffer et al. (159) reported an incidence of 0.12% for patients with structurally normal hearts. The incidence was higher (0.89%) for patients with structural heart disease undergoing ablation.

SPECIAL CONSIDERATIONS FOR PEDIATRICS

Age (Infants)

There are three special considerations in infants that make their management different from that of the older child or adult when considering catheter ablation for the management of tachyarrhythmias. First, the risk of a sustained re-entrant primary atrial tachycardia, such as atrial fibrillation, is very close to zero in the small structurally normal heart, making the risk of sudden death in infants with WPW very low (17,160). Second, in approximately 40% of infants, accessory pathway function will spontaneously disappear by 1 year of age (17,18). Finally, the known risks of any catheterization, combined with the specific risks of catheter ablation in this age group (5,12,161–163), suggest that pharmacologic control should be aggressively pursued prior to ablation. This last issue deserves further discussion.

In humans, myocardial cell division probably occurs through approximately 6 months of age (164). Although this finding could potentially protect the myocardium from long-term complications secondary to early injury, the observation has been made that ventriculotomy scars produced in newborn puppies (165) and RF ablation lesions in immature lambs (6) appear to increase in size during subsequent development. In addition, in

contrast to mature ablation scars from adult animals, late lesions from the neonatal lambs were often histologically invasive and poorly demarcated from the surrounding tissue (6). The potential clinical importance of these results is underscored by a reported sudden death 2 weeks after an accessory pathway ablation in a 5-week-old, 3.2-kg infant (5,70). An echocardiogram from the infant at the time of a brief resuscitation, and autopsy findings, revealed relatively large lesions extending into the left ventricle from the intended mitral groove ablation site. Another heightened risk in infants is coronary artery damage due to the potentially close proximity of the coronaries to the ablation catheter and the reduced capacity for protective cooling during RF application in any small coronary artery. Although most reports of coronary damage in the literature have been limited to the posterior septum or a nondominant right coronary (13,15,16), complete occlusion of the left circumflex artery has been reported in a 5-week-old, 5.0-kg infant undergoing RF ablation of a left lateral accessory pathway (14).

Despite these disturbing cases, nonpharmacologic therapy will be necessary in a small subset of the infants with Accessory posture-mediated tachycardia (162,166). Until accurate methods are available to assess lesion size in real time, alternative methodologies should be used in all infants. Early data on the effects of cryotherapy suggest that this form of energy may be much less harmful to coronary arteries, even when in very close contact (167), because of the differing effects of cold and heat on connective tissue and the vascular inflammatory response. Coronary artery flow also protects the vessel through local warming during cryotherapy, similar to how flow protects through local cooling during RF energy application. If technical or other considerations require the use of RF energy, considerable caution should be used. RF lesion size is related to catheter tip size, RF power, tip temperature, and lesion duration (168,169). Thus, the following technical modifications should be adopted: (i) Deliver energy in as atrial a location as possible, (ii) use a 5 Fr catheter tip, (iii) use *low-temperature mapping* (50°C to 55°C) to identify the correct location prior to higher temperature RF application (37), (iv) use a lower-temperature setpoint of 60°C for the ablation lesion, and (v) use shorter-duration lesions (seven to ten times the time to effect, with a maximum of 30 to 40 seconds). The future development of real-time ultrasonographic or other modality monitoring of lesion size may also help reduce the procedural risks (170).

Size

Patient size by itself does not appear to affect the success rate of catheter ablation but has distinctly influenced the catheter approach. Some have advocated using the standard retrograde approach to left-sided accessory pathways but with two modifications: First, a smaller catheter (5 or 6 Fr), and second, fewer catheters, one for the ablation and one additional diagnostic catheter, both modifications designed to avoid vascular complications. Others researchers, including our own group (70), have worried about producing inadvertent ventricular lesions and have found that manipulation of the ablation catheter inside small ventricles is more difficult, leading to the use of the transseptal approach to all left-sided pathways, as described above. In fact, using the atrial approach, smaller patient size may actually make catheter manipulation easier, as discussed below.

Pre-excitation Syndromes in Patients with Structural Congenital Heart Disease

Though not only a pediatric issue, the combination of structural heart disease and arrhythmias will clearly be encountered often by the pediatric electrophysiologist. In agreement with previous studies (171,172), a review of this issue in unselected patients with congenital heart disease at the Children's Hospital in Boston found that pre-excitation syndromes are statistically increased in patients with Ebstein malformation, L-transposition of the great arteries, and hypertrophic myopathy (131). Of course, pre-excitation also occurs in other patients with congenital heart disease, but with an incidence not statistically higher than the general population.

Ebstein Malformation

The association of WPW with Ebstein disease and with the left-sided tricuspid valve in L-transposition probably has its basis in the embryology of tricuspid valve formation (173–175). The leaflets of the AV valves normally develop through a process of undermining, or delamination, of the interior surface of the embryonic ventricular myocardium. Separation of the atrium from the ventricle occurs through completion of this process and encroachment of fibrous tissue from the AV sulcus. The mitral valve and the anterior leaflet of the tricuspid valve are fully delaminated early in development; however, the posterior and septal leaflets of the tricuspid valve are not fully formed even by 3 months' gestation (175). Ebstein disease appears to occur when there is arrested development of tricuspid valve formation sometime between delamination of the anterior and the posterior leaflets. The high prevalence of pre-excitation combined with anatomic findings of accessory connections in a number of selected cases of Ebstein (174,176) suggests that the arrested valve development results in remnants of muscular or specialized tissue connections that cross the AV groove. In fact, multiple pathways are common in these patients, often with a combination of a posteroseptal pathway and one or more additional free wall pathways.

The electrophysiology of the accessory pathways in patients with congenital heart disease is not particularly unique. Bidirectional, antegrade only, and retrograde only pathways have all been reported. Furthermore, these patients have the same range of tachyarrhythmias found in patients with structurally normal hearts: Orthodromic and antidromic AV reciprocating tachycardia and other SVTs (AVNRT, atrial flutter/fib, and so on) with bystander participation of an antegrade-conducting AP. However, the physiologic and clinical implications of the tachycardia may be markedly different in patients with congenital heart disease.

Abnormal hemodynamics, increased incidence of isolated atrial and ventricular ectopy, sometimes poor tolerance of antiarrhythmic therapy, and the need for surgical repair that accompanies congenital heart disease all contribute to an increased need for aggressive arrhythmia management in this patient population. However, abnormal anatomy and atypical conduction systems may also enhance the difficulty and risks of either surgical or catheter ablation. Although difficult, RF catheter ablation results have been good enough to recommend the procedure first, for all patients requiring subsequent surgical repair to avoid postoperative arrhythmias and second, most symptomatic patients older than 1 year of age with significant structural lesions. A review of the reported cases of RF ablation in patients with congenital heart disease reveals that most of the patients have Ebstein malformation of a right-sided tricuspid valve (69,91,177–179). However, a significant portion have more complex anatomy with AV valve discordance (right atrium to left ventricle, left atrium to right ventricle—S,L,L or I,D,D) and often heterotaxy. Multiple pathways are extremely common in this group, occurring in between 30% and 80% of patients (69,176–178,180), compared with 5% to 10% in patients without congenital heart disease (69,91,181–183). It

is interesting to note that similar to the patients with Ebstein, patients with AV discordance had all of their accessory pathways associated with the tricuspid valve regardless of atrial situs, atrioventricular relationship, or valve function. This finding is in contrast to the more random location of accessory pathways reported for patients without congenital heart disease (69,91,181–186). Hypertrophic cardiomyopathy is the exception where pathways are more likely to be on the normal left-sided mitral valve.

Some aspects of the procedure in patients with Ebstein malformation are of special note. First, differentiation of atrial and ventricular signals and precise localization of the AV groove can be difficult, leading to a lack of specificity for what appear to be excellent signals in predicting a successful ablation site. In fact, very early ventricular activations, which might be termed pseudo-AP potentials, can often be seen near the AV groove (Fig. 17.17). This issue is particularly important for older patients

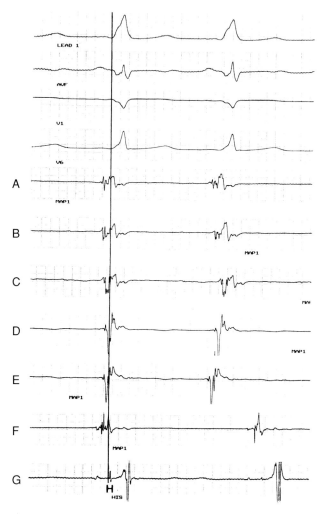

FIGURE 17.17 Electrograms near the accessory pathway with Ebstein malformation. Electrograms **A** through **F** were recorded with the distal pair of an ablating catheter very near the point of successful ablation shown in **F**. Note early ventricular activation in **A** through **D**, despite lack of success. Electrograms in **D** and **E** were not significantly different, but **E** had transient success. **F**, the point of permanent success, probably has the earliest activation; however, the differences are much more clear in retrospect. The *dark vertical line* marks the point of earliest surface QRS activation for all electrograms. **G** shows the position of the atrial and His electrograms. Pathway location was posterior septal.

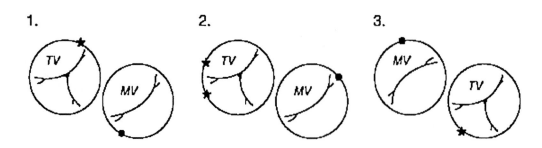

1.

2.

3.

DORV {I,D,A}, situs inversus, pulmonary stenosis, PAPVC, dextrocardia

TGA {I,D,D}, situs inversus, subpulmonary stenosis

DORV {S,L,L}, situs inversus, pulmonary stenosis, straddling mitral valve

● HIS Bundle
★ Accessory Pathway

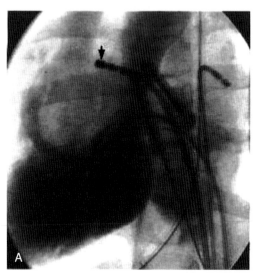

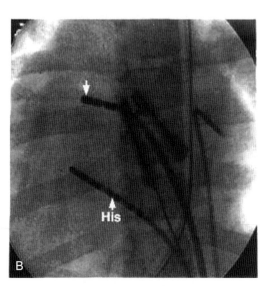

FIGURE 17.18 A: A drawing demonstrating the locations of the mitral valve (MV), tricuspid valve (TV), the His bundle, and accessory pathways in three patients with pre-excitation syndromes and atrioventricular discordance. Patient 1 corresponds with **A** and **B**. The angiogram in the anteroposterior projection (**B**) illustrates the importance of defining the anatomy of the AV valves. The decapolar catheter (*bottom white arrow* in **B**) was advanced from the left-sided inferior vena cava across the mitral valve and positioned with the second pair of electrodes at the His bundle. The mapping catheter (*black arrow* in **A**, *upper white arrow* in **B**) was advanced from the inferior vena cava across the atrial septum to the right-sided (anatomic) left atrium and positioned at the location of the accessory pathway, which in this case was at the superior and anterior portion of the left-sided tricuspid valve. The unmarked catheter is an atrial pacing catheter in the left-sided right atrium. DORV, double-outlet right ventricle; PAPVC, partial anomalous pulmonary venous connection; TGA, transposition of the great arteries.

who have large hearts with poorly defined AV grooves. The true AV groove is best identified by the right coronary artery. Use of a right coronary electrode wire can be considered (181–187) but may be difficult owing to a diminutive right coronary artery, and may need to be in place for long periods when multiple pathways are present. A safer recommended alternative is continual display of the relevant coronary angiogram using a real-time biplane image storage and display system. As with any AP, searching for balanced atrial and ventricular electrograms during mapping is important. Despite these maneuvers, it may still be very difficult to define the AV groove in these patients, requiring more test applications of the ablation modality to identify the correct location. Catheter stabilization for free wall pathways in the largest hearts is difficult and is not sufficiently

improved through the use of a long sheath or a variety of approaches (70). One observation that is difficult to prove statistically is that the smaller chamber size in smaller patients with structural heart disease is a technical asset in catheter ablation. In one series (177), a total of seven procedures lasting an average of 4.1 hours were required to ablate seven of nine accessory connections in six patients <40 kg, whereas seven procedures lasting an average of 6.5 hours were used to ablate only three of seven connections in four patients who weighed >40 kg.

As expected, it appears to be impossible to approach the ventricular side of the tricuspid valve in patients with Ebstein's malformation. No specific reports have noted the use of *nonstandard* ablation technologies for the patient with Ebstein's, but a few observations can be made. Coronary damage has been reported on multiple occasions in patients with Ebstein's, probably owing to the thin RV wall and often diminutive right coronary artery. Consequently, despite the tendency to use higher-power active or passive cooling ablation systems for difficult cases, such technologies should be used only when an adequate distance between the catheter tip and the artery has been documented. The definition of adequate here depends on the size of the nearby coronary artery—the larger the size, the safer the ablation. Furthermore, strong consideration should be given to the use of cryotherapy, at least as a mapping tool. Safety will be enhanced, and the adhesion of the catheter may be particularly useful in the larger patients.

When multiple pathways are present, persistence may be the electrophysiologist's best weapon for successful ablation. In general, 80% to 90% of patients can be rendered arrhythmia free by the procedure, with relatively infrequent major complications, such as permanent AV block (69,89,177,178). However, recurrence rates have been reported as high as 40%, particularly when multiple pathways are present (69,89,177,178).

Corrected Transposition

Ablation procedures in patients with AV discordance (S,L,L or I,D,D) require special considerations. First, detailed echocardiography and angiography are instrumental in defining the complex anatomy of the atria, the AV ring, and the coronary sinus so that the cameras and catheters can be positioned appropriately (Fig. 17.18). Second, careful attention must be given to locating the normal conduction system. Virtually all patients with AV discordance have had their accessory pathway associated with the tricuspid valve, whereas the His bundle has been associated more closely with the mitral valve. As predicted by Ho and Andersen (188), the normal conduction axis is often located at an anterior position along the AV groove. Once the normal and abnormal conduction fibers are located, electrophysiologic study and RF ablation of the accessory pathways can proceed with less risk of damage to the normal conduction system. Mapping and ablation requires a detailed knowledge of the anatomy and often innovative approaches. For instance, for cases of atrial inversion (*right atrium* on the left, and vice versa) with AV discordance (I,D,D), an atrial approach to the right-sided tricuspid valve may require a *reverse* transseptal procedure from the left-sided IVC and right atrium to the right-sided left atrium. If present, the coronary sinus in such cases will also be reversed. AVNRT may also be present in these patients, requiring identification of the slow pathway of an AV node, which is typically along the anterior mitral annulus. Clearly, the need for a detailed understanding of the anatomy in these cases cannot be overemphasized. Ablation technologies similar to those recommended above for Ebstein's patients, including cryoablation as the preferred energy source, are applicable to AV discordance patients as well.

Double AV Nodes

In hearts with discordant AV connections (S,L,L or I,D,D), the AV node is typically situated superior and anterior in the atrial wall near the anterolateral quadrant of the mitral valve (173,188). A second AV node, which is often present more inferiorly in the normal area of the triangle of Koch, can also link to the ventricular conduction fibers posteriorly, usually inferior to a ventricular septal defect. If the posterior and anterior ventricular bundle branches link together, a conduction sling, sometimes referred to as a Mönckeberg sling, is formed (Fig. 17.19) (173,189,190). These anatomic findings provide the substrate for a host of different modes of ventricular excitation or pre-excitation and AV reciprocating tachycardias.

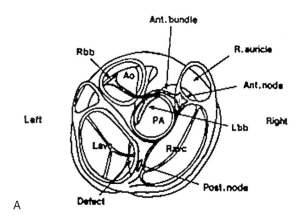

A

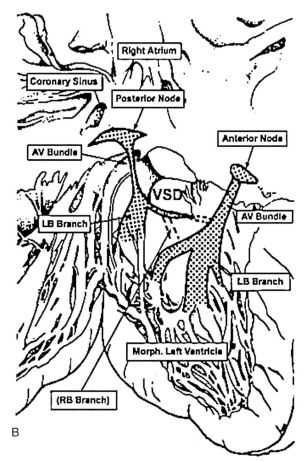

B

FIGURE 17.19 A: Diagram of the base of the heart and the atrioventricular (AV) conduction system in L-transposition of the great arteries (corrected) as seen from above. Note the bicommissural mitral valve on the right and the tricommissural tricuspid valve on the left. The AV node may either lie posteriorly (Post. node) in the septum in a somewhat normal location, anteriorly on the right-sided mitral valve (Ant. bundle), or in both places. Ao, aorta; (From Anderson RH, Arnold R, Wilkinson JL. The conducting system in congenitally corrected transposition. *Lancet* 1973;1:1286–1288, with permission.)
B: Diagram of the conduction system from a patient with corrected transposition in a crisscross heart, with AV valve anatomy similar to that shown in A. Note the dual conduction system with both the posterior and anterior AV nodes penetrating into the ventricles, and near connection of the conduction systems within the ventricle. LB, left bundle; RB, right bundle; morph., morphologic; VSD, ventricle septal defect; Rbb, right bundle branch; Lbb, left bundle branch; Ant., anterior; R., right; Post., posterior.

However, prior to our reports, there had been no electrophysiologic documentation of this phenomenon (191,192).

In 2001, we reported seven such cases, all of whom had AV discordance (2-S,L,L and 1-I,D,D) and characteristics consistent with the diagnosis of two separate AV nodes (twin or double) (191). Five of the seven also had a malaligned AV septal defects. The electrophysiologic findings included (a) the existence of two discrete non–pre-excited QRS morphologies, each with an associated His-bundle electrogram and normal HV interval; (b) decremental as well as adenosine-sensitive anterograde and retrograde conduction; and (c) inducible AV reciprocating tachycardia with anterograde conduction over one AV node and retrograde conduction over the alternate AV node. Ventricular premature beats placed into tachycardia when the His was refractory could pre-excite the atrium, indicating that the tachycardia involved two AV connections. In all cases, applications of RF energy at the site of the bidirectional pathway resulted in transient *junctional* acceleration with an identical QRS morphology to that generated by anterograde conduction over the targeted AV node, and modified or eliminated antegrade and retrograde conduction at that site. Although there is a possibility that one or the other of these pathways was a *Mahaim-type* AV fiber, their locations and the presence of near-normal HV intervals, retrograde conduction, *orthodromic* tachycardia, and *junctional*-type acceleration during RF ablation all favor a second AV node. The precise cause may make little difference for the management of such patients, but the phenomenon is important to be aware of to avoid damage to the better of the two conduction systems during ablation procedures performed prior to surgery in these patients with complex anatomy.

Clearly, an extensive understanding of the anatomy and electrophysiology should be obtained in such patients before proceeding to mapping and ablation. Furthermore, the lack of clarity in defining the anatomy of AV conduction in these patients suggests that ablation should first be undertaken using cryotherapy, proceeding to RF energy only if unsuccessful or after a recurrence. The one caveat to this recommendation is that low-power RF application may be helpful in identifying the location of the anterior and posterior AV nodes through their acceleration response when heated.

Summary—Pre-excitation and Congenital Heart Disease

Based on our own observations and those in the literature, a few recommendations concerning catheter ablation in patients with congenital defects can be made: (a) An attempt should be made to carefully identify the location of the normal AV conducting system, particularly in patients with AV discordance; (b) the anatomic tricuspid valve is the most likely location for accessory connections; (c) smaller patient size may be an asset; (d) an atrial approach should probably be attempted first for connections around the tricuspid annulus (right or left sided); (e) the true AV groove should be well identified, using either atrial and ventricular electrogram balance, a coronary angiogram, or if available, a coronary mapping wire in larger patients; and (f) whenever possible, cryoenergy is the preferred ablation technology to minimize the risk to the AV conduction system and adjacent small coronary arteries. With these caveats in mind, it appears that despite the difficulties of unusual anatomic landmarks and abnormally positioned conduction systems, most accessory pathways in patients with structural congenital heart disease can be safely and effectively ablated.

SUMMARY

Children are usually smaller than adults, but in general, ablation techniques used in adults should not simply be miniaturized to fit the size of the pediatric patient. Multiple factors, including the distribution of arrhythmia mechanisms, ongoing myocardial development, potentially increased risk of vascular injury and AV node damage, as well as the effects of smaller cardiac size, should all influence the ablation technique. An overriding theme in the child should be that safety takes precedence over efficacy. Thus, variations of technique should include the decision to ablate, the energy source and its delivery, the catheter approach to the heart and the AV ring, and the follow-up. For instance, because of its strong safety profile and despite lower efficacy, the use of cryotherapy may be even better suited to ablation in children than in adults. Attention to these factors is probably most important in infants, a group who differ both quantitatively and qualitatively from adults. In addition, the pediatric patient is obviously more likely to have the simultaneous presence of structural congenital heart disease, which in itself has various implications for the decision to ablate and the procedure technique. Alternatively, there are numerous similarities between adult and pediatric patients. Specifically, regardless of age, it seems clear that a variety of techniques and approaches are necessary to successfully ablate APs in all locations around the AV groove.

References

1. Wolferth CC, Wood FC. The mechanism of production of short PR intervals and prolonged QRS complexes in patients with presumably undamaged hearts: Hypothesis of an accessory pathway of auriculoventricular conduction (bundle of Kent). *Am Heart J* 1932;8,297–311.
2. Wolff L, Parkinson J, White PD. Bundle branch block with short P-R interval in healthy young people prone to paroxysmal tachycardia. *Am Heart J* 1930;5:685.
3. Sealy WC, Hattler BG, Blumenschein SD, et al. Surgical treatment of Wolff-Parkinson-White syndrome. *Ann Thorac Surg* 1969;8:1.
4. Haines DE, Watson DD. Tissue heating during radiofrequency catheter ablation: A thermodynamic model and observation in isolated perfused and superfused canine right ventricular free wall. *Pacing Clin Electrophysiol* 1989;12:962–976.
5. Erickson CC, Walsh EP, Triedman JK, et al. Efficacy and safety of radiofrequency ablation in infants and young children <18 months of age. *Am J Cardiol* 1994;74:944–947.
6. Saul JP, Hulse JE, Papagiannis J, et al. Late enlargement of radiofrequency lesions in infant lambs. Implications for ablation procedures in small children. *Circulation* 1994;90:492–499.
7. Van Hare GF, Lesh MD, Scheinman M, et al. Percutaneous radiofrequency catheter ablation for supraventricular arrhythmias in children. *J Am Coll Cardiol* 1991;17:1613–1620.
8. Kugler JD, Danford DA, Deal BJ, et al. Radiofrequency catheter ablation for tachyarrhythmias in children and adolescents. The Pediatric Electrophysiology Society. *N Engl J Med* 1994;330:1481–1487.
9. Friedman RA, Walsh EP, Silka MJ, et al. NASPE Expert Consensus Conference: Radiofrequency catheter ablation in children with and without congenital heart disease. Report of the writing committee. North American Society of Pacing and Electrophysiology. *Pacing Clin Electrophysiol* 2002;25:1000–1017.
10. Blaufox AD, Denslow S, Felix GL, et al., Participating Members of the Pediatric Electrophysiology Society. Radiofrequency catheter ablation in

Registry infants: When is it done and how do they fare [abstract]? *Circulation* 2000;102:II698.

11. Blaufox AD, Paul T, Saul JP. Radiofrequency catheter ablation in small children: Relationship of complications to application dose. *Pacing Clin Electrophysiol* 2004;27:224–229.

12. Blaufox AD, Felix GL, Saul JP. Pediatric Catheter Ablation Registry. Radiofrequency catheter ablation in infants </=18 months old: When is it done and how do they fare?: Short-term data from the pediatric ablation registry. *Circulation* 2001;104:2803–2808.

13. Paul T, Bokenkamp R, Mahnert B, et al. Coronary artery involvement early and late after radiofrequency current application in young pigs. *Am Heart J* 1997;133:436–440.

14. Paul T, Kakavand B, Blaufox AD, et al. Complete occlusion of the left circumflex coronary artery after radiofrequency catheter ablation in an infant. *J Cardiovasc Electrophysiol* 2003;14:1004–1006.

15. Bertram H, Bokenkamp R, Peuster M, et al. Coronary artery stenosis after radiofrequency catheter ablation of accessory atrioventricular pathways in children with Ebstein's malformation. *Circulation* 2001;103:538–543.

16. Blaufox AD, Saul JP. Acute coronary artery stenosis during slow pathway ablation for atrioventricular nodal reentrant tachycardia in a child. *J Cardiovasc Electrophysiol* 2004;15:97–100.

17. Deal BJ, Keane JF, Gillette PC, et al. Wolff-Parkinson-White syndrome and supraventricular tachycardia during infancy: Management and follow-up. *J Am Coll Cardiol* 1985;5:130–135.

18. Benson DW Jr, Dunnigan A, Benditt DG. Follow-up evaluation of infant paroxysmal atrial tachycardia: Transesophageal study. *Circulation* 1987;75:542–549.

19. Perry JC, Garson A Jr. Supraventricular tachycardia due to Wolff-Parkinson-White syndrome in children: Early disappearance and late recurrence [see comments]. *J Am Coll Cardiol* 1990;16:1215–1220.

20. Klein GJ, Yee R, Sharma AD. Longitudinal electrophysiologic assessment of asymptomatic patients with the Wolff-Parkinson-White electrocardiographic pattern [see comment]. *N Engl J Med* 1989;320:1229–1233.

21. Zardini M, Yee R, Thakur RK, et al. Risk of sudden arrhythmic death in the Wolff-Parkinson-White syndrome: Current perspectives. *Pacing Clin Electrophysiol* 1994;17:966–975.

22. Bromberg BI, Lindsay BD, Cain ME, et al. Impact of clinical history and electrophysiologic characterization of accessory pathways on management strategies to reduce sudden death among children with Wolff-Parkinson-White syndrome. *J Am Coll Cardiol* 1996;27:690–695.

23. Zipes DP, Garson A Jr. 26th Bethesda conference: Recommendations for determining eligibility for competition in athletes with cardiovascular abnormalities. Task Force 6: Arrhythmias. *Med Sci Sports Exerc* 1994;26(suppl):S276–283.

24. Vedel J, Frank R, Fontaine G, et al. Bloc auriculo-ventriculaire intra-Hisien definitif induit au cours d'une exploration endoventriculaire droite. *Arch Mal Coeur* 1979;72:107–112.

25. Scheinman MM, Morady F, Hess DS, et al. Catheter-induced ablation of the atrioventricular junction to control refractory supraventricular arrhythmias. *JAMA* 1982;248:851–855.

26. Scheinman MM, Evans-Bell T. Catheter ablation of the atrioventricular junction: A report of the percutaneous mapping and ablation registry. *Circulation* 1984;70:1024–1029.

27. Warin JF, Haissaguerre M, D'Ivernois C, et al. Catheter ablation of accessory pathways: Technique and results in 248 patients. *Pacing Clin Electrophysiol* 1990;13:1609–1614.

28. Sebag C, Lavergne T, Millat B. Rupture of the stomach and the esophagus after attempted transcatheter ablation of an accessory pathway by direct current shock. *Am J Cardiol* 1989;63:890–891.

29. Gillette PC, Garson A Jr, Porter JC, et al. Junctional automatic ectopic tachycardia: New proposed treatment by transcatheter His bundle ablation. *Am Heart J* 1983;106:619–623.

30. Smith RT Jr, Gillette PC, Massumi A, et al. Transcatheter ablative techniques for treatment of the permanent form of junctional reciprocating tachycardia in young patients. *J Am Coll Cardiol* 1986;8:385–390.

31. Cunningham D, Rowland E, Rickards AF. A new low energy power source for catheter ablation. *Pacing Clin Electrophysiol* 1986;9:1384–1390.

32. Cosman ER, Nashold BS, Ovelman-Levitt J. Theoretical aspects of radiofrequency lesions in the dorsal root entry zone. *Neurosurgery* 1984;15:945–950.

33. Huang SK, Bharati S, Graham AR, et al. Closed chest catheter desiccation of the atrioventricular junction using radiofrequency energy—a new method of catheter ablation. *J Am Coll Cardiol* 1987;9:349–358.

34. Borggrefe M, Budde T, Podczeck A, et al. High frequency alternating current ablation of an accessory pathway in humans. *J Am Coll Cardiol* 1987;10:576–582.

35. Haines DE, Verow AF. Observations on electrode-tissue interface temperature and effects on electrical impedance during radiofrequency ablation of ventricular myocardium. *Circulation* 1990;82:1034–1038.

36. Calkins H, Prystowsky E, Carlson M, et al. Temperature monitoring during radiofrequency catheter ablation procedures using closed loop control. Atakr Multicenter Investigators Group. *Circulation* 1994;90:1279–1286.

37. Cote JM, Epstein MR, Triedman JK, et al. Low-temperature mapping predicts site of successful ablation while minimizing myocardial damage. *Circulation* 1996;94:253–257.

38. Nakagawa H, Yamanashi WS, Pitha JV, et al. Comparison of in vivo tissue temperature profile and lesion geometry for radiofrequency ablation with a saline-irrigated electrode versus temperature control in a canine thigh muscle preparation. *Circulation* 1995;91:2264–2273.

39. Langberg JJ, Gallagher M, Strickberger SA, et al. Temperature-guided radiofrequency catheter ablation with very large distal electrodes. *Circulation* 1993;88:245–249.

40. Bergau D, Brucker GG, Saul JP. Porous metal tipped catheter produces larger radiofrequency lesions through tip cooling [abstract]. *Circulation* 1993;88:I164.

41. Whayne JG, Nath S, Haines DE. Microwave catheter ablation of myocardium in vitro. Assessment of the characteristics of tissue heating and injury. *Circulation* 1994;89:2390–2395.

42. Agnoletti G, Borghi A, Vignati G, et al. Fontan conversion to total cavopulmonary connection and arrhythmia ablation: Clinical and functional results. *Heart* 2003;89(2):193–198.

43. Gaita F, Haissaguerre M, Giustetto C, et al. Safety and efficacy of cryoablation of accessory pathways adjacent to the normal conduction system. *J Cardiovasc Electrophysiol* 2003;14:825–829.

44. Gaita F, Montefusco A, Riccardi R, et al. Cryoenergy catheter ablation: A new technique for treatment of permanent junctional reciprocating tachycardia in children. *J Cardiovasc Electrophysiol* 2004;15:263–268.

45. Lowe MD, Meara M, Mason J, et al. Catheter cryoablation of supraventricular arrhythmias: A painless alternative to radiofrequency energy. *Pacing Clin Electrophysiol* 2003;26(pt 2):500–503.

46. Skanes AC, Yee R, Krahn AD, et al. Cryoablation of atrial arrhythmias. *Card Electrophysiol Rev* 2002;6(4):383–388.

47. Skanes AC, Dubuc M, Klein GJ, et al. Cryothermal ablation of the slow pathway for the elimination of atrioventricular nodal reentrant tachycardia. *Circulation* 2000;102:2856–2860.

48. Miyazaki A, Blaufox AD, Fairbrother DL, et al. Prolongation of the fast pathway effective refractory period during cryoablation in children: A marker of slow pathway modification. *Heart Rhythm* 2005;2:1179–1185.

49. Miyazaki A, Blaufox AD, Fairbrother DL, et al. Cryoablation for septal tachycardia substrates in pediatric patients: Mid-term results. *J Am Coll Cardiol* 2005;45:581–588.

50. Rodriguez LM, Leunissen J, Hoekstra A, et al. Transvenous cold mapping and cryoablation of the AV node in dogs: Observations of chronic lesions and comparison to those obtained using radiofrequency ablation. *J Cardiovasc Electrophysiol* 1998;9:1055–1061.

51. Dubuc M, Roy D, Thibault B, et al. Transvenous catheter ice mapping and cryoablation of the atrioventricular node in dogs. *Pacing Clin Electrophysiol* 1999;22:1488–1498.

52. Lustgarten DL, Bell S, Hardin N, et al. Safety and efficacy of epicardial cryoablation in a canine model. *Heart Rhythm* 2005;2(1):82–90.

53. Skanes AC, Jones DL, Teefy P, et al. Safety and feasibility of cryothermal ablation within the mid- and distal coronary sinus. *J Cardiovasc Electrophysiol* 2004;15:1319–1323.

54. Khairy P, Chauvet P, Lehmann J, et al. Lower incidence of thrombus formation with cryoenergy versus radiofrequency catheter ablation. *Circulation* 2003;107:2045–2050.

55. Kugler JD, Danford DA, Houston K, et al. Radiofrequency catheter ablation for paroxysmal supraventricular tachycardia in children and adolescents without structural heart disease. Pediatric EP Society, Radiofrequency Catheter Ablation Registry. *Am J Cardiol* 1997;80:1438–1443.

56. Schaffer MS, Silka MJ, Ross BA, et al. Inadvertent atrioventricular block during radiofrequency catheter ablation. Results of the Pediatric Radiofrequency Ablation Registry. Pediatric Electrophysiology Society. *Circulation* 1996;94:3214–3220.

57. Bokenkamp R, Wibbelt G, Sturm M, et al. Effects of intracardiac radiofrequency current application on coronary artery vessels in young pigs. *J Cardiovasc Electrophysiol* 2000;11:565–571.

58. Nakagawa H, Chandrasekaren K, Pitha J, et al. Early detection of coronary artery injury produced by radiofrequency ablation within the coronary sinus using intravascular ultrasound imaging. *Circulation* 1995;92:I610.

59. Haines DE. Thermal ablation of perfused porcine left ventricle in vitro with the neodymium-YAG laser hot tip catheter system. *Pacing Clin Electrophysiol* 1992;15:979–985.

60. Svenson RH, Littmann L, Colavita PG, et al. Laser photoablation of ventricular tachycardia: Correlation of diastolic activation times and photoablation effects on cycle length and termination–observations supporting a macroreentrant mechanism. *J Am Coll Cardiol* 1992;19:607–613.

61. Wu G, Svenson RH, Littmann L, et al. Laser photoablation of experimental post-infarction ventricular tachycardia guided by three dimensional activation mapping. *Lasers Surg Med* 1997;20(2):119–130.

62. Lesh MD, Diederich C, Guerra PG, et al. An anatomic approach to prevention of atrial fibrillation: Pulmonary vein isolation with through-the-balloon ultrasound ablation (TTB-USA). *Thorac Cardiovasc Surg* 1999;47(suppl 3):347–351.

63. Blaufox AD, Numan MT, Laohakunakorn P, et al. Catheter tip cooling during radiofrequency ablation of intra-atrial reentry: Effects on power, temperature, and impedance. *J Cardiovasc Electrophysiol* 2002;13:783–787.

64. Love BA, Collins KK, Alexander ME, et al. Early results of radiofrequency ablation for intraatrial reentry tachycardia in congenital heart disease using electroanatomic mapping [abhstract]. *Circulation* 2000;102:II698.

65. Love BA, Collins KK, Walsh EP, et al. Electroanatomic characterization of conduction barriers in sinus/atrially paced rhythm and association with intra-atrial reentrant tachycardia circuits following congenital heart disease surgery. *J Cardiovasc Electrophysiol* 2001;12:17–25.

66. Triedman JK. Arrhythmias in adults with congenital heart disease. *Heart* 2002;87(4):383–389.

67. Triedman JK, Alexander ME, Love BA, et al. Influence of patient factors and ablative technologies on outcomes of radiofrequency ablation of intra-atrial re-entrant tachycardia in patients with congenital heart disease. *J Am Coll Cardiol* 2002;39:1827–1835.

68. Triedman JK, DeLucca JM, Alexander ME, et al. Prospective trial of electroanatomically guided, irrigated catheter ablation of atrial tachycardia in patients with congenital heart disease. *Heart Rhythm* 2005;2:700–705.

69. Jackman WM, Wang XZ, Friday KJ, et al. Catheter ablation of accessory atrioventricular pathways (Wolff-Parkinson-White syndrome) by radiofrequency current [see comments]. *N Engl J Med* 1991;324:1605–1611.

70. Saul JP, Hulse JE, De W, et al. Catheter ablation of accessory atrioventricular pathways in young patients: Use of long vascular sheaths, the transseptal approach and a retrograde left posterior parallel approach. *J Am Coll Cardiol* 1993;21:571–583.

71. Beukema WP, Van Dessel PF, van Hemel NM, et al. Radiofrequency catheter ablation of accessory pathways associated with a coronary sinus diverticulum. *Eur Heart J* 1994;15:1415–1418.

72. Chiang CE, Chen SA, Yang CR, et al. Major coronary sinus abnormalities: Identification of occurrence and significance in radiofrequency ablation of supraventricular tachycardia. *Am Heart J* 1994;127:1279–1289.

73. Chiang CE, Chen SA, Yang CR, et al. Radiofrequency ablation of posteroseptal accessory pathways in patients with abnormal coronary sinus. *Am Heart J* 1993;126:1213–1216.

74. Giorgberidze I, Saksena S, Krol RB, et al. Efficacy and safety of radiofrequency catheter ablation of left-sided accessory pathways through the coronary sinus. *Am J Cardiol* 1995;76:359–365.

75. Huang SK, Graham AR, Bharati S, et al. Short and long-term effects of transcatheter ablation of the coronary sinus by radiofrequency energy. *Circulation* 1988;78:416–427.

76. Langberg JJ, Griffin JC, Herre JM, et al. Catheter ablation of accessory pathways using radiofrequency energy in the canine coronary sinus. *J Am Coll Cardiol* 1989;13:491–496.

77. Lesh MD, van Hare G, Kao AK, et al. Radiofrequency catheter ablation for Wolff-Parkinson-White syndrome associated with a coronary sinus diverticulum. *Pacing Clin Electrophysiol* 1991;14:1479–1484.

78. Sanchez-Quintana D, Ho SY, Cabrera JA, et al. Topographic anatomy of the inferior pyramidal space: Relevance to radiofrequency catheter ablation. *J Cardiovasc Electrophysiol* 2001;12:210–217.

79. Shinbane JS, Lesh MD, Stevenson WG, et al. Anatomic and electrophysiologic relation between the coronary sinus and mitral annulus: Implications for ablation of left-sided accessory pathways. *Am Heart J* 1998;135:93–98.

80. Tebbenjohanns J, Pfeiffer D, Jung W, et al. Radiofrequency catheter ablation of a posteroseptal accessory pathway within a coronary sinus diverticulum. *Am Heart J* 1993;126:1216–1219.

81. Khanal S, Ribeiro PA, Platt M, et al. Right coronary artery occlusion as a complication of accessory pathway ablation in a 12-year-old treated with stenting. *Catheter Cardiovasc Interv* 1999;46(1):59–61.

82. Kuck K, Schluter M, Gursoy S. Preservation of atrioventricular nodal conduction during radiofrequency current catheter ablation of midseptal accessory pathways. *Circulation* 1992;86:1743–1752. Ref Type: Generic.

83. Schlüter M, Siebels J, Duckeck W, et al. Catheter approaches to radiofrequency current ablation of posteroseptal accessory pathways [abstract]. *J Am Coll Cardiol* 1992;19:27A.

84. Atienza F, Arenal A, Torrecilla EG, et al. Acute and long-term outcome of transvenous cryoablation of midseptal and parahisian accessory pathways in patients at high risk of atrioventricular block during radiofrequency ablation. *Am J Cardiol* 2004;93:1302–1305.

85. Lanzotti ME, De PR, Tritto M, et al. Successful treatment of anteroseptal accessory pathways by transvenous cryomapping and cryoablation. *Ital Heart J* 2002;3(2):128–132.

86. Lee AW, Crawford FA Jr, Gillette PC, et al. Cryoablation of septal pathways in patients with supraventricular tachyarrhythmias. *Ann Thorac Surg* 1989;47(4):566–568.

87. Stobie EP, Green GMS. Cryoablation for septal accessory pathways: Has the next ice age arrived? *J Cardiovasc Electrophysiol* 2003;14:830–831.

88. Laohaprasitiporn D, Walsh EP, Saul JP, et al. Predictors of permanence of successful radiofrequency lesions created with controlled catheter tip temperature. *Pacing Clin Electrophysiol* 1997;20(pt 1):1283–1291.

89. Tanel RE, Walsh EP, Triedman JK, et al. Five-year experience with radiofrequency catheter ablation: Implications for management of arrhythmias in pediatric and young adult patients. *J Pediatr* 1997;131:878–887.

90. Van Hare GF, Javitz H, Carmelli D, et al. Prospective assessment after pediatric cardiac ablation: Demographics, medical profiles, and initial outcomes. *J Cardiovasc Electrophysiol* 2004;15:759–770.

91. Calkins H, Langberg J, Sousa J, et al. Radiofrequency catheter ablation of accessory atrioventricular connections in 250 patients. Abbreviated therapeutic approach to Wolff-Parkinson-White syndrome. *Circulation* 1992;85:1337–1346.

92. Van Hare GF, Javitz H, Carmelli D, et al. Prospective assessment after pediatric cardiac ablation: Recurrence at 1 year after initially successful ablation of supraventricular tachycardia. *Heart Rhythm* 2004;1(2):188–196.

93. Van Hare GF, Carmelli D, Smith WM, et al. Prospective assessment after pediatric cardiac ablation: Design and implementation of the multicenter study. *Pacing Clin Electrophysiol* 2002;25:332–341.

94. Danford DA, Kugler JD, Deal B, et al. The learning curve for radiofrequency ablation of tachyarrhythmias in pediatric patients. *Am J Cardiol* 1995;75:587–590.

95. Kugler JD, Danford DA, Houston KA, et al. Pediatric radiofrequency catheter ablation registry success, fluoroscopy time, and complication rate for supraventricular tachycardia: Comparison of early and recent eras. *J Cardiovasc Electrophysiol* 2002;13:336–341.

96. Critelli G, Gallagher JJ, Thiene G. The permanent form of junctional reciprocating tachycardia. In: Benditt DG, Benson DW, eds. *Cardiac Preexcitation Syndromes, Origins, Evaluation and Treatment*. Boston: Martinus Nijhoff, 1986:233–254.

97. Ticho BS, Saul JP, Hulse JE, et al. Variable location of accessory pathways associated with the permanent form of junctional reciprocating tachycardia and confirmation with radiofrequency ablation. *Am J Cardiol* 1992;70:1559–1564.

98. Fishberger SB, Colan SD, Saul JP, et al. Myocardial mechanics before and after ablation of chronic tachycardia. *Pacing Clin Electrophysiol* 1996;19:42–49.

99. Haissaguerre M, Montserrat P, Warin JF, et al. Catheter ablation of left posteroseptal accessory pathways and of long RP tachycardias with a right endocardial approach. *Eur Heart J* 1991;12:845–859.

100. Ticho BS, Walsh EP, Saul JP. Ablation of permanent junctional reciprocating tachycardia. In: Huang SK, ed. *Radiofrequency Catheter Ablation of Cardiac Arrhythmias: Basic Concepts and Clinical Applications*. Mt. Kisko, NY: Futura Publishing, 1994:397–409.

101. Gaita F, Haissaguerre M, Giustetto C, et al. Catheter ablation of permanent junctional reciprocating tachycardia with radiofrequency current. *J Am Coll Cardiol* 1995;25:648–654.

102. Morady F, Scheinman MM, Kou WH, et al. Long-term results of catheter ablation of a posteroseptal accessory atrioventricular connection in 48 patients. *Circulation* 1989;79:1160–1170.

103. Haissaguerre M, Warin JF, Lemetayer P, et al. Closed-chest ablation of retrograde conduction in patients with atrioventricular nodal reentrant tachycardia. *N Engl J Med* 1989;320:426–433.

104. Huang SK, Bharati S, Graham AR, et al. Chronic incomplete atrioventricular block induced by radiofrequency catheter ablation. *Circulation* 1989;80:951–961.

105. Jackman WM, Beckman KJ, McClelland JH, et al. Treatment of supraventricular tachycardia due to atrioventricular nodal reentry by radiofrequency catheter ablation of slow-pathway conduction. *N Engl J Med* 1992;327.

106. Wong T, Segal OR, Markides V, et al. Cryoablation of focal atrial tachycardia originating close to the atrioventricular node. *J Cardiovasc Electrophysiol* 2004;15:838.

107. Wathen M, Natale A, Wolfe K, et al. An anatomically guided approach to atrioventricular node slow pathway ablation. *Am J Cardiol* 1992;70:886–889.

108. Benito F, Sanchez C. Radiofrequency catheter ablation of accessory pathways in infants. *Heart* 1997;78:160–162.

109. Solomon AJ, Tracy CM, Swartz JF, et al. Effect on coronary artery anatomy of radiofrequency catheter ablation of atrial insertion sites of accessory pathways. *J Am Coll Cardiol* 1993;21:1440–1444.

110. Chatelain P, Zimmermann M, Weber R, et al. Acute coronary occlusion secondary to radiofrequency catheter ablation of a left lateral accessory pathway. *Eur Heart J* 1995;16:859–861.

111. Garson A Jr, Smith RT, Moak JP, et al. Atrial automatic ectopic tachycardia in children. In: Touboul P, Waldo AL, eds. *Atrial Arrhythmias: Current Concepts and Management*. St. Louis, MO: Mosby–Year Book, 1990:282–287.

112. Walsh EP, Saul JP, Hulse JE, et al. Transcatheter ablation of ectopic atrial tachycardia in young patients using radiofrequency current [see comments]. *Circulation* 1992;86:1138–1146.

113. Walsh EP. Ablation of ectopic atrial tachycardia in children. In: Huang SK, ed. *Radiofrequency Catheter Ablation of Cardiac Arrhythmias: Basic Concepts and Clinical Applications*. Mt. Kisko, NY: Futura Publishing, 1994:421–443.

114. Walsh EP, Saul JP, Triedman JK, et al. Natural and unnatural history of ectopic atrial tachycardia: One institution's experience [abstract]. *Pacing Clin Electrophysiol* 1994;17:746.
115. Tracy CM, Swartz JF, Fletcher RD, et al. Radiofrequency catheter ablation of ectopic atrial tachycardia using paced activation sequence mapping [see comments]. *J Am Coll Cardiol* 1993;21:910–917.
116. Silka MJ, Gillette PC, Garson A Jr, et al. Transvenous catheter ablation of a right atrial automatic ectopic tachycardia. *J Am Coll Cardiol* 1985;5:999–1001.
117. Haissaguerre M, Hocini M, Sanders P, et al. Catheter ablation of long-lasting persistent atrial fibrillation: Clinical outcome and mechanisms of subsequent arrhythmias. *J Cardiovasc Electrophysiol* 2005;16:1138–1147.
118. Haissaguerre M, Sanders P, Hocini M, et al. Pulmonary veins in the substrate for atrial fibrillation: The "venous wave" hypothesis. *J Am Coll Cardiol* 2004;43:2290–2292.
119. Hsu LF, Jais P, Hocini M, et al. Incidence and prevention of cardiac tamponade complicating ablation for atrial fibrillation. *Pacing Clin Electrophysiol* 2005;28(suppl 1):S106–S109.
120. Ko JK, Deal BJ, Strasburger JF, et al. Supraventricular tachycardia mechanisms and their age distribution in pediatric patients. *Am J Cardiol* 1992;69:1028–1032.
121. Dunnigan A, Benson DW, Benditt DG. Atrial flutter in infancy: Diagnosis, clinical features, and treatment. *Pediatrics* 1985;75:725–729.
122. Nanthakumar K, Lau YR, Plumb VJ, et al. Electrophysiological findings in adolescents with atrial fibrillation who have structurally normal hearts. *Circulation* 2004;110:117–123.
123. Cosio FG, Arribas F, Lopez-Gil M, et al. Atrial flutter mapping and ablation: II. Radiofrequency ablation of atrial flutter circuits. *Pacing Clin Electrophysiol* 1996;19:965–975.
124. Kalman JM, Olgin JE, Saxon LA, et al. Electrocardiographic and electrophysiologic characterization of atypical atrial flutter in man: Use of activation and entrainment mapping and implications for catheter ablation. *J Cardiovasc Electrophysiol* 1997;8:121–144.
125. Manolis AS, Vassilikos V, Maounis TN, et al. Radiofrequency ablation in pediatric and adult patients: Comparative results. *J Interv Card Electrophysiol* 2001;5:443–453.
126. Garson A Jr, Bink-Boelkens M, Hesslein PS, et al. Atrial flutter in the young: A collaborative study of 380 cases. *J Am Coll Cardiol* 1985;6:871–878.
127. Fishberger SB, Wernovsky G, Gentles TL, et al. Factors that influence the development of atrial flutter after the Fontan operation. *J Thorac Cardiovasc Surg* 1997;113:80–86.
128. Bink-Boelkens MT, Meuzelaar KJ, Eygelaar AA. Arrhythmias after repair of secundum atrial septal defect: The influence of surgical modification. *Am Heart J* 1988;115:629–633.
129. Rhodes LA, Walsh EP, Gamble WJ, et al. Benefits and potential risks of atrial antitachycardia pacing after repair of congenital heart disease. *Pacing Clin Electrophysiol* 1995;18(pt 1):1005–1016.
130. Triedman JK, Saul JP, Weindling SN, et al. Radiofrequency ablation of intraatrial reentrant tachycardia after surgical palliation of congenital heart disease. *Circulation* 1995;91:707–714.
131. Saul JP, Walsh EP, Triedman JK. Mechanisms and therapy of complex arrhythmias in pediatric patients. *J Cardiovasc Electrophysiol* 1995;6:1129–1148.
132. Triedman JK, Alexander ME, Love BA, et al. Influence of patient factors and ablative technologies on outcomes of radiofrequency ablation of intra-atrial re-entrant tachycardia in patients with congenital heart disease. *J Am Coll Cardiol* 2002;39:1827–1835.
133. Triedman JK, Bergau DM, Saul JP, et al. Efficacy of radiofrequency ablation for control of intraatrial reentrant tachycardia in patients with congenital heart disease. *J Am Coll Cardiol* 1997;30:1032–1038.
134. Collins KK, Love BA, Walsh EP, et al. Location of acutely successful radiofrequency catheter ablation of intraatrial reentrant tachycardia in patients with congenital heart disease. *Am J Cardiol* 2000;86:969–974.
135. Gillette PC. Diagnosis and management of postoperative junctional ectopic tachycardia. *Am Heart J* 1989;118:192–194.
136. Villain E, Vetter VL, Garcia JM, et al. Evolving concepts in the management of congenital junctional ectopic tachycardia. A multicenter study [see comments]. *Circulation* 1990;81:1544–1549.
137. Sholler GF, Walsh EP, Saul JP, et al. Evaluation of a staged treatment protocol for postoperative rapid junctional ectopic tachycardia [abstract]. *Circulation* 1998;78:II597.
138. Balaji S, Sullivan I, Deanfield J, et al. Moderate hypothermia in the management of resistant automatic tachycardias in children. *Br Heart J* 1991;66(3):221–224.
139. Bash SE, Shah JJ, Albers WH. Hypothermia for the treatment of postsurgically accelerated junctional ectopic tachycardia. *J Am Coll Cardiol* 1987;10:1095–1099.
140. Till JA, Rowland E. Atrial pacing as an adjunct to the management of post-surgical His bundle tachycardia. *Br Heart J* 1991;66(3):225–229.
141. Walsh EP, Saul JP, Sholler GF, et al. Evaluation of a staged treatment protocol for rapid automatic junctional tachycardia after operation for congenital heart disease. *J Am Coll Cardiol* 1997;29:1046–1053.
142. Perry JC, Fenrich AL, Hulse JE, et al. Pediatric use of intravenous amiodarone: Efficacy and safety in critically ill patients from a multicenter protocol. *J Am Coll Cardiol* 1996;27:1246–1250.
143. Figa FH, Gow RM, Hamilton RM, et al. Clinical efficacy and safety of intravenous amiodarone in infants and children. *Am J Cardiol* 1994;74:573–577.
144. Balaji S, Gillette PC, Case CL. Successful radiofrequency ablation of permanent junctional reciprocating tachycardia in an 18-month-old child. *Am Heart J* 1994;127:1420–1421.
145. Ehlert FA, Goldberger JJ, Deal BJ, et al. Successful radiofrequency energy ablation of automatic junctional tachycardia preserving normal atrioventricular nodal conduction. *Pacing Clin Electrophysiol* 1993;16(pt 1):54–61.
146. Rychik J, Marchlinski FE, Sweeten TL, et al. Transcatheter radiofrequency ablation for congenital junctional ectopic tachycardia in infancy. *Pediatr Cardiol* 1997;18:447–450.
147. Van Hare GF, Velvis H, Langberg JJ. Successful transcatheter ablation of congenital junctional ectopic tachycardia in a ten-month-old infant using radiofrequency energy. *Pacing Clin Electrophysiol* 1990;13:730–735.
148. Young ML, Mehta MB, Martinez RM, et al. Combined alpha-adrenergic blockade and radiofrequency ablation to treat junctional ectopic tachycardia successfully without atrioventricular block. *Am J Cardiol* 1993;71:883–885.
149. Fishberger SB, Rossi AF, Messina JJ, et al. Successful radiofrequency catheter ablation of congenital junctional ectopic tachycardia with preservation of atrioventricular conduction in a 9-month-old infant. *Pacing Clin Electrophysiol* 1998;21(pt 1):2132–2135.
150. Morady F, Kadish AH, DiCarlo L, et al. Long-term results of catheter ablation of idiopathic right ventricular tachycardia. *Circulation* 1990;82:2093–2099.
151. Langberg JJ, Desai J, Dullet N, et al. Treatment of macroreentrant ventricular tachycardia with radiofrequency ablation of the right bundle branch. *Am J Cardiol* 1989;63:1010.
152. Laohakunakorn P, Paul T, Knick B, et al. Ventricular tachycardia in non-postoperative pediatric patients: Role of radiofrequency catheter ablation. *Pediatr Cardiol* 2003;24(2):154–160.
153. Stevenson WG, Khan H, Sager P, et al. Identification of reentry circuit sites during catheter mapping and radiofrequency ablation of ventricular tachycardia late after myocardial infarction. *Circulation* 1993;88(pt 1):1647–1670.
154. Biblo LA, Carlson MD. Transcatheter radiofrequency ablation of ventricular tachycardia following surgical correction of tetralogy of Fallot. *Pacing Clin Electrophysiol* 1994;17:1556–1560.
155. Burton ME, Leon AR. Radiofrequency catheter ablation of right ventricular outflow tract tachycardia late after complete repair of tetralogy of Fallot using the pace mapping technique. *Pacing Clin Electrophysiol* 1993;16:2319–2325.
156. Chinushi M, Aizawa Y, Kitazawa H, et al. Successful radiofrequency catheter ablation for macroreentrant ventricular tachycardias in a patient with tetralogy of Fallot after corrective surgery. *Pacing Clin Electrophysiol* 1995;18(pt 1):1713–1716.
157. Goldner BG, Cooper R, Blau W, et al. Radiofrequency catheter ablation as a primary therapy for treatment of ventricular tachycardia in a patient after repair of tetralogy of Fallot. *Pacing Clin Electrophysiol* 1994;17:1441–1446.
158. Moak JP. Radiofrequency ablation of arrhythmias in the pediatric patient. *Curr Opin Cardiol* 1996;11(1):81–92.
159. Schaffer MS, Gow RM, Moak JP, et al. Mortality following radiofrequency catheter ablation (from the Pediatric Radiofrequency Ablation Registry). Participating members of the Pediatric Electrophysiology Society. *Am J Cardiol* 2000;86:639–643.
160. Mantakas ME, McCue CM, Miller WW. Natural history of Wolff-Parkinson-White syndrome in infants and children: A review and a report of 28 cases. *Am J Cardiol* 1978;41:1097–1103.
161. Kugler JD. Radiofrequency catheter ablation for supraventricular tachycardia. Should it be used in infants and small children [editorial comment]? *Circulation* 1994;90:639–641.
162. Case CL, Gillette PC, Oslizlok PC, et al. Radiofrequency catheter ablation of incessant, medically resistant supraventricular tachycardia in infants and small children. *J Am Coll Cardiol* 1992;20:1405–1410.
163. Case CL, Gillette PC. Indications for catheter ablation in infants and small children with reentrant supraventricular tachycardia [letter]. *J Am Coll Cardiol* 1996;27:1551–1552.
164. Zak R. Development and proliferative capacity of cardiac muscle cells. *Circ Res* 1974;35(2 suppl II):17–26.
165. Denfield SW, Kearney DL, Michael L, et al. Developmental differences in canine cardiac surgical scars. *Am Heart J* 1993;126:382–389.
166. Erickson CC, Carr D, Greer GS, et al. Emergent radiofrequency ablation of the AV node in a neonate with unstable, refractory supraventricular tachycardia. *Pacing Clin Electrophysiol* 1995;18:1959–1962.
167. Finelli A, Rewcastle JC, Jewett MA. Cryotherapy and radiofrequency ablation: Pathophysiologic basis and laboratory studies. *Curr Opin Urol* 2003;13(3):187–191.

168. Haines DE. The biophysics of radiofrequency catheter ablation in the heart: The importance of temperature monitoring. *Pacing Clin Electrophysiol* 1993;16:586–591.

169. Haines DE, Watson DD, Verow AF. Electrode radius predicts lesion radius during radiofrequency energy heating. Validation of a proposed thermodynamic model. *Circ Res* 1990;67(1):124–129.

170. Chu E, Fitzpatrick AP, Chin MC, et al. Radiofrequency catheter ablation guided by intracardiac echocardiography. *Circulation* 1994;89:1301–1305.

171. Schiebler GL, Adams P Jr, Anderson RC. The Wolff-Parkinson-White syndrome in infants and children: A review and a report of 28 cases. *Pediatrics* 1959;24:585–603.

172. Schiebler GL, Adams P Jr, Anderson RC, et al. Clinical study of twenty-three cases of Ebstein's anomaly of the tricuspid valve. *Circulation* 1959;19:187.

173. Anderson RH, Becker AE, Arnold R, et al. The conducting tissues in congenitally corrected transposition. *Circulation* 1974;50:911–923.

174. Symons JC, Shinebourne EA, Joseph MC, et al. Criss-cross heart with congenitally corrected transposition: Report of a case with d-transposed aorta and ventricular preexcitation. *Eur J Cardiol* 1977;5:493.

175. Van Mierop LHS, Kutsche LM, Victoria BF. Ebstein's anomaly. In: Adams FH, Emmanouilides GC, Riemenschneider TA, eds. *Heart Disease in Infants, Children and Adolescents.* Baltimore: Williams & Wilkins, 1989:361–363.

176. Lev M, Gibson S, Miller RA. Ebstein's disease with Wolff-Parkinson-White syndrome: Report of a case with a histopathologic study of possible conduction pathways. *Am J Cardiol* 1955;49:724–741.

177. Levine JC, Walsh EP, Saul JP. Radiofrequency ablation of accessory pathways associated with congenital heart disease including heterotaxy syndrome. *Am J Cardiol* 1993;72:689–693.

178. Van Hare GF, Lesh MD, Stanger P. Radiofrequency catheter ablation of supraventricular arrhythmias in patients with congenital heart disease: Results and technical considerations. *J Am Coll Cardiol* 1993;22:883–890.

179. Kuck KH, Schluter M, Geiger M, et al. Radiofrequency current catheter ablation of accessory atrioventricular pathways. *Lancet* 1991;337:1557–1561.

180. Smith WM, Gallagher JJ, Kerr CR, et al. The electrophysiologic basis and management of symptomatic recurrent tachycardia in patients with Ebstein's anomaly of the tricuspid valve. *Am J Cardiol* 1982;49:1223–1234.

181. Lesh MD, Van Hare GF, Schamp DJ, et al. Curative percutaneous catheter ablation using radiofrequency energy for accessory pathways in all locations: Results in 100 consecutive patients. *J Am Coll Cardiol* 1992;19:1303–1309.

182. Twidale N, Wang X, Beckman KJ, et al. Factors associated with recurrence of accessory pathway conduction after radiofrequency catheter ablation. *Pacing Clin Electrophysiol* 1991;14:2042–2048.

183. Gallagher JJ, Pritchett ELC, Sealy WC, et al. The preexcitation syndromes. *Prog Cardiovasc Dis* 1978;20:285–327.

184. Cox JL, Gallagher JJ, Cain ME. Experience with 118 consecutive patients undergoing operation for the Wolff-Parkinson-White syndrome. *J Thorac Cardiovasc Surg* 1985;90:490–501.

185. Gillette PC, Garson A Jr, Kugler JD, et al. Surgical treatment of supraventricular tachycardia in infants and children. *Am J Cardiol* 1980;46:281–284.

186. Ott DA, Gillette PC, Garson A Jr, et al. Surgical management of refractory supraventricular tachycardia in infants and children. *J Am Coll Cardiol* 1985;5:124–129.

187. Weston LT, Hull RW, Laird JR. A prototype coronary electrode catheter for intracoronary electrogram recording. *Am J Cardiol* 1992;70:1492–1493.

188. Ho SY, Anderson RH. Embryology and anatomy of the normal and abnormal conduction system. In: Gillette PC, Garson A Jr, eds. *Pediatric Arrhythmias: Electrophysiology and Pacing.* Philadelphia: WB Saunders, 1990:2–27.

189. Wenink ACG. Congenitally complete heart block with an interrupted Mönckeberg sling. *Eur J Cardiol* 1979;9(2):89–99.

190. Bharati S, Rosen K, Steinfield L, et al. The anatomic substrate for preexcitation in corrected transposition. *Circulation* 1980;62:831–842.

191. Epstein MR, Saul JP, Weindling SN, et al. Atrioventricular reciprocating tachycardia involving twin atrioventricular nodes in patients with complex congenital heart disease. *J Cardiovasc Electrophysiol* 2001;12:671–679.

192. Walsh EP, Saul JP, Triedman JK, et al. Ablation of the "second conducting system": Mahaim fibers and "double AV nodes" in congenital heart disease [abstract]. *Circulation* 1994;90:I100.

193. Anderson RH, Arnold R, Wilkinson JL. The conducting system in congenitally corrected transposition. *Lancet* 1973;1,1286–1288.

CHAPTER 18 ■ PEDIATRIC HEART TRANSPLANTATION

MARK M. BOUCEK, MD, FRANCESCO PARISI, MD, AND ROBERT E. SHADDY, MD

Pediatric heart transplantation has been practiced for over 20 years. With the advent of the T-cell activation inhibitors such as cyclosporine, heart transplant success rates for pediatric and adult patients have improved to the point that the initially restricted ages and indications have expanded considerably. Infant heart transplantation has been performed for >15 years (1), and infants, children, and adolescents with complex cardiac anatomic lesions are now routinely successfully transplanted (2,3). There have been additional immune pharmacologic agents discovered since cyclosporine, and novel new agents are in investigational stages. The increasing experience and newer drugs promise even better long-term results. Currently the half-life (50% still alive) for children transplanted in the early 1980s is approximately 12 to 14 years (4). Decades-long survival seems likely.

Over 250 heart transplant procedures are performed annually in pediatric patients in the United States. It has been estimated that upwards of 1,000 infants and children and adolescents could benefit from heart transplantation each year. The rate-limiting step to making heart transplantation more widely available is donor availability. Matching of appropriate donors to recipients is a more complicated problem in pediatrics with fewer recipients awaiting transplant at any given time compared with adults. Thus the logistics of matching the size, blood type, and location of donor and recipient are logistically more complex.

Organ transplantation in the United States is sanctioned by congressional mandate through the National Organ Transplant Act (NOTA). NOTA created the framework for the Organ Procurement and Transplant Network (OPTN). The contractor for the OPTN is the United Network for Organ Sharing (UNOS). The process of organ donor identification is required for all hospitals, and the management of organ donors is by government-regulated local agencies called organ procurement organizations (OPOs). The decision to donate organs remains a voluntary process involving donor and family wishes. The current UNOS allocation algorithm has three status categories based on medical urgency. These categories are status IA, IB, and II. Status IA is for the sickest patients needing an urgent transplantation for survival. Waiting mortality is approximately 25% for status I patients and remains a significant problem in all age groups (5). The synchronization of recipient need, donor availability, consent for organ donation, and finally, organ transplantation is a modern medical miracle that represents the ultimate in human sharing.

At present, 1-year survival >80% and 5-year survival >65% can be expected following pediatric heart transplantation (Fig. 18.1). Morbidity other than hypertension is uncommon and catch-up growth and hemodynamic rehabilitation to normal childhood functional status is the likely outcome. The quality of life can be normal. Heart transplantation remains the only hope for children with lethal cardiomyopathy, some forms of complex congenital heart disease, and some infants and children with failed surgical interventions. This chapter discusses the indications for heart transplantation, various phases of the transplant process (preoperative, early postoperative, and late postoperative), the immunosuppressive drugs, the role of heart and lung transplantation, and the issue of retransplantation.

PRETRANSPLANT EVALUATION

A large amount of historical, anatomic, hemodynamic, metabolic, immunologic, and psychosocial information is required before deciding whether or not a child is an acceptable transplant candidate (Table 18.1). A comprehensive history and physical examination is mandatory, including age, height, weight, and body surface area. Since pediatric heart donors are matched with recipient size, accurate measurements of the recipient are critical and need to be continually updated in those patients who wait long periods of time and undergo changes in their height or weight. Cardiac diagnoses, including all previous surgeries, need to be meticulously delineated, with particular attention to venous and arterial connections, since the surgeon will need this information to devise a surgical plan in those with complex congenital heart disease with abnormal connections. The use of extended donor heart and vessel retrieval and creative intraoperative techniques has resulted in successful orthotopic heart transplantation in children with abnormal situs and/or significant systemic and pulmonary venous anomalies (2,6). Immunization status should

TABLE 18.1
ROUTINE PRETRANSPLANT EVALUATION
Comprehensive history and physical examination, including: Age, height, weight, body surface area   Diagnoses   Past medical history   Medications   Allergies   Immunization record
Laboratory data   Liver and kidney function tests   Urinalysis   Glomerular filtration rate   Prothrombin time/partial thromboplastin time   Complete blood count and differential   PPD skin test   Serologies for human immunodeficiency virus, hepatitis, cytomegalovirus, Epstein–Barr virus, *Toxoplasmosis gondii*, syphilis   ABO type   Panel reactive antibody
Consulation with dental service, or other services as indicated   Cardiopulmonary data   Cardiac catheterization and angiography   Echocardiogram   Radionuclide angiography   Endomyocardial biopsy   Electrocardiogram   Chest radiograph   Pulmonary function tests   VO$_2$ max
Psychosocial evaluation   Possible relocation   Long-term supportive care   Parental substance abuse   History of neglect or abuse

be determined, and if incomplete and prior to listing for transplant, immunizations may be given as indicated by age (7). A history of malignancy, once considered to be an absolute contraindication to transplantation, may not preclude transplantation in selected patients (8). A thorough laboratory evaluation is necessary to determine liver and kidney function since

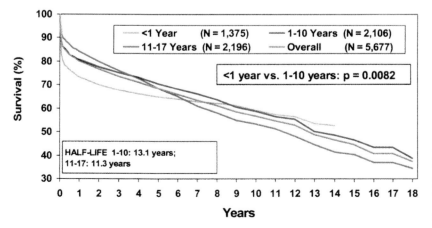

FIGURE 18.1 Actuarial survival for pediatric heart transplant recipients (UNOS/ISHLT 1982–2003) overall and by age at transplant. (From Boucek MM, Edwards LB, Keck BM, et al. Registry of the ISHLT: 8th Official Pediatric Report-2005. *J Heart Lung Transplant* 2005;24:968–982, with permission.)

severe, irreversible liver or kidney dysfunction would generally exclude the child from consideration for transplantation. An equally extensive infectious disease evaluation is necessary to exclude active infection, to determine potential latent infections such as cytomegalovirus (CMV) or Epstein-Barr virus (EBV) and to provide baseline data on susceptibilities that can be followed serially after transplant. An accurate and documented blood type is critical since this is the main compatibility factor used for donor/recipient matching.

Evaluation of the immune system is an important part of the pretransplant evaluation. Although it is common to check recipient and donor HLA status, this information is not normally part of the decision-making process when determining donor suitability. Retrospective studies have suggested that HLA compatibility is rare but may lessen rejection and improve graft survival in heart transplantation (9). In part, because of the constraints of cold ischemic time (usually about 4 hours) and the ongoing organ donor shortage, prospective HLA matching is not routinely used in heart transplantation. Panel reactive antibodies (PRA), a laboratory measure of preformed anti-human antibodies, are assayed to determine whether the recipient has any, circulating HLA alloantibodies. Because circulating donor-specific HLA alloantibodies may decrease graft survival, patients with a significantly elevated PRA before transplantation often undergo a prospective crossmatch between donor and recipient before acceptance of a donor organ (10,11). However, this can severely limit the donor pool available to a recipient, and there is evidence that patients with elevated PRAs have a higher degree of allograft loss and a higher mortality after transplantation despite a compatible cross-match (12). Because of the significant difficulties associated with finding a compatible crossmatch in patients with elevated PRAs, multiple treatment modalities, including intravenous immunoglobulin, plasmapheresis, cyclophosphamide, and more recently, rituximab, have been used with variable degrees of success to try to decrease the PRA of highly sensitized patients (13–15).

With the exception of some infants with congenital heart disease (e.g., hypoplastic left heart syndrome [HLHS]), most children will require a cardiac catheterization before heart transplantation. Cardiac catheterization and angiography should be performed as part of the pretransplant evaluation by someone experienced in the diagnosis and treatment of pediatric cardiovascular disease and heart transplantation. Especially in patients with complex congenital heart disease, hemodynamic and anatomic assessment is critical for appropriate pretransplant evaluation. In addition to precise anatomic and hemodynamic definition, it is necessary to determine whether other pharmacologic, catheter interventional, or surgical options may be necessary prior to transplantation. Patients with univentricular physiology, particularly those who have undergone multiple palliative procedures, are a unique group of patients whose pretransplant evaluation can be very complicated. For example, children after the Fontan operation may have many complications such as dysrhythmias, protein-losing enteropathy, cirrhosis, and/or low cardiac output that may bring them to transplant consideration.

Assessment of pulmonary artery anatomy, pressures and, when possible, pulmonary vascular resistance is critically important in the pretransplant evaluation of most children being assessed for heart transplantation. Severe, fixed elevation of the pulmonary vascular resistance is a contraindication to heart transplantation because of concerns of acute posttransplant donor right ventricular failure. Both elevated transpulmonary pressure gradient and elevated pulmonary vascular resistance have been identified as risk factors for early mortality after heart transplantation (16). A multi-institutional analysis of risk factors for mortality in children >1 year of age at the time of transplantation did not find elevated pulmonary vascular resistance to be a risk factor (17). The current selection criteria exclude those patients with significantly elevated nonreactive pulmonary vascular resistance (3). In these patients who are denied orthotopic heart transplantation, other options such as heterotopic heart transplantation, heart/lung transplantation, or lung transplantation with repair of the congenital heart defect may need to be considered (18,19). Accurate evaluation of the degree of pulmonary hypertension may not be possible in those patients with either discontinuous pulmonary arteries, multiple sources of pulmonary blood flow, or in those with multiple branch pulmonary artery stenoses. Various agents have been shown to have both acute and chronic beneficial effects in lowering transpulmonary gradients and pulmonary artery pressures in adults and children. Response to these agents, including intravenous nitroglycerin, nitroprusside, prostaglandin E_1, dobutamine, enoximone, milrinone, in addition to inhaled nitric oxide, has been shown to predict outcome after heart transplantation (20–24). Children with restrictive cardiomyopathy appear to be at higher risk for development and rapid progression of significant pulmonary hypertension, and thus require careful monitoring and possibly early consideration for heart transplantation (25).

Assessment of anatomy and function by a complete echocardiogram is a necessary part of the pretransplant evaluation. Cardiac MRI may also be beneficial for defining anatomy and physiology. Radionuclide angiography may be superior to echocardiography in terms of quantitating the degree of systemic ventricular dysfunction. Endomyocardial biopsy may be indicated in certain instances, for example, to exclude active myocarditis or myocardial infiltrative diseases. Electrocardiograms and 24-hour continuous ambulatory electrocardiograms may be important in determining underlying rhythm, evidence of ischemia or previous infarction, and abnormal rhythms or intervals. A chest radiograph may be very useful for measuring the degree of recipient cardiomegaly to help in determining size limitations in potential donors. In older children, pulmonary function tests may be important, especially if there is any concern of chronic lung disease.

Psychosocial evaluation is a critical part of the pretransplant evaluation. A stable family support system that is emotionally and intellectually able to provide medications and posttransplant care is crucial to the success of the heart transplant. In many instances, it is necessary for the family to relocate to be in close proximity to the transplant center for the entire waiting period before transplantation and for 3 to 6 months after the transplant. This often provides additional stressors to the family. It is uncommon to have an absolute psychosocial contraindication to pediatric heart transplantation. However, a family history of noncompliance, substance abuse, or child abuse or neglect may be a relative contraindication to transplantation. In some instances in which the patient's parents have been determined to be incapable of handling the responsibility of caring for the child before and after transplantation, it has been necessary for a relative to take over those responsibilities (7). Financial needs and resources can vary considerably and should be thoroughly evaluated.

PRETRANSPLANT MANAGEMENT

Once a patient is under consideration for transplantation, every effort must be made to stabilize or improve the patient's clinical status. Since the waiting time for donors is unpredictable, patients may wait for long periods of time, during which time ongoing pharmacologic, catheter interventional, and occasional surgical treatments must be used as needed. Patients may deteriorate rapidly while waiting for a suitable donor, in which case, more invasive measures may be necessary to bridge the patient to transplantation.

Neonates represent a large proportion of children transplanted in this country. The great majority of these infants have ductal-dependent lesions (e.g., HLHS) and thus are critically ill, chronically instrumented, and usually in an intensive care unit (ICU) awaiting transplantation (26,27). Waiting times for donors for these infants increased at many institutions from the early to the mid 1990s, increasing the challenges and problems associated with keeping these infants stable, sometimes for several months, before a suitable donor becomes available (28). Management of these infants has improved, and they can now be stabilized for several months while awaiting transplantation (29). Initial efforts must be directed toward opening and maintaining patency of the ductus arteriosus through the use of continuous infusion of prostaglandin E_1. Once unrestricted ductal patency is achieved, therapy must then be directed toward maintaining adequate systemic blood flow through proper manipulation of the pulmonary vasculature. Through a mechanism of pulmonary vasoconstriction, supplemental nitrogen can be used to maintain adequate systemic cardiac output for an extended period of time without adverse effects on the pulmonary vasculature (30,31). Some infants with HLHS have undergone percutaneous or surgical stenting of the ductus arteriosus to maintain ductal patency (32,33). Up to 50% of infants with HLHS may develop a critical restriction at the atrial septal defect (ASD) level. These infants have excessive cyanosis and hemodynamic instability and represent a high-risk group of infants who can be stabilized with interventional catheter procedures (34). Palliative surgery for a critically restrictive ASD in HLHS is risky and generally not performed.

Patients with congestive heart failure secondary to ventricular dysfunction represent a significant proportion of children who are referred for heart transplantation. The natural history of dilated cardiomyopathy in children is quite variable; thus the optimal therapy for dilated cardiomyopathy and timing for transplantation in these children is unknown. Large, multicenter, randomized studies in adults with chronic heart failure have shown a significant improvement in left ventricular performance, symptoms, and survival in patients receiving ACE inhibitors and beta-blockers such as carvedilol or metoprolol when compared with placebo controls (35–38). Addition of beta-blockers to chronic heart failure therapy in some children may improve ventricular function, symptoms, and survival, thus delaying or even precluding the need for transplantation, although further study is needed (39–44). Extracorporeal membrane oxygenation has been used successfully in children as a bridge to transplantation, but remains problematic owing to the complications of sepsis, bleeding, and neurologic injury (45). Presently available ventricular assist devices are physically restricted to older children (46,47).

Donor Issues

Because of the ongoing donor shortage for pediatric heart transplantation in this country, transplant cardiologists have made great efforts to maximize donor usage. Although optimal donors have normal cardiac anatomy and function, ideal size and blood type match, and minimal cold ischemic time, many successful pediatric heart donors have been used that did not meet these ideal criteria (1). Some degree of both systolic and diastolic dysfunction in the donor heart can be tolerated (1,48). Studies have shown successful pediatric heart transplant outcomes after donor ischemic times as long as 8 hours, with no significant differences in outcomes between those with donor ischemic times >8 hours and those with donor ischemic times ≤90 minutes (49). Although the mechanism is unclear, the use of advanced-age donor hearts (>40 years of age) carries a significantly higher 1-year posttransplant mortality than use of younger donor hearts (50). Most recently, there is increased interest and investigation into the use of non–heart beating heart donors as an additional source of donors for both adults and children (51). The increasing number of donors remains an important goal to ensure that sick patients in need of transplant have that opportunity. Based on the success of cardiac donation following SIDS, non–heart beating donation may become an important pathway to increase potential pediatric heart donors.

ABO-Incompatible Heart Transplantation

The need for matching donors and recipients can lead to donor hearts that are not used and recipients who die waiting. Blood group matching is considered critical for heart transplantation. Since infants usually lack preformed blood group antibodies, ABO-incompatible heart transplants have been successfully performed in infants <1 year old, and occasionally older patients (52). Those infants who received an ABO-incompatible graft fail to develop antibodies against the incompatible blood group epitope from the donor, while making antibodies normally to other incompatible blood groups. For example, a recipient whose blood type was O received a heart from a B donor and later made antibody to blood group A but not to blood group B. This observation has been used as an example of B-cell tolerance (53). Tolerance is the holy grail of successful transplantation. The demonstration of B-cell tolerance in infants has encouraged the hope that perhaps T-cell tolerance is also possible in infants. Tolerance would allow for transplantation without threat of rejection or the risk of immunosuppression.

POSTOPERATIVE MANAGEMENT

General Considerations

The postoperative course after heart transplantation can be complicated by numerous unique issues. Potential complications relate both to the donor and the recipient. Myocardial injury and cause of death, donor versus recipient size, donor heart ischemic time, blood and tissue compatibility, infectious status of both donor and recipient, recipient diagnosis, and recipient clinical and psychosocial conditions may affect myocardial performance and postoperative course.

The effects of brain injury and death on myocardial performance have been investigated (48,54). The process of brain death leads to myocardial dysfunction and is often due to multiple factors. Brain death itself may cause myocardial dysfunction, the donor cause of death (sepsis, trauma, etc.) can directly depress myocardial contractility, and the high catecholamine environment of stress or the pharmacologic support of the donor can lead to receptor down-regulation. Although no specific correlation with survival has been demonstrated, it is common for many centers to accept some degree of donor systolic or diastolic dysfunction, either or both of which are often reversible after transplantation. Donor ischemic time in pediatric heart transplantation has been reported by many centers to increase the postoperative need for inotropic support but to not be a risk factor for 1-year mortality (4,49,55).

As described above, ABO-incompatible heart transplants, although not a usual practice, have been successful in the first year of life before the onset of isohemagglutinin production. This practice requires particular attention to postoperative management including specific immunosuppression and transfusion protocols (52,56). In the adolescent age group, the number of patients with congenital heart disease who become transplant candidates after a long surgical and transfusional history is increasing. These patients represent an increasingly sensitized heart transplant population who require special consideration and often require preoperative and postoperative immunomodulatory treatment (15). In addition, this group of patients with congenital heart disease present unique perioperative problems related to their specific morphology, previous surgical procedures, and reconstructive surgery. Heart transplantation in children with an anatomic or physiologic single lung has been successfully performed, but pulmonary artery reconstruction increases risk for mortality (57–59). Heart transplantation for structural congenital heart disease with single ventricle physiology is associated with substantial early mortality, and transplantation after the acutely failing Fontan's may be prohibitively risky (60). In addition, a history of cardiac failure may, in many recipients, cause elevated pulmonary vascular resistances, which, while generally reversible, can represent a major complication in the immediate postoperative period. Finally, the transplanted heart is denervated and the direct coupling between cardiac and vascular systems is disturbed. Heart rate response as an additional form of myocardial reserve thus may be impaired.

Practical Considerations

Most patients can be supported with catecholamine infusions after transplant surgery and often benefit from an elevated heart rate to compensate diastolic filling abnormalities. Temporary pacing is often employed. Milrinone is often used to reduce pulmonary and systemic resistance and potentially provides a non–adrenergic-receptor–dependent form of inotropic support. The donor right ventricle is not prepared to deal with the elevation of pulmonary vascular resistances, and thus some degree of right ventricular failure is common and usually lasts from 3 to 5 days. Many agents, such as prostaglandins, prostacyclin, nitroprusside, inhaled nitric oxide, and others have been proven to be effective in these patients (24). In rare instances, right heart failure may be so severe that extracorporeal membrane oxygenation (ECMO) is required to support the circulation. Hemodynamic parameters, such as right-sided filling pressures and functional right ventricular assessment with echocardiography, can be used to follow the course of right ventricular recovery and direct appropriate weaning from supportive measures.

The early posttransplant period (<30 days) is the most hazardous. Primary graft failure and early morbidity are largely explained by recipient issues that increase perioperative risk (61). Review of the UNOS/International Society of Heart and Lung Transplantation (ISHLT) Scientific Registry details several significant risk factors for 1-year mortality:

1. Congenital diagnosis, on ECMO (relative risk: 4.16)
2. Congenital diagnosis, no ECMO (relative risk: 2.19)
3. ECMO, diagnosis other than congenital (relative risk: 1.9)
4. Year of transplant: 1995 versus 1998 (relative risk: 1.9)
5. Year of transplant: 1996 versus 1998 (relative risk: 1.62)
6. Hospitalized (including ICU) (relative risk: 1.55)
7. Year of transplant 1997 versus 1998 (relative risk: 1.5)
8. On ventilator (relative risk: 1.35)
9. Female recipient (relative risk: 1.22).

A preventive therapy with selective vasodilators as well as the availability of mechanical assist devices during and after heart transplantation can reduce deleterious effects of both transitional pulmonary hypertension and primary graft failure (62).

Immunosuppression is started in the perioperative period. Many institutions begin calcineurin inhibitors (cyclosporine or tacrolimus) just before the transplant operation. High-dose corticosteroids are given intraoperatively and continued for 48 hours, after which they can be discontinued or decreased to a low-dose maintenance regimen. Additional immunosuppressive medications may be given postoperatively in the form of polyclonal antibodies directed toward multiple T-cell epitopes (Atgam, ATG), or either chimeric or humanized monoclonal antibodies directed toward the interleukin-2 (IL-2) activation pathway (CD25) (63). This induction therapy may provide potential benefits by preventing early acute rejection episodes and allowing delayed administration of calcineurin inhibitors or steroid avoidance. Because they are very well tolerated, anti–IL-2 receptor antibodies are increasingly used in preference to rabbit-antithymocyte globulin, but the former have not yet been proven to be more effective or to be less toxic than polyclonal agents (64). Other maintenance immunosuppressants include azathioprine or mycophenolate mofetil, and in a few selected cases, rapamycin. Data from the Pediatric Heart Transplant Study, a research study group of 23 North American centers, show that approximately two thirds of recipients are free from rejection by 1 month after transplantation, but this has fallen to under one third by 1 year. The peak hazard, or instantaneous risk, for rejection is around 1 to 2 months after transplantation (65). Older age at transplantation represents the strongest predictor of risk for first rejection and a risk for an increased number of episodes of rejection within the first 6 months after transplantation.

Institutional preference usually dictates whether endomyocardial biopsy or echocardiography is used as the primary rejection-surveillance tool. Because of the inconvenience, greater technical challenges, and possible increased morbidity of biopsy in smaller children, there has been much interest in evaluating the role of echocardiography in children undergoing transplantation (66–71). Many quantitative echocardiographic parameters have been investigated, including various measures of systolic and diastolic function, changes in left ventricular wall thickness and mass, and development of mitral regurgitation or pericardial effusion. Doppler studies and tissue characterization have also been evaluated. Despite this interest, the controversy over the role of echocardiography is far from resolved. Furthermore, if the gold standard for diagnosing allograft rejection after heart transplantation is still considered the endomyocardial biopsy (72–75), the value of routine surveillance biopsies is also controversial in children. In fact, many centers have discontinued routine surveillance biopsies after the first or second year from transplantation. The need for noninvasive diagnosis of rejection has stimulated the ongoing search for bio-humoral markers, such as B-type natriuretic peptide, vascular endothelial growth factors (VEGF), or enzyme-linked immunosorbent assay (ELISA)-detected anti-HLA antibodies. The clinical relevance is still to be defined for all these markers (76–78).

Clinical evaluation of rejection is important but can be misleading, particularly in pediatric patients where infectious issues can mimic the presentation of rejection. The characteristic infiltration of the donor heart by lymphocytes leads to the diagnosis of rejection on endomyocardial biopsy (79). However, as many as 10% to 20% of rejection episodes that impair graft function lack the typical lymphocyte infiltration, some of which have been labelled "vascular or humoral rejection," despite that lack of convincing evidence for either a vascular or antibody etiology (80). Patients who have been transfused or palliated with human allografts at the time of previous surgery may become sensitized to a wide variety of human leukocyte antigens (81). These patients are at increased risk of allograft rejection. Preoperative and postoperative strategies to reduce this risk include treatment with intravenous immunoglobulin, agents that may inhibit the production of antibodies by B cells, and plasmapheresis. Arrhythmias also may be a marker for rejection. The surface electrocardiogram may suggest atrial flutter or atrioventricular dissociation, but this observation may be attributed to the fact the recipient atrial tissue contracts independently of the donor atrial tissue, and there may be two p waves present on the surface electrocardiogram that are not synchronous. The vast majority of initial rejection episodes can be successfully reversed by high-dose corticosteroids alone or in conjunction with anti–T-cell antibodies. Intravenous methylprednisolone (10 to 30 mg/kg every 12 hours) is the first line in rejection therapy. Repeat episodes of rejection can be more difficult to treat and can result in graft loss and patient death.

Immunosuppressive Medications

Immunosuppression is considered a necessary evil for successful transplantation. Ideally, manipulation of immune mechanisms to promote tolerance to foreign antigens is the goal of immunosuppression. In fact, tolerance may require stimulation of certain immune pathways rather than immunosuppression. An unintended consequence of immunosuppression may be to inhibit the active immune process of tolerance. A class of T cells, designated T_{REG}, can prevent exuberant immune reaction, are critical to recognition and tolerance of "self," could play a critical role in immune tolerance after transplantation, and may be suppressed by current medications used posttransplant (82). The data on long-term outcome posttransplant for infants suggests a window of opportunity for successful transplantation in infancy that may involve tolerizing mechanisms. The clinical experience and laboratory data following ABO-incompatible transplantation in infancy demonstrate tolerance at least in the B-cell lineage. T cells are also likely involved in the ABO-incompatible experience and support the idea that tolerance could be a realistic goal for infants after unmatched transplantation.

The class of drugs that inhibit T-cell activation are still the mainstay of immunosuppressive therapy. Cyclosporine was the first drug of this class to reach clinical utility in the early 1980s and in effect began the modern era of solid organ transplantation. Cyclosporine can be given initially intravenously in a dose of 0.03 to 0.1 mg/kg/hr. When oral medications can be tolerated, the usual dose is approximately three times the intravenous dose or 2 to 6 mg/kg/day divided every 8 hours in infants and every 12 hours in older children. Blood levels of cyclosporine must be monitored to ensure efficacy and avoid toxicity. The therapeutic dose for blood levels for the active compound, cyclosporine A, range from 100 to 350 ng/mL. Higher blood levels are usually maintained in the first year posttransplant and tapered based on time posttransplant and clinical course. The bioavailability of cyclosporine is variable, particularly in children, although the microemulsion preparations have improved bioavailability (83). Multi-institutional studies comparing cyclosporine with tacrolimus have shown no clear clinical or survival advantage for either in heart transplant recipients, and the selection of a primary calcineurin inhibitor is often institutional specific. (84). Drug and food interactions are common with immunosuppressive agents and should be carefully evaluated when starting new drugs, even antibiotics or foods such as grapefruit.

Tacrolimus acts at a different site in the IL-2 activation pathway of lymphocytes. Like cyclosporine, it can be given intravenously in a dosage of 0.03 of 0.05 mg/kg/hr. When given orally, the dosage is usually 0.05 to 0.1 mg/kg/day divided twice daily. Trough blood levels must be monitored. The usual therapeutic range is 5–15 ng/mL. The third agent in this class (T-cell activation inhibitors) is rapamycin (sirolimus). Rapamycin acts at a more distal site (TOR receptor) in the lymphocyte activation cascade by blocking transcription of activation genes. It may be more efficacious than either cyclosporine or tacrolimus, and combinations with cyclosporine have been promising in early clinical trials (85). Rapamycin can inhibit smooth muscle proliferation and may have another advantage by inhibiting the process of coronary vasculopathy (86). The dosing and monitoring of rapamycin in pediatric patients is not well defined. The usual dosage is 1 to 2 mg/m²/day with levels of 2 to 10 ng/mL at present in heart transplant. Rapamycin is most often used in combination with a calcineurin inhibitor. However, rapamycin may be less nephrotoxic over the long term and has been tried as the sole T-cell activation inhibition in liver, renal, and most recently, heart transplant recipients, with encouraging early results (87–89).

Antiproliferative Agents

Historically, the most commonly used agent to block immune cell proliferation was azathioprine. It is a nonselective inhibitor causing nonspecific bone marrow suppression. The usual dosage is 2 mg/kg/day as a single daily dose, and drug effect is monitored by the white blood count. The white blood count is usually maintained at >4,000/mL and <12,000/mL. Mycophenolic acid in the form of mycophenolate mofetil (MMF) inhibits the de novo pathway for purine synthesis. Since lymphocytes lack the salvage pathway, MMF can selectively block lymphocyte proliferation without the side effects of nonspecific bone marrow suppression. The improved selectivity compared with azathioprine may provide more effective immunosuppression (90). Because of these benefits, MMF is rapidly replacing azathioprine in many transplant protocols. Comparative studies in adult heart transplantation indicate an efficacy benefit for MMF over azathioprine (91). The usual dosage of MMF in children is 25 to 50 mg/kg/day, but absorption varies widely and higher doses may be required. In adults and adolescents, the dosage of MMF is 3 gm/day divided twice daily. Blood levels are still not widely available but are useful owing to interindividual variability. The effective blood level for mycophenolic acid has been reported as 3–7 ng/mL (92). Methotrexate and cyclophosphamide have also been used in transplant recipients as adjunctive therapy for chronic/recurrent rejection (93,94).

Nonspecific Immunosuppression

Corticosteroids are potent immunosuppressive agents and are the first line of rejection therapy. Many centers also use corticosteroids as part of routine immunosuppression. In pediatric patients, the side effects of corticosteroids have encouraged many programs to attempt to discontinue routine oral steroids (95). The favorable experience in pediatric heart transplant with a corticosteroid-free maintenance protocol has led to its use with other pediatric solid organ transplant recipients. For rejection, methylprednisolone is given in a dosage of 10 to 30 mg/kg every 12 hours intravenously for six to eight doses. A tapering dose may then be used to return to usual maintenance oral doses of prednisone or discontinued depending on the policy of each individual program. The dosage for maintenance oral prednisone is in the range of 0.1 to 1 mg/kg/day.

All the current immunosuppressive medications do not lead to tolerance in humans, although they can lead to tolerance in experimental models. The transplanted graft must work for many decades in pediatric recipients. To reduce the burden of immunosuppressive drugs, the drive to develop tolerizing protocols for infants and children is pressing. Recent studies with ABO incompatible transplantation in infants and the description of T_{REG} have invigorated the search for tolerizing protocols in pediatric heart transplantation.

LATE FOLLOW-UP

The number of pediatric heart transplants performed worldwide markedly increased in the late 1980s and has since plateaued (4). The 5- to 10-year survival after pediatric heart transplantation can be achieved with good quality of life, although long-term concerns remain regarding rejection, infection, cardiac allograft vasculopathy (CAV), and complications of chronic immunosuppression, including malignancy, hypertension, renal insufficiency, as well as compliance with therapy (96). Data from the Registry of the ISHLT show a different late survival for young-childhood-age recipients and adolescent recipients: When looking at conditional survival (i.e., subsequent survival for recipients who survived at least 1 year after transplant), both the infants (age <1 year) and children (age 1 to 10 years) show a significantly lower risk of late mortality than adolescents (age 11 to 17 years). The conditional graft half-life was 17.5 years for childhood-age recipients and 13.7 years for adolescent recipients. In addition to immunologic factors that favor transplantation in the first year of life (97), reduced compliance to therapies in adolescent-age patients may play a key role in determining these results. Many centers have reported that incomplete adherence with immunosuppressive therapy is the leading cause of late death in the adolescents. In this section we will discuss some of the important facets of long-term follow-up of pediatric heart transplant recipients, including routine health care maintenance issues and potential complications that may occur.

Health Care Maintenance

Transplantation programs have recommended that in the unimmunized child, immunizations should follow the usual schedule for polio (using killed virus), diphtheria, pertussis, tetanus, hepatitis B, and *Haemophilus influenzae*, beginning between the third and fourth postoperative month (98).

Pneumococcal vaccine is also recommended (99). The use of live viral vaccines is still debated. These vaccines are usually avoided, despite the apparent ability of pediatric heart transplant recipients to effectively overcome viral infections. Particularly, the measles, mumps, and rubella vaccine is deferred in most centers. Generally, to reduce the risk of morbidity and mortality from these preventable diseases, it is important that physicians caring for pediatric transplant recipients update the immunization status of their patients. As with all children, pediatric heart transplant recipients can have fevers and require prompt evaluation for these. Fortunately, most acute febrile illnesses in these patients are not serious and can be managed safely in an outpatient setting (100).

Quality of Life and Rehabilitation

Children have very good quality of life and rehabilitation after heart transplantation. Key pediatric issues after transplantation include psychosocial support for patients and families with regard to school, growth, development, and future expectations (101). Heart transplantation in children aged 5 to 18 years seems to be associated with an ongoing deficit in parent-perceived physical health status (102). Most children grow at a normal rate after transplantation, showing normal onset and progression of puberty. However, catch-up growth may not be observed. This seems related to the types of heart disease, the age at transplantation, and the immunosuppressive regimen (103–105). Most children and adolescents have the capacity for healthy cognitive and psychological functioning after heart transplantation. Nevertheless, approximately 20% of pediatric heart recipients have abnormal neurologic examinations and 25% have emotional adjustment difficulties (106). Adolescent poor compliance or noncompliance represents part of these difficulties. Some centers have reported an incidence of noncompliance as high as 20% in their pediatric heart transplant population. Late rejection, associated with poor outcome, is often associated with nonadherence and adolescent age (107). Older children return to school and a more normal lifestyle after transplantation and express an improvement in the quality of their lives. Rehabilitation of the pediatric heart transplant recipient depends on the age of the patient and the degree of illness before and after transplantation. Exercise capacity in infants and children after cardiac transplantation is within low-normal parameters. The persistence of some chronotropic incompetence may contribute to the lesser exercise capacity (108). Exercise should be encouraged in this population. Benefits include improved blood glucose control, increase in bone density, and potential psychological enrichment. Return to age-appropriate activities including a physical education class can be achieved in most patients within the first 6 months after transplantation (109). Patients with neurologic deficits may require special treatment programs.

Arrhythmias

Significant arrhythmias after transplantation are relatively uncommon and when they occur may be indicative of graft problems such as rejection. Onset of supraventricular and ventricular tachyarrhythmias correlate highly with rejection (110). Ventricular arrhythmias also may be indicative of CAV. Posttransplantation symptomatic sinus bradycardia and heart block requiring pacemaker placement have been described in a few children (111).

Rejection

One of the most important factors in reducing the risk of and morbidity from rejection is to maintain regular and frequent routine office visits for all pediatric heart transplant patients. Evidence of rejection in infants and small children ranges from no symptoms to a wide variety of nonspecific symptoms including tachycardia, tachypnea, lethargy, irritability, poor feeding, and fever. Physical signs are similar to those in adults, including jugular venous distention, organomegaly, new murmur, and gallop rhythm. Children who have no rejection in the first year posttransplantation may be at lower risk for hemodynamically compromising rejection late after transplantation. Also biopsy-negative rejection—at times presenting with severe left ventricular dysfunction and negative cellular infiltration on biopsy—can occur late after transplantation. These patients can improve with augmented immunosuppression including plasmapheresis, cyclophosphamide, and agents suppressing antibody production, but their long-term outcome remains guarded (112). Either cellular or humoral rejection can present as recurrent or refractory: In these cases, treatment strategies can include several immunosuppressant combinations and total lymphoid irradiation (113). Generally, late rejection can be an ominous sign and may be predictive of graft loss. Episodes of late rejection with or without hemodynamic compromise always raise the concern of noncompliance.

Infection

Pediatric heart transplant recipients are at risk for serious and opportunistic infections, including bacterial, viral (especially cytomegalovirus [CMV]), and protozoal (*Pneumocystis*) infections, particularly in the first 6 months after heart transplantation when immunosuppression is greatest. Because of the significant postoperative risk of infection, many centers use some form of prophylaxis against fungal (nystatin), CMV (acyclovir or ganciclovir in recipients who receive organs from CMV-positive donors), and/or protozoal (trimethoprim/sulfamethoxazole) infections, although exact indication and duration of prophylaxis are unknown. The Pediatric Heart Transplant Study Group reported the time-related risk of serious infection and death in a large pediatric heart transplant population from 22 participating centers in the United States (114). The most common types of infections were bacterial in 60%, followed by CMV (18%), other viral infections (13%), fungal (7%), and protozoal (2%). The peak hazard for bacterial and fungal infections was in the first month after transplantation, whereas the peak hazard for viral infection was in the second month after transplantation, with the most common virus being CMV. Availability of ganciclovir, development of assays for rapid diagnosis of active infection, such as PP65 antigenemia test and polymerase chain reaction detection of viral genome, have reduced the risk of CMV disease. Identification of viral genome, particularly adenovirus, in the myocardium of pediatric transplant recipients appears to be predictive of adverse clinical events, including CAV and graft loss (115). The risk of all types of infections is very low by 6 months posttransplantation, but a low risk persists indefinitely. Exposure to pets is controversial, but most centers recommend avoidance of cat feces because of the risk of toxoplasmosis and avoidance of reptiles because of the risk of *Salmonella*. Although infective endocarditis is a rare complication after heart transplantation, many centers recommend endocarditis prophylaxis long-term after heart transplantation before dental, upper respiratory, gastrointestinal, and genitourinary tract procedures that are likely to cause bacteremia.

Malignancy, Epstein-Barr Virus Infection, and Posttransplant Lymphoproliferative Disorders

An increased risk of malignancy is a well-recognized complication after organ transplantation. In pediatric heart transplant recipients, the incidence of neoplasms appears to be equal to or greater than that observed in adult recipients (116). The vast majority are lymphoproliferative disorders and are associated with primary infection with Epstein-Barr virus. The pathology of early-onset disease is usually polymorphic, whereas late expression, usually >3 years, is often monomorphic and lymphomatous (65). Lymphoma accounts for about 8% of the deaths occurring 5 years after transplantation. First-line treatment remains the reduction of immunosuppression with good results in almost 50% of cases. Monomorphic disease may require treatment with conventional chemotherapeutic agents. More recently, other therapies have been proposed. As >90% of lymphoproliferative disorders are of recipient B-cell origin after heart transplantation, the use of monoclonal antibodies directed against B-cell antigen (rituximab) has been successful (117,118). The development of quantitative Epstein-Barr virus polymerase chain reaction on peripheral blood samples represents the most useful technique for diagnosing and monitoring disorders driven by this virus. The development of very high viral loads should alert the physician to look for signs or symptoms of disease, even in the asymptomatic patient. Another novel approach is cellular immunotherapy, whereby the patient is given infusion of Epstein-Barr virus–specific cytotoxic T cells. This strategy has already been successfully applied in bone marrow transplant recipients (119). Reports of malignant neoplasia other than lymphoma are rare in transplanted children. These include squamous cell carcinomas and other skin cancers. Therefore, children should be advised to avoid excessive sun exposure and use sunscreen.

Chronic Rejection and Cardiac Allograft Vasculopathy

CAV is the major factor limiting long-term survival after pediatric heart transplantation. CAV is manifested pathologically by a diffuse and accelerated form of coronary disease consisting of myointimal proliferation that is concentric and involves the entire length of the vessel, including intramyocardial branches. Eventually, luminal occlusion occurs. There may also be a pronounced inflammatory component (120). The cause of CAV remains obscure, but most investigators agree that CAV is primarily an immune-mediated disease and thus can be considered the major manifestation of chronic rejection. Immunologic events interact with nonimmunologic risk factors, such as donor age and hypertension, graft ischemia/reperfusion injury, in addition to recipient hypertension, hyperlipidemia, obesity, diabetes, smoking, race, and gender (121). CMV infection after transplantation also has been associated with the development of CAV. The final common pathway of these mechanisms is endothelial activation, a prothrombotic environment, and endothelial damage with subsequent diffuse intimal proliferation. Identification of specific risk factors for development of disease in children has recently been investigated (122). The major risk factors were older recipient and donor age and two or more episodes of rejection in the first year. Late rejection episodes and late pacemaker requirement appear to be other independent predictors of CAV in children (123). Patients suffering from severe late rejection or presenting with

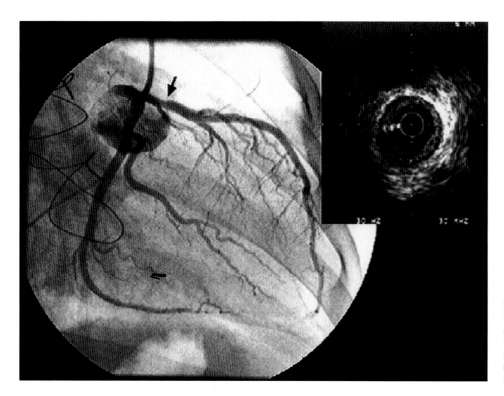

FIGURE 18.2 Selected posttransplantation left coronary angiogram demonstrating proximal left anterior descending (LAD) lesion which appeared minimal by angiography but demonstrated prominent intimal thickening on intravascular ultrasonography (*inset*).

symptoms of high-grade atrioventricular block must be monitored aggressively and should be evaluated closely for the presence or development of CAV.

The incidence of CAV in children is less than that in adults (75% of pediatric patients CAV-free at 7 years after transplant), but recipient age has been significantly related to freedom from CAV (4). Infant recipients appear to have the lowest risk of CAV. It is possible that pediatric recipients have less CAV than adults because of fewer persisting donor factors or because of fewer nonimmune risk factors. However, the actual incidence of CAV in children is probably being underestimated because of the lack of reliable methods for diagnosing and monitoring the disease. Therefore, few data are currently available regarding natural history of the disease in children. Because the cardiac allograft is not innervated, angina is an uncommon presenting symptom of CAV. Clinical symptoms are generally limited to congestive heart failure with allograft dysfunction, silent myocardial infarction, or sudden death. Coronary angiography is still the first modality for diagnosing CAV, although it is well appreciated that this modality underestimates the incidence and severity of disease. Dobutamine stress echocardiography is a safe, noninvasive technique that may be useful in diagnosing and following CAV in children (124,125). More recently, intravascular ultrasound appears more sensitive than angiography in detecting CAV, also in pediatric heart recipients, but prospective multicenter studies are needed to know how to best use this technique in this patient population (126,127) (Fig. 18.2). The ideal management of CAV is unknown; intervention or surgical management has had limited utility whereas medical management appears to have some promise. Coronary interventional procedures can be safely used in pediatric heart transplant recipients for palliation of CAV (128). Medical treatment has primarily been directed toward attempts to decrease the progression of the disease by using preventive measures and manipulation of immunosuppression. A reduction in the incidence of CAV has been found after treatment with pravastatin in adult patients (129). In pediatric patients, pravastatin and atorvastatin as well have been found safe and effective for reducing total cholesterol and low-density lipoprotein, but long-term studies are required to evaluate the effect on the incidence of CAV (130,131). Nevertheless, the clinical use of statins is now common in most pediatric heart transplant centers. More recently, a new class of immunosuppressants, proliferation signal inhibitors, sirolimus and everolimus, have been studied. A recent multicenter trial in adult heart transplant recipients has provided evidence that everolimus can reduce both the incidence and severity of CAV in de novo heart transplant recipients (132). No data are yet available in the pediatric population. However, the mainstay of therapy for established, severe CAV remains retransplantation.

Complications of Immunosuppression

Because two of the main functions of the immune system are fighting infection and tumor surveillance, all immunosuppressants put the patient at risk for infection and malignancy. Additionally, individual immunosuppressant medications have significant adverse effects, even when properly used in appropriate doses. Hypertension is a common complication after transplantation and may represent in part an adverse effect of cyclosporine, particularly when used in combination with routine prednisone. Catastrophic neurologic complications have resulted from severe postoperative hypertension and require urgent treatment. Chronic hypertension appears to be less prevalent in pediatric heart transplant recipients than in adults, but it is still a problem requiring treatment, even in centers using a steroid-sparing maintenance immunosuppressive protocol. Antihypertensive therapy in these children should be similar to that used for adults, including calcium channel blockers and angiotensin-converting enzyme inhibitors.

Neurotoxicity is another recognized complication of cyclosporine, occurring in as many as 10% to 25% of patients, with a peak in the early postoperative period. Symptoms include tremors, restlessness, dysesthesias of the palms and soles, seizures, and altered mental status. Cyclosporine and tacrolimus (calcineurin inhibitors) may cause acute and chronic renal insufficiency, and monitoring for renal insufficiency in children should be lifelong. The vast majority of published reports do not provide evidence for differences in calcineurin inhibitor doses and blood levels between patients who maintain normal renal function and those who develop renal dysfunction. Recently, it has been suggested that individual susceptibility, which includes $TGF\beta_1$ gene polymorphism, could play a role in the long-term outcome of renal function in patients with calcineurin inhibitor–based immunosuppression (133). Strategies to minimize long-term exposure to calcineurin inhibitors may reduce the prevalence of renal insufficiency in this vulnerable population (134,135). These strategies include reduction of calcineurin inhibitors dosage, replacement of azathioprine by mycophenolate mofetil, and the use of antiproliferative agents like sirolimus and everolimus (136).

A high prevalence of lipoprotein abnormalities has been described among pediatric heart transplant recipients (137). Again, the use of cyclosporine and steroids has been associated with this disorder. Therefore, the increasing use of lipid-lowering agents also in pediatric patients appears justified. Posttransplant diabetes mellitus is present in approximately 2% of pediatric recipients with cyclosporine-based immunosuppression, but in 8% of recipients with tacrolimus-based immunosuppression (138,139). Diabetes may be related to reversible insulin resistance. Tacrolimus levels, HLA-DR mismatch, and older age at transplant may predispose to posttransplant diabetes. Gastrointestinal complications can also occur during the follow-up of pediatric heart transplant recipients. They include cholelithiasis, intestinal pneumatosis, and colitis (140–142). Rapamycin reportedly has less nephrotoxicity than cyclosporine or tacrolimus but has been associated with severe stomatitis and frequent elevations in cholesterol and lipid profiles (143). Rapamycin has growth factor antagonist properties and may cause marrow suppression, particularly when used in combination with other agents that can suppress the marrow such as tacrolimus or MMF.

Miscellaneous

Infants with hypoplastic left heart syndrome who undergo heart transplantation require extended reconstruction of their aortic arch. Of these, as many as 20% will develop coarctation of the aorta that may require treatment. Although surgical repair may be necessary in complex obstructive lesions, balloon coarctation angioplasty is a safe and effective treatment in most situations (144). Tricuspid regurgitation secondary to valve damage from endomyocardial biopsies is an uncommon but potentially hemodynamically significant complication. Attempts to minimize the number of biopsies, careful placement of the biopsy catheter, or the use of a long sheath may reduce the incidence of this complication. Anemia is highly prevalent in children after heart transplantation. The cause of this is uncertain, but usually is not secondary to iron deficiency (145).

Retransplantation

Experience with pediatric cardiac retransplantation is limited. Nevertheless, in the most recent summary of the Registry of the ISHLT, the number of patients undergoing retransplantation has increased to 6% for recipients between 11 and 17 years of age (4). The most common indications for retransplantation are CAV, followed by acute rejection, chronic rejection, and intraoperative donor organ failure. Elective retransplantation can be performed with acceptable mortality. The intermediate outcome is similar to that of children undergoing primary cardiac transplantation (146). When retransplantation is performed in the setting of early primary graft failure, the results are quite poor, and the appropriateness of this strategy is questionable in light of the limited donor supply (147). Although at present retransplant is uncommon, it would seem reasonable to expect the numbers to increase in the growing number of long-term survivors following primary transplantation. Encouragingly, the outcomes following retransplantation after a long intertransplant interval are equivalent to the outcomes following primary transplant (146). The medical and pharmacologic issues after retransplant mimic those following primary transplant.

Heterotopic and Heart–Lung Transplantation

Experience with heterotopic heart transplantation in children is limited. The main indications for this procedure are primarily the presence of fixed high pulmonary vascular resistance that precludes orthotopic heart transplantation, although some consider availability of an undersized donor or expectation of a certain degree of recipient heart recovery to be indications as well. One and 5-year actuarial survival rates have been reported to be as high as 83% and 66%, respectively. Thus, in selected patients, heterotopic heart transplantation may be considered an alternative, particularly when pulmonary vascular resistance is excessively high for orthotopic heart transplantation. Another alternative in this situation is heart–lung transplantation. The volume of pediatric heart–lung transplantation decreased significantly in the 2000s both in frequency and in survival rates (4). Thus the ongoing role of this procedure in the management of irreversible pediatric cardiopulmonary disease seems uncertain. In effect, the poor late survival after heart–lung transplant tracks the poor late survival seen after lung transplant alone. Another alternative that has met with some success in the setting of excessively high, fixed pulmonary vascular resistance in those patients with unrepaired congenital heart lesions is the performance of single-lung transplantation and repair of the congenital heart lesion.

References

1. Boucek MM, Kanakriyeh MS, Mathis CM, et al. Cardiac transplantation in infancy: Donors and recipients. Loma Linda University Pediatric Heart Transplant Group [see comments]. *J Pediatr* 1990;116(2): 171–176.
2. Mayer JE Jr. Cardiac transplantation for neonates with hypoplastic left heart syndrome [editorial comment]. *Ann Thorac Surg* 1990;50:864–865.
3. Webber SA, Fricker FJ, Michaels M, et al. Orthotopic heart transplantation in children with congenital heart disease. *Ann Thorac Surg* 1994;58: 1664–1669.
4. Boucek MM, Edwards LB, Keck BM, et al. Registry of the International Society for Heart and Lung Transplantation: Eighth official pediatric report—2005. *J Heart Lung Transplant* 2005;24:968–982.

5. McGiffin DC, Naftel DC, Kirklin JK, et al. Pediatric Heart Transplant Study Group. Predicting outcome after listing for heart transplantation in children: Comparison of Kaplan-Meier and parametric competing risk analysis. *J Heart Lung Transplant* 1997;16:713–722.

6. Chartrand C, Dumont L, Stanley P. Pediatric cardiac transplantation. *Transplant Proc* 1989;21:3349–3350.

7. Addonizio LJ. Cardiac transplantation in the pediatric patient. *Prog Cardiovasc Dis* 1990;33(1):19–34.

8. Levitt G, Bunch K, Rogers CA, et al. Cardiac transplantation in childhood cancer survivors in Great Britain. *Eur J Cancer* 1996;32A:826–830.

9. Opelz G, Wujciak T. The influence of HLA compatibility on graft survival after heart transplantation. The Collaborative Transplant Study [see comments]. *N Engl J Med* 1994;330:816–819.

10. Jacobs JP, Quintessenza JA, Boucek RJ, et al. Pediatric cardiac transplantation in children with high panel reactive antibody. *Ann Thorac Surg* 2004;78:1703–1709.

11. Smith JD, Danskine AJ, Laylor RM, et al. The effect of panel reactive antibodies and the donor specific crossmatch on graft survival after heart and heart-lung transplantation. *Transplant Immunol* 1993;1(1):60–65.

12. Kobashigawa JA, Sabad A, Drinkwater D, et al. Pretransplant panel reactive-antibody screens. Are they truly a marker for poor outcome after cardiac transplantation? *Circulation* 1996;94(suppl):II294–297.

13. Tyan DB, Li VA, Czer L, et al. Intravenous immunoglobulin suppression of HLA alloantibody in highly sensitized transplant candidates and transplantation with a histoincompatible organ. *Transplantation* 1994;57:553–562.

14. McIntyre JA, Higgins N, Britton R, et al. Utilization of intravenous immunoglobulin to ameliorate alloantibodies in a highly sensitized patient with a cardiac assist device awaiting heart transplantation. Fluorescence-activated cell sorter analysis. *Transplantation* 1996;62:691–693.

15. Shaddy RE, Fuller TC. The sensitized pediatric heart transplant candidate: Causes, consequences, and treatment options. *Pediatr Transplant* 2005;9(2):208–214.

16. Kirklin JK, Naftel DC, Kirklin JW, et al. Pulmonary vascular resistance and the risk of heart transplantation. *J Heart Transplant* 1988;7(5):331–336.

17. Shaddy RE, Naftel DC, Kirklin JK, et al. Outcome of cardiac transplantation in children. Survival in a contemporary multi-institutional experience. Pediatric Heart Transplant Study. *Circulation* 1996;94(suppl): II69–73.

18. Khaghani A, Santini F, Dyke CM, et al. Heterotopic cardiac transplantation in infants and children [see comments]. *J Thorac Cardiovasc Surg* 1997;113:1042–1048; discussion 1048–1049.

19. Spray TL, Mallory GB, Canter CE, et al. Pediatric lung transplantation for pulmonary hypertension and congenital heart disease. *Ann Thorac Surg* 1992;54(2):216–223; discussion 224–225.

20. Murali S, Uretsky BF, Armitage JM, et al. Utility of prostaglandin E1 in the pretransplantation evaluation of heart failure patients with significant pulmonary hypertension [see comments]. *J Heart Lung Transplant* 1992;11(pt 1):716–723.

21. Zales VR, Pahl E, Backer CL, et al. Pharmacologic reduction of pretransplantation pulmonary vascular resistance predicts outcome after pediatric heart transplantation. *J Heart Lung Transplant* 1993;12(pt 1):965–972; discussion 972–973.

22. Gajarski RJ, Towbin JA, Bricker JT, et al. Intermediate follow-up of pediatric heart transplant recipients with elevated pulmonary vascular resistance index. *J Am Coll Cardiol* 1994;23:1682–1687.

23. Kieler-Jensen N, Lundin S, Ricksten SE. Vasodilator therapy after heart transplantation: Effects of inhaled nitric oxide and intravenous prostacyclin, prostaglandin E1, and sodium nitroprusside. *J Heart Lung Transplant* 1995;14:436–443.

24. Shaddy RE. Pulmonary hypertension in pediatric heart transplantation. *Prog Pediatr Cardiol* 2000;11(2):131–136.

25. Denfield SW, Rosenthal G, Gajarski RJ, et al. Restrictive cardiomyopathies in childhood. Etiologies and natural history. *Tex Heart Inst J* 1997;24(1):38–44.

26. Boucek RJ Jr, Chrisant MR. Cardiac transplantation for hypoplastic left heart syndrome. *Cardiol Young* 2004;14(suppl 1):83–87.

27. Chrisant MR, Naftel DC, Drummond-Webb J, et al. Fate of infants with hypoplastic left heart syndrome listed for cardiac transplantation: A multicenter study. *J Heart Lung Transplant* 2005;24:576–582.

28. Sable CA, Shaddy RE, Suddaby EC, et al. Impact of prolonged waiting times of neonates awaiting heart transplantation. *J Perinatol* 1997;17(6):481–488.

29. Mitchell MB, Campbell DN, Clarke DR, et al. Infant heart transplantation: Improved intermediate results. *J Thorac Cardiovasc Surg* 1998;116(2):242–252.

30. Day RW, Tani LY, Minich LL, et al. Congenital heart disease with ductal-dependent systemic perfusion: Doppler ultrasonography flow velocities are altered by changes in the fraction of inspired oxygen. *J Heart Lung Transplant* 1995;14:718–725.

31. Bourke KD, Sondheimer HM, Ivy DD, et al. Improved pretransplant management of infants with hypoplastic left heart syndrome enables discharge to home while waiting for transplantation. *Pediatr Cardiol* 2003;24:538–543.

32. Ruiz CE, Gamra H, Zhang HP, et al. Brief report: Stenting of the ductus arteriosus as a bridge to cardiac transplantation in infants with the hypoplastic left-heart syndrome. *N Engl J Med* 1993;328:1605–1608.

33. Boucek MM, Mashburn C, Chan KC. Catheter-based interventional palliation for hypoplastic left heart syndrome. *Semin Thorac Cardiovasc Surg Pediatr Card Surg Annu* 2005;8:72–77.

34. Canter CE, Moorehead S, Huddleston CB, et al. Restrictive atrial septal communication as a determinant of outcome of cardiac transplantation for hypoplastic left heart syndrome. *Circulation* 1993;88(pt 2):II456–460.

35. Bristow MR, Gilbert EM, Abraham WT, et al. Carvedilol produces dose-related improvements in left ventricular function and survival in subjects with chronic heart failure. MOCHA Investigators. *Circulation* 1996;94:2807–2816.

36. Packer M, Colucci WS, Sackner-Bernstein JD, et al. Double-blind, placebo-controlled study of the effects of carvedilol in patients with moderate to severe heart failure. The PRECISE Trial. Prospective Randomized Evaluation of Carvedilol on Symptoms and Exercise [see comments]. *Circulation* 1996;94:2793–2799.

37. Effect of metoprolol CR/XL in chronic heart failure: Metoprolol CR/XL Randomised Intervention Trial in Congestive Heart Failure (MERIT-HF). *Lancet* 1999;353:2001–2007.

38. Packer M, Fowler MB, Roecker EB, et al. Effect of carvedilol on the morbidity of patients with severe chronic heart failure: Results of the carvedilol prospective randomized cumulative survival (COPERNICUS) study. *Circulation* 2002;106:2194–2199.

39. Shaddy RE, Tani LY, Gidding SS, et al. Beta-blocker treatment of dilated cardiomyopathy with congestive heart failure in children: A multi-institutional experience. *J Heart Lung Transplant* 1999;18:269–274.

40. Bruns LA, Chrisant MK, Lamour JM, et al. Carvedilol as therapy in pediatric heart failure: An initial multicenter experience. *J Pediatr* 2001;138(4):505–511.

41. Gachara N, Prabhakaran S, Srinivas S, et al. Efficacy and safety of carvedilol in patients with dilated cardiomyopathy: A preliminary report. *Indian Heart J* 2001;53(1):74–78.

42. Azeka E, Franchini Ramires JA, et al. Delisting of infants and children from the heart transplantation waiting list after carvedilol treatment. *J Am Coll Cardiol* 2002;40:2034–2038.

43. Shaddy RE, Curtin EL, Sower B, et al. The Pediatric Randomized Carvedilol Trial in Children with Heart Failure: Rationale and design. *Am Heart J* 2002;144(3):383–389.

44. Rusconi P, Gomez-Marin O, Rossique-Gonzalez M, et al. Carvedilol in children with cardiomyopathy: 3-year experience at a single institution. *J Heart Lung Transplant* 2004;23:832–838.

45. Gajarski RJ, Mosca RS, Ohye RG, et al. Use of extracorporeal life support as a bridge to pediatric cardiac transplantation. *J Heart Lung Transplant* 2003;22:28–34.

46. Ibrahim AE, Duncan BW, Blume ED, et al. Long-term follow-up of pediatric cardiac patients requiring mechanical circulatory support. *Ann Thorac Surg* 2000;69:186–192.

47. Duncan BW. Mechanical circulatory support for infants and children with cardiac disease. *Ann Thorac Surg* 2002;73:1670–1677.

48. Paul JJ, Tani LY, Shaddy RE, et al. Spectrum of left ventricular dysfunction in potential pediatric heart transplant donors. *J Heart Lung Transplant* 2003;22:548–552.

49. Scheule AM, Zimmerman GJ, Johnston JK, et al. Duration of graft cold ischemia does not affect outcomes in pediatric heart transplant recipients. *Circulation* 2002;106(suppl):I163–167.

50. Chin C, Miller J, Robbins R, et al. The use of advanced-age donor hearts adversely affects survival in pediatric heart transplantation. *Pediatr Transplant* 1999;3(4):309–314.

51. Singhal AK, Abrams JD, Mohara J, et al. Potential suitability for transplantation of hearts from human non-heart-beating donors: Data review from the Gift of Life Donor Program. *J Heart Lung Transplant* 2005;24:1657–1664.

52. West LJ, Pollock-Barziv SM, Dipchand AI, et al. ABO-incompatible heart transplantation in infants. *N Engl J Med* 2001;344:793–800.

53. Fan X, Ang A, Pollock-Barziv SM, et al. Donor-specific B-cell tolerance after ABO-incompatible infant heart transplantation. *Nat Med* 2004;10:1227–1233.

54. Odim J, Laks H, Banerji A, et al. Does duration of donor brain injury affect outcome after orthotopic pediatric heart transplantation? *J Thorac Cardiovasc Surg* 2005;130:187–193.

55. Morgan JA, John R, Park Y, et al. Successful outcome with extended allograft ischemic time in pediatric heart transplantation. *J Heart Lung Transplant* 2005;24:58–62.

56. Dellgren G, Coles JG. Pediatric heart transplantation: Improving results in high-risk patients. *Semin Thorac Cardiovasc Surg Pediatr Card Surg Annu* 2001;4:103–114.

57. Chen JM, Davies RR, Mital SR, et al. Trends and outcomes in transplantation for complex congenital heart disease: 1984 to 2004. *Ann Thorac Surg* 2004;78:1352–1361; discussion 1352–1361.

58. Groetzner J, Reichart B, Roemer U, et al. Cardiac transplantation in pediatric patients: Fifteen-year experience of a single center. *Ann Thorac Surg* 2005;79:53–60; discussion 61.

59. Lamour JM, Hsu DT, Quaegebeur JM, et al. Heart transplantation to a physiologic single lung in patients with congenital heart disease. *J Heart Lung Transplant* 2004;23:948–953.

60. Michielon G, Parisi F, Squitieri C, et al. Orthotopic heart transplantation for congenital heart disease: An alternative for high-risk Fontan candidates? *Circulation* 2003;108(suppl 1):II140–149.

61. Huang J, Trinkaus K, Huddleston CB, et al. Risk factors for primary graft failure after pediatric cardiac transplantation: Importance of recipient and donor characteristics. *J Heart Lung Transplant* 2004;23:716–722.

62. Schindler E, Muller M, Akinturk H, et al. Perioperative management in pediatric heart transplantation from 1988 to 2001: Anesthetic experience in a single center. *Pediatr Transplant* 2004;8(3):237–242.

63. Boucek MM, Pietra B, Sondheimer H, et al. Anti-T-cell-antibody prophylaxis in children: Success with a novel combination strategy of mycophenolate mofetil and antithymocyte serum. *Transplant Proc* 1997;29(8A): 16S–20S.

64. Di Filippo S. Anti-IL-2 receptor antibody vs polyclonal anti-lymphocyte antibody as induction therapy in pediatric transplantation. *Pediatr Transplant* 2005;9:373–380.

65. Webber SA. The current state of, and future prospects for, cardiac transplantation in children. *Cardiol Young* 2003;13(1):64–83.

66. Boucek MM, Mathis CM, Boucek RJ Jr, et al. Prospective evaluation of echocardiography for primary rejection surveillance after infant heart transplantation: Comparison with endomyocardial biopsy. *J Heart Lung Transplant* 1994;13(pt 1):66–73.

67. Asante-Korang A, Fickey M, Boucek MM, et al. Diastolic performance assessed by tissue Doppler after pediatric heart transplantation. *J Heart Lung Transplant* 2004;23:865–872.

68. Levi DS, DeConde AS, Fishbein MC, et al. The yield of surveillance endomyocardial biopsies as a screen for cellular rejection in pediatric heart transplant patients. *Pediatr Transplant* 2004;8(1):22–28.

69. Boucek RJ Jr, Boucek MM, Asante-Korang A. Advances in methods for surveillance of rejection. *Cardiol Young* 2004;14(suppl 1):93–96.

70. Mooradian SJ, Goldberg CS, Crowley DC, et al. Evaluation of a noninvasive index of global ventricular function to predict rejection after pediatric cardiac transplantation. *Am J Cardiol* 2000;86(3):358–360.

71. Kimball TR, Semler DC, Witt SA, et al. Noninvasive markers for acute heart transplant rejection in children with the use of automatic border detection. *J Am Soc Echocardiogr* 1997;10:964–972.

72. Chin C, Naftel DC, Singh TP, et al. Risk factors for recurrent rejection in pediatric heart transplantation: A multicenter experience. *J Heart Lung Transplant* 2004;23:178–185.

73. Wagner K, Oliver MC, Boyle GJ, et al. Endomyocardial biopsy in pediatric heart transplant recipients: a useful exercise? (Analysis of 1,169 biopsies.) *Pediatr Transplant* 2000;4(3):186–192.

74. Kirklin JK. Is biopsy-proven cellular rejection an important clinical consideration in heart transplantation? *Curr Opin Cardiol* 2005;20(2): 127–131.

75. Rosenthal DN, Chin C, Nishimura K, et al. Identifying cardiac transplant rejection in children: Diagnostic utility of echocardiography, right heart catheterization and endomyocardial biopsy data. *J Heart Lung Transplant* 2004;23:323–329.

76. Lindblade CL, Chun DS, Darragh RK, et al. Value of plasma B-type natriuretic peptide as a marker for rejection in pediatric heart transplant recipients. *Am J Cardiol* 2005;95:909–911.

77. Abramson LP, Pahl E, Huang L, et al. Serum vascular endothelial growth factor as a surveillance marker for cellular rejection in pediatric heart transplantation. *Transplantation* 2002;73(1):153–156.

78. Di Filippo S, Girnita A, Webber SA, et al. Impact of ELISA-detected anti-HLA antibodies on pediatric cardiac allograft outcome. *Hum Immunol* 2005;66:513–518.

79. Billingham ME, Cary NR, Hammond ME, et al. A working formulation for the standardization of nomenclature in the diagnosis of heart and lung rejection: Heart Rejection Study Group. The International Society for Heart Transplantation. *J Heart Transplant* 1990;9:587–593.

80. Zales VR, Crawford S, Backer CL, et al. Spectrum of humoral rejection after pediatric heart transplantation. *J Heart Lung Transplant* 1993;12: 563–571; discussion 572.

81. Shaddy RE, Hunter DD, Osborn KA, et al. Prospective analysis of HLA immunogenicity of cryopreserved valved allografts used in pediatric heart surgery. *Circulation* 1996;94:1063–1067.

82. Wood KJ, Sakaguchi S. Regulatory T cells in transplantation tolerance. *Nat Rev Immunol* 2003;3(3):199–210.

83. Barone G, Chang CT, Choc MG Jr, et al. The pharmacokinetics of a microemulsion formulation of cyclosporine in primary renal allograft recipients. The Neoral Study Group. *Transplantation* 1996;61:875–880.

84. Reichart B, Meiser B, Vigano M, et al. European Multicenter Tacrolimus (FK506) Heart Pilot Study: One-year results—European Tacrolimus Multicenter Heart Study Group. *J Heart Lung Transplant* 1998;17:775–781.

85. Keogh A, Richardson M, Ruygrok P, et al. Sirolimus in de novo heart transplant recipients reduces acute rejection and prevents coronary artery disease at 2 years: A randomized clinical trial. *Circulation* 2004;110: 2694–2700.

86. Gregory CR. Immunosuppressive approaches to the prevention of graft vascular disease. *Transplant Proc* 1998;30:878–880.

87. Fairbanks KD, Eustace JA, Fine D, et al. Renal function improves in liver transplant recipients when switched from a calcineurin inhibitor to sirolimus. *Liver Transplant* 2003;9:1079–1085.

88. Knechtle SJ, Pirsch JD, Fechner JH Jr, et al. Campath-1H induction plus rapamycin monotherapy for renal transplantation: Results of a pilot study. *Am J Transplant* 2003;3:722–730.

89. Hunt J, Lerman M, Magee MJ, et al. Improvement of renal dysfunction by conversion from calcineurin inhibitors to sirolimus after heart transplantation. *J Heart Lung Transplant* 2005;24:1863–1867.

90. Kobashigawa J, Miller L, Renlund D, et al. A randomized active-controlled trial of mycophenolate mofetil in heart transplant recipients. Mycophenolate Mofetil Investigators. *Transplantation* 1998;66:507–515.

91. Eisen HJ, Kobashigawa J, Keogh A, et al. Three-year results of a randomized, double-blind, controlled trial of mycophenolate mofetil versus azathioprine in cardiac transplant recipients. *J Heart Lung Transplant* 2005;24:517–525.

92. Oellerich M, Armstrong VW, Schutz E, et al. Therapeutic drug monitoring of cyclosporine and tacrolimus. Update on Lake Louise Consensus Conference on cyclosporin and tacrolimus. *Clin Biochem* 1998;31(5): 309–316.

93. Ross HJ, Gullestad L, Pak J, et al. Methotrexate or total lymphoid radiation for treatment of persistent or recurrent allograft cellular rejection: A comparative study. *J Heart Lung Transplant* 1997;16:179–189.

94. Shaddy RE, Bullock EA, Tani LY, et al. Methotrexate therapy in pediatric heart transplantation as treatment of recurrent mild to moderate acute cellular rejection. *J Heart Lung Transplant* 1994;13:1009–1013.

95. Boucek RJ Jr, Boucek MM. Pediatric heart transplantation. *Curr Opin Pediatr* 2002;14:611–619.

96. Sigfusson G, Fricker FJ, Bernstein D, et al. Long-term survivors of pediatric heart transplantation: A multicenter report of sixty-eight children who have survived longer than five years [see comments]. *J Pediatr* 1997;130:862–871.

97. Ibrahim JE, Sweet SC, Flippin M, et al. Rejection is reduced in thoracic organ recipients when transplanted in the first year of life. *J Heart Lung Transplant* 2002;21:311–318.

98. Neu A, Fivush BA. Recommended immunization practices for pediatric renal transplant recipients. *Pediatr Transplant* 1998;2:263–269.

99. Stovall SH, Ainley KA, Mason EO Jr, et al. Invasive pneumococcal infections in pediatric cardiac transplant patients. *Pediatr Infect Dis J* 2001;20:946–950.

100. Crandall WV, Norlin C, Bullock EA, et al. Etiology and outcome of outpatient fevers in pediatric heart transplant patients. *Clin Pediatr (Phila)* 1996;35(9):437–442.

101. Kichuk-Chrisant MR. Children are not small adults: Some differences between pediatric and adult cardiac transplantation. *Curr Opin Cardiol* 2002;17(2):152–159.

102. Hirshfeld AB, Kahle AL, Clark BJ 3rd, et al. Parent-reported health status after pediatric thoracic organ transplant. *J Heart Lung Transplant* 2004;23:1111–1118.

103. de Broux E, Huot CH, Chartrand S, et al. Growth after pediatric heart transplantation. *Transplant Proc* 2001;33:1735–1737.

104. Hathout EH, Chinnock RE. Growth after heart transplantation. *Pediatr Transplant* 2004;8(2):97–100.

105. Cohen A, Addonizio LJ, Softness B, et al. Growth and skeletal maturation after pediatric cardiac transplantation. *Pediatr Transplant* 2004;8(2): 126–135.

106. DeMaso DR, Douglas Kelley S, Bastardi H, et al. The longitudinal impact of psychological functioning, medical severity, and family functioning in pediatric heart transplantation. *J Heart Lung Transplant* 2004;23:473–480.

107. Ringewald JM, Gidding SS, Crawford SE, et al. Nonadherence is associated with late rejection in pediatric heart transplant recipients. *J Pediatr* 2001;139(1):75–78.

108. Abarbanell G, Mulla N, Chinnock R, et al. Exercise assessment in infants after cardiac transplantation. *J Heart Lung Transplant* 2004;23:1334–1338.

109. Fricker F. Should physical activity and/or competitive sports be curtailed in pediatric heart transplant recipients? *Pediatr Transplant* 2002;6:267–269.

110. Collins KK, Thiagarajan RR, Chin C, et al. Atrial tachyarrhythmias and permanent pacing after pediatric heart transplantation. *J Heart Lung Transplant* 2003;22:1126–1133.

111. Chinnock RE, Torres VI, Jutzy RV, et al. Cardiac pacemakers in pediatric heart transplant recipients: Incidence, indications, and associated factors. Pediatric Heart Transplant Group—Loma Linda. *Pacing Clin Electrophysiol* 1996;19:26–30.

112. Pahl E, Crawford SE, Cohn RA, et al. Reversal of severe late left ventricular failure after pediatric heart transplantation and possible role of plasmapheresis. *Am J Cardiol* 2000;85:735–739.

113. Asano M, Gundry SR, Razzouk AJ, et al. Total lymphoid irradiation for refractory rejection in pediatric heart transplantation. *Ann Thorac Surg* 2002;74:1979–1985.

114. Schowengerdt KO, Naftel DC, Seib PM, et al. Infection after pediatric heart transplantation: Results of a multiinstitutional study. The Pediatric Heart Transplant Study Group. *J Heart Lung Transplant* 1997;16:1207–1216.

115. Shirali GS, Ni J, Chinnock RE, et al. Association of viral genome with graft loss in children after cardiac transplantation. *N Engl J Med* 2001;344:1498–1503.

116. Boyle GJ, Michaels MG, Webber SA, et al. Posttransplantation lymphoproliferative disorders in pediatric thoracic organ recipients. *J Pediatr* 1997;131(2):309–313.

117. Herman J, Vandenberghe P, van den Heuvel I, et al. Successful treatment with rituximab of lymphoproliferative disorder in a child after cardiac transplantation. *J Heart Lung Transplant* 2002;21:1304–1309.

118. Webber S, Fine R, McGhee W, et al. Anti-CD20 monoclonal antibody (rituximab) for pediatric post-transplant lymphoproliferative disorders: A preliminary multicenter experience [abstract]. *Am J Transplant* 2001;1(suppl 1):469.

119. Khanna R, Bell S, Sherritt M, et al. Activation and adoptive transfer of Epstein-Barr virus-specific cytotoxic T cells in solid organ transplant patients with posttransplant lymphoproliferative disease. *Proc Natl Acad Sci USA* 1999;96:10391–10396.

120. Billingham ME. Histopathology of graft coronary disease. *J Heart Lung Transplant* 1992;11(pt 2):S38–44.

121. Costanzo MR, Naftel DC, Pritzker MR, et al. Heart transplant coronary artery disease detected by coronary angiography: A multiinstitutional study of preoperative donor and recipient risk factors. Cardiac Transplant Research Database. *J Heart Lung Transplant* 1998;17:744–753.

122. Pahl E, Naftel DC, Kuhn MA, et al. The impact and outcome of transplant coronary artery disease in a pediatric population: A 9-year multi-institutional study. *J Heart Lung Transplant* 2005;24:645–651.

123. Webber SA, Naftel DC, Parker J, et al. Late rejection episodes more than 1 year after pediatric heart transplantation: Risk factors and outcomes. *J Heart Lung Transplant* 2003;22:869–875.

124. Pahl E, Crawford SE, Swenson JM, et al. Dobutamine stress echocardiography: Experience in pediatric heart transplant recipients. *J Heart Lung Transplant* 1999;18:725–732.

125. Di Filippo S, Semiond B, Roriz R, et al. Non-invasive detection of coronary artery disease by dobutamine-stress echocardiography in children after heart transplantation. *J Heart Lung Transplant* 2003;22:876–882.

126. Kuhn MA, Jutzy KR, Deming DD, et al. The medium-term findings in coronary arteries by intravascular ultrasound in infants and children after heart transplantation. *J Am Coll Cardiol* 2000;36(1):250–254.

127. Costello JM, Wax DF, Binns HJ, et al. A comparison of intravascular ultrasound with coronary angiography for evaluation of transplant coronary disease in pediatric heart transplant recipients. *J Heart Lung Transplant* 2003;22:44–49.

128. Shaddy RE, Revenaugh JA, Orsmond GS, et al. Coronary interventional procedures in pediatric heart transplant recipients with cardiac allograft vasculopathy. *Am J Cardiol* 2000;85:1370–1372.

129. Kobashigawa JA, Moriguchi JD, Laks H, et al. Ten-year follow-up of a randomized trial of pravastatin in heart transplant patients. *J Heart Lung Transplant* 2005;24:1736–1740.

130. Chin C, Gamberg P, Miller J, et al. Efficacy and safety of atorvastatin after pediatric heart transplantation. *J Heart Lung Transplant* 2002;21:1213–1217.

131. Penson MG, Fricker FJ, Thompson JR, et al. Safety and efficacy of pravastatin therapy for the prevention of hyperlipidemia in pediatric and adolescent cardiac transplant recipients. *J Heart Lung Transplant* 2001;20:611–618.

132. Eisen HJ, Tuzcu EM, Dorent R, et al. Everolimus for the prevention of allograft rejection and vasculopathy in cardiac-transplant recipients. *N Engl J Med* 2003;349:847–858.

133. Di Filippo S, Zeevi A, McDade KK, et al. Impact of TGFbeta1 gene polymorphisms on late renal function in pediatric heart transplantation. *Hum Immunol* 2005;66(2):133–139.

134. Alonso EM. Long-term renal function in pediatric liver and heart recipients. *Pediatr Transplant* 2004;8(4):381–385.

135. Boyer O, Le Bidois J, Dechaux M, et al. Improvement of renal function in pediatric heart transplant recipients treated with low-dose calcineurin inhibitor and mycophenolate mofetil. *Transplantation* 2005;79:1405–1410.

136. Groetzner J, Kaczmarek I, Meiser B, et al. Sirolimus and mycophenolate mofetil as calcineurin inhibitor-free immunosuppression in a cardiac transplant patient with chronic renal failure. *J Heart Lung Transplant* 2004;23:770–773.

137. Chin C, Rosenthal D, Bernstein D. Lipoprotein abnormalities are highly prevalent in pediatric heart transplant recipients. *Pediatr Transplant* 2000;4(3):193–199.

138. Paolillo JA, Boyle GJ, Law YM, et al. Posttransplant diabetes mellitus in pediatric thoracic organ recipients receiving tacrolimus-based immunosuppression. *Transplantation* 2001;71(2):252–256.

139. Hathout EH, Chinnock RE, Johnston JK, et al. Pediatric post-transplant diabetes: Data from a large cohort of pediatric heart-transplant recipients. *Am J Transplant* 2003;3:994–998.

140. Rakhit A, Nurko S, Gauvreau K, et al. Gastrointestinal complications after pediatric cardiac transplantation. *J Heart Lung Transplant* 2002;21:751–759.

141. Sakopoulos AG, Gundry S, Razzouk AJ, et al. Cholelithiasis in infant and pediatric heart transplant patients. *Pediatr Transplant* 2002;6(3):231–234.

142. Fleenor JT, Hoffman TM, Bush DM, et al. Pneumatosis intestinalis after pediatric thoracic organ transplantation. *Pediatrics* 2002;109(5):E78.

143. Chueh SC, Kahan BD. Dyslipidemia in renal transplant recipients treated with a sirolimus and cyclosporine-based immunosuppressive regimen: Incidence, risk factors, progression, and prognosis. *Transplantation* 2003;76(2):375–382.

144. Shirali GS, Cephus CE, Kuhn MA, et al. Posttransplant recoarctation of the aorta: A twelve year experience. *J Am Coll Cardiol* 1998;32(2):509–514.

145. Embleton ND, O'Sullivan JJ, Hamilton JR, et al. High prevalence of anemia after cardiac transplantation in children. *Transplantation* 1997;64:1590–1594.

146. Kanter KR, Vincent RN, Berg AM, et al. Cardiac retransplantation in children. *Ann Thorac Surg* 2004;78:644–649; discussion 644–649.

147. Mahle WT, Vincent RN, Kanter KR. Cardiac retransplantation in childhood: Analysis of data from the United Network for Organ Sharing. *J Thorac Cardiovasc Surg* 2005;130:542–546.

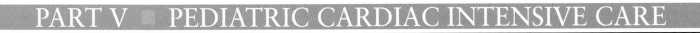

PART V ■ PEDIATRIC CARDIAC INTENSIVE CARE

CHAPTER 19 ■ PHYSIOLOGY OF THE PRETERM AND TERM INFANT

TIMOTHY M. HOFFMAN, MD, AND STEPHEN E. WELTY, MD

Approach to the care of the neonate with congenital heart disease is multidisciplinary. Whether the neonates are cared for in a dedicated cardiac intensive care unit with neonatology consultation or are cared for in the neonatal intensive care unit with cardiology consultation, a firm understanding of neonatal physiology and development is imperative to provide state-of-the-art interdisciplinary care. This chapter provides a unique perspective of the neonate via a multiorgan system approach. Cardiac lesion-specific data are outlined throughout the textbook; therefore, this chapter will not include a discussion of these conditions. Instead, this chapter focuses on the complex interactions of multiple organ systems in neonates who also have congenital heart disease. In addition, an overview of lung development and the management of a patent ductus arteriosus in premature infants is presented.

TRANSITIONAL CIRCULATION

With the onset of spontaneous respiration, the low-resistance placenta is removed from the circulation, thus increasing systemic vascular resistance. Expansion of the lungs elicits an immediate decrease in the pulmonary vascular resistance owing to the physical recruitment of pulmonary vasculature and via the vasodilation of the pulmonary arteriolar bed because of elevated oxygen content. In turn, the shift of the systemic and pulmonary vascular resistances causes a reversal of flow of the ductus arteriosus from right to left to predominantly left to right. In theory, this change from fetal circulation causes an increase in pulmonary blood flow and a decrease in systemic venous return owing to the lack of umbilical venous flow. Left atrial pressure increases and will eventually exceed the pressure in the right atrium. This pressure change may lead to closure of the foramen ovale flap against the crista dividens, eliminating shunting at the atrial level. All of these alterations may be influenced by disease processes that influence the systemic and pulmonary vascular resistances, inhibiting the usual transition to adult circulation (1,2). Additionally, after the initial precipitous fall in pulmonary vascular resistance, it continues to fall gradually in the first 48 hours of life and takes several weeks to fall to adult levels. In a normal neonate, the ductus generally closes functionally within several days of life.

PATENT DUCTUS ARTERIOSUS

Classic studies by Gittenberger-De Groot (3) have described the sequence of events that occur in infants that lead to functional and anatomic closure of the ductus arteriosus in infants. The molecular events explaining closure and the predisposition of the ductus to remain patent in premature infants have been described (4–8). Ductal closure is dependent on initial ductal constriction, which is associated with the media of the structure developing hypoxia. Hypoxia mediates a series of molecular events that then lead to disruption of the internal elastic lamina and endothelial cell. Smooth muscle cells proliferate, forming intimal mounds that impinge on the ductal lumen, ultimately leading to its anatomic closure. In premature infants, ductal constriction is essential for anatomic closure of the ductus arteriosus. But this alone may not be sufficient for ductal closure. Hypoxia in the muscular media may not occur, and the postconstriction sequence fails to follow. Thus, premature infants may present with a symptomatic patent ductus arteriosus (PDA), especially those who are <30 weeks gestation.

The incidence of PDA in premature infants is inversely related to gestational age. In a recent multicenter trial of indomethacin prophylaxis in premature infants weighing <1,000 g, the incidence of PDA in the placebo group was 50% (9). Premature infants with a PDA may present with classic findings of a left-to-right shunting lesion. In this case, infants may have a systolic murmur, increased left precordial activity, sometimes with a thrill, bounding pulses, and a wide pulse pressure that also may be evident on umbilical arterial waveform tracings. Unfortunately, many infants with a physiologically significant PDA may not have these findings. Thus there should be a high index of suspicion for a PDA even without classic physical findings in a premature infant who has lung disease. Doppler-echocardiography is the gold standard for diagnosing a PDA and should be done before treatment decisions are made.

The physiology of the PDA is secondary to overperfusion of the lung and possibly underperfusion of the systemic circulation. Infants' lungs are fully recruited at rest so that any increase in flow from left-to-right shunts predictably increases fluid filtration in the lung (10). Increased fluid filtration will lead to pulmonary edema if it exceeds the ability of the lymphatics to remove fluid, and pulmonary edema is frequently associated with pulmonary overcirculation from a PDA. The PDA may also steal from the systemic circulation. Animal studies have shown that even small shunts underperfuse systemic organs (10). Studies in extremely premature infants with a hemodynamically significant PDA observed that although total left ventricular output was increased, flow was decreased in the abdominal aorta, celiac, mesenteric, and renal arteries, whereas there were no differences in the anterior cerebral artery flow (11). Although the changes in acute physiology are concerning, the effect of PDA on the outcome of premature infants and the management of PDA is controversial (12,13).

Various approaches to the PDA in premature infants have included expectant management and treatment of congestive symptoms (14), to aggressive management with PDA ligation in the first day of life (15). Although there is no consensus for treatment of premature infants with a PDA, most centers now use one of two approaches. Indomethacin is the primary medical therapy for closure of the PDA. Indomethacin prophylaxis is given to infants born at <27 to 28 weeks gestation at 24-hour intervals during the first 3 days of life. This approach decreases the occurrence of a clinically significant ductus and lessens the need for surgical ligation. This strategy does not significantly change the incidence of other clinically relevant outcomes in these infants. The prophylaxis approach means that infants who would not develop a clinically significant PDA will undergo indomethacin treatment, but this approach has also been found to be safe, despite some short-term effects on renal function (16). Another approach for the premature infant with a PDA is to treat with indomethacin as soon as signs and symptoms are present, before the development of congestive symptoms. Using this approach, most premature infants with PDA are treated around 72 hours of life and, typically, higher doses of indomethacin are used. Despite these approaches, extremely premature infants with PDA may need ligation. In infants <27 to 28 weeks gestation, it is optimal to document closure at around 1 week of life, and if the ductus is not closed, ligation should probably be performed.

LUNG DEVELOPMENT

Lung development from the embryonic phase to the alveolar phase has been studied in humans and in many mammals (17–20). Furthermore, the molecular basis for lung development continues to be elucidated, and a discussion of the mechanisms for lung development is beyond the scope of this chapter. However, since lung development proceeds through postnatal life for several years, understanding the effects on lung development of congenital heart disease, its treatment, and supportive medical care for lung disease is important. Overall lung development can be optimized in infants with respiratory disease and heart disease whether they are born prematurely or not.

Infants born as early as 23 weeks gestation can survive. At 23 weeks gestation, infants are still in the canalicular phase of lung development, which continues through 26 weeks gestation. Despite the relatively immature lung architecture, including no identifiable alveoli and a thickened alveolar interstitium with a double capillary network, the lung can subserve enough air exchange function for the infant to survive. The saccular phase of lung development extends from 27 to 36 weeks gestation, and the alveolar phase starts at 37 weeks and proceeds through approximately 3 years of postnatal age. In infants born prematurely without heart disease, supportive care with mechanical ventilation and supplemental oxygen frequently injures the lung and predisposes the infant to the development of chronic bronchopulmonary dysplasia (BPD) (21). Furthermore, perinatal inflammation of the lung is frequently observed in premature infants, which also can injure the lung profoundly (22). The injury caused by lung support and/or inflammation leads to an arrest of lung development, and the lung function abnormalities can persist for years (23,24). Thus in infants, especially premature infants who have heart disease and require supportive care delivered to the respiratory system, therapies should be pursued that limit lung injury and thereby limit aberrations in lung development, similar to treatment strategies being explored in infants born prematurely who do not have heart disease.

The most important intervention to improve the outcomes of premature infants is the administration of antenatal steroids to mothers who are at risk of delivering a premature infant. The landmark study by Liggins and Howie (25) demonstrated a beneficial effect of antenatal steroids given to mothers who delivered infants at <34 weeks gestation. These results have been verified by many other randomized, double-blinded, placebo-control trials. Although the initial studies focused on decreasing the incidence of respiratory distress, there was also evidence that antenatal corticosteroid (ACS) administration decreased mortality and other morbidities in premature infants (26–28). ACS administration enhanced lung and circulatory development, so much so that an NIH consensus statement stated strongly that ACS should be given to mothers with threatened premature delivery at between 24 and 34 weeks gestation (29). Details for ACS administration can be found in the NIH consensus statement. There is no present evidence that supports repeat ACS administration to those mothers who do not deliver within 1 week of steroid administration (30).

Surfactant administration has been shown to improve outcomes in premature infants. Exogenous surfactant has been given in prophylactic and rescue modes. In the prophylaxis studies of premature infants who were at high risk of having respiratory distress syndrome (RDS), surfactant administration was given within 15 to 20 minutes of birth. This led to lower mortality rates and less morbidity than was seen in infants who were given surfactant after the diagnosis of RDS was established (selective) (31). These differences are less relevant in more mature infants. Thus, infants born after 30 weeks of gestation can be assessed for development of RDS, and if RDS is present, surfactant should be delivered in the rescue mode (32).

Other therapeutic measures in premature infants that help to prevent development of BPD include (a) monitoring to prevent hyperoxemia and minimize exposure to supplemental oxygen and mechanical ventilation, (b) fluid restriction in the first few days of life (33), and (c) the institution of aggressive and early parenteral and enteral nutrition. The combination of therapies just discussed is supported in premature infants without congenital heart disease. However, there are no reports regarding the impact of congenital heart disease on lung development in premature infants, or on postnatal lung development in term infants. Acute management of premature infants with congenital heart disease is thus extrapolated from what has been observed in premature infants without heart disease.

PULMONARY HYPERTENSION

Abnormalities of smooth muscle development frequently influence acute cardiopulmonary physiology in newborn infants. Pulmonary hypertension is frequently present when there is abnormal smooth muscle development. Pulmonary hypertension presenting in the newborn period is classified into three separate categories based on the underlying mechanisms for the development of the disorder. The three categories include underdevelopment, maldevelopment, and maladaptive forms. In this classification only underdevelopment and maldevelopment pulmonary hypertension are associated with abnormalities of smooth muscle development. In fetal development, airway branching and smooth muscle development occur in parallel in an environment where pulmonary vascular resistance is high and blood flow is low. In normal lung development, smooth muscle development around the vasculature extends to the level of the respiratory bronchiole. When the fetus is compromised by poor placental function and high placental vascular resistance, smooth muscle development is altered so that it extends farther out the pulmonary vasculature and is thicker. The thickening occurs as a combination of intimal and adventitial thickening, which gives rise to maldevelopment pulmonary hypertension (34). Underdevelopment pulmonary hypertension is associated with pulmonary hypoplasia, which leads to a decreased cross-sectional surface area of the pulmonary vascular bed. In addition, underdevelopment pulmonary hypertension is frequently associated with maldevelopment of the pulmonary vasculature (35).

Infants with maldevelopment pulmonary hypertension frequently present with evidence of poor placental function and poor adaptation to their extrauterine environment. Evidence for poor placental function may present as a poorly nourished infant with evidence of fetal weight loss. The perinatal period is often associated with marked fetal distress because labor taxes the function of the compromised placenta. Thick meconium may be noted, and the infant may be depressed or asphyxiated at birth. Even without these adverse perinatal events, the abnormal pulmonary vascular bed may not allow the normal rapid initial drop in pulmonary vascular resistance and subsequent increase in pulmonary blood flow, which are essential for appropriate cardiopulmonary physiology and adaptation to an adult-type circulation in series with high pulmonary blood flow and air exchange in the lung.

RESPIRATORY PHYSIOLOGY

In the fetus, the organ of respiration is the placenta and the lung is a high-resistance, minimal flow, liquid-filled organ. Furthermore, the fetal lung secretes fluid into the airway (36). During late gestation, surfactant production increases in preparation for the lung becoming the organ of respiration, and the molecular processes essential for fluid absorption are induced (37). This induction is enhanced by labor. At delivery, with the onset of regular respirations, optimal air exchange physiology occurs when lung volume is adequate and pulmonary vascular resistance drops, allowing the resultant increase in blood flow.

Disorders of transition occur when any one of the three critical steps do not occur or are delayed. The three disorders of transition are (i) transient tachypnea of the newborn, which occurs when the removal of lung water is delayed; (ii) respiratory distress syndrome, formerly known as hyaline membrane disease; and (iii) pulmonary hypertension of the newborn, which occurs when the normal drop in pulmonary vascular resistance does not occur or is delayed. Each of these disorders has a characteristic physiology that leads to alterations in air exchange. In most cases, the primary aberration is hypoxemia, even though the physiology by which this aberration occurs is different.

To understand respiratory physiology of the newborn, it is critical to understand some of the physical properties of the lung that determine ventilation. The equation of motion describes the properties of the lung important for proper ventilation:

$$\Delta P = \frac{1}{c}V + R\dot{V} + I\ddot{V}$$

where P stands for the pressure applied to the respiratory system; C is compliance, which is defined as the change in volume divided by the change in pressure, describing the elastance of the respiratory system; V is volume; R is resistance; $\dot{V}$ is flow; I is inertance; and $\ddot{V}$ is acceleration. Thus, properties of the lung can be divided into the static properties of the lung, which are measured when there is no flow and are dependent on the compliance term in the equation of motion; and the resistive properties of the lung, which are measured when there is flow and are dependent on the resistance term in the equation of motion and inertance, which in most cases is thought to be negligible relative to the static and resistive properties and is therefore ignored. In well newborn infants the compliance is normal and the resistance is low so that minimal effort or energy is needed to provide reasonable ventilation to the respiratory system independent of whether the infant is doing the work or if the infant requires mechanical ventilation.

In infants with primary lung disease, the most common biochemical derangement is arterial hypoxemia. The mechanisms for significant hypoxemia in infants with lung disease are primarily ventilation–perfusion abnormalities and/or right-to-left shunting (both intrapulmonary and extrapulmonary). The sum of the shunt fraction and the ventilation–perfusion inequalities is the venous admixture. The venous admixture is higher in newborns even without lung disease (38,39). In parenchymal lung disease, the venous admixture increases dramatically and arterial hypoxemia may become profound. Furthermore, the relative proportion of the shunt fraction and V/Q abnormalities is dynamic such that as ventilation of the lung improves, it has been shown that the shunt fraction and low V/Q compartments may be affected independently or in tandem. The primary strategy in infants with lung disease is to improve the function of the low V/Q compartment. Administration of supplemental oxygen may improve the oxygen concentration in the terminal air units and may relieve hypoxic pulmonary vasoconstriction, in which case improvement in oxygenation occurs by decreasing the size of the shunt compartment with no effect on the low V/Q compartment. Improving the ventilation to the low V/Q compartment of the lung frequently addresses both the shunt compartment and the low V/Q compartment. In this case, these strategies may recruit the shunt compartment by improving ventilation, raising the partial pressure of oxygen, and relieving hypoxic pulmonary vasoconstriction. The same strategies may recruit the former low V/Q compartment into the normal V/Q compartment at the same time. Thus while administration of supplemental oxygen is relatively safe and may decrease the shunt compartment, supportive strategies to safely increase ventilation to the most diseased areas of the lung may affect the shunt compartment and low V/Q compartment simultaneously.

The most appropriate strategies to support the respiratory system in the diseased lung depend on the physical properties of the lung, including the static properties and the resistive properties. It is appropriate to bear in mind that supportive measures that improve the function of the diseased lung do not improve the underlying disorder. In fact, supplemental oxygen is toxic, and the application of positive pressure to the lung causes injury (40). When positive pressure is administered, the strategy used should be tailored to the abnormalities in the lung. In lung diseases dominated by low respiratory system compliance, such as RDS or hyaline membrane disease, the airways and airspaces fill and empty quickly so that if mechanical ventilation is used, a fast rate/low tidal volume ventilation strategy should be used and has been associated with better outcomes (41). In diseases dominated by high airway resistance, a ventilator strategy using a slower rate with slightly higher tidal volume ventilation is more successful. Examples of such diseases include meconium aspiration and bronchopulmonary dysplasia. In infants with RDS, the safest and most efficient technique to improve lung physiology is by increasing the mean airway pressure, and the safest and most efficient technique to increase mean airway pressure is to increase the end pressure (42). In fact, many infants with RDS can be managed with continuous positive airway pressure (CPAP) only, which is the preferable mode in relatively mature infants (43,44).

CARDIOPULMONARY INTERACTION

The pulmonary vasculature in the lung of infants is fully recruited at rest and is particularly predisposed to the development of pulmonary edema when flow is increased via anatomic left-to-right shunts. The rate of fluid filtration (Q_f) in the lung or any other organ or vascular bed is governed by the Frank-Starling equation:

$$Q_f = K_f [(P_{mv} - P_{pmv}) - \sigma(\pi_{mv} - \pi_{pmv})]$$

where K_f is hydraulic conductance, P_{mv} is hydrostatic pressure in the microvasculature, P_{pmv} is hydrostatic pressure in the perimicrovascular space, σ (sigma) is the reflection coefficient, p_{mv} is oncotic pressure in the microvasculature, and π_{pmv} is oncotic pressure in the perimicrovascular space.

Abnormalities in K_f and P_{mv} are the dominant variables in fluid filtration. K_f is a function of the number and size of the pores in the endothelial cell layer. Disorders that injure endothelial cells markedly increase K_f and fluid filtration (45). When K_f is increased and leads to pulmonary edema, it is characterized as permeability pulmonary edema. There are many disorders that increase K_f and lead to pulmonary edema, but the most common disorders confronted in the newborn period include RDS and sepsis, both of which are frequently associated with lung inflammation and a component of lung edema secondary to inflammatory injury (46,47). Unfortunately, mechanical ventilation has the potential to induce lung inflammation; thus careful supportive care to limit lung inflammation is imperative.

High-pressure pulmonary edema is common in the newborn period, since the lung of the newborn is fully recruited at rest, left-to-right shunts increase fluid filtration substantially (48,49), and elevations of left atrial pressure also increase filtration. The equation for P_{mv} is as follows:

$$P_{mv} = P_{LA} + c(P_{PA} - P_{LA})$$

where c is equal to a constant between 0 and 1 and PA and LA are pulmonary arterial and left atrial, respectively. This equation illustrates the significant impact of elevated P_{LA} in lung fluid filtration. P_{LA} (or pulmonary venous pressure) can be particularly elevated in some forms of congenital heart disease (e.g., obstructed anomalous pulmonary venous connection, mitral valve disease, or hypoplastic left heart syndrome). Fluid accumulation in the lung can occur only when fluid filtration exceeds lymphatic function that returns filtered fluid to the venous circulation ($Q_f > Q_L$). Q_L is dependent on intrinsic contractility of the lymphatics in the lung and on the right atrial pressure. Right atrial pressure may be elevated in infants with lung disease, enhancing fluid accumulation in the lung, and the pressures at which lymphatic flow is impaired are lower in the fetus and newborn than in older patients. In summary, infants with lung disease and/or heart diseases are more predisposed to develop pulmonary edema than any other age group because increases in flow are invariably associated with increased microvascular pressure and developmentally impaired lymphatic function is frequently incapable of meeting the demands of increased fluid filtration.

The effects of pulmonary edema on respiratory physiology are dependent on the location of the edema fluid. Typically fluid filtration occurs in the alveolar capillary, but hydrostatic forces in the lung favor fluid accumulation in the extra-alveolar interstitium (50). The extra-alveolar interstitium contains airways so that fluid can compress the airways leading to constriction and increased airway resistance (51). This explains

the finding of cardiac asthma and increased airway resistance with pulmonary edema. Decreased respiratory system compliance can also occur with pulmonary edema, primarily when accumulation occurs in the alveolar space and impairs surfactant function. It is difficult to filter fluid to the extent that fluid accumulates in the alveolar space because respiratory epithelial cells are excellent barriers to fluid egress and they actively pump fluid from the alveolar space into the interstitium (52). The extra-alveolar interstitium can accumulate excessive fluid before it egresses into the alveolar space. However, the lung is more susceptible to alveolar fluid accumulation when increased fluid filtration is associated with injury to respiratory epithelial cells.

Treatment for pulmonary edema is almost entirely supportive and includes measures to lower P_{mv} or to support the respiratory system by applying positive pressure. Measures to decrease P_{mv} include reducing pulmonary blood flow by decreasing left-to-right shunts or by decreasing circulating blood volume. Decreasing fluid administration is a reasonable short-term maneuver to decrease fluid filtration, but only if the fluid restriction does not impair the delivery of adequate nutrition. Therapy with diuretics may also reduce P_{mv} by decreasing circulating blood volume. Although equipotent doses of diuretics improve lung function by decreasing lung water, furosemide has the additional effect of pulmonary dilation (53), which lowers P_{mv} further. Thus this diuretic is more effective for pulmonary edema than are equipotent doses of other diuretics. Pulmonary edema may accumulate to the extent that pressure support to the lung is necessary. The delivery of positive pressure does not decrease fluid accumulation in the lung. It simply improves the acute physiology, usually by improving V/Q mismatching (54,55) by improving ventilation to the low V/Q compartment in the lung. Decreasing pulmonary edema by decreasing K_f or by improving lymphatic function would be optimal, but measures to consistently achieve these improvements have not been described.

Abnormalities of pulmonary vascular physiology are confined primarily to inappropriate vasoconstriction. Persistent pulmonary hypertension in the newborn occurs when the normal decrease in pulmonary vascular resistance that occurs at birth does not occur and can be a result of underdevelopment, maldevelopment, or maladaptive forms of pulmonary vascular disease as described previously. Pulmonary hypertension in the newborn frequently presents with significant hypoxia because of right-to-left shunting at the fetal shunt pathways at the atrial and ductal levels. Pulmonary constriction is usually on the arterial side of the circuit so that therapies that dilate the pulmonary circuit may improve hypoxemia without increasing fluid filtration if the venous circuit is normal.

Pulmonary hypertension was the most common reason for placing infants on extracorporeal life support because specific pulmonary vasodilators had not been identified. However, inhaled nitric oxide has unequivocally improved the abnormal pulmonary physiology observed in infants with pulmonary hypertension. In several large randomized trials, nitric oxide was effective at reducing the incidence of death or the need for extracorporeal support (56). Inhaled nitric oxide was approved for use in infants with hypoxic respiratory failure in 1997 and was restricted to infants at or beyond 34 weeks gestation. The use of this drug has meant that supportive treatments previously used to support these infants, including treatment with high concentrations of oxygen and/or induced alkalosis, are contraindicated. Typical indications for the use of inhaled nitric oxide in term or near-term infants are respiratory failure as indicated by an oxygenation index of >20 to 25 (OI = FiO$_2$ × mean airway pressure × 100/PaO$_2$) and evidence of pulmonary hypertension from Doppler-echocardiography. Supportive efforts with mechanical ventilation and/or administration of surfactant that improve lung inflation improve the efficacy of inhaled nitric oxide (57). Nitric oxide is started at 20 ppm and is decreased in 50% decrements when supplemental oxygen requirements decrease substantially, usually to <50%. When the dose of nitric oxide is 5 ppm, further decrements must be done cautiously as rebound pulmonary hypertension has been described in this range (58). Infants <34 weeks gestation may also present with hypoxic respiratory failure, and recent trials have been published suggesting that these infants may also benefit from treatment with nitric oxide (59–61). However, nitric oxide therapy has not yet been approved for these infants.

RESPIRATORY SYNCYTIAL VIRUS

Infections caused by respiratory syncytial virus (RSV) create significant morbidity and mortality for patients at high risk including premature infants, infants with BPD, and infants with complicated hemodynamically significant congenital heart disease. The overall hospitalization rate for patients <1 year of age with RSV is 2% annually. Those at high risk experience approximately five times the rate of admissions for RSV-related illness as compared with those not at high risk (62–65). No active immunization program has ever been shown to be efficacious for RSV (66,67); however, passive immunity with palivizumab has been shown to decrease RSV infections in high-risk infants. Palivizumab is a monoclonal antibody directed against the F protein of RSV (68,69). Palivizumab has been shown to decrease RSV-related hospitalizations in patients with hemodynamically significant congenital heart disease (70). Monthly intramuscular injections (15 mg/kg) during RSV season in this patient population yielded a 45% reduction in RSV-related hospitalizations, a 56% reduction in total days of RSV related hospitalizations, and a 73% reduction in RSV hospitalization days with increased supplemental oxygen (70). Evidence exists in patients who receive palivizumab and then undergo surgery involving cardiopulmonary bypass that the levels of monoclonal antibody decrease dramatically. Therefore, after surgery involving cardiopulmonary bypass, dosing should be repeated at a safe time in the postoperative period.

NEUROLOGY

Many institutions arrange for a head ultrasound study on patients prior to intervention for critical congenital heart disease. The head ultrasound is used to determine anatomic issues, hemorrhage, ischemia, hydrocephalus, and atrophy. Although this test is routinely performed, it is often replaced by other imaging studies if there is an abnormality. Cranial ultrasound in patients with congenital heart disease has shown abnormalities in as many as 42% of those screened (71). Findings included widened ventricular and/or subarachnoid spaces, lenticulostriate vasculopathy, calcification of basal nuclei, and ischemia. Patients with left-sided obstructive lesions seem to have a higher incidence of brain abnormalities (71). There is increasing concern that certain lesions may impact cerebral blood flow not only postnatally but also during fetal development. Cerebrovascular resistance is lower than normal in fetuses with hypoplastic left heart syndrome where cerebral perfusion occurs retrogradely via the ductus

arteriosus (72). In patients with right-sided lesions, the cerebrovascular resistance is higher than in those with left-sided obstructive lesions (72). This may have implications for neurologic development and subsequent susceptibility to adverse sequelae.

A recent study suggested that 19% of neurologic events occur preoperatively in patients with congenital heart disease (73). Predictive factors for a neurologic event, namely seizure, abnormal tone, or choreoathetosis, include an abnormal preoperative imaging study and an Apgar score of <7 at 5 minutes of life (73). Magnetic resonance imaging (MRI) studies done preoperatively, acutely postoperatively (within weeks of surgery), and then several months postoperatively have shown abnormalities. Preoperatively, patients mainly had periventricular leukomalacia (PVL) and infarct. Shortly after surgery, MRI examinations showed new PVL in 48%, new infarct in 19%, and a new parenchymal hemorrhage in 33% (74). Late MRI did show resolution of the findings in a subset of patients. Among 82 neonates who had undergone cardiac surgery, 54% had PVL, but in older infants the incidence was only 4% (75). Early postoperative hypoxemia and hypotension (mainly diastolic) were noted to be risk factors (75).

Among survivors of congenital heart disease surgery, there are well-known late sequelae that may include learning disabilities, behavioral abnormalities, and attention deficit disorders (76,77). Many issues may lead to these findings including neuroprotection during cardiac surgery, use of deep hypothermic circulatory arrest, and postoperative decreased perfusion from low cardiac output syndrome. With the application of perioperative noninvasive real-time neurologic monitoring, interdisciplinary teams caring for the patient may be able to intervene and prevent brain injury.

GASTROINTESTINAL SYSTEM

The development of the gastrointestinal system occurs as early as the fourth week of gestation. Mesenteric vascular system development parallels that of the intestine. Regulation of the mesenteric blood flow occurs at the arteriolar and precapillary level. Feeding causes hyperemia and as documented in animal studies (78), the neonate has lower intestinal vascular resistance than the fetus (79). Therefore, mesenteric blood flow is greater in the neonate than in the fetus until the second to fourth postnatal weeks, when intestinal resistance increases with a corresponding decrease in blood flow and oxygen delivery. Of potential importance to those patients with critical congenital heart disease, mild hypoxia triggers dilation of the vascular bed and perfusion increases whereas severe hypoxia (PO_2 of ≤40 mm Hg) causes vasoconstriction, tissue hypoxia, and potential ischemia (80).

The cause of necrotizing enterocolitis (NEC) remains poorly understood, especially in term infants. Studies have shown that most term newborns who develop NEC have underlying congenital disorders that are commonly either heart disease or endocrine disorders (81). A case-control study of neonates with congenital heart disease showed that hypoplastic left heart syndrome (odds ratio 3.8) and truncus arteriosus or aortopulmonary window (odds ratio 6.3) were independently associated with development of NEC (82). Additionally, in the same cohort, earlier gestational age at birth (36.7 weeks ± 2.7 weeks), prematurity, and episodes of shock or low cardiac output were all risk factors (82). There was no documented mortality difference in patients who developed NEC versus those who did not; however, the hospital stay was significantly higher in those who developed NEC. In patients with congenital heart disease who develop NEC, it is felt that mesenteric ischemia associated with a low perfusion state is the cause; however, infectious associations are difficult to elucidate (83). Cardiac lesions that elicit a difficult balance between pulmonary and systemic blood flow (Q_p:Q_s) whereby systemic perfusion can be limited owing to a shift in the systemic and pulmonary vascular resistances pose a difficult dilemma to the intensivist regarding if and when to feed preoperatively and postoperatively.

Many patients with congenital heart disease also have heterotaxy (situs abnormalities). Situs inversus totalis is associated with intra-abdominal anomalies in more than half of the patients. These may include duodenal atresia, biliary atresia, gastroschisis with malrotation, and tracheoesophageal fistula. Hiatal and diaphragmatic hernias are commonly noted in patients with right isomerism. Patients with left isomerism may have malrotation and biliary atresia (84). Intestinal malrotation may lead to gastrointestinal complications and require emergent surgery. It is debatable whether an elective Ladd's procedure is warranted in all patients with malrotation once the cardiac condition is stabilized or appropriately palliated. Upper gastrointestinal contrast procedures likely should be recommended in all patients with heterotaxy and cardiac lesions to evaluate for intestinal malrotation (85).

RENAL SYSTEM

The glomerular filtration rate (GFR) in term neonates is 20 mL/minute times 1.73 m^2, which is generally twice that of premature newborns (86). GFR improves over the first several weeks of life in all newborns, but the velocity at which it improves is less in premature infants. In term newborns, the GFR doubles in the first 2 weeks of life (87,88). These differences in GFR values among varying gestational age newborns affect the administration of medications that are primarily eliminated in the renal system. Digoxin dosages should be decreased for preterm infants. Creatinine is the most commonly used marker for renal function; however, in neonates interpretation must take into account several caveats (89). The creatinine level is falsely elevated at birth, reflecting maternal levels. Over the first several weeks of life in term neonates, creatinine decreases rapidly to expected levels (0.40 mg/dL). In those with extreme prematurity, a transient increase is noted over the first 4 days followed by a steady decrease over the next month of life. In premature infants, the transient rise in creatinine is caused by reabsorption of creatinine across renal tubules (90).

Because of the unique vascular supply of the renal medulla, the kidney is susceptible to hypoxic-ischemic injury. In congenital heart disease that presents with either decreased systemic blood flow in critical left-sided obstructive disease or a shift in Q_p:Q_s with resultant decreased systemic oxygen delivery, renal function may be altered. Prolonged ischemia may result in impairment in sodium and water reabsorption as well as decreased GFR (91). Similarly, use of angiotensin-converting enzyme (ACE) inhibitors may lower systemic blood pressure to the extent that hypoperfusion to the kidney occurs (92). Renal perfusion pressure may drop below the autoregulatory threshold and thus promote acute renal failure. Caution in dosing and monitoring of effects of ACE inhibitors in neonates is important to avoid adverse renal effects.

Many institutions advocate using umbilical catheters in newborns with critical congenital heart disease for access, monitoring, and acquisition of blood samples. Arterial lines have been associated with aortic and renal arterial complications including thrombosis. No definitive study has shown whether high or low umbilical arterial line placement affects the incidence of thrombotic complications; in fact, conflicting data exist (93,94). Both abdominal coarctation and renal artery stenosis have been reported as long-term complications of umbilical arterial lines. Umbilical venous lines are placed with the tip in the inferior vena cava cephalad to the hepatic and portal veins. Complications of these lines include thrombosis of the portal or hepatic venous systems or inferior vena caval thrombus. Renal vein thrombosis may occur and could manifest itself with symptoms of oliguria, anuria, hematuria, thrombocytopenia, acidosis, and hemolytic anemia (95). Hypertension can occur late after renal vein thrombosis, but the magnitude of hypertension is much less than in those with umbilical artery thrombosis.

CARDIAC INTERVENTION IN THE PREMATURE OR LOW-BIRTH-WEIGHT NEONATE

Recent reports suggest that aggressive attempts to treat congenital heart disease in either premature or low-birth-weight infants are appropriate. Delaying surgery or cardiac catheter intervention for weight gain lead to longer hospital stays and increased morbidity.

Many studies have evaluated the subgroup of patients <2,500 g who have congenital heart disease. In one report (96), the mortality rate for closed procedures was 10.4% versus 5.4% for the comparison group. Similarly, the mortality rate for open heart procedures in those <2,500 g was 25.4% versus 10.5% for term counterparts. The actuarial survival rate at 10 years was 51%. Another study examined palliations versus complete biventricular repair in the same weight cutoff and noted that a higher mortality rate was seen in premature infants (versus those with low birth weight) and in those who had undergone palliations (97). A contemporary study (98) showed that overall surgical mortality in those <2,500 g (either palliation or definitive repair) was 18%. Definitive repair was associated with better outcomes with 13% mortality versus 28% mortality in those who underwent palliative surgery. Medium-term follow-up indicated that survival was 87% in those with corrective surgery and 54% in the palliation group. Obviously, morbidity is higher in the entire low-birth-weight group compared with term infants. Statistical analysis showed that early outcome was independent of age, weight, prematurity, use of cardiopulmonary bypass, and type of intervention. The authors concluded that primary correction has an early survival benefit over palliation. These results were similarly noted in a series of 60 patients <2,500 g with 35 who had cardiopulmonary bypass (99). Overall results showed acute deaths being 15% and survival at 60 months to be 70% for the entire group.

Similar conclusions have been made for the very low birth weight infant (<1,500 g). Complete repair has been advocated for these patients since delays for weight gain have been shown to be associated with no long-term benefit and increased preoperative morbidity. Additionally, complete surgical correction is preferred over prolonged medical management or other palliative procedures (100).

Aggressive surgical strategies for the low or very low-birth-weight neonate have prompted cardiac catheterization in the same group. A recent study compared those <1,500 g who had undergone catheterization in a case-control study with the comparison population weighing between 2 and 3 kg (101). In essence, success rates, complication rates, incidence of blood transfusions, and incidence of major complications were the same for each group. The procedures in the very low birth weight infant are rare, yet pose an impetus for equipment alterations and safety considerations in the catheterization lab for these patients.

INTERDISCIPLINARY APPROACH

This unique patient population merits the same interdisciplinary approach provided to children and adults with congenital heart disease. A firm understanding of neonatal physiology and organ system development is imperative to ensure the highest quality of care. The future of this field may involve an evolution of multiple services that may lead to specific neonatal cardiac services that will promote research and enhance care.

References

1. Rudolph AM. The changes in the circulation after birth: Their importance in congenital heart disease. *Circulation* 1970;41:343–359.
2. Teitel DF, Iwamaoto HS, Rudolph AM. Effects of birth related events on central flow patterns. *Pediatr Res* 1987;22:557–566.
3. Gittenberger-De Groot AC. Persistent ductus arteriosis: Most probably a primary congenital malformation. *Br Heart J* 1977;39:610–618.
4. Waleh N, Seidner S, McCurnin D, et al. The role of monocyte-derived cells and inflammation in baboon ductus arteriosus remodeling. *Pediatr Res* 2005;57(2):254–262.
5. Keller RL, Clyman RI. Persistent Doppler flow predicts lack of response to multiple courses of indomethacin in premature infants with recurrent patent ductus arteriosus. *Pediatrics* 2003;112(pt 1):583–587.
6. Kajino H, Goldbarg S, Roman C, et al. Vasa vasorum hypoperfusion is responsible for medial hypoxia and anatomic remodeling in the newborn lamb ductus arteriosus. *Pediatr Res* 2002;51(2):228–235.
7. Clyman RI, Seidner SR, Kajino H, et al. VEGF regulates remodeling during permanent anatomic closure of the ductus arteriosus. *Am J Physiol Regul Integr Comp Physiol* 2002;282(1):R199–R206.
8. Kajino H, Chen YQ, Chemtob S, et al. Tissue hypoxia inhibits prostaglandin and nitric oxide production and prevents ductus arteriosus reopening. *Am J Physiol Regul Integr Comp Physiol* 2000;279(1):R278–R286.
9. Schmidt B, Roberts RS, Fanaroff A, et al. Indomethacin prophylaxis, patent ductus arteriosus, and the risk of bronchopulmonary dysplasia: Further analyses from the Trial of Indomethacin Prophylaxis in Preterms (TIPP). *J Pediatr* 2006;148:730–734.
10. Alpan G, Scheerer R, Bland R, et al. Patent ductus arteriosus increases lung fluid filtration in preterm lambs. *Pediatr Res* 1991;30:616–621.
11. Shimada S, Kasai T, Konishi M, et al. Effects of patent ductus arteriosus on left ventricular output and organ blood flows in preterm infants with respiratory distress syndrome treated surfactant. *J Pediatr* 1994;125:270–277.
12. Laughon MM, Simmons MA, Bose CL. Patency of the ductus arteriosus in the premature infant: Is it pathologic? Should it be treated? *Curr Opin Pediatr* 2004;16(2):146–151.
13. Fowlie PW, Davis PG. Prophylactic intravenous indomethacin for preventing mortality and morbidity in preterm infants. *Cochrane Database Syst Rev* 2002;(3):CD000174.
14. Cotton RB, Stahlman MT, Bender HW, et al. Randomized trial of early closure of symptomatic patent ductus arteriosus in small preterm infants. *J Pediatr* 1978;93:647–651.
15. Cassady G, Crouse DT, Kirklin JW, et al. A randomized, controlled trial of very early prophylactic ligation of the ductus arteriosus in babies who weighed 1000 g or less at birth. *N Engl J Med* 1989;320:1511–1516.
16. Clyman RI. Recommendations for the postnatal use of indomethacin: An analysis of four separate treatment strategies [editorial]. *J Pediatr* 1996;128(pt 1):601–607.
17. Langston C, Kida K, Reed M, et al. Human lung growth in late gestation and in the neonate. *Am Rev Respir Dis* 1984;129:607–613.
18. Langston C. Normal and abnormal structural development of the human lung. *Prog Clin Biol Res* 1983;140:75–91.
19. Langston C, Thurlbeck WM. Lung growth and development in late gestation and early postnatal life. *Perspect Pediatr Pathol* 1982;7:203–235.
20. Ten Have-Opbroek AA. Lung development in the mouse embryo. *Exp Lung Res* 1991;17(2):111–130.
21. Northway WH Jr, Rosan RC, Porter DY. Pulmonary disease following respirator therapy of hyaline-membrane disease. Bronchopulmonary dysplasia. *N Engl J Med* 1967;276:357–368.
22. Viscardi RM, Muhumuza CK, Rodriguez A, et al. Inflammatory markers in intrauterine and fetal blood and cerebrospinal fluid compartments are associated with adverse pulmonary and neurologic outcomes in preterm infants. *Pediatr Res* 2004;55:1009–1017.
23. Doyle LW, Faber B, Callanan C, et al. Bronchopulmonary dysplasia in very low birth weight subjects and lung function in late adolescence. *Pediatrics* 2006;118(1):108–113.
24. Doyle LW. Respiratory function at age 8–9 years in extremely low birth-weight/very preterm children born in Victoria in 1991–1992. *Pediatr Pulmonol* 2006;41:570–576.
25. Liggins GC, Howie RN. A controlled trial of antepartum glucocorticoid treatment for prevention of the respiratory distress syndrome in premature infants. *Pediatrics* 1972;50:515–525.
26. Crowley PA. Antenatal corticosteroid therapy: A meta-analysis of the randomized trials, 1972 to 1994. *Am J Obstet Gynecol* 1995;173(1):322–335.
27. Wright LL, Verter J, Younes N, et al. Antenatal corticosteroid administration and neonatal outcome in very low birth weight infants: The NICHD Neonatal Research Network. *Am J Obstet Gynecol* 1995;173(1):269–274.
28. Horbar JD. Antenatal corticosteroid treatment and neonatal outcomes for infants 501 to 1500 gm in the Vermont-Oxford Trials Network. *Am J Obstet Gynecol* 1995;173(1):275–281.
29. Effect of corticosteroids for fetal maturation on perinatal outcomes. NIH Consens Statement 1994;12(2):1–24.
30. Antenatal corticosteroids revisited: Repeat courses—National Institutes of Health Consensus Development Conference Statement, August 17–18, 2000. *Obstet Gynecol* 2001;98(1):144–150.
31. Pollock JS, Forstermann U, Tracey WR, et al. Nitric oxide synthase isozymes antibodies. *Histochem J* 1995;27:738–744.
32. Soll RF. Synthetic surfactant for respiratory distress syndrome in preterm infants. *Cochrane Database Syst Rev* 2000;(2):CD001149.
33. Bell EF, Acarregui MJ. Restricted versus liberal water intake for preventing morbidity and mortality in preterm infants. *Cochrane Database Syst Rev* 2001;(3):CD000503.
34. Reid LM. Structure and function in pulmonary hypertension. New perceptions. *Chest* 1986;89(2):279–288.
35. Geggel RL, Murphy JD, Langleben D, et al. Congenital diaphragmatic hernia: Arterial structural changes and persistent pulmonary hypertension after surgical repair. *J Pediatr* 1985;107:457–464.
36. Bland RD. Dynamics of pulmonary water before and after birth. *Acta Paediatr Scand Suppl* 1983;305:12–20.
37. Bland RD, Bressack MA, McMillan DD. Labor decreases the lung water content of newborn rabbits. *Am J Obstet Gynecol* 1979;135(3):364–367.
38. Landers S, Hansen TN, Corbet AJ, et al. Optimal constant positive airway pressure assessed by arterial alveolar difference for CO_2 in hyaline membrane disease. *Pediatr Res* 1986;20:884–889.
39. Hansen TN, Corbet AJ, Kenny JD, et al. Effects of oxygen and constant positive pressure breathing on aADCO2 in hyaline membrane disease. *Pediatr Res* 1979;13:1167–1171.
40. Hansen TN, Gest AL. Oxygen toxicity and other ventilatory complications of treatment of infants with persistent pulmonary hypertension. *Clin Perinatol* 1984;11:653–672.
41. Multicentre randomised controlled trial of high against low frequency positive pressure ventilation. Oxford Region Controlled Trial of Artificial Ventilation OCTAVE Study Group. *Arch Dis Child* 1991;66(7 Spec No):770–775.
42. Stewart AR, Finer NN, Peters KL. Effects of alterations of inspiratory and expiratory pressures and inspiratory/expiratory ratios on mean airway pressure, blood gases, and intracranial pressure. *Pediatrics* 1981;67(4):474–481.
43. Alba J, Agarwal R, Hegyi T, et al. Efficacy of surfactant therapy in infants managed with CPAP. *Pediatr Pulmonol* 1995;20(3):172–176.
44. Mandy GT, Moise AA, Smith EO, et al. Endotracheal continuous positive airway pressure after rescue surfactant therapy. *J Perinatol* 1998;18:444–448.
45. Parker JC, Townsley MI. Evaluation of lung injury in rats and mice. *Am J Physiol Lung Cell Mol Physiol* 2004;286(2):L231–L246.

46. Carlton DP, Albertine KH, Cho SC, et al. Role of neutrophils in lung vascular injury and edema after premature birth in lambs. *J Appl Physiol* 1997;83:1307–1317.

47. Calkins CM, Bensard DD, Partrick DA, et al. Altered neutrophil function in the neonate protects against sepsis-induced lung injury. *J Pediatr Surg* 2002;37:1042–1047.

48. Nelin LD, Weardden ME, Welty SE, et al. The effect of blood flow and left atrial pressure in the DLCO in lambs and sheep. *Resp Physiol* 1992;88:333–342.

49. Means LJ, Hanson WL, Mounts KO, et al. Pulmonary capillary recruitment in neonatal lambs. *Pediatr Res* 1993;34:596–599.

50. Michel RP, Zocchi L, Rossi A, et al. Does interstitial lung edema compress airways and arteries? A morphometric study. *J Appl Physiol* 1987;62(1):108–115.

51. Sasidharan P, Heimler R. Alterations in pulmonary mechanics after transfusion in anemic preterm infants. *Crit Care Med* 1990;18:1360–1362.

52. Pitkanen OM, O'Brodovich HM. Significance of ion transport during lung development and in respiratory disease of the newborn. *Ann Med* 1998;30(2):134–142.

53. Demling RH, Will JA. The effect of furosemide on the pulmonary transvascular fluid filtration rate. *Crit Care Med* 1978;6(5):317–319.

54. Demling RH, Edmunds LH Jr. Effect of continuous positive airway pressure on extravascular lung water. *Surg Forum* 1973;24:226–228.

55. Wickerts CJ, Berg B, Blomqvist H. Influence of positive end-expiratory pressure on extravascular lung water during the formation of experimental hydrostatic pulmonary oedema. *Acta Anaesthesiol Scand* 1992;36(4):309–317.

56. Finer NN, Barrington KJ. Nitric oxide for respiratory failure in infants born at or near term. *Cochrane Database Syst Rev* 2006;(4):CD000399.

57. Inhaled nitric oxide in full-term and nearly full-term infants with hypoxic respiratory failure. The Neonatal Inhaled Nitric Oxide Study Group. *N Engl J Med* 1997;336:597–604.

58. Davidson D, Barefield ES, Kattwinkel J, et al. Safety of withdrawing inhaled nitric oxide therapy in persistent pulmonary hypertension of the newborn. *Pediatrics* 1999;104(pt 1):231–236.

59. Kinsella JP, Cutter GR, Walsh WF, et al. Early inhaled nitric oxide therapy in premature newborns with respiratory failure. *N Engl J Med* 2006;355:354–364.

60. Ballard RA, Truog WE, Cnaan A, et al. Inhaled nitric oxide in preterm infants undergoing mechanical ventilation. *N Engl J Med* 2006;355:343–353.

61. Van Meurs KP, Wright LL, Ehrenkranz RA, et al. Inhaled nitric oxide for premature infants with severe respiratory failure. *N Engl J Med* 2005;353:13–22.

62. Heilman CA. Respiratory syncytial and parainfluenza viruses. *J Infect Dis* 1990;161:402–406.

63. Hall CB, Kopelman AE, Douglas RG Jr, et al. Neonatal respiratory syncytial virus infection. *N Engl J Med* 1979;300:393–396.

64. Groothius JR, Gutierrez KM, Lauer BA. Respiratory syncytial virus infection in children with bronchopulmonary dysplasia. *Pediatrics* 1988;82:199–203.

65. MacDonald NE, Hall CB, Suffin SC, et al. Respiratory syncytial virus infection in infants with congenital heart disease. *N Engl J Med* 1982;207:397–400.

66. Kim HW, Canchola JG, Brandt CD, et al. Respiratory syncytial virus disease in infants despite prior administration of antigenic inactivated vaccine. *Am J Epidemiol* 1969;89:422–434.

67. Openshaw PJM, Cully FJ, Olszewska W. Immunopathogenesis of vaccine-enhanced RSV disease. *Vaccine* 2002;20:S27–S31.

68. Prince GA, Hemmin VG, Horswood RL, et al. Immunoprophylaxis and immunotherapy of respiratory syncytial virus infection in the cotton rat. *Virus Res* 1985;3:193–206.

69. Johnson S, Oliver C, Prince GA, et al. Development of a humanized monoclonal antibody (MEDI-493) with potent in vitro and in vivo activity against respiratory syncytial virus (RSV). *J Infec Dis* 1997;176:1215–1224.

70. Feltes TF, Cabalka AK, Meissner C, et al. Palivizumab prophylaxis reduces hospitalization due to respiratory syncytial virus in young children with hemodynamically significant congenital heart disease. *J Pediatr* 2003;143:532–540.

71. Te Pas AB, van Wezel-Meijler G, Bokenkamp-Gramann R, et al. Preoperative cranial ultrasound findings in infants with major congenital heart disease. *Acta Pediatrica* 2005;94;1597–1603.

72. Kaltman JR, Di H, Tian Z, et al. Impact of congenital heart disease on cerebrovascular blood flow dynamics in the fetus. *Ultrasound Obstet Gynecol* 2005;25(1):32–36.

73. Chock VY, Reddy VM, Bernstein D, et al. Neurologic events in neonates treated surgically for congenital heart disease. *J Perinatol* 2006;26(4):237–242.

74. Mahle WT, Tavani F, Zimmerman RA, et al. An MRI study of neurological injury before and after congenital heart surgery. *Circulation* 2002;106(suppl 1):I109–114.

75. Galli KK, Zimmeran RA, Jarvik GP, et al. Periventricular leukomalacia is common after neonatal cardiac surgery. *J Thorac Cardiovasc Surg* 2004;127:692–704.

76. McKenzie ED, Andropoulos DB, DiBardino D, et al. Congenital heart surgery 2005: The brain: Its the heart of the matter. *Am J Surg* 2005;190(2):289–294.

77. Wernovsky G, Shillingford AJ, Gaynor JW. Central nervous system outcomes in children with complex congenital heart disease. *Curr Opin Cardiol* 2005;20(2):94–99.

78. Crissinger KD, Burney DL. Influence of luminal nutrient composition on hemodynamics and oxygenation in developing piglet intestine. *Am J Physiol* 1992;263(pt 1):G254–260.

79. Martinussen M, Brubakk AM, Vi T, et al. Mesenteric blood flow velocity and its relation to transitional circulatory adaptation in appropriate for gestational age preterm infants. *Pediatr Res* 1996;39(2):275–280.

80. Nowicki PT, Miller CE, Haun SE. Effects of arterial hypoxia and isoproterenol on in vitro postnatal intestinal circulation. *Am J Physiol* 1988;255(pt 2):H1144–148.

81. Bolisetty S, Lui K, Oei J, et al. A regional study of underlying congenital diseases in term neonates with necrotizing enterocolitis. *Acta Paediatr* 2000;89:1226–1230.

82. McElhinney DB, Hedrick HL, Bush DM, et al. Necrotizing enterocolitis in neonates with congenital heart disease: Risk factors and outcomes. *Pediatrics* 2000;106:1080–1087.

83. Fatica C, Gordon S, Mossad E, et al. A cluster of necrotizing enterocolitis in term infants undergoing open heart surgery. *Am J Infect Control* 2000;28(2):130–132.

84. Lee SE, Kim HY, Jung SE, et al. Situs anomalies and gastrointestinal abnormalities. *J Pediatr Surg* 2006;41:1237–1242.

85. Chang J, Brueckner M, Touloukian RJ. Intestinal rotation and fixation abnormalities in heterotaxia: Early detection and management. *J Pediatr Surg* 1993;28:1281–1284.

86. Guignard JP, Torrado A, Da Cunha O, et al. Glomerular filtration rate in the first three weeks of life. *J Pediatr* 1975;87(2):268–272.

87. Bueva A, Guignard JP. Renal function in preterm neonates. *Pediatr Res* 1994;36:572–577.

88. Vanpee M, Blennow M, Linne T, et al. Renal function in very low birth weight infants: Normal maturity reached during early childhood. *J Pediatr* 1992;121(pt 1):784–788.

89. Guignard JP, Drukker A. Why do newborn infants have a high plasma creatinine? *Pediatrics* 1999;103(4):e49.

90. Matos P, Duarte-Silva M, Drukker A, et al. Creatinine reabsorption by the newborn rabbit kidney. *Pediatr Res* 1998;44:639–641.

91. Myers BD, Moran SM. Hemodynamically mediated acute renal failure. *N Engl J Med* 1986;314:97–105.

92. Rasoulpour M, Marinelli KA. Systemic hypertension. *Clin Perinatol* 1992;19(1):121–137.

93. Harris MS, Little GA. Umbilical artery catheters: High, low or no. *J Perinat Med* 1978;6(1):15–21.

94. Seibert JJ, Northington FJ, Miers JF, et al. Aortic thrombosis after umbilical artery catheterization in newborns: Prevalence of complications on long-term follow-up. *AJR Am J Roentgenol* 1991;156:567–569.

95. Mocan H, Beattie TJ, Murphy AV. Renal venous thrombosis in infancy: Long-term follow-up. *Pediatr Nephrol* 1991;5(1):45–49.

96. Dees E, Lin H, Cotton RB, et al. Outcome of preterm infants with congenital heart disease. *J Pediatr* 2000;137:653–659.

97. Malec E. Werynski P, Mroczek T, et al. Results of surgical treatment of congenital heart defects in infants below 2,500 grams. *Przegl Lek* 2000;57(4):187–190.

98. Bove T, Francois K, De Groote K, et al. Outcome analysis of major cardiac operations in low weight neonates. *Ann Thorac Surg* 2004;78(1):181–187.

99. Oppido G, Napoleone CP, Formigari R, et al. Outcome of cardiac surgery in low birth weight and premature infants. *Eur J Cardiothorac Surg* 2004;26(1):44–53.

100. Reddy VM, Hanley FL. Cardiac surgery in infants with very low birth weight. *Sem Pediatr Surg* 2000;9(2):91–95.

101. Sutton N, Lock JE, Geggel RL. Cardiac catheterization in infants weighing less than 1,500 grams. *Catheter Cardiovasc Interv* 2006;68;948–956.

CHAPTER 20 ■ CARDIAC INTENSIVE CARE

GIL WERNOVSKY, MD, ANTHONY C. CHANG, MD, MBA, DAVID L. WESSEL, MD,
AND CHITRA RAVISHANKAR, MBBS

During the last three decades, the development of surgical and catheter techniques for the diagnosis and treatment of critical heart disease in children has been paralleled by major advances in the field of pediatric intensive care. Increasingly, children with congenital heart disease (CHD) are now managed in units specifically dedicated to pediatric intensive care or pediatric cardiac intensive care in particular, rather than in surgical units that primarily care for adults following surgical management of acquired heart disease. This approach is based on the premise that children with CHD represent an extremely heterogeneous population due to the variety of anatomic defects and secondary physiologic derangements that are infrequently encountered in adult patients.

Optimal care of these neonates, infants, and children requires an understanding of the subtleties of complex congenital cardiac anomalies, respiratory mechanics, and physiology; the transitional circulation of the neonate; pharmacologic and mechanical support of the circulation; the effects of cardiopulmonary bypass (CPB) on the heart, lungs, brain, and abdominal organs; airway management; mechanical ventilation; and multiorgan system failure. Pediatric cardiologists are assuming a more central role in the intensive care management of these patients as more complex therapeutic options have become available.

PERIOPERATIVE CONSIDERATIONS

Special Considerations for the Neonate

Although most pediatric patients who undergo cardiac surgery are diagnosed and treated preoperatively as outpatients, the neonate with significant, unrepaired CHD frequently requires preoperative assessment and management in an intensive care unit (ICU) setting. The disappointing cumulative morbidity and mortality rates associated with palliative operations (followed by later repair) compared with early corrective procedures have become apparent during the past decade. Primary corrective surgery for CHD has had a significant impact on both the mortality of the underlying defect and on the secondary effects of the CHD on the development of other organ systems. Nowhere has this impact been more dramatic than among neonates (1).

Expanding the scope of reparative operations to the neonate has altered the demographic makeup of cardiac patients scheduled for surgery and in the ICU. Of the >2,000 combined annual admissions to the Cardiac ICUs at Children's Hospital in Boston and Children's Hospital in Philadelphia, 25% are neonates (<30 days of age) transferred prior to and cared for after surgery, and >50% are <1 year of age. Optimal management requires a multidisciplinary team approach, combining the disciplines of cardiology, cardiac surgery, cardiac anesthesia, neonatology, intensive care, and nursing.

Care of the critically ill neonate requires an appreciation of the special structural and functional features of immature organs, the interactions of the "transitional" neonatal circulation, and the secondary effects of the congenital heart lesion on other organ systems. The neonate appears to respond more quickly and profoundly to physiologically stressful circumstances, which may be expressed in terms of rapid changes in pH, lactate acid, glucose, and temperature. Neonates have diminished fat and carbohydrate reserves. The higher metabolic rate and oxygen consumption of the neonate accounts for the rapid appearance of hypoxia when these patients become apneic. Immaturity of the liver and kidney may be associated with reduced protein synthesis and glomerular filtration such that drug metabolism is altered and hepatic synthetic function is reduced. These issues may be compounded by the normal increased total body water of the neonate compared with that of the older patient, along with the propensity for the capillary system of the neonate to leak fluid from the intravascular space. This is especially prominent in the lung of the neonate, where the pulmonary vascular bed is nearly fully recruited at rest and lymphatic recruitment required to handle increased mean capillary pressures associated with increases in pulmonary blood flow (PBF) may be unavailable.

The neonate may be more likely to maintain blood pressure when there exists a state of impending shock, luring the practitioner into a false sense of security immediately prior to circulatory collapse. Systemic blood pressure is not always a reliable indicator of the adequacy of preload or satisfactory oxygen delivery. The neonatal myocardium is less compliant than that of the older child, is less tolerant of increases in afterload, and is less responsive to increases in preload. The potential for sustained or labile increases in pulmonary vascular resistance (PVR) is common in neonates, and concern over inciting pulmonary hypertensive events has deterred some clinicians from pursuing a reparative approach in neonates. Finally, the extreme stress responses demonstrated in response to CPB must be considered in the overall approach to the management of these patients (2).

These factors do not preclude intervention in the neonate but simply dictate that extraordinary vigilance be applied to the care of these children, and that management plans emerge to account for the immature physiology. Whereas the neonate may be more labile than the older child, there is ample evidence that this age group is more resilient to metabolic or ischemic injury. In fact, the neonate may be particularly capable of coping with some forms of stress. Tolerance of hypoxia in the neonate is characteristic of many species, and the "plasticity" of the neurologic system in the newborn is well described (3). For example, neonates with obstructive left heart lesions frequently present with profound metabolic acidosis and shock, but can be effectively resuscitated without major organ system impairment or sequelae in many cases (4). The elasticity and mobility of vascular structures in the neonate improve the technical aspects of surgery. Reparative operations in neonates take best advantage of normal postnatal changes, allowing more normal growth and development in crucial areas such as myocardial muscle, pulmonary parenchyma, and coronary and pulmonary angiogenesis. Neonatal repair may prevent irreversible secondary organ damage arising from unrepaired or palliated approaches. Postoperative pulmonary hypertensive events are more common in the infant who has been exposed to weeks or months of high pulmonary pressure and flow. This observation seems especially true in such lesions as truncus arteriosus, complete atrioventricular septal defects (AVSDs), and transposition of the great arteries (TGA) with ventricular septal defect. Finally, cognitive and psychomotor abnormalities associated with months of hypoxemia or abnormal hemodynamics may be attenuated by early repair.

Optimal perioperative care involves the following: (a) initial stabilization, airway management, and establishment of vascular access; (b) a complete and thorough noninvasive delineation of the anatomic defect(s); (c) resuscitation with evaluation and treatment of secondary organ dysfunction, particularly of the brain, kidneys, and liver; (d) cardiac catheterization if necessary, typically for physiologic assessment, interventional procedures such as balloon atrial septostomy or valvotomy, or anatomic definition not visible by echocardiography (e.g., coronary artery distribution in pulmonary atresia with intact ventricular septum (IVS) or delineation of aorticopulmonary collaterals in tetralogy of Fallot with pulmonary atresia); and (e) surgical management when cardiac, pulmonary, renal, and central nervous systems are optimized. Crucial in this process is the continued communication among medical, surgical, and nursing disciplines.

Manipulation of Pulmonary Vascular Resistance

Manipulation of the PVR allows some measure of control of cardiac output and intracardiac shunting, depending on the specific anatomic defect and pathophysiology. A thorough understanding of the effects of the pharmacologic and ventilatory manipulation of PVR is crucial in the care of children with complex CHD. For example, in some "right-sided" lesions (e.g., Ebstein's malformation), manipulations to decrease PVR may increase PBF, decrease right heart afterload, and improve cardiac output; similar manipulations in patients with large left-to-right shunt lesions or single ventricle will increase PBF excessively and result in decreased systemic cardiac output and oxygen delivery. Also, many medical conditions and procedures necessary in ICU management increase PVR, which may be particularly deleterious in children with complex CHD because of increased reactivity and resistance of the pulmonary vasculature. These include sympathetic stimulation, endotracheal suctioning, encroachments on lung volumes that produce atelectasis (surgical retraction, pneumothoraces, pleural and peritoneal fluid collections, abdominal packing), CPB, alveolar hypoxia, and hypoventilation. Appropriate ventilation of children with CHD is very important, because it is subject to precise manipulation in the ICU and is crucial for determining PVR via airway pressure, lung volumes, $PaCO_2$, pH, and FiO_2.

Ventilatory Control of Pulmonary Vascular Resistance

Pulmonary vascular resistance can be controlled independently of systemic vascular resistance (SVR) by manipulating various aspects of ventilation (Table 20.1), whereas specific pharmacologic control of PVR is difficult because no specific

TABLE 20.1

MANIPULATIONS ALTERING PVR

Increase PVR	Decrease PVR
Hypoxia	Oxygen
Hypercarbia/acidosis	Hypocarbia/alkalosis
Hyperinflation	Normal FRC
High hematocrit	Low hematocrit
Atelectasis	Nitric oxide

PVR, pulmonary vascular resistance; FRC, functional residual capacity.

pulmonary vasoactive drugs have been available until the recent introduction of nitric oxide (Table 20.1). Even with selective infusions of rapidly metabolized vasoactive drugs into the pulmonary circulation, systemic drug concentrations and systemic hemodynamic effects can be appreciable. In contrast, high levels of inspired oxygen, especially 100% O_2, decrease elevated PVR in infants without changing (or slightly increasing) SVR, whereas inspired oxygen concentrations of $\leq 21\%$ increase PVR. The effectiveness of oxygen as a pulmonary vasodilator after CPB, however, is less certain (6). Hypoventilation, with associated acidosis and hypercapnia, also increases PVR. In contrast, hyperventilation to a pH of >7.50 reliably decreases PVR in infants with dynamically vasoconstricted small vessels. In neonates with severe pulmonary hypertension, this degree of hyperventilation increases effective PBF and decreases right-to-left shunting, thereby increasing the PaO_2. Although prolonged hyperventilation to decrease PVR may theoretically cause problems from decreased cerebral blood flow, clinical experimental studies in hyperventilated infants show minimal evidence of cerebral damage.

The pattern of ventilation and use of positive end-expiratory pressure (PEEP) also can alter PVR. PVR is lowest at normal functional residual capacity (FRC). PVR increases at low lung volumes (collapsed alveoli) (7). If atelectasis and pulmonary edema are corrected by PEEP, the PVR may decrease. However, high levels of PEEP may increase PVR, primarily by hyperinflating the alveoli. Different patterns of ventilation may further reduce PVR by stimulating production of prostacyclin in the pulmonary vasculature. In children with the Fontan circulation, positive pressure ventilation with increased mean airway pressure may limit ventricular filling and thus adversely affect cardiac output. Early extubation usually improves hemodynamics in the awake patient.

Anesthesia, Drugs, and Pulmonary Circulation

The effects of various anesthetic agents on PVR are poorly understood. Ketamine and nitrous oxide increase PVR in adults but do not affect the PVR of infants with normal or elevated PVR when ventilation and FiO_2 are held constant. However, some have observed an increase in PVR with ketamine given to sedated children spontaneously breathing room air during cardiac catheterization. Stress responses in the pulmonary circulation of patients with CHD are of primary concern during the perioperative period. Large doses of potent narcotics (e.g., fentanyl) attenuate pulmonary vascular responses to noxious stimuli such as endotracheal suctioning without changing the baseline PVR (8). Reactive hypertensive responses in the pulmonary bed are partially mediated by the sympathoadrenal axis and thus are attenuated by an adequate depth of anesthesia, usually without changing the baseline PVR.

Pulmonary Vasodilators

Children with many forms of CHD are prone to develop perioperative elevations in PVR. This may particularly complicate the postoperative course, when transient myocardial dysfunction may require a reduction in right ventricular afterload (9,10). Success using vasodilators for treatment of pulmonary hypertension has had mixed results because of systemic vasodilating effects that may predominate and limit effectiveness. Tolazoline, prostaglandin E1, prostacyclin, sodium nitroprusside, and dobutamine have all been suggested as useful pharmacologic treatments for pulmonary hypertension.

Several factors peculiar to CPB may increase PVR: microemboli, pulmonary leukosequestration, excess thromboxane production, atelectasis, hypoxic pulmonary vasoconstriction, and adrenergic events have all been suggested to play a role in producing postoperative pulmonary hypertension. Postoperative pulmonary vascular reactivity has been related not only to the presence of preoperative pulmonary hypertension and left-to-right shunts, but also to the duration of total CPB. The elimination or attenuation of acute postoperative pulmonary hypertensive events has been only partly addressed by surgery at earlier ages, pharmacologic intervention, and other postoperative management strategies. However, recent developments in vascular biology have offered new insights into the possible causes and correction of post-CPB pulmonary hypertension.

Acetylcholine (ACH) relaxes preconstricted vascular smooth muscle by binding to muscarinic receptors on the endothelial cell, causing release of a potent vasodilating substance termed endothelium-derived relaxing factor (EDRF). The active component of EDRF has recently been identified as nitric oxide (11). Nitric oxide is thought to diffuse from the endothelium to adjacent smooth muscle and produce relaxation by activating guanylate cyclase and increasing intracellular cyclic guanosine monophosphate (cGMP). This response is dependent on an intact, functioning endothelium.

Pulmonary vascular endothelial dysfunction may be a contributing factor in post-CPB pulmonary hypertension. Structural damage to the pulmonary endothelium is demonstrable after CPB, and the degree of pulmonary hypertension is correlated to the extent of endothelial damage after CPB. The decreased PBF on CPB may result in postoperative impairment of endothelial function and inability to release nitric oxide. To overcome this, gaseous nitric oxide can be delivered to the pulmonary circulation by direct inhalation to produce pulmonary vasodilation.

Although the effects of inhaled nitric oxide gas in humans were studied in the 1970s, the use of nitric oxide to treat pulmonary hypertension awaited the demonstration in 1987 that nitric oxide was an important EDRF (11,12). The feasibility of using inhaled nitric oxide in animal models of pulmonary hypertension has been demonstrated using awake animals with hypoxia, acidosis, and thromboxane- or protamine-induced pulmonary hypertension. The first published experience (in 1991) with nitric oxide treatment of pulmonary hypertension in humans was provided by Pepke-Zaba et al. (12a) in adults with primary pulmonary hypertension, where PVR declined by 5% to 68%; pulmonary artery pressure was not reported. Recent reports suggest a therapeutic role for inhaled nitric oxide in the treatment of persistent pulmonary hypertension of the neonate (13). Children with pulmonary hypertension and CHD with relative selectivity for the pulmonary circulation vasodilate in response to inhaled nitric oxide (5). This is effective after CPB, when response to ACH is

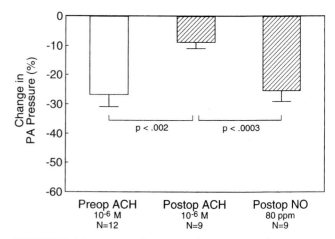

FIGURE 20.1 Percentage change in pulmonary vascular resistance (PVR) with 10^{-6} M dose of acetylcholine (ACH) in preoperative (Preop) and postoperative (Postop) patients. The vasodilating response to ACH is attenuated in postoperative patients, but the capacity for vasodilation, as indicated by the response to inhaled nitric oxide (NO) is retained. (Modified from Wessel DL, Adatia I, Giglia TM, et al. Use of inhaled nitric oxide and acetylcholine in the evaluation of pulmonary hypertension and endothelial function after cardiopulmonary bypass. *Circulation* 1993;88:2128–2138, with permission.)

minimal (Fig. 20.1). This suggests that CPB is responsible for transient pulmonary endothelial dysfunction. Inhaled nitric oxide may be an important addition to the diagnostic and therapeutic tools in the treatment of pulmonary hypertension or respiratory failure.

Nitric oxide (NO) is a vasodilator that can be delivered selectively by inhalation and distributed across the alveoli to the pulmonary vascular smooth muscle (14,15). Because of its rapid inactivation by hemoglobin, inhaled NO can achieve selective pulmonary vasodilation and lower pulmonary artery pressure in a number of diseases without the unwanted effect of systemic hypotension. Inhaled NO has had a dramatic impact in a number of complex heart defects in children (16–21). Descriptions of its use after repair of obstructed total anomalous pulmonary venous connection (TAPVC), the Fontan procedure and after ventricular septal defect repair have been reported, along with a variety of other anatomical lesions. In a study by Atz et al., 20 infants presenting with isolated TAPVC were monitored for pulmonary hypertension in the postoperative period. A mean percentage decrease of 42% in pulmonary vascular resistance and 32% in mean pulmonary artery pressure was demonstrated with 80 PPM of NO. There was no significant change in heart rate, systemic blood pressure, or vascular resistance. Possible toxicities of inhaled NO include methemoglobinemia, production of excess nitrogen dioxide, peroxynitrite, or injury to the pulmonary surfactant system. Abrupt withdrawal of NO can lead to rebound pulmonary hypertension (19). Appreciation of the transient characteristics of withdrawal of NO may facilitate weaning from NO. The withdrawal response to NO may be attenuated by pretreatment with the phosphodiesterase type 5 inhibitor sildenafil (20). Sildenafil (Viagra™) is a selective phosphodiesterase type 5 inhibitor. Phosphodiesterase type 5 breaks down cyclic guanosine monophosphate (cyclic GMP). Sildenafil produces acute and relatively selective pulmonary vasodilatation and acts synergistically with nitric oxide (22). Preliminary reports suggest that sildenafil may have useful effects in pulmonary hypertension particularly in attenuating rebound effects after discontinuing inhaled nitric oxide and in the chronic therapy of pulmonary hypertension. Sildenafil is well tolerated and available as an oral preparation, which makes it particularly attractive in patients with pulmonary hypertension whose symptoms do not warrant a continuous intravenous infusion (23).

Airway Management and Mechanical Ventilation

Intubation of the trachea in an awake neonate or infant with CHD may elicit major hemodynamic and metabolic responses. Appropriate anesthetic and muscle relaxant techniques are therefore warranted to secure the airway under most circumstances. This substantially facilitates the procedure, especially in a fragile postoperative patient, but demands an appropriate level of expertise in anesthetic principles and practice for the practitioners.

Ventilation and respiratory mechanics exert strong influences on the hemodynamics of children with CHD, especially after palliative or reparative operations. The uncertainties of gas exchange during spontaneous breathing in the immediate postoperative period can be minimized by use of mechanical ventilation, end-expiratory pressure, and manipulation of PCO_2 and pH to influence cardiovascular function. General anesthesia, residual neuromuscular blockade, mid-sternal or thoracotomy incisions, lung retraction, atelectasis, and increased lung water from left-to-right shunt lesions all may reduce postoperative FRC and vital capacity. Acute lung injury from CPB, left main stem bronchomalacia (from long-standing left atrial (LA) or left pulmonary artery enlargement), phrenic nerve dysfunction from intraoperative injury, and abnormalities of PBF may also occur. These factors may have a profound impact on gas exchange, lung compliance, ventilation/perfusion abnormalities, and intrapulmonary shunts.

Reduction in FRC decreases lung compliance and decreases pulmonary venous oxygenation. Stiff, "wet" lungs of hypoxic patients are associated with an unusual work of breathing, which in turn may substantially increase oxygen consumption. Mechanical ventilation with positive pressure reverses these pathophysiologic processes and will substantially reduce the work of breathing. Although early postoperative extubation can be successfully accomplished for closed procedures and for children with less complex disease repaired during CPB, the advantages of postoperative positive pressure ventilation have been increasingly apparent for neonates with complex disease as well as in adults following CPB.

To ensure selected preset mechanical minute ventilation, even through changing pulmonary mechanics, several issues require emphasis. Nasotracheal intubation may be preferred if it provides greater stability of the airway than orotracheal intubation. A close-fitting endotracheal tube should be selected that permits air to leak at pressures of 25 to 35 cm H_2O.

Ventilator tubing with an internal diameter of 15 to 25 mm and a wall thickness of 2.4 mm minimizes the compressible volume within the breathing system. Tubing lengths of approximately 40 cm with water traps to remove condensed water vapor (which otherwise collects in the tubing lumen and impedes gas flow) result in a system-compressible volume of less than 1.0 to 1.5 mL/cm H_2O.

Compressible volume considerations are especially important in the neonate where the delivered tidal volume (typically 12 to 15 mL/kg) begins to approach the compressible volume (1.5 mL/cm H_2O of peak pressure). Thus, a 3-kg neonate who generates a peak inspiratory pressure of 30 cm H_2O during a delivered tidal volume of 45 mL will also have 45 mL of compressible volume. One adjusts for this by setting the ventilator

(volume-preset mode) at 90 mL. When the compressible volume substantially exceeds the delivered tidal volume (as in smaller neonates with a less compliant lung), other modes of ventilation (such as time-cycled pressure-limited ventilation as used in many neonatal ICUs) may be more appropriate.

An important consideration in the neonate or young infant is the modification of volume-limited ventilators to allow for continuous flow, which eliminates the work of breathing required to open the inspiratory valve on these machines. This modification requires larger-bore tubing to minimize expiratory retard in continuous-flow circuits. Larger-bore tubing, however, reintroduces the hazards of larger compression volumes, which in neonates may approximate or exceed the actual delivered tidal volume. Consequently, sudden changes in lung compliance may result in a significant loss of minute ventilation in the neonate despite the use of volume-preset ventilators. Unlike the older child, the neonate may lose considerable tidal volume when lung compliance changes suddenly and peak inspiratory pressure increases. Equipping the ventilator to sound an alarm when specified peak inspiratory pressures are exceeded is thus very important.

Volume-preset mechanical ventilators are commonly used to provide mechanical ventilation in children with CHD. Warm, filtered, humidified gas is delivered by the ventilator. In the control mode of ventilation, the ventilator will deliver a preset volume through the system at specific unvarying times without the opportunity for additional patient breaths. The intermittent mandatory ventilation (IMV) mode requires modification with a reservoir in the inspiratory loop; additional spontaneous breaths are thus allowed and can be coordinated with the patient's inspiratory effort to deliver a preset volume, synchronized to allow spontaneous breaths to occur in addition to and exclusive of a predetermined minimum number of mechanical ventilator volume preset breaths (SIMV).

The mechanical ventilator frequency is typically set at 12 to 20 breaths per minute, the higher values used in neonates. Initially a tidal volume is selected that, by inspection, produces significant movement of the chest wall. The peak inspiratory pressure generated frequently exceeds 25 cm H_2O. Alveoli are recruited largely during peak inspiration and are distended by end-expiratory pressure. Subsequent adjustments, usually in rate rather than tidal volume, are then guided by the pH and $PaCO_2$.

Alternatively, the inspiratory pressure can be preset and the delivered tidal volume allowed to vary with both the selected pressure limit and the total lung compliance of the patient (pressure-control mode). The patient's spontaneous breaths are allowed in this mode of ventilation and can be assisted when sufficient negative pressure is generated by a respiratory effort that triggers positive-pressure augmentation of the spontaneous breath (pressure-support mode). Varying levels of pressure support also can be combined with volume-preset IMV modes of ventilation to facilitate weaning, by maximizing synchrony while ensuring a minimum number of adequate mechanical breaths. Pressure regulated volume control ventilation or PRVC combines the features of both volume and pressure-limited ventilation. This mode uses a decelerating inspiratory flow waveform to deliver a set tidal volume during the selected inspiratory time and at a set frequency. Airway pressure is limited below a selected high pressure threshold, and may vary as mush as 3 cm H_2O from the previous breath. Thus the ventilator is continuously adapting the inspiratory pressure to changes in airway compliance and resistance.

Caution must be exercised while suctioning the airway in infants in the immediate postoperative period. Increasing airway pressure, diminished motion of the chest wall, visible blood (or blood-tinged secretions), or large amounts of normal-appearing secretions in the artificial airway are clear indications to perform this maneuver. Suctioning of the airway is a stressful event that can have a serious adverse effect on hemodynamics. Consequently, one may choose to extend the anesthetic period through the first postoperative night in selected patients in an attempt to blunt the pulmonary hypertensive response to this and other external stimuli.

Postoperatively, mechanical ventilation is continued until (a) hemostasis is complete; (b) atrial-derived rhythm or pacemaker-protected heart rate is within the 95% confidence limits for age; (c) adequate cardiac output is established (strong peripheral pulses, capillary refill of <3 seconds with warm distal extremities, etc.); (d) the arterial waveform suggests adequate stroke volume; (e) normothermia has been achieved; and (f) there is no evidence of metabolic acidosis, uncontrolled seizures, or thick copious secretions. The mandatory rate of mechanical ventilation is usually decreased until spontaneous breathing begins, noting the patient's respiratory rate and effort, along with the hemodynamic effects of weaning. Guided by physical examination, hemodynamic criteria, and arterial blood gas measurements, mechanical ventilatory breath frequency is usually reduced to <5 to 10 breaths per minute before the child is extubated. Measurement of airway resistance and work of breathing may be a helpful predictor of those infants who will not permit successful weaning from mechanical ventilation. Other modes of ventilatory support may be introduced to the SIMV mean (e.g., pressure-support mode) to overcome natural and artificial airway resistance, permit synchronized support, and decrease the work of breathing while encouraging spontaneous respiratory effort and diaphragmatic function.

If a postoperative patient fails to tolerate spontaneous respiration and weaning from mechanical ventilation using the techniques described above, a search for any residual hemodynamic cause must be initiated. Intraoperatively placed intracardiac monitoring catheters and/or echocardiography serve to identify residual structural abnormalities remaining after surgery, or those that have arisen as a result of palliation or repair. If these data are inconclusive, cardiac catheterization may be indicated. Noncardiovascular causes of respiratory failure can be broadly grouped into neuromuscular and central nervous system (CNS) disorders, airway abnormalities proximal to the alveoli, alveolar disease, and compression of lung volume by extrapulmonary factors (pleural effusion, pneumothorax, etc.). Depression of the respiratory center occurs most commonly as a result of the administration of analgesics, sedative hypnotics, or anesthetics. Hypoxic-ischemic injury to the respiratory center is an unusual cause for disordered respiratory control but occasionally can be a contributing factor.

Special Physiologic Considerations

Single-Ventricle Physiology

A wide variety of anatomic lesions, usually associated with atresia of an atrioventricular (AV) or semilunar valve, share the common physiology of complete mixing of the systemic and pulmonary venous return (Table 20.2). In these conditions, the total ventricular output is divided between two competing parallel circuits; the pulmonary artery and aortic oxygen saturations are equal. The relative proportion of the ventricular output to either the pulmonary or systemic vascular bed is determined by the relative resistance to flow in the two circuits.

TABLE 20.2

NON-SPECIFIC CAUSES OF LCOS

Inflammation
Ischemia-reperfusion injury
Lack of atrioventricular synchrony
Brady-or trachyarrhythmia
Hypothyroidism

Resistance to pulmonary flow is determined (a) by the degree of subvalvar or valvar pulmonary obstruction; (b) by the pulmonary arteriolar resistance; and (c) more distally by the pulmonary veins and left atrial (LA) pressures. The LA pressure is in part determined by the volume of PBF entering the LA and the relative degree of restriction to outflow through the left AV valve and atrial septum.

Resistance to systemic flow is determined by the presence of (a) anatomic obstructive lesions (subaortic obstruction, aortic valve stenosis, arch hypoplasia, and coarctation) and (b) systemic arteriolar resistance.

With the newborn's first breaths, there is an immediate decrease in PVR and a relative increase in PBF. The PVR continues to decrease with time, with an increasing proportion of ventricular output committed to the lungs. The normal homeostatic mechanisms to improve systemic output will result in an increased stroke volume and increase in heart rate. The single-ventricle physiology of a newborn with hypoplastic left heart syndrome typifies the pathophysiology and management of all lesions with complete mixing and will be discussed for illustrative purposes (Fig. 20.2).

The "Ideal" Anatomy and Physiology

An acceptable balance between the pulmonary and systemic output provides enough pulmonary flow for adequate oxygen delivery to prevent acidosis without an excessive volume load to the single ventricle (Fig. 20.2A). Anatomically, there would be a widely patent ductus arteriosus with no aortic arch narrowing, providing no restriction to systemic blood flow (SBF) and normal coronary perfusion. The foramen ovale would be mildly restrictive, providing some limitation to PBF. This would result in mild right ventricular volume overload without tricuspid regurgitation, normal SBF, and a pulmonary-to-systemic flow ($Q_p{:}Q_s$) ratio of approximately 1.0. Assuming a mixed venous oxygen saturation of 65% and a pulmonary venous oxygen saturation of 95%, arterial oxygen saturation will be 80%.

The Decreasing Pulmonary Vascular Resistance Physiology

The normal decrease in PVR over the first few hours to days of life results in elevated PBF relative to SBF (Fig. 20.2B). As SBF decreases, stroke volume and heart rate increase as a mechanism to preserve cardiac (systemic) output. There may be enhancement of the renin–angiotensin system and elevated circulating catecholamines. As the $Q_p{:}Q_s$ ratio approaches 2.0, the right ventricle becomes more volume overloaded with mildly elevated end-diastolic and LA pressures. The neonate may show signs of tachypnea or respiratory distress, and hepatomegaly may be present. The greater proportion of pulmonary venous return in the mixed ventricular blood results in elevated systemic arterial oxygen saturation (85%), and visible cyanosis may be mild or absent. Not infrequently, these infants are discharged from the nursery as normal newborns.

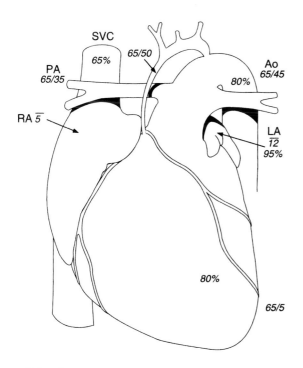

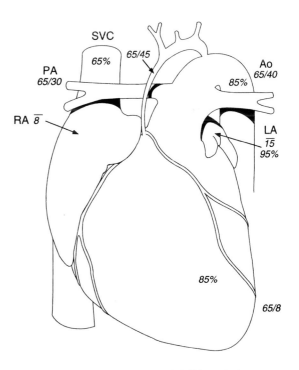

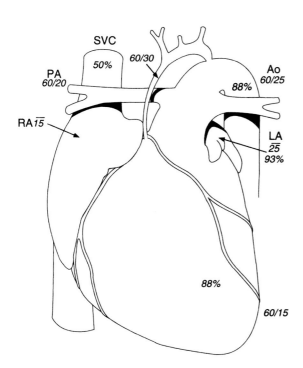

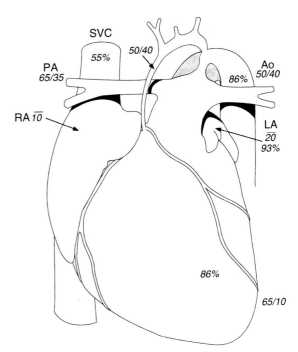

FIGURE 20.2 A–D: The heterogeneous preoperative physiology in hypoplastic left heart syndrome. See text for details and discussion. Ao, aorta; LA, left atrium; RA, right atrium; PA, pulmonary artery; PVR, pulmonary vascular resistance; Q_p/Q_s, pulmonary to systemic flow ratio; SVC, superior vena cava.

The Low Pulmonary Vascular Resistance Physiology

The natural history at this point is one of a continued, gradual decrease in PVR with a resultant increase in PBF and relative decrease in SBF (Fig. 20.2C). Because total ventricular output is limited by heart rate and stroke volume, with a continued increase in Q_p:Q_s ratio, there is the onset of clinically apparent congestive heart failure, right ventricular dilation and dysfunction, progressive tricuspid regurgitation, poor peripheral perfusion with metabolic acidosis, decreased urine output, and pulmonary edema. Arterial oxygen saturation approaches 90%.

The Closing Ductus Physiology

Alternatively, a sudden deterioration takes place with rapidly progressive congestive failure and shock as the ductus arteriosus constricts (Fig. 20.2D). There is decreased SBF and increased PBF, which is largely independent of the PVR. The peripheral pulses are weak to absent. Renal, hepatic, coronary, and CNS perfusion is compromised, possibly resulting in acute tubular necrosis, necrotizing enterocolitis, or cerebral infarction or hemorrhage. A vicious cycle also may result from inadequate retrograde perfusion of the ascending aorta (coronary blood supply), with further myocardial dysfunction and continued compromise of coronary blood flow. The Q_p:Q_s ratio approaches infinity as Q_s nears zero. Thus, one has the paradoxical presentation of profound metabolic acidosis in the face of a relatively high PO_2 (70 to 100 mm Hg).

Management

The arterial blood gas may represent the single best indicator of hemodynamic stability. Arterial oxygen saturation of 80% with normal pH typically indicates a Q_p:Q_s ratio of close to 1.0 with adequate peripheral perfusion, whereas elevated oxygen saturation (>90%) with acidosis represents significantly increased pulmonary and decreased systemic flow with probable myocardial dysfunction and secondary effects on other organ systems. Resuscitation of these neonates involves pharmacologic maintenance of ductal patency with prostaglandin E1, maneuvers to increase pulmonary resistance and decrease systemic resistance, and inotropic support if needed. Large doses of inotropic agents may have a deleterious effect, depending on the relative effects on the systemic and pulmonary vascular beds. Preferential selective elevations of systemic vascular tone will secondarily increase PBF, and careful monitoring of mean arterial blood pressure and arterial oxygen saturation is warranted. However a majority of these neonates with high oxygen saturation can maintain reasonable systemic perfusion as assessed by acid-base status and end-organ function with minimal intervention other than continuation of prostaglandin infusion.

Although most neonates with high O_2 saturation are stable, some with excessive pulmonary blood flow or a high Q_p:Q_s can develop systemic hypoperfusion with associated hypotension, metabolic and lactic acidosis, and end-organ dysfunction. These infants require sedation, paralysis, and controlled minute ventilation. The pulmonary vascular resistance in the newborn is sensitive to alveolar oxygen, carbon dioxide and pH. Hypoxia (14% to 20% FiO_2), and increasing arterial PCO_2 by hypoventilation or hypercarbia (2% to 5% $FiCO_2$) are described strategies for decreasing pulmonary blood flow in single ventricle patients (24). In order to compare the effect of hypoxia (17% FiO_2) and hypercarbia (2.7% $FiCO_2$) on oxygen delivery, 10 infants with hypoplastic left heart syndrome were evaluated preoperatively in a randomized, crossover trial under conditions of anesthesia, paralysis, and fixed minute ventilation. Arterial (SaO_2) and superior vena caval (SvO_2) co-oximetry and cerebral oxygen saturation (ScO_2) measurements were made at the end of each condition (10 minutes per condition) and recovery period (15 to 20 minutes). ScO_2 was measured using NIRS or near infrared spectroscopy. Both hypoxia and hypercarbia decreased SaO_2 and Q_p:Q_s. Both ScO_2 and arteriovenous oxygen difference remained unchanged with hypoxia, whereas hypercarbia increased both ScO_2 and SvO_2, and narrowed the arteriovenous oxygen difference. Thus, inspired gas mixtures can be used to improve systemic blood flow in single ventricle patients with excessive pulmonary blood flow. These patients should undergo early surgical intervention to restrict pulmonary blood flow with an aorto-pulmonary.

The neonate who presents in shock in the first weeks of life has duct-dependent CHD until proven otherwise. Too often, valuable time is lost at initial presentation with diagnostic testing to "rule out sepsis." Although sepsis must be considered and treated empirically, resuscitation will frequently be ineffective if the ductus arteriosus is not reopened with prostaglandin. The presentation of shock, acidosis, and a failed hyperoxia challenge (failure to increase the arterial PaO_2 >150 torr in 100% inspired oxygen) is typical for duct-dependent, left-sided obstructive heart disease; prostaglandin therapy should be strongly considered even before echocardiographic confirmation of the anatomic defect. Monitoring of vital signs, establishment of vascular access, and attention to the airway (due to prostaglandin-related apnea) are mandatory.

Initial Management in Transposition of the Great Arteries

In neonates with TGA, usually with an IVS, a very low arterial PO_2 (15 to 20 torr) with high PCO_2 (despite adequate chest motion and ventilation) and metabolic acidosis are markers for severely decreased effective PBF and require urgent attention. The initial management of the severely hypoxemic patient with TGA includes both ensuring adequate mixing between the two parallel circuits and maximizing mixed venous oxygen saturation.

Maximizing Intercirculatory Mixing

In patients who do not respond with an increased arterial oxygen saturation to the opening of the ductus arteriosus with prostaglandin (usually these neonates have very restrictive atrial defects or pulmonary hypertension), the foramen ovale should be emergently enlarged by balloon atrial septostomy. This can be done in the catheterization laboratory. However, bedside echocardiography is generally successful for catheter guidance. Hyperventilation and treatment with sodium bicarbonate are important maneuvers to promote alkalosis, lower PVR, and increase PBF, which increases atrial mixing following septostomy.

Maximizing Mixed Venous Oxygen Saturation

In d-TGA, most SBF is the recirculated systemic venous return. In the presence of poor mixing, much can be gained by increasing the mixed venous oxygen saturation, which is the major determinant of systemic arterial oxygen saturation. These maneuvers include decreasing oxygen consumption (muscle relaxants, sedation, mechanical ventilation, normothermia) and improving oxygen delivery (increasing cardiac output with inotropic agents, increasing oxygen carrying capacity by treating anemia). Coexisting causes of pulmonary venous desaturation (e.g., pneumothorax) should also be sought and treated. Increasing the fraction of inspired oxygen to 100% will have little effect on the arterial PO$_2$, unless it serves to lower PVR and increase PBF.

If severe hypoxemia persists despite the above maneuvers, mechanical support with extracorporeal membrane oxygenation or early arterial switch surgery may be indicated.

Tetralogy of Fallot Spells

When an acute increase in right ventricular outflow obstruction (or a decrease in SVR) occurs in patients with tetralogy of Fallot, right-to-left shunting of systemic venous return across the VSD increases, and hypercyanotic spells may occur. These spells characteristically occur as a result of the combination of (a) irritability, (b) profound cyanosis, (c) hyperpnea, and (d) syncope. Initial management of these patients is geared toward maintaining SVR, minimizing PVR, and providing sedation with minimal myocardial depression. Hypercyanotic spells are initially treated with 100% oxygen by face mask, a knee-chest position, and morphine sulfate (0.1 mg/kg). This regimen usually causes the dynamic infundibular stenosis to relax while maintaining SVR.

Deeply cyanotic and lethargic patients are given intravenous crystalloid infusions to augment circulating blood volume. Continued severe hypoxemia may then be treated first with a vasopressor (e.g., phenylephrine) to increase SVR, and rarely with judicious use of a short-acting beta-blocker (e.g., esmolol) to slow the heart rate. If a hypercyanotic spell persists despite treatment, immediate surgical management of the anomaly is indicated; the child should be anesthetized with intravenous narcotics and the lungs ventilated in a way that maintains a normal SVR with a low PVR. In this extreme situation, temporary support of the circulation with epinephrine or phenylephrine may be beneficial in supporting left ventricular (LV) function and SVR when the PBF is severely limited. Extracorporeal oxygenation may be indicated in severe cases when corrective or palliative surgery is not possible.

POSTOPERATIVE CONSIDERATIONS

Ideal postoperative care of the patient following either reparative or palliative operations requires a thorough understanding and systematic evaluation of the following: (a) the underlying anatomic defect, (b) the pathophysiology of the preoperative state (including secondary effects on other organ systems from altered cardiac output preoperatively), (c) the anesthetic regimen used during surgery, (d) CPB issues (e.g., duration of bypass and circulatory arrest), (e) the details of the operative procedure and any concerns of the surgeon regarding the potential for residual defects, and (f) data available from monitoring catheters, echocardiography, and cardiac catheterization. Optimal management of these critically ill children can best be achieved through a harmonious team approach, combining the expertise of cardiologists, cardiac surgeons, anesthesiologists, intensivists, nurses, and respiratory therapists.

In general, when the clinical course, postoperative hemodynamic measurements, or laboratory data do not correspond to the expected postoperative recovery, it is prudent to suspect both the accuracy of the preoperative diagnosis and the adequacy of the surgical repair, rather than to presume that the preoperative diagnoses and surgical repair were entirely complete and

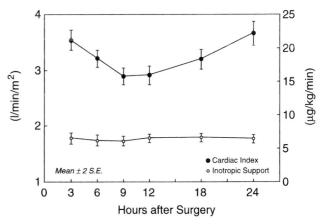

FIGURE 20.3 Serial measurements of cardiac index obtained by thermodilution in 118 neonates following the arterial switch operation (ASO) for d-transposition of the great arteries (TGA). The x-axis displays hours after removal of the aortic cross clamp. The leftward y-axis (•) depicts the cardiac index; the rightward y-axis (○) the dosage of dopamine. Cardiac index decreased by 25% during the first postoperative night, which was not due to a significant change in the amount of inotropic support. Cardiac index decreased below 2.0 L/min/m^2 in 28 patients (24%). (Modified from Wernovsky G, Wypij D, Jonas RA, et al. Postoperative course and hemodynamic profile after the arterial switch operation in neonates and infants: A comparison of low-flow bypass and circulatory arrest. Circulation 1995;92:2226–2235, with permission.)

that the patient is failing for some ill-defined reason (such as "low–cardiac output syndrome"). Decreased cardiac output occurs following CPB (10) but usually can be anticipated and adequately managed (Fig. 20.3). When significant residual anatomic defects are suspected, complete investigation, including echocardiography or catheterization, should be pursued. Reintervention (surgical or catheter) to correct residual anatomic problems is then undertaken if indicated. Information obtained through invasive monitoring is essential to make these assessments and to guide diagnostic and therapeutic interventions.

Pain Control and Sedation

Stress responses to pain and other noxious stimuli are profound in even the youngest neonates, regardless of conceptual age (25). These hormonal and metabolic stress responses are pathologic and probably deleterious (26). Regardless of which medications are chosen, it is important on physiologic grounds alone to give children of all ages adequate anesthesia or analgesia for suppression of the responses to noxious stimulation. Studies in neonates confirm this requirement, which in the past had been neglected in premature neonates and young infants undergoing procedures such as ligation of a patent ductus arteriosus.

Some intravenous and intramuscular anesthetics provide a larger margin of safety for induction of anesthesia and sedation in the immature and compromised cardiovascular system of neonates and infants with severe cardiac disease. However, very high transient arterial, cardiac, and brain concentrations of intravenous agents can occur when normal intravenous doses of drugs are given as a rapid infusion in children with known right-to-left shunts because mixing, uptake, and metabolism in the pulmonary circulation are bypassed. For example, in dogs with right-to-left shunts, a 1 mg/kg bolus of intravenous lidocaine resulted in arterial drug concentrations above those reported to cause irreversible myocardial toxicity.

Routinely administered bolus doses of lidocaine used for dysrhythmias or intubation, or other drugs such as barbiturates, beta-blockers, or calcium channel blockers, may be potentially toxic to children with substantial right-to-left shunts, and the doses should be adjusted appropriately and titrated to effect.

Postoperative Sedation and Analgesia

The infant and neonate respond to stressful perioperative stimuli with altered hemodynamics and stress hormone levels (25). The postoperative myocardium that has been exposed to the effects of CPB, aortic cross clamping, deep hypothermia, or myocardial ischemic damage may not be capable of increasing stroke volume during a bradycardic episode or of maintaining cardiac output during an acute increase in afterload following surgical procedures. This is especially true if myocardial performance is impaired by a ventriculotomy as required for repair of a variety of CHDs.

In an infant with a healthy heart and normal cardiovascular reserve, a painful or stressful stimulus may produce tachycardia, hypertension, and a transient decrease in arterial PO_2 (27). However, in a postoperative cardiac surgical patient, the tachycardia may evolve into a hemodynamically compromising tachyarrhyarrthmia, and the hypertension may represent a critical and intolerable increase in ventricular afterload or may complicate hemostasis. Hypoxemia may be profound and prolonged if the child has cyanotic heart disease or opportunities for intermittent right-to-left shunting during periods of agitation when intrathoracic pressure and right ventricular afterload are increased.

This sensitivity to stimuli and lability in hemodynamic response may be expressed as sudden death during the first postoperative night following apparently successful and uncomplicated congenital heart surgery. This appears to be true, especially among patients with labile pulmonary artery hypertension and in palliated single ventricle patients where the balance between systemic and PVR plays an important role in hemodynamic stability.

These observations have motivated some to extend anesthesia through the first postoperative night in selected patients using continuous infusions of fentanyl (5 mcg/kg/h) following intraoperative anesthetic doses (50 to 100 mcg/kg) (10,26). This approach has been applied in the past to patients with unstable hemodynamics and to all neonates after CPB; doses of fentanyl as high as 10 to 15 mcg/kg/h have been used especially in neonates with labile pulmonary hypertension. The objective is to minimize hemodynamic lability in unstable patients during the first postoperative night when cardiac output reaches its nadir and myocardial reserve is diminished. Precise control of PCO_2 and pH, and hence PVR, is more easily achieved in a paralyzed and heavily sedated patient. However in the current era many centers routinely use low-dose fentanyl at 1–2 mcg/kg/hour without any obvious adverse effect on outcomes.

For less labile patients who can be awakened in the immediate postoperative period, providing adequate analgesia is an important aspect of care. Traditional pratice employs analgesia and sedation on an as-needed basis, although continuous infusions of narcotics or benzodiazepines may be used in the immediate postoperative period as well. Regional anesthetic techniques (using epidural anesthetics or narcotics) can provide excellent analgesia, as well as providing synergistic control of postoperative hypertension (e.g., following surgical therapy for coarctation of the aorta). Older patients may benefit from patient-controlled analgesia regimens that provide better pain control with safeguards against oversedation.

Specific Agents

Ketamine. When intravenous access or lack of patient cooperation is a problem, intramuscular ketamine (3 to 5 mg/kg) is generally well tolerated in sick infants and children with cyanosis or congestive heart failure. Because of the potential effects of ketamine on airways, ventilation, and secretions, it should be given in combination with an antisialagogue (e.g., atropine) while the airway and ventilation are carefully maintained, especially in children with decreased oxygen reserve. Ketamine can be mixed with atropine and succinylcholine in the same syringe; the final volume is relatively small. Injection of this mixture allows rapid control of the airway.

Although increased PVR has been reported with ketamine use in adults, 2 mg/kg intravenously in premedicated infants and young children usually does not increase pulmonary artery pressure or PVR, even when the baseline PVR is elevated. If hypoventilation or apnea occurs after an intravenous dose of ketamine, undesirable increases in PVR can occur because of the associated changes in PaO_2 and $PaCO_2$. Little change in cardiac output, heart rate, or arterial pressure is seen after intravenous ketamine in infants and small children with CHD. Despite reports of ketamine having a negative inotropic effect on isolated heart muscle in animal studies (at very high doses), the ejection fraction of children with CHD is typically well preserved after ketamine. Furthermore, arterial saturation is improved when ketamine is used to induce anesthesia in cyanotic patients. Clinical experience with using ketamine has been excellent for sick infants and children with most forms of heart disease, including those with limited PBF and cyanosis. Ketamine is also useful for sedation and for anesthesia for cardiac catheterization of children with CHD, although a delayed recovery time compared with drugs such as propofol has been reported. In older children and adults, delirium and excessive catecholamine production may be a limiting factor in the use of ketamine.

Narcotics. High-dose narcotics provide excellent cardiovascular stability in children with CHD who may require anesthesia for invasive procedures in the ICU. Up to 1 mg/kg morphine, when given slowly and over a prolonged period of time, provides reasonable cardiovascular stability in children; however, as in adults, histamine release can occur and cause hypotension. The more potent narcotics, fentanyl (10 to 50 μg/kg) and sufentanil (5 to 10 μg/kg), given more slowly, provide better stability of the cardiovascular system on induction of anesthesia when used with pancuronium in very sick infants with CHD. Pancuronium is commonly used when anesthesia is provided with high-dose narcotics; other muscle relaxants may induce hemodynamic instability when given rapidly in large doses during critical situations. Doses of these agents that blunt systemic and pulmonary stress responses in younger and sicker children are well tolerated. Changes in pulmonary and systemic hemodynamics are insignificant in infants with a bolus of fentanyl of 25 μg/kg, but mild hypotension and bradycardia have been reported with the shorter-acting synthetic narcotic alfentanil.

Used with 100% oxygen, these high-dose narcotics are safe and result in increased arterial oxygenation in cyanotic children. Fentanyl doses as low as 5 μg/kg/h may be sufficient for effective maintenance of anesthesia in neonates and have proven invaluable in the maintenance of anesthesia in the ICU (10,28). The high-dose narcotic technique is most suitable for sick infants and older children in whom postoperative mechanical ventilation is planned.

Lower doses of narcotics (e.g., morphine 0.05 to 0.1 mg/kg or fentanyl 1 to 2 μg/kg) are very useful for pain control and sedation in the ICU setting. Respiratory depression may result in decreased minute ventilation and CO_2 retention in the spontaneously breathing patient; appropriate monitoring of vital signs and pulse oximetry is recommended.

Other Intravenous Agents. The benzodiazepine derivatives (e.g., midazolam or diazepam) can be very useful for sedation when titrated in small doses (0.05 to 0.1 mg/kg). Lack of vascular damage and pain on injection make the water-soluble midazolam a more useful benzodiazepine than diazepam, particularly because it has a shorter duration of action. Myocardial depression with midazolam is minor except when used in conjunction with narcotics in patients whose cardiovascular tone is supported largely by high sympathetic output. Larger doses of midazolam (0.2 to 0.3 mg/kg) may be used to achieve anesthesia and facilitate tracheal intubation.

Published studies of the effects of other intravenous agents in small children with CHD are sparse. Some centers use thiopental (1 to 5 mg/kg) for the induction of anesthesia to secure the airway in small children, although thiopental is used less for neonates and young infants. In the older age group, thiopental does not reduce the arterial oxygenation of cyanotic patients. However, the myocardial depression associated with thiopental has made it an uncommon choice for short-term sedation or anesthesia except to facilitate intubation of the hypertensive child with increased intracranial pressure and good myocardial function. Rectal barbiturates, notably methohexital, may be an acceptable induction agent in an otherwise uncooperative child with less severe CHD and good cardiac reserve, but absorption of the drug is variable, myocardial depression is possible, and its use in a critical care setting is uncommon. New nonsteroidal anti-inflammatory agents such as ketorolac (1 mg/kg) offer improved analgesia in postoperative patients with less respiratory depression and little effect on gastrointestinal motility. Other agents that are occasionally used for sedation such as pentobarbital, chloral hydrate, propofol, and more recently dexmedetomidine are beyond the scope of this chapter.

Muscle Relaxants. Dosage requirements for pancuronium are unchanged in children with CHD and intracardiac shunts; it produces no significant heart rate or blood pressure changes when given slowly to these patients. However, a bolus dose of pancuronium can produce tachycardia and hypertension in children through its sympathomimetic effect, which is sometimes desirable to support the cardiac output of infants with relatively fixed stroke volumes. If tachycardia is undesirable, metocurine (Metubine), which causes minimal change in heart rate, blood pressure, or cardiac rhythm in small children (even at doses of 0.5 mg/kg), is often appropriate. For patients in whom a short-acting, nondepolarizing muscle relaxant is desirable, atracurium or vecuronium have few cardiovascular side effects in children when given in low doses.

If the depolarizing agent succinylcholine is given to children with CHD, atropine also should be given to avoid associated bradycardia or sinus arrest. Although not reported as a clinical problem in normal children, simultaneous use of the potent narcotics and succinylcholine without atropine should be avoided in children with compromised cardiovascular function because of the potential for severe bradycardia with this combination of drugs. Significant hyperkalemia is a contraindication for the use of depolarizing muscle relaxants.

Monitoring

Accurate measurement of systemic and pulmonary arterial (PA) pressure, ventricular filling pressures, urine output, alveo-

lar gas exchange, cardiac output, SVR, and PVR allows precise pharmacologic and ventilatory support in the perioperative period. The neonate and infant in particular have wider swings in physiologic variables such as heart rate, temperature, glucose metabolism, SVR, and PVR compared with adults, and they frequently require more physiologic monitoring, not less.

Many different invasive catheters have become the mainstay of postoperative care. Invasive monitoring catheters have two general functions: assessment of the surgical repair and "on-line" assessment of hemodynamics. Accurate measurement of systemic blood pressure, ventricular filling pressures, urine output, alveolar gas exchange, cardiac output, SVR, and PVR allows for precise pharmacologic and ventilatory support in the perioperative period. However, although these catheters are generally safe (29) they are associated with a number of risks and should be chosen on an individual basis.

In general, most patients are invasively monitored in the perioperative period using arterial and urinary catheters, electrocardiographic (ECG) monitoring, end-tidal CO_2 monitoring, pulse oximetry, and intracardiac monitoring catheters. Following surgery, one or two right atrial (RA) catheters are typically placed through the RA appendage (frequently in the site used for venous cannulation on CPB), and an LA catheter may be placed into the right superior pulmonary vein or LA appendage. If necessary, a PA catheter is inserted through a purse-string suture in the right ventricular outflow tract, and may be a single-lumen pressure catheter or a double-lumen catheter with a thermistor for measurement of cardiac output and core temperature (Fig. 20.4). RA catheters are used to assess the central venous pressure and for measurement of RA oxygen saturation. The RA saturation may not truly reflect the "mixed venous" saturation if the tip of the catheter is close to the renal vein flow (falsely high), coronary sinus ostium or hepatic venous flow (falsely low); radiographic confirmation of tip position is important in correctly interpreting the data. Saline contrast injections through the RA catheter during echocardiography may detect right-to-left intracardiac shunting. RA catheters may be used for vasoactive and inotropic medications, and they also may be used for parenteral nutrition if care is taken to prevent contamination. LA catheters (infrequently used) provide indirect data on the function of the systemic ventricle and may be used for contrast (saline) injections during echocardiography to detect residual left-to-right shunts. Inspection of the pressure tracing allows assessment of the function of the systemic AV valve and may be helpful in distinguishing various arrhythmias with loss of AV synchrony (Fig. 20.5). The LA catheter is usually removed on the first or second postoperative day; RA catheters may be left in place for up to 2 weeks if necessary. Complications (1% rate) of these catheters include bleeding, entrapment, fragmentation, transient arrhythmias, and infection (29).

In the past, PA catheters, in particular, were relied upon both for monitoring of PA pressure and PVR, as well as assessment of the adequacy of the surgical repair (30,31). Adequate, short-acting sedation was frequently necessary to obtain stable hemodynamics during catheter withdrawal (Fig. 20.6) (usually on the first postoperative day). However, the increasing use of intraoperative transesophageal echocardiography has all but obviated the need for transthoracic PA catheters (32), which had the highest incidence of complications of the transthoracic lines (29). Hemodynamically significant shunts or outflow tract obstruction can be accurately identified before leaving the operating room, and surgical revision performed if necessary (32).

Continuous monitoring of PA pressure is still helpful in a small number of patients at risk for reactive pulmonary hypertension following surgical repair of certain congenital lesions (e.g., obstructed total anomalous pulmonary venous connection,

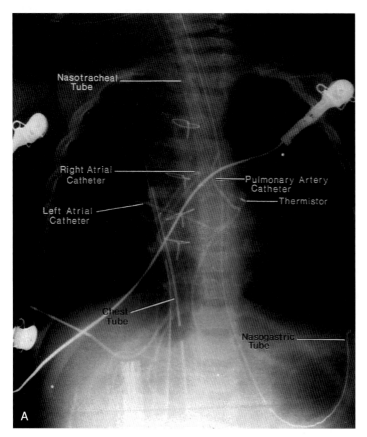

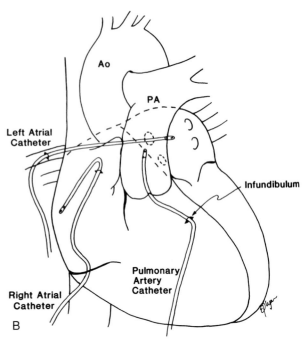

FIGURE 20.4 Postoperative chest radiograph (**A**) and schematic drawing (**B**) of intracardiac line placement. Double-lumen pulmonary artery catheters equipped with a thermistor may be used (**B**), rather than two separate catheters (**A**). Ao, aorta; PA, pulmonary artery.

mitral stenosis). These catheters also allow continuous assessment of the effects of respiratory and pharmacologic manipulations on the pulmonary vascular bed.

Finally, a double-lumen PA catheter equipped with a thermistor allowing measurement of cardiac output (following injection of cold saline in the right atrium) and calculation of pulmonary and systemic resistance in the absence of residual intracardiac shunt was used in therapeutic trials such as the Boston Circulatory Arrest trial. This is now rarely used.

Arterial Catheters

Continuous monitoring of intra-arterial systemic pressure is routinely used. Blood pressure measurements by cuff and auscultation are unreliable in an unstable child, and automated Doppler techniques lack accuracy and reliability during low-flow states. Arterial catheters allow beat-to-beat analysis of the arterial waveform and can provide insight into specific disease states such as cardiac tamponade (narrow pulse pressure with pulsus paradoxus) or a large run-off lesion such as a Blalock–Thomas–Taussig shunt or aortic regurgitation (widened pulse pressure). Pronounced phasic variations in a patient receiving positive-pressure ventilation coupled with low atrial pressures are typical for significant hypovolemia.

The radial artery is the most frequently used site for arterial access. In patients with arch obstruction or who have had Blalock–Thomas–Taussig shunts, the site of arterial access must be chosen carefully and the data interpreted appropriately. Too often, valuable time is lost in resuscitating patients when loss of a

blood pressure trace is ascribed to a "dampened" arterial line; a dampened wave form is more frequently due to a low-output state. Palpation of either the femoral or carotid pulse is an often forgotten alternative. One or two judicious chest compressions will restore the waveform in a pulseless patient and confirm low cardiac output; appropriate resuscitative measures should then be used.

Other Monitoring

Continuous monitoring of the heart rate and QRS morphology is standard practice in most ICUs. Indwelling urinary (Foley) catheters are useful for continuous, hourly assessment of urine output. Transcutaneous oxygen saturation monitors and end-tidal CO_2 monitoring aid in the management of any patient with unstable respiratory status or labile PVR with intracardiac shunts. These monitors are particularly useful in cases where parallel pulmonary and systemic circulations are supplied by a single ventricle, because variations in SVR and PVR may occur rapidly with resulting changes in arterial saturation. Also, alterations in arterial oxygen saturation owing to pneumothorax, unrecognized extubation, or ventilator failure are rapidly identified. Failure to obtain an adequate signal may be a sign of inadequate peripheral perfusion.

The saturation in the superior vena cava (SVC) approximates the pulmonary artery saturation closely enough that the SVC saturation is used as a surrogate for the mixed venous saturation. In patients with biventricular repair, saturations obtained from a right atrial catheter provide an indirect

BASELINE RHYTHM
(COMPLETE HEART BLOCK)

CI = 2.2 liters/min/m²

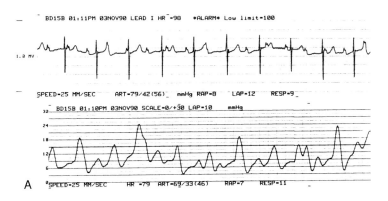

EPICARDIAL PACING:
VVI PACING

CI = 2.5 liters/min/m²

EPICARDIAL PACING:
A-V SEQUENTIAL PACING

CI = 3.4 liters/min/m²

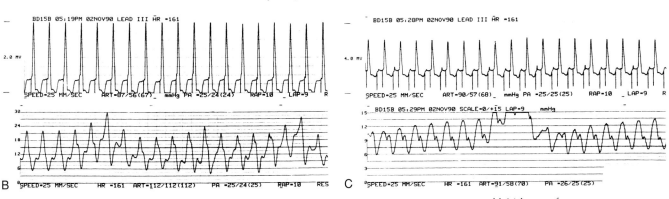

FIGURE 20.5 Hemodynamic effects of pacing (using temporary wires) in a 1-year-old 24 hours after inlet ventricular septal defect closure with complete heart block. *Upper panels* show ECG obtained from bedside monitor; *lower panel* is left atrial (LA) pressure (LAP) tracing from transthoracic catheter. **A:** Complete heart block with AV dissociation and a ventricular escape rate of 98 beats/min; note cannon waves in LA waveform. Blood pressure was 69/33 (mean 46) mm Hg with a mean LA pressure of 10 mm Hg and a thermodilution cardiac index (CI) of 2.2 L/min/m². **B:** Institution of ventricular (VVI) pacing resulted in an increase in blood pressure to 87/56 (mean 67) mm Hg, a mean LA pressure of 12 mm Hg, and a CI of 2.5 L/min/m². **C:** Re-establishment of atrial-ventricular (A-V) synchrony with dual-chamber pacing resulted in a blood pressure of 91/58 (mean 70) mm Hg, an LA pressure of 9 mm Hg (with a more normal waveform), and a CI of 3.4 L/min/m². ART, arterial pressure; RAP, right atrial pressure; RESP, breaths/min; HR, heart rate.

assessment of cardiac output and oxygen delivery and are a useful trend to follow. In patients with single ventricle physiology, a catheter in the SVC is required to measure a "mixed" venous saturation (33,34). Some centers use an optical catheter in the SVC to continuously monitor systemic venous oxygen saturation after the Norwood operation (34,35).

Serum lactate is another surrogate marker of adequate oxygen delivery. Several studies have suggested the usefulness of serum lactate in predicting outcome after open-heart surgery (36–38). An elevated serum lactate represents anaerobic metabolism, which occurs with inadequate oxygen delivery or impaired oxygen utilization. Although absolute values of serum lactate vary from lesion to lesion and are dependant on a host of intraoperative factors (e.g., DHCA, blood transfusion, etc.), a steadily falling lactate is a reassuring finding, while elevations in serum lactate may suggest inadequate oxygen delivery.

Temporary epicardial pacing wires are typically placed on the anterior surface of the right ventricle and, increasingly, on the right atrium as well. Atrial wires may be used to increase heart rate in the presence of sinus node dysfunction while allowing the ventricles to contract through the AV node and the normal His–Purkinje system. Rapid atrial pacing, occasionally with interposed premature beats, is very effective in converting many types of supraventricular tachycardias to normal sinus rhythm at the bedside, without the need for synchronized DC cardioversion. In addition to the therapeutic uses, epicardial atrial wires may be used to record both unipolar and bipolar atrial electrograms for diagnostic purposes. Epicardial ventricular wires are useful in cases of AV node disease (complete heart block), although cardiac output may not be as effective when the ventricles contract desynchronously, i.e., with the right ventricle contracting prior to the left ventricle, rather

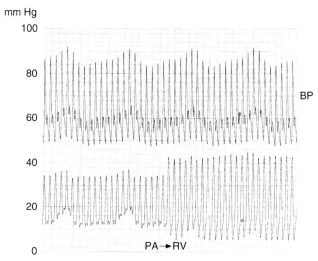

FIGURE 20.6 Hemodynamic monitoring in a 6-month-old child following complete repair for double-outlet right ventricle with pulmonary stenosis. The VSD was closed with a patch, subpulmonary muscle bundles were resected, and a pulmonary commissurotomy was performed. Simultaneous right atrial and pulmonary artery oxygen saturations were 63% and 68%, respectively. Continuous pressure monitoring of the arterial blood pressure (BP, **above**) and pulmonary artery (PA) catheter during withdrawal into the right ventricle (RV, **below**) is shown. A 10 mm Hg peak systolic ejection gradient across the RV outflow tract is demonstrated. Note the phasic variation in the pressure tracings due to positive pressure mechanical ventilation, and the easily visible change in the pressure waveform when the PA catheter crosses the pulmonary valve. Echocardiography at hospital discharge demonstrated no residual VSD, an RV outflow gradient of <15 mm Hg, and an estimated RV pressure (using a mild tricuspid regurgitation jet) of 35 to 40 mm Hg.

than through the His–Purkinje system and without AV synchrony. Dual-chamber pacing is particularly useful in cases of complete heart block. In patients at risk for complete heart block, the temporary wires should be checked for threshold and sensitivity after arrival in the ICU, and a temporary pacemaker should be kept at the bedside.

Near Infrared Spectroscopy (NIRS) allows evaluation of O_2 delivery at the tissue level, allowing regional O_2 delivery monitoring, but does not replace traditional evaluation methods.

Low–Cardiac Output States

Despite improvements in myocardial protection, surgical and cardiopulmonary bypass techniques, many young patients experience a fall in cardiac output with associated tissue edema and end-organ dysfunction referred to as low cardiac output syndrome (LCOS) after surgery for congenital heart disease. LCOS typically occurs between 6 and 18 hours after surgery (10,39,40). In a study of 139 children undergoing biventricular repair, 25% had cardiac index (CI) <2 L per min per m^2 (40). In this study, CI of <2 L per min per m^2 strongly correlated with mortality. Similarly, in the Boston circulatory arrest study, 25% of neonates had CI <2 L per min per m^2 on the first postoperative night after the arterial switch operation (10). LCOS was associated with an elevated systemic vascular resistance of 25% and a rise in pulmonary vascular resistance of nearly 40% from baseline values (Fig. 20.7). Similarly, in the PRIMACORP trial (Prophylactic Intravenous use of Milri-

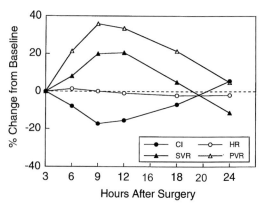

FIGURE 20.7 Decrease in cardiac index (CI) associated with a rise in systemic (SVR) and pulmonary vascular resistance (PVR) in newborns after the arterial switch operation. During the study period, heart rate (HR) remained unchanged, and inotropic and sedation were held constant. (Modified with permission from Wernovsky G, Wypij D, Jonas RA, et al. Postoperative course and hemodynamic profile after the arterial switch operation in neonates and infants: A comparison of low-flow cardiopulmonary bypass versus circulatory arrest. *Circulation* 1995;92:2226–2235).

none After Cardiac OpeRation in Pediatrics), the incidence of LCOS in the placebo group was 25.9% and occurred in the first 6 to 18 hours after surgery. Nearly half of the patients with clinical LCOS had a widened (>30%) arterial-mixed venous oxygen difference. Consistent with previous studies, the lowest mixed venous saturations occurred in the first 6 to 18 hours after surgery. Compared to neonates and infants, LCOS is less commonly seen in older children but may occur following any complex operation with long myocardial ischemic times or in patients of any age with pre-existing ventricular dysfunction, atrioventricular valve regurgitation, arrhythmias, or following operations that adversely change loading conditions of the myocardium.

Etiology

Causes of low cardiac output syndrome (LCOS) after cardiac surgery are multifactorial. They include factors related to CPB such as myocardial ischemia during aortic cross clamping, hypothermia, reperfusion injury, activation of inflammatory, and complement cascades and alterations in systemic and pulmonary vascular reactivity (41). Nonspecific and lesion specific causes of LCOS are listed in Tables 20.2 and 20.3. However, before implicating myocardial dysfunction as the cause of LCOS, it is imperative to rule out residual surgically remedial structural defects, as medical management is unlikely to reverse the low cardiac output state in the presence of an anatomical problem. Specific examples include residual aortic arch obstruction after the Norwood operation, presence of a significant left-to-right shunting due to a residual VSD or previously unrecognized muscular VSD after repair of tetralogy of Fallot. To mitigate LCOS inflammatory response, high dose (10–30 mg/kg) solumedrol is routinely given at CPB initiation.

Use of Modified Ultrafiltration (MUF)

Ultrafiltration is a technique that removes plasma water and low molecular weight solutes using hydrostatic forces across a semi permeable membrane (Figure 20.8). Elliott et al. introduced a technique of ultrafiltration after separation from CPB, which

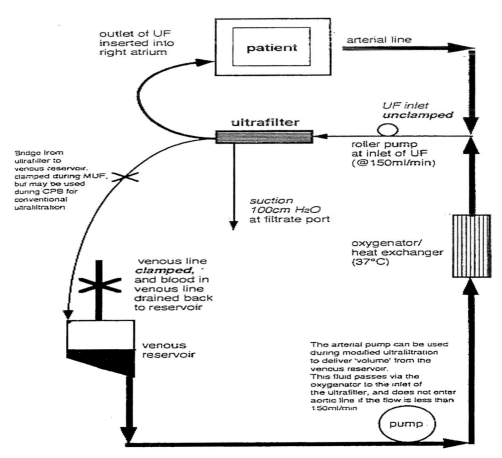

FIGURE 20.8 Courtesy of Elliott MJ: Ultrafiltration and modified ultrafiltration in pediatric open-heart operations. *Ann Thorac Surg* 1993;56:1516–1522.

they termed modified ultrafiltration (42,43). Early studies on the use of MUF reported a decrease in the amount of total body water that accumulates after CPB. MUF removes not only plasma water, but also solutes of <50 kDa, including a number of inflammatory mediators such as IL-6 and endothelin-1, thus attenuating the inflammatory cascade activated by CPB. Use of MUF has been shown to decrease total body water accumulation and postoperative blood loss, decrease the incidence of pleural effusions after cavopulmonary connection and the Fontan procedure, improve left ventricular systolic function, improve lung compliance, and decrease the duration of postoperative ventilation (44).

Volume therapy (increased preload) is commonly necessary, followed by appropriate use of inotropic and afterload-reducing agents (45). Atrial pressure and the ventricular response to changes in atrial pressure must be evaluated. Ventricular response is judged by observing systemic arterial pressure and waveform, heart rate, skin color and peripheral extremity temperature, peripheral pulse magnitude, urine flow, core body temperature, and acid–base balance.

Selected children with low cardiac output due to postoperative right ventricular dysfunction may benefit from strategies that allow right-to-left shunting at the atrial level. A typical example follows repair of tetralogy of Fallot, when the hypertrophied, noncompliant right ventricle has undergone a ventriculotomy and may be further compromised by an increased volume load from pulmonary regurgitation secondary to a transannular patch across the right

ventricular outflow tract. In these children it is useful to leave the foramen ovale patent, permitting right-to-left shunting of blood, preserving cardiac output and oxygen delivery despite the attendant transient cyanosis. If the foramen is not patent or is surgically closed, right ventricular dysfunction can lead to reduced LV filling, low cardiac output, and, ultimately, LV dysfunction. In infants and neonates with repaired truncus arteriosus, the same concerns apply and may even be exaggerated if right ventricular afterload is elevated because of pulmonary artery hypertension. This concept has been extended to older patients with single-ventricle physiology who undergo the Fontan operation. If an atrial septal communication or fenestration is left at the time of the Fontan procedure, the resulting right-to-left shunt helps to preserve cardiac output. These children have fewer postoperative complications (44,46).

Pharmacologic Support

Although pharmacologic support can be grouped into three broad categories—catecholamines, phosphodiesterase inhibitors, and other afterload-reducing agents—some agents may have multiple effects.

Catecholamines

Catecholamines, either endogenous (e.g., dopamine or epinephrine) or synthetic (e.g., isoproterenol or dobutamine),

TABLE 20.3

LESION-SPECIFIC CAUSES OF LCOS

1. Changes in loading conditions
   - decreased preload and increased afterload (after repair of systemic atrioventricular valve regurgitation)
   - increased volume load (systemic-to-pulmonary artery shunt, pulmonary regurgitation)
2. Ventriculotomy
3. Coronary reimplantation (after the arterial switch operation or Ross)
4. Denervation (orthotopic heart transplantation)

have been the mainstay of therapy to improve cardiac output. The catecholamines act by stimulating myocardial surface β receptors, leading to increased adenylate cyclase and intracellular cyclic adenosine monophosphate (cAMP). Catecholamines have different actions on the adrenergic receptors (Table 20.3).

In patients with heart failure, down-regulation and desensitization of β receptors as a result of either antecedent congestive heart failure or sustained use of catecholamines can decrease the efficiency of these agents. Furthermore, endogenous norepinephrine may be decreased in chronic heart failure and limit the efficacy of certain catecholamines.

Deleterious effects of catecholamines, as a result of their nonspecific actions on adrenergic receptors include (a) excessive chronotropy, which increases myocardial oxygen consumption, (b) atrial and ventricular dysrhythmias, and (c) increase in afterload from activation of peripheral α receptors, leading to increased impedance and decreased cardiac output. Additional noncardiac side effects of catecholamines include electrolyte and glucose derangements, increase in PVR, depression of ventilatory response to hypoxemia and hypercarbia, and limb ischemia.

Dopamine

Mechanism of Action. Dopamine, an endogenous precursor of norepinephrine, increases myocardial contractility via several mechanisms:

1. By directly stimulating postsynaptic β_1-adrenergic receptors and thus leading to increased intracellular cAMP, increased intracellular calcium, and positive inotropic and chronotropic effects
2. By increasing the release of norepinephrine from presynaptic sympathetic storage sites in the myocardium
3. By decreasing enzymatic degradation and reuptake of norepinephrine

Dopamine has vasoconstrictive properties via its action on postsynaptic α_1 and α_2 receptors as well as vasodilatory effects on the renal, coronary, cerebral, and splanchnic vascular beds through its action on DA_1 receptors.

Dose-response data in animals suggest that younger animals, when compared with more mature animals, respond with less effectiveness to equivalent doses of dopamine. This difference may be secondary to a higher dopamine clearance rate, decreased myocardial adrenergic innervation and releasable norepinephrine, reduced myocardial β_1-adrenergic receptor density, different maturation of peripheral α and myocardial β_2 receptors, as well as DA_1 receptors, and the observation that the neonatal myocardium functions at near peak capacity with little systolic end-diastolic reserve. Additionally, because both

hypoxia and chronic congestive heart failure can reduce β_1 receptor density, children with CHD may have a decreased response to dopamine (47).

Pharmacokinetics. Pharmacokinetic studies in children have shown a wide interindividual variation, but a linear correlation between infusion rate and plasma dopamine concentration has been demonstrated (47). There appears to be an age-dependent effect on dopamine clearance.

Indications. Mild to moderate hypotension, especially where renal perfusion and mobilization and excretion of excessive extravascular water have occurred, is important following CPB.

Clinical Use. Clinical studies suggest that adults respond to dopamine by increasing cardiac index with minimal increase in heart rate or blood pressure at a low dose (<10 μg/kg/min), whereas infants and premature neonates (48) respond to dopamine with increases in cardiac index, as well as heart rate and systemic blood pressure. Although one study (49) showed that critically ill neonates and infants have greater responsiveness to dopamine than previously appreciated (with hemodynamic responses to infusion rates as low as 0.8 to 1 μg/kg/min), others have noted a decreased sensitivity to dopamine (50). The response to dopamine after cardiac surgery may be different than seen in patients with congestive heart failure. Dopamine may have negative myocardial consequences in the postischemic myocardium, secondary to an unfavorable demand: supply ratio. Lang et al. (51) noted a significant increase in cardiac output in children following CPB only when an infusion of >15 μg/kg/min was given. Other investigators noted that dopamine was increasingly efficacious in combination with nitroprusside. Last, although dopamine has been noted to increase glomerular filtration rate and renal blood flow, it does not appear to be superior to dobutamine for conserving renal function in children after CPB.

Dobutamine

Mechanism of Action. Dobutamine, a synthetic sympathomimetic amine (52) and an analogue of isoproterenol, is mainly a β_1 receptor agonist. Unlike dopamine, it does not release endogenous norepinephrine stores and has little effect on the peripheral vasculature.

Pharmacokinetics. Although one study showed a linear correlation between infusion rate and plasma levels of dobutamine, a more recent report indicated that dobutamine pharmacokinetics may not follow a simple linear model. There also appear to be altered dobutamine pharmacokinetics when it is administered concomitantly with dopamine.

Indications. Dobutamine is used for treatment of myocardial dysfunction (e.g., acute myocarditis or anthracycline-induced cardiomyopathy) not accompanied by severe hypotension. In sepsis with myocardial dysfunction, dobutamine may be beneficial in conjunction with a vasoconstrictor such as norepinephrine; in sepsis without cardiac failure, however, dobutamine is seldom the first agent of choice.

Clinical Use. Studies in adults have shown that dobutamine increases cardiac output with relatively low chronotropic activity and arrhythmogenic potential. In addition, dobutamine seems to be able to maintain favorable hemodynamic changes over a period of days to weeks (53). Compared with dopamine, dobutamine appears to lower ventricular filling pressures as well as PVR and SVR more effectively (53). As with dopamine, the hemodynamic effects of dobutamine can be augmented further with concomitant use of an afterload-reducing agent such as nitroprusside.

Hemodynamic studies of dobutamine in children and neonates have shown an increase in cardiac index and a decrease in SVR with doses as low as 2.5 μg/kg/min, without a significant increase in heart rate. Experience with dobutamine in children after open heart surgery is limited, but studies have shown that tachycardia can be a limiting factor in its use (54). Dobutamine has been largely replaced with milrimone.

Isoproterenol

Mechanism of Action. Isoproterenol, a synthetic analog of norepinephrine, is a pure β agonist that stimulates myocardial β_1 receptors, thus leading to increase in inotropy and chronotropy, and peripheral β_2 receptors, resulting in vasodilation.

Pharmacokinetics. There are few data on pharmacokinetics of isoproterenol in the pediatric population. One study showed that postoperative cardiac patients had lower clearance compared with asthmatic patients.

Indications. Isoproterenol is especially effective for treatment of sinus bradycardia or transient AV block. It also can be useful in treating low cardiac output in pulmonary hypertension of the newborn or following cardiac surgery. Isoproterenol should be avoided in hypertrophic cardiomyopathy because the outflow tract obstruction gradient may be exacerbated with its use.

Clinical Use. There are few data on the use of isoproterenol in newborn animals. There are sporadic reports of transient myocardial ischemia in pediatric patients with asthma. Other undesirable cardiac effects include unfavorable redistribution of cardiac output, ventricular dysrhythmias, tachycardia, and hypotension, all of which may compromise coronary blood flow.

Although isoproterenol was found to be particularly effective for inotropic support in children after surgery for tetralogy of Fallot (55), its effectiveness could be affected by prior use of propranolol. Currently, isoproterenol may be of some benefit in patients with abnormal heart rate responses (e.g., following heart transplantation or cavopulmonary connections) or with heart failure and pulmonary hypertension.

Epinephrine

Mechanism of Action. Epinephrine is an endogenous catecholamine released from the adrenal medulla and derived from norepinephrine. It acts on α, β_1, and β_2 receptors.

Pharmacokinetics. One study on the pharmacokinetics of epinephrine in children showed linear pharmacokinetics but noted that clearance was lower than in adults (56). Endotracheal administration of epinephrine in children can be effective in emergency situations.

Indications. Epinephrine is efficacious for low cardiac output accompanied by hypotension, especially cardiogenic or septic shock not responsive to dopamine (57). Epinephrine also can be effective in asystolic arrest, although there is current controversy regarding its appropriate dose.

Clinical Use. At low doses (0.05 to 0.1 μg/kg/min), there are both β_1 and β_2 receptor activation; at higher doses (1 μg/kg/min), however, there are significant β receptor–mediated vasoconstriction and tissue ischemia. Significant hemodynamic changes have been noted to occur at only twice basal levels of epinephrine. The hemodynamic effects of epinephrine in adult patients after cardiac surgery has been well studied (58). Epinephrine is currently used as advance therapy in the treatment of low cardiac output syndrome after open heart surgery in children, after administration of dopamine and phosphodiesterase inhibitors.

Vasopressin

Arginine vasopressin (AVP) is an endogenous hormone with both osmoregulatory and vasomotor activities. The hallmarks of vasodilatory shock are a triad of hypoperfusion, lactic acidosis, and profound vasodilatory hypotension unresponsive to catecholamine vasopressors. This state occurs in postcardiotomy shock in which inflammatory mediators from cardiopulmonary bypass contribute to this loss of vascular tone. This state of vasodilatory shock is often associated with a deficiency in arginine vasopressin pressin or AVP. Arginine vasopressin is a potent vasoconstrictor that has been used under these circumstances with resolution of shock in some cases (62). Although no vasoconstrictor effects are demonstrable in hemodynamically normal subjects, AVP is a potent pressor in states where arterial pressure is threatened. AVP appears to act synergistically with catecholamine vasopressors to make them effective in this clinical situation. The ususal recommended dose is 0.0003–0.002 units/kg/minute. There is very limited experience in children, however early use of AVP may have a beneficial effect in refractory postoperative hypotension.

Phosphodiesterase Inhibitors

Because of the undesirable side effects associated with the use of high dose catecholamines, afterload reducing agents such as amrinone and milrinone are being increasingly used in the postoperative period (55). They are nonglycoside, noncatecholamine inotropic agents with additional vasodilatory and lusitropic properties. These drugs inhibit phosphodiesterase type III, the enzyme that metabolizes cyclic adenosine monophosphate (cyclic AMP). By increasing intracellular cyclic AMP, they increase intracellular calcium, thus, enhancing myocardial contractility. In addition, they also enhance diastolic relaxation of the myocardium by increasing the rate of re-uptake of calcium after systole, thus, providing a "lusitropic" effect. These drugs also act synergistically with β agonists and have fewer side effects (Fig. 20.9).

Katz et al. (60) showed that amrinone had no inotropic effects in fetal and neonatal preparations of rat myocardial cells and avian, cat, and rabbit papillary muscles. Other studies have shown negative inotropic effects in newborn canine muscle as well as in neonatal piglet hearts. There appear to be differences between the immature and adult myocardium in the handling of amrinone (61).

Pharmacokinetics. Studies in adults have shown a correlation between cardiac index and serum amrinone level. Neonates and infants require a higher loading dose (3 to 4.5 μg/kg) than adults to achieve adequate serum levels. Clinical experience with amrinone suggests that a continuous infusion of 5 to 15 μg/kg/min is effective (Fig. 20.10). In preliminary animal studies, there is an apparent dose-related correlation between plasma concentration of milrinone and both increase in cardiac index and decrease in pulmonary capillary wedge pressure (62). The dose

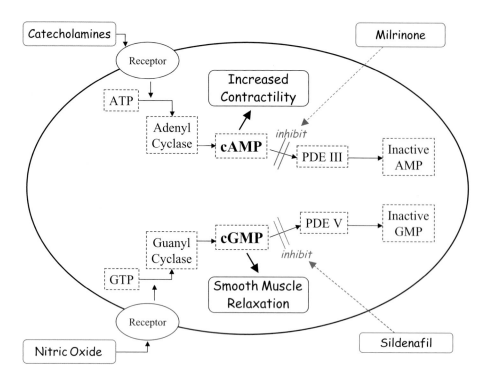

FIGURE 20.9 This figure depicts the mechanism of action of phosphodiesterase inhibitors (PDE) at the cellular level and the synergistic effects of catecholamines and PDE III. ATP, adenosine triphosphate; c-AMP, cyclic adenosine monophosphate; GTP, guanosine triphosphate; cGMP, guanosine monophosphate.

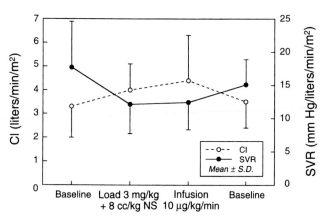

FIGURE 20.10 Hemodynamic effects of amrinone in nine infants after repair of transposition of the great arteries ($n = 7$) and complete AV septal defect ($n = 2$). After baseline measurements of right and left atrial pressures, systemic blood pressure and thermodilution cardiac output, 3 μg/kg of amrinone and 8 mL/kg of normal saline (NS) were administered; the NS was given to increase left atrial pressure back to baseline values. Repeat measurements were made, followed by an infusion of 10 μg/kg for 30 minutes. A final set of hemodynamic measurements was obtained 1 hour after discontinuation of the amrinone. Cardiac index improved significantly ($p < 0.05$ compared with baseline) following the loading dose, isotonic volume infusion, and continuous infusion of amrinone, falling back to baseline values after discontinuation of amrinone. The systemic vascular resistance (SVR) decreased significantly ($p < 0.05$) as well, remaining significantly below baseline values 1 hour after discontinuation of the amrinone infusion. (Modified from Lang P, Wessel DL, Wernovsky G, et al. Hemodynamic effects of amrinone in infants after cardiac surgery. In: Crupi G, Parenzan L, Anderson RH, eds. Perspectives In Pediatric Cardiology. Vol. 2, Pediatric cardiac surgery, part 2. Mt Kisco, NY: Futura, 1989:292–295, with permission.)

recommended in adults with normal renal function is 50 μg/kg bolus given over 10 minutes with a maintenance infusion of 0.4 to 1.2 μg/kg/min titrated to a desired hemodynamic response, and duration of hemodynamic effects is more prolonged following higher (50 or 75 μg/kg) bolus doses. The major route of elimination for milrinone is renal. Short-term intravenous administration of milrinone has been well tolerated (63).

Indications. Indications include low cardiac output with myocardial dysfunction and elevated SVR not accompanied by severe hypotension.

Clinical Use. Hemodynamic assessment of amrinone in adults has shown that it increases cardiac index and peak rate of LV pressure increase (dP/dt) while decreasing LV end-diastolic pressure, pulmonary capillary pressure, and RA pressure in congestive heart failure (64) and in patients after cardiac surgery (65). Furthermore, amrinone has been found to increase cardiac index and lower SVR further when added to dobutamine (66).

The use of amrinone after cardiac surgery in the pediatric patient population increases cardiac index and decreases SVR without a significant increase in heart rate (67–69). Despite successful application of amrinone treatment in adults and children (70) with myocardial failure, some have avoided its use owing to concerns of potential side effects and its relatively long biologic half-life. However, following successful clinical trials, phosphodiesterase inhibitors have now become the second-line drug (after dopamine) in the treatment of low cardiac output in neonates, infants, and children following CPB in many institutions. Side effects have been minimal and are typically the need for isotonic volume infusions (5 to 15 mL/kg) following bolus (>2 mg/kg) administration and occasional thrombocytopenia following prolonged (>7 to 10 days) use (especially with amrinone).

A comparison between milrinone and dobutamine suggested that milrinone was superior in decreasing SVR for any given increase in dP/dt, whereas direct comparison between milrinone and nitroprusside showed that in equally hypotensive doses, milrinone was superior in increasing the peak positive rate of pressure development (+dP/dt) as well as the stroke work of the left ventricle. Furthermore, milrinone does not increase myocardial oxygen consumption and is a coronary vasodilator. Lastly, improvement in indices of diastolic performance is observed in patients with congestive heart failure following administration of milrinone. Clinical trials of milrinone in children following cardiac surgery have yielded findings similar to those with amrinone (Fig. 20.11) (23,45,50,71–73).

Milrinone

Clinical Use. Milrinone, a 2-methyl, 5-carbonitrile congener of amrinone is approximately 15 times more potent than its parent compound, amrinone (74). In a pharmacodynamic study evaluating the hemodynamic effects of intravenous milrinone in 10 neonates with established LCOS after cardiac surgery (mean cardiac index of 2 L/min/m^2), Chang and colleagues showed that milrinone lowered filling pressures, systemic and pulmonary artery pressures, and systemic and pulmonary vascular resistances, while improving cardiac index (45) (Fig. 20.12). The results of the PRIMACORP (Prophylactic Intravenous Use of Milrinone after Cardiac Surgery in Pediatrics) trial were recently published (72,73). In this multicenter pediatric trial, patients were randomly assigned. In a 1:1:1 ratio within 90 minutes after arriving in the intensive care unit, to receive either low-dose intravenous milrinone (25 µg/kg bolus over 60 minutes followed by 0.25 µg/kg/min infusion for 35 hours), high-dose milrinone (75 µg/kg bolus over 60 minutes followed by 0.75 µg /kg per min infusion for 35 hours), or placebo. The prophylactic use of high dose milrinone resulted in a 64% relative risk reduction in the development of LCOS (Fig. 20.11). Consistent with previous studies, the lowest mixed venous saturations and highest lactate values occurred in the first 12 hours after surgery. Patients who developed LCOS had a significantly lower urine output (1.9 vs. 2.5 mL/kg/h, $p = 0.002$), longer duration of mechanical ventilation (3.1 versus 1.4 days, $p = 0.01$) and longer length of stay (11.3 vs. 8.9 days, $p = 0.016$). There were no significant differences in the incidence of adverse events (hypotension, arrhythmia, and thrombocytopenia) with milrinone compared with placebo.

Unlike amrinone, milrinone does not have a negative inotropic effect on the neonatal myocardium, and is also free of thrombocytopenic effects (75). In many centers, milrinone is the first line of therapy for children with LCOS following cardiac surgery, as well as for children with cardiomyopathy awaiting heart transplantation. A combination of Dopamine (3 to 5 µg/kg/min) and Milrinone (0.5 to 1 µg/kg/min) has become standard therapy for all neonates and young infants undergoing bypass, and for many older children following complex biventricular repair or staged reconstruction (e.g., Fontan procedure).

Side Effects. Unlike catecholamines, the phosphodiesterase inhibitor amrinone improves myocardial performance without increased myocardial oxygen consumption (76), tachycardia, arrhythmias, or afterload.

Unlike amrinone, milrinone has not been shown to have negative inotropic effects on the neonatal myocardium (75) and also appears to be free of thrombocytopenic effects (71).

Other Afterload-Reducing Agents

Vasodilator therapy improves low cardiac output principally by decreasing impedance to ventricular ejection. These effects are especially helpful after cardiac surgery in children and in adults when SVR is particularly elevated (10).

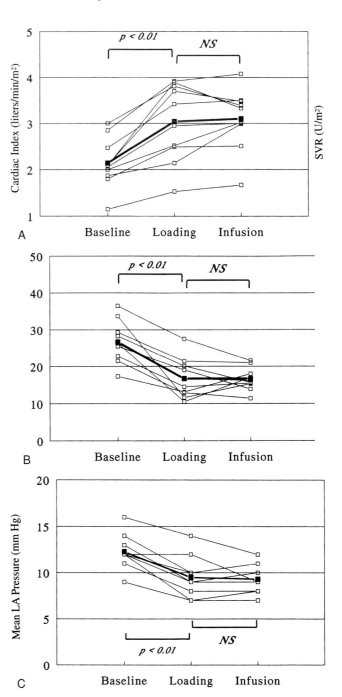

FIGURE 20.11 Hemodynamic effects of milrinone in 10 neonates with low (<3 L/min/m^2) cardiac index after repair of transposition of the great arteries ($n = 6$), tetralogy of Fallot ($n = 2$), total anomalous pulmonary venous return ($n = 1$), and truncus arteriosus ($n = 1$). After baseline measurements of right and left atrial pressures, systemic blood pressure and thermodilution cardiac output, 50 µg/kg of milrinone was given intravenously over 15 minutes. Repeat measurements were made, followed by an infusion of 0.5 µg/kg for 30 minutes. Cardiac index (A) increased significantly following the loading dose and was maintained during continuous infusion. The improved cardiac index was associated with a significant decrease in systemic vascular resistance (SVR) (B) and left atrial pressure (C). NS, not significant. (Modified from Chang AC, Atz AM, Wernovsky G, et al. Milrinone: Systemic and pulmonary hemodynamic effects in neonates after cardiac surgery. *Crit Care Med* 1995;33:1907–1914, with permission.)

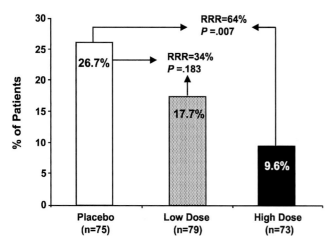

FIGURE 20.12 Development of low cardiac output syndrome (LCOS)/death in the first 36 hours after placebo, low dose and high dose milrinone. (Modified from Hoffman TM, Wernovsky G, Atz AM, et al. Efficacy and safety of milrinone in preventing low cardiac output syndrome in infants and children after corrective surgery for congenital heart disease. *Circulation* 2003;107:996–1002. RRR, relative risk ratio.

Sodium Nitroprusside

Mechanism of Action. The most widely used afterload-reducing agent is the nitrovasodilator sodium nitroprusside (77). Sodium nitroprusside acts as a nitric oxide donor, increasing intracellular cGMP, which effects relaxation of vascular smooth muscle in both arterioles and veins. The overall effect is a decrease in atrial filling pressure and SVR with a concomitant increase in cardiac output. Nitroprusside reduces SVR more than dobutamine.

Pharmacokinetics. Vasodilation occurs within minutes with intravenous nitroprusside administration. The principal metabolites of sodium nitroprusside are thiocyanate and cyanide; thiocyanate toxicity is unusual in children with normal hepatic and renal function, and monitoring of cyanide and thiocyanate concentrations in children may not be correlated with clinical signs of toxicity.

Indications and Clinical Use. Nitroprusside is useful in patients with low cardiac output following cardiac surgery, in patients with aortic or mitral insufficiency, and in patients with systemic ventricular dysfunction. In children after cardiac surgery, nitroprusside increases cardiac output and decreases filling pressure without inducing tachycardia. Historically, nitroprusside was used in the treatment of pulmonary hypertension following congenital heart surgery, but its use as an antihypertensive agent is currently limited to the treatment of systemic hypertension, including that observed after surgical repair of coarctation of the aorta.

Additional Vasodilators and Antihypertensive Agents

Many other agents have been used as arterial and venous vasodilators to treat hypertension, reduce ventricular afterload and SVR, and improve cardiac output. A second nitrovasodila-

TABLE 20.4

COMPLETE INTRACARDIAC MIXING

Anatomy	Preoperative	Postoperative
Variations of single left ventricle		
Tricuspid valve atresia		
Normally related great arteries	Yes	Yes
Double-inlet left ventricle	Yes	Yes
Normally related great arteries (Holmes' heart)	Yes	Yes
Transposed great arteries[a]	Yes[b]	Yes
Malaligned complete atrioventricular septal defect with hypoplastic right ventricle	Yes	Yes
Pulmonary atresia with intact ventricular septum	Yes	Variable[b]
Variations of single right ventricle		
Mitral valve atresia		
Hypoplastic left heart syndrome	Yes	Yes
Double-outlet right ventricle	Yes	Yes
Aortic valve atresia		
Hypoplastic left heart syndrome	Yes	Yes
With large VSD and normal LV size	Yes	Variable[b]
Malaligned complete atrioventricular septal defect with hypoplastic left ventricle	Yes	Yes
Heterotaxy syndromes—typically with pulmonary stenosis or atresia—asplenia or polyspenia	Yes	Yes
Two-ventricle hearts with potential single-ventricle physiology		
Tetralogy of Fallot with pulmonary atresia	Yes	Variable[b]
Truncus arteriosus	Yes[b]	No

VSD, ventricular septal defects; LV, left ventricle.
[a]Streaming may result in incomplete mixing.
[b]Single-ventricle physiology will pertain to postoperative patients with systemic to pulmonary artery shunts or following pulmonary artery banding, although two-ventricle repairs with normal series circulation or partial repairs with incomplete mixing are possible in certain anatomic subtypes.
Modified from Wernovsky G, Bove EL. Single ventricle lesions. In: Chang AC, Hanley Fl, Wernovsky G, et al., eds. *Pediatric Cardiac Intensive Care*. Baltimore: Williams & Wilkins, 1998:271–287, with permission.

tor, nitroglycerin, principally a venous dilator, also has rapid onset of action and a short half-life (about 2 minutes). Tolerance may develop after several days of continuous infusion. Nitroglycerin is used extensively in adult cardiac units for patients with ischemic heart disease. Experience in pediatric patients is more limited. Vasodilators have been used for myocardial ischemia in the setting of acute Kawasaki's disease. Hydralazine is more typically used for acute hypertension (especially after repair of coarctation of the aorta). Its relatively long half-life limits its use in postoperative patients with labile hemodynamics. The angiotensin-converting enzyme inhibitor enalaprilat similarly has a relatively long half-life (2 to 4 hours), which limits its use in the acute setting. Beta-blockers (e.g., propranolol, esmolol, labetalol), although excellent in reducing blood pressure, may have deleterious effects on ventricular function. Calcium channel blockers (e.g., verapamil) may cause acute and severe hypotension and bradycardia in the neonate. All intravenous vasodilators must be used cautiously in patients with moderate to severe lung disease; their use has been associated with increased intrapulmonary shunting and acute reductions of PaO_2.

Nesiritide is a synthetic intravenous form of brain natriuretic peptide (BNP) which has recently been used in the treatment of decompensated heart failure in adults due to its beneficial effects on the renal, neurohormonal and cardiovascular systems (78,79). Exogenous administration of Nesiritide results in natriuresis, diuresis, vasodilation, and increased renal blood flow. This has been shown to increase cardiac output and urine output, as well as improve symptomatology in the adult heart failure patient. However, there are limited data regarding its use in the pediatric patient population, with the majority focusing on its use in postoperative patients (80–83). The dose used in infants and children has ranged from 0.005 to 0.03 μg/kg/min. A bolus dose of 1 μg/kg/min has been used in some patients prior to initiation of a continuous infusion. Most pediatric investigators have focused on functional outcomes. In addition, concerns raised regarding its adverse effects on renal function in the adult population highlight the importance of proper patient selection in the use of this medication (84).

Phenoxybenzamine is a potent, long acting α-blocker that has been advocated as part of the postoperative management of infants after the Norwood operation. It is used to lower the systemic vascular resistance and produce a more "balanced" circu-

lation (34,35). In a prospective, nonrandomized trial by Tweddell et al., infants who received phenoxybenzamine after the Norwood operation had higher systemic oxygen delivery and a more stable postoperative course compared with historical controls. Many centers have incorporated this approach in the postoperative care of infants after the Norwood operation (35). The usual dose is 0.25 mg/kg administered on initiation of cardiopulmonary bypass with or without an infusion of 0.25 to 1 mg/kg/day after separation from cardiopulmonary bypass.

Transient hypothyroidism is well described in adults and children after cardiopulmonary bypass. In a study by Bettendorf et al., thyroid function tests were evaluated in 139 children undergoing cardiac surgery with cardiopulmonary bypass. There was a significant decrease in both T3 (triiodothyronine) and T4 (thyroxine), and a low TSH (thyroid stimulating hormone) consisting with sick euthyroid syndrome-type 2 (85). The mechanism of hypothyroidism is not fully characterized but is likely related to hemodilution, endogenous release of mediators such as glucocorticoids, tumor necrosis factor and cytokines such as IL-6, and exogenous factors such as dopamine infusion and iodine skin preparations. Thyroid hormones increase cardiac contractility and lower systemic vascular resistance.

Some investigators have recently evaluated the role of triiodothyronine (T3) infusion as an inotrope after cardiac surgery in children and the initial experience appears favorable (86–88). In a prospective randomized study, 28 children with documented low T3 levels after cardiac surgery were randomized to receive either T3 or placebo (86). A small subset of neonates had improved inotropic scores and therapeutic intervention scores. In another randomized double-blind controlled trial of T3 treatment in 42 infants undergoing the Norwood operation or repair of interrupted aortic arch and ventricular septal defect closure, T3 resulted in a higher systolic blood pressure and more rapid achievement of negative fluid balance (88). In this study, there was no improvement in cardiac index. No serious adverse effects were noted in this fragile patient population at a dose of 0.05 μg/kg/h). An ongoing trial called the triiodothyronine for infants and children undergoing cardiopulmonary bypass (TRICC) study is a multicenter, randomized clinical trial that is designed to study the safety and efficacy of T3 children <2 years undergoing surgery for congenital heart disease (87).

Levosimendan (87a), a Ca sensitizing agent that binds to Troponin C improves contractile efficiency and reduces after load. Pediatric experience is limited.

Arrhythmias after CPB

Arrhythmias occur in >25% of patients after CPB. Risk factors include longstanding volume overload, ventricular hypertrophy, myocardial ischemia, ventriculotomy, multiple suture lines, and electrolyte disturbances. The majority of arrhythmias occur within the first 48 hours of surgery and include bradyarrhythmias, such as sinus bradycardia, and complete heart block and tachyarrhythmias such as supraventricular tachycardia, atrial flutter, atrial fibrillation, junctional ectopic tachycardia (JET), and ventricular tacycardia. JET is common after pediatric cardiac surgery, particularly in young infants after repair of tetralogy of Fallot, closure of ventricular septal defects and atrioventricular canal defects (89–91). Strategies for management of JET include adequate analgesia and sedation, avoidance of hyperthermia and induced hypothermia, minimizing exogenous catecholamines, using medications such as amiodarone and procainamide, and atrial pacing. Atrioventricular synchrony using atrial and/or atrioventricular

TABLE 20.5

ADRENERGIC RECEPTORS: LOCATION AND ACTION

Receptors	Location	Action
α_1	Postsynaptic	Vasoconstriction
α_2	Presynaptic	Inhibits NE release
	Postsynaptic	Vasoconstriction
β_1	Myocardium	Increases inotropy
	SA node	Increases chronotropy
	AV node	Increases conduction
β_2	Arterioles (mesentery, skeletal muscle)	Vasodilation
	Bronchioles	Bronchodilation
DA_1	Postsynaptic (vascular smooth muscle)	Vasodilation
DA_2	Presynaptic	Inhibits NE release

NE, norepinephrine; SA, sinoatrial; AV, atrioventricular.

sequential pacing augments cardiac output and it is particularly important in the treatment of arrhythmias such as JET and complete heart block.

Fluid Overload after CPB

Despite the advances in intraoperative strategies, including the routine use of MUF after CPB, fluid overload and renal dysfunction are major contributors to morbidity after neonatal and infant surgery. The relative increase in total body water accumulation is more significant in neonates, and is directly proportional to the duration of CPB. Its etiologies include both capillary leak and transient postoperative renal dysfunction. In the PRIMACORP trial, the creatinine clearance (mL/min per 1.73 m^2) was significantly less in neonates (mean 37.2) compared with infants aged 1 to 4.8 months (mean 59.2) and older children aged 4.8 months through 6 years (mean 84.5). In neonates, diuresis typically peaks on the second to fourth postoperative day. Intermittent diuretic therapy is perhaps just as efficient as a continuous infusion, though the latter may be better tolerated in the hemodynamically unstable patient (92). "Renal dose dopamine" is commonly used in clinical practice, however according to a recent meta-analysis, the renal protective effect of dopamine is equivocal (93).

Recent animal and clinical studies in adults suggest a role for fenoldopam, a dopamine 1 receptor agonist, in improving renal function after ischemia and reperfusion (94). It has been used in adults as anti-hypertensive therapy, however there is minimal experience in children after cardiac surgery (95).

Mechanical Support

When conventional measures such as fluid resuscitation, inotropic support, and afterload reduction fail, institution of mechanical support may be lifesaving (96).

Indications for mechanical support are as follows:

- Inability to wean off CPB
- Ventricular dysfunction
- Cardiopulmonary arrest
- Pulmonary hypertension refractory to medical therapy
- Occluded systemic-to-pulmonary artery shunt
- Intractable arrhythmias with hemodynamic compromise
- Short Term (<30 days)
    - Intraaortic balloon pump
    - ECMD
    - VAP on centrifugal pump
- Long Term (>30 days)
    - Pulsatile devices
    - Axial devices

Experience with the intra-aortic balloon pump (IABP) in pediatric patients is limited. The mechanism of action of IABP is inflating a balloon situated in the descending aorta, inflated during diastole to augment coronary blood flow and deflating it during systole to decrease LV afterload. IABP has limited effectiveness in most pediatric and neonatal patients because of the small size of the patient and because the relatively rapid heart rate minimizes the opportunity for diastolic augmentation. Sporadic reports include successful use in a neonate as small as 2 kg and in a pediatric patient after a Fontan operation. However, overall hospital survival has been disappointing. Complications from the IABP include limb ischemia, vessel dissection, thrombocytopenia, and infection.

Extracorporeal membrane oxygenation (ECMO) has become the most widely used mode of mechanical cardiopul-

monary support for children with CHD, both before and after cardiac surgery (96,97). Although venous–arterial ECMO is necessary for cardiac dysfunction unresponsive to conventional pharmacologic therapy or in patients with coexisting pulmonary disease, venous–venous ECMO can be appropriate therapy for patients with predominant pulmonary disease such as pneumonitis or adult respiratory distress syndrome. Patients must be considered to have "reversible" or "correctable" cardiac or pulmonary disease to be considered candidates for ECMO support. In particular, postoperative patients should have hemodynamically significant residual lesions ruled out prior to initiation of ECMO support. Patients who are too critically ill to undergo evaluation should be thoroughly investigated while cycling from ECMO support with echocardiography (transthoracic or transesophageal), cardiac catheterization, or both.

Reported hospital survival rates in children receiving ECMO after heart surgery have ranged between 35% and 60% (98–102). The highest survival rates are reported in postoperative patients with a biventricular repair or those placed on support primarily for pulmonary disease. The lowest survival rates have been in patients with single-ventricle lesions or pulmonary hypertension (103,104). This is a significantly lower survival rate than seen in other uses of ECMO. Neonatal respiratory distress syndrome can be successfully managed with ECMO in >90% of patients. Most deaths in patients with cardiac disease are attributable to irreversible cardiac failure, hemorrhage, or neurologic damage. The effect of ECMO on hospital mortality postcardiotomy is unequivocal, and even more obvious when it is used as rescue therapy during cardiopulmonary resuscitation (105–107). Children with cardiac disease represent a heterogeneous group and it is not prudent to impose strict indications or contraindications for ECMO support.

The majority of the pediatric experience consists of use of ECMO. However, with the advent of new technology, ventricular assist devices (VAD) are being increasingly used in infants, children and young adults for resuscitation, as a bridge to transplantation and as a bridge to recovery (108,109).

A Comparison of ECMO Versus VAD Support

Despite recent advances in VAD technology, ECMO remains the most common circulatory assist system in use for pediatric patients. The advantages of ECMO include its familiarity among practitioners, ability to provide biventricular support and respiratory support, universal availability across all pediatric age groups, and relative low cost. Unlike adults in whom pure left ventricular failure is the common indication for mechanical circulatory support, cardiopulmonary support is more commonly required in children due to a combination of pulmonary dysfunction, pulmonary hypertension, and right ventricular dysfunction. This is particularly true in the immediate postoperative period. ECMO is obviously the mechanical support of choice for rapid deployment during cardiopulmonary arrest. However, ECMO has a number of disadvantages, including the need for a dedicated team of ECMO specialists, immobilization, requirement for intensive care monitoring, risks of bleeding, thrombosis, infection, and multiorgan failure. These attendant disadvantages increase over time and hamper the use of ECMO for long-term support. The short-term VADs with a roller pump or centrifugal pump have many of the disadvantages of ECMO including shorter duration of use, occasional thrombus in the circuit and nonpulsatile flow. Advantages include easy implantation, fast set-up time, low priming volume, low-level anticoagulation, and lower cost.

The advantages of long-term implantable VAD include less trauma to blood cells (lack of membrane oxygenator) thus decreasing the need for anticoagulation, and decreased risk of infection compared to ECMO where the system is more open with multiple access ports. Implantable VADs also allow greater mobility for cardiac rehabilitation and have chronic support capability as bridge to transplantation. The disadvantages of VAD include the need for transthoracic cannulation, while ECMO can be initiated with peripheral cannulation. In addition, biventricular support with VAD requires four cannulas, whereas ECMO provides biventricular support with two cannulas. VAD does not provide respiratory support and cannot be used in the presence of respiratory failure.

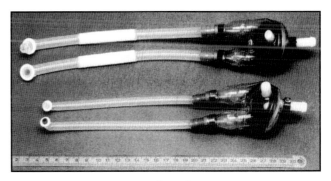

FIGURE 20.13 The Berlin Heart VAD.

Short-Term Mechanical Assist Device

Historically, the centrifugal pump VAD has been the mainstay of pediatric VAD support (110). This device evolved as the need for a mechanical support device superior to conventional ECMO became necessary, especially for patients with isolated ventricular failure. With this VAD, an extracorporeal centrifugal pump produces a vortex continuous nonpulsatile flow, which creates a negative pressure that enables blood to move. The BP-50 and BP-80 models have volumes of 50 mL and 80 mL respectively. Heparin-bonded tubing can be used to minimize the need for anticoagulation. Compared to roller pumps, there is less trauma to red blood cells and less pronounced inflammatory response. Cannulation is performed via the left atrium and aorta (left ventricular assist) or right atrium and pulmonary artery (right ventricular assist). In a study of 34 children, average age 60 days, 63% were successfully decannulated and 31% survived to discharge (110a).

Long-Term Mechanical Assist Devices

The pediatric experience with long-term pulsatile devices has been growing (111–114). Advantages of these devices include their chronic support capability, ease of use, capability for biventricular support without an oxygenator, mobility for cardiac rehabilitation, need for low-level anticoagulation, and pulsatile flow nature with the pulsatile devices. Disadvantages include a propensity to have thromboembolic complications, difficulty of implantation/explantation, cumulative cost, exteriorization of the cannulae, ventricular apical cannulation in most patients, increased risk of presensitization, and size limitation especially with biventricular support. Infection is also a serious complication, the risk can be minimized by immobilization of the driveline as close to the exit site as possible with a binder.

Pulsatile Devices

1. Berlin Heart or EXCOR: for neonates and infants
2. Thoratec, Heartmate, Abiomed for adolescents and young adults
3. Axial Devices: Heartmate II and DeBakey

The Berlin heart is a paracorporeal pneumatically driven pulsatile device that has been available for use in a miniaturized version since 1992 (111,112). The inlet is cannulation via the ventricular apex, and the outlet is to the aorta or pulmonary artery with both cannulas exteriorized. The polyurethane pumps have a wide range of stroke volumes of 10, 12, 15, 25, 30, 50 and 80 mL (Fig. 20.13). Three membranes provide stability and the system is heparin coated. Silicon cannulas connect the blood pump to the patient. The pumps are driven by a pulsatile pneumatic system. A rechargeable battery can provide up to five hours of independent power supply. This device can provide univentricular support (right or left) or biventricular support. The MEDOSHIA VAD is another pulsatile, paracorporeal pneumatically driven VAD with limited pediatric experience in Europe (113). Prolonged support allows extubation and bridging to transplant.

Thoratec Pulsatile Device. There is some pediatric experience in adolescents with the use of the Thoratec ventricular assist device (114). This is a pneumatically powered pulsatile VAD that consists of a flexible seam-free segmented sac within a ridged polycarbonate housing. There are tilting disc valves in the inlet and outlet portions. The inlet is cannulation via the left atrium or ventricular apex and the outlet is to the aorta with both cannulas exteriorized. The stroke volume is 65 ml with a maximum output of 7 L/min. Three modes exist: fixed rate, synchronous, or fill-to-empty.

Axial Flow Devices

Although the pediatric experience with axial flow devices such as the DeBakey device is limited to a few adolescents, its smaller size holds promise for future pediatric use (115,116). This class of devices consists of relatively small axial pumps that involve an impeller with its housing that is entirely implantable. The advantages of such an axial system are the relative ease of implantation, decreased infection, and its continuous flow provides unloading throughout the cardiac cycle. Its disadvantage is the need for a large-sized ventricular apical cannulation, and higher incidence of hemolysis.

Management Principles after VAD Placement

In the immediate postoperative period, patients on VAD need to be fully ventilated and oxygenated. It is also important to remember that output from the VAD is dependant on both preload and afterload. Although most children with end-stage cardiomyopathy or congenital heart disease have biventricular dysfunction, the ventricular unloading provided by the "left" or "systemic" VAD has generally made biventricular assist uncommon. It is important to appreciate that the right ventricular output is the preload to the left ventricular assist device (LVAD). Inadequate filling of LVAD may be from low intravascular volume, tamponade, right ventricular dysfunction, pulmonary hypertension, and arrhythmias. Monitoring of central venous pressure is critical in these patients, and there should be frequent echocardiographic assessment of right ventricular function and estimated right ventricular pressure. Right ventricular dysfunction and elevated pulmonary vascular resistance must be treated in a timely fashion with pharmacological agents such as milrinone, isoproterenol, prostacycline, or inhaled nitric oxide. Anticoagulation is necessary after VAD therapy. Heparin is used acutely, followed with aspirin. Long term anticoagulation is accomplished with coumadin alone or in combination with aspirin, dipyramidine, or clopidogrel. If it clots, replace the pump head.

With the long-term VADs, majority of patients including infants can be extubated. Older children and adolescents can be ambulatory and eventually regain near normal activity with good nutrition and physical rehabilitation.

Survival with VAD as a bridge to transplantation approaches 75% in children (108,117,118). A majority of the pediatric VAD experience is in older children and adolescents. However with the availability of the Berlin heart and the Medos HIA, infants and young children can also be successfully bridged to transplantation.

Lesion-Specific Care

In addition to the general principles of postoperative care outlined above, each surgical repair brings a special set of concerns and investigations necessary for thorough and successful postoperative management. Also, some postinterventional catheterization patients require stabilization and management in the ICU (Table 20.6). The individual anatomic lesions and general principles of surgical management are discussed elsewhere in the text.

Atrial Septal Defect

Postoperative problems after secundum atrial septal defect (ASD) repair are extremely uncommon. Transient atrial dysrhythmias or sinus node dysfunction may occur in 5% of children. Patients with primum ASDs typically have a cleft mitral valve; postoperative function should be assessed by auscultation, inspection of the LA pressure waveform, and echocardiography. If significant mitral valve reconstruction has been performed, acute hypertension (secondary to abrupt awakening from anesthesia, pain, etc.) should be avoided and treated because acute increases in LV pressure may result in dehiscence of the valvuloplasty sutures. Sinus venosus ASDs may require more extensive atrial patching because there is frequently anomalous pulmonary venous drainage. If the superior vena cava (SVC) is transected and anastomosed to the RA appendage (Warden technique), evaluation should include ruling out SVC and right pulmonary venous obstruction. Sinus node dysfunction may occur following this type of repair as well, and temporary atrial pacing may be necessary.

Ventricular Septal Defect

Postoperative evaluation should include assessment for residual or previously undiagnosed shunt (auscultation, invasive monitoring, echocardiography, or catheterization if indicated) and assessment of the conduction system (postoperative 12-lead ECG in all patients and continuous bedside ECG monitoring). Aortic regurgitation, more common in subpulmonary defects, should be ruled out by auscultation, palpation of peripheral pulses, and inspection of the pulse pressure, and with echocardiography.

Tetralogy of Fallot

The postoperative evaluation should include (a) assessment for residual shunt (auscultation, invasive monitoring, echocar-

TABLE 20.6

DOSES OF INOTROPES AND VASODILATORS

Agent	Usual dose range (IV)
Catecholamines	
Dopamine	2–20 μg/kg/min
Dobutamine	2–20 μg/kg/min
Epinephrine	0.01–0.5 μg/kg/min
Norepinephrine	0.1–0.5 μg/kg/min
Phenylephrine	0.1–0.5 μg/kg/min
Isoproterenol	0.01–0.5 μg/kg/min
Vasopressin	0.0003–0.002 units/kg/min
Phosphodiesterase Inhibitors	
Amrinone	1–3 mg/kg loading dose
	5–20 μg/kg/min
Milrinone	100–250 μg/kg load on CPB
	25–75 μg/kg load off CPB
	0.25–1.0 μg/kg/min
Afterload-reducing agents	
Sodium Nitroprusside	0.5–5 μg/kg/min
Other agents	
T3 (Triiodothyronine)	0.05–0.15 μg/kg/hour
Phenoxybenzamine	0.25 mg/kg on initiation of CPB (cardiopulmonary bypass)

diography, or catheterization if indicated); (b) residual right ventricular outflow tract obstruction (auscultation, PA catheter pullback, echocardiography, or catheterization if indicated); and (c) conduction abnormalities (postoperative 12-lead ECG, bedside monitoring). A complete right bundle branch block pattern is extremely common following repair using a right ventriculotomy. Ventricular ectopy is more common in patients repaired at a relatively older age (119). A relatively small residual left-to-right shunt or right ventricular outflow tract gradient may be poorly tolerated early in the postoperative period (120), especially in patients with coexisting pulmonary regurgitation and right ventricular dysfunction. Hypocalcemia should be closely monitored in patients with coexisting DiGeorge syndrome.

Complete Atrioventricular Septal Defect

The postoperative evaluation should include (a) assessment for residual shunt (auscultation, invasive monitoring, echocardiography, or catheterization if indicated); (b) function of the left-sided AV (mitral) valve (auscultation, invasive monitoring [inspection of the LA waveform, pulmonary artery pressure]); (c) conduction abnormalities (postoperative 12-lead ECG, bedside monitoring); and (d) evaluation for subaortic obstruction (auscultation and echocardiography). Transient sinus node dysfunction occurs with a surprisingly high frequency, especially in patients with trisomy 21.

d-Transposition of the Great Arteries: Arterial Switch

The postoperative evaluation should include (a) assessment of LV function (indices of systemic cardiac output, LA pressure); (b) great vessel anastomoses (auscultation, echocardiography if indicated); (c) function of the neoaortic valve (auscultation, inspection of pulse pressure with echocardiography); and (d) ischemia and conduction abnormalities (postoperative 12-lead ECG, bedside monitoring). Residual left-to-right shunt should be investigated in patients with a coexisting VSD. LV dysfunction may be a sign of myocardial ischemia owing to coronary insufficiency or acute dysfunction caused by an "unprepared" left ventricle. Arrhythmias, especially on weaning from CPB, are frequently a marker for coronary insufficiency and should be promptly investigated and treated. Serial 12-lead ECGs are valuable in following ischemic changes. The left ventricle is frequently poorly compliant following the arterial switch, and acute increases in preload may be followed by significant increases in LA pressure, pulmonary edema, and a decrease in cardiac output. Volume infusions should be given slowly, and afterload reduction is particularly helpful in the immediate postoperative period in these patients. Acute LV failure owing to an unprepared left ventricle is uncommon in the first few weeks of life, but can occur in older infants. Mechanical support may be life saving in these patients. Hemodynamically significant great vessel anastomosis obstruction or neoaortic regurgitation are extremely uncommon early postoperative problems.

d-Transposition of the Great Arteries: Atrial Switch

The postoperative evaluation should include (a) assessment of cardiac rhythm (12-lead ECG, bedside monitoring); (b) systemic (right) ventricular and (tricuspid) AV valve function (auscultation, indices of cardiac output, invasive monitoring); (c) assessment for systemic venous pathway obstruction (clinical examination, echocardiography if indicated); (d) assessment for pulmonary venous pathway obstruction (chest radiograph for pulmonary edema, arterial blood gases, echocardiography if indicated); and (e) evaluation for subpulmonary stenosis (auscultation, echocardiography if indicated). Only 80% of patients following atrial correction are in normal sinus rhythm at hospital discharge. Temporary atrial pacing wires are extremely valuable in the early postoperative period, both for diagnostic and therapeutic purposes. Systemic ventricular dysfunction and tricuspid regurgitation are uncommon early problems after atrial level correction, but may progress with time. Systemic venous pathway obstruction (usually the SVC) is more common with the Mustard operation, whereas pulmonary venous pathway obstruction appears more commonly after the Senning repair.

Total Anomalous Pulmonary Venous Connection

Infradiaphragmatic anomalous drainage of the pulmonary veins frequently presents shortly after birth with severe respiratory distress, hypoxemia, and suprasystemic pulmonary artery pressures owing to severe pulmonary venous obstruction; repair is usually performed on an emergent basis. Paroxysmal, severe pulmonary hypertensive crises have been minimized by (a) the use of neuromuscular blockade and high-dose narcotic (e.g., fentanyl) infusions through the first postoperative day, (b) inhaled nitric oxide if necessary, and (c) early diagnosis and repair (prior to the development of significantly suprasystemic PVR). Other postoperative problems include residual pulmonary venous obstruction, low cardiac output, and arrhythmias.

Truncus Arteriosus

The postoperative evaluation should include (a) assessment for residual shunt (as above), (b) assessment of function of the truncal (neoaortic) valve, (c) residual right ventricular

outflow tract obstruction (as above), and (d) conduction abnormalities (postoperative 12-lead ECG, bedside monitoring). As with tetralogy repair, complete right bundle branch block pattern is to be expected because the repair includes a right ventriculotomy. Older patients (>3 months) are more likely to have paroxysmal pulmonary hypertension than those repaired in the neonatal period. Hypocalcemia should be closely monitored in patients with coexisting DiGeorge syndrome.

Coarctation of the Aorta

The postoperative assessment includes evaluation for residual arch obstruction (femoral pulses, four extremity blood pressures) and (b) management of postoperative hypertension. Pain control and sedation and continuous infusions of arterial vasodilators (e.g., sodium nitroprusside) are important in the treatment of severe hypertension in the immediate postoperative period. Significant paroxysmal increases in blood pressure may produce tension on the arterial suture line and increase the potential for bleeding. Intravenous beta-blockers such as esmolol or labetalol may be necessary. For persistent hypertension, oral angiotensin-converting enzyme inhibitors or beta-blockers (121) may be necessary. Other potential postoperative problems include injury to the phrenic or recurrent laryngeal nerve, sepsis, stroke (possibly owing to transiently increased intracranial pressure), spinal cord or intestinal ischemia, and chylothorax.

Single Ventricle: Parallel Circulation with Complete Mixing

The physiology of a parallel circulation (e.g., Norwood operation, pulmonary atresia lesions with systemic-to-pulmonary shunts or collaterals) is discussed above (Table 20.2). Goals of the initial surgical procedure include (a) providing unobstructed SBF, (b) providing unobstructed pulmonary venous return to the single ventricle, usually via atrial septectomy, and (c) providing limited PBF without pulmonary artery distortion (122). The postoperative evaluation should assess all aspects of the specific procedure that have been used. The evaluation after a Norwood palliation for hypoplastic left heart syndrome must be much more extensive than following a shunt for single ventricle with pulmonary atresia. The patient with either excessive cyanosis (oxygen saturation <65% to 70%) or relatively high (>85% to 88%) oxygen saturations must have the repair and postoperative physiology carefully evaluated.

Low Cardiac Output. A low cardiac output syndrome may occur in the first 24 to 48 hours after surgery, with typical findings of tachycardia, hypotension, oliguria, and metabolic acidosis. In addition to standard monitoring, many centers have recently advocated intermittent measurement of the mixed venous oxygen saturation following stage I surgery, typically in the SVC. The arterial-venous oxygen saturation difference (A-V ΔO_2) is a sensitive predictor of low SBF and inadequate oxygen delivery (35,36,123,124), an A-V ΔO_2 of >40% to 50% suggests advanced low cardiac output and inadequate tissue delivery of oxygen.

The patient with evidence of low SBF requires immediate attention and evaluation of the potential cause(s). Low systemic cardiac output may be due to (a) globally decreased ventricular output (poor pump performance), (b) elevated Q_p:Q_s ratio (adequate pump performance with maldistribution of flow), or (c) AV valve regurgitation (adequate pump performance with large regurgitant fraction with or without maldistribution of flow).

TABLE 20.7

CARDIAC CATHETERIZATION PROCEDURES THAT MAY REQUIRE ICU MANAGEMENT

Procedure	Representative lesion(s)	Potential complications
Diagnostic catheterization	Congenital heart disease	Blood loss requiring transfusion Air embolism Stroke, cerebral vascular accident Myocardial perforation and tamponade Femoral vessel occlusion Arrhythmias: ventricular and supraventricular tachycardia, ventricular fibrillation, complete heart block
Coil embolization	Aortopulmonary collaterals Blalock–Taussig's shunts Anomalous coronary arteries Hepatic hemangiomas	Fever Excessive hypoxemia Systemic embolization Hepatic necrosis
Transcatheter device closure	Patent ductus arteriosus Atrial septal defect Ventricular septal defect	Air or device embolization Interference with atrioventricular or semilunar valve function, ventricular arrhythmias, complete heart block Pulmonary artery tear and bleeding Unilateral pulmonary edema False aneurysm Cardiac arrest
Balloon dilations/intravascular stents	Pulmonary artery stenosis Blalock–Taussig's shunt Pulmonary valve stenosis Aortic valve stenosis Mitral valve stenosis Coarctation of the aorta	Pulmonary artery tear and bleeding Thrombosis Pulmonary edema Pulmonary insufficiency Aortic regurgitation Ventricular fibrillation (neonate) Mitral insufficiency Pulmonary hypertension Aortic dissection Hypertension False aneurysms Stent embolization
Atrial septotomy/blade atrial septectomy	Right ventricular conduit Transposition of the great arteries, mitral stenosis (atresia) and restrictive atrial septum	Perforation of the heart and tamponade Air embolus Complete heart block Supraventricular tachycardia
Radiofrequency mapping and ablation	Anomalous conduction pathways	Thromboembolus from long sheath and prolonged ablation procedure
Myocardial biopsy	Cardiomyopathy or transplant	Myocardial perforation Complete heart block

The combination of echocardiography to evaluate ventricular and AV valve function and measurement of the A-V ΔO_2 to evaluate the $Q_p:Q_s$ ratio is important in establishing the cause of the low cardiac output and rationally directing therapy. The patient with globally depressed function may best benefit from increasing inotropic support, whereas the patient with adequate pump function but a high $Q_p:Q_s$ ratio will best benefit from maneuvers to increase the PVR and decrease SVR.

The patient who is "too pink" with a parallel circulation typically has PBF (Q_p) far in excess of SBF (Q_s). This may result in inadequate systemic perfusion, renal dysfunction, and an inability to wean the patient from mechanical ventilation. In children palliated with left-sided obstructive lesions (e.g., Norwood procedure), arch obstruction must be ruled out because distal obstruction will force more blood through the shunt and increase Q_p at the expense of Q_s. Subambient oxygen (FiO$_2$ 17% to 19%), permissive hypercapnia, or the addition of carbon dioxide to the inspired gas mixture may be useful to temporarily increase the PVR and decrease Q_p (24,124–126). An alternative strategy is to lower SVR and thus produce a more "balanced" circulation. Phenoxybenzamine, a potent, long acting α-blocker is routinely used by some centers in the post-operative period after the Norwood operation (34,35).

Hypoxemia. The differential diagnosis of excessive cyanosis includes (a) pulmonary venous desaturation (pneumothorax, pleural effusion, pulmonary edema, pneumonia, infection); (b) systemic venous desaturation (anemia, high oxygen consumption states, low cardiac output); and (c) decreased PBF (elevated PVR, pulmonary venous hypertension, restrictive

ASD, pulmonary artery distortion, a physically small or stenotic systemic-to-pulmonary artery shunt).

Single Ventricle: Bidirectional Cavopulmonary (Glenn) Anastomosis

Interim palliation with a bidirectional Glenn shunt has been used increasingly in the past decade. Following this procedure, the PBF is obligate. The SVC return passes through the lungs (in the absence of decompressing venous collaterals) (127). Thus, the PBF equals the brachiocephalic arterial flow, which is typically about half the total ventricular output (somewhat more than half in infants, and less than half in adults). The Q_p:Q_s ratio is therefore approximately 0.5. This results in a decrease in the ventricular volume load, improved ventricular function, and improved AV valve function.

Patients with clinical signs of significantly elevated SVC pressure (upper extremity plethora and edema) may have obstruction at the anastomosis, distal pulmonary artery distortion, or elevations in PVR. Significant elevations of pressure in the SVC may limit cerebral blood flow (which may be further decreased by hyperventilation and alkalosis used to decrease PVR). The etiology should be promptly investigated, including early catheterization if necessary. Transient postoperative hypertension has been frequently observed (127) and may be owing to pain, catecholamine secretion, or intracranial hypertension. Aggressive lowering of the blood pressure may thus adversely affect the cerebral perfusion pressure, and vasodilators should be used cautiously. Excessive cyanosis (oxygen saturations <70% to 75%) should be investigated promptly, especially in infants, where a greater proportion of systemic output dedicated to the upper half of the body should result in oxygen saturations closer to 80% to 85%. Causes include pulmonary or excessive systemic venous desaturation or decreased PBF due to decompressing venous collaterals, an undiagnosed contralateral (usually left) SVC, or a baffle leak (if the intracardiac orifice of the SVC has been patch closed [hemi-Fontan]). Transient (or rarely, permanent) sinus node dysfunction is common and responds well to chronotropic agents or temporary atrial pacing.

The Glenn circulation is unique in that the cerebral and pulmonary circulations are connected in series, and their auto regulatory mechanisms are in direct competition with each other. It is well known that hypercarbia causes vasodilation in the cerebral vessels, while inducing vasoconstriction in the pulmonary vascular bed, and hyperoxia has the opposite effect. Some elegant studies have demonstrated that hypercarbia after the bidirectional cavopulmonary connection increases cerebral blood flow and systemic oxygenation despite a small increase in pulmonary artery pressure (128–130).

Single Ventricle: Fontan Operation. The many modifications of the Fontan operation in the past three decades (including conduits, atriopulmonary connections, cavopulmonary connections and the recent use of adjustable atrial defects (131) or fixed fenestrations (47,132) in the intraatrial baffle), combined with improved patient selection and postoperative management, have reduced the operative mortality to <5% in many centers (45,133–136). Postoperative management must be specifically tailored to the preoperative anatomy and physiology, as well as the specific type of surgical procedure performed, but in general is geared toward optimizing cardiac output at the lowest central venous pressure possible. Physiologic RA and LA catheters are invaluable in the management of these patients.

Low cardiac output may be due to inadequate preload. This may be a sign of hypovolemia (low RA and LA pressures), elevated PVR (low LA and high RA pressures), or anatomic obstruction in the systemic venous pathway. Low cardiac output in the face of high LA pressure is an ominous sign and may be due to ventricular dysfunction, loss of AV synchrony, AV valve regurgitation, or ventricular outflow obstruction (e.g., subaortic stenosis).

Significant arrhythmias, especially those with loss of AV synchrony (e.g., junctional ectopic tachycardia), are tolerated particularly poorly in this patient population. With progressive tachycardia there is usually continued hemodynamic deterioration. Frequently it is difficult to decide if the arrhythmia is a result of poor hemodynamics or its cause. Prompt investigation of the surgical repair, including catheterization and angiography, is indicated in the patient with low cardiac output.

Mechanical positive-pressure ventilation with increased mean airway pressures may adversely affect PVR and ventricular filling (137). Early institution of spontaneous ventilation may improve hemodynamics in the awake patient. In our experience, physiologic (3 to 5 cm H_2O) PEEP is generally well tolerated, does not significantly affect PVR or cardiac output, and may improve oxygenation by reducing areas of microatelectasis and improving ventilation–perfusion matching.

Excessive cyanosis following the Fontan procedure may be due to a leak in the intracardiac baffle or pulmonary venous desaturation. In patients with fenestrated baffles, low mixed venous saturation, additional baffle leaks, and decompressing venous collaterals must be excluded. The duration and frequency of pleural and pericardial effusions, typically the most frequent postoperative problem requiring prolonged hospitalization, have been reduced recently with the use of modified ultrafiltration (45), "baffle fenestrations," and the "adjustable atrial septal defect." Drainage catheters, with appropriate replacement of intravascular volume, electrolytes, protein, and immunoglobulins, are necessary in cases of prolonged drainage.

Other potential postoperative problems include arrhythmia (138) (particularly sinus node dysfunction, atrial flutter, and junctional ectopic tachycardia), acute liver dysfunction, protein-losing enteropathy, and CNS complications (139).

SPECIFIC SYSTEM-RELATED PROBLEMS

Central Nervous System

Children with complex congenital cardiac malformations, particularly those requiring cardiac surgery as neonates and infants have a significantly higher incidence of academic difficulties, behavioral abnormalities, fine and gross motor problems, problems with visual-motor integration and executive planning, speech delays, inattention and hyperactivity (140–143). As these children get older, they have a greater need for special services compared to the general population. More than a decade ago, emphasis was placed on the role of intraoperative factors in neurodevelopmental disabilities. Much has been learned in the intervening years regarding the multifactorial causes of abnormal school-age development such as prenatal, perioperative, socioeconomic, and genetic influences. The incidence of these abnormalities may range from infrequent to ubiquitous. Children with more "significant" cardiac disease such as obstructed total anomalous pulmonary venous connection, hypoplastic left heart syndrome etc have a higher incidence of neurodevelopmental disabilities, with perhaps only one third of those tested having no dysfunction in any domain. While most of these abnormalities are relatively mild, and may only be detected by formal testing, they result in a so-called "high-prevalence, low severity" developmental "signature."

Genetic and Environmental Factors

Socioeconomic status is perhaps the strongest predictor of neurodevelopmental outcome. Multiple studies have shown the relationship between socioeconomic status and/or parental intelligence and outcome in children with congenital cardiac disease. Children with syndromes with known and unknown chromosomal abnormalities such as Down, DiGeorge, Williams, Trisomy 13 and 18, CHARGE and VACTERL syndromes, frequently have coexisting congenital cardiac disease. Down syndrome is universally associated with mental retardation and other neurologic impairment; 22q11 deletion has been shown to result in the phenotype of DiGeorge or velo-cardio-facial syndrome, with many of these children having abnormalities of the outflow tract such as tetralogy of Fallot, interrupted aortic arch, and truncus arteriosus. Although some of the developmental abnormalities may be related to the underlying cardiac disease and its treatment, and some speech delay may be attributed to palatal abnormalities, recent reports suggest that there is an increased incidence of abnormalities of the white matter, as well as predisposition to psychiatric abnormalities such as schizophrenia. Apolipoprotein E which is important in the regulation of cholesterol metabolism is thought to effect neurological recovery following a variety of central nervous system injuries. Gaynor et al. have recently reported that genetic polymorphisms of apolipoprotein E were related to abnormal neurological development and a small head circumference in children aged one year who underwent surgery as neonates or young infants (158).

Congenital Cerebral Disease

There is an increased incidence of structural abnormalities of the brain in children with structural cardiac abnormalities. Many children with multiple congenital anomalies or chromosomal abnormalities will have developmental delay as a significant component of late morbidity. Microcephaly which is independently associated with later developmental delays occurs frequently at birth in children with congenital heart disease, approaching one-fourth of children in some reports (144). The "operculum" denotes the region of the brain that covers the insulae relie, and is made up of frontal, temporal, and parietal cortical convolutions. The operculum is thought to be related to oral-motor coordination, taste and speech, particularly expressive language. In magnetic resonance imaging (MRI) and computer tomographic imaging (CT) studies of neonates with complex congenital cardiac malformations, underdevelopment of the operculum or "open operculum" may be seen in nearly a quarter of the patients. This may be one of the factors responsible for the high prevalence of feeding problems, expressive language delay and oral-motor apraxia in these children. Periventricular leukomalacia (PVL) or white matter injury, a common finding in premature infants, has been increasingly recognized in full term neonates with congenital cardiac disease. Mahle et al. studied 24 neonates preoperatively with MRI of the brain, and noted PVL in 4 neonates (145). In a larger

study of 105 children, MRI of the brain in the early postoperative period revealed PVL in slightly over half of the neonates in the study, but rarely in older children (146). In prematures infants, severe PVL has been associated with cerebral palsy, while mild degrees of injury have been associated with motor difficulties, and behavioral disorders. Other congenital anomalies of the brain such as holoprosencephaly and agenesis of the corpus callosum have also been described in children with complex congenital cardiac disease.

Preoperative Factors

These neonates frequently require continuous prostaglandin infusion, some require mechanical ventilation, or invasive interventions such as balloon atrial septostomy. All of these interventions carry risks to the central nervous system, especially the potential for paradoxical embolus to the brain in the presence of right-left intracardiac shunt. Many of these patients also have oxygen saturations that are below normal, potentially compromising the delivery of oxygen to the brain. In a study by Licht et al. cerebral blood flow was on average less than half that seen in normal term neonates, under conditions of general anesthesia and mechanical ventilation with normocapnia (146). The cerebral vascular response to increased inspired carbon dioxide was preserved, suggesting normal autoregulation.

Intraoperative Factors

Variations in intraoperative support is one of the few modifiable risk factors to improve long-term neurological outcomes. The conduct of cardiopulmonary bypass (CPB) has been the subject of active research. Potentially modifiable technical features of CPB are shown in Table 20.1. Much has been written on the potentially deleterious effects of deep hypothermic circulatory arrest (DHCA). Though it is generally agreed that prolonged periods of DHCA may have adverse neurological outcomes, it is increasingly clear that the effects of short duration of DHCA are inconsistently related to adverse outcomes, that the effect is not linear with a cut-off point in the range of 40 minutes, and that the effects are most likely modifiable by other patient-related, pre- and postoperative factors. Innovative techniques have been developed to provide continuous cerebral perfusion during complex reconstruction of the aortic arch or intracardiac repair. It must be pointed out that the avoidance of DHCA by necessity increases the duration of CPB, which has consistently been shown to have an adverse effect on short-term and long-term outcomes.

The Boston Circulatory Arrest Study is a landmark study with multiple reports from Bellinger, Newburger and Jonas et al. (147–153). In this cohort, 171 children with d-transposition of great arteries were assigned an intraoperative support strategy of predominantly DHCA or predominantly low-flow cardiopulmonary bypass during the arterial switch operation. Earlier reports suggested that the group as a whole was performing below expectations in many aspects of evaluation, with worse outcomes for the DHCA group in the areas of postoperative seizures, motor skills at 1 year, as well as behavior, speech and language at 4 years. Neurodevelopmental testing at 8 years revealed scores for Intelligence Quotient for the cohort as a whole was closer to normal, at 98 versus the population mean of 100. The group demonstrated significant deficits in visual-spatial and visual-memory skills, and they had difficulty coordinating skills in order to perform complex operations. Those assigned to the

DHCA group scored worse on motor and speech functioning, while patients in the low-flow CPB group demonstrated worse scores for impulsivity and behavior. More than one third of these patients received remedial school services, and about 10% repeated a grade. The results serve to show that multiple factors influence developmental outcome in school-age children. Influence of factors which may seem important on early testing, may be attenuated or abolished during longer-term follow-up, as other factors assume a more important role.

Postoperative Factors

The central nervous system may be particularly vulnerable during the period of LCOS that follows cardiac surgery. Seizures occur in the immediate postoperative period in up to 20% of neonates, depending on method of detection (154–156). Clinical seizures are significantly less prevalent than those detected on continuous electroencephalographic monitoring (154). Risk factors are younger age, longer periods of DHCA, and presence of coexisting abnormalities of the central nervous system. Perioperative seizures are a marker for early central nervous system injury, and have previously been reported to be associated with worse scores on developmental testing in children with transposition studied in the Boston Circulatory Arrest Trial (156). However recent data may show less of an impact than previously identified. In addition to the factors described above, the immediate postoperative period typically requires invasive monitoring, central venous access, and mechanical ventilation. These factors may adversely affect the central nervous system, including the risk of paradoxical embolus from central and peripheral intravenous access in patients with residual intracardiac shunts, fever, hyperglycemia, and swings in cerebral blood flow brought on by acute changes in mechanical ventilation. In the Boston Circulatory Arrest Trial longer hospital and intensive care unit length of stay was associated with worse developmental outcome at 8 years (157). Following discharge, some patients remain at risk for ongoing injury to the central nervous system. Many patients have chronic hypoxemia due to ongoing palliation and/or intentional intracardiac right-to-left shunting. The presesnce of hypoxemia probably has a role in neurodevelopmental impairment; however, it is difficult to measure its effect in isolation.

It is interesting to examine the developmental abnormalities seen in groups of children with hypoplastic left heart syndrome undergoing staged reconstruction, and compare them to the findings after heart transplantation in infancy for the same disease (140,159). The patterns of dysfunction are remarkably similar, despite the markedly different strategies of treatment, suggesting factors other than the surgical approach and techniques used for intraoperative support may play a significant role in long-term outcome in these patients.

Choreoathetosis is an enigmatic and sometimes devastating complication that has been described following cardiac surgery using CPB both with and without DHCA. Factors that have been implicated in the development of choreoathetosis include age beyond infancy, chronic preoperative hypoxemia, depth of hypothermia, and the use of DHCA (148). The duration and rapidity of core cooling on CPB may result in uneven brain cooling, especially in the deep areas of the basal ganglia and mid-brain. Finally, the presence of systemic-to-pulmonary collaterals may potentially result in a "cerebral steal" (from the head and neck vessels into the low-resistance pulmonary vascular bed), contributing to uneven or inadequate brain cooling during core cooling on CPB.

Thus neurodevelopmental abnormalities are widely prevalent in children with complex cardiac disease, and affect the quality of life of school-age children and their families.

Pulmonary

Diaphragmatic paresis (no motion) or paralysis (paradoxical motion) may precipitate and promote respiratory failure, particularly in the neonate or young infant who relies on diaphragmatic function for breathing more than older infants and children (who can recruit accessory and intercostal muscles if diaphragmatic function proves inadequate). Injury to the phrenic nerve, usually the left, may occur during operations that involve dissection of the branch pulmonary arteries well out to the hilum (e.g., tetralogy of Fallot, arterial switch operation), arch reconstruction from the midline (e.g., Norwood operation), manipulation of the SVC (Glenn shunts), takedown of previous systemic-to-pulmonary shunts, or after percutaneous central venous access. Phrenic injury may occur more frequently at reoperation, when adhesions and scarring may obscure landmarks. Topical cooling with ice during deep hypothermia also may cause transient phrenic palsy. Increased work of breathing on low ventilator settings, increased PCO_2, and a chest radiograph revealing an elevated hemidiaphragm are suggestive of diaphragmatic dysfunction. The chest radiograph may be misleading, however, if the film is taken during peak positive-pressure ventilation. Ultrasonography and/or fluoroscopy are useful for identifying diaphragmatic motion or paradoxical excursion. Recovery of diaphragmatic contraction usually occurs. However, if a patient fails to tolerate repeated extubations despite maximal cardiovascular and nutritional support, and diaphragmatic dysfunction persists with volume loss in the affected lung, the diaphragm can be surgically plicated. Negative pressure ventilation has been a useful adjunct in the treatment of these infants and may shorten the period of intubation and positive-pressure ventilation.

Diminished conductance or increased airway resistance arises from several pathologic changes alone or in combination: secretions, either excessive in quantity or viscosity; swelling of the mucosa owing to hyperemia or edema, most often resulting from trauma or infection; hyperactive bronchial smooth muscle; or extrinsic compression by neighboring structures or diminished forces pulling the conducting passages open. Patients who have secretions from the tracheal aspirate showing many visible organisms and polymorphonuclear cells on microscopy, together with fever, an elevated white cell count, and consolidation on the chest radiograph, should be treated with appropriate antibiotics.

Postextubation stridor may be due to mucosal swelling of the large airway. A nebulized, inhaled α agonist (e.g., racemic epinephrine) promotes vasoconstriction and decreases hyperemia and, possibly, edema. If reintubation is necessary, a smaller endotracheal tube should be used if possible. An evaluation for vocal cord dysfunction should be considered, especially in patients with surgery near the recurrent laryngeal nerve (e.g., Norwood procedure for hypoplastic left heart syndrome).

Bronchospasm may be treated by inhaled or systemically administered bronchodilators, but must be used with caution in light of their chronotropic and tachyarrhythmic potential. If all of these maneuvers fail to improve the patient, the minimum tidal volume and frequency that provide sufficient mechanical minute ventilation to satisfactorily supplement spontaneous ventilation and minimize over-inflation of the lungs are determined and used during the recovery phase.

Pulmonary edema, pneumonia, and atelectasis are the most common causes of lower airway and alveolar abnormalities that interfere with gas exchange. If a bacterial pathogen is identified, therapy includes antibiotics. If the cause is pulmonary edema, maintenance of good hemodynamics is required, as are low pulmonary venous pressures. If a cardiogenic basis for increased extrapulmonary water exists, treatable residual defects should be excluded, fluid should be restricted, and inotropic and diuretic therapy begun. For infants, fluid restriction is frequently incompatible with adequate nutrition and, therefore, an aggressive diuretic regimen is preferable to restriction of caloric intake. Adjustment of end-expiratory pressure and mechanical ventilation serve as supportive therapies until the alveoli and pulmonary interstitium are cleared of the fluid that interferes with gas entry. PEEP redistributes interstitial lung water from the alveolar-capillary space to peribronchial and hilar spaces, improving lung compliance and gas exchange.

Pleural effusions, and less often ascites, may occur in patients after a Fontan operation or reparative procedures requiring a right ventriculotomy (e.g., tetralogy of Fallot, truncus arteriosus) with transient right ventricular dysfunction. Fluid in the pleural space or peritoneum and intestinal distention compete with intrapulmonary gas for thoracic space. Evacuation of the pleural space or drainage of ascites and decompression of the intestinal lumen allow the intrapulmonary gas volume to increase.

Renal

In adults, renal failure after cardiac surgery has been associated with mortality as high as 90%. Risk factors for postoperative renal failure include preoperative renal dysfunction, prolonged bypass time (>180 minutes), and low cardiac output. In addition to relative ischemia and nonpulsatile flow on CPB, an angiotensin II–mediated renal vasoconstriction and delayed healing of renal tubular epithelium has been proposed as one mechanism for renal failure. Postoperative sepsis and nephrotoxic drugs may cause further damage to the kidneys.

Renal failure may occur in children after open heart surgery and can also carry an associated high mortality rate. Acute tubular necrosis is suggested by urine sodium of >20 mEq/L, the presence of granular casts or tubular epithelium in the urine, and a urine osmolality that is close to the serum osmolality. Metabolic derangements secondary to renal failure such as acidosis, hyponatremia, hyperkalemia, and hypocalcemia as well as impairment in gas exchange can complicate the postoperative management. Support for the myocardium should be directed toward improving cardiac output and renal blood flow without causing further renal vasoconstriction. In addition, drugs that are excreted by the kidney should have dosages decreased, and drugs that are nephrotoxic should be discontinued if possible.

Mechanical support in patients with renal failure includes peritoneal dialysis, hemodialysis, and continuous arteriovenous hemofiltration. Criteria for dialysis may be somewhat subjective but can include (a) blood urea nitrogen >100 mg/dL; (b) life-threatening electrolyte imbalance, especially hyperkalemia; (c) intractable metabolic acidosis; (d) fluid imbalance causing pulmonary compromise; or (e) fluid restrictions limiting caloric intake.

Recently, continuous arteriovenous hemofiltration (160) has been used to manage acute renal failure in children after CPB. Paret et al. (161) described a successful experience (ten children) with continuous arteriovenous hemofiltration (at 20 to 100 mL/h for 5 hours to 8 days), which resulted in correction of hypervolemia and an increase in caloric intake.

Gastrointestinal

Following cardiac surgery in neonates and children, adequate nutrition is exceedingly important but frequently overlooked. These critically ill children often have decreased caloric intake and increased energy demand after surgery. The neonate in particular has limited metabolic and fat reserves. Total parenteral nutrition can provide adequate nutrition in the early hypercatabolic phases of the immediate postoperative period. The gastrointestinal tract also can be particularly sensitive to stresses such as hypoperfusion and hypoxia sometimes encountered in the postoperative period after cardiac surgery, and enteral feeds should be reinstituted slowly.

Although gastrointestinal complications are rare in adults after cardiac surgery, the mortality rate can approach 40%. Upper gastrointestinal bleeding and ulcer formation may occur following the stress of cardiac surgery in children and adults. There are limited reports of the efficacy of histamine H_2 antireceptors, sucralfate, or oral antacids in pediatric cardiac patients, although their use is common in many ICUs. Hepatic failure may occur after cardiac surgery and is typically characterized by elevated liver enzymes and difficulties with hemostasis. Necrotizing enterocolitis, although typically a disease of premature infants, is seen with a surprisingly high frequency in neonates with CHD. Risk factors include (a) left-sided obstructive lesions with mesenteric hypoperfusion following ductus arteriosus constriction, (b) umbilical or femoral arterial catheterization, (c) angiography, (d) hypoxemia, and (e) lesions with wide pulse pressures (e.g., systemic to pulmonary shunts, patent ductus arteriosus, and severe aortic regurgitation) producing retrograde flow in the mesenteric vessels during diastole. Frequently, multiple risk factors exist in the same patient, making a specific etiology difficult to establish. Treatment includes continuous nasogastric suction, parenteral nutrition, and broad-spectrum antibiotics; bowel exploration or resection may be necessary in severe cases.

Infection

Low-grade (<38.5°C) fever during the immediate postoperative period is common and may be present for ≤3 to 4 days, even without a demonstrable infectious cause. However, there are several reports of increased susceptibility to infection after CPB. CPB may activate complement and other mediators of inflammation but can also lead to derangements of the immune system and increase the likelihood of infection. A centrally mediated etiology of fever following CPB has been postulated.

Sepsis after cardiac surgery in adults is associated with a high mortality rate and can be correlated with higher APACHE (acute physiology and chronic health evaluation) scores. Despite the recent increased use of broad-coverage, third-generation cephalosporins, these agents did not seem to be more effective in decreasing postoperative infections (162). Early removal of indwelling catheters in the postoperative patient may potentially reduce the incidence of sepsis. The safe in situ period for catheters has not been clearly established, but should probably not be greater than 10 to 14 days. Last, in the presence of fever, broad-spectrum antibiotics can be initiated while awaiting blood, urine, and tracheal culture results.

Mediastinitis occurs in ≤2% of patients undergoing cardiac surgery. Risk factors may include delayed sternal closure, early re-exploration for bleeding, or reoperation. Mediastinitis is characterized by persistent fever, purulent drainage from the sternotomy wound, instability of the sternum, and leukocytosis. *Staphylococcus* is the most common offending organism. Delayed diagnosis of mediastinitis can lead to a mortality rate as high as 25%. Treatment usually involves debridement and irrigation with aggressive parenteral antibiotic therapy.

Postpericardiotomy Syndrome

Postpericardiotomy syndrome was first noted in 1952 with the advent of surgery for mitral stenosis, but was initially thought to represent the reactivation of rheumatic fever. In 1958, Engle et al. (163) recognized that the syndrome could be seen in any patient in whom the pericardial sac was opened. Postpericardiotomy syndrome is not common in the infant and toddler but occurs with surprising frequency in the older child and adolescent. The condition is more often mild than severe, and when mild, may be overlooked. Possible causes include viral infection and an autoimmune reaction.

The child may complain of anterior precordial chest pain, which increases on deep inspiration. A pericardial friction rub may be present. Chest radiography may reveal pleural effusions and cardiac enlargement (secondary to a pericardial effusion). The white blood cell count is frequently elevated with a left shift, and the erythrocyte sedimentation rate will be elevated. Blood cultures are negative. The ECG shows nonspecific abnormalities of the T waves, typically flattening in lead I and the lateral chest leads. Only with a large pericardial effusion will the voltages decrease. Echocardiography identifies the pericardial effusion and helps to monitor its course.

Because the illness is usually self-limited, therapy is generally limited to bed rest and anti-inflammatory agents, either salicylates (aspirin, 100 mg/kg in four divided doses for about 1 month, then tapered over 1 to 2 months), nonsteroidal anti-inflammatory agents, or, in more severe cases, steroids (prednisone, 2 mg/kg/day for 1 week and gradually tapered over 2 to 3 weeks). Some patients will develop a pericardial effusion postoperatively without other signs or symptoms of postpericardiotomy syndrome.

The persistence of pericardial effusion is of most concern because of the possibility of life-threatening tamponade. Cardiac tamponade is characterized by (a) an elevation of intracardiac filling pressures, (b) progressive limitation of ventricular diastolic filling, and (c) a reduction of stroke volume and cardiac output. Children with sizable pericardial effusions frequently have nausea and vomiting or abdominal pain as a chief complaint, along with tachycardia and signs of diminished cardiac output. If echocardiography demonstrates a large pericardial effusion and clinical signs of cardiovascular compromise are present, the effusion should be drained. While preparing for pericardial drainage, 10 to 20 mL/kg of isotonic saline or albumin should be administered, and in certain cases (e.g., patients on anticoagulation) blood should be made available and surgeons notified of the procedure. Simple pericardiocentesis generally is effective, but persistent effusions occasionally require the placement of an indwelling drainage catheter (164) or surgical pericardiectomy.

Pericardiocentesis

An intravenous line and reliable blood pressure monitoring must be in place. The patient should sit at about a 30- to 45-degree angle, breathing supplemental oxygen in most cases. The young child generally will require intravenous sedation or even anesthesia to prevent movement during needle or catheter placement. Sedative and anesthetic agents must be used cautiously because the abrupt cessation of endogenous catecholamine production in the suddenly sedated or anesthetized patient may lower blood pressure, heart rate, and cardiac output dramatically. Moreover, any need for assisted positive-pressure ventilation may be particularly deleterious in the setting of tamponade. The relative risks of these medications must be weighed against the risks of inserting a needle into the pericardial space of a struggling infant or child. Afterload reducing agents should be avoided.

Echocardiography is extremely useful in guiding needle placement, allowing for more accurate direction of advancement of the needle and as a guide to the depth of effusion from the skin and the width of the effusion. After subcutaneous anesthesia and using a sterile technique, the needle should be inserted just below the xiphoid process at about 30 to 45 degrees from the perpendicular, with the tip aimed at the mid-clavicular line (based on echocardiographic findings). A syringe should be attached to the needle with continuous aspiration as the needle is advanced. Once pericardial fluid is present in the syringe, a hemostat may be clamped at the skin surface to prevent further penetration. The addition of an ECG lead to the aspiration needle is usually not necessary, and may make the procedure more cumbersome. Fluid should be removed until it no longer comes out easily. If the fluid is thick or prolonged drainage is anticipated, a temporary drainage catheter should be placed. A guide wire is placed through the needle in a similar manner to that of the Seldinger technique used for venous access, and a pigtail-type catheter can be positioned over the wire and connected to continuous suction (84).

Further Directions

While the past decades have seen gratifying progress in the field of pediatric cardiac intensive care medicine, many challenges and opportunities remain. It is clear that the majority of neonates, infants, children, and young adults with congenital or acquired heart disease are now *expected* to survive. It is also clear that some long term morbidities are related to events in the intensive care unit. We must reduce ICU morbidities to the lowest possible level, including nosocomial infections and other complications related to patient safety, as well as pay more attention to resource utilization.

Single center trials will be augmented with collaborative, hypothesis-driven multicenter trials. Advances in biotechnology and computing will improve our monitoring capabilities, gradually shifting to continuous, real-time assessment of clinical and laboratory parameters (such as arterial blood gases) that have been traditionally measured intermittently. The growing population of adults with congenital heart disease, a continued emphasis on neonatal and fetal intervention, as well as ongoing advances in mechanical support of the failing circulation is likely to change the patient mix in many units.

A combination of mandated reduced working hours for trainees, and in some countries, staff physicians, has resulted in limited human resources in an increasingly demanding and technology-based field, in which multidisciplinary care is needed. As a field, we need to better define what training is necessary to provide intensive care to pediatric and young adult patients with cardiovascular disease, both for the individual practitioners as well as the ideal skill mix for the team of caregivers.

References

1. Castañeda AR, Mayer JE Jr, Jonas RA, et al. The neonate with critical congenital heart disease: Repair—a surgical challenge. *J Thorac Cardiovasc Surg* 1989;98:869–875.
2. Anand KJS, Hansen DD, Hickey PR. Hormonal-metabolic stress responses in neonates undergoing cardiac surgery. *Anesthesiology* 1990;73:661–670.
3. Lenn NJ. Plasticity and responses of the immature nervous system to injury. *Semin Perinatol* 1987;11:117–131.
4. Mahle WT, Clancy RR, Moss E, et al. Functional and cognitive outcome in school-age and adolescent children with hypoplastic left heart syndrome. *Pediatrics* 2000;105:1082–1089.
5. Wessel DL, Adatia I, Giglia TM, et al. Use of inhaled nitric oxide and acetylcholine in the evaluation of pulmonary hypertension and endothelial function after cardiopulmonary bypass. *Circulation* 1993;88:2128–2138.
6. Giglia T, Wessel D. Effects of oxygen on pulmonary and systemic hemodynamics in infants after cardiopulmonary bypass (abstract). *Circulation* 1990;82:III-78.
7. West JB, Dollery CT, Naimark A. Distribution of blood flow in isolated lung: Relation to vascular and alveolar pressures. *J Appl Physiol* 1964;19:713–924.
8. Hickey PR, Hansen DD, Wessel DL, et al. Blunting of stress responses in the pulmonary circulation of infants by fentanyl. *Anesth Analg* 1985;64:1137–1142.
9. Hickey PR, Hansen DD. Pulmonary hypertension in infants: Postoperative management. In: Yacoub M, ed. *Annual of Cardiac Surgery.* London: Current Science, 1989:16–22.
10. Wernovsky G, Wypij D, Jonas RA, et al. Postoperative course and hemodynamic profile after the arterial switch operation in neonates and infants: A comparison of low-flow cardiopulmonary bypass and circulatory arrest. *Circulation* 1995;92:2226–2235.
11. Palmer RMJ, Ferrige AG, Moncada S. Nitric oxide release accounts for the biologic activity of endothelium-derived relaxing factor. *Nature* 1987;327:524–526.
12. Ignarro L, Buga G, Woods K, et al. Endothelium-derived relaxing factor produced and released from artery and vein is nitric oxide. *Proc Natl Acad Sci USA* 1987;84:9265–9269.
12a. Pepke-Zaba J, Higenbottam TW, Dinh-Xuan AT, et al. Inhaled nitric oxide as a cause of selective pulmonary vasodilation in pulmonary hypertension. *Lancet* 1991;338:1173–1174.
12b. Wessel DL, Adatia I, Van Marter LJ, et al. Improved oxygenation in a randomized trial of inhaled nitric oxide for persistent pulmonary hypertension of the newborn. *Pediatrics* 1997;100:1–7.
13. Journois D, Pouard P, Mauriat P, et al. Inhaled nitric oxide as a therapy for pulmonary hypertension after operations for congenital heart defects. *J Thorac Cardiovasc Surg* 1994;107:1129–1135.
14. Luciani GB, Chang AC, Starnes VA. Surgical repair of transposition of the great arteries in neonates with persistent pulmonary hypertension. *Ann Thorac Surg* 1996; 61:800–805.
15. Adatia I, Perry S, Moore P, et al. Inhaled nitric oxide and hemodynamic evaluation of patients with pulmonary hypertension before transplantation. *J Am Coll Cardiol* 1995;25:1652–1664.
16. Yahagi N, Kumon K, Tanigami H, et al. Inhaled nitric oxide for the postoperative management of Fontan-type operations. *Ann Thorac Surg* 1994;57:1371–1372.
17. Atz AM, Munoz RA, Adatia I, et al. Diagnostic and therapeutic uses of inhaled nitric oxide in neonatal Ebstein's anomaly. *Am J Card* 2003;91:906–908.
18. Atz AM, Adatia I, Wessel DL. Rebound pulmonary hypertension after inhalation of nitric oxide. *Ann Thorac Surg* 1996;62:1759–1764.
19. Atz AM, Wessel DL. Sildenafil ameliorates effects of inhaled nitric oxide withdrawal. *Anesthesiol* 1999;91:307–310.
20. Adatia I. Recent advances in pulmonary vascular disease. *Curr Opin Pediatr* 2002;14:292–297.
21. Prasad S, Wilkinson J, Gatzoulis MA. Sildenafil in primary pulmonary hypertension. *N Eng J Med* 2000;343:1342–1343.
22. Abrams D, Schulze-Nieck I, Magee AG. Sildenafil as a selective pulmonary vasodilator in childhood primary pulmonary hypertension. *Heart* 2000;84:e4–e5.
23. Tabbutt S, Ramamoorthy C, Montenegro LM, et al. Impact of inspired gas mixtures on preoperative infants with hypoplastic left heart syndrome during controlled ventilation. *Circulation* 2001;104:1159–1164.
25. Anand KJS, Hickey PR. Pain and its effects in the human neonate and fetus. *N Engl J Med* 1987;317:1321–1329.
26. Anand KJS, Hickey PR. Halothane-morphine compared with high-dose sufentanil for anesthesia and postoperative analgesia in neonatal cardiac surgery. *N Engl J Med* 1992;326:1–9.
27. Tanner GE, Angers DG, Barash PG. Effect of left-to-right, mixed left-to-right, and right-to-left shunts on inhalational anesthetic induction in children. *Anesth Analg* 1985;64:101–107.

28. Katz R, Kelly HW. Pharmacokinetics of continuous infusions of fentanyl in critically ill children. *Crit Care Med* 1993;21:995–1000.
29. Gold JP, Jonas RA, Lang P, et al. Transthoracic intracardiac monitoring lines in pediatric surgical patients: a ten-year experience. *Ann Thorac Surg* 1986;42:185–191.
30. Lang P, Chipman CW, Siden H, et al. Early assessment of hemodynamic status after repair of tetralogy of Fallot: A comparison of 24 hour (ICU) and 1 year postoperative data in 98 patients. *Am J Cardiol* 1982;50:795–799.
31. Vincent RN, Lang P, Chipman CW, et al. Assessment of hemodynamic status in the intensive care unit immediately after closure of ventricular septal defect. *Am J Cardiol* 1985;55:526–529.
32. Rosenfeld HM, Gentles TL, Wernovsky G, et al. Evaluation of intraoperative transesophageal echocardiography during congenital heart surgery. *Pediatr Cardiol* 1998;19:346–351.
33. Rossi AF, Sommer RJ, Litvin A, et al. Usefulness of intermittent monitoring of mixed venous oxygen saturation after stage 1 palliation for hypoplastic left heart syndrome. *Am J Cardiol* 1994;73:1118–1123.
34. Hoffman GM, Ghanayem NS, Kampine JM, et al. Venous saturation and anaerobic threshold in neonates after the Norwood procedure for hypoplastic left heart syndrome. *Ann Thorac Surg* 2000;70:1515–1521.
35. Hoffman GM, Tweddell JS, Ghanayem NS, et al. Alteration of the critical arteriovenous oxygen saturation relationship by sustained after load reduction after the Norwood procedure. *J Thorac Cardiovasc Surg* 2004;127:738–745.
36. Siegel LB, Dalton HJ, Hertzog JH, et al. Initial postoperative serum lactate levels predict survival in children after open-heart surgery. *Intensive Care Med* 1996;22:1418–1423.
37. Duke T, Butt W, South M, et al. Early markers of major adverse events in children after cardiac operations. *J Thorac Cardiovasc Surg* 1997;114:1042–1051.
38. Cheifetz IM, Kern FH, Schulman SR, et al. Serum lactates correlate with mortality after operations for complex congenital heart disease. *Ann Thorac Surg* 1997;64:735–738.
39. Wessel DL. Managing low cardiac output syndrome after congenital heart surgery. *Crit Care Med* 2001;29(suppl):220–230.
40. Kirklin JK, Westaby S, Blackstone EH, et al. Complement and the damaging effects of cardiopulmonary bypass. *J Thorac Cardiovasc Surg* 1983;86:845–857.
41. Hovels-Gurich HH, Vazquez-Jimenez JF, Silvestri A, et al. Production of proinflammatory cytokines and myocardial dysfunction after arterial switch operation in neonates with transposition of the great arteries. *J Thorac Cardiovasc Surg* 2002;124:811–820.
42. Naik SK, Knight A, Elliott MJ. A randomized study of a modified technique of ultrafiltration during pediatric open-heart surgery. *Circulation* 1991;84(Suppl 3):422–431.
43. Elliott MJ. Ultrafiltration and modified ultrafiltration in pediatric open heart operations. *Ann Thorac Surg* 1993;56:1518–1522.
44. Koutlas TC, Gaynor JW, Nicolson SC, et al. Modified ultrafiltration reduces postoperative morbidity after cavopulmonary connection. *Ann Thorac Surg* 1997;64:37–42.
45. Chang AC, Atz AM, Wernovsky G, et al. Milrinone: Systemic and pulmonary hemodynamic effects in neonates after cardiac surgery. *Crit Care Med* 1995;23:1907–1914.
46. Bridges ND, Lock JE, Castañeda AR. Baffle fenestration with subsequent transcatheter closure: Modification of the Fontan operation for patients at increased risk. *Circulation* 1990;82:1681–1689.
47. Padbury JF, Agata Y, Baylen BG, et al. Pharmacokinetics of dopamine in critically ill newborn infants. *J Pediatr* 1990;117:472–476.
48. Seri I, Tulassay T, Kiszel J, et al. Cardiovascular response to dopamine in hypotensive preterm neonates with severe hyaline membrane disease. *Eur J Pediatr* 1984;142:3–9.
49. Padbury J, Agata Y, Baylen B, et al. Dopamine pharmacokinetics in critically ill newborn infants. *J Pediatr* 1986;110:293–298.
50. Maill-Allen VM, Whitelaw AG. Response to dopamine and dobutamine in the preterm infant less than 30 weeks gestation. *Crit Care Med* 1989;17:1166–1169.
51. Lang P, Williams RG, Norwood WI, et al. The hemodynamic effects of dopamine in infants after corrective cardiac surgery. *J Pediatr* 1980;96:630–634.
52. Sonnenblick EH, Frishman WH, LeJemtel TH. Dobutamine: A new synthetic cardioactive sympathetic amine. *N Engl J Med* 1979;300:17–23.
53. Loeb HS, Bredakis J, Gunnar RM. Superiority of dobutamine over dopamine for augmentation of cardiac output in patients with chronic low output cardiac failure. *Circulation* 1977;55:375–382.
54. Bohn DJ, Poirier CS, Edmonds JF. Hemodynamic effects of dobutamine after cardiopulmonary bypass in children. *Crit Care Med* 1980;8:367–371.
55. Jaccard C, Berner M, Touge JC, et al. Hemodynamic effect of isoprenaline and dobutamine immediately after correction of tetralogy of Fallot.

Relative importance of inotropic and chronotropic action in supporting cardiac output. *J Thorac Cardiovasc Surg* 1984;87:862–869.

56. Fisher EG, Schwartz PH, Davis AL. Pharmacokinetics of exogenous epinephrine in critically ill children. *Crit Care Med* 1993;21:111–117.

57. Moran JL, O'Fathartaigh MS, Peisach AR, et al. Epinephrine as an inotropic agent in septic shock: A dose-profile analysis. *Crit Care Med* 1993;21:70–77.

58. Royster RL, Butterworth JF, Prielipp RC, et al. A randomized, blinded, placebo-controlled evaluation of calcium chloride and epinephrine for inotropic support after emergence from cardiopulmonary bypass. *Anesth Analg* 1992;74:3–13.

59. Rosenzweig EB, Starc TJ, Chen JM, et al. Intravenous arginine-vasopressin in children with vasodilatory shock after cardiac surgery. *Circulation* 1999;100:182–186.

60. Katz AM, McCall D, Messineo FC, et al. Comments on "cardiotonic activity of amrinone-win 40680 (5-amino-3-48-bypyridin-6(1H)-one)". *Circ Res* 1980;46:887–888.

61. Alousi A, Johnson D. Pharmacology of the bipyridines: Amrinone and milrinone. *Circulation* 1986;73:10–24.

62. Benotti JR, Hood WB. Dose-ranging study of intravenous milrinone to determine efficacy and pharmacokinetics. In: Braunwald E, Sonnenblick EH, Chakrin LW, eds. *Milrinone: Investigation of New Therapy for Congestive Heart Failure.* New York: Raven Press, 1984:95–107.

63. Anderson JL, Baim DS, Fein SA. Efficacy and safety of sustained (48 hours) intravenous infusion of milrinone in patients with severe congestive heart failure: A multicenter study. *J Am Coll Cardiol* 1987;9:711–722.

64. LeJemtel T, Keung E, Sonnenblick EH. Amrinone: A new nonglycosidic, nonadrenergic cardiotonic agent effective in the treatment of intractable myocardial failure in man. *Circulation* 1979;59:1098–1104.

65. Goenen M, Pedermonte O, Baele P. Amrinone in the management of low cardiac output after open heart surgery. *Am J Cardiol* 1990;56:33B–38B.

66. Gage J, Rutman H, Lucido D. Additive effects of dobutamine and amrinone on myocardial contractility and ventricular performance in patients with severe heart failure. *Circulation* 1986;74:367–373.

67. Lang P, Wessel DL, Wernovsky G, et al. Hemodynamic effects of amrinone in infants after cardiac surgery. In: Crupi G, Parenzan L, Anderson RH, eds. *Perspectives in Pediatric Cardiology.* Vol. 2. *Pediatric Cardiac Surgery*, Part 2. Mount Kisco, NY: Futura Publishing, 1989:292–295.

68. Skippen P, Taylor R, Bohn D. Amrinone in infants and children after cardiac surgery. *Crit Care Med* 1990;18(suppl):268S.

69. Sorensen GK, Ramamoorthy C, Lynn AM, et al. Hemodynamic effects of amrinone in children after Fontan surgery. *Anesth Analg* 1996;82: 241–246.

70. Ovadia M, Thoele D, Gersony W. Amrinone: Efficacy and safety in infants and children. *Circulation* 1988;78:II-293.

71. Ramamoorthy C, Anderson GD, Williams GD, et al. Pharmacokinetics and side effects of milrinone in infants and children after open heart surgery. *Anesth Analg* 1998;86:283–289.

72. Hoffman TM, Wernovsky G, Atz AM, et al. Prophylactic intravenous use of milrinone after cardiac operation in pediatrics (PRIMACORP) study. *Am Heart J* 2002;143:15–21.

73. Hoffman TM, Wernovsky G, Atz AM, et al. Efficacy and safety of milrinone in preventing low cardiac output syndrome in infants and children after corrective surgery for congenital heart disease. *Circulation* 2003;107:996–1002.

74. Colucci WS, Wright RF, Braunwald E. New positive inotropic agents in the treatment of congestive heart failure. *N Engl J Med* 1975;314:349–358.

75. Ross-Ascuitto NT, Ascuitto RJ, Ramage D. Positive inotropic, vasodilatory and chronotropic effects of milrinone on the post-ischemic neonatal pig heart. *Am J Cardiol* 1989;64:414.

76. Benotti J, Grossman W, Braunwald E. Effects of amrinone on myocardial energy metabolism and hemodynamics in patients with severe congestive heart failure due to coronary artery disease. *Circulation* 1980;62:28–34.

77. Palmer RE, Lasseter KC. Sodium nitroprusside. *N Engl J Med* 1975;292: 294–299.

78. Mills RM, LeJemtel TH, Horton DP, et al. Sustained hemodynamic effects of an infusion of nesiritide (human b-type natriuretic peptide) in heart failure: A randomized, double-blind, placebo-controlled clinical trial. Natrecor Study Group. *J Am Coll Cardiol* 1999;34:155–162.

79. Colucci WS, Elkayam U, Horton DP, et al. Intravenous nesiritide, a natriuretic peptide in the treatment of decompensated congestive heart failure. Nesiritide Study Group. *N Engl J Med* 2000;343:246–253.

80. Marshall J, Berkenbosch JW, Russo P, et al. Preliminary experience with nesiritide in the pediatric population. *J Intensive Care Med* 2004;19: 164–170.

81. Sehra R, Underwood K. Nesiritide use for critically ill children awaiting cardiac transplantation. *Pediatr Cardiol* 2006;27:47–50.

82. Mahle WT, Cuadrado AR, Kirshbom PM, et al. Nesiritide in infants and children with congestive heart failure. *Ped Crit Care Med* 2005;6:543–546.

83. Jeffries JL, Dreyer WJ, Kim JJ, et al. A prospective evaluation of nesiritide in the treatment of pediatric heart failure. *Pediatr Cardiol* 2006;27: 402–407.

84. Sackner-Bernstein JD, Skopicki HA, Aaranson KD. Risk of worsening renal function with nesiritide in patients with acutely decompensated heart failure. *Circulation* 2005;111:1487–1491.

85. Bettendorf M, Schmidt KG, Grulich-Henn J, et al. Tri-iodothyronine treatment in children after cardiac surgery: A double-blind, randomized, placebo-controlled study. *Lancet* 2000;356:529–534.

86. Chowdhury D, Ojamaa K, Parnell VA, et al. A prospective randomized clinical study of thyroid hormone treatment after operations for complex congenital heart disease. *J Thorac Cardiovasc Surg* 2001;122:1023–1025.

87. Portman MA, Fearneyhough RN, Karl TR, et al. The triiodothyronine for infants and children undergoing cardiopulmonary bypass (TRICC) study: Design and rationale. *Am Heart J* 2004;148:393–398.

87a. Wessel DL. Testing new drugs for heart failure in children. *Pediatr Crit Care Med* 2006;7:493–494.

88. Mackie AS, Booth KL, Newburger JW, et al. A randomized, double-blind, placebo-controlled pilot trial of triiodothyronine in neonatal heart surgery. *J Thorac Cardiovasc Surg* 2005;130:810–816.

89. Braunstein PW, Sade RM, Gillette PC, et al. Life-threatening postoperative junctional ectopic tachycardia. *Ann Thorac Surg* 1992,53:726–728.

90. Perry JC, Fenrich AL, Hulse JE, et al. Pediatric use of intravenous amiodarone: Efficacy and safety in critically ill patients from a multicenter protocol. *J Am Coll Cardiol* 1996;27:1246–1250.

91. Hoffman TM, Bush DM, Wernovsky G, et al. Postoperative junctional ectopic tachycardia in children: Incidence, risk factors, and treatment. *Ann Thorac Surg* 2002;74:1607–1611.

92. Van der Vorst MM, Ruys-Dudok VI, Kist-van Holthe JE, et al. Continuous intravenous furosemide in hemodynamically unstable children after cardiac surgery. *Int Care Med* 2001;27:711–715.

93. Marik PE. Low-dose dopamine: A systematic review. *Intensive Care Med* 2002;28:877–883.

94. Hughes AD, Sever PS. Action of fenoldopam, a selective dopamine (DA1) receptor agonist, on isolated human arteries. *Blood Vessels* 1989;26: 119–127.

95. Costello JM, Thiaragarajan RR, Dionne RE, et al. Initial experience with fenoldopam after cardiac surgery in neonates with an insufficient response to conventional diuretics. *Pediatr Crit Care Med* 2006;7:28–33.

96. Nido PJ. Extracorporeal membrane oxygenation for cardiac support in children. *Ann Thorac Surg* 1996;61:336–339.

97. Duncan BW, Hraska V, Jonas RA, et al. Mechanical circulatory support in children with cardiac disease. *J Thorac Cardiovasc Surg* 1999;117:529–542.

98. Spray T. Extracorporeal membrane oxygenation for pediatric cardiac support. *Cardiac Surg State Art Rev* 1993;7:177–188.

99. Duncan BW, Bohn DJ, Atz AM, et al. Mechanical circulatory support for the treatment of children with acute fulminant myocarditis. *J Thorac Cardiovasc Surg* 2001;122:440–448.

100. Duncan BW. Mechanical circulatory support for infants and children with cardiac disease. *Ann Thorac Surg* 2002;73:1670–1677.

101. Kolovos NS, Bratton SL, Moler FW, et al. Outcome of pediatric patients treated with extracorporeal life support after cardiac surgery. *Ann Thorac Surg* 2003;76:1435–1442.

102. Morris MC, Ittenbach RF, Godinez RI, et al. Risk factors for mortality in 137 pediatric cardiac intensive care unit patients managed with extracorporeal membrane oxygenation. *Crit Care Med* 2004;32:1061–1069.

103. Hintz SR, Benitz WE, Colby CE, et al. Utilization and outcomes of neonatal cardiac extracorporeal life support: 1996–2000. *Pediatr Crit Care Med* 2005;6:33–38.

104. Hoskote A, Bohn D, Gruenwald C, et al. Extracorporeal life support after staged palliation of a functional single ventricle: Subsequent morbidity and survival. *J Thorac Cardiovasc Surg* 2006;131(5):1114–1121.

105. Ravishankar C, Dominguez TE, Kreutzer J, et al. Extracorporeal membrane oxygenation after stage I reconstruction for hypoplastic left heart syndrome. *Pediatr Crit Care Med* 2006;7(4):319–323.

106. Del Nido PJ, Dalton HJ, Thomson AE, et al. Extracorporeal membrane oxygenator rescue in children during cardiac arrest after cardiac surgery. *Circulation* 1992;86:II300–II304.

107. Duncan BW, Ibrahim AE, Hraska V, et al. Use of rapid-deployment extracorporeal membrane oxygenation for the resuscitation of pediatric patients with heart disease after cardiac arrest. *J Thorac Cardiovasc Surg* 1998;116:305–311.

108. Jacobs JP, Ojito JW, McConaghey TW, et al. Rapid cardiopulmonary support for children with complex congenital heart disease. *Ann Thorac Surg* 2000;70:742–750.

109. Chang AC, McKenzie ED. Mechanical cardiopulmonary support in children and young adults: Extracorporeal membrane oxygenation, ventricular assist devices, and long-term support devices. *Pediatr Cardiol* 2005;26:2–28.

110. Blume ED, Naftel DC, Bastardi HJ, et al. Outcomes of children bridged to heart transplantation with ventricular assist devices: A multi-institutional study. *Circulation* 2006;113(19):2313–2319.

110a. Thuys CA, Mullaly RJ, Horton SB, et al. Centrifugal ventricular assist in children under 6 kg. *Euro J Cardiothoracic Surg* 1998;13:130–134.

111. Karl TR, Sano S, Horton S, et al. Centrifugal pump left heart assist in pediatric cardiac operations. Indication, technique, and results. *J Thorac Cardiovasc Surg* 1991;102:624–630.

112. Hetzer R, Loebe M, Potapov EV, et al. Circulatory support with pneumatic paracorporeal ventricular assist device in infants and children. *Ann Thorac Surg* 1998;66:1498–1506.

113. Ishino K, Loebe M, Uhlemann F, et al. Circulatory support with paracorporeal pneumatic ventricular assist device (VAD) in infants and chidren. *Euro J Cardiothorac Surg* 1997;11:965–972.

114. Konertz W, Hotz H, Schneider M, et al. Clinical experience with the MEDOS HIA-VAD system in infants and children. *Ann Thorac Surg* 1997;63:1138–1144.

115. Wieselthaler GM, Schima H, Hiesmayr M, et al. First clinical experience with the DeBakey VAD continuous-axial-flow pump for bridge to transplantation. *Circulation* 2000;101:356–359.

116. Padalino MA, Ohye RG, Chang AC, et al. Bridge to transplant using the MicroMed DeBakey ventricular assist device in a child with idiopathic dilated cardiomyopathy. *Ann Thorac Surg* 2006;81(3):1118–1121.

117. Sharma MS, Webber SA, Gandhi SK, et al. Pulsatile paracorporeal assist devices in children and adolescents with biventricular failure. *ASAIO J* 2005;51:490–494.

118. Hetzer R, Potapov EV, Stiller B, et al. Improvement in survival after mechanical circulatory support with pneumatic pulsatile ventricular assist devices in pediatric patients. *Ann Thorac Surg* 2006;82(3):917–924; discussion 924–5.120.

119. Walsh EP, Rockenmacher S, Keane JF, et al. Late results in patients with tetralogy of Fallot repaired during infancy. *Circulation* 1988;77: 1062–1067.

120. Wernovsky G, Spray TL. Tetralogy of Fallot. In: Chang AC, Hanley FL, Wernovsky G, et al., eds. *Pediatric Cardiac Intensive Care*. Baltimore: Williams & Wilkins, 1998:257–265.

121. Gidding SS, Rocchini AP, Beekman R, et al. Therapeutic effect of propranolol on paradoxical hypertension after repair of coarctation of the aorta. *N Engl J Med* 1985;312:1224–1228.

122. Wernovsky G, Bove EL. Single ventricle lesions. In: Chang AC, Hanley FL, Wernovsky G, et al., eds. *Pediatric cardiac intensive care*. Baltimore: Williams & Wilkins, 1998:271–287.

123. Riordan CJ, Randsbaek F, Storey JH, et al. Balancing pulmonary and systemic arterial flows in parallel circulations: The value of monitoring system venous oxygen saturations. *Cardiol Young* 1997;7:74–79.

124. Riordan CJ, Randsbaek F, Storey JH, et al. Effects of oxygen, positive end-expiratory pressure, and carbon dioxide on oxygen delivery in an animal model of the univentricular heart. *J Thorac Cardiovasc Surg* 1996;112: 644–654.

125. Chang AC, Zucker HA, Hickey PR, et al. Pulmonary vascular resistance in infants after cardiac surgery: Role of carbon dioxide and hydrogen ion. *Crit Care Med* 1995;23:568–574.

126. Reddy VM, Liddicoat JR, Fineman JR, et al. Fetal model of single ventricle physiology: Hemodynamic effects of oxygen, nitric oxide, carbon dioxide, and hypoxia in the early postnatal period. *J Thorac Cardiovasc Surg* 1996;112:437–449.

127. Chang AC, Hanley FL, Wernovsky G, et al. Early bidirectional cavopulmonary shunt in young infants: Postoperative course and early results. *Circulation* 1993;88:149–158.

128. Bradley SM, Simsic JM, Mulvihill DM. Hyperventilation impairs oxygenation after bidirectional superior cavopulmonary connection. *Circulation* 1998;98:II372–II377.

129. Bradley SM, Simsic JM, Mulvihill DM. Hypoventilation improves oxygenation after bidirectional superior cavopulmonary connection. *J Thorac Cardiovasc Surg* 2003;126:1033–1039.

130. Hoskote A, Li J, Hickey C, et al. The effects of carbon dioxide on oxygenation and systemic, cerebral, and pulmonary vascular hemodynamics after the bidirectional superior cavopulmonary anastomosis. *J Am Coll Cardiol* 2004;44:1501–1509.

131. Laks H, Pearl JM, Haas GS, et al. Partial Fontan: Advantages of an adjustable interatrial communication. *Ann Thorac Surg* 1991;52: 1084–1095.

132. Bridges ND, Mayer JE Jr, Lock JE, et al. Effect of baffle fenestration on outcome of the modified Fontan operation. *Circulation* 1992;86: 1762–1769.

133. Gentles TL, Mayer JE Jr, Gauvreau K, et al. Fontan operation in five hundred consecutive patients: Factors influencing early and late outcome. *J Thorac Cardiovasc Surg* 1997;114:376–391.

134. Knott-Craig C, Danielson G, Schaff H, et al. The modified Fontan operation: An analysis of risk factors for early postoperative death or takedown in 702 consecutive patients from one institution. *J Thorac Cardiovasc Surg* 1995;109:1237–1243.

135. Mitchell ME, Ittenbach RF, Gaynor JW, et al. Intermediate outcomes after the Fontan procedure in the current era. *J Thorac Cardiovasc Surg* 2006; 131(1):172–180.

136. Petrossian E, Reddy VM, Collins KK, et al. The extracardiac conduit Fontan operation using minimal approach extracorporeal circulation: Early and midterm outcomes. *J Thorac Cardiovasc Surg* 2006;132(5): 1054–1063.

137. Penny DJ, Hayek Z, Redington AN. The effects of positive and negative extrathoracic pressure ventilation on pulmonary blood flow after the total cavopulmonary shunt procedure. *Int J Cardiol* 1991;30: 128–130.

138. Cohen MI, Wernovsky G, Vetter VL, et al. Sinus node dysfunction following systematically staged Fontan. *Circulation* 1998;96(suppl):II352–II359.

139. du Plessis AJ, Chang AC, Wessel DL, et al. Cerebrovascular accidents following the Fontan operation. *Pediatr Neurol* 1995;12:230–236.

140. Mahle WT, Clancy RR, Moss EM, et al. Neurodevelopmental outcome and lifestyle assessment in school-aged and adolescent children with hypoplastic left heart syndrome. *Pediatrics* 2000;105(5):1082–1089.

141. Goldberg CS, Schwartz EM, Brunberg JA, et al. Neurodevelopmental outcome of patients after the fontan operation: A comparison between children with hypoplastic left heart syndrome and other functional single ventricle lesions. *J Pediatr* 2000;137(5):646–652.

142. Limperopoulos C, Majnemer A, Shevell M. Neurodevelopmental status of newborns and infants with congenital heart defects before and after open heart surgery. *J Pediatr* 2000;137(5):638–645.

143. Wernovsky G. Current insights regarding neurological and developmental abnormalities in children and young adults with complex congenital cardiac disease. *Cardiol Young* 2006;16:92–104.

144. Wernovsky G, Shillingford AJ, Gaynor JW. Central nervous system outcomes in children with complex congenital heart disease (review). *Curr Opin Cardiol* 2005;20(2):94–99.

145. Mahle WT, Tavani F, Zimmerman RA, et al. An MRI study of neurological injury before and after congenital heart surgery. *Circulation* 2002;106(12 Suppl 1):I109–I114.

146. Licht DJ, Wang J, Silvestre DW, et al. Preoperative cerebral blood flow is diminished in neonates with severe congenital heart defects. *J Thorac Cardiovasc Surg* 2004;128(6):841–849.

147. Bellinger DC, Jonas RA, Rappaport LA, et al. Developmental and neurologic status of children after heart surgery with hypothermic circulatory arrest or low-flow cardiopulmonary bypass. *N Engl J Med* 1995;332: 549–555.

148. Wernovsky G, Jonas RA, Hickey PR, et al. Clinical neurologic and developmental studies after cardiac surgery utilizing hypothermic circulatory arrest and cardiopulmonary bypass. *Cardiol Young* 1993;3:308–316.

149. Newburger JW, Jonas RA, Wernovsky G, et al. A comparison of the perioperative neurologic effects of hypothermic circulatory arrest versus low-flow cardiopulmonary bypass in infant heart surgery. *N Engl J Med* 1993;329:1057–1064.

150. Bellinger DC, Rappaport LA, Wypij D, et al. Patterns of developmental dysfunction after surgery during infancy to correct transposition of the great arteries. *J Dev Behav Pediatr* 1997;18:75–83.

151. Bellinger DC, Wypij D, Kuban KCK, et al. Developmental and neurological status of children at four years of age after heart surgery with hypothermic circulatory arrest or low-flow cardiopulmonary bypass. *Circulation* 1999;100:526–532.

152. Bellinger DC, Wypij D, duDuplessis AJ, et al. Neurodevelopmental status at eight years in children with dextro-transposition of the great arteries: The Boston Circulatory Arrest Trial. *J Thorac Cardiovasc Surg* 2003; 126(5):1385–1396.

153. Wypij D, Newburger JW, Rappaport LA, et al. The effect of duration of deep hypothermic circulatory arrest in infant heart surgery on late neurodevelopment: The Boston Circulatory Arrest Trial. *J Thorac Cardiovasc Surg* 2003;126:1397–1403.

154. Clancy RR, Legido A, Lewis D. Occult neonatal seizures. *Epilepsia* 1988;29:256–261.

155. Ehyai A, Fenichel GM, Bender HWJ. Incidence and prognosis of seizures in infants after cardiac surgery with profound hypothermia and circulatory arrest. *JAMA* 1984;252:3165–3167.

156. Rappaport LA, Wypij D, Bellinger DC, et al. Relation of seizures after cardiac surgery in early infancy to neurodevelopmental outcome. *Circulation* 1998;97:773–779.

157. Newburger JW, Wypij D, Bellinger DC, et al. Length of stay after infant heart surgery is related to cognitive outcome at age 8 years. *J Pediatr* 2003;143(1):67–73.

158. Gaynor JW, Gerdes M, Zackai EH, et al. Apolipoprotein E genotype and neurodevelopmental sequelae of infant cardiac surgery. *J Thorac Cardiovasc Surg* 2003;126(6):1736–1745.

159. Freier MC, Babikian T, Pivonka J, et al. A longitudinal perspective on neurodevelopmental outcome after infant cardiac transplantation. *J Heart Lung Transplant* 2004;23(7):857–864.

160. Lamer C, Valleaux T, Plaisance P, et al. Continuous arteriovenous hemodialysis for acute renal failure after cardiac operations. *J Thorac Cardiovasc Surg* 1990;99:175–176.

161. Paret G, Cohen AJ, Bohn DJ, et al. Continuous arteriovenous hemofiltration after cardiac operations in infants and children. *J Thorac Cardiovasc Surg* 1992;104:1222–1230.

162. Prophylactic parenteral cephalosporins in surgery. Are the newer agents better? *JAMA* 1984;252:3277–3279.

163. Ito T, Engle MA, Goldberg HP. Postpericardiotomy syndrome following surgery for nonrheumatic heart disease. *Circulation* 1958;17:549.

164. Lock JE, Bass JL, Kulik TJ, et al. Chronic percutaneous pericardial drainage with modified pigtail catheters in children. *Am J Cardiol* 1984;53:1179–1182.

CHAPTER 21 ■ CARDIAC MECHANICAL SUPPORT THERAPIES

ELIZABETH D. BLUME, MD, AND PETER C. LAUSSEN, MBBS

Mechanical circulatory assistance in the pediatric patient plays an important short-term role in the setting of reversible myocardial failure such as that seen with fulminant myocarditis (24,39) or in the perioperative period (31,65,84,107,121), and may also serve as an effective long-term bridge to cardiac transplantation in chronic cardiomyopathy (45,48,81,87). There is a growing consensus that in any center undertaking complex congenital cardiac surgery, a mechanical circulatory support device (MCSD) program that includes at least extracorporeal membrane oxygenation (ECMO) capability be readily available. However, there have been no prospective randomized trials comparing the indications for, modes of, and success from MCSD use in infants and children. Consequently, there remains considerable interinstitutional variability in MCSD utility and outcome. In general, institutions with a well-established ECMO service for either respiratory or cardiac failure are more likely to use this form of support for a child with a failing circulation whereas institutions that have close collaboration with adult implantable ventricular assist device (VAD) programs may be more likely to use other forms of MSCD, especially in the older, larger patient. Surgeon preference, case mix, surgical techniques, and cardiopulmonary bypass (CPB) management are additional confounding factors that make institutional comparisons difficult. Fortunately, considerable information from national and international registries for ECMO and VAD do provide a framework for MSCD decision making.

ANATOMIC AND PHYSIOLOGIC DIFFERENCES IN CHILDREN

The greatest challenge to the design and implementation of safe pediatric circulatory support systems is accommodating for a wide range of patient sizes, from newborns to young adults. For example, MCSDs that employ a flexible membrane pump, such as the paracorporeal pneumatic devices, rely on a number of pump sizes to cover the pediatric spectrum. This, along with maintaining a supply of variously sized cannulae and control systems, substantially increases both developmental and inventory expense. Furthermore, the diverse anatomic variations encountered in complex congenital heart disease challenge the design of such devices. For example, abnormalities of visceroatrial situs, such as situs inversus and abnormalities of the location of the cardiac apex (dextrocardia), may complicate the application of many existing pump designs. The design of circulatory support devices for children must take into account other unique physiologic factors. The susceptibility to anticoagulation-related complications is particularly notable in infants and children, as evidenced by the important risk of intracranial hemorrhage during infant

ECMO support (61,62). Newborns are known to manifest an exaggerated systemic inflammatory response (5,15,50,67,104) after cardiopulmonary bypass and during ECMO support, which may induce multisystem organ dysfunction. Other factors have developmental components as well, such as changes in pharmacokinetics of anticoagulant medications. The ideal mechanical circulatory support system for children, therefore, must provide maximal biocompatibility, resulting in minimal activation of systemic inflammatory cascades and avoidance of high-dose, multiagent anticoagulation. During mechanical circulatory support, children are also vulnerable to infectious complications, which are a frequent cause of mortality (27,30,36). Thus, implantable systems that do not require multiple skin penetrations for drive lines or other device components are an important goal. Since urgent institution of support may be required to treat cardiac arrest after cardiac surgery or acute myocarditis, some device designs must allow for rapid deployment (35,40). Finally, the use of MCSD in children for long-term, permanent use as an alternative to heart transplantation, so-called destination therapy, has not been explored. One could imagine this possibility in the future, however, if technological advances could overcome the issues of growth and development.

DURATION OF SUPPORT

Table 21.1 summarizes the various types of MCSDs currently available for pediatric patients in the United States. The design of these MCSDs can be functionally categorized based on the anticipated duration of their use. Short-term (days to weeks) support devices include cardiopulmonary bypass (CPB), extracorporeal membrane oxygenation (ECMO), intra-aortic balloon pump (IABP) counterpulsation, and centrifugal ventricular assist devices. Longer-term (weeks to months) support may be accomplished by pulsatile paracorporeal or implantable ventricular assist devices (VADs) and axial flow implantable VADs. These systems will be further explored.

SHORT-TERM MODES OF MECHANICAL CIRCULATORY SUPPORT

Cardiopulmonary Bypass

The first use of MCSDs for children was in the 1950s, shortly after the first successful use of the adult heart-lung machine. In 1953, Gibbon (70) repaired an atrial septal defect using the adult CPB system. At the same time, Lillehei et al. (88) began

TABLE 21.1

TYPES OF MECHANICAL CIRCULATORY SUPPORT FOR CHILDREN

Support name	Type	Clinical experience and age supported
Short-term support		
ECMO	Extracorporeal, centrifugal	Extensive pediatric, all ages
Bio-Pump*[a]	Extracorporeal, centrifugal	Extensive pediatric, all ages
Intra-aortic balloon pump	Extracorporeal, counterpulsation	Limited pediatric, older children
Abiomed BVS 5000*[b]	Extracorporeal, pneumatic	Limited pediatric, older children
Chronic support		
Thoratec*[c]	Paracorporeal, pneumatic	Limited pediatric, older children
Heartmate V-E*[d]	Implantable, electric	Limited pediatric, older children
Medos HIA-VAD[e]	Paracorporeal, pneumatic	Increasing pediatric, all ages
Berlin Heart EXCOR[f]	Paracorporeal, pneumatic	Increasing pediatric, all ages
DeBakey VAD Child*[g]	Implantable, axial flow	Limited pediatric, 5–12 yrs

*FDA approved in the United States.
Note: [a]Bio-Pump (Medtronic Bio-Medicus, Minneapolis, MN).
[b]ABIOMED BVS 5000 (ABIOMED, Inc., Danvers, MA);
[c]Thoratec VAD, Thoratec, Corp., Pleasanton, CA;
[d]HeartMate LVAS, Thoratec, Corp., Pleasanton, CA;
[e]MEDOS HIA, (MEDOS Medizintechnik AG, Stolberg Germany)
[f]Berlin Heart EXCOR, (Berlin Heart AG, Berlin, Germany);
[g]Debakey VAD Child, (MicroMed Technology, Inc. Houston, Texas).

using crosscirculation to repair congenital heart lesions in children. Kirklin et al. (80) developed a pump oxygenator, which required much less prime volume than the earlier versions. The next major improvements came in the 1970s, with the description of deep hypothermic circulatory arrest in infants by Castañeda et al. (23) and Barratt-Boyes (8), which allowed surface cooling and shorter CPB times. Over the next several decades, incremental improvements in CPB technology and operative techniques contributed to a significant reduction in mortality rates associated with pediatric cardiac surgery. Nonetheless, the potential morbidity following the use of CPB in infants and children continues to be a significant limitation to mechanical circulatory support.

Although an in-depth discussion of the mechanisms and techniques of CPB is beyond the scope of this chapter (78), it is worth understanding the overall principles of CPB to assess other mechanical circulatory support devices, such as ECMO and VADs, and to note specific differences from adult CPB. The CPB circuit has several components including arterial and venous cannulae, circuit reservoir, pump, oxygenator, and heat exchanger. CPB is an open mechanical support system, allowing for blood, air, and particulate matter to be returned to the circuit reservoir via cardiotomy suckers. This is an important contradistinction to ECMO and VAD circuits, which are both closed systems; any air entering the closed circuit will cause an air lock, and these circuits do not have a reservoir volume to compensate for changes in circulating blood volume. Most pediatric systems use a *roller pump* with flow rates governed by the internal diameter of the tubing, the amount of occlusion of the roller, and the revolutions per minute (rpm) of the pump head. Typically the membrane-type *oxygenator* systems have a microporous membrane with a hollow fiber or folded membrane, which must function efficiently at a wide variety of pump flow rates. Some considerations for cannulation for CPB

are unique to congenital heart surgery. Venous cannulation in neonates and infants may be single or multiple depending on the anatomy and bypass technique. Obstruction to venous return is more likely due to the small vessel size and will increase venous pressures, thereby decreasing perfusion pressure to the cerebral and splanchnic circulations. In particular, an elevated SVC pressure will reduce cerebral blood flow, increase the risk of cerebral edema, and reduce the rate of cerebral cooling. Systemic-to-pulmonary shunts such as a patent ductus arteriosus and aortopulmonary collateral vessels must be controlled when initiating bypass to prevent excessive pulmonary flow with resultant increased blood return to the heart, myocardial distention, systemic hypoperfusion, and uneven cooling or rewarming.

Pump flow rates are generally higher in neonates and infants, reflecting their increased metabolic rate. During bypass, there is no one measure or index that ensures adequate perfusion. Generally flow rates of 100 to 150 mL/kg/minute, or indexed flows to 2.2 to 2.5 L/minute/m², should provide adequate flow at normothermia. Venous oxygen saturation of >75% suggests adequate perfusion. However, these values may be misleading in patients with poor venous drainage, severe hemodilution, and malposition of the aortic cannula or in the presence of a large left-to-right shunt. On-line continuous monitoring of blood gas and saturation of oxygen is important to identify trends in oxygen extraction.

During hypothermia, there are two broad bypass management strategies. The first is deep hypothermia (<20°C) with low/intermittent flow or circulatory arrest (DHCA). DHCA provides optimal operating conditions for intracardiac repairs with an empty, relaxed heart and reduces the duration on bypass and exposure of circulating blood to foreign surfaces. Prolonged ischemia to the brain is a major disadvantage and is both time and temperature dependent. Low-flow deep hypothermic bypass is preferable with improved neurologic protection. Flow rates between 30 and 50 mL/kg/min are often referred to as low flow, but optimal flow rates during low-flow bypass are not firmly established. The second CPB strategy is moderate hypothermia with normal or increased pump flow. Bicaval cannulation is generally used with this mode of CPB with reduced risk of cerebral ischemia at the expense of prolonged CPB.

It is well recognized that the exposure of blood elements to the nonepithelialized cardiopulmonary bypass circuit, along with ischemic-reperfusion injury, induces a systemic inflammatory response (5,15,50,67,104). The effects of the interactions of blood components with the extracorporeal circuit is magnified in children owing to the large bypass circuit surface area and priming volume relative to patient blood volume. Humoral responses include activation of complement, kallikrein, eicosanoid, and fibrinolytic cascades. Cellular responses include platelet activation and an inflammatory response with an adhesion molecule cascade stimulating neutrophil activation and release of proteolytic and vasoactive substances (52,120).

Clinical consequences to the inflammatory response include increased interstitial fluid and generalized capillary leak, as well as potential multiorgan dysfunction. Total lung water is increased with an associated decrease in lung compliance and increase in the alveolar to arterial oxygen (A-aO$_2$) gradient. Myocardial edema results in impaired ventricular systolic and diastolic function. A secondary fall in cardiac output by 20% to 30% is common in neonates during the first 6 to 12 hours following surgery, contributing to decreased renal function and oliguria (124). Sternal closure may be delayed owing to mediastinal edema and associated cardiorespiratory compromise when closure is attempted. Ascites, hepatic congestion, and bowel edema may affect mechanical ventilation, cause a prolonged ileus, and delay feeding. A coagulopathy post-CPB may contribute to delayed hemostasis.

Evolving strategies that limit the effect of endothelial injury resulting from the systemic inflammatory response include limiting both the time spent on bypass and use of deep hypothermic circulatory arrest (DHCA). Hypothermia, steroids, and aprotinin (a serine protease inhibitor) may also limit activation of the inflammatory response. The use of antioxidants such as mannitol, altering prime composition to maintain hematocrit and oncotic pressure, and ultrafiltration during rewarming or immediately after bypass are also used to limit the clinical consequences of the inflammatory response (43,69,76).

Hypothermia and Cerebral Protection

Techniques of deep hypothermia with or without circulatory arrest have extended the safe duration of cardiopulmonary bypass in children, particularly in neonates and infants, and enable improved surgical conditions and patient outcomes. As mortality has decreased, an increasing emphasis has been placed on improving patient morbidity following repair. The consequences of deep hypothermia and low perfusion have become particularly scrutinized.

The brain is very sensitive to ischemia, creating special concerns about the deleterious effects of CPB. Hypothermia is the principle method used for cerebral protection during CPB, effecting both pressure-flow and metabolism-flow cerebral autoregulation (38,46,57). Reductions in oxygen consumption and metabolic rate during deep hypothermia partially explain the increased tolerance to cerebral ischemia produced by hypothermia. Other factors possibly contributing to the protective effects of hypothermia include altered cellular metabolism with an increase in high-energy phosphates and

intracellular pH, reduced neurotransmitter release, and that the neonatal and infant brain may be more tolerant of cerebral ischemia than that of the adult.

Despite precautions, diffuse cerebral abnormalities may occur in patients after open heart surgery including global and watershed injuries related to hypoperfusion or hypoxemia and multifocal lesions presumed secondary to embolic events (37,51,112). The early clinical manifestations of neurologic injury in children include seizures, stroke, choreoathetosis (21), and coma. Subtle long-term behavioral, developmental, and motor abnormalities have been associated with neurologic injury during hypothermic CPB, regardless of strategy, which supports the importance of early developmental intervention. The Boston Circulatory Arrest Study (99) demonstrated a strong association between the duration of circulatory arrest and the occurrence of postoperative seizures, which are becoming more likely beyond 40 minutes of circulatory arrest. Analysis of developmental outcomes at 1 year of age in these patients indicated a significant association between the occurrence of postoperative seizures and a lower psychomotor development (11). The risk of neurologic abnormalities increased with the duration of circulatory arrest. Data at 4 and 8 years follow-up in these patients indicated a spectrum of both motor and language delays or abnormalities, which also correlated with the presence of postoperative seizures (10,12). Recently, genetic polymorphisms have been recognized that may predispose to impairments in the ability for neurons to repair (49).

Although hypothermia is the principle method for providing protection during CPB, the means by which hypothermia is induced and maintained is critical. Because of the large body surface area-to-mass ratio in neonates and infants, a 2°C to 3°C reduction in core temperature is common prior to bypass. Respiratory alkalosis secondary to mechanical ventilation reduces cerebral blood flow and should be avoided. Cannula position is important as noted above; obstruction to systemic venous return by a venous cannula decreases cerebral perfusion pressure, and an obstructive or malpositioned aortic cannula will also decrease cerebral blood flow and effective cooling. Shunts and collateral vessels must be controlled when initiating bypass to prevent excessive runoff to the lungs and return to the heart, resulting in myocardial distention, systemic hypoperfusion, and uneven cooling or rewarming. Once on bypass, rapid cooling should be avoided because this results in uneven cooling of the brain; cooling times of 20 to 25 minutes have been advocated for infants and neonates requiring CPB and DHCA. Possible pharmacologic manipulations include using vasodilating drugs to facilitate cooling and rewarming. Steroids are commonly administered to stabilize membranes and possibly reduce cerebral edema.

The use of crystalloid pump primes may be associated with an increase in total body water after hypothermic CPB in neonates and infants, secondary to a reduction in plasma oncotic pressure. This contributes to postoperative capillary leak and potentially delayed recovery. There is intercenter variability in the target hematocrit during hypothermic CPB, but maintaining a hematocrit of approximately 30% appears to be optimal with respect to altered blood viscosity during hypothermia while maintaining oncotic pressure and oxygen-carrying capacity (68). The blood gas strategy during hypothermic CPB is also an important consideration (37,86). Carbon dioxide (CO$_2$) is a potent cerebral vasodilator in both awake and anesthetized patients with or without CPB. During CPB and hypothermia, cerebral blood flow continues to increase with PaCO$_2$. However, this response is attenuated in neonates and infants during deep hypothermia and reflects cold-induced vasoparesis. During hypothermia, the solubility

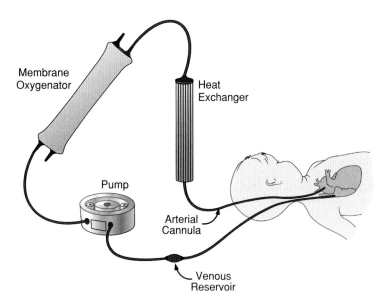

Membrane Oxygenator

Heat Exchanger

Pump

Arterial Cannula

Venous Reservoir

FIGURE 21.1 Extracorporeal membrane oxygenator circuit with membrane gas exchange device and roller pump.

of CO_2 increases and the neutral pH of both water and blood are reset in the alkaline direction. In the alpha-stat strategy, no compensation is made for the alkaline shift. The alpha-stat strategy theoretically maintains a more normal intracellular pH and therefore electrochemical neutrality with preserved enzymatic function. Furthermore, the uncoupling of flow metabolism is less pronounced, thereby limiting luxuriant cerebral flow during CPB. However, in the context of low mean perfusion pressure, flow, and temperature, cerebral perfusion may be inadequate to meet metabolic demands and cerebral cooling may be nonhomogeneous. In contrast, the pH strategy aims to maintain a normal pH over varying temperatures, thus CO_2 must be added to the oxygenator gas mixture during deep hypothermia. The increased cerebral blood flow associated with pH-stat regulation may result in an increased risk of air or particulate emboli to the brain. Clearly, this is a concern in congenital heart disease patients who have intracardiac and extracardiac communications and the need for intracardiac surgical repairs. Additionally, pH-stat strategies increase cerebral blood volume, which may result in hyperemia and edema particularly during reperfusion. Luxuriant cerebral flow and perfusion have the advantage of enhancing global cerebral cooling and reducing cerebral steal from aortopulmonary shunts. Hypothermia causes a left shift of the oxyhemoglobin curve and is further shifted to the left by an alkaline pH. Thus off-loading of oxygen into the tissues is impaired unless the left shift is counteracted by more acidotic pH such as provided by the pH strategy.

Extracorporeal Membrane Oxygenation

ECMO was first introduced as a form of respiratory support in children with severe lung disease and is currently the most common approach to pediatric cardiac support today (Fig. 21.1). Indications have evolved to effectively provide biventricular support and oxygenation in pediatric patients who have a failing circulation. Reduction in the need for ECMO as respiratory support is most notable in neonates as a result of newer therapies such as inhaled nitric oxide, high frequency oscillatory ventilation, surfactant therapy, and permissive hypercapnia (44,77,95,125). Patients who now receive ECMO for respiratory support have usually failed multiple medical therapies,

and survival in these high risk neonates has declined over recent years. Cumulative data reported by the Extracorporeal Life Support Registry (ELSO) (44) from 140 centers through to January 2006 provide important insight into the outcomes and changing landscape of ECMO. In the 2006 report, 77% of all neonates who were placed on ECMO for respiratory support survived to hospital discharge. The outcome for older patients is considerably lower, with the reported cumulative survival for pediatric and adult patients placed on ECMO for respiratory support being 55%. Table 21.2 outlines the survival in the respiratory group by diagnostic category.

In contrast to respiratory ECMO, the use of ECMO for the treatment of circulatory failure following congenital cardiac surgery or as a bridge to cardiac transplantation has increased over the past decade (2,13,17,18,41,60,63,78,82,84,90,108, 121,122). Despite the increased enthusiasm for cardiac ECMO support of the circulation, the survival to hospital discharge as reported by ELSO (44) (38% for neonates and 44% for pediatric patients), has not increased and remains lower than the outcomes following ECMO used for respiratory failure (Fig. 21.2). The average duration for cardiac ECMO runs reported to ELSO over the past 15 years has increased slightly from approximately 4 to 5 days to between 5 to 7 days, with the

TABLE 21.2

SURVIVAL FOLLOWING ECMO CANNULATION IN NEONATES BY RESPIRATORY DIAGNOSTIC GROUP COMPARED WITH CARDIAC NEONATES

Diagnosis	Survived (%)
Meconium aspiration syndrome	94
Primary pulmonary hypertension	79
Sepsis	75
Air leak syndrome	70
Congenital diaphragmatic hernia	53
Cardiac disease	37

Data from ELSO, Extracorporeal Life Support Organization, international summary, July 2006.

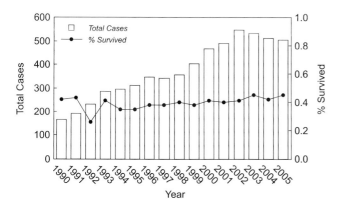

FIGURE 21.2 Cardiac extracorporeal membrane oxygenation (ECMO) volume and survival over time. The use of cardiac ECMO in the United States has increased dramatically over time, although overall survival rates continue to be stable. (Data adapted from the ELSO [Extracorporeal Life Support Organization] Registry Report, International Summary, July 2006.)

longest reported being 78 days (44). These data highlight the fact that ECMO should be viewed as a short-term circulatory support device.

There are significant differences between ECMO used for circulatory support and that used for respiratory support. Many cardiac ECMO patients are post-cardiotomy, and cannot be weaned from CPB. In these cases, residual hemodynamic lesions, underlying pathophysiology, and end-organ dysfunction play important roles in increased risk for adverse events. ECMO facilitates ventricular recovery by reducing myocardial wall tension, increasing coronary perfusion pressure and providing adequate systemic perfusion with oxygenated blood (2,18,63,78,84). ECMO is the preferred means of mechanical support in infants where myocardial failure can be either uni- or bi-ventricular and associated with respiratory insufficiency or pulmonary hypertension. In contrast to the concept of "resting the lungs" for patients who are placed on ECMO for respiratory failure and lung injury, it is important that the heart regain contractile function and conduction so as to prevent involution of the myocardial mass. This requires serial evaluation with echocardiography (90) to prevent overdistension of the heart. As noted above, the ECMO circuit is a "closed" circuit with limited ability to handle any air in the venous limb of the ECMO circuit, and careful de-airing of the venous cannula during initiation is essential.

Indications for ECMO

Indications for cardiac ECMO are similar to indications for all MCSD (Table 21.3). It can be an effective bridge to recovery, to transplantation, or to longer-term mechanical support.

Preoperative Stabilization. For complex congenital lesions: ECMO has been beneficial for critically ill pediatric cardiac patients prior to cardiac surgery (60), enabling resuscitation, optimization, and prevention of end-organ dysfunction. Some indications include severe low cardiac output states from left-sided obstructive lesions (e.g., critical aortic stenosis), pulmonary hypertension (e.g., obstructed total anomalous pulmonary venous drainage), or severe hypoxemia (e.g., transposition of the great arteries).

Post-cardiotomy. There is limited utility for ECMO as a bridge to recovery of ventricular function and overall survival

TABLE 21.3

INDICATIONS FOR MECHANICAL CIRCULATORY SUPPORT IN INFANTS AND CHILDREN

- Preoperative stabilization for complex congenital heart disease
- Post-cardiotomy
- In-hospital cardiac arrest resuscitation
- Bridge to cardiac transplantation
- Support during high-risk procedures

when patients fail to wean from CPB in the operating room (41,108,121). Unrecognized residual or irreparable defects are major factors determining successful outcome in this circumstance. Careful assessment in the operating room with echocardiography and measurements of oxygen saturations and intracardiac pressures may help identify correctable anatomic defects. Early transport to the cardiac catheterization laboratory must be considered to rule out residual defects (17). A major complication for this group transitioned directly to ECMO from CPB is hemorrhage. A lower activated clotting time (ACT) is used in this circumstance, often needing small increments of protamine (1 mg/kg) until a target ACT of 160 to 180 seconds is achieved. Infusions of antifibrinolytic drugs such as aprotinin (bolus 30,000 IU/kg, infusion 10,000 IU/kg/hour), tranexamic acid (bolus 100 mg/kg, infusion 10 mg/kg/hour), or epsilon aminocaproic acid (bolus 100 mg/kg, infusion 30 mg/kg/hour) should also be considered. Exploration of the chest is usually necessary, particularly if the bleeding persists at >10 to 15 mL/kg/hour or problems with ECMO flow are encountered from tamponade-like effect.

Ideally, only children with potentially reversible myocardial injury who cannot be weaned from CPB should be considered candidates for ECMO, although this may be extremely difficult to determine in the operating room immediately following cardiac surgery.

Considerations include preoperative condition, intraoperative course and the likelihood of becoming a suitable transplant candidate. When a patient is placed on ECMO in the operating room, it is important that discussions with the family to be clear and direct. If no recovery of myocardial function occurs within 2 to 3 days (41), listing for cardiac transplantation, or withdrawal from support must be considered.

ECMO is an effective option for patients who, following a period of relative stability after CPB, have low-output compromise (Table 21.4). Because patients were stable enough to wean off CPB, bleeding is less of an issue. For this group, cannulation can be undertaken through the chest at the bedside; however, if sufficiently stable, neck or femoral sites are preferable. Myocardial or respiratory failure contributing to a low output state, hypoxemia, or pulmonary hypertension are the major indications in this group, and survival rates as high as 60% to 70% have been reported provided ECMO is instituted rapidly and effectively (13,18,41,44,78,84,90,108,121).

In-Hospital Cardiac Arrest Resuscitation. Survival in this group of pediatric patients cannulated following cardiac arrest is poor (9% and 31%) (97,104,114,128). The duration of

TABLE 21.4

SURVIVAL FOLLOWING ECMO CANNULATION BY CARDIAC PROCEDURE

Procedure	% Total reported cardiac ECMO	% Survived
Anomalous venous return repair	2.5	44
Aortic outflow repair	1.3	32
AV canal repair	1.5	41
Bidirectional Glenn's shunt	0.5	32
Fontan's procedures	2.3	26
Heart transplant	5.7	43
Mitral valve repair	1.9	42
Rastelli's repair	0.9	36
Stage 1 palliation (Norwood's)	5.1	29
Tetralogy repair	3.5	44
VSD repair	2.1	32

AV, atrioventricular; VSD, ventricular septal defect.

resuscitation is an important determinant of outcome, and a critical threshold of 15 minutes has been reported (97,104). There are, however, reports of the successful use of ECMO to support children during active resuscitation and chest compressions (31,35,40,62,65). To avoid significant delays, a rapid response ECMO system has been established at some institutions to initiate ECMO during active resuscitation efforts (35,40). As a guideline, ECMO should be considered in patients in this circumstance who have suffered a witnessed arrest, who received rapid institution of effective and monitored CPR, who have no apparent recovery of cardiac function within 5 to 10 minutes of initiating resuscitation or after two to three rounds of resuscitation medications, and who have no obvious contraindications for ECMO.

The aim of a rapid-response system is to provide systemic perfusion and oxygen delivery as soon as possible to prevent end-organ injury. Ideally, this should be within 30 minutes of starting resuscitation, although it may take longer if cannulation is complicated. In postoperative cardiac patients, atrial and aortic cannulation via a reopened sternotomy is usually the access mode of choice. In other patients, experienced practitioners can rapidly gain access via the neck vessels. Groin vessel cannulation has been reported, even in the infant (16). It is important to provide effective and monitored resuscitation during cannulation, and there will be times during cannulation that chest compressions will be briefly discontinued. Mild hypothermia should be induced during resuscitation and continued once ECMO has been started to possibly provide end-organ and specifically neurologic protection. Because the aim of ECMO is to provide systemic perfusion as soon as possible, there is usually insufficient time to blood prime the ECMO circuit. This means that infants and small children are extremely hemodiluted once ECMO flow is initiated, but after flow is established, blood products can be added or the priming crystalloid can be removed via hemofiltration.

Determining the relative contraindications to ECMO support during active resuscitation is difficult. Patients with repaired two-ventricle defects who have a sudden or unexpected event leading to cardiac arrest are good candidates for early initiation of ECMO during resuscitation because effec-

tive CPR is more likely to maintain perfusion and oxygen delivery during chest compressions, decreasing the risk for end-organ injury. In contrast, patients with cavopulmonary connections, i.e., Fontan's or bidirectional Glenn's (BDG) anastomoses, have been difficult to resuscitate using ECMO (18). First, these patients may have occluded or abnormal venous and arterial access, thereby limiting possible cannulation sites; and second, an inability to maintain adequate systemic oxygen delivery during CPR and cerebral venous hypertension during CPR with chest compressions may hinder neurologic outcome. Other complicated groups include patients with pulmonary hypertension and those with systemic outflow obstruction. These patients, similar to the cavopulmonary connection group, are at significant risk for inadequate oxygen delivery during CPR, contributing to subsequent end-organ injury.

Bridge to Cardiac Transplantation. Patients who present with acute fulminant myocarditis can be successfully managed with ECMO. They may present in full cardiac arrest, low cardiac output state, or with hemodynamically unstable dysrhythmias including ventricular tachycardia or heart block. Prompt institution of ECMO often allows sufficient resuscitation and stabilization to prevent end-organ injury and enable the myocardium to rest and potentially recover. After instituting ECMO, it is essential that the heart be fully decompressed, and urgent left atrial vent placement is often necessary (17). Although the recovery of electrical activity within the first few hours should be expected, the heart may not begin to eject for the first 24 to 36 hours after starting ECMO. If recovery of ventricular function is not evident within 2 to 3 days, consideration of transition to an alternative longer-term support with a VAD should be considered.

ECMO can be viewed as a short-term bridge to cardiac transplantation because of the limited donor availability and the time-related risks for complications, such as infection, as well as bleeding, end-organ impairment, problems secondary to immobilization, and difficulties in maintaining adequate nutrition. In our experience at Children's Hospital, Boston, the median time spent on ECMO awaiting heart transplantation has been 164 hours (range 21 to 556 hours), however only 50% of listed patients have been effectively bridged.

Our current practice for a patient who is resuscitated with ECMO includes transition to a longer-term mechanical support device (MCSD) to bridge to transplant in the older patients. As newer, smaller devices become available, this strategy will no doubt be used for the younger patients as well.

ECMO has either been used to effectively support the failing heart following transplantation, immediately after transplantation because of primary graft failure, during periods of acute rejection (6,114). Inflammation and myocardial edema are similar to that seen with fulminant myocarditis. ECMO can allow the transplanted heart to decompress while antirejection therapy is increased. In our experience, survival to discharge for this indication has been 64%, and the median duration of ECMO support has been 4 days.

ECMO Support During High Risk Procedures.

As the complexity and interventions during cardiac catheterization in patients with complex congenital heart disease have continued to expand, patients may be at increased risk for sudden unexpected adverse events. These may range from complications associated with specific intervention to dysrhythmias and low cardiac output states related to wires and catheters within the heart. ECMO support during resuscitation from an acute event during catheterization is beneficial, but there are important technical and resuscitative considerations (3). Percutaneous cannulation for ECMO can be rapidly achieved using existing catheter access, but staff must be familiar with the technique for upsizing from the catheter sheath to large-bore ECMO cannulae. The catheterization laboratory environment is a challenge, and resuscitation to ECMO must be well organized to be effective. Often there are conflicting or simultaneous considerations during resuscitation including ongoing chest compressions, cannulation for ECMO, and ongoing efforts to stabilize the complication with methods such as balloon occlusion of a ruptured vessel.

It is possible to anticipate hemodynamic instability during catheterization in some patients, particularly those with dysrhythmias induced during electrophysiologic studies and radiofrequency ablation (22). The cannulation and support of the circulation using ECMO will enable safe and successful completion of the procedure.

Technical Considerations of ECMO

Children with complex structural cardiac defects may have associated abnormalities of systemic venous damage (e.g., heterotaxy syndromes) or have undergone previous cardiac catheterization or catheter placement that may have caused femoral vessel occlusion. It is essential, therefore, that the venous and arterial anatomy be well known, including the patency of individual vessels, and be well documented to prevent inappropriate cannulation attempts. Arteriovenous cannulation is usually employed for cardiac ECMO (26,66,74,83), although venovenous bypass can be used in patients who require ventilatory support only. Venous cannulation and ECMO flow via the jugular vein using a double-lumen catheter can also provide hemodynamic support in select neonates who have a ductus-dependent circulation, such as hypoplastic left heart syndrome.

The daily management of a patient on ECMO requires attention to cardiorespiratory function, end-organ perfusion and injury, evolving complications such as bleeding or sepsis, and the mechanics of the ECMO circuit (68). Assessing flow and systemic perfusion adequacy after initiation of ECMO is essential, and well-defined protocols must be in place (Table 21.5). ECMO flow rates in infants and small children typically range

TABLE 21.5

ECMO CIRCUIT GUIDELINES, CHILDREN'S HOSPITAL, BOSTON

Weight (kg)	2–15	16–20	21–35	36–60	>60	STAT >15 kg
Circuit	Neonatal	Pediatric	Pediatric	Adult	Adult	STAT
Membrane, m²	0.8–1.5	2.5	3.5	4.5	4.5	Optima
Prime						
5% albumin (mL)	50	100	100	100	100	100
RBCs (mL)	500	1,000	1,000	1,500	1,500	1,000
FFP (mL)	200	400	400	500	500	400
Cryo (units)	2	3	3	4	4	3
Platelets (units)	2	4	4	6	6	6
Medications						
Heparin (units)	500	500	500	800	800	500
THAM (mL)	100	200	300	300	300	200
Calcium (mg)	1,500	3,000	3,000	4,000	4,000	3,000
Flow						
Minimum (mL/min)	100	200	250	300	600	500
Maximum (L/min)	1.8	4.5	5.5	6.5	6.5	8.0
Sweep gas range (L/min)	1–4.5	2–8	2–11	2–13	2–13	0.5–20
Membrane volume (mL)	174	455	575	665	1,330	260
Circuit volume (mL)	580	1,500	1,600	2,500	3,200	1,000

RBCs, red blood cells; FFP, fresh frozen plasma; Cryo, cryoprecipitate.

from 100 to 150 mL/kg/minute during full circulatory support. Inadequate flow states and/or significant persistent hypotension despite adequate circuit flow may be due to ECMO-related problems with cannula size, cannula position, and venous drainage, or to patient-related factors such as vasodilation and low systemic vascular resistance secondary to sepsis. Venous cannula malposition or inadequate size will limit venous drainage and should be addressed with repositioning or upsizing of existing cannulae. Addition of a second venous drain may be necessary. Elevated postmembrane pressures (i.e., >250 mm Hg) may reflect malposition of the arterial cannula or a cannula that is too small and needs to be replaced. Elevated premembrane pressures (i.e., >350 mm Hg) at normal flows without change in postmembrane pressure or evidence of blood-to-gas leak imply membrane oxygenator dysfunction and may require oxygenator replacement. Extensive thrombus evident within the circuit or development of a consumptive coagulopathy with hypofibrinogenemia and thrombocytopenia are indications for circuit replacement. Blood products are administered to keep the hematocrit between 35% and 45% and the platelet count >100,000/mm³.

Considerations for cannulation and flow rates once on ECMO may be specific to the underlying cardiac defect or surgical repair. For example, the management of an aortopulmonary shunt in patients with single-ventricle physiology may require circuit flows ≥200 mL/kg/minute to maintain adequate systemic perfusion while accounting for runoff into the pulmonary circulation.

Echocardiography, especially transesophageal imaging (90), and occasionally cardiac catheterization (17) are used to assess cardiac anatomy and function and to detect residual lesions. Additionally, assessment of left atrial hypertension by clinical findings, chest radiograph, and echocardiography is critical. Venting the left atrium may be necessary to lower left atrial pressure and decrease left ventricular wall stress, thereby minimizing ongoing myocardial injury. Placement of a left atrial vent can be accomplished by direct placement through an open chest or by a transcatheter approach (17). If a patient fails to wean from ECMO or there is delay in anticipated recovery of myocardial function, the possibility of a residual surgical problem must always be considered. This is usually difficult to diagnose by echocardiography alone, and cardiac catheterization (i.e., diagnostic and/or interventional) should be considered.

OTHER SHORT-TERM MECHANICAL CIRCULATORY SUPPORT DEVICES

ECMO has limitations as an effective bridge to transplantation and precludes chronic ambulatory use. In patients unable to be weaned from ECMO who are listed for transplant, transition to a chronic circulatory support device can be done successfully.

Centrifugal Assist Pump

The centrifugal assist device (Bio-Pump, Medtronic Bio-Medicus, Minneapolis, MN) has been the principle means for providing support of the circulation without an oxygenator membrane. This centrifugal pump provides flow by power applied to a rotating magnet coupled to an opposing magnet on a cone-shaped impeller. There are no valves and no obligatory volume displacement by the pump, which results in nonpulsatile flow that is both preload- and afterload-sensitive with priming volumes of ≤100 mL (29,32,72,73,75,79,87,111). The various sizes of cone heads available allow this device to be used by various-sized patients from infants through to adults.

Reports using the Bio-Pump predominately as a left ventricular support device have demonstrated survival rates of 40% to 70% (29,32,72,73,75,79,87,111) when used as a bridge to recovery. Central nervous system complications, both short- and long-term, tend to be less prevalent compared with a concurrent group of patients supported with ECMO (29,34). The absence of an oxygenator and reduced lengths of tubing remove an important substrate for cerebral embolic events while the generally reduced level of anticoagulation used during VAD support may decrease the incidence of hemorrhage. The centrifugal pump VAD enables only short-term support as a bridge to recovery or transplantation. The complications related to this nonpulsatile extracorporeal circuit are similar to those encountered with longer-term ECMO use, and patients are unable to ambulate. This is an important consideration when longer-term support with recovery of end-organ function, improved nutrition, and ability for rehabilitation and ambulation are necessary prior to transplantation.

Intra-aortic Balloon Counter Pulsation (IABP)

Intra-aortic balloon counter pulsation (IABP) is used for the treatment of left ventricular failure in adults. When used in infants and children, however, results have been disappointing, with survival rates <50% (1,9,25,33,92,94,101, 102,106). Effective timing of inflation and deflation is more difficult in children because of their relatively rapid heart rates and the variable delay between aortic valve closure and the appearance of the arterial tracing. At heart rates >160 beats per minute (bpm), the IABP is often reduced to a 1:2 or even 1:4 pumping frequency to facilitate cycle timing, at the same time decreasing its effectiveness to 50% to 80% (1,94,101). Both coronary flow augmentation during diastole (balloon inflation) and afterload reduction during systole (balloon deflation) are likely to be decreased because the aorta is typically more distensible in infants and in children. Additionally, the effect of diastolic augmentation of flow to normal coronary arteries, as seen in most pediatric patients, is limited. The extensive development of aortopulmonary collateral vessels, that accompanies cyanotic heart disease may complicate shunting of blood into the pulmonary circulation during balloon inflation, reducing augmentation of coronary blood flow.

The smallest balloon system available for children is 2.5 mL, which can be used for neonates as small as 2 kg (33). In general, a balloon volume of 0.5 mL/kg is recommended. The incidence of vascular complications such as limb ischemia bleeding, or emboli, is similar to that in children, in the adult population, 10% to 20%. Other potential complications are infection, renal dysfunction, mesenteric occlusion or embolism, and cerebrovascular accidents (9,106).

IABP may have a role in the temporary support of the adolescents and adults with single ventricle physiology and poor systolic function during procedures or as a short-term bridge. Technical improvements may have an impact in the pediatric population. These include smaller sized catheters, improved tracking, more rapid inflation heart rate deflation, and the use of echocardiography for cycle timing (92).

LONG-TERM MECHANICAL CIRCULATORY SUPPORT FOR CHILDREN

The use of long-term mechanical circulatory support in children has increased over the past decade as waiting times for pediatric cardiac allografts have increased and understanding of recovery of cardiac function has improved. In adults on chronic term devices, normalization of cardiac output provided by chronic and implantable VADs allows a period of improvement in end-organ function that, combined with patient ambulation and cardiac rehabilitation, optimize the patient's condition prior to transplant. The use of adult devices in larger children and adolescents has proved successful. Additionally, technology advances (19) have allowed the possibility of mechanical support as a bridge to transplant or recovery for longer periods of time.

The experience with VAD support in infants and children is increasing (4,14,28,42,47,53–56,58,59,64,71,85,89,91,93, 97,98,105,109,110,115–118,123) but remains relatively small, mainly owing to size and technical limitations. A benefit is the ability to ambulate while wearing the device, which cannot be accomplished currently with ECMO and centrifugal VADs. Another advantage of VADs is superior ventricular unloading (53), a prerequisite for myocardial rest and potential recovery. As with ECMO, the selection of appropriate candidates is crucial and surgical problems or residual defects should be excluded where possible. Although ECMO can be instituted by peripheral cannulation of neck or femoral vessels, VADs require direct cannulation of the heart through a sternotomy.

Clinical Criteria for VAD Placement

VADs can successfully support the circulation and bridge patients to cardiac transplant by improving the patient's cardiac output and oxygen delivery. Therefore, the primary indication for VAD is in patients who have unacceptable symptoms or signs of low cardiac output state. In addition to improved oxygen delivery, pulmonary capillary wedge pressure, and pulmonary vascular resistance decrease, congestive heart failure symptoms diminish, and nutrition and physical rehabilitation markedly improve in many cases. Thus, VADs have the potential to improve pretransplant status. Evidence for developing end-organ dysfunction despite maximal medical interventions is an indication for VAD in transplant-eligible or listed patients. This includes the obvious symptoms of persistent congestive heart failure and biochemical evidence for renal and hepatic dysfunction. In children the symptoms may be less obvious; abdominal pain, vomiting, or anorexia may be early signs of low cardiac output, and if they persist, will lead to poor nutrition. Early use of VAD in this circumstance will improve nutrition, which in turn will improve recovery after cardiac transplant.

Patients with structurally normal hearts who develop heart failure from acquired heart disease such as myocarditis or who have idiopathic cardiomyopathy are successfully supported and bridged to transplantation with VADs. Compared with patients with structurally normal hearts, the use of chronic MSCD in children with congenital heart disease has not been as favorable, with only approximately 30% successfully bridged to transplant in the congenital group in one study (Fig. 21.3). Reoperative status, complex anatomy, nutritional issues, and chronic nature of the diseases are all contributing factors. Patients with single-ventricle defects or those who have undergone cavopulmonary procedures are particularly challenging to support with VAD because of issues related to cannula position (98,105).

In contrast to the ECMO experience, the outcomes for children placed on VADs have improved over recent years. Smaller single-center studies (4,28,55,71) and device registry data (58) report an approximately 60% successful bridge to transplantation in pediatric patients supported with VAD. Improved outcomes in the most recent era (14) may be related to an increasing experience with the surgical techniques and perioperative care, better patient selection, and earlier introduction of support before irreversible end-organ injury develops, and the application and development of device technology over time.

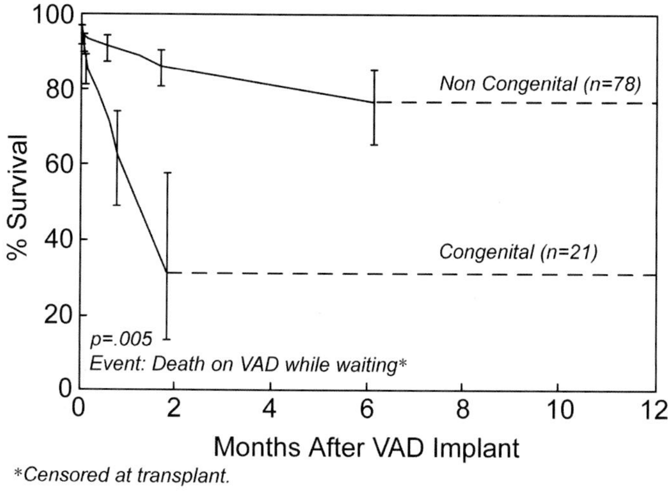

FIGURE 21.3 Congenital heart disease outcomes are poor. Survival following ventricular assist device (VAD) implantation in pediatric patients with congenital heart disease is significantly worse than in children implanted with structurally normal hearts. (From Blume ED, Naftel DC, Bastardi HJ, et al., for the Pediatric Heart Transplant Study Investigators. Outcomes of children bridged to heart transplantation with ventricular assist devices: A multi-institutional study. *Circulation* 2006;113:2313–2319, reproduced with permission.)

TABLE 21.6

ADVERSE EVENTS IN PEDIATRIC PATIENTS
(1993–2003, *n* = 99) SUPPORTED BY SHORT-TERM
VENTRICULAR ASSIST DEVICE COMPARED WITH
PEDIATRIC PATIENTS IMPLANTED WITH CHRONIC
PULSATILE DEVICE

	Chronic (n = 70)	Short term (n = 26)	*p*
Stroke*	9 (13%)	9 (35%)	0.02
Infection#	29 (41%)	2 (12%)	0.004
Reoperative bleeding	22 (31%)	11 (42%)	0.32
Hemolysis	13 (19%)	2 (1%)	0.17
Thrombus	8 (11%)	4 (15%)	0.64

Blume ED, Naftel DC, Bastardi HJ, et al., for the Pediatric Heart
Transplant Study Investigators. Outcomes of children bridged to heart
transplantation with ventricular assist devices: A multi-institutional
study. *Circulation* 2006;113:2313–2319, with permission.

Adverse Events Related to VAD Support

The adverse event profile and hazard function for death in
children are shown in Table 21.6 and Figure 21.4, and are
similar to those reported from the larger mechanical circulatory support device database of adult outcomes (109). Substantial morbidity is associated with the use of VADs. Prevention requires meticulous attention to detail, with the major
morbidity related to problems with chronic anticoagulation,
neurologic complications, and infection (Table 21.6). Neurologic complications in that series (14) included a 20% incidence of stroke, often fatal or leading to withdrawal of support. Stroke rate was statistically different between
short-term devices (35%) and those intended for long-term
support (13%, *p* = 0.02). Protocols or recommendations for
anticoagulation management vary between devices and centers and include a combination of heparin, coumadin, and
antiplatelet drugs. Close monitoring of heparin level, coagulation profiles, INR, and of platelet function are all critical,
e.g., maintaining an anti–factor Xa level 0.4 to 0.7 or PTT

1.5 to 2 times normal with an ATIII level >75%, INR 3.0 to
3.5, and platelet mapping with arachidonic acid suppression
>80%. Additionally, pediatric research efforts must address
biocompatibility issues to mitigate risks arising from
blood–prosthetic surface interactions in these devices, which
may be unique to children.

Use of Current VAD Systems in Children

As noted previously and in Figure 21.3, the use of VADs in
children has continued to expand. The currently available
devices for children and adolescents in the United States are
shown in Table 21.1. The Pediatric Heart Transplant Study
Group reported the experience from 24 pediatric heart transplant institutions over the decade of 1993 to 2003, in which
99 pediatric patients received VAD support as a bridge to
transplantation (14). In this study, which included 2,375 pediatric patients listed for transplant, the percentage of patients
transplanted with VAD technology implanted increased from
3.2% of all transplants between 1993 and 1999, to 6.6% of
all transplants between 2000 and 2003 (Fig. 21.5). This
increasing use of VADs in pediatric patients is multifactorial
and includes center experience, regulatory issues, and development of smaller technology. There continues to be a large gap,
however, in the critical need for smaller devices and the development side. Of the 99 patients retrospectively reviewed with
a median age of 13.3 years (range 2 days to 17.9 years), 78%
had cardiomyopathy with 22 patients with congenital heart
disease. The status prior to implantation included 34 inotrope
dependent, 41 requiring ventilatory support, and 26 on
another form of mechanical circulatory support such as
ECMO (87), intra-aortic balloon pump (81), and cardiopulmonary bypass (84).

Of the 99 patients studied, there were 70 patients supported with a chronic pulsatile adult device (median age 14
years, median BSA 1.6) with a mean time of implantation of
70 days (range 1 to 465 days). One third of pediatric patients
in this study required biventricular support, which is proportionately higher than comparable adult populations. In contrast to the adult data, there was no discernible difference in
outcome between the LVAD and BiVAD patients following
implantation. This may be secondary to the type of disease,
with children having less focal ischemic disease and more

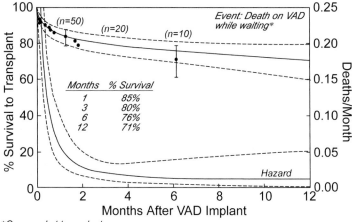

*Censored at transplant.

FIGURE 21.4 Overall survival following ventricular assist device
(VAD) implant. Of the 99 pediatric patients implanted with VAD,
percent survival to transplant is seen. In addition, the hazard
curve shows the highest risk of death in the first 2 weeks following
implantation. (From Blume ED, Naftel DC, Bastardi HJ, et al., for
the Pediatric Heart Transplant Study Investigators. Outcomes of
children bridged to heart transplantation with ventricular assist
devices: A multi-institutional study. *Circulation* 2006;113:2313–
2319, reproduced with permission.)

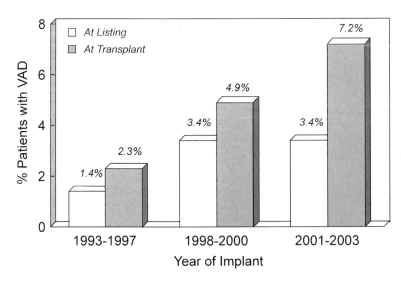

FIGURE 21.5 Ventricular assist device (VAD) use in children by era. VAD use in children as a bridge to transplant has increased over the last decade for children at listing as well as at the time of transplant. (From Blume ED, Naftel DC, Bastardi HJ, et al., for the Pediatric Heart Transplant Study Investigators. Outcomes of children bridged to heart transplantation with ventricular assist devices: a multi-institutional study. *Circulation* 2006;113:2313–2319, reproduced with permission.)

global myopathic-type disorders. Another observation, however, is that the use of biventricular support decreases with VAD implantation volume. This suggests that as pediatric centers gain experience and potentially assess right ventricular function more aggressively in the operating room, left ventricular support alone may be an option in more of the young patients. Of those 70 children supported on an adult pulsatile device, 60 (86%) were successfully bridged to transplant. Comparing pretransplant and posttransplant outcomes of the pediatric VAD group to >1200 patients listed for transplantation as Status 1 (on inotropic support without mechanical support), there was no statistically significant difference. The hazard curve for death following implantation was highest at 2 weeks following implantation (Fig. 21.4). This early mortal-

ity improved over the years, making era of implant the most significant predictor of outcome in this group. Figure 21.6 shows the era effect by competing outcomes analysis of all 99 patients in this study, again suggesting a learning curve in pediatric patients and improved patient selection. The 5-year survival following transplant for patients on VAD support at time of transplant is comparable with those who did not require a VAD (77% versus 73%, $p = 0.8$).

In sharp contrast to ECMO and the short-term support devices, 84% of pediatric patients supported by adult VAD systems were extubated and 73% were ambulatory at the time of transplant. Risk factors for death following pediatric VAD implantation in this study included era of implant, diagnosis of congenital heart disease, and gender.

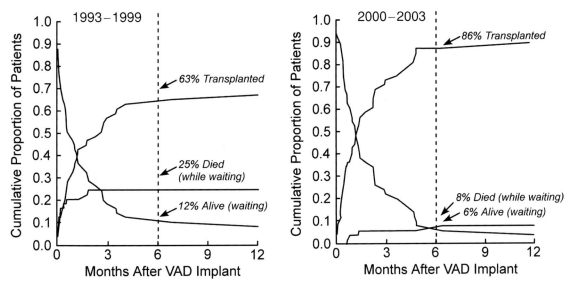

FIGURE 21.6 Era effect of outcome following pediatric ventricular assist device (VAD) implantation. Competing outcomes analysis shows the early mortality improving over time comparing the 1993–1999 (**left**) era with the current 2000–2003 era (**right**). (From Blume ED, Naftel DC, Bastardi HJ, et al., for the Pediatric Heart Transplant Study Investigators. Outcomes of children bridged to heart transplantation with ventricular assist devices: a multi-institutional study. *Circulation* 2006;113:2313–2319, reproduced with permission.)

Pulsatile VADs for Neonates, Infants, and Small Children

Currently there are two pulsatile VAD systems that are suitable for the entire age range of pediatric patients: MEDOS HIA VAD (MEDOS Medizintechnik AG, Stolberg, Germany) and the Berlin Heart VAD (Berlin Heart AG, Berlin, Germany). In particular, both devices can be used in neonates and infants, and for this reason, are currently the only alternatives for longer-term VAD support in these patients. Both are paracorporeal systems that use pneumatically driven, thin-membrane pumps to provide pulsatile flow. Both systems are available in various pump sizes (10 to 80 mL), with the smallest pump sizes suitable for infant support. A measured amount of compressed air delivered through a pneumatic line compresses the ventricular chamber or bladder, thereby enforcing ejection of blood (Fig. 21.7). Diastolic pump filling is achieved by negative pressure suction. In general, pump rates are kept low, 60 to 80 bpm and negative pressure 40 to 60 mm Hg, to allow for complete filling, and the systolic drive pressure is 20 to 30 mm Hg more than the patient's systolic pressure. The power source generates positive and negative pressures to move the membrane that separates a blood chamber from an air chamber. This membrane appearance can be evaluated at the bedside to ensure minimal wrinkling (Table 21.7). Insufficient filling (more wrinkles noted in convex position) prompts an assessment of preload, intrathoracic pressures, and/or tamponade, or an increase of the diastolic drive pressure (i.e., more negative). In the case of inadequate ejection or stroke volume (wrinkles in concave position), assessment should be made of possible sources of increased pulmonary or systemic vascular resistance (afterload) owing to inadequate sedation, ventilatory status, and infection. Additional support of the circulation with vasodilators and/or inotropes to augment stroke volume should be considered.

Because of the high resistance of the small-bore cannulae in small children, positive pressures ≤350 mm Hg and negative suction of 100 mm Hg at pumping rates of ≤180 bpm may be necessary, increasing the power requirements for the driving unit considerably, although at these maximal settings, there may be considerable blood trauma and hemolysis. It is critical

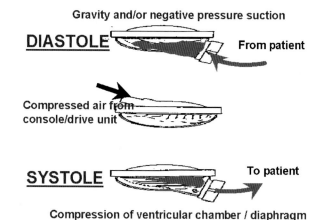

FIGURE 21.7 Mechanics of pneumatically driven, pulsatile, paracorporeal systems. Blood from the patient enters the pump in diastole, in the presence of gravity and/or negative pressure suction, resulting in a concave membrane. Compressed air from the console then enters from the drive unit, resulting in the convex membrane and resulting in systolic ejection of the blood back to the patient.

TABLE 21.7

ALGORITHM FOR PULSATILE VAD PUMP TROUBLESHOOTING

A. Inadequate filling (wrinkles in convex position)
- Assess preload, monitor:
  - □ CVP, RAp, LAp
  - □ Heart rate, arterial blood pressure
  - □ Maintain adequate preload; volume available at bed space
- Assess changes in intrathoracic pressure with ventilation
- Tamponade: inadequate membrane filling
  - □ Increased filling pressure (increased CVP)
  - □ Tachycardia
  - □ Hypotension
- Consider adjusting diastolic pressure
- Consider adjusting systolic ejection time

B. Inadequate ejection (wrinkles in concave position)
- Increased PVR and SVR (afterload)
  - □ Assess hemodynamics
  - □ Consider inotropic support and afterload reduction
  - □ Consider other factors leading to increased PVR and SVR (i.e., level of sedation, mechanical ventilation, sepsis)
- Consider adjusting systolic drive pressure
- Consider adjusting systolic ejection time

CVP, central venous pressure; RAp, right arterial pressure; LAp, left arterial pressure; PVR, pulmonary vascular resistance; SVR, systemic vascular resistance.

---

to reevaluate the cannula position and cardiac function either by echocardiography or cardiac catheterization. The changes in setting of the pulsatile devices should be reassessed with changes such as intubation or extubation, and once the patient is ambulatory. Otherwise, settings will remain relatively stable throughout the patient's course. The polyurethane inlet and outlet valves are trileaflet and function well to prevent regurgitation, but they remain a potential nidus for thrombus formation, which requires at least twice daily assessment.

In a report of 68 children (average age 12 years) supported by the Berlin Heart (54,55), the mean duration of support was 35 days with a range of 0 to 420 days. Forty-two patients (62%) were successfully transplanted or weaned to recovery. Patients could be mobile with the Berlin Heart but had to manage movement of a large console while ambulating. The most frequent cause of death was vasodilatory shock associated with multisystem organ failure and/or sepsis. Hemorrhagic complications were the second most frequent causes of death. The current worldwide experience with the Berlin Heart VAD in pediatric patients now exceeds 200 patients (Dr. Peter Goettel, Berlin Heart AG, Berlin, Germany, personal communication).

Axial-Flow VAD for Children

A further development in pediatric circulatory support has been the development of an implantable axial-flow device, DeBakey VAD *Child* (MicroMed Cardiovascular Inc., Houston, TX), which was granted humanitarian device exemption (HDE) status by the Food and Drug Administration and became available for use in small children in 2004. This pediatric device uses the same continuous axial-flow pump used in

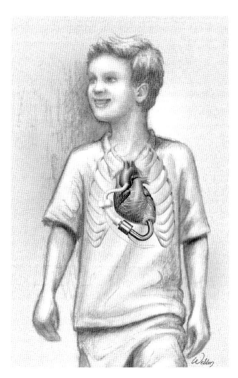

FIGURE 21.8 MicroMed DeBakey VAD *Child* was the first humanitarian device exemption (HDE) approval granted for a device labeled specifically for children. (Reproduced with permission from B. S. Russell Micromed Cardiovascular, Inc.)

the adult version with design modifications aimed at reducing the lateral space requirements for device implantation (Fig. 21.8). Under the current HDE, the VAD *Child* is used to provide temporary left ventricular support as a bridge to cardiac transplantation for children from 5 to 16 years of age with a BSA of 0.7 m² to 1.5 m² and is designed to be fully implantable in this size range. Although the clinical experience is still limited (47,93), this device has been used successfully in a small number of children since its introduction.

The current U.S. experience with VAD in children remains relatively small primarily because of technical considerations and concerns regarding suitability of children with congenital heart disease, at least for univentricular support. Nevertheless, VAD support has been successful as a bridge to transplantation in children and enables recovery of end-organ function, improvement in nutritional status, elimination of fluid overload, and rehabilitation of critically ill patients. An important component of these benefits is the ability of the device to allow for ambulation, which cannot be currently accomplished with ECMO and centrifugal VADs.

The paracorporeal pulsatile VADs and the continuous axial-flow devices have not been approved for routine use in the United States, but anecdotal experience continues to increase with application through the Federal Drug Administration (FDA) regulatory review process. Registry data collection has begun through a contract with the National Heart, Lung, and Blood Institute at the National Institute of Health (NHLBI), and clinical and engineering colleagues have collaborated (7,100,119) to move the field forward. A multicenter trial is necessary to determine utility, efficacy, and safety, including issues of patient mobility and quality of life.

References

1. Akomea-Agyin C, Kejriwal NK, Franks R, et al. Intraaortic balloon pumping in children. *Ann Thorac Surg* 1999;67:1415–1420.
2. Alexi-Meskishvili V, Nurnberg JH, Werner H, et al. Long-term extracorporeal membrane oxygenation in a newborn child after arterial switch operation. *Cardiovasc Surg* 1996;4(2):258–260.
3. Allan CK, Thiagarajan RR, Armsby LR, et al. Emergent use of extracorporeal membrane oxygenation during pediatric cardiac catheterization. *Pediatr Crit Care Med* 2006;7(3):212–219.
4. Arabia FA, Tsau PH, Smith RG, et al. Pediatric bridge to heart transplantation: Application of the Berlin Heart, Medos and Thoratec ventricular assist devices. *J Heart Lung Transplant* 2006;25(1):16–21.
5. Ashraf SS, Tian Y, Zacharrias S, et al. Effects of cardiopulmonary bypass on neonatal and paediatric inflammatory profiles. *Eur J Cardiothorac Surg* 1997;12:862–868.
6. Bae JO, Frischer JS, Waich M, et al. Extracorporeal membrane oxygenation in pediatric cardiac transplantation. *J Pediatr Surg* 2005;40:1051–1056.
7. Baldwin JT, Borovetz HS, Duncan BW, et al. The National Heart, Lung, and Blood Institute Pediatric Circulatory Support Program. *Circulation* 2006;113:147–155.
8. Barratt-Boyes B. Complete correction of cardiovascular malformations in the first two years of life using profound hypothermia. In: Barratt-Boyes BG, Neutze JM, Harris EA, eds. *Heart Disease in Infancy*. Edinburgh: Churchill Livingstone; 1973:35.
9. Beckman CB, Geha AS, Hammond GL, et al. Results and complications of intraaortic balloon counterpulsation. *Ann Thorac Surg* 1977;24:550–559.
10. Bellinger D, Jonas RA, Rappaport L. Developmental and neurologic status of children after heart surgery with hypothermic circulatory arrest or low-flow cardiopulmonary bypass. *New Eng J Med* 1995;332:540–555.
11. Bellinger DC, Wernovsky G, Rappaport LA, et al. Cognitive development of children following early repair of transposition of the great arteries using deep hypothermic circulatory arrest. *Pediatrics* 1991;87:701.
12. Bellinger DC, Wypij D, duDuplessis AJ, et al. Neurodevelopmental status at eight years in children with dextro-transposition of the great arteries: The Boston Circulatory Arrest Trial. *J Thorac Cardiovasc Surg* 2003;126:1385–1396.
13. Black MD, Coles JG, Williams WG, et al. Determinants of success in pediatric cardiac patients undergoing extracorporeal membrane oxygenation. *Ann Thorac Surg* 1995;60:133–138.
14. Blume ED, Naftel DC, Bastardi HJ, et al. For the Pediatric Heart Transplant Study Investigators. Outcomes of children bridged to heart transplantation with ventricular assist devices: A multi-institutional study. *Circulation* 2006;113:2313–2319.
15. Blume ED, Nelson DP, Gauvreau K, et al. Soluble adhesion molecules in infants and children undergoing cardiopulmonary bypass. *Circulation* 1997;96(suppl):II352–II357.
16. Booth KL, Guleserian KJ, Mayer JE, et al. Extracorporeal membrane oxygenation support of a neonate with percutaneous femoral arterial cannulation. *Ann Thorac Surg* 2006;81:1514–1516.
17. Booth KL, Roth SJ, Perry SB, et al. Cardiac catheterization of patients supported by extracorporeal membrane oxygenation. *J Am Coll Cardiol* 2002;40:1681–1686.
18. Booth KL, Roth SJ, Thiagarajan RR, et al. Extracorporeal membrane oxygenation support of the Fontan and bidirectional Glenn circulations. *Ann Thorac Surg* 2004;77:1341–1348.
19. Borovetz HS, Badylak S, Boston JR, et al. Towards the development of a pediatric ventricular assist device. *Cell Transplant* 2006;15(suppl 1):S69–S74.
20. Bowen FW, Carboni AF, O'Hara ML, et al. Application of "double bridge mechanical" resuscitation for profound cardiogenic shock leading to cardiac transplantation. *Ann Thorac Surg* 2001;72:86–90.
21. Brunberg JA, Doty DB, Reilly EL. Choreoathetosis in infants following cardiac surgery with deep hypothermic and circulatory arrest. *J Pediatr* 1974;84:232.
22. Carmichael TB, Walsh EP, Roth SJ. Anticipatory use of venoarterial extracorporeal membrane oxygenation for a high-risk interventional cardiac procedure. *Respir Care* 2002;47:1002–1006.
23. Castaneda AR, Lamberti J, Sade RM, et al. Open heart surgery during the first three months of life. *J Thoarac Cardiovasc Surg* 1974;68:719–731.
24. Chang AC, Hanley FL, Weindling SN, et al. Left heart support with a ventricular assist device in an infant with acute myocarditis. *Crit Care Med* 1992;20:712–715.

25. Chatterjee S, Rosensweig J. Evaluation of intra-aortic balloon counterpulsation. *J Thorac Cardiovasc Surg*, 1971;61:405–410.

26. Cheung PY, Vickar DB, Hallgren RA, et al. Carotid artery reconstruction in neonates receiving extracorporeal membrane oxygenation: A 4-year follow-up study. Western Canadian ECMO Follow-Up Group. *J Pediatr Surg* 1997;32:560–564.

27. Coffin SE, Bell LM, Manning M, et al. Nosocomial infections in neonates receiving extracorporeal membrane oxygenation. *Infect Control Hosp Epidemiol* 1997;18(2):93–96.

28. Coskun O, Parsa A, Weitkemper H, et al. Heart transplantation in children after mechanical circulatory support: Comparison of heart transplantation with ventricular assist devices and elective heart transplantation. *ASAIO J* 2005;51:495–497.

29. Costa RJ, Chard RB, Nunn GR, et al. Ventricular assist devices in pediatric cardiac surgery. *Ann Thorac Surg* 1995;60:S536–S538.

30. del Nido PJ, Armitage JM, Fricker FJ, et al. Extracorporeal membrane oxygenation support as a bridge to pediatric heart transplantation. *Circulation* 1994;90(pt 2):II66–II69.

31. del Nido PJ, Dalton HJ, Thompson AE, et al. Extracorporeal membrane oxygenator rescue in children during cardiac arrest after cardiac surgery. *Circulation* 1992;86(suppl II):II300–II304.

32. del Nido PJ, Duncan BW, Mayer JE Jr, et al. Left ventricular assist device improves survival in children with left ventricular dysfunction after repair of anomalous origin of the left coronary artery from the pulmonary artery. *Ann Thorac Surg* 1999;67:169–172.

33. del Nido PJ, Swan PR, Benson LN, et al. Successful use of intraaortic balloon pumping in a 2-kilogram infant. *Ann Thorac Surg* 1988;46:574–576.

34. Dela Cruz TV, Stewart DL, Winston SJ, et al. Risk factors for intracranial hemorrhage in the extracorporeal membrane oxygenation patient. *J Perinatol* 1997;17(1):18–23.

35. Dembitsky WP, Moreno-Cabral RJ, Adamson RM, et al. Emergency resuscitation using portable extracorporeal membrane oxygenation. *Ann Thorac Surg* 1993;55:304–309.

36. Douglass BH, Keenan AL, Purohit DM. Bacterial and fungal infection in neonates undergoing venoarterial extracorporeal membrane oxygenation: An analysis of the registry data of the extracorporeal life support organization. *Artif Organs* 1996;20(3):202–208.

37. du Plessis AJ, Jonas RA, Wypij D, et al. Perioperative effects of alpha-stat versus pH-stat strategies for deep hypothermic cardiopulmonary bypass in infants. *J Thorac Cardiovasc Surg* 1997;114:991–1001.

38. du Plessis AJ. Neurologic complications of cardiac disease in the newborn. *Clin Perinat* 1997;24:807–825.

39. Duncan BW, Bohn DJ, Atz AM, et al. Mechanical circulatory support for the treatment of children with acute fulminant myocarditis. *J Thorac Cardiovasc Surg* 2001;122:440–448.

40. Duncan BW, Ibrahim AE, Hraska V, et al. Use of rapid-deployment ECMO for the resuscitation of pediatric patients with heart disease after cardiac arrest. *J Thorac Cardiovasc Surg* 1998;116:305–311.

41. Duncan BW. Mechanical circulatory support in children with cardiac disease. *J Thorac Cardiovasc Surg* 1999;117:529–542.

42. Eghtesady P, Nelson D, Schwartz SM, et al. Heparin-induced thrombocytopenia complicating support by the Berlin Heart. *ASAIO J* 2005;51:820–825.

43. Elliot M. Modified ultrafiltration and open heart surgery in children. *Paediatr Anaesth* 1999;9:1–5.

44. Extracorporeal Life Support Organization. ECLS Registry Report: International summary, July 2006, Ann Arbor, Michigan.

45. Fiser WP, Yetman AT, Gunselman RJ, et al. Pediatric arteriovenous extracorporeal membrane oxygenation (ECMO) as a bridge to cardiac transplantation. *J Heart Lung Transplant* 2003;22:770–777.

46. Fox LS, Blackstone EH, Kirklin JW, et al. Relationship of brain blood flow and oxygen consumption to perfusion flow rate during profoundly hypothermic cardiopulmonary bypass. *J Thorac Cardiovasc Surg* 1984;87:658–664.

47. Fraser CD Jr, Carberry KE, Owens WR, et al. Preliminary experience with the MicroMed DeBakey pediatric ventricular assist device. *Semin Thorac Cardiovasc Surg Pediatr Card Surg Annu* 2006;109–114.

48. Gajarski RJ, Mosca RS, Ohye RG, et al. Use of extracorporeal life support as a bridge to pediatric cardiac transplantation. *J Heart Lung Transplant* 2003;22:28–34.

49. Gaynor JW, Gerdes M, Zackai EH, et al. Apolipoprotein E genotype and neurodevelopmental sequelae of infant cardiac surgery. *J Thorac Cadiovasc Surg* 2003;126:1736.

50. Gessler P, Pfenninger J, Pfammatter JP, et al. Inflammatory response of neutrophil granulocytes and monocytes after cardiopulmonary bypass in pediatric cardiac surgery. *Intensive Care Med* 2002;28:1786–1791.

51. Greeley WJ, Kern FH, Ungerleider RM, et al. The effect of hypothermic cardiopulmonary bypass and total circulatory arrest on cerebral metabolism in neonates, infants and children. *J Thorac Cardiovasc Surg* 1991;101:783–794.

52. Hall RI, Smith MS, Rocker G. Systemic inflammatory response to cardiopulmonary bypass: Pathophysiological, therapeutic and pharmacological considerations. *Anesth Analg* 1997;85:766–782.

53. Havemann L, McMahon CJ, Ganame J, et al. Rapid ventricular remodeling with left ventricular unloading postventricular assist device placement: New insights with strain imaging. *J Am Soc Echocardiogr* 2006;19(3):355.e9–355.e11.

54. Hetzer R, Alexi-Meskishvili V, Weng Y, et al. Mechanical cardiac support in the young with the Berlin Heart EXCOR pulsatile ventricular assist device: 15 years' experience. *Semin Thorac Cardiovasc Surg Pediatr Card Surg Annu* 2006;99–108.

55. Hetzer R, Potapov EV, Stiller B, et al. Improvement in survival after mechanical circulatory support with pneumatic pulsatile ventricular assist devices in pediatric patients. *Ann Thorac Surg* 2006;82:917–924.

56. Hetzer R, Muller J, Weng Y, et al. Cardiac recovery in dilated cardiomyopathy by unloading with a left ventricular assist device. *Ann Thorac Surg* 1999;68:742–749.

57. Hickey PR, Andersen NP. Deep hypothermic circulatory arrest: A review of pathophysiology and clinical experience as a basis for anesthetic management. *J Cardiothorac Anesth* 1987;1:137.

58. Hill JD, Reinhartz O. Clinical outcomes in pediatric patients implanted with Thoratec ventricular assist device. *Semin Thorac Cardiovasc Surg Pediatr Card Surg Annu* 2006;115–122.

59. Huang SC, Wu ET, Ko WJ, et al. Clinical implication of blood levels of B-type natriuretic peptide in pediatric patients on mechanical circulatory support. *Ann Thorac Surg* 2006;81:2267–2272.

60. Hunkeler NM, et al. Extracorporeal life support in cyanotic congenital heart disease before cardiovascular operation. *Am J Cardiol* 1992;69:790.

61. Ibrahim AE, Duncan BW, Blume ED, et al. Long-term follow-up of pediatric cardiac patients requiring mechanical circulatory support. *Ann Thorac Surg* 2000;69:186–192.

62. Ibrahim AE, Duncan BW. Long-term follow-up of children with cardiac disease requiring mechanical circulatory support. In: Duncan BW, eds. *Mechanical Circulatory Support for Cardiac and Respiratory Failure in Pediatric Cardiac Patients*. New York: Marcel Dekker Inc, 2001:205–220.

63. Ishino K, Alexi-Meskishvili V, Hetzer R. Myocardial recovery through ECMO after repair of total anomalous pulmonary venous connection: The importance of left heart unloading. *Eur J Cardiothorac Surg* 1997;11:585–587.

64. Ishino K, Loebe M, Uhlemann F, et al. Circulatory support with paracorporeal pneumatic ventricular assist device (VAD) in infants and children. *Euro J Cardiothorac Surg* 1997;11:965–972.

65. Jacob JP, Ojito JW, McConaghey TW, et al. Rapid cardiopulmonary support for children with complex congenital heart disease. *Ann Thorac Surg* 2000;70:742–750.

66. Jaggers JJ, Forbess JM, Shah AS, et al. Extracorporeal membrane oxygenation for infant postcardiotomy support: Significance of shunt management. *Ann Thorac Surg* 2000;69:1476–1483.

67. Jensen E, Andreasson S, Bengtsson A, et al. Influence of two different perfusion systems on inflammatory response in pediatric heart surgery. *Ann Thorac Surg* 2003;75:919–925.

68. Jonas RA, Wypij D, Roth SJ, et al. The influence of hemodilution on outcome after hypothermic cardiopulmonary bypass: Results of a randomized trial in infants. *J Thorac Cardiovasc Surg* 2003;126:1765–1774.

69. Journois D, Israel-Biet D, Pouard P, et al. High-volume, zero-balanced hemofiltration to reduce delayed inflammatory response to cardiopulmonary bypass in children. *Anesth* 1996;85:965–976.

70. Gibbon JH Jr. Application of a mechanical heart and lung apparatus to cardiac surgery. *Minn Med* 1954;37:171–185.

71. Kaczmarek I, Sachweh J, Groetzner J, et al. Mechanical circulatory support in pediatric patients with the MEDOS assist device. *ASAIO J* 2005;51:498–500.

72. Karl TR, Horton SB. Centrifugal pump ventricular assist device in pediatric cardiac surgery. In: Duncan BW, ed. *Mechanical Support for Cardiac and Respiratory Failure in Pediatric Patients*. New York: Marcel Dekker Inc, 2001:21–47.

73. Karl TR, Sano S, Horton S, et al. Centrifugal pump left heart assist in pediatric cardiac operations. Indication, technique, and results. *J Thorac Cardiovasc Surg* 1991;102:624–630.

74. Karl TR, Iyer KS, Sano S, et al. Infant ECMO cannulation technique allowing preservation of carotid and jugular vessels. *Ann Thorac Surg* 1990;50:488–489.

75. Karl TR. Extracorporeal circulatory support in infants and children. *Semin Thorac Cardiovasc Surg* 1994;6:154–160.

76. Keenan HT, Thiagarajan R, Stephens KE, et al. Pulmonary function after modified venovenous ultrafiltration in infants: A prospective, randomized trial. *J Thorac Cardiovas Surg* 2000;119:501–505.

77. Kennaugh JM. Impact of new treatments for neonatal pulmonary hypertension on extracorporeal membrane oxygenation use and outcome. *J Perinatol* 1997;17(5):366–369.

78. DiNardo JA. Physiology and Techniques of Extracorporeal Circulation in the Pediatric Patient. In: Lake CL, ed. *Pediatric Cardiac Anesthesia*. Philadelphia, PA: Lippincott Williams & Wilkins, 2005:228–250.

79. Kesler KA, Pruitt AL, Turrentine MW, et al. Temporary left-sided mechanical cardiac support during acute myocarditis. *J Heart Lung Transplant* 1994;13:268–270.

80. Kirklin JW, Dushane JW, Patrick RT, et al. Intracardiac surgery with the aid of a mechanical pump-oxygenator system (Gibbon type): Report of eight cases. *Mayo Clin Proc* 1955;30:201–206.

81. Kirshbom PM, Bridges ND, Myung RJ, et al. Use of extracorporeal membrane oxygenation in pediatric thoracic organ transplantation. *J Thorac Cardiovasc Surg* 2002;123:130–136.

82. Klein MD, Shaheen KW, Whittlesey GC, et al. Extracorporeal membrane oxygenation for the circulatory support of children after repair of congenital heart disease. *J Thorac Cardiovasc Surg* 1990;100:498–505.

83. Klein MD, Lessin MS, Whittlesey GC, et al. Carotid artery and jugular vein ligation with and without hypoxia in the rat. *J Pediatr Surg* 1997; 32:565–570.

84. Kulik TJ, Moler FW, Palmisano JM, et al. Outcome-associated factors in pediatric patients treated with extracorporeal membrane oxygenator after cardiac surgery. *Circulation* 1996;94(suppl):II63–II68.

85. Laliberte E, Cecere R, Tchervenkov C, et al. The combined use of extracorporeal life support and the Berlin Heart pulsatile pediatric ventricular assist device as a bridge to transplant in a toddler. *J Extra Corpor Technol* 2004;36(2):158–161.

86. Laussen PC. Optimal blood gas management during deep hypothermic pediatric cardiac surgery: Alpha-stat is easy, but pH-stat may be preferable. *Paediatr Anaesth* 2002;12(3):199–204.

87. Levi D, Marelli D, Plunkett M, et al. Use of assist devices and ECMO to bridge pediatric patients with cardiomyopathy to transplantation. *J Heart Lung Transplant* 2002;21:760–770.

88. Lillehei CW, Varco RL, Cohen M, et al. The first open-heart repairs of ventricular septal defect, atrioventricular communis, and tetralogy of Fallot using extracorporeal circulation by cross-circulation: A 30-year follow-up. *Ann Thoracic Surg* 1986;41:4–21.

89. Loebe M, Muller J, Hetzer R. Ventricular assistance for recovery of cardiac failure. *Curr Opin Cardiol* 1999;14(3):234–248.

90. Marcus B. Successful use of transesophageal echocardiography during extracorporeal membrane oxygenation in infants after cardiac operations. *J Thorac Cardiovasc Surg* 1995;109:846–848.

91. Merkle F, Boettcher W, Stiller B, et al. Pulsatile mechanical cardiac assistance in pediatric patients with the Berlin Heart ventricular assist device. *J Extra Corpor Technol* 2003;35:115–120.

92. Minich LL, Tani LY, McGough EC, et al. A novel approach to pediatric intraaortic balloon pump timing using M-mode echocardiography. *Am J Cardiol* 1997;80:367–369.

93. Morales DL, Dibardino DJ, Mckenzie ED, et al. Lessons learned from the first application of the DeBakey VAD Child: An intracorporeal ventricular assist device for children. *J Heart Lung Transplant* 2005;24:331–337.

94. Moran JM, Opravil M, Gorman AJ, et al. Pulmonary artery balloon counterpulsation for right ventricular failure: II. Clinical experience. *Ann Thorac Surg* 1984;38:254–259.

95. Moront MG, Katz NM, Keszler M, et al. Extracorporeal membrane oxygenation for neonatal respiratory failure. A report of 50 cases. *J Thorac Cardiovasc Surg* 1989;97:706–714.

96. Morris MC, Wernovsky G, Nadkarni VM. Survival outcomes after extracorporeal cardiopulmonary resuscitation instituted during active chest compressions following refractory in-hospital pediatric cardiac arrest. *Pediatr Crit Care Med* 2004;5(5):440–446.

97. Muller J. Weaning from mechanical cardiac support in patients with idiopathic dilated cardiomyopathy [see comments]. *Circulation* 1997;96: 542–549.

98. Nathan M, Baird C, Fynn-Thompson F, et al. Successful implantation of a Berlin Heart biventricular assist device in a failing single ventricle. *J Thorac Cardiovasc Surg* 2006;131:1407–1408.

99. Newburger JW, Jonas RA, Wernovsky G, et al. A comparison of the perioperative neurologic effects of hypothermic circulatory arrest versus lowflow cardiopulmonary bypass in infant heart surgery. *N Engl J Med* 1993;329:1057–1064.

100. Nose Y. Food and Drug Administration workshop on regulatory process for pediatric mechanical circulatory support devices. *Artif Organs* 2006;30(6):409–410.

101. Pantalos GM, Minich LL, Tani LY, et al. Estimation of timing errors for the intraaortic balloon pump use in pediatric patients. *ASAIO J* 1999; 45(3):166–171.

102. Park JK, Hsu DT, Gersony WM. Intraaortic balloon pump management of refractory congestive heart failure in children. *Pediatr Cardiol* 1993;14(1): 19–22.

103. Parra DA, Totapally BR, Zahn E, et al. Outcome of cardiopulmonary resuscitation in a pediatric cardiac intensive care unit. *Crit Care Med* 2000;28:3296–3300.

104. Pasnik J, Siniewicz K, Moll JA, et al. Effect of cardiopulmonary bypass on neutrophil activity in pediatric open-heart surgery. *Arch Immunol Ther Exp (Warsz)* 2005;53(3):272–277.

105. Pekkan K, Frakes D, De Zelicourt D, et al. Coupling pediatric ventricle assist devices to the Fontan circulation: Simulations with a lumpedparameter model. *ASAIO J* 2005;51:618–628.

106. Pinkney KA, Minich LL, Tani LY, et al. Current results with intraaortic balloon pumping in infants and children. *Ann Thorac Surg* 2002;73: 887–891.

107. Raithel SC, et al. Extracorporeal membrane oxygenation in children after cardiac surgery. *Circulation* 1992;86(suppl):II305–II310.

108. Rogers AJ, Trento A, Siewers RD, et al. Extracorporeal membrane oxygenation for postcardiotomy cardiogenic shock in children. *Ann Thorac Surg* 1989;47:903–906.

109. Rose EA, Gelijns AC, Moskowitz AJ, et al. Long-term mechanical left ventricular assistance for end-stage heart failure. *N Engl J Med* 2001;345: 1435–1443.

110. Schmitz C, Welz A, Dewald O, et al. Switch from a BIVAD to a LVAD in a boy with Kawasaki disease. *Ann Thorac Surg* 2000;69:1270–1271.

111. Ashton RC, Oz MC, Michler RE, et al. Left ventricular assist device options in pediatric patients. *ASAIO J* 1995;41:M277–M280.

112. Slogoff ST, Girgis KZ, Keats AS. Etiologic factors in neuro-psychiatric complications associated with cardiopulmonary bypass. *Anesth Analg* 1982;61:903–911.

113. Slomin AD, Patel KM, Ruttimann UE, et al. Cardiopulmonary resuscitation in pediatric intensive care units. *Crit Care Med* 1997;25:1951–1955.

114. Smoot L, O'Brien P, Blume ED, et al. Perioperative mechanical support in pediatric heart transplantation. *Circulation* 1999;100(suppl).

115. Stiller B, Dahnert I, Weng Y, et al. Children may survive severe myocarditis with prolonged use of biventricular assist devices. *Heart* 1999;82: 237–240.

116. Stiller B, Lemmer J, Merkle F, et al. Consumption of blood products during mechanical circulatory support in children: Comparison between ECMO and a pulsatile ventricular assist device. *Intensive Care Med* 2004;30:1814–1820.

117. Stiller B, Weng Y, Hubler M, et al. Pneumatic pulsatile ventricular assist devices in children under 1 year of age. *Eur J Cardiothorac Surg* 2005;28: 234–239.

118. Uber BE, Webber SA, Morell VO, et al. Hemodynamic guidelines for design and control of a turbodynamic pediatric ventricular assist device. *ASAIO J* 2006;52(4):471–478.

119. Undar A. Outcomes of the First International Conference on Pediatric Mechanical Circulatory Support Systems and Pediatric Cardiopulmonary Perfusion. *ASAIO J* 2006;52(1):1–3.

120. Verrier EW, Boyle EM. Endothelial cell injury in cardiovascular surgery: An overview. *Ann Thoracac Surg* 1997;64:S2–S8.

121. Walters HL 3rd, Hakimi M, Rice MD, et al. Pediatric cardiac surgical ECMO: Multivariate analysis of risk factors for hospital death. *Ann Thorac Surg* 1995;60:329–336; discussion 336–337.

122. Weinhaus L, Canter C, Noetzel M, et al. Extracorporeal membrane oxygenation for circulatory support after repair of congenital heart defects. *Ann Thorac Surg* 1989;48:206–212.

123. Weiss WJ. Pulsatile pediatric ventricular assist devices. *ASAIO J* 2005; 51(5):540–545.

124. Wernovsky G, Wypij D, Jonas RA. Postoperative course and hemodynamic profile after the arterial switch operation in neonates and infants: A comparison of low-flow cardiopulmonary bypass versus circulatory arrest. *Circulation* 1995;92:2226–2235.

125. Wilson JM, Bower LK, Thompson JE, et al. ECMO in evolution: The impact of changing patient demographics and alternative therapies on ECMO. *J Pediatr Surg* 1996;31:1116–1122; discussion 1122–1123.

126. Zaritsky A. Outcome following cardiopulmonary resuscitation in the pediatric intensive care unit. *Crit Care Med* 1997;25:1937.

CHAPTER 22 ■ CARDIOPULMONARY AND RIGHT-LEFT HEART INTERACTIONS

ANDREW N. REDINGTON, MD, FRCS

The singular function of the right ventricle, left ventricle, and the lungs will be discussed elsewhere. Nonetheless, particularly in the field of congenital heart disease, we are becoming increasingly aware of the importance of the interactions between them. There is continual cross talk between the two sides of the heart, and in turn, the ventricles are continually responding to subtle changes occurring within the thorax as a whole. In this chapter, these interactions, and their modification by congenital heart disease and its surgical repair, will be discussed.

COMPARISON OF RIGHT AND LEFT HEART HEMODYNAMICS

The average cardiac output from the right ventricle must, of course, essentially equal the cardiac output from the left heart. Nonetheless, the mechanism by which this is achieved is very different. The right ventricle performs approximately one quarter of the external mechanical work compared with its left ventricular counterpart. External mechanical work is a function of stroke volume and developed ventricular pressure, and is more accurately described as the area enclosed by the ventricular pressure–volume curve. Figure 22.1 shows a schematic comparison of left and right ventricular pressure–volume curves. Not only is the developed pressure substantially lower in the right ventricle, but its trapezoidal shape still further reduces the amount of work performed on the circulation to generate the cardiac output. The left ventricle essentially works

as a square wave pump, its stroke work being reasonably well represented as a direct product of its stroke volume and developed pressure (stroke work = stroke volume × peak left ventricular pressure − minimum left ventricular pressure). Because of its ability to eject blood into the pulmonary circulation during both pressure rise and pressure fall (1), the external work performed by the right ventricle cannot be described using such a simple derivation. Furthermore, it can be seen that small changes in hemodynamics might impose a major change to global workload of the right ventricle. Indeed, small changes in right ventricular afterload can lead to major changes in workload and the shape of the pressure–volume characteristics to mirror the left ventricle (2).

The trapezoidal shape of the right ventricular pressure–volume relationship is exquisitely matched to the low hydraulic impedance imposed by the pulmonary vascular bed. Unlike the systemic vascular resistance, which reflects a dynamic balance between vasodilator and vasoconstrictor influences, the pulmonary vascular bed appears to be maximally vasodilated. The low pulmonary vascular resistance requires a healthy endothelium and normal lung function for its integrity. In health, additional inhaled nitric oxide, for example, fails to lower the pulmonary vascular resistance, suggesting pulmonary endothelial vasodilatory capacity is at its maximum (3). This is a markedly different mechanism to that of the systemic vascular bed where a wide portfolio of vasodilatory substances can lower its resistance. The pulmonary vascular bed is also uniquely affected by external factors. The status of lung inflation, even the normal circulation, has major effects on the pulmonary vascular resistance and hemodynamic function. Normal respiration, ventilating around functional residual capacity, minimizes the pulmonary vascular resistance. Underinflation of the lungs leads to an increased pulmonary vascular resistance, as a result of atelectasis and secondary alveolar hypoxemia, and overinflation of the lungs leads to an increase, secondary to alveolar stretch and direct vascular compression (Fig. 22.2) (4). Both should be avoided whenever right ventricular afterload needs to be minimized.

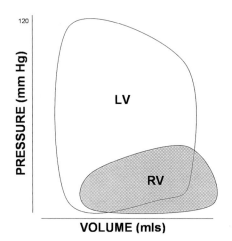

FIGURE 22.1 Schematic representations of right (*shaded*) and left ventricular pressure–volume relationships. The external stroke work of the right ventricle (RV; area enclosed by loop) is markedly lower than the left ventricle (LV) (see text for details).

CARDIOPULMONARY INTERACTIONS IN THE NORMAL CIRCULATION

Descent of the diaphragm during normal inspiration leads to a modest fall in pleural pressure (3 to 5 cm of water) (5) and a concomitant rise in intra-abdominal pressure. These two changes lead to increased venous return and an increased right ventricular stroke volume, in accord with the Frank Starling mechanism. There is thus a waxing and waning of cardiac output of approximately 10% to 15% during the cardiac cycle (6).

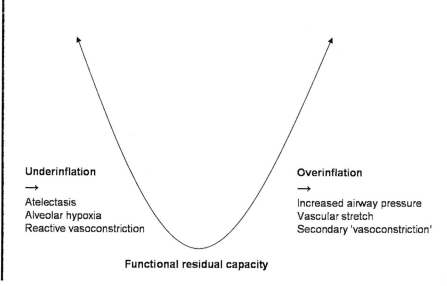

FIGURE 22.2 Effect of lung inflation on pulmonary vascular resistance. Resistance is at its nadir when the lung is at functional residual capacity.

The classic experiments of Cournand in the 1940s (7) were interpreted as confirmation that right heart filling and cardiac output were related to intrathoracic pressure. Positive-pressure ventilation via a mask in conscious volunteers led to a fall in cardiac output of approximately 10% to 15%. This was initially thought to be entirely due to changes in systemic venous return (and reduced ventricular preload) imposed by a raised mean intrathoracic pressure. It has subsequently become clear that reduced preload, as a result of increased airway pressure, is not the whole story. In an elegant series of experiments in dogs, Henning (8) showed that restoration of preload during positive-pressure ventilation failed to restore cardiac output to its baseline levels. The persistent reduction in right ventricular stroke volume, despite normalized preload, suggested an adverse effect on intrinsic right ventricular performance. It was hypothesized that the right ventricle shows signs of reduced systolic function, even under the circumstances of a modest hemodynamic burden imposed by lung hyperinflation, as a result of increased afterload occurring via the mechanism described in Figure 22.2. No matter what the mechanism, however, the functional implications of these changes are not simply theoretic. In a study of children undergoing cardiac catheterization performed by Shekerdemian et al. (9), a negative-pressure cuirass device was used to mimic normal ventilation to compare the effects of positive-pressure and negative-pressure ventilation on cardiac output. In essentially normal children having undergone closure of a small arterial duct, for example, there is an approximate 16% fall in cardiac output, simply as a result of a modest rise in mean airway pressure (to approximately 8 cm of water) secondary to positive-pressure ventilation. These adverse hemodynamic effects of increased right ventricular afterload (negative cardiopulmonary interactions) become even more important when the right heart circulation is affected by congenital heart disease.

Cardiopulmonary Interactions in Congenital Heart Disease

Given that normal right heart function is dependent on a low right ventricular afterload, normal ventricular preload, and maintained right ventricular systolic function, it would be surprising if congenital heart diseases did not have major effects on its performance. This is indeed the case.

Reduced Right Ventricular Contractile Performance

It has long been known that right ventricular ischemia, in the setting of atherosclerotic coronary disease, is an extremely poorly tolerated hemodynamic burden (10). This, in part, is related to adverse right-left heart interactions (see below), but illustrates the importance of right ventricular contractile performance, even in the presence of a relatively normal pulmonary vascular bed. A more common scenario in congenital heart disease is the adverse effect of cardiopulmonary bypass on right heart function. Brookes et al. (11) showed that even a brief period of cardiopulmonary bypass and cardioplegic arrest, during coronary bypass surgery, leads to a significant decline in right ventricular systolic performance, as assessed by end-systolic elastance. This translates to an even greater dependence on cardiopulmonary interactions in children undergoing congenital heart surgery. Shekerdemian (9), in the study described above, showed that positive-pressure ventilation had an even greater adverse effect in such patients. Compared with negative-pressure ventilation, there was on average a 25% fall in cardiac output with positive-pressure ventilation in children on the intensive care unit after simple right heart surgery (ventricular septal defect [VSD], atrial septal defect [ASD], etc.).

CARDIOPULMONARY INTERACTIONS AND THE ABNORMAL RIGHT HEART

The potential for beneficial and adverse cardiopulmonary interactions is greater when the right heart is intrinsically abnormal because of congenital anomalies or is primarily affected by surgery. There are two circumstances in which these concepts are exemplified, those patients with abnormal right ventricular diastolic function and those with exclusion of the right ventricle from the venopulmonary circulation.

Abnormal Right Ventricular Diastolic Function

It is now known that restrictive right ventricular physiology is a common sequel of surgery for hypoplasia of the right heart, e.g., pulmonary atresia with intact ventricular septum (12), and after repair of tetralogy of Fallot, for example. The characteristic physiology of these patients is the presence of antegrade diastolic pulmonary blood flow during atrial systole. This occurs when the resistance to right ventricular filling exceeds the pulmonary vascular resistance. Atrial contraction ejects blood through the tricuspid valve, but there is little or no right ventricular filling as the blood passes through the right ventricle (which acts as a passive conduit) to the pulmonary artery. Consequently, up to one third of the antegrade pulmonary blood flow, and therefore cardiac output, is dependent on atrial systole. Furthermore, this flow is generated by only modest pressure transients (1 or 2 mm Hg) between the right atrium and the pulmonary artery in diastole. Clearly a low pulmonary vascular resistance is crucial for this source of cardiac output to be maintained. An important element of the total pulmonary resistance, as discussed above, is the mean airway pressure. Indeed, antegrade diastolic flow is often entirely abrogated during positive-pressure inspiration. Conversely, negative-pressure ventilation may have a major beneficial effect on cardiac output. In postoperative tetralogy patients, positive-pressure ventilation reduces cardiac output by >30% compared with that achieved during negative-pressure ventilation with a cuirass device (13).

The influence of cardiopulmonary interaction is even more impressive when one considers right heart bypass procedures. Here, resting and exercise pulmonary blood flow is markedly dependent on the work of breathing. In our earlier Doppler studies, the phase relationship between ventilation and pulmonary blood flow was shown clearly in both the venopulmonary and atriopulmonary Fontan circulations (14,15). Subsequently, MRI studies have suggested that well over one third of the cardiac output occurs as a direct result of the work of breathing (16). This may be even more important during exercise (17), particularly in those with total cavopulmonary anastomosis. Positive-pressure ventilation in the Fontan circulation has long been known to adversely affect cardiac output. In early studies of the use of positive end-expiratory pressure, a linear relationship between positive end-expiratory pressure and cardiac output was demonstrated (18). Unsurprisingly, negative-pressure ventilation under these circumstances can lead to a marked increase in cardiac output compared with positive-pressure ventilation. In a separate series of studies, Shekedemian et al. (19) showed the profound effects of positive and negative pressure ventilation on the pattern of pulmonary blood flow in the Fontan circuit (Fig. 22.3) as well as on total cardiac output measured by respiratory mass spectrometry.

These studies and others have reinforced the desirability of normal ventilation in such circulations, and this, wherever possible, should be established as early as possible after surgery. In those requiring positive-pressure ventilation, efforts to reduce the mean airway pressure will reap benefits in terms of changes in cardiac output. Thus, minimizing positive end-expiratory pressure, shortening the inspiratory time, and reducing the airway pressure plateau time will all help to reduce the hemodynamic burden on the right heart. Clearly this must not be at the expense of alveolar ventilation (to

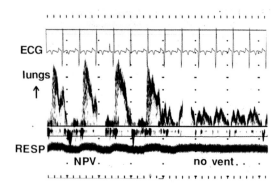

FIGURE 22.3 The effects of negative-pressure ventilation (NPV) on the pattern of pulmonary blood flow after total cavopulmonary connection. Each negative pressure breath is associated with massive augmentation of pulmonary blood flow, an effect abolished when the ventilator is switched off (no vent).

avoid hypercapnic pulmonary vasoconstriction) or alveolar inflation (to avoid hypoxemic vasoconstriction).

Exclusion of the Right Ventricle

Because of the very marked changes in right ventricular hemodynamics imposed by progressive pulmonary hypertension or right ventricular outflow tract obstruction, the effects of subtle changes in airway pressure on right ventricular intrinsic contractile performance are much less marked. Indeed, one can consider the pressure–volume relationships of the hypertensive right ventricle to be similar to those of the normal left ventricle (2). Consequently, while changes in preload will continue to occur, the effects of afterload are much less marked. Also, it should not be forgotten that the adverse effects of positive-pressure ventilation on the right heart are in contradistinction to those on the left heart, particularly the failing left ventricle.

CARDIOPULMONARY INTERACTIONS AND THE LEFT HEART

Although the manifestations are different, the left ventricle is also subject to cardiopulmonary interactions and the effect of mean airway pressure on its function. Although in general the effects of increased mean airway pressure are largely adverse on the right heart, they are largely beneficial on the left heart. This is because the total afterload of the left ventricle (transmural pressure) is reduced by increased mean airway pressure (20). Although essentially insignificant to the normal left ventricle, such changes can provide beneficial effects, for example, in dilated cardiomyopathy. Indeed, continuous positive airway pressure (CPAP) has a multitude of beneficial effects to the failing left heart (21). By increasing alveolar pressure, the transalveolar gradient for edema formation is reduced. Furthermore, the afterload of the left ventricle is also reduced, improving its ejection fraction and stroke volume. Although relatively infrequently used in pediatric practice, CPAP masks have proven to be particularly useful in the dilated cardiomyopathy of ischemic and acquired heart disease in adults (22), and such therapy merits further investigation in children.

RIGHT-LEFT HEART INTERACTIONS

It has been traditional to examine left and right ventricular function as separate entities. Nonetheless, the last two decades have seen an explosion in our understanding of the ways in which the two sides of the heart interrelate and contribute to each other. Not only is this a manifestation of its shared cavity, the pericardium, but also the recognition of shared myofibers that can neither be defined as exclusively left or right ventricular (23). Thus, the function of the left ventricle has profound effects on the function of the right ventricle, and vice versa, both in health and disease.

The Effects of the Left Ventricle on the Right Ventricle

The classic experiment of Damiano et al. in 1991 (24) confirmed the presence of substantial cross talk between the ventricles in health. Albeit in an experimental model, the effects of left ventricular performance on right ventricular force generation were clearly demonstrated. In their exquisite study, the electrically isolated but mechanically contiguous ventricles were examined during individual chamber pacing (Fig. 22.4). Under these circumstances, pacing the right ventricle led to virtually no mechanical effects on the left side of the heart. Pacing the electrically isolated left ventricle, however, led to almost normal right ventricular pressure development. It appears, therefore, that the geometric change, consequent on left ventricular shortening, imposes a major mechanical effect on the right ventricle. The crescent-shaped free wall, wrapped around the ventricular septum and contiguous with the left ventricular free wall, is presumably deformed to generate a right ventricular pressure. This effect appears to be largely independent of the right ventricular free wall function. In another set of experiments, Hoffman et al. (25) showed that replacement of the right ventricular free wall with a noncontractile patch was still associated with significant right ventricular pressure generation during left ventricular contraction. Overall, it has been estimated that over one third of the work performed by the right ventricle is a direct consequence of left ventricular shortening. It might be possible to harness this ventricular-ventricular cross talk to improve biventricular function. In animal experiments, aortic constriction, leading to an increase in left ventricular afterload and work, was shown to increase right ventricular stroke volume, again as a result of the cross talk phenomenon (26).

The Effects of the Right Ventricle on the Left Ventricle

In the experiments by Hoffman et al. (25) described above, the effect of left ventricular shortening on right ventricular (RV) pressure development in a model of RV free wall replacement was described. This experiment also showed that as the size of the artificial right ventricle was increased, there appeared to be an adverse effect on left ventricular mechanical function. As the right ventricle dilated, left ventricular pressure development fell. Whether this was a parallel effect (reflecting adverse ventricular cross talk) or a series effect (reflecting reduced cardiac output from the right ventricle and therefore reduced preload to the left

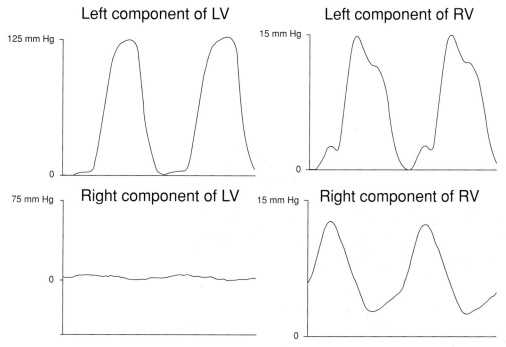

FIGURE 22.4 This study demonstrates the passive effect of active contraction of the contralateral ventricle (see text for details). Ventricular-ventricular interaction is shown clearly in the top right-hand panel. There is almost normal right ventricular pressure development when the left ventricle (LV) contracts, even though the right ventricle (RV) is electrically isolated. (Redrawn from Damiano RJ Jr, La Follette P Jr, Cox JL, et al. Significant left ventricular contribution to right ventricular systolic function. *Am J Physiol* 1991;261(pt 2):H1514–H1524, with permission.)

ventricle) could not be determined in these experiments. In the mid-1990s, Brooks et al. (27) aimed to dissect out these influences in a porcine model. Isolated right ventricular ischemia was used to induce acute right heart dilation, during which right and left ventricular contractile performance was measured using end-systolic elastance derived from pressure–volume analysis. It was shown that right ventricular dilation imposes adverse effects on left ventricular mechanical performance directly, presumably owing to geometric changes influencing left ventricular contractile efficiency. These effects were more manifest when the pericardium was intact, supporting this hypothesis.

It would be naive to assume that all of these effects are manifestations purely of systolic interactions. Independent of major changes in contractile performance, adverse diastolic ventricular-ventricular interaction is frequently encountered. Primarily a manifestation of septal shift toward the left ventricle in early diastole, pulmonary hypertension, for example, leads to reduced left ventricular early diastolic filling velocities and increased dependence on atrial systole (28).

The superimposition of congenital heart disease and the effects of surgical correction further amplify these ventricular-ventricular effects and will be discussed below.

Right-Left Heart Interactions in Congenital Heart Disease

It is likely that all congenital heart diseases have more or less subtle abnormalities of ventricular-ventricular interaction. However there are some major, clinically significant interactions that bear more detailed analysis. These can loosely be described as functional and geometric and will be discussed in detail below.

Functional Interactions

Surgery to the right ventricular outflow tract almost invariably leads to some degree of residual pulmonary regurgitation, and it is now well known that this ventricular volume load leads to right ventricular dilation in most patients. The effects of pulmonary regurgitation after repair of tetralogy of Fallot are probably the best described example of this phenomenon. Although our understanding of the effects of right heart dilation under these circumstances have evolved over the last 15 years, it is only in the last 5 years that the biventricular effects

of this problem have become apparent. Several studies have now shown a loose but linear relationship between right ventricular ejection fraction and left ventricular ejection fraction late after repair of tetralogy of Fallot (29,30). Furthermore, those with overt biventricular dysfunction have a worse outcome compared with those without (30). Not only are ventricular-ventricular interactions important in terms of global function, but abnormalities of ventricular-ventricular timing may also have significant adverse effects. D'Andrea et al. (31) have explored this phenomenon in a recent study analyzing the dyssynchrony between the ventricles. They studied the onset of right and left ventricular contraction in patients after repair of tetralogy of Fallot, showing a worse exercise tolerance and an increased frequency of arrhythmia in those with significant ventricular-ventricular delay.

It is likely that subtle regional abnormalities will also have significant biventricular effects. Regional wall motion abnormalities have been described in virtually all congenital heart diseases (32,33). They are also almost always associated with decreased global performance and therefore likely biventricular effects. It remains to be seen whether this intraventricular and interventricular incoordination will be responsive to interventions such as biventricular pacing, but early data appear promising (34).

Geometric Interactions

Unlike the more directly functional interaction described above, acute changes in geometry can modify functional performance of both sides of the heart, particularly in congenital heart disease. Acute right heart dilation not only affects right ventricular performance, but also induces left ventricular dysfunction via systolic and diastolic interactions (see above).

More chronic geometric changes can lead to unique abnormalities in the setting of congenital heart disease. The systemic right ventricle is particularly susceptible to such changes. Here, the morphologic tricuspid valve is the systemic atrioventricular valve and is characterized by its septal papillary muscle and chordal attachments. It is now well recognized both under the circumstances of surgical repair of simple transposition and in the setting of congenitally corrected transposition that septal shift makes a significant contribution to the development of tricuspid regurgitation in these hearts. Conversely, efforts to modify this septal shift can produce profound improvements in the degree of tricuspid incompetence. Figure 22.5 shows just such a change. The right-hand panel from this

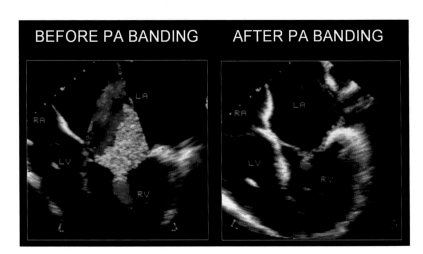

BEFORE PA BANDING   AFTER PA BANDING

FIGURE 22.5 The acute effects of pulmonary artery (PA) banding on tricuspid valve regurgitation in congenitally corrected transposition. Left ventricular (LV) hypertension induces septal shift toward the systemic right ventricle (RV), leading to restoration of tricuspid leaflet apposition by its effect on its septal attachments. As a result, the left atrial (LA) size is markedly reduced. RA, right atrium.

patient with congenitally corrected transposition shows a dilated right atrium and hugely dilated morphologic left atrium as a result of severe tricuspid valve incompetence. The left-hand panel shows minimal tricuspid incompetence in the same heart, just 20 seconds later. The reduction in tricuspid regurgitation and the remarkable change in left atrial size have occurred as a consequence of pulmonary artery banding. Elevation of left ventricular pressure to modify septal geometry restored tricuspid valve competence in this patient. This phenomenon has been demonstrated in patients after the Mustard procedure (35) as well as in patients undergoing left ventricular retraining in the setting of congenitally corrected transpositions. It is beyond the scope of this chapter to discuss the advisability, prerequisites, and methods for evaluation of left ventricular retraining under such circumstances, but by its

effects on tricuspid incompetence, pulmonary artery banding alone may be destination therapy for some of these patients.

CONCLUSIONS

Important cardiopulmonary and ventricular-ventricular interactions are intrinsic to normal cardiovascular physiology. The consequences of these effects are amplified by disease in the structural normal heart and may be profound when the heart is modified by congenital anomalies. Our understanding of the effects of congenital heart disease on cardiopulmonary and ventricular-ventricular interactions continues to evolve, but we have learned that description of functional performance in any patient is incomplete without their consideration.

References

1. Redington AN, Gray HH, Hodson ME, et al. Characterisation of the normal right ventricular pressure-volume relation by biplane angiography and simultaneous micromanometer pressure measurements. *Br Heart J* 1988; 59(1):23–30.
2. Redington AN, Rigby ML, Shinebourne EA, et al. Changes in the pressure-volume relation of the right ventricle when its loading conditions are modified. *Br Heart J* 1990;63(1):45–49.
3. Brett SJ, Chambers J, Bush A, et al. Pulmonary response of normal human subjects to inhaled vasodilator substances. *Clin Sci (Lond)* 1998 95:621–627.
4. Steingrub JS, Tidswell M, Higgins TL. Hemodynamic consequences of heart-lung interactions. *J Intensive Care Med* 2003;18(2):92–99.
5. Bromberger-Barnea B. Mechanical effects of inspiration on heart functions: A review. *Fed Proc* 1981;40:2172–2177.
6. Norgard G, Vik-Mo H. Effects of respiration on right ventricular size and function: An echocardiographic study. *Pediatr Cardiol* 1992;13(3):136–140.
7. Cournand A, Riley RL, Breed ES, et al. Measurement of cardiac output in man using the technique of catheterization of the right auricle or ventricle. *J Clin Invest* 1945;24(1):106–116.
8. Henning RJ. Effects of positive end-expiratory pressure on the right ventricle. *J Appl Physiol* 1986;61:819–826.
9. Shekerdemian LS, Bush A, Lincoln C, et al. Cardiopulmonary interactions in healthy children and children after simple cardiac surgery: The effects of positive and negative pressure ventilation. *Heart* 1997;78:587–593.
10. Pfisterer M. Right ventricular involvement in myocardial infarction and cardiogenic shock. *Lancet* 2003;362:392–394.
11. Brookes C, Ravn H, White P, et al. Acute right ventricular dilatation in response to ischemia significantly impairs left ventricular systolic performance. *Circulation* 1999;100:761–767.
12. Redington AN, Rigby ML, Hayes A, et al. Right ventricular diastolic function in children. *Am J Cardiol* 1991;67:329–330.
13. Cullen S, Shore D, Redington A. Characterization of right ventricular diastolic performance after complete repair of tetralogy of Fallot. Restrictive physiology predicts slow postoperative recovery. *Circulation* 1995;91:1782–1789.
14. Redington AN, Penny D, Shinebourne EA. Pulmonary blood flow after total cavopulmonary shunt. *Br Heart J* 1991;65(4):213–217.
15. Penny DJ, Redington AN. Doppler echocardiographic evaluation of pulmonary blood flow after the Fontan operation: The role of the lungs. *Br Heart J* 1991;66(5):372–374.
16. Fogel MA, Weinberg PM, Hoydu A, et al. The nature of flow in the systemic venous pathway measured by magnetic resonance blood tagging in patients having the Fontan operation. *J Thorac Cardiovasc Surg* 1997; 114:1032–1041.
17. Rosenthal M, Bush A, Deanfield J, et al. Comparison of cardiopulmonary adaptation during exercise in children after the atriopulmonary and total cavopulmonary connection Fontan procedures. *Circulation* 1995;91:372–378.
18. Williams DB, Kiernan PD, Metke MP, et al. Hemodynamic response to positive end-expiratory pressure following right atrium-pulmonary artery bypass (Fontan procedure). *J Thorac Cardiovasc Surg* 1984;87:856–861.
19. Shekerdemian LS, Bush A, Shore DF, et al. Cardiopulmonary interactions after Fontan operations: Augmentation of cardiac output using negative pressure ventilation. *Circulation* 1997;96:3934–3942.

20. Pinsky MR, Summer WR, Wise RA, et al. Augmentation of cardiac function by elevation of intrathoracic pressure. *J Appl Physiol* 1983;54:950–955.
21. Bradley TD, Logan AG, Kimoff RJ, et al.; CANPAP Investigators. Continuous positive airway pressure for central sleep apnea and heart failure. *N Engl J Med* 2005;353:2025–2033.
22. Mehta S, Liu PP, Fitzgerald FS, et al. Effects of continuous positive airway pressure on cardiac volumes in patients with ischemic and dilated cardiomyopathy. *Am J Respir Crit Care Med* 2000;161(1):128–134.
23. Anderson RH, Ho SY, Sanchez-Quintana D, et al. Heuristic problems in defining the three-dimensional arrangement of the ventricular myocytes. *Anat Rec A Discov Mol Cell Evol Biol* 2006;288:579–586.
24. Damiano RJ Jr, La Follette P Jr, Cox JL, et al. Significant left ventricular contribution to right ventricular systolic function. *Am J Physiol* 1991; 261(pt 2):H1514–H1524.
25. Hoffman D, Sisto D, Frater RW, et al. Left-to-right ventricular interaction with a noncontracting right ventricle. *J Thorac Cardiovasc Surg* 1994;107: 1496–1502.
26. Karunanithi MK, Michniewicz J, Young JA, et al. Effect of acutely increased left ventricular afterload on work output from the right ventricle in conscious dogs. *J Thorac Cardiovasc Surg* 2001;121:116–124.
27. Brookes CI, White PA, Bishop AJ, et al. Validation of a new intraoperative technique to evaluate load-independent indices of right ventricular performance in patients undergoing cardiac operations. *J Thorac Cardiovasc Surg* 1998;116:468–476.
28. Stojnic BB, Brecker SJ, Xiao HB, et al. Left ventricular filling characteristics in pulmonary hypertension: A new mode of ventricular interaction. *Br Heart J* 1992;68(1):16–20.
29. Davlouros PA, Kilner PJ, Hornung TS, et al. Right ventricular function in adults with repaired tetralogy of Fallot assessed with cardiovascular magnetic resonance imaging: Detrimental role of right ventricular outflow aneurysms or akinesia and adverse right-to-left ventricular interaction. *J Am Coll Cardiol* 2002;40:2044–2052.
30. Ghai A, Silversides C, Harris L, et al. Left ventricular dysfunction is a risk factor for sudden cardiac death in adults late after repair of tetralogy of Fallot. *J Am Coll Cardiol* 2002;40:1675–1680.
31. D'Andrea A, Caso P, Sarubbi B, et al. Right ventricular myocardial activation delay in adult patients with right bundle branch block late after repair of Tetralogy of Fallot. *Eur J Echocardiogr* 2004;5(2):123–131.
32. Penny DJ, Redington AN. Angiographic demonstration of incoordinate motion of the ventricular wall after the Fontan operation. *Br Heart J* 1991;66(6):456–459.
33. Millane T, Bernard EJ, Jaeggi E, et al. Role of ischemia and infarction in late right ventricular dysfunction after atrial repair of transposition of the great arteries. *J Am Coll Cardiol* 2000;35:1661–1668.
34. Dubin AM, Janousek J, Rhee E, et al. Resynchronization therapy in pediatric and congenital heart disease patients: An international multicenter study. *J Am Coll Cardiol* 2005;46:2277–2283.
35. van Son JA, Reddy VM, Silverman NH, et al. Regression of tricuspid regurgitation after two-stage arterial switch operation for failing systemic ventricle after atrial inversion operation. *J Thorac Cardiovasc Surg* 1996;111: 342–347.

CHAPTER 23 ■ CARDIAC TRAUMA

GARY A. SMITH, MD, DrPH

Traumatic injury to the heart occurs when energy is transferred to the heart in amounts or at rates that exceed the tissue's threshold to withstand it, resulting in structural damage or functional abnormality. The transfer of injurious energy is most commonly associated with blunt trauma, penetrating trauma, or contact with electrical current. Most medical knowledge about cardiac trauma in children is extrapolated from studies of adults. Relatively little direct information is available regarding cardiac injuries in children.

BLUNT CARDIAC INJURY

Blunt trauma accounts for the vast majority of injuries to children and is the chief cause of cardiac trauma in the pediatric age group. The incidence of cardiac injury in blunt trauma among children has been reported to be from 0% to 43% (1). Blunt cardiac injuries are often unsuspected injuries associated with multiple system trauma. Clinical manifestations of cardiac trauma vary depending on the location of injury. They are often nonspecific and include shock, cardiovascular instability, dysrhythmias, chest pain, and changes in mentation. In victims of multiple trauma, all of these findings can be easily attributed to other serious injuries to the head, abdomen, or extremities.

Parmley et al. (2) performed autopsies on a large series of motor vehicle crash victims and found that blunt cardiac injury was one of the most frequently missed diagnoses. This finding has been corroborated by others. Having a high level of suspicion for blunt cardiac injury is necessary for early diagnosis and intervention. The autopsy series of Parmley et al. described various mechanisms of nonpenetrating cardiovascular injury (Table 23.1).

Most blunt cardiac injuries from direct chest impact among children are the result of a motor vehicle crash (3). Blunt blows with weapons, fists, and animal kicks; blunt collisions during sports; and falls from heights also cause direct-impact cardiac injuries.

TABLE 23.1

MECHANISMS OF BLUNT CARDIAC TRAUMA

Direct impact
Acceleration–deceleration
Compression
Hydraulic ram effect
Concussion
Blast
Combination

Adapted from Parmley LF, Manion WC, Mattingly TW. Nonpenetrating traumatic injury of the heart. *Circulation* 1958;18:371–396, with permission.

Because the heart is suspended from the great vessels, acceleration–deceleration injuries occur as the heart moves like a pendulum in the thorax. Traction on the great vessels can cause tears at their points of fixation.

Compression of the chest can crush the heart or cause damage through increased intrathoracic and intracardiac pressures. Cardiac rupture is more likely if compression occurs during maximum filling of the chambers. Rib fractures and contusions of the chest wall are not always seen, especially in children owing to their highly compliant chest walls. Abdominal and lower extremity compression also can force blood back to the heart, causing damage through a hydraulic ram effect.

In cardiac concussion (commotio cordis), there is functional abnormality without visible myocardial damage. These cardiac electrical conduction abnormalities can be fatal. Cardiac concussion causes sudden death in motor vehicle crash victims who sustain blunt chest trauma. Commotio cordis is the most common cause of traumatic death in youth baseball, estimated to cause two to three deaths annually in the United States. Fatal sports-related commotio cordis has been reported from blows to the chest by objects such as a softball, hard baseball, lacrosse ball, or hockey puck, and some sports require protective equipment (4). See Table 23.2 for features differentiating cardiac concussion from cardiac contusion (5).

Two other mechanisms of blunt cardiac injury have been described: Blast injury and a combination injury, which involves more than one of the above mechanisms.

The types of anatomic injuries resulting from these various mechanisms in blunt cardiac trauma include pericardial injury, myocardial contusion, cardiac rupture, septal disruption, ventricular aneurysm, injury to the heart valves and supporting structures, and injury to the great vessels, brachiocephalic arteries, venae cavae, and coronary arteries (Table 23.3).

Pericardial Injury

Blunt pericardial injuries range from contusion to rupture and are usually associated with myocardial injury. Isolated pericardial injuries are rare. Pericardial lacerations and pericardial rupture are rarely significant injuries unless cardiac herniation occurs through a pericardial tear. Cardiac herniation can result in severe circulatory compromise and rapid death. Cardiac tamponade is a common complication of myocardial injury but is not likely with isolated pericardial injury.

Traumatic pericarditis can develop after pericardial contusion. A chronic pericarditis after cardiac trauma can last 1 to 4 weeks. The clinical features are single or recurrent pericardial or pleural effusions, similar to the postpericardiotomy syndrome.

The frequency of pericardial injury associated with blunt chest trauma is unknown. Asymptomatic pericardial effusions have been demonstrated by cardiac ultrasonographic examination following blunt chest trauma. Pericardial lacerations

TABLE 23.2

DIFFERENTIAL FEATURES OF CARDIAC CONCUSSION AND CONTUSION

Feature	Concussion	Contusion
Force	Sharp, not necessarily violent	Generally violent
Direction of force	Sternum to vertebra	Of no significance
Onset	Immediate	Gradual
Course	Transitory	Persisting
Loss of consciousness	Usually	Not characteristic
Disturbances of rhythm and conduction	Characteristic, immediate	Absent or delayed
Changes in ST segment and T waves	Nonspecific	Anatomically localized injury or ischemia

Adapted from Abrunzo TJ. Commotio cordis: The single most common cause of traumatic death in youth baseball. *Am J Dis Child* 1991;145:1279–1282; and Michelson WB. CPK-MB isoenzyme determinations: Diagnostic and prognostic value in evaluation of blunt chest trauma. *Ann Emerg Med* 1980;9:562–567, with permission.

were frequently found in dogs following sublethal blunt chest trauma. The most frequent manifestations of traumatic pericarditis include pericardial friction rub and nonspecific electrocardiographic (ECG) ST-T wave changes and diffuse low voltages.

Traumatic cardiac tamponade rarely presents with all the classic Beck's triad features of hypotension, distant heart sounds, and elevated central venous pressure with neck vein distension. An echocardiogram is the most sensitive diagnostic test for cardiac tamponade and can be used in the emergency department for selected trauma patients. A diagnostic and therapeutic pericardiocentesis also can be used for patients with suspected cardiac tamponade. However, false-negative pericardiocentesis results have been observed in 25% to 80% of patients who have blood in the pericardium (6).

Treatment of traumatic pericarditis is based on symptoms. If pericardial effusion or associated pleural effusions are clinically significant, pericardiocentesis or thoracocentesis is indicated. Chronic pericarditis or postpericardiotomy syndrome is treated with anti-inflammatory agents.

Most pericardial lacerations are incidentally found during thoracotomy being performed for other indications and are not repaired unless the defect is large enough to pose a risk of cardiac herniation. Large pericardial lacerations that are difficult to repair may be managed by pericardiectomy.

TABLE 23.3

TYPES OF BLUNT CARDIAC INJURIES

Pericardial injury
Myocardial injury
   Myocardial contusion
   Cardiac rupture
   Septal disruption
   Ventricular aneurysm
Injury to heart valves and supporting structures
Injury to great vessels, brachiocephalic arteries, vena cavae, and coronary arteries

Adapted from Liedtke AJ, DeMuth WE Jr. Nonpenetrating cardiac injuries: A collective review. *Am Heart J* 1973;86:687–697, with permission.

Myocardial Contusion

Myocardial contusion in the general population is most often a result of direct blunt force to the chest during motor vehicle crashes, industrial injuries, farm injuries, or sports injuries. The reported incidence of myocardial contusion associated with major trauma varies between 3% and 76% depending on the study population and the diagnostic criteria (7,8). Approximately one third of children with cardiac contusion may have no external evidence of chest injury. ECG abnormalities and dysrhythmias are less common in these children than in adults who have cardiac contusion.

The first reported case of autopsy-proven myocardial contusion was in 1764; it described a boy struck in the chest by a plate (9). Recognition of cardiac contusion is difficult because of nonspecific clinical findings and lack of an accurate diagnostic test (3). The findings of cardiac contusion are easily attributed to other serious injuries that are often present. Predicting which cases will be clinically significant has not been possible, thus complicating the discussion about appropriate management of myocardial contusion. The diagnosis of myocardial contusion should be considered in any child with significant blunt chest or multiple system trauma.

Most cases of myocardial contusion are mild and asymptomatic, and go unrecognized, but complications can be serious. Complications of myocardial contusion include dysrhythmias, conduction disturbances, cardiac failure, aneurysms, pseudoaneurysms, myocardial wall thinning, cardiac rupture, and cardiac arrest. Most are late findings. Underlying cardiac disease, including ischemia, cardiomyopathy, or congenital heart disorders, increases the risk of complications from blunt cardiac injury. The pathologic findings of myocardial contusion include myocardial hemorrhage, myocardial fiber necrosis, and later fibrous scar formation.

The diagnosis of myocardial contusion can generally be made in patients with blunt chest trauma if the ECG demonstrates a dysrhythmia or changes compatible with ischemia or contusion, the creatine phosphokinase–muscle band (CPK-MB) fraction is >5% of the total CPK, and the echocardiogram is abnormal (10). However, ECG findings in cardiac contusion are nonspecific, and false-positive results can occur. Because CPK-MB is also present in skeletal muscle, pancreas, and bowel, extensive skeletal muscle or abdominal trauma can cause elevation of CPK-MB. In addition, CPK-MB has been shown to have a low sensitivity and specificity for cardiac injury in some studies (11,12). Lactate dehydrogenase isoenzymes and serum glutamic oxalotransaminase are of no value in the diagnosis of cardiac contusion. Troponin I and T have been shown to be accurate indicators of myocardial injury that may aid in the diagnosis of myocardial contusion (13–15).

The echocardiogram may be more useful than serial ECGs or cardiac isoenzyme measurements in evaluating blunt cardiac injuries because it can detect pericardial effusion, valvular dysfunction, septal defects, enlarging chambers, and wall motion abnormalities and can be used to determine ejection fraction. Echocardiographic abnormalities are detected in 20% to 47% of patients following blunt trauma (16). Transesophageal echocardiography may offer advantages over transthoracic echocardiography, especially in obese patients. The proximity of the esophagus to the thoracic aorta and atrioventricular (AV) valves allows clearer visualization of injuries to these structures. In the absence of ECG abnormalities or cardiac isoenzyme elevation, cardiac dysmotility on echocardiogram is not associated with adverse patient outcome (17).

Gated radionuclide angiography is a useful method for detecting abnormalities of cardiac function. It has been applied in the evaluation of blunt cardiac trauma to detect diminished ejection fractions, hypokinetic wall segments, and ventricular aneurysms. The most common finding it identified in adult patients with blunt chest trauma was mild hypokinesis of the right ventricular wall with diminished ejection fraction. Unfortunately, gated radionuclide angiography is not predictive of morbidity and mortality in cardiac contusion.

Following blunt chest trauma, patients with abnormal ECGs require admission, continuous cardiac monitoring, and evaluation of cardiac isoenzymes. Cardiac monitoring should continue until abnormal ECGs have reverted to normal for at least 24 hours, cardiac isoenzymes have normalized, and stabilization of other major injuries has been achieved. The main treatment goal is avoidance of death caused by dysrhythmias or hemodynamic compromise.

Cardiac Rupture

Although an uncommon injury, cardiac rupture is estimated to cause 10% to 15% of adult motor vehicular crash fatalities. Two thirds of deaths owing to cardiac rupture occur at the scene (18). Cardiac rupture occurs most commonly in young male drivers suffering precordial steering wheel impact during a crash (19). Ventricular rupture is more common than atrial rupture, and the thin-walled anteriorly positioned right ventricle is more commonly ruptured than the left ventricle. Multiple chamber rupture is not uncommon in these cases, as is combined cardiac rupture and aortic rupture, reflecting the large amount of force involved in these injuries (2).

Ventricular rupture can result from direct cardiac compression or from an indirect hydraulic ram effect that occurs during abdominal or extremity compression. During late diastole, compressing a distended noncompliant ventricle can tear AV valves, chambers, septa, and other cardiac structures. Atrial rupture appears to involve compression of the filled chamber as well as torsion when the AV valves are closed and the chamber is filled during late systole. The atrial appendages are the thinnest portions and most prone to atrial rupture. Delayed ruptures are extremely rare and may follow infarction associated with trauma and gradual softening of the ischemic tissues or rupture of a myocardial aneurysm or pseudoaneurysm (19).

The clinical manifestation of myocardial rupture is usually tamponade, although approximately one third of patients will have exsanguinating hemorrhage through associated pericardial lacerations. The association of cardiac tamponade with cardiac rupture limits the rate of exsanguination and increases the chances of survival for these patients.

The first surgical repair of blunt cardiac rupture was reported by Des Forges et al. (20) in 1955 involving a 4-cm right atrial laceration. Until then, cardiac rupture had been considered universally lethal. Surviving ventricular rupture secondary to blunt chest trauma is rare. In 1990 the first pediatric survivor was preceded by only three reported adult cases (21).

Septal Disruption

The interventricular septum ruptures most commonly in the muscular portion near the apex, which is the thinnest area of the septum. Any portion of the muscular septum can rupture, even in multiple sites, with concomitant injury to the conduction system. Echocardiography should demonstrate the abnormality. Cardiac catheterization can be performed to determine the magnitude of left-to-right shunt, measure pulmonary artery pressures, and evaluate ventricular function. Ventricular septal defects with significant left-to-right shunts require surgical closure.

Ventricular Aneurysm

Posttraumatic ventricular aneurysms usually occur as a complication of coronary artery injury, most commonly of the left anterior descending coronary artery (22). In a world literature review by Grieco et al. (22) in 1989, 32 cases of left ventricular aneurysm following blunt chest trauma were reported. Patients ranged in age from 3 to 59 years. Motor vehicle crashes were the principal mechanism of injury. The most common presenting symptoms were congestive heart failure (ten patients), palpitations or dysrhythmias (nine patients), and arterial embolus (five patients). Seven patients had mild constitutional complaints or were asymptomatic. Time of diagnosis ranged from 5 days to 18 years (median time 3 months) postinjury. Ventricular aneurysmectomy is recommended to avoid lethal complications (22).

Injury to Heart Valves and Supporting Structures

Heart valve rupture from blunt chest trauma occurs infrequently. Nine percent of adult fatalities from blunt chest trauma had cardiac valve injury in the autopsy series by Parmley et al. (2), and nearly all of these cases had other associated cardiac injuries. The aortic valve is the most frequently injured valve followed by the mitral and tricuspid valves.

Valvular injury results from a rapid increase in intracardiac pressure against a closed valve. During late diastole to early systole, the filled chambers experience their highest normal intraluminal pressures. With additional external pressure from forceful compression of the chest, abnormally high pressure is exerted on a closed heart valve. The timing of chest trauma in the cardiac cycle appears to determine which valve is injured. The greater left heart pressure gradients may contribute to the higher frequency of injury to the aortic and mitral valves. Another mechanism by which the aortic valve can be injured is the hydraulic ram effect that occurs when the aortic blood flow reverses during abdominal and lower extremity compression (23).

Presenting signs and symptoms of valvular injury depend on which valve is involved, the degree of valvular insufficiency, and the presence of other associated cardiac structural damage. Surgical valve replacement is generally required for the more severe injuries. Helpful diagnostic tests are the chest radiograph and ECG. The most useful test is Doppler echocardiography, which can identify disrupted blood flow or valvular dysfunction in addition to other associated structural defects.

Great Vessel Injury

Great vessel injury can occur with blunt trauma. The aorta is the most commonly injured great vessel. Injury to the pulmonary artery is rarely reported. Although aortic rupture from blunt trauma can occur with falls, crush injuries, and blast injuries, nearly 70% of cases in the general population occur with motor vehicle crashes. The mechanism of aortic rupture involves the shearing stress of sudden deceleration or sudden increases in intraluminal pressure. Ejected passengers, pedestrians struck by vehicles, and persons who fall from heights have higher risk for aortic rupture than victims of deceleration vehicular collisions. Aortic injury can occur with either horizontal or vertical deceleration (23).

The aorta most commonly ruptures when acceleration–deceleration forces pull a mobile aortic segment away from a point of fixation. The sites usually ruptured are the aortic isthmus, fixed by the brachiocephalic arteries; the ascending aorta, fixed to the heart at the aortic root; and the descending aorta, fixed at the diaphragm. Tears of the ascending aorta carry a high risk of immediate mortality and are frequently associated with myocardial contusion and aortic valve injuries (2). Autopsy studies show that tears in the aortic isthmus and ascending aorta occur in 45% and 20% of cases of aortic rupture, respectively, but clinical studies show about 90% of aortic tears at the aortic isthmus. Overall, 80% to 90% of persons with motor vehicle–related aortic rupture are dead at the scene (6). Of the 10% to 20% who survive long enough for diagnosis and intervention, 30% die within 6 hours and 50% within 24 hours.

More common than aortic rupture and transmural aortic tears are superficial aortic tears into the intima and media with blunt trauma. These are generally without serious consequence and are often undiagnosed. Partial tears are infrequent and usually are located posteriorly. Multiple tears occur in 15% to 20% of cases. Traumatic aortic dissection is rare, occurring when the subadventitial layer remains intact and contains a periaortic hematoma (23).

Presenting complaints and physical findings may not accurately predict the presence or absence of aortic rupture. Symptoms may be absent, and visible external injury is not seen in about one third of cases. Symptoms of aortic rupture include dyspnea, back pain, dysphagia and hoarseness, upper extremity hypertension, or an upper and lower extremity blood pressure differential similar to that seen with aortic coarctation. An aortic insufficiency heart murmur may be heard.

Chest radiographs may show mediastinal widening, a right-sided aortic root prominence, loss of aortic arch sharpness, or rightward deviation of the trachea. Less common radiographic findings include downward displacement of the left mainstem bronchus, rightward deviation of the esophageal nasogastric tube, left hemothorax, the apical cap sign, and first rib fracture. Aortography is considered to be the gold standard and is indicated in all cases of suspected aortic rupture, even if plane radiographs are normal (6). Transesophageal echocardiography, CT scanning, and magnetic resonance imaging also are useful in diagnosing rupture of the aorta.

Brachiocephalic Arteries

The second most common vascular injury with blunt trauma is injury of the brachiocephalic arteries. The mechanism of injury includes horizontal and vertical deceleration, chest compression, crush, distraction, and hyperextension of the shoulder. The resulting arterial injury is similar to that of the aorta. Massive bleeding or ischemia are rare complications (23).

Vena Caval Injury

Similar to aortic injury, vena caval injury is infrequent with nonpenetrating trauma. The abdominal segment of the inferior vena cava is more frequently injured than the chest segment. Because the thin-walled veins do not vasoconstrict like transected arteries after injury, severe hemorrhage and high mortality are usual with vena caval injuries. Mortality is higher in abdominal than in chest segment vena caval injury. Blunt trauma can cause avulsion or tear of the inferior vena cava near the right atrium that can extend into the right atrium. Therefore, associated cardiac injury is common when inferior vena caval injuries are located near the heart (23).

Plane chest radiography is not helpful. The emergent nature of these injuries does not allow time for venography. Therefore, rapid surgical exploration and repair is indicated when vena caval injury is suspected (23).

Coronary Artery Injury

Coronary artery injury from blunt trauma is rare. The study by Parmley et al. (2) of 547 patients who died from blunt chest trauma reported only 10 coronary artery lacerations and no cases of intraluminal thrombosis, even in areas of cardiac contusion. The incidence of coronary artery injury in nonfatal trauma cases is unknown. The most commonly injured coronary artery is the left anterior descending coronary artery. Consequences of coronary artery injury are myocardial infarction, hemopericardium, cardiac tamponade, and coronary artery and ventricular aneurysms and pseudoaneurysms (23).

A review of the English-language medical literature by Neiman and Hui (24) in 1992 reported 40 cases of myocardial infarction associated with blunt cardiac trauma. The pathophysiologic mechanism underlying acute myocardial infarction following blunt chest injuries has not been clearly established. Suggested mechanisms include transient coronary artery spasm, thrombus formation within the coronary artery, coronary artery dissection, or hemorrhage into an atheromatous plaque.

Definitive diagnosis of coronary artery injury is accomplished by angiography. These injuries are underdiagnosed because chest pain associated with blunt chest injury is often attributed to concomitant chest wall contusion, pericarditis, pulmonary contusion, rib fractures, or other associated injuries that are not routinely evaluated by coronary angiography. Coronary angiography is indicated for all blunt cardiac trauma patients with angina or myocardial infarction to determine the status of the coronary arteries and to locate surgically correctable lesions.

PENETRATING CARDIAC INJURY

Although blunt trauma accounts for most injuries among the pediatric population, penetrating trauma is increasing among young adults, teenagers, and even younger children. The ratio of gunshot to stab wounds is also increasing (25,26). With the concomitant improvement in emergency medical services, more patients with penetrating cardiac wounds are now reaching hospital emergency departments.

The first description of penetrating cardiac wounds is found in the Edwin Smith Papyrus, written in 3000 BC. Homer also described penetrating cardiac trauma in The Iliad. Baron Larrey, Napoleon's surgeon, is credited with performing the first pericardiocentesis in 1829. It was common wisdom for years that nothing could be done for wounds to the heart until von Rehn performed the first successful cardiorrhaphy in 1896 for a 22-year-old man with a 1.5-cm stab wound to the right ventricle. This was only 13 years following the statement by Dr. Theodore Billroth that, "A surgeon who tries to suture a wound of the heart deserves to lose the esteem of his colleagues" (27).

The mortality risk for penetrating cardiac trauma is related to a number of factors, including the cause of injury, size of the wound, location of the wound, any associated noncardiac injuries, and length of time from injury to initiation of resuscitative measures.

Gunshot wounds cause much more extensive tissue destruction than stab wounds owing to transfer of large amounts of kinetic energy to the tissues. Not only does a bullet cause greater disruption of myocardium and internal structures of the heart, but the rent in the pericardium is larger, which makes tamponade less likely and exsanguination more rapid. For these reasons, the mortality rate of gunshot wounds to the heart is approximately twice that of stab wounds.

A stab wound is more likely to result in cardiac tamponade than a gunshot wound. More than 80% of stab wounds to the heart present with cardiac tamponade, whereas only 20% of gunshot wounds present in this fashion. Stab wounds are the most common cause of acute tamponade (27,28). The retention of blood within the pericardial sac prevents rapid exsanguination, providing more time for the patient to reach medical care and receive life-saving cardiorrhaphy. This has led some to consider hemopericardium as a mixed blessing. However, if allowed to progress, hemopericardium can lead to fatal cardiac tamponade. Because of its thicker myocardial wall, stab wounds to the left ventricle that measure <1 cm will often spontaneously seal. Stab wounds to the right ventricular wall, however, usually result in cardiac tamponade because the thinner myocardial wall does not usually spontaneously seal. The thinness of atrial walls decreases the likelihood of spontaneous sealing; however, the low intrachamber pressures counterbalance this factor (27).

As is the case with blunt cardiac trauma, the anatomic position of cardiac structures determines their likelihood of injury owing to penetrating trauma. Those structures located more anteriorly are more likely to be injured. In decreasing order of frequency, penetrating cardiac injuries involve the right ventricle, left ventricle, right atrium, and left atrium. For the same reason, the left anterior descending coronary artery is more frequently injured than the right coronary artery (28). Multiple chamber injury has a high mortality rate (29).

Penetrating cardiac injury can occur owing to iatrogenic causes. These injuries most often occur during diagnostic procedures, invasive monitoring, or other therapeutic interventions (26). Other causes of penetrating injury to the heart include ice picks, nonbullet projectiles, swallowed sewing needles, and inward displacement of fractured ribs with chest trauma (30).

Cardiac injury should be presumed to be present until proven otherwise in patients presenting with penetrating wounds of the precordium, neck, axilla, back, or upper abdomen. Beck's triad is frequently absent in patients with cardiac tamponade, and determination of jugular venous distension is particularly difficult in young children because of their short necks. Additionally, if there is hypovolemia owing to acute blood loss, increased central venous pressure may not be seen with cardiac tamponade (27).

Penetrating injuries to the chest are frequently associated with intra-abdominal injury. Ten percent to 30% of patients with penetrating cardiac wounds also have intra-abdominal injury. This is important because mortality is greater for patients with penetrating cardiac injury associated with intra-abdominal injury than for those with cardiac injury alone (27).

Approximately 60% to 80% of patients with penetrating cardiac wounds die prior to reaching a hospital. For those who arrive in the emergency department with vital signs, or for those who had vital signs at the scene and lost them en route to the hospital, resuscitative intervention must be immediate (31). Diagnostic tests, such as a chest radiograph, are of little use. Emergency department echocardiography is available at some trauma centers, which has decreased the time to diagnosis of penetrating cardiac injury and has improved survival. Pericardiocentesis can rule in, but not rule out, cardiac tamponade because of the high frequency of false-negative results. Performing a subxiphoid pericardial window has been recommended by some to diagnose hemopericardium in selected stable trauma patients.

Initial emergency management of penetrating cardiac trauma is the same for children and adults, following the principles of (a) maintaining a patent airway with adequate oxygenation and ventilation, (b) preservation of adequate tissue perfusion through rapid intravenous or intraosseous administration of fluids and blood, and (c) control of hemorrhage (6).

As with adults, children with a penetrating cardiac wound should receive emergency thoracotomy in the emergency department whenever they are too unstable to be transported to the operating room. Pericardiocentesis must be viewed as a temporizing measure until thoracotomy and definitive cardiorrhaphy can be performed. Emergency department thoracotomy was first described by Beall et al. (32) in 1966 for immediate resuscitation of moribund patients with penetrating chest injuries. The purpose of emergency department thoracotomy is reversal of cardiac tamponade, control of hemorrhage, open chest cardiac massage, and temporary cross-clamping of the descending aorta to redistribute blood flow to the coronary and cerebral circulations (32). Indications for emergency department thoracotomy in patients with blunt chest trauma are controversial because reported survival rates for both pediatric and adult patients are 0% to 2% with this procedure (33). This is unfortunate, because the vast majority of trauma deaths in the pediatric age group are due to blunt injury.

ELECTRICAL INJURY

The first human fatality caused by alternating current (250 volts) was reported in 1879. Among all age groups, >1,000 people die each year in the United States because of electrocution on the work site or in the home, and 150 to 300 others die annually from lightning strikes. These deaths are primarily due to fatal cardiac dysrhythmia (34).

Injury from Man-made Electricity

Ohm's law (amperage = voltage/resistance) describes the inverse relationship between current (A) and tissue resistance (R) and the direct relationship between current (A) and voltage (V). Damage to human tissue from electricity is related to the amount and duration of current that passes through it. In electrical injuries, only voltage is known. The amount of current involved (and resulting tissue damage) is variable, because tissue resistance varies. Overall, bone provides the greatest resistance

TABLE 23.4

FACTORS AFFECTING SEVERITY OF ELECTRICAL INJURIES

Frequency
Voltage
Amperage
Resistance
Pathway
Duration

Adapted from Cooper MA, Andrews CJ, Holle RL, et al. Lightning injuries. In: Auerbach PS, ed. *Wilderness Medicine*. 4th ed. St. Louis, MO: Mosby, 2001, with permission.

to current flow, followed in descending order by fat, tendons, skin, muscle, vasculature, and nerves (35). Skin resistance is the most important factor determining the probability of cardiac injury from electrocution. Skin resistance can vary dramatically, depending on skin thickness, vascularity, and, most important, moisture. Although the resistance of dry skin may be 100,000 ohms, that of moist skin may be as little as 1,000 ohms. This hundredfold change in skin resistance may mean the difference between a painful electrical shock and the conduction of enough current to cause cardiac dysrhythmia (35).

Alternating current is a greater hazard than direct current. Alternating current can cause tetanic contraction of muscles. Because the forearm flexors are stronger than the extensors, this may prevent the child from being able to let go of an electrical source that he or she has grasped. Additionally, the heart is more sensitive to alternating current than direct current. Cardiac dysrhythmias are more likely to occur from household current at 60 Hz than electrical current of higher frequency. The path of the electrical current through the body also is a determinant of the likelihood of cardiac dysrhythmia. Current passing through the thorax is more likely to cause a dysrhythmia (36). See Table 23.4 for factors influencing electrical injury severity (34).

The mechanism by which electricity injures the heart is unknown. Proposed mechanisms include direct myocardial muscle damage, coronary artery endarteritis, and coronary artery spasm. Myocardial ischemia, resulting from decreased coronary perfusion during electrically induced dysrhythmia, also has been proposed as a mechanism of cardiac damage. The only reported pathologic finding at autopsy is petechial hemorrhages in the myocardium (36). Sudden death owing to low-voltage (110 to 380 volts) alternating current found in the household is usually secondary to ventricular fibrillation. Following electrical injury, nonspecific ST-segment and T-wave changes are the most common abnormalities observed on ECG (36).

The use of CPK-MB isoenzyme levels in the diagnosis of myocardial infarction after electrical injury is complicated by the extensive skeletal muscle damage that normally occurs with these injuries. Skeletal muscle damaged by electricity will release large amounts of CPK, including the CPK-MB isoenzyme fraction. Skeletal muscle biopsy adjacent to the site of electrical injury demonstrates an increased production of CPK, as well as increased CPK-MB activity. This increased enzymatic activity is hypothesized to have been stimulated by the electrical injury. The utility of troponin levels in lightning injuries is unknown. The effects of cardiopulmonary resuscitation, as well as direct current countershock during resuscitative attempts, also potentially confuse the picture (36).

Initial emergency management of patients injured by electricity includes attention to the airway; breathing, and circulation and treatment of any cardiac dysrhythmias following pediatric advanced life support (PALS) and advanced cardiac life support (ACLS) protocols. Asymptomatic patients with normal ECGs following electrical injury from low-voltage alternating household current do not require routine cardiac monitoring or admission to the hospital (35,37).

Injury from Lightning

Each second, there are an estimated 100 lightning strikes to the earth's surface worldwide. Lightning is responsible for more deaths in the United States than any other natural disaster. Lightning-related injuries are most common during the summer, when there is more thunderstorm activity. Only 20% to 30% of people struck by lightning die, and they are usually the ones who experience immediate cardiopulmonary arrest. However, survivors often suffer from serious sequelae (34).

Lightning-related injuries differ in a number of ways from injuries owing to man-made electricity. Lightning strikes involve brief, massive surges of unidirectional current with an associated shock wave. Current magnitude often exceeds 100,000 amperes, and >30,000,000 volts is seen. The 8,000°C temperature of a lightning stroke is threefold to fourfold higher than that seen with high-voltage man-made current, but contact is extremely brief. Lightning typically flashes over the body, causing only minor or superficial burns. This contrasts with the deep and extensive burns associated with high-voltage alternating current. See Table 23.5 for a

TABLE 23.5

LIGHTNING VERSUS HIGH-VOLTAGE ELECTRICAL INJURY

Factor	Lightning	High voltage
Energy level	30,000,000 V, 50,000 A	Usually much lower
Time of exposure	Brief, instantaneous	Prolonged
Pathway	Flashover orifice	Deep, internal
Burns	Superficial, minor	Deep, major injury
Cardiac	Primary and secondary arrest, asystole	Fibrillation
Renal	Rare myoglobinuria or hemoglobinuria	Myoglobinuric renal failure common
Fasciotomy	Rarely if ever necessary	Common, early, and extensive
Blunt injury	Explosive thunder effect	Falls, being thrown

Adapted from Cooper MA, Andrews CJ, Holle RL, et al. Lightning injuries. In: Auerbach PS, ed. *Wilderness Medicine*. 4th ed. St. Louis, MO: Mosby, 2001, with permission.

comparison of electrical injuries owing to lightning and high-voltage current (34).

The electrical surge associated with a lightning strike is thought to cause widespread myocardial depolarization with subsequent asystole. Ventricular fibrillation also has been commonly reported. Respiratory arrest frequently occurs in lightning strike victims, and the associated hypoxia can prevent cardiac recovery from the initial electrically induced cardiac asystole or other dysrhythmia (34,38).

Myocardial necrosis has been found at autopsy following fatal lightning injury. Myocardial damage may be reflected by ECG abnormalities demonstrating an acute myocardial infarction pattern. Nonspecific ST-T wave changes also have been reported. ECG abnormalities may develop up to several days following the injury (38). Resolution of most ECG changes occurs within a few days, although abnormalities have been reported to last for months (34).

Initial emergency management of children struck by lightning is the same as for those with electrical injuries from man-made sources. Maintenance of a patent airway with adequate oxygenation and ventilation is the highest priority, as well as treatment of cardiac dysrhythmias following PALS and ACLS guidelines (34,38). Any child found with linear or punctate burns, clothes exploded off, tympanic membrane rupture, confusion, outdoor location of discovery, or pathognomonic feathering burns should be managed medically as a lightning strike victim. In the case of multiple casualties in a lightning strike, contrary to standard triage guidelines, resuscitation attempts should be directed first toward those who appear dead. Those who are apneic and asystolic may respond to resuscitative efforts, whereas those with spontaneous respirations are likely to already be recovering (34).

References

1. Baum VC. Cardiac trauma in children. *Paediatr Anaesth* 2002;12(2):110–117.
2. Parmley LF, Manion WC, Mattingly TW. Nonpenetrating traumatic injury of the heart. *Circulation* 1958;18:371–396.
3. Dowd MD, Krug S. Pediatric blunt cardiac injury: Epidemiology, clinical features, and diagnosis. *J Trauma* 1996;40:61–67.
4. Bliss D, Silen M. Pediatric thoracic trauma. *Crit Care Med* 2002;30:S409–S415.
5. Abrunzo TJ. Commotio cordis: The single, most common cause of traumatic death in youth baseball. *Am J Dis Child* 1991;145:1279–1282.
6. *Advanced Trauma Life Support Manual.* Chicago: American College of Surgeons, 1993.
7. Tenzer ML. The spectrum of myocardial contusion: A review. *J Trauma* 1985;25:620–627.
8. Roddy MG, Lange PA, Klein BL. Cardiac trauma in children. *Clin Pediatr Emerg Med* 2005;6(4):234–243.
9. Akenside M. Account of blow upon heart and its effects. *Philos Trans R Soc Lond Biol* 1764:353.
10. Fabian TC, Mangiante EC, Patterson CR, et al. Myocardial contusion in blunt trauma: Clinical characteristics, means of diagnosis, and implications for patient management. *J Trauma* 1988;28:50–57.
11. Bertinchant JP, Polge A, Mohty D, et al. Evaluation of incidence, clinical significance, and prognostic value of circulating troponin I and T elevation in hemodynamically stable patients with suspected myocardial contusion after blunt chest trauma. *J Trauma* 2000;48:924–931.
12. Nagy KK, Krosner SM, Roberts RR, et al. Determining which patients require evaluation for blunt cardiac injury following blunt chest trauma. *World J Surg* 2001;25:108–111.
13. Towbin JA. Cardiac troponin I. A new diagnostic gold standard of cardiac injury in children? *J Pediatr* 1997;130:853–854.
14. Hirsch R, Landt Y, Porter S, et al. Cardiac troponin I in pediatrics: Normal values and potential use in the assessment of cardiac injury. *J Pediatr* 1997;130:872–877.
15. Rajan GP, Zellweger R. Cardiac troponin I as a predictor of arrhythmia and ventricular dysfunction in trauma patients with myocardial contusion. *J Trauma* 2004;57:801–808.
16. Hiatt JR, Yeatman LA Jr, Child JS. The value of echocardiography in blunt chest trauma. *J Trauma* 1988;28:914–922.
17. Turturro MA. Emergency echocardiography. *Emerg Med Clin North Am* 1992;10:47–57.
18. Scorpio RJ, Wesson DE, Smith CR, et al. Blunt cardiac injuries in children: A postmortem study. *J Trauma* 1996;41:306–309.
19. Pevec WC, Udekwu AO, Peitzman AB. Blunt rupture of the myocardium. *Ann Thorac Surg* 1989;48:139–142.
20. Desforges G, Ridder WP, Lenoci RJ. Successful suture of ruptured myocardium after nonpenetrating injury. *N Engl J Med* 1955;252:567–569.
21. Mozzetti MD, Devin JB, Susselman MS, et al. A pediatric survivor of left ventricular rupture after blunt chest trauma. *Ann Emerg Med* 1990;19:386–389.
22. Grieco JG, Montoya A, Sullivan HJ, et al. Ventricular aneurysm due to blunt chest injury. *Ann Thorac Surg* 1989;47:322–329.
23. Godwin JD, Tolentino CS. Thoracic cardiovascular trauma. *J Thorac Imaging* 1987;2:32–44.
24. Neiman J, Hui WKK. Posteromedial papillary muscle rupture as a result of right coronary artery occlusion after blunt chest injury. *Am Heart J* 1992;123:1694–1699.
25. Centers for Disease Control and Prevention. Rates of homicide, suicide, and firearm-related death among children in 26 industrialized countries. *JAMA* 1997;277:289–295.
26. Hall JR, Reyes HM, Meller JL, et al. The new epidemic in children: Penetrating injuries. *J Trauma* 1995;39:487–491.
27. Karrel R, Shaffer MA, Franaszek JB. Emergency diagnosis, resuscitation, and treatment of penetrating cardiac trauma. *Ann Emerg Med* 1982;11:504–517.
28. Asfaw I, Arbulu A. Penetrating wounds of the pericardium and heart. *Surg Clin North Am* 1977;57:37–48.
29. Asensio JA, Berne JD, Demetriades D, et al. One hundred five penetrating cardiac injuries: A 2-year prospective evaluation. *J Trauma* 1998;44:1073–1082.
30. Haller JA, Shermeta DW. Major thoracic trauma in children. *Pediatr Clin North Am* 1975;22:341–347.
31. Tyburski JG, Astra L, Wilson RF, et al. Factors affecting prognosis with penetrating wounds of the heart. *J Trauma* 2000;48:587–591.
32. Beall AC Jr, Diethrich EB, Crawford HW, et al. Surgical management of penetrating cardiovascular trauma. *Am J Surg* 1966;112:686–692.
33. Lorenz HP, Steinmetz B, Liberman J, et al. Emergency thoracotomy: Survival correlates with physiologic status. *J Trauma* 1992;32:780–788.
34. Cooper MA, Andrews CJ, Holle RL, et al. Lightning injuries. In: Auerbach PS, ed. *Wilderness Medicine.* 4th ed. St. Louis, MO: Mosby, 2001:73–111.
35. Fatovich DM, Lee KY. Household electrical shocks: Who should be monitored? *Med J Aust* 1991;155:301–303.
36. Solem L, Fischer RP, Strate RG. The natural history of electrical injury. *J Trauma* 1977;17:487–492.
37. Garcia CT, Smith GA, Cohen DM, et al. Electrical injuries in a pediatric emergency department. *Ann Emerg Med* 1995;26:604–608.
38. Andrews CJ, Cooper MA, Darveniza M, et al. *Lightning Injuries: Electrical, Medical, and Legal Aspects.* Boca Raton, FL: CRC Press, 1992.

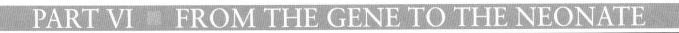

PART VI ■ FROM THE GENE TO THE NEONATE

CHAPTER 24 ■ MOLECULAR DETERMINANTS OF CARDIAC DEVELOPMENT AND DISEASE

DEEPAK SRIVASTAVA, MD, AND H. SCOTT BALDWIN, MD

The heart has for centuries been the fascination of anatomists, embryologists, biologists, and physicians. As the organ most essential for life, the heart is the first organ to form in an embryo and must function to support the rapidly growing embryo before it has the opportunity to shape itself into a four-chambered organ. The combination of the complex morphogenetic events necessary for cardiogenesis and the superimposed hemodynamic influences may contribute to the exquisite sensitivity of the heart to perturbations. This phenomenon is reflected in the estimated 10% incidence of severe cardiac malformations observed in spontaneously aborted fetuses. The fraction of congenital heart malformations that is hemodynamically compatible with the intrauterine circulation (1% of population) composes the spectrum of congenital heart defects (CHDs) that is the subject of this pediatric cardiology textbook.

In addition to the nearly 1% of children with CHD (1), an additional 1% to 2% of the population harbor more subtle cardiac developmental anomalies that become apparent only as age-dependent phenomena reveal the underlying pathology. With >1 million survivors of congenital heart disease (CHD) in the United States, it is becoming apparent that genetic disruptions that predispose to developmental defects can have ongoing consequences in maintenance of specific cell types and cellular processes over decades (2). A more precise understanding of the causes of CHD is imperative for the recognition and potential intervention of progressive degenerative conditions among survivors of CHD.

The anatomic features of most CHD in humans have been carefully catalogued. Although CHD was classified in the 18th and 19th centuries based on embryologic considerations, the advent of palliative procedures and clinical management led to a descriptive nomenclature founded on anatomic and physiologic features that governed surgical and medical therapy. However, seemingly unrelated CHDs could be argued to share common embryologic origins from a mechanistic standpoint, suggesting that the causes of CHDs may be better understood by considering their developmental bases. Recent advances in genetics and molecular biology have stimulated a renaissance in seeking an embryologic framework for understanding CHDs as alterations and null mutations in a wide array of genes have targeted the heart and vascular system and established abnormalities in cardiovascular ontogeny as a primary cause of embryonic demise (3). The ability to go beyond descriptions of the anatomic defects to developing an understanding of the genes responsible for distinct steps of cardiac morphogenesis has raised the prospects that the future of pediatric cardiology will involve more directed therapeutic and preventive measures.

Although human genetic approaches have been important in understanding CHDs, detailed molecular analysis of cardiac development in humans has been difficult. The recognition that cardiac genetic pathways are highly conserved across vastly diverse species from flies to man has resulted in an explosion of information from studies in more tractable and accessible biologic models. The fruit fly (Drosophila) has been a source of discovery for genes involved in early cardiac determination events. Although no biologic system is ideal for studying human disease, Drosophila has several advantages: It has a simple genome and usually has a single copy of genes that often have three or four homologues in vertebrates; genetic studies are facilitated by the rapid breeding times; and, most important, its DNA can be chemically mutated in a random fashion followed by phenotypic analysis and reverse genetics to identify the DNA mutation associated with distinct developmental defects. Similar chemical mutagenesis efforts have been successful in another model system, the zebrafish. Zebrafish have the added advantages of being vertebrates; having a more complex two-chambered heart; and, because the embryos grow in water, having a heart that is easily visible and not necessary for survival during the period of cardiac development. Although genetic approaches are not feasible in chick embryos, they have four-chambered hearts, and the embryos are easily accessible within the egg for surgical and molecular manipulation during cardiogenesis. Such approaches have been useful in cell fate analyses and defining the role of populations of cells during development. Finally, use of the laboratory mouse, a mammal with a cardiovascular system nearly identical to humans, has been invaluable in understanding the mechanisms underlying human disease. Advances in technology have made it possible to mutate or delete specific genes in the mouse genome and study the effects of such mutations in mice heterozygous or homozygous for the disrupted gene of interest. Thus, each biologic system offers unique opportunities to develop a deeper understanding of cardiogenesis.

In adults, heart disease is the number one killer of men and women in the United States, with an additional 5 million people surviving with insufficient cardiac function (4). Deciphering nature's secrets of heart formation might lead to novel approaches to repair or regenerate damaged heart muscle. Recent evidence has begun to support this idea and has led to heightened interest in the early events involved in cardiac cell fate decisions and cardiomyocyte differentiation, migration, and survival. The potential of stem cells in regenerative medicine is enormous, and insights into the natural process of cardiogenesis from progenitor cells during embryogenesis will form the basis of reprogramming cells for therapeutic use (3).

In this chapter, anatomic, molecular, and clinical aspects of cardiac embryology will be interwoven to develop a framework in which to consider the causes of human congenital cardiac defects. Clinical lessons combined with experimental studies in mice, fish, and flies have led to a model suggesting that unique regions of the heart have been added in a modular fashion during evolution. In this model, defects in particular regions of the heart would arise from unique genetic and environmental effects during specific developmental windows of time. To simplify the complex events of cardiogenesis, unique regions of the developing heart will be considered individually in the context described above. In addition to the classic review of cardiac development by DeHaan in 1966 (5), more recent publications provide additional details into anatomic events that are required for normal cardiac morphogenesis (6–8). The primary focus of this chapter will be to highlight recent work that has identified the molecular processes controlling these critical morphologic events.

ORIGIN OF CARDIOMYOCYTE PRECURSORS

Despite decades of cell lineage tracings and descriptive embryology of the heart's origins, only recently has a more complete and accurate picture of cardiogenesis emerged (reviewed in [7]). Two distinct mesodermal heart fields that share a common origin appear to contribute cells to the developing heart in a temporally and spatially specific manner. The well-studied primary heart field is derived from cells in the anterior lateral plate mesoderm that align in a crescent shape at approximately embryonic (E) day 7.5 in the mouse embryo, roughly corresponding to week 2 of human gestation (Fig. 24.1). By mouse E8.0, or 3 weeks in humans, these cells coalesce along the ventral midline to form a primitive heart tube, which consists of an interior layer of endocardial cells and an exterior layer of myocardial cells, separated by extracellular matrix necessary for reciprocal signaling between the two layers.

Previous lineage tracings using dye-labeling techniques suggested that cells along the anterior-posterior axis of the heart tube were destined to contribute to specific chambers of the future heart (reviewed in [9]). However, such studies could not determine the clonal contributions of individual cells (10). More recent studies using Cre-lox technologies to mark progenitor cells and all their descendents indicate—in stark contrast to previous models—that the heart tube derived from the primary heart field may predominantly provide a scaffold that enables a second population of cells to migrate and expand into cardiac chambers (7). These additional cells arise from an area often referred to as the secondary heart field (SHF), or anterior heart field, based on its location anterior and medial to the crescent-shaped primary heart field (11–13) (Fig. 24.1). Both heart fields appear to be regulated by complex positive and negative signaling networks involving members of the bone morphogenetic protein (Bmp), sonic hedgehog (Shh), fibroblast growth factor (Fgf), Wnt, and Notch proteins. Such signals often arise from the adjacent endoderm, although the precise nature and role of these signals remain unknown (reviewed in [14–17]). SHF cells remain in an undifferentiated progenitor state until incorporation into the heart, and this may in part be due to closer proximity to inhibitory Wnt signals emanating from the midline.

As the heart tube forms, the SHF cells also migrate into the midline and position themselves dorsal to the heart tube in the pharyngeal mesoderm. On rightward looping of the heart tube, SHF cells cross the pharyngeal mesoderm into the anterior and posterior portions, populating a large portion of the outflow tract, future right ventricle, and atria (18) (Fig. 24.1). Precursors of the left ventricle are sparsely populated by the SHF and appear to be derived largely from the primary heart field. In contrast to the primary heart field, SHF cells do not differentiate into cardiac cells until they are positioned within the heart. Once within the heart, primary and secondary heart field cells appear to proliferate in response to endocardial

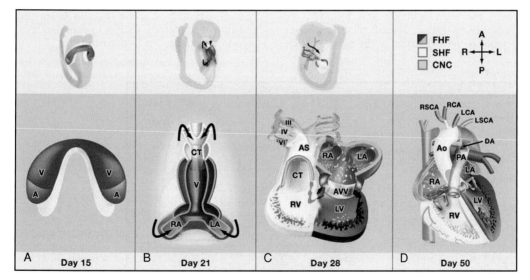

FIGURE 24.1 Mammalian heart development. Oblique views of whole embryos and frontal views of cardiac precursors during human cardiac development are shown. **A:** First heart field (FHF) cells form a crescent shape in the anterior embryo with second heart field (SHF) cells medial and anterior to the FHF. **B:** SHF cells lie dorsal to the straight heart tube and begin to migrate (*arrows*) into the anterior and posterior ends of the tube to form the right ventricle (RV), conotruncus (CT), and part of the atria (A). **C:** Following rightward looping of the heart tube, cardiac neural crest (CNC) cells also migrate (*arrow*) into the outflow tract from the neural folds to septate the outflow tract and pattern the bilaterally symmetric aortic arch artery arteries (III, IV, and VI). **D:** Septation of the ventricles, atria, and atrioventricular valves (AVV) results in the four-chambered heart. Ao, aorta; AS, aortic sac; DA, ductus arteriosus; LA, left atrium; LCA, left carotid artery; LSCA, left subclavian artery; LV, left ventricle; PA, pulmonary artery; RA, right atrium; RCA, right carotid artery; RSCA, right subclavian artery; V, ventricle.

derived signals such as neuregulin and epicardial signals dependent on retinoic acid, although the mechanisms through which these noncell autonomous events occur remain poorly understood (19,20).

TRANSCRIPTIONAL REGULATION OF CARDIAC PRECURSORS

Regulation of the SHF involves numerous signaling and transcriptional cascades (Fig. 24.2). Factors secreted from the anterior portion of the heart tube may serve as chemoattractant signals to induce the migration of SHF cells, although the nature of such molecules remains unknown (13). Islet1 (Isl1), a LIM-domain transcription factor involved in pancreatic development, is necessary for development of the SHF (18). Progeny of Isl1+ cells contribute to most of the heart except the left ventricle, but Isl1 expression is extinguished as progenitor cells begin to express markers of cardiac differentiation. The mechanisms through which Isl1 regulates SHF progenitor cells are being explored, with a significant advance coming from the recent discovery that expression of a forkhead protein essential for SHF development, Foxh1, is dependent on Isl1 (21). Interestingly, Isl1+ cells mark niches of undifferentiated cardiac progenitor cells in the postnatal heart (22), suggesting that understanding the regulation of SHF-derived progenitor pools may be useful in developing approaches for cardiac repair (discussed below).

Discovery of the SHF led to the reinterpretation of findings in mice lacking critical regulatory proteins and in transgenic mice harboring enhancers of genes expressed in the heart. As the molecular aspects of cardiogenesis were first being discovered approximately a decade ago, right ventricle–specific enhancers were repeatedly found for various genes that were expressed more widely in the developing heart (reviewed in [23]). Subsequently, the right ventricle was found to be enriched in a transcription factor, Hand2 (also known as dHAND), that is required for expansion of the right ventricle

(24). This observation further supported the concept that separable regulatory pathways control the development of the right and left ventricles from the crescent-shaped lateral mesoderm precursors. Since we now know that Hand2 is highly expressed in the SHF, the right ventricular hypoplasia that results from disruption of Hand2 likely represents a failure of SHF cells to expand into the right ventricle (24,25). Similarly, right ventricular hypoplasia in mice lacking Mef2c (26), now a known target of Isl1, Gata4, Foxh1, and Tbx20 in the SHF (27), may also represent a defect of SHF development. Indeed, many of the central transcriptional regulators of cardiac development in the primary heart field, including Nkx2-5 and Gata4, are found in the SHF and may primarily target SHF development (28) (Fig. 24.2). As such, pathways regulating the determination and differentiation of SHF cells may provide the foundation for efforts to induce the cardiac lineage from progenitor cells.

The significance of SHF transcriptional regulation is highlighted by the human cardiac defects observed in DiGeorge syndrome, the most common human deletion syndrome. The transcription factor TBX1 is the cause of cardiac and craniofacial disorders in this syndrome, which typically involves a deletion on chromosome 22q11 (29–32). TBX1 is another central transcriptional regulator of the secondary heart field and is necessary for proper development of cardiac outflow tract myocardium (33,34). The secreted morphogen Sonic hedgehog (Shh) is required to maintain Tbx1 expression in the SHF via a group of forkhead-containing transcription factors that directly regulate Tbx1 (35,36). Correspondingly, mice lacking Shh, Foxc1 and Foxc2, and Tbx1 share similar cardiac outflow tract defects (36,37). Tbx1 not only regulates outflow tract myocardium, but also regulates production of growth factors such as fibroblast growth factor 8 (Fgf8), which are secreted and act via receptors on adjacent neural crest-derived cells to affect their differentiation (33,38,39). Whether members of the pathway involving TBX1 or the Isl1-dependent pathway described above (Fig. 24.2) contribute to sporadic outflow tract defects similar to those seen in 22q11 deletion syndrome remains to be determined.

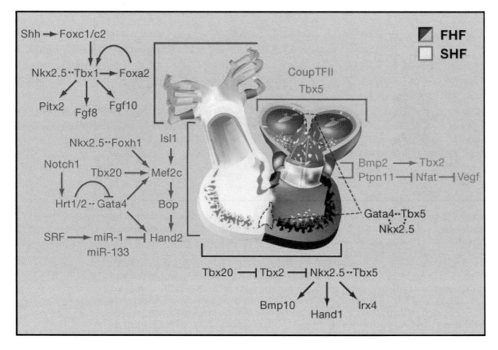

FIGURE 24.2 Pathways regulating region-specific cardiac morphogenesis. A partial list of transcription factors, signaling proteins, and miRNAs that can be placed in pathways that influence the formation of regions of the heart. Positive influences are indicated by *arrowheads*, and negative effects by *bars*. Physical interactions are indicated by direct contact of factors. In some cases relationships of proteins are unknown. Pathways regulating neural crest cells have been reviewed elsewhere (170). FHF, first heart field; SHF, second heart field.

While Hand2 and the closely related gene Hand1 are expressed in the SHF, they are also present in the primary heart field, with Hand1 being most enriched in the left ventricle (40). Hand1 expression is dependent on Nkx2.5 in the left ventricle, suggesting that Nkx2.5 plays a critical role in not only the SHF but also the primary heart field (41). Although disruption of tinman, the Nkx2.5 orthologue in flies, results in complete loss of cardial cells (42), deletion of Nkx2.5 in mice causes a less severe defect with lethality at E9.5 after initial formation of the heart tube (43,44). However, loss of Nkx2.5 and Hand2, thereby effectively eliminating Hand1 and Hand2 expression, results in complete failure of ventricular expansion in mice (25). Similar but slightly less severe defects were observed with conditional disruption of Hand1 and Hand2 (45). Consistent with an evolutionarily conserved role of Hand in ventricular expansion, zebrafish and fruitflies lacking the single Hand orthologue present in these species fail to expand the pool of comparable ventricular precursors (46,47).

The preservation of atrial precursors in mouse and fish Hand mutants suggested that a separate progenitor population may contribute to the atria. Indeed, mice lacking the nuclear receptor CoupTFII have a specific loss of atrial myocytes (48), as do mice lacking the T-box–containing transcription factor Tbx5 (49). Distinct aspects of atrial versus ventricular gene expression appear to be in part regulated by Irx4, a member of the Iroquois family of transcription factors (50).

Epigenetic factors may also contribute to cardiomyocyte differentiation and chamber morphogenesis. Disruption of the chromatin remodeling protein Smyd1 (also known as Bop) results in a phenotype reminiscent of Hand2 mutants: a small right ventricular segment and poor development of the left ventricular myocardium (51). Smyd1 contains a SET domain that harbors methyltransferase activity and a MYND domain that recruits histone deacetylase (HDAC) activity that together are responsible for transcriptional repression of target genes (51). Smyd1 activity is necessary for Hand2 expression in cardiac precursors, likely through an intermediate that is not yet known. Interestingly, Smyd1 is a direct target of Mef2c (52), suggesting that a transcriptional cascade involving Isl1, Mef2c, Smyd1, and Hand proteins regulates the development of ventricular cardiomyocytes (Fig. 24.2). A direct role for HDACs in cardiac development was also demonstrated by a failure of ventricular growth in compound mutant mice lacking HDAC5 and HDAC9 (53). These and other pathways in the heart appear to be regulated by a muscle-specific member of the SWI/SNF complex, Baf60c (54), suggesting that transcriptional activity of cardiac DNA-binding proteins is highly regulated through epigenetic events.

MicroRNA Regulation of Cardiomyocyte Differentiation

Although transcriptional and epigenetic events regulate many critical cardiac genes, translational control by small noncoding RNAs, such as microRNAs (miRNAs), has recently emerged as another mechanism to fine-tune dosages of key proteins during cardiogenesis (55,56). MicroRNAs are genomically encoded 20–22 nucleotide RNAs that target mRNAs for translational inhibition or degradation by many of the same pathways as small interfering RNA (siRNA) (57,58). More than 400 human microRNAs have been identified (59), but in only a few cases are the biologic function and mRNA targets known.

In particular, the microRNA-1 family (miR-1-1 and miR-1-2) is highly conserved from worms to humans and is specifically expressed in the developing cardiac and skeletal muscle

progenitor cells as they differentiate (55). Both are highly expressed in the SHF-derived cells of the cardiac outflow tract. Interestingly, expression of these microRNAs is directly controlled by well-studied transcriptional regulatory networks that promote muscle differentiation. Cardiac expression is dependent on serum response factor (SRF), and skeletal muscle expression requires the myogenic transcription factors MyoD and Mef2. Consistent with a role in differentiation, overexpression of miR-1 in the developing mouse heart results in a decrease in ventricular myocyte expansion, with fewer proliferating cardiomyocytes remaining in the cell cycle. In vivo validation of Hand2 as a miR-1 target suggests that tight regulation of Hand2 protein levels may be involved in controlling the balance between cardiomyocyte proliferation and differentiation. Both miR-1 and another miRNA, miR-133a, are transcribed in a polycistronic message, therefore sharing common regulation, and both are co-expressed in heart and skeletal muscle. As in cardiac muscle, miR-1 promotes the differentiation of skeletal myoblasts in culture, but interestingly, miR-133a has the opposite effect, inhibiting differentiation and promoting the proliferation of myoblasts (60).

Defects caused by mutations in miRNA genes range from benign to severe. Although no miRNA mutations have yet been described in mammals, disruption of individual miRNA genes in worms and flies has caused relatively mild phenotypes consistent with the role of miRNAs in adjusting the precise dose of proteins. However, disruption of the single fly orthologue of miR-1 had catastrophic consequences, resulting in uniform lethality at embryonic or larval stages with a frequent defect in maintaining cardiac gene expression (56). In a subset of flies lacking miR-1, a severe defect of cardiac progenitor cell differentiation provided loss-of-function evidence that miR-1 was involved in muscle differentiation events, similar to the gain-of-function findings in mice. In flies, miR-1 regulates the Notch signaling pathway by directly targeting mRNA of the Notch ligand, Delta (56), potentially explaining the involvement of miR-1 in deriving differentiated cardiac cells from an equivalency group of progenitor cells (61) (Fig. 24.3). Thus, miR-1 seems to be a muscle-specific microRNA that directs progenitor cells toward a cardiac cell fate by regulating central mediators of determination and differentiation.

Complex Regulation of Cardiac Morphogenesis

Although the pathways regulating individual cell lineages contributing to the heart are deeply understood, the subsequent complex events involved in integrating multiple cell types, formation of chambers, and patterning of the distinct regions of the heart are also now being elucidated. From an evolutionary standpoint, it appears that as organisms became more complex, a more elaborate cardiovascular system was required. Distinct cardiac chambers began to develop and adopted specialized functions. Fish, which have a circulatory system that functions in series, developed separate atrial and ventricular chambers with a single inflow and outflow tract. The single ventricle pumps blood to the body via the gills, and no separation of deoxygenated and oxygenated blood is necessary. The amphibious frog adopted an intermediate three-chambered heart. In contrast, terrestrial vertebrates required complete separation of oxygenated and deoxygenated blood after birth, necessitating two separate atrial and ventricular chambers along with two distinct inflow and outflow tracts. These evolutionary observations suggest that the heart was built in modules that were added as they became necessary. The discovery

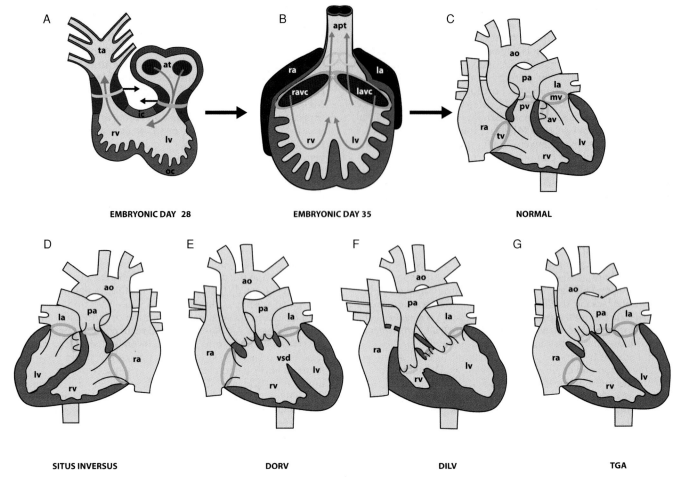

FIGURE 24.3 Normal and abnormal cardiac morphogenesis associated with left-right signaling. **A:** As the linear heart tube loops rightward with inner curvature (ic) remodeling and outer curvature (oc) proliferation, the endocardial cushions (*dark blue*) of the inflow (*green*) and outflow (*light blue*) tracts become adjacent to one another. Subsequently, the atrioventricular septum (AVS) shifts to the right, while the aortopulmonary trunk shifts to the left. **B:** The inflow tract is divided into the right (ravc) and left atrioventricular canal (lavc) by the atrioventricular septum (*asterisk*). The outflow tract, known as the truncus arteriosus (ta), becomes the aortopulmonary trunk (apt) on septation. **C:** Ultimately, the left (la) and right atrium (ra) are aligned with the left ventricle (lv) and right ventricle (rv), respectively. The lv and rv become aligned with the aorta (ao) and pulmonary artery (pa), respectively, after 180-degree rotation of the great vessels. **D:** If the determinants of the left-right axis are coordinately reversed, then a condition known as situs inversus results. **E:** If the apt fails to shift to the left, then a condition known as double-outlet right ventricle (DORV) results, in which the right ventricle is aligned with both the aorta and pulmonary artery. **F:** Likewise, if the AVS fails to shift to the right, both atria communicate with the left ventricle in a condition known as double-inlet left ventricle (DILV). **G:** Transposition of the great arteries (TGA) results if the apt fails to twist, resulting in communication of the rv with ao and lv with pa. av, aortic valve; mv, mitral valve; pv, pulmonary valve; vsd, ventricular septal defect.

of distinct heart fields as described above and evidence of modular gene expression in the heart supports such a notion.

Dorsal-Ventral Polarity

Beyond the asymmetric addition of SHF cells along the anterior-posterior axis, a discrete dorsal-ventral (DV) polarity occurs in the primitive heart tube. As the heart tube loops to the right, the ventral surface of the tube rotates to become the outer curvature of the looped heart, and the dorsal surface forms the inner curvature. The outer curvature becomes the site of active growth, whereas remodeling of the inner curvature is essential for the ultimate alignment of the inflow and outflow tracts of

the heart. A model in which individual chambers "balloon" from the outer curvature in a segmental fashion has been proposed (62). Consistent with this model, numerous genes, including the transcription factor Hand1 and the sarcomeric protein Serca2, are expressed specifically on the outer curvature of the heart (41,63). Hand2 is expressed on the inner and outer curvature, but protein production of Hand2 in the inner curvature may be repressed by miRNA regulation, as miR-1 is first detected in the inner but not outer curvature at E8.5 (55). Also, through a complex transcriptional network, the unique identity of inner curvature cells is determined by Tbx2-mediated repression of genes typically found on the outer curvature (64). Another Tbox transcription factor, Tbx20, serves to repress

Tbx2 activity in the outer curvature as it expands into the cardiac chambers, thereby establishing the regional patterning of expanding or remodeling myocardium (65–67). Remodeling of the inner curvature allows migration of the inflow tract to the right and the outflow tract to the left, facilitating proper alignment and separation of right- and left-sided circulations. In addition to its role in repressing Tbx2, Tbx20 affects expansion of both the primary and secondary heart field–derived cells and is necessary for outflow tract development, possibly via regulation of Nkx2.5 and Mef2c (65).

Left-Right Asymmetry and Cardiac Looping

Rightward looping of the heart tube with the caudal portion of the tube moving to a more anterior and dorsal position is the first obvious sign of the break in left-right (LR) symmetry. The cellular mechanisms that drive cardiac looping remain poorly understood, but it has been postulated that differential rates of proliferation of cardioblasts, regional differences in intracardiac actin bundles, or altered cell adhesion across the heart tube may be involved. When considering the mechanisms for cardiac looping, it is important to distinguish between the process of looping and the directionality of looping (68). Directionality of looping reflects overall asymmetry throughout the embryo, which is superimposed on the morphogenetic mechanisms for looping.

It has been proposed that abnormalities in the process of cardiac looping underlie a number of CHDs. Folding of the heart tube positions the inflow cushions adjacent to the outflow cushions and involves extensive remodeling of the inner curvature of the looped heart tube. In the primitive looped heart, the segments of the heart are still in a linear pattern and must be repositioned considerably for alignment of the atrial chambers with the appropriate ventricles and the ventricles with the aorta and pulmonary arteries. The atrioventricular septum (AVS) begins to divide the common atrioventricular canal (AVC) into a right and left AVC that subsequently shifts to the right to position the AVS over the ventricular septum (Fig. 24.3). This allows the right AVC and the left AVC to be aligned with the right and left ventricles, respectively. Simultaneously, the conotruncal region becomes septated into the aorta and pulmonary trunks as the conotruncus moves toward the left side of the heart such that the conotruncal septum is positioned over the AVS (Fig. 24.3). The rightward shift of the AVS and leftward shift of the conotruncus converts the single-inlet, single-outlet heart into a four-chambered heart that has separate atrial inlets and ventricular outlets (reviewed in [69]).

Arrest or incomplete movement of the AVS or conotruncus might result in malalignment of the inflow and outflow tracts (Fig. 24.3). A scenario in which the AVS fails to shift to the right would result in communication of the right and left AVCs with the left ventricle, a condition known as double-inlet left ventricle (DILV). Incomplete shifting may be the basis for "unbalanced" AVC defects where the right AVC only partly communicates with the right ventricle. Similarly, if the conotruncal septum fails to shift to the left, both the aorta and pulmonary artery would arise from the right ventricle causing a double-outlet right ventricle (DORV). From this embryologic perspective, it is not surprising that double-outlet left ventricles and double-inlet right ventricles are rarely, if ever, seen clinically. In contrast, any abnormality in cardiac looping can be associated with DILV or DORV, along with other manifestations of improper alignment of specific regions of the heart.

The elegant molecular network regulating LR asymmetry of the body plan has been reviewed (70) and will not be summarized here. However, it is worth highlighting several clues about the relationship between LR asymmetry and proper alignment of the cardiac chambers. The cascade of LR signals including Sonic hedgehog (Shh) and Nodal converge on the transcription factor Pitx2 (71). Pitx2 is initially LR asymmetric in the linear heart tube, but this asymmetry is translated into a dorsal-ventral polarity in the looped heart tube. Because Pitx2 regulates cell proliferation via cyclin D2 and also controls cell migration events (72), it is a potential link between signals regulating the direction and process of cardiac looping. Within certain subdomains, regulation of Pitx2 by Tbx1 integrates transcriptional pathways controlling morphogenesis and LR asymmetry (73).

How do the insights into LR asymmetry impact our understanding of CHDs? It is likely that patients with situs inversus totalis have a well-coordinated reversal of LR asymmetry and thus have a lower incidence of defects in visceral organogenesis. However, most patients with LR defects have visceroatrial heterotaxy and thus have randomization of cardiac, pulmonary, and gastrointestinal situs where coordinated signaling is absent. Such patients can have defects in almost all aspects of cardiogenesis. Often either the right or left side predominates with patients either having bilateral right-sidedness (asplenia syndrome) or bilateral left-sidedness (polysplenia syndrome). In such cases, features of the right or left side of the lungs, heart, and gut are duplicated. Disruption of cascades determining either the left or right side of the embryo might result in asplenia or polysplenia syndromes, respectively. Indeed, mutations in LR pathway members are found in some patients with heterotaxy (74). Familial cases of heterotaxy have also led to identification of mutations in a zinc-finger transcription factor, ZIC3, that result in LR axis abnormalities (75).

Cardiac Outflow Tract Regulation

Congenital cardiac defects involving the cardiac outflow tract, aortic arch, ductus arteriosus, and proximal pulmonary arteries account for 20% to 30% of all CHDs. This region of the heart undergoes extensive and rather complex morphogenetic changes with contributions from neural crest cells and the SHF, as discussed above. The cardiac outflow tract can be divided into the muscularized conus and the adjacent truncus arteriosus, collectively termed the conotruncus, as it arises from the primitive right ventricle. The conotruncus normally shifts to the left to override the forming ventricular septum. The truncus arteriosus then becomes septated by mesenchymal cells into the aorta and pulmonary arteries with a muscular ridge forming between the two vessels known as the conotruncal septum (Fig. 24.4). However, at this stage, the aorta communicates with the right ventricle and the pulmonary artery with the left ventricle. Subsequent rotation of the two vessels in a spiraling fashion places the aorta in a more dorsal and leftward position and the pulmonary artery in a more ventral and rightward location. This spiraling event achieves the normal alignment of the aorta and pulmonary artery to the left and right ventricles, respectively.

Abnormalities in septation or incomplete spiraling of the conotruncus result in many CHDs. For example, the conotruncal septum between the aorta and pulmonary artery forms in tetralogy of Fallot (TOF), but because of malalignment of the great vessels, the conotruncal septum and aorta are shifted to the right. This results in an overriding aorta and failure of the conotruncal septum to connect to the muscular ventricular septum, resulting in a ventricular septal defect (Fig. 24.3). Similarly, any malalignment of the conotruncus results in an obligatory ventricular septal defect that, unlike muscular VSDs, does not have the potential to close spontaneously after birth.

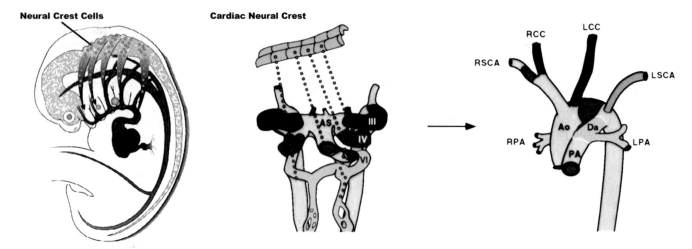

FIGURE 24.4 Cardiac neural crest contributions to aortic arch development. Cardiac neural crest cells arise from the neural folds and migrate into the outflow tract of the heart and aortic arch arteries. They are involved in remodeling the arch arteries, with derivatives color-coded by their arch artery origins. Ao, aorta; AS, atrial septum; Da, descending aorta; LCC, left common carotid; LPA, left pulmonary artery; LSCA, left subclavian artery; RCC, right common carotid; RSCA, right subclavian artery.

A structure referred to as the aortic sac lies distal to the conotruncus and gives rise to six bilaterally symmetric vessels known as aortic arch arteries. The aortic arch arteries arise sequentially along the anterior-posterior (AP) axis, each traversing a pharyngeal arch before joining the paired dorsal aortae (Fig. 24.4). The first and second arch arteries involute, and the fifth arch artery never fully forms. The third, fourth, and sixth arch arteries undergo extensive remodeling to ultimately form distinct regions of the mature aortic arch and proximal pulmonary arteries. Most of the right-sided dorsal aorta and aortic arch arteries undergo programmed cell death leading to a left-sided aortic arch. The third aortic arch artery contributes to the proximal carotid arteries and right subclavian artery. The left fourth aortic arch artery forms the transverse aortic arch between the left common carotid and left subclavian arteries. Finally, the sixth arch artery contributes to the proximal pulmonary artery and the ductus arteriosus (76). Extrapolating from their embryologic origins, it is believed that aberrant right subclavian arteries and other subtle arch anomalies are the result of third aortic arch defects; interrupted aortic arch from fourth arch defects; and patent ductus arteriosus and proximal pulmonary artery hypoplasia/discontinuity from defects in sixth arch artery development.

Mesenchyme cells originating from the crest of the neural folds are essential for proper septation and remodeling of the outflow tract and aortic arch (reviewed in [77]). Such neural crest-derived cells migrate away from the neural folds and retain the ability to differentiate into multiple cell types (Fig. 24.4). The migratory path and ultimate fate of these cells depends on their relative position of origin along the anterior-posterior axis and are partly regulated by the Hox code (78). Neural crest cells differentiate and contribute to diverse embryonic structures, including the cranial ganglia, peripheral nervous system, adrenal glands, and melanocytes. Neural crest cells that arise from the otic placode to the third somite migrate through the developing pharyngeal arches and populate the mesenchyme of each of the aortic arch arteries and the mesenchyme necessary to septate the outflow tract septum (Fig. 24.4). Because of their migratory path and role, this segment of the neural crest is often referred to as the cardiac neural crest.

Mutations in many signaling cascades affect neural crest migration or development, including the endothelin and semaphorin pathways, and cause outflow tract defects similar to those observed in humans (77). Embryos deficient in cardiac neural crest cell migration or differentiation display various cardiac outflow tract and aortic arch defects resembling those in humans. These include tetralogy of Fallot, persistent truncus arteriosus, double-outlet right ventricle, ventricular septal defects, and defects of aortic arch patterning. Thus, abnormalities in neural crest migration or differentiation likely underlie many of the conotruncal and aortic arch defects seen in humans. Indeed, human mutations of the neural crest–enriched transcription factor TFAP2β result in persistent patency of the ductus arteriosus, a specialized aortic arch vessel essential for fetal cardiac physiology (79) (Fig. 24.4). It is likely that other genetic mutations affect specific regions of the aortic arch.

Disruption of SHF development by mutation of genes such as Tbx1, Fgf8, and Islet1 results in defects similar to those observed with neural crest disruption (Fig. 24.2), including persistent truncus arteriosus (failure of outflow septation), malalignment of the outflow tract of the heart with the ventricular chambers, and ventricular septal defects (18,32,38,39). Since SHF-derived myocardial cells neighbor neural crest–derived cells and secrete growth factors such as Fgf8 in a Tbx1-dependent manner that influence neural crest cells (33), reciprocal interactions between the SHF and neural crest–derived cells in the outflow tract are likely essential for normal development. Consistent with this, humans with deletion or mutation of *TBX1* (80), expressed in the SHF, appear to have cell-autonomous defects of SHF development and non–cell-autonomous anomalies of neural crest–derived tissues. It will be interesting to determine if many human cardiac outflow tract defects are a direct result of SHF migration, differentiation, or proliferation.

Cardiac Valve Formation

Appropriate placement and function of cardiac valves is essential for chamber septation and for unidirectional flow of blood through the heart. A molecular network involving Bmp2 and Tbx2 defines the position of the valves relative to the chambers (64,81,82). During early heart tube formation, "cushions" of extracellular matrix (ECM) between the endocardium and myocardium presage valve formation at each end of the heart tube. Reciprocal signaling, mediated in part by TGF-β family members, between the myocardium and endocardium in the cushion region induces a transformation of endocardial cells into mesenchymal cells that migrate into the ECM cushion (83–85). These mesenchymal cells differentiate into the fibrous tissue of the valves and are involved in septation of the common atrioventricular canal into right- and left-sided orifices.

Although the processes regulating early epithelial to mesenchymal transition (EMT) in the atrioventricular canal have been extensively investigated as described above, our understanding of the mechanisms regulating later stages of semilunar valve development are still primarily limited to morphogenic descriptions. This is due, in part, to the fact that this period of development has been essentially inaccessible to experimental manipulation because gene perturbation studies result in embryonic demise in the midgestation mouse embryo. However, based on studies of normal mouse and human embryos (86,87), investigators have demonstrated that the endocardial cushions form condensed mesenchymal protrusions, the primitive valves. These condensed mesenchymal protrusions subsequently elongate to provide the true cardiac valve leaflets (Fig. 24.5). The elongation of primitive valves appears to be a result of restricted proliferation of endocardial cells overlying the mesenchymal projections on the vascular side of the valve and selective cell death under the expanding endocardial rim. The growth of the endocardial edge and evacuation of apoptotic cells underneath the proliferating endocardial rim sculpt the swollen mesenchymal primitive valves into a typical excavated shape and result in morphogenesis of the sinuses of valsalva.

Recent studies using immunohistochemistry and electron microscopy described late gestational and postnatal valve development in chicken and mouse (88), with a remarkably similar progression of developmental events seen in human fetuses (89). These studies document progression of remodeling and compartmentalization of the valve leaflet from a disorganized matrix of proteoglycans with little detectable elastin, and small amounts of disorganized collagen and relative uniform distribution of vascular interstitial cells (VICs), to a highly stratified ECM. The ECM contains three organized layers of fibrosa (arterial aspect primarily composed of collagens), spongiosa (central aspect, primarily glycosaminogly-cans), and ventricularis (ventricular aspect with elastin fibers) with compartmentalization of VICs resulting in increased cell density in the fibrosa and ventricularis. Notably, this process is not only conserved across species but extends well after birth into postnatal life. Interestingly, the fetal VIC activation that occurs throughout development is similar to the valve changes occurring in pathologic conditions (90,91), suggesting that analogous molecular mechanisms likely direct both normal developmental and pathologic interstitial cell activation (91). Furthermore, recent experiments have suggested that a small population of VICs may reside as a progenitor cell population that retains the ability to differentiate into either endothelial or interstitial cells in the valve leaflet (92).

A few mouse mutants escape early embryonic demise and are thus informative in unraveling the mechanisms of late gestational and early postnatal semilunar valve pathology. Most of these mouse models display normal EMT but then evolve a hyperplastic valve phenotype that suggests aberrations in valve remodeling. One common feature of many of these defects is perturbations that either enhance or attenuate RAS-MAPK signaling (reviewed in [93,94]). Gitler et al. (95) showed that hyperplastic aortic valve defects in neurofibromatosis 1 (NF1) mutant embryos, previously attributed to defects in cardiac neural crest cells, result from a primary defect in outflow tract and atrioventricular canal endocardium. These defects were at least partially due to elevations in endocardial MAPK signaling secondary to the loss of NF1 suppression of *Ras-Erk* signaling, resulting in increased proliferation and decreased apoptosis (96). Consistent with this, patients with NF1 mutations develop pulmonary stenosis and hypertension but rarely defects in the AVC (97). NF1 loss of function is mimicked by gain of function mutations in the tyrosine phosphatase Shp2/PTPN11, which causes an increase in Ras-Erk activation, increased proliferation, and decreased apoptosis, resulting in semilunar valve and atrioventricular valve hyperplasia (98,99). Autosomal dominant gain of function mutations in Shp2 cause Noonan syndrome, characterized by pulmonary stenosis, hypertrophic cardiomyopathy, and occasional atrioventricular valve defects (100,101). Most recently, hypomorphic mutations in SOS1, an essential RAS guanine nucleotide-exchange factor (Ras-Gef), result in enhanced RAS-ERK activation and can account for as many as 20% of the cases of Noonan syndrome not explained by Shp2 mutations (102,103).

Recent evidence implicates EGF signaling as an important regulator of late valve remodeling. Loss or attenuation of EGFR/ErbB1 signaling results in preferential hypercellularity

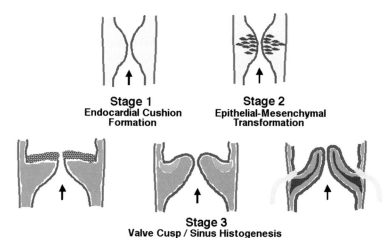

Stage 1
Endocardial Cushion Formation

Stage 2
Epithelial-Mesenchymal Transformation

Stage 3
Valve Cusp / Sinus Histogenesis

FIGURE 24.5 Summary of the critical stages in semilunar valve formation. Initially, regional swellings of extracellular matrix (ECM) form the endocardial cushions, which provide valvelike action ensuring that initial blood flow is unidirectional in the developing embryo. Subsequently, endothelial cells undergo a mesenchymal transformation and populate the endocardial cushions. Finally, the endothelial cells on the arterial face proliferate and the ECM is remodeled to begin valve cusp histogenesis. Subsequently, a selected population of mesenchymal cells is thought to undergo apoptosis simultaneously with continued remodeling of the ECM to form the sinuses, which will eventually become the origin of the proximal coronary arteries. The *black arrows* denote the direction of blood flow.

of semilunar but not AV valves (104). The hyperplastic semilunar valve phenotype is augmented when crossed to mice heterozygous for a null mutation in Shp2 (105). Deletion of the EGF ligand, heparin binding (HB)-EGF, results in increased endocardial cushion size and cell proliferation of both semilunar and AV valves (106,107). These mice show prolonged Smad 1/5/8 phosphorylation and loss of phospolipase E (108), a downstream component of EGF and Ras signaling, and are similar to mice with a null mutation in inhibitory Smad6 (109). In contrast, mice lacking the Erb3 receptor die in midgestation of heart failure from hypoplastic semilunar and AV valve primordial (110). Null mutations in other EGFR ligands (EGF, ampiregulin, TGF-α) have no effect on valve formation. Finally, mice lacking Ephrin B2 also have thickened valves, and although the mechanism for this remains unclear, it will be interesting to determine how these signaling pathways intersect (111). The exact mechanism of regulation is likely to be context dependent and receptor specific and may involve the intersection of multiple growth factor signaling pathways.

In contrast to the thickened leaflets described above, disruption of signaling pathways converging on the transcription factor Nfatc revealed a requirement of this calcium-activated regulator. Nfatc is expressed specifically in the forming embryonic valves, and targeted deletion of Nfatc in mice results in absence of cardiac valve formation (112,113). Signaling via the phosphatase, calcineurin, results in nuclear translocation of Nfatc and is similarly involved in cardiac valve formation, in part through regulation of vascular endothelial growth factor (Vegf) expression in the endocardium (114).

The Notch signaling pathway is required for cell fate and differentiation decisions throughout the embryo (61), but only recently have Notch proteins been implicated in vertebrate cardiac development. In fish and frogs, Notch appears to be involved in development of the endocardial cushions that contribute to valve tissue (115). In humans, heterozygous NOTCH1 mutations disrupt normal development of the aortic valve and occasionally the mitral valve (116) (Table 24.1).

The severity of valve disease associated with NOTCH1 mutations in humans varies widely from mild disease in which the aortic valve has two rather than three leaflets (bicuspid aortic valve) to severe defects in valve patency in utero, resulting in left ventricular growth failure. Consistent with this genetic finding, 15% of "normal" relatives of children with hypoplastic left heart syndrome (HLHS) have subclinical bicuspid aortic valves (117,118), suggesting that disruption of the NOTCH signaling cascade may underlie a spectrum of aortic valve disease. Although not specifically affecting valves, human mutations in JAGGED1, a NOTCH ligand, also cause outflow tract defects associated with the autosomal dominant disease, Alagille syndrome (119–121). The hairy-related family of transcriptional repressors (Hrt1, Hrt2, and Hrt3) may mediate the Notch signal during valve and myocardial development; however, their targets for repression remain unknown (122) (reviewed in [123]).

GENETICS OF HUMAN SEPTAL DEFECTS

Recent findings with the cardiac transcription factors NKX2.5, TBX5, and GATA4 exemplify the synergy between human genetics and studies of model organisms for understanding the etiologic factors of human CHD (Table 24.1). Numerous point mutations have been identified in NKX2.5 in families with atrial septal defects and progressive cardiac conduction abnormalities (124). Retrospective analysis of mice heterozygous for Nkx2.5 disruption revealed a similar phenotype and progressive apoptotic loss of conduction cells, suggesting a likely mechanism for the human phenotype (125,126).

Humans with Holt–Oram syndrome, caused by mutations in TBX5, have cardiac anomalies similar to those with NKX2.5 mutations (atrial and ventricular septal defects) as well as limb abnormalities (127,128). Intriguingly, mutations

---

TABLE 24.1

GENETIC CAUSES OF CONGENITAL HEART DISEASE

Genetic mutation	Syndrome name	Cardiac disease
Nonsyndromic		
NKX2-5	—	Atrial septal defect, ventricular septal defect, electrical conduction defect
GATA4	—	Atrial septal defect, ventricular septal defect
MHC	—	Atrial septal defect
NOTCH1	—	Aortic valve disease
Syndromic		
TBX5	Holt–Oram	Atrial septal defect, ventricular septal defect, electrical conduction defect
TBX1	DiGeorge	Cardiac outflow tract defect
TFAP2β	Char	Patent ductus arteriosus
JAG1	Alagille	Pulmonary artery stenosis, tetralogy of Fallot
PTPN11	Noonan's	Pulmonary valve stenosis
Elastin	William	Supravalvar aortic stenosis
Fibrillin	Marfan	Aortic aneurysm

Narrowing of vessels or valves is indicated as stenosis; patent ductus arteriosus represents persistence of a fetal vessel connecting the aorta and pulmonary artery that normally closes after birth; tetralogy of Fallot describes a misalignment of the aorta and pulmonary artery with the ventricular chambers such that the aorta communicates with both chambers.

responsible for defects in the heart and limbs are clustered in different regions of the protein, suggesting that TBX5 engages different downstream genes or cofactors in these tissues that depend on unique structural motifs in the protein. One potential cofactor is NKX2-5, as the two physically interact and cooperate to activate common target genes (129).

Like the NKX2.5 and TBX5 mutations, mutations in the zinc-finger–containing protein GATA4 cause similar atrial and ventricular septal defects in autosomal dominant nonsyndromic human pedigrees (130). GATA4 or related proteins are essential for cardiogenesis in flies, fish, and mice (131–134). Like NKX2.5, GATA4 and TBX5 also form a complex to regulate downstream genes, such as myosin heavy chain. Consistent with an important role for such combinatorial interactions, a familial GATA4 point mutation disrupts GATA4's ability to interact with TBX5 (116). Conversely, several human TBX5 mutations disrupt TBX5 interaction with GATA4, suggesting that the two cooperate in cardiac septation events (130). GATA4, TBX5, and NKX2-5 may form a common complex that is necessary for proper cardiac septation (Fig. 24.2). Disruption of any one of the three proteins or their interactions can result in atrial or ventricular septal defects. Although the compendium of septal genes regulated by these transcription factors is unknown, it is intriguing that mutations in human myosin heavy chain (MHC), a direct target of GATA4, TBX5, and NKX2-5, also cause atrial septal defects (135). This observation suggests a possible mechanism by which these genes cause septation defects.

THE EPICARDIUM, CORONARY VASCULARIZATION, AND CONDUCTION SYSTEM MORPHOGENESIS

The origin of coronary vascular endothelium and formation of the coronary vessels has been an area of intense investigation (reviewed in [136]). Several theories have evolved to explain coronary morphogenesis, which range from the sprouting of vessels from the aorta into developing myocardium to outgrowth of the endocardial lining of the heart to the epicardial vessels. Such theories have evolved from descriptive examination of the coronary ontogeny of various animals as well as human embryos. A critical component from most of these reports was the observation that coronary vessel formation was coordinately related to epicardial formation.

Several investigators have demonstrated that the epicardium originates as a villous projection of mesothelial cells in the area of the sinus venosus termed the proepicardial organ. This cluster of cells extends to the atrioventricular region and migrates out over the myocardial surface to completely encase the heart (137–141). In vitro data initially suggested that this villous or mesothelial projection might be the source of the coronary arteries (142). The correlation between epicardial formation and coronary ontogeny has been clarified in three definitive series of experiments. Using retroviral tagging of cells initially infected while in the pre-epicardial mesothelium, Mikawa and Fischman (143) were able to document that coronary smooth muscle cells, perivascular fibroblasts, and coronary endothelial cells all derive from independent precursors that arise outside the heart and that the endothelium of the coronary arteries and endocardium have different clonal origins. In complementary experiments, Poelmann et al. (144) used quail epicardial and liver tissue transplanted into chicken so that endothelial cells of quail origin

could be identified. These experiments also demonstrate that the entire coronary endothelial vasculature originated from an extracardiac source. In addition, this approach suggested that endothelial cells originating from the liver mesenchyme and located within this mesothelial projection or epicardial primordium used the subepicardial matrix to completely vascularize the developing heart. This subepicardial matrix is rich in fibronectin and vitronectin, a conducive ECM for vascular development E104-15. In a definitive set of experiments using retroviral injections directly into the proepicardial organ as well as proepicardial transplants, Mikawa and Gourdie (145) were able to demonstrate that this cluster of extracardiac cells contained differentiated endothelial cells, smooth muscles, and perivascular cells that would ultimately serve as the source of precursors for the coronary vascular bed. These experiments were later confirmed and expanded using a novel in vitro assay of epicardial differentiation (146). All of these experiments provide compelling evidence that coronary artery formation appears to be primarily a vasculogenic process. The coronary angioblasts originate from precursors located within the extracardiac pre-epicardial mesothelium and subsequently organize within the subepicardial matrix into the coronary vascular network.

Whereas distal coronary development occurs by vasculogenesis, proximal coronary artery morphogenesis appears to result from an angiogenic process. Although traditionally the proximal coronary arteries were described as an outgrowth from the aorta to the epicardial surface of the heart, several investigators have recently shown that in fact the angiogenic process is in the reverse direction. Angiogenic sprouts from the subepicardial endothelial plexus form endothelial strands that grow into the aorta and develop multiple communications with all three cusps of the developing aortic valve (147–149). However, lumens develop only in facing semilunar sinuses with resorption of the strands to the nonfacing or noncoronary cusp (144). These observations have obvious implications for determining the factors that direct coronary artery anatomy in congenital heart diseases.

Despite the centrality of electrophysiologic abnormalities to congenital heart diseases, very little is known about development of the cardiac conduction system (reviewed in [150,151]). A central controversy has revolved around whether primary conduction tissue differentiates from contractile myocytes or whether it is derived from "invading" neural crest. Using retroviral lineage tracing similar to that described above for defining the source of the coronary vasculature, Gourdie et al. (152) were able to show that pulse-generating conduction cells were derived from local recruitment of differentiated myocytes along the developing coronary artery system. This same group has gone on to demonstrate that endothelin produced by the developing coronary vasculature is a primary mediator of this recruitment of myocytes to the conduction lineage (153). Thus, initial development of the distal conduction system is independent of neural crest. However, the neural crest cells may exert a later, indirect effect on conduction system development via their role in maintaining the coronary vasculature (154,155). Establishment of epicardial to endocardial gradients of key channels is also important for appropriate depolarization and is in part regulated by the transcription factor Irx5 (156). Networks of transcription factors involving Nkx, T-box, and Irx family members appear to control discrete aspects of the cardiac conduction system and are disrupted in human arrhythmias (49,157). These observations pave the way for a more detailed evaluation of the factors that regulate normal and potentially abnormal development of the conduction system.

ADULT CONSEQUENCES OF CARDIAC MALFORMATIONS

As human survivors of cardiac malformations ranging from simple atrial septal defects to more complex heart disease enter their third and fourth decades of life, new cardiac disease processes are becoming apparent, including abnormal conduction of electricity within the heart and diminished contractile function of the heart. The cause of these secondary defects had in the past been ascribed to abnormal hemodynamics, but recent evidence suggests that the same genes that cause early morphologic defects in heart development might later be directly involved in cardiac dysfunction and cell lineage disturbances in adulthood (2).

For example, human and mouse mutations in *NKX2.5* not only cause a developmental atrial septal defect, but also progressively disrupt electrical conduction through the cardiac chambers and can result in sudden death later in life (124,157). The atrioventricular (AV) node, which serves as the essential site of electrical communication between the atria and ventricles, is smaller than normal in adult Nkx2.5 mouse mutants; over time, the specialized muscle-derived conduction cells are lost and replaced by fibrotic tissue, resulting in progressive defects in electrical conduction (126).

Another example of a congenital heart malformation causing disease later in life involves the aortic valve. Worldwide, 1% of the population is born with a bicuspid aortic valve, typically silent in childhood (1). However, one third of bicuspid aortic valves develop premature age-dependent calcific stenosis, resulting in poorly mobile, nonfunctioning valves, often in the fifth, sixth, or seventh decades of life (158). As a result, calcific aortic stenosis is the third leading cause of heart disease in adults and requires >30,000 surgical valve replacements per year in the United States. The recent discovery that NOTCH1 mutations in humans cause bicuspid aortic valves and later calcification provides firm genetic evidence that the early developmental and later degenerative disease share a common genetic cause (116). Some family members with NOTCH1 mutations had normal tricuspid valves but still developed calcification, supporting the idea that the premature and severe calcification was primarily due to the genetic mutation itself rather than to hemodynamic effects on the valve leaflets.

Calcified human valves are characterized by ectopic osteoblast-specific gene expression suggesting a cell fate change of mesenchymal or inflammatory cells (158,159). Notch1 can repress a central transcriptional regulator of osteoblast cell fate, Runx2/Cbfa1 (160), suggesting a potential mechanism through which NOTCH1 normally suppresses calcification in the valve tissue (116). It will be interesting to determine if polymorphisms in *NOTCH1* are associated with altered risk of aortic valve or even vascular calcification, given the similar osteoblast gene expression in atherosclerotic vascular smooth muscle (161). If so, it is attractive to imagine effective preventive interventions over decades with pharmaceuticals, such as statins, to lower levels of cholesterol, a well-known risk factor for calcification (162).

CARDIAC STEM CELL AND REGENERATIVE APPROACHES

The notion that genes involved in the early formation of the heart may be redeployed to help protect, repair, or regenerate cardiac muscle has been a driving force in efforts to understand early developmental pathways (163). Two recent examples highlight the potential utility of this approach.

Several reports describing niches of small, noncardiomyocyte populations in the postnatal heart that on isolation in culture can differentiate into cardiac muscle and endothelial cells have generated considerable excitement that the heart, like other organs, may have a resident pool of progenitor cells. Some controversy exists regarding the markers of these cells with partially nonoverlapping reports of Sca-1-, c-kit-, or Abcg2-positive progenitors (164–166). A fourth population of progenitors expressing the developmental transcription factor Isl1 suggests an important connection between postnatal progenitor cells and an early developmental pathway regulating cardiomyocyte precursors (22). As described earlier, Isl1 is expressed in SHF cells before they differentiate into myocytes and is downregulated on expression of sarcomeric proteins. Cell fate studies suggest that cells derived from Isl1$^+$ progenitors populate most of the right ventricle and outflow tract and Isl1 is required for the formation of these regions (18); some cells derived from these Isl1$^+$ cells also contribute to the atria and left ventricle. In mice and humans, niches of Isl1$^+$ cells are detectable in the early postnatal heart and may be remnants of developmental progenitor cells among terminally differentiatiated myocytes (22). It will be interesting to determine if these cells have the potential to differentiate into cardiomyocytes, endothelial cells, and conduction system cells, consistent with SHF contributions.

Deeper understanding of the regulatory networks governing SHF proliferation and differentiation may allow expansion of the postnatal pool of Isl1 progenitors for therapeutic purposes. Interestingly, Shh, a regulator of pluripotency in some settings (167,168), is an early regulator of the SHF and controls expression of Tbx1 in the cardiac progenitors (35,36). Whether Shh regulates the postnatal Isl1 progenitors remains to be determined. It will also be interesting to investigate whether use of Isl1 as a marker of cardiac progenitor cells in differentiating embryonic stem cells may provide an intermediate population that could be efficiently induced to differentiate into cardiomyocytes by cardiogenic transcription factors or miRNAs.

SUMMARY

The field of cardiac developmental biology has progressed rapidly over the last decade, and the heart is now one of the best-understood organs at the molecular, physiologic, and anatomic levels. Advances in human genetic tools have also led to a deeper understanding of the importance of developmental pathways in human disease. Congenital heart disease can now be conceived as not only a defect of morphogenesis, but in some cases, a failure of differentiation among subsets of lineages that contribute to the heart. We are now embarking on a phase in which knowledge of developmental pathways and high-throughput methods of genotyping rare and common gene variants should allow rigorous investigation into the causes of human heart disease. With the increasing recognition that CHD has a significant genetic contribution, we can now imagine that genetic variation underlies both the morphogenetic defect and the predisposition to long-term consequences that will affect clinical outcomes for the millions of CHD survivors. Thus, vigorous efforts to identify genetic variation associated with CHD and outcome will be essential as therapeutic or preventive measures to alter the course of disease may be possible throughout childhood and in the adult. It may even be conceivable to eventually predict genetic risk among parents and focus preventive strategies on those at greatest risk to transmit disease vertically. The efficacy of folic acid in prevention of neural tube defects provides hope for similar prevention of congenital heart disease (169,170).

As the next phase of disease-related biology evolves, parallel advances in stem cell biology should usher in an era of new approaches. It is exciting to imagine future technologies that may enable generation of disease-specific embryonic stem cell lines for mechanistic studies of disease etiology and development of patient-specific stem cells for ultimate treatment modalities. Although it may become possible to guide stem or progenitor cells into a cardiac lineage based on our knowledge of early developmental pathways, many hurdles must be overcome for therapeutic use. Issues such as stem cell expansion, delivery, incorporation, electrical coupling, and safety remain to be addressed. Despite these significant challenges, there is reason for optimism as we continue to unravel the mysteries surrounding the lineage determination, differentiation, and morphogenesis of cardiac cells.

References

1. Hoffman JI, Kaplan S. The incidence of congenital heart disease. *J Am Coll Cardiol* 2002;39:1890–1900.
2. Srivastava D. Heart disease: An ongoing genetic battle? *Nature* 2004; 429:819–822.
3. Srivastava D, Ivey KN. Potential of stem cell-based therapies for heart disease. *Nature* 2006;441:1097–1099.
4. AHA. *Heart Disease and Stroke Statistics—2004 Update*. Dallas, TX: 2004.
5. DeHaan RL. Morphogenesis of the vertebrate heart. In: DeHaan RL, Ursprung H, eds. *Organogenesis*. New York: Holt, Reinhart & Winston, 1965:377–420.
6. Srivastava D. Making or breaking the heart: From lineage determination to morphogenesis. *Cell* 2006;126:1037–1048.
7. Buckingham M, Meilhac S, Zaffran S. Building the mammalian heart from two sources of myocardial cells. *Nat Rev Genet* 2005;6:826–835.
8. Olson EN. Gene regulatory networks in the evolution and development of the heart. *Science* 2006;313:1922–1927.
9. Srivastava D, Olson EN. A genetic blueprint for cardiac development. *Nature* 2000;407:221–226.
10. Meilhac SM, Esner M, Kelly RG, et al. The clonal origin of myocardial cells in different regions of the embryonic mouse heart. *Dev Cell* 2004;6: 685–698.
11. Kelly RG, Brown NA, Buckingham ME. The arterial pole of the mouse heart forms from Fgf10-expressing cells in pharyngeal mesoderm. *Dev Cell* 2001;1:435–440.
12. Waldo KL, Kumiski DH, Wallis KT, et al. Conotruncal myocardium arises from a secondary heart field. *Development* 2001;128:3179–3188.
13. Mjaatvedt CH, Nakaoka T, Moreno-Rodriguez R, et al. The outflow tract of the heart is recruited from a novel heart-forming field. *Dev Biol* 2001; 238(1):97–109.
14. Zaffran S, Frasch M. Early signals in cardiac development. *Circ Res* 2002;91(6):457–469.
15. Schultheiss TM, Burch JB, Lassar AB. A role for bone morphogenetic proteins in the induction of cardiac myogenesis. *Genes Dev* 1997;11(4): 451–462.
16. Schneider VA, Mercola M. Wnt antagonism initiates cardiogenesis in *Xenopus laevis*. *Genes Dev* 2001;15(3):304–315.
17. Marvin MJ, Di Rocco G, Gardiner A, et al. Inhibition of Wnt activity induces heart formation from posterior mesoderm. *Genes Dev* 2001; 15(3):316–327.
18. Cai CL, Liang X, Shi Y, et al. Isl1 identifies a cardiac progenitor population that proliferates prior to differentiation and contributes a majority of cells to the heart. *Dev Cell* 2003;5:877–889.
19. Garratt AN, Ozcelik C, Birchmeier C. ErbB2 pathways in heart and neural diseases. *Trends Cardiovasc Med* 2003;13(2):80–86.
20. Stuckmann I, Evans S, Lassar AB. Erythropoietin and retinoic acid, secreted from the epicardium, are required for cardiac myocyte proliferation. *Dev Biol* 2003;255(2):334–349.
21. von Both I, Silvestri C, Erdemir T, et al. Foxh1 is essential for development of the anterior heart field. *Dev Cell* 2004;7:331–345.
22. Laugwitz KL, Moretti A, Lam J, et al. Postnatal isl1$^+$ cardioblasts enter fully differentiated cardiomyocyte lineages. *Nature* 2005;433:647–653.
23. Firulli AB, Olson EN. Modular regulation of muscle gene transcription: A mechanism for muscle cell diversity. *Trends Genet* 1997;13(9):364–369.
24. Srivastava D. The bHLH proteins, dHAND and eHAND in cardiac development. In: Harvey RP, Olson EN, Schulz RA, et al., eds. *Genetic Control of Heart Development*. Strasbourg: HFSP, 1997.
25. Yamagishi H, Yamagishi C, Nakagawa O, et al. The combinatorial activities of Nkx2.5 and dHAND are essential for cardiac ventricle formation. *Dev Biol* 2001;239(2):190–203.
26. Lin Q, Srivastava D, Olson E. A transcriptional pathway for cardiac development. *Cold Spring Harb Symp Quant Biol* 1997;62:405–411.
27. Dodou E, Verzi MP, Anderson JP, et al. Mef2c is a direct transcriptional target of ISL1 and GATA factors in the anterior heart field during mouse embryonic development. *Development* 2004;131:3931–3942.
28. Zeisberg EM, Ma Q, Juraszek AL, et al. Morphogenesis of the right ventricle requires myocardial expression of Gata4. *J Clin Invest* 2005;115: 1522–1531.
29. Lindsay EA, Botta A, Jurecic V, et al. Congenital heart disease in mice deficient for the DiGeorge syndrome region. *Nature* 1999;401:379–383.
30. Lindsay EA, Vitelli F, Su H, et al. Tbx1 haploinsufficiency in the DiGeorge syndrome region causes aortic arch defects in mice. *Nature* 2001;410: 97–101.
31. Merscher S, Funke B, Epstein JA, et al. TBX1 is responsible for cardiovascular defects in velo-cardio-facial/DiGeorge syndrome. *Cell* 2001;104: 619–629.
32. Jerome LA, Papaioannou VE. DiGeorge syndrome phenotype in mice mutant for the T-box gene, Tbx1. *Nat Genet* 2001;27(3):286–291.
33. Hu T, Yamagishi H, Maeda J, et al. Tbx1 regulates fibroblast growth factors in the anterior heart field through a reinforcing autoregulatory loop involving forkhead transcription factors. *Development* 2004;131:5491–5502.
34. Xu H, Morishima M, Wylie JN, et al. Tbx1 has a dual role in the morphogenesis of the cardiac outflow tract. *Development* 2004;131:3217–3227.
35. Garg V, Yamagishi C, Hu T, et al. Tbx1, a DiGeorge syndrome candidate gene, is regulated by sonic hedgehog during pharyngeal arch development. *Dev Biol* 2001;235(1):62–73.
36. Yamagishi H, Maeda J, Hu T, et al. Tbx1 is regulated by tissue-specific forkhead proteins through a common Sonic hedgehog-responsive enhancer. *Genes Dev* 2003;17(2):269–281.
37. Kume T, Jiang H, Topczewska JM, et al. The murine winged helix transcription factors, Foxc1 and Foxc2, are both required for cardiovascular development and somitogenesis. *Genes Dev* 2001;15:2470–2482.
38. Abu-Issa R, Smyth G, Smoak I, et al. Fgf8 is required for pharyngeal arch and cardiovascular development in the mouse. *Development* 2002;129: 4613–4625.
39. Frank DU, Fotheringham LK, Brewer JA, et al. An Fgf8 mouse mutant phenocopies human 22q11 deletion syndrome. *Development* 2002;129: 4591–4603.
40. Srivastava D. HAND proteins: Molecular mediators of cardiac development and congenital heart disease. *Trends Cardiovasc Med* 1999;9(1–2): 11–18.
41. Biben C, Harvey RP. Homeodomain factor Nkx2-5 controls left/right asymmetric expression of bHLH gene eHAND during murine heart development. *Genes Dev* 1997;11:1357–1369.
42. Bodmer R. The gene tinman is required for specification of the heart and visceral muscles in *Drosophila*. *Development* 1993;118:719–729.
43. Lyons I, Parsons LM, Hartley L, et al. Myogenic and morphogenetic defects in the heart tubes of murine embryos lacking the homeo box gene Nkx2-5. *Genes Dev* 1995;9:1654–1666.
44. Tanaka M, Chen Z, Bartunkova S, et al. The cardiac homeobox gene Csx/Nkx2.5 lies genetically upstream of multiple genes essential for heart development. *Development* 1999;126:1269–1280.
45. McFadden DG, Barbosa AC, Richardson JA, et al. The Hand1 and Hand2 transcription factors regulate expansion of the embryonic cardiac ventricles in a gene dosage-dependent manner. *Development* 2005;132:189–201.
46. Yelon D, Ticho B, Halpern ME, et al. The bHLH transcription factor hand2 plays parallel roles in zebrafish heart and pectoral fin development. *Development* 2000;127:2573–2582.
47. Han Z, Yi P, Li X, et al. Hand, an evolutionarily conserved bHLH transcription factor required for *Drosophila* cardiogenesis and hematopoiesis. *Development* 2006;133:1175–1182.
48. Pereira FA, Qiu Y, Zhou G, et al. The orphan nuclear receptor COUP-TFII is required for angiogenesis and heart development. *Genes Dev* 1999;13: 1037–1049.
49. Bruneau BG, Nemer G, Schmitt JP, et al. A murine model of Holt-Oram syndrome defines roles of the T-box transcription factor Tbx5 in cardiogenesis and disease. *Cell* 2001;106:709–721.
50. Bao ZZ, Bruneau BG, Seidman JG, et al. Regulation of chamber-specific gene expression in the developing heart by Irx4. *Science* 1999;283: 1161–1164.
51. Gottlieb PD, Pierce SA, Sims RJ, et al. Bop encodes a muscle-restricted protein containing MYND and SET domains and is essential for cardiac differentiation and morphogenesis. *Nat Genet* 2002;31(1):25–32.
52. Phan D, Rasmussen TL, Nakagawa O, et al. BOP, a regulator of right ventricular heart development, is a direct transcriptional target of MEF2C in the developing heart. *Development* 2005;132:2669–2678.

53. Chang S, McKinsey TA, Zhang CL, et al. Histone deacetylases 5 and 9 govern responsiveness of the heart to a subset of stress signals and play redundant roles in heart development. *Mol Cell Biol* 2004;24:8467–8476.

54. Lickert H, Takeuchi JK, Von Both I, et al. Baf60c is essential for function of BAF chromatin remodelling complexes in heart development. *Nature* 2004;432:107–112.

55. Zhao Y, Samal E, Srivastava D. Serum response factor regulates a muscle-specific mircroRNA that targets *Hand2* during cardiogenesis. *Nature* 2005;436:214–220.

56. Kwon C, Han Z, Olson EN, et al. MicroRNA1 influences cardiac differentiation in *Drosophila* and regulates Notch signaling. *Proc Natl Acad Sci USA* 2005;102:18986–18991.

57. He L, Hannon GJ. MicroRNAs: Small RNAs with a big role in gene regulation. *Nat Rev Genet* 2004;5:522–531.

58. Ambros V. The functions of animal microRNAs. *Nature* 2004;431:350–355.

59. Cummins JM, He Y, Leary RJ, et al. The colorectal microRNAome. *Proc Natl Acad Sci USA* 2006;103:3687–3692.

60. Chen JF, Mandel EM, Thomson JM, et al. The role of microRNA-1 and microRNA-133 in skeletal muscle proliferation and differentiation. *Nat Genet* 2006;38(2):228–233.

61. Artavanis-Tsakonas S, Rand MD, Lake RJ. Notch signaling: Cell fate control and signal integration in development. *Science* 1999;284:770–776.

62. Moorman AF, Christoffels VM. Cardiac chamber formation: Development, genes, and evolution. *Physiol Rev* 2003;83:1223–1267.

63. Tucker A, Matthews K, Sharpe P. Transformation of tooth type induced by inhibition of BMP signaling. *Science* 1998;282:1136–1138.

64. Harrelson Z, Kelly RG, Goldin SN, et al. Tbx2 is essential for patterning the atrioventricular canal and for morphogenesis of the outflow tract during heart development. *Development* 2004;131:5041–5052.

65. Takeuchi JK, Mileikovskaia M, Koshiba-Takeuchi K, et al. Tbx20 dose-dependently regulates transcription factor networks required for mouse heart and motoneuron development. *Development* 2005;132:2463–2474.

66. Singh MK, Christoffels VM, Dias JM, et al. Tbx20 is essential for cardiac chamber differentiation and repression of Tbx2. *Development* 2005;132:2697–2707.

67. Stennard FA, Costa MW, Lai D, et al. Murine T-box transcription factor Tbx20 acts as a repressor during heart development, and is essential for adult heart integrity, function and adaptation. *Development* 2005;132:2451–2462.

68. Brown NA, Wolpert L. The development of handedness in left/right asymmetry. *Development* 1990;109:1–9.

69. Mjaatvedt CH, Yamamura H, Wessels A, et al. Mechanisms of segmentation, septation, and remodeling of the tubular heart: Endocardial cushion fate and cardiac looping. In: Harvey RP, Rosenthal N, eds. *Heart Development*. San Diego: Academic Press, 1999:530.

70. Palmer AR. Symmetry breaking and the evolution of development. *Science* 2004;306:828–833.

71. Piedra ME, Icardo JM, Albajar M, et al. Pitx2 participates in the late phase of the pathway controlling left-right asymmetry. *Cell* 1998;94(3):319–324.

72. Kioussi C, Briata P, Baek SH, et al. Identification of a Wnt/Dvl/beta-Catenin → Pitx2 pathway mediating cell-type-specific proliferation during development. *Cell* 2002;111:673–685.

73. Nowotschin S, Liao J, Gage PJ, et al. Tbx1 affects asymmetric cardiac morphogenesis by regulating Pitx2 in the secondary heart field. *Development* 2006;133:1565–1573.

74. Kosaki R, Gebbia M, Kosaki K, et al. Left-right axis malformations associated with mutations in ACVR2B, the gene for human activin receptor type IIB. *Am J Med Genet* 1999;82(1):70–76.

75. Gebbia M, Ferrero GB, Pilia G, et al. X-linked situs abnormalities result from mutations in ZIC3. *Nat Genet* 1997;17(3):305–308.

76. Sadler TW, ed. *Langman's Medical Embryology*. Baltimore: Williams & Wilkins. 1995.

77. Hutson MR, Kirby ML. Neural crest and cardiovascular development: A 20-year perspective. *Birth Defects Res C Embryo Today* 2003;69(1):2–13.

78. Le Douarin NM, Creuzet S, Couly G, et al. Neural crest cell plasticity and its limits. *Development* 2004;131:4637–4650.

79. Satoda M, Zhao F, Diaz GA, et al. Mutations in TFAP2B cause Char syndrome, a familial form of patent ductus arteriosus. *Nat Genet* 2000;25(1):42–46.

80. Yagi H, Furutani Y, Hamada H, et al. Role of TBX1 in human del22q11.2 syndrome. *Lancet* 2003;362:1366–1373.

81. Beis D, Bartman T, Jin SW, et al. Genetic and cellular analyses of zebrafish atrioventricular cushion and valve development. *Development* 2005;132:4193–4204.

82. Ma L, Lu MF, Schwartz RJ, et al. Bmp2 is essential for cardiac cushion epithelial-mesenchymal transition and myocardial patterning. *Development* 2005;132:5601–5611.

83. Gaussin V, Van de Putte T, Mishina Y, et al. Endocardial cushion and myocardial defects after cardiac myocyte-specific conditional deletion of the bone morphogenetic protein receptor ALK3. *Proc Natl Acad Sci USA* 2002;99:2878–2883.

84. Kim RY, Robertson EJ, Solloway MJ. Bmp6 and Bmp7 are required for cushion formation and septation in the developing mouse heart. *Dev Biol* 2001;235(2):449–466.

85. Brown CB, Boyer AS, Runyan RB, et al. Requirement of type III TGF-beta receptor for endocardial cell transformation in the heart. *Science* 1999;283:2080–2082.

86. Hurle JM, Icardo JM, Ojeda JL. Compositional and structural heterogenicity of the cardiac jelly of the chick embryo tubular heart: A TEM, SEM and histochemical study. *J Embryol Exp Morphol* 1980;56:211–223.

87. Maron BJ, Hutchins GM. The development of the semilunar valves in the human heart. *Am J Pathol* 1974;74(2):331–344.

88. Hinton RB Jr, Lincoln J, Deutsch GH, et al. Extracellular matrix remodeling and organization in developing and diseased aortic valves. *Circ Res* 2006;98:1431–1438.

89. Aikawa E, Whittaker P, Farber M, et al. Human semilunar cardiac valve remodeling by activated cells from fetus to adult: Implications for postnatal adaptation, pathology, and tissue engineering. *Circulation* 2006;113:1344–1352.

90. Rabkin E, Aikawa M, Stone JR, et al. Activated interstitial myofibroblasts express catabolic enzymes and mediate matrix remodeling in myxomatous heart valves. *Circulation* 2001;104:2525–2532.

91. Rabkin-Aikawa E, Farber M, Aikawa M, et al. Dynamic and reversible changes of interstitial cell phenotype during remodeling of cardiac valves. *J Heart Valve Dis* 2004;13:841–847.

92. Paruchuri S, Yang JH, Aikawa E, et al. Human pulmonary valve progenitor cells exhibit endothelial/mesenchymal plasticity in response to vascular endothelial growth factor-A and transforming growth factor-beta2. *Circ Res* 2006;99:861–869.

93. Yutzey KE, Colbert M, Robbins J. Ras-related signaling pathways in valve development: Ebb and flow. *Physiology (Bethesda)*. 2005;20:390–397.

94. Gelb BD, Tartaglia M. Noonan syndrome and related disorders: Dysregulated RAS-mitogen activated protein kinase signal transduction. *Hum Mol Genet* 2006;15(spec no 2):R220–R226.

95. Gitler AD, Zhu Y, Ismat FA, et al. Nf1 has an essential role in endothelial cells. *Nat Genet* 2003;33(1):75–79.

96. Lakkis MM, Epstein JA. Neurofibromin modulation of ras activity is required for normal endocardial-mesenchymal transformation in the developing heart. *Development* 1998;125:4359–4367.

97. Lin AE, Birch PH, Korf BR, et al. Cardiovascular malformations and other cardiovascular abnormalities in neurofibromatosis 1. *Am J Med Genet* 2000;95(2):108–117.

98. Tartaglia M, Gelb BD. Noonan syndrome and related disorders: Genetics and pathogenesis. *Annu Rev Genomics Hum Genet* 2005;6:45–68.

99. Araki T, Mohi MG, Ismat FA, et al. Mouse model of Noonan syndrome reveals cell type- and gene dosage-dependent effects of Ptpn11 mutation. *Nat Med* 2004;10:849–857.

100. Tartaglia M, Mehler EL, Goldberg R, et al. Mutations in PTPN11, encoding the protein tyrosine phosphatase SHP-2, cause Noonan syndrome. *Nat Genet* 2001;29(4):465–468.

101. Tartaglia M, Kalidas K, Shaw A, et al. PTPN11 mutations in Noonan syndrome: Molecular spectrum, genotype-phenotype correlation, and phenotypic heterogeneity. *Am J Hum Genet* 2002;70:1555–1563.

102. Roberts AE, Araki T, Swanson KD, et al. Germline gain-of-function mutations in SOS1 cause Noonan syndrome. *Nat Genet* 2007;39(1):70–74.

103. Tartaglia M, Martinelli S, Stella L, et al. Diversity and functional consequences of germline and somatic PTPN11 mutations in human disease. *Am J Hum Genet* 2006;78(2):279–290.

104. Sibilia M, Wagner B, Hoebertz A, et al. Mice humanised for the EGF receptor display hypomorphic phenotypes in skin, bone and heart. *Development* 2003;130:4515–4525.

105. Chen B, Bronson RT, Klaman LD, et al. Mice mutant for Egfr and Shp2 have defective cardiac semilunar valvulogenesis. *Nat Genet* 2000;24(3):296–299.

106. Iwamoto R, Yamazaki S, Asakura M, et al. Heparin-binding EGF-like growth factor and ErbB signaling is essential for heart function. *Proc Natl Acad Sci USA* 2003;100:3221–3226.

107. Jackson LF, Qiu TH, Sunnarborg SW, et al. Defective valvulogenesis in HB-EGF and TACE-null mice is associated with aberrant BMP signaling. *EMBO J* 2003;22:2704–2716.

108. Tadano M, Edamatsu H, Minamisawa S, et al. Congenital semilunar valvulogenesis defect in mice deficient in phospholipase C epsilon. *Mol Cell Biol* 2005;25:2191–2199.

109. Galvin KM, Donovan MJ, Lynch CA, et al. A role for smad6 in development and homeostasis of the cardiovascular system. *Nat Genet* 2000;24(2):171–174.

110. Erickson SL, O'Shea KS, Ghaboosi N, et al. ErbB3 is required for normal cerebellar and cardiac development: A comparison with ErbB2-and heregulin-deficient mice. *Development* 1997;124:4999–5011.

111. Cowan CA, Yokoyama N, Saxena A, et al. Ephrin-B2 reverse signaling is required for axon pathfinding and cardiac valve formation but not early vascular development. *Dev Biol* 2004;271(2):263–271.

112. Ranger AM, Grusby MJ, Hodge MR, et al. The transcription factor NF-ATc is essential for cardiac valve formation. *Nature* 1998;392:186–190.

113. de la Pompa JL, Timmerman LA, Takimoto H, et al. Role of the NF-ATc transcription factor in morphogenesis of cardiac valves and septum. *Nature* 1998;392:182–186.

114. Chang CP, Neilson JR, Bayle JH, et al. A field of myocardial-endocardial NFAT signaling underlies heart valve morphogenesis. *Cell* 2004;118: 649–663.

115. Timmerman LA, Grego-Bessa J, Raya A, et al. Notch promotes epithelial-mesenchymal transition during cardiac development and oncogenic transformation. *Genes Dev* 2004;18(1):99–115.

116. Garg V, Muth AN, Ransom JF, et al. Mutations in NOTCH1 cause aortic valve disease. *Nature* 2005;437:270–274.

117. Cripe L, Andelfinger G, Martin LJ, et al. Bicuspid aortic valve is heritable. *J Am Coll Cardiol* 2004;44(1):138–143.

118. Loffredo CA, Chokkalingam A, Sill AM, et al. Prevalence of congenital cardiovascular malformations among relatives of infants with hypoplastic left heart, coarctation of the aorta, and d-transposition of the great arteries. *Am J Med Genet A* 2004;124(3):225–230.

119. Li L, Krantz ID, Deng Y, et al. Alagille syndrome is caused by mutations in human Jagged1, which encodes a ligand for Notch1. *Nat Genet* 1997; 16(3):243–251.

120. Oda T, Elkahloun AG, Pike BL, et al. Mutations in the human Jagged1 gene are responsible for Alagille syndrome. *Nat Genet* 1997;16(3): 235–242.

121. Krantz ID, Smith R, Colliton RP, et al. Jagged1 mutations in patients ascertained with isolated congenital heart defects. *Am J Med Genet* 1999; 84(1):56–60.

122. Nakagawa O, Nakagawa M, Richardson JA, et al. HRT1, HRT2, and HRT3: A new subclass of bHLH transcription factors marking specific cardiac, somitic, and pharyngeal arch segments. *Dev Biol* 1999;216(1):72–84.

123. Kokubo H, Miyagawa-Tomita S, Johnson RL. Hesr, a mediator of the Notch signaling, functions in heart and vessel development. *Trends Cardiovasc Med* 2005;15(5):190–194.

124. Schott JJ, Benson DW, Basson CT, et al. Congenital heart disease caused by mutations in the transcription factor NKX2-5. *Science* 1998;281:108–111.

125. Biben C, Weber R, Kesteven S, et al. Cardiac septal and valvular dysmorphogenesis in mice heterozygous for mutations in the homeobox gene Nkx2-5. *Circ Res* 2000;87:888–895.

126. Jay PY, Harris BS, Maguire CT, et al. Nkx2-5 mutation causes anatomic hypoplasia of the cardiac conduction system. *J Clin Invest* 2004;113: 1130–1137.

127. Basson CT, Bachinsky DR, Lin RC, et al. Mutations in human TBX5 cause limb and cardiac malformation in Holt-Oram syndrome. *Nat Genet* 1997;15(1):30–35.

128. Mori AD, Bruneau BG. TBX5 mutations and congenital heart disease: Holt-Oram syndrome revealed. *Curr Opin Cardiol* 2004;19(3):211–215.

129. Hiroi Y, Kudoh S, Monzen K, et al. Tbx5 associates with Nkx2-5 and synergistically promotes cardiomyocyte differentiation. *Nat Genet* 2001; 28(3):276–280.

130. Garg V, Kathiriya IS, Barnes R, et al. GATA4 mutations cause human congenital heart defects and reveal an interaction with TBX5. *Nature* 2003;424:443–447.

131. Molkentin JD, Lin Q, Duncan SA, et al. Requirement of the transcription factor GATA4 for heart tube formation and ventral morphogenesis. *Genes Dev* 1997;11:1061–1072.

132. Kuo CT, Morrisey EE, Anandappa R, et al. GATA4 transcription factor is required for ventral morphogenesis and heart tube formation. *Genes Dev* 1997;11:1048–1060.

133. Reiter JF, Kikuchi Y, Stainier DY. Multiple roles for Gata5 in zebrafish endoderm formation. *Development* 2001;128:125–135.

134. Gajewski K, Zhang Q, Choi CY, et al. Pannier is a transcriptional target and partner of Tinman during *Drosophila* cardiogenesis. *Dev Biol* 2001; 233(2):425–436.

135. Ching YH, Ghosh TK, Cross SJ. Mutation in myosin heavy chain 6 causes atrial septal defect. *Nat Genet* 2005;37(4):423–428.

136. Noden DM, Poelmann RE, Gittenberger-de-Groot AC. Cell origins and tissue boundaries during outflow tract development. *Trends Cardiovasc Med* 1995;5:69–75.

137. Shimada Y, Ho E, Toyota N. Epicardial covering over myocardial wall in the chicken embryo as seen with the scanning electron microscope. *Scan Electron Microsc* 1981(pt 2):275–280.

138. Viragh S, Challice CE. The origin of the epicardium and the embryonic myocardial circulation in the mouse. *Anat Rec* 1981;201(1):157–168.

139. Viragh S, Gittenberger-de Groot AC, Poelmann RE, et al. Early development of quail heart epicardium and associated vascular and glandular structures. *Anat Embryol* 1993;188(4):381–393.

140. Komiyama M, Ito K, Shimada Y. Origin and development of the epicardium in the mouse embryo. *Anat Embryol* 1987;176(2):183–189.

141. Hiruma T, Hirakow R. Epicardial formation in embryonic chick heart: Computer-aided reconstruction, scanning, and transmission electron microscopic studies. *Am J Anat* 1989;184(2):129–138.

142. Bolender LM, Olson D, Markwald RR. Coronary vessel vasculogenesis. *Ann N Y Acad Sci* 1990;588:340–344.

143. Mikawa T, Fischman DA. Retroviral analysis of cardiac morphogenesis: Discontinuous formation of coronary vessels. *Proc Natl Acad Sci USA* 1992;89:9504–9508.

144. Poelmann RE, Gittenberger-de Groot AC, Mentink MM, et al. Development of the cardiac coronary vascular endothelium, studied with antiendothelial antibodies, in chicken-quail chimeras. *Circ Res* 1993;73(3):559–568.

145. Mikawa T, Gourdie RG. Pericardial mesoderm generates a population of coronary smooth muscle cells migrating into the heart along with ingrowth of the epicardial organ. *Dev Biol* 1996;174(2):221–232.

146. Dettman RW, Denetclaw W Jr, Ordahl CP, et al. Common epicardial origin of coronary vascular smooth muscle, perivascular fibroblasts, and intermyocardial fibroblasts in the avian heart. *Dev Biol* 1998;193(2):169–181.

147. Bogers AJ, Gittenberger-de Groot AC, Dubbeldam JA, et al. The inadequacy of existing theories on development of the proximal coronary arteries and their connexions with the arterial trunks. *Int J Cardiol* 1988;20(1): 117–123.

148. Bogers AJ, Gittenberger-de Groot AC, Poelmann RE, et al. Development of the origin of the coronary arteries, a matter of ingrowth or outgrowth? *Anat Embryol* 1989;180(5):437–441.

149. Waldo KL, Willner W, Kirby ML. Origin of the proximal coronary artery stems and a review of ventricular vascularization in the chick embryo. *Am J Anat* 1990;188(2):109–120.

150. Mikawa T. Cardiac lineages. In: Harvey RP, Rosenthal N, eds. *Heart Development*. San Diego: Academic Press, 1999:19–33.

151. Gourdie RG, Kubalak S, Mikawa T. Conducting the embryonic heart: Orchestrating development of specialized cardiac tissues. *Trends Cardiovasc Med* 1999;9(1–2):18–26.

152. Gourdie RG, Mima T, Thompson RP, et al. Terminal diversification of the myocyte lineage generates Purkinje fibers of the cardiac conduction system. *Development* 1995;121:1423–1431.

153. Gourdie RG, Wei Y, Kim D, et al. Endothelin-induced conversion of embryonic heart muscle cells into impulse-conducting Purkinje fibers. *Proc Natl Acad Sci USA* 1998;95:6815–6818.

154. Waldo KL, Kumiski DH, Kirby ML. Association of the cardiac neural crest with development of the coronary arteries in the chick embryo. *Anat Rec* 1994;239(3):315–331.

155. Hood LC, Rosenquist TH. Coronary artery development in the chick: Origin and deployment of smooth muscle cells, and the effects of neural crest ablation. *Anat Rec* 1992;234(2):291–300.

156. Costantini DL, Arruda EP, Agarwal P, et al. The homeodomain transcription factor Irx5 establishes the mouse cardiac ventricular repolarization gradient. *Cell* 2005;123:347–358.

157. Pashmforoush M, Lu JT, Chen H, et al. Nkx2-5 pathways and congenital heart disease: Loss of ventricular myocyte lineage specification leads to progressive cardiomyopathy and complete heart block. *Cell* 2004;117:373–386.

158. Rajamannan NM, Gersh B, Bonow RO. Calcific aortic stenosis: From bench to the bedside—emerging clinical and cellular concepts. *Heart* 2003;89:801–805.

159. O'Brien JR, Etherington MD, Brant J, et al. Decreased platelet function in aortic valve stenosis: High shear platelet activation then inactivation. *Br Heart J* 1995;74:641–644.

160. Ducy P, Zhang R, Geoffroy V, et al. Osf2/Cbfa1: A transcriptional activator of osteoblast differentiation. *Cell* 1997;89:747–754.

161. Steitz SA, Speer MY, Curinga G, et al. Smooth muscle cell phenotypic transition associated with calcification: Upregulation of Cbfa1 and downregulation of smooth muscle lineage markers. *Circ Res* 2001;89:1147–1154.

162. Rajamannan NM, Subramaniam M, Springett M, et al. Atorvastatin inhibits hypercholesterolemia-induced cellular proliferation and bone matrix production in the rabbit aortic valve. *Circulation* 2002;105:2660–2665.

163. Parmacek MS, Epstein JA. Pursuing cardiac progenitors: Regeneration redux. *Cell* 2005;120:295–298.

164. Oh H, Bradfute SB, Gallardo TD, et al. Cardiac progenitor cells from adult myocardium: Homing, differentiation, and fusion after infarction. *Proc Natl Acad Sci USA* 2003;100:12313–12318.

165. Beltrami AP, Barlucchi L, Torella D, et al. Adult cardiac stem cells are multipotent and support myocardial regeneration. *Cel.* 2003;114:763–776.

166. Martin CM, Meeson AP, Robertson SM, et al. Persistent expression of the ATP-binding cassette transporter, Abcg2, identifies cardiac SP cells in the developing and adult heart. *Dev Biol* 2004;265(1):262–275.

167. Yoon YS, Wecker A, Heyd L, et al. Clonally expanded novel multipotent stem cells from human bone marrow regenerate myocardium after myocardial infarction. *J Clin Invest* 2005;115(2):326–338.

168. Ahn S, Joyner AL. In vivo analysis of quiescent adult neural stem cells responding to Sonic hedgehog. *Nature* 2005;437:894–897.

169. Mitchell LE, Adzick NS, Melchionne J, et al. Spina bifida. *Lancet* 2004; 364:1885–1895.

170. Stoller JZ, Epstein JA. Cardiac neural crest. *Semin Cell Dev Biol* 2005; 16:704–715.

CHAPTER 25 ■ EPIDEMIOLOGY AND PREVENTION OF CONGENITAL HEART DEFECTS

LORENZO D. BOTTO, MD, ELIZABETH GOLDMUNTZ, MD, AND ANGELA E. LIN, MD

THE CONTRIBUTION OF EPIDEMIOLOGY TO PEDIATRIC CARDIOLOGY

Following the birth of a child with a congenital heart defect, an anxious parent unknowingly asks the crucial questions that crystallize the related epidemiology and public health issues: "What will happen to my child?" (outcomes), "why did this happen?" (causation), and "will it happen again?" (risk assessment and prevention). These questions are the focus of much clinical and basic research. This chapter describes the ongoing contribution by epidemiology to answer these questions, with an emphasis on current developments and remaining data gaps (Table 25.1). Currently, major gaps remain, particularly in identifying causes and effective primary prevention. However, substantial progress is being made, particularly through interdisciplinary collaboration between basic scientists, clinicians, and epidemiologists.

The emphasis of epidemiology on individuals in the context of populations is key to translating basic and clinical findings into effective treatment and prevention in the community. For example, epidemiologic studies help characterize in human populations the contribution of candidate genes identified in high-risk families or experimental models. They also help characterize environmental risk factors and protective factors as well as their impact (1). And, from a public health perspective, epidemiologic studies help monitor the health of the population, detect health disparities, and evaluate interventions.

In this discussion of impact, causation, and prevention, key references will be supplemented with selected review papers, where further references may be found.

IMPACT AND OUTCOMES: A LIFESPAN PERSPECTIVE

Improving technology and emerging challenges are forcing reassessment of the outcomes and impact of congenital heart defects (Fig. 25.1). For example, better and more widespread noninvasive diagnostics (e.g., ultrasonography) are increasing prenatal and postnatal identification of an expanding range of

---

TABLE 25.1

PARENTS' QUESTIONS AND THEIR EPIDEMIOLOGIC CORRELATES IN PEDIATRIC CARDIOLOGY

Question	Focus	Current areas of epidemiologic studies	Population aspects
What will happen to my child?	Outcomes	Prenatal survival, association with extracardiac malformations, likelihood of syndromes Neurodevelopmental outcome Quality of life, cost of living, employment, independent living; role in the community and family.	Surveillance, population-based prevalence, morbidity, mortality Disparities (by socioeconomic status, insurance status, minority status)
Why did this happen?	Causes	Contribution of mendelian conditions, genotype–phenotype correlations Role of common polymorphisms and gene-environment interactions Effect of common exposures and family history	Detection of teratogen-induced epidemics Gene characterization in populations (genotype frequencies, interactions, attributable fractions) Likely or common risk factors, even if associated with low relative risks
Will it happen again?	Prevention	Altering behavior related to known teratogens, including chronic illness and medications Effect of multivitamin supplementation Recurrence prevention Prevention of complications	Trends of common risk factors in population groups Disparities in preventive services Comprehensive periconceptional care

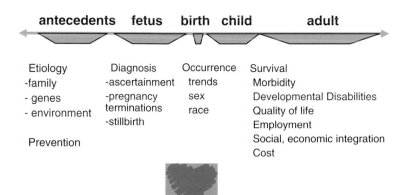

FIGURE 25.1 Epidemiologic issues in the lifespan.

conditions. Improving survival focuses increasing attention to the multifaceted needs of adolescents and adults with congenital heart defects, including their quality of life and social integration (2,3). Also, with improving technology and treatment options comes the need to monitor aggressively for the potential for health outcome disparities.

CLASSIFICATION OF HEART DEFECTS IN EPIDEMIOLOGY

The method of grouping heart defects determines in part a study's approach and can shape its findings. As such, classification of heart defects continues to be a challenge to investigators. A broad goal of classification is to cluster defects to obtain homogeneous groups of adequate size for the analysis of interest. What constitutes a homogeneous group typically depends on the goal of the study. For example, the World Health Organization's ICD system has been helpful for general comparisons (frequency, causes of death) among countries with different health systems but is not specifically targeted to outcome or etiologic studies. For this reason, international collaborations of surgeons and clinicians have developed a comprehensive system for outcomes studies after cardiac surgery (4) and for risk stratification studies (5–8). Crucially, mapping strategies between different classifications systems are also being developed (7,9).

In epidemiology, the focus of etiologic studies is finding associations. A key tension for the investigator is between defining groups so narrowly that each group has too few cases or so broadly that, by lumping heterogeneous conditions, associations may be diluted or missed altogether. Case homogeneity can be increased by grouping cases based on developmental relationships rather than anatomic findings alone (10–12). One such pathogenetic classification of heart defects (Table 25.2), based on developmental relationships, has been developed and is regularly revised by Dr. E. B. Clark (11); this classification has been used in several large epidemiologic studies (1,13–15). For some phenotypes, such as the left heart defects, their grouping in etiologic investigations is supported by accumulating epidemiologic and genetic data (16–19). On the other hand, conotruncal anomalies, often lumped in etiologic analyses, may in fact include conditions that are heterogeneous in their causes and development (1,11,20,21).

Finding such commonalities among types of heart defects requires large epidemiologic studies. When large studies are available, one approach focuses on defining pure groups of heart defects, that is, simple phenotypes in individuals without extracardiac anomalies or syndromes. This is the approach used in studies from the National Birth Defects Prevention Study in the United States. Such pure groups can be composed of simple phenotypes (e.g., isolated coarctation of the aorta), plus common associations (e.g., coarctation of the aorta plus aortic stenosis). Common associations can also be studied on their own, if the study is sufficiently large. For example, secundum atrial septal defects and perimembranous ventricular septal defect occur frequently together more commonly than by chance. If there are risk factors preferentially associated with this pattern of septal defects, then they may be best detected by evaluating this phenotype in isolation. Although the approach focuses on pure groups, it does not exclude evaluating other phenotypes in a pooled analysis. Rather, it considers the pooled analysis as more appropriate in a second stage but not as the first or only approach. This approach is most practical in large studies of cases with accurate clinical description of both the baby and the heart.

OCCURRENCE AND OUTCOMES

Occurrence: The Present

The best epidemiologic measure of occurrence is debated, though prevalence is generally preferable (22) and will be used here. Incidence reflects the number of new cases over time among an initially diseasefree cohort of at-risk individuals. Such diseasefree cohort is that of all conceptuses, which is unknown because of the indefinite, but likely considerable, number of early pregnancy losses (22). Prevalence, on the other hand, reflects the occurrence of disease at a point in time in a defined population. Based on the population, different prevalence rates can be derived, including prevalence among infants, newborns, stillbirths, fetuses at a certain gestational age, or a combination of these. In practice, incidence better measures disease development and impact but is not known. Prevalence, although underestimating the global impact of heart defects, can be more reliably defined and is commonly used in epidemiologic studies.

Estimating the prevalence of congenital heart defects is challenging. The range of published estimates is wide (23–25), including, as shown in Table 25.3, even recent studies (26–37). A crucial question is what part of such rate variations is due to methodology (e.g., diagnosis and reporting) and what part is due to biology (e.g., true differences in occurrence rates). Many factors can influence local estimates, including diagnostic practices, case definitions, case classification, inclusion of pregnancy

TABLE 25.2

PATHOGENETIC CLASSIFICATION OF HEART DEFECTS

Ectomesenchymal tissue migration
Conotruncal septation defects
    Subarterial ventricular septal defect
    Double-outlet right ventricle
    Tetralogy of Fallot
    Pulmonary atresia with ventricular septal defect
    Aortopulmonary window
    Truncus arterious
Abnormal conotruncal cushion position
    d-Transposition of the great arteries
Branchial arch defects
    Interrupted aortic arch type B
    Double aortic arch
    Right aortic arch with mirror-image branching

Abnormal intracardiac blood flow
Perimembranous ventricular septal defect
Left heart defects
    Bicuspid aortic valve
    Aortic valve stenosis
    Coarctation of the aorta
    Interrupted aortic arch type A
    Hypoplastic left heart, aortic atresia/mitral atresia
Right heart defects
    Bicuspid pulmonary valve
    Secundum atrial septal defect
    Pulmonary valve stenosis
    Pulmonary valve atresia with intact ventricular septum

Cell death abnormalities
    Muscular ventricular septal defect
    Ebstein's malformation

Extracellular matrix abnormalities
Endocardial cushion defects
    Ostium primum atrial septal defect
    Inflow/inlet ventricular septal defect
    Atrioventricular septal defect
Dysplastic pulmonary or aortic valve

Abnormal targeted growth
    Anomalous pulmonary venous return

Abnormal situs and looping
    Heterotaxy, other situs anomalies, L-loop

(Modified from Clark EB. In: *Moss and Adams' Heart Disease in Infants, Children, and Adolescents*, 6th ed. Philadelphia: Lippincott Williams & Wilkins, 2001, with permission.)

terminations, timing of diagnosis (fetal, birth, or childhood), length of follow-up, and reporting procedures (23–25,38). Because of the many factors involved, understanding how prevalence is derived in specific studies is crucial for their interpretation.

Table 25.4 summarizes data from three studies that, jointly, provide some guidance to estimating and interpreting occurrence information. One is the Baltimore-Washington Infant Study (BWIS), a population-based study of live births with heart defects conducted in the 1980s, with follow-up through 1 year of age (15). Although designed as an etiologic case-control study, the study also allowed investigators to estimate

prevalence because of the high quality of ascertainment. The second study, which spans through the 1990s, is based on the congenital defect monitoring program in metropolitan Atlanta (MACDP), run by the U.S. Centers for Disease Control and Prevention. The approach is similar to BWIS (active ascertainment from multiple sources, follow-up period through early infancy, similar case classification), but the study also included affected stillbirths and pregnancy terminations (13). The third, more recent set of estimates, from Norway, exemplifies an innovative approach that combines systematic assessment with prenatal diagnosis (39). Specifically, these researchers used echocardiography to systematically evaluate a large, unselected cohort of pregnancies, first at midgestation, then postnatally, with follow-up through 2 years of life (39).

Prevalence of heart defects in the aggregate was 9 per 1,000 (1 in 110 births) in the Atlanta study. By comparison, in the Norwegian study prevalence was 14.6 per 1,000 (about 50% higher), and in the BWIS it was 4.8 per 1,000 (about 50% lower). Much of such variation is likely due to methods and timing. For example, ultrasonography is commonly cited as a major factor explaining both the higher prevalence reported in more recent studies compared with older studies and the increasing time trends seen in studies spanning decades of observations (13,23–25,40). In the Norwegian study, the higher overall rate of occurrence of heart defects may also have derived from systematic prenatal assessment and the inclusion of some cases associated with chromosomal anomalies (e.g., Down or Turner syndromes) that have a high fetal mortality.

A closer examination of the distribution of heart defect types indicates that, in general, the variation in overall prevalence is driven largely by common and generally mild conditions (13,23,24). In Table 25.4, for example, rates of ventricular and atrial septal defects accounted for much of the overall rate variations among the three studies (in addition, a sample of small ventricular septal defects was excluded by the BWIS (41). For septal defects, the potential for variable ascertainment and reporting is particularly great because of the high frequency of clinically mild forms. For example, systematic Doppler ultrasonography at birth identified ventricular septal defects in 2% of 1,028 systematically examined newborns in Japan (42). Most were small muscular defects, and only about half had an associated murmur at hospital discharge (42). In the Norwegian study, nearly all (96%) of the ventricular septal defects were considered minor (39).

Mild pulmonic or aortic stenosis and isolated bicuspid aortic valve are other common conditions for which ascertainment has likely increased considerably in the last few decades (13,43). As illustrated in Figure 25.2, in one population-based study, birth prevalence increased steeply from the 1970s through 1990s for the milder right-sided obstructive defects (13). Whereas there was a steep increase for peripheral pulmonic stenosis, for valvar pulmonic stenosis the rate increase was moderate, and for pulmonary atresia with intact septum there was no material change (13).

By contrast (Table 25.4), prevalence estimates for the clinically more significant heart defects tend to be more stable across studies and over time (13,15,23,24,44,45). For such serious heart defects, significant differences may still occur and may be related to factors such as the extent of fetal assessment (Table 25.4).

Summary

Provided that methodologic issues are appreciated, these data on occurrence can be globally summarized as indicating a prevalence of approximately 3 per 1,000 for clinically severe conditions, 6 per 1,000 when including also moderately serious

TABLE 25.3

ESTIMATED FREQUENCY OF CONGENITAL HEART DEFECTS: STUDIES AFTER 1980

Group	Author	Year of publication	Population studied	Rate per 1,000	Births	Age	Population-based	Location	Diagnosis
Fetal deaths[a]	Ursell et al.	1985	412	24	SA	GA 8–28 weeks	No	United States (New York City)	Autopsy
	Chinn et al.	1989	400	13	SA SB	GA 9–40 weeks	No	United States (Seattle)	Autopsy
	Stoll et al.	1989	105,374	34.5	SB	GA ≥26 weeks	Yes	France (Strasbourg)	Autopsy
Births[c]	Fyler et al.	1980	1,083,083	2.1	L	≤1 y	Yes	United States (New England)	PE (rare), cath, surgery, autopsy; included myocardial disease
	Grabitz et al.	1988	103,411	5.5	L	≤1 y	Yes	Canada (Alberta)	PE, cath, surgery, autopsy, echo added
	Stoll et al.	1989	105,374	7.6	T	≤1 y	Yes	France (Strasbourg)	Cath, surgery, autopsy, echo
	Fixler et al.	1990	379,561	6.6	L	4–17 y	Yes	United States (Texas)	PE by cardiologist, cath, surgery, autopsy, echo
	Tikkanen et al.	1990	132,993	3.1	T	≤1 y	Yes	Finland	Cath, surgery, autopsy, echo
	Pradat et al.	1992	573,422	2.8	T	≤1 y	Yes	Sweden	PE, cath, surgery, autopsy, echo
	Kidd et al.	1993	343,521	4.3	L	≤1 y	Yes	Australia	PE, echo
	Ferencz et al.	1993	906,646	4.8	L	≤1 y	Yes	United States (Baltimore-Washington)	Cath, surgery, autopsy, echo
	Samanek et al.	1994	664,218	6.6	L	≤5 y	Yes	Czech Republic	PE, cath, surgery, autopsy, echo in all, nuclear scan
	Bower et al.	1994	233,502	7.6	T	≤6 y	Yes	Australia	Cath surgery autopsy echo; included complete heart block
	Abu-Harb et al.	1994	230,654	4.6	L	≤1 y	Autopsy	United Kingdom (Northern England)	Cath, surgery, autopsy, echo
	Lin et al.	1999	126,689	3.3	L, TOP	GA 20 weeks–≤5 hospital discharge days	Hospital	United States (Boston)	Cath, surgery, autopsy, fetal and postnatal echo
	Botto et al.	2001	937,195	6.2 (1968–1997) 9 (1995–1997)	T	GA 20 weeks–2 y	Yes	United States (Atlanta)	Cath, surgery, autopsy, echo
	Bosi et al.	2003	480,793	5.1	L	GA 28 weeks–2 y	Yes	Italy (Emilia-Romagna)	Cath, surgery, autopsy, echo
	Pradat et al.	2003	4.4 million	California 3.2 France 2.9 Sweden 2.5	T	GA 20/28 weeks–1 y	Yes	United States (California), France, Sweden	Cath, surgery, autopsy, echo
	Tanner et al.	2005	521,619	5.7	L	≤1 y	Yes	United Kingdom (Northern England)	Cath, surgery, autopsy, echo
	Tegnander et al.[d]	2006	30,149	14.6	T	GA 18 weeks–2 y	Hospital	Norway	Second-trimester ultrasonography (postnatal verification in 97%)

(continued)

TABLE 25.3

ESTIMATED FREQUENCY OF CONGENITAL HEART DEFECTS: STUDIES AFTER 1980 (CONTINUED)

Group	Author	Year of publication	Population studied	Rate per 1,000	Births	Age	Population-based	Location	Diagnosis
Children	Roy et al.	1994	32,926	8	—	1–16 y	Yes	Canada (Maritime Provinces)	PE, cath, surgery, autopsy, echo
Adults	Eichhorn et al.	1990	11,450	14	—	Male, 38.4 y; Female, 37.4 y, mean	Yes	Switzerland (Zurich)	Echo with Doppler in all; reported incidence of new CHD; included mild anomalies
	Warnes et al.[e]	2001	Based on census birth rate data	1.5 complex, 2.5 moderate, 2.2 simple	—	Adult	Yes	United States	Extrapolation of Fyler et al., 1980

All studies used some type of case classification, which refers to the assignment of a single unifying diagnosis for each heart.
SA, spontaneous abortion; GA, gestational age; SB, stillbirths; L, live births; PE, physical examination; cath, catheterization; echo, echocardiography; T, total births; TOP termination of pregnancy.
From References 26 to 37, with permission. Also see Rosenthal (ref. 25) and Hoffman and Kaplan (ref. 23) for summary of earlier studies (Table 48.2, Prevalence of congenital heart disease. In: Garson A Jr, Bricker JT, Fisher DJ, Neish SR, eds. *The Science and Practice of Pediatric Cardiology*. Vols. 1 and 2. 2nd ed. Baltimore: Williams & Wilkins, 1998:1092.)
[a]Frequency of CHD reported as "% in autopsy series with a CHD."
[b]Rates reported as cases per 1,000. Table lists studies of at least 100,000 births, with the exception of fetal (autopsy) series.
[c]See text for discussion of birth prevalence versus incidence.
[d]Cohort of births followed from midgestations (18 weeks) through 2 years of life.
[e]Estimates of prevalence of simple CHD in adulthood were extrapolated from birth prevalence studies.

TABLE 25.4

RATES OF CONGENITAL HEART DEFECTS IN THREE RECENT STUDIES FROM THE UNITED STATES AND NORWAY

Group	BWIS, USA 1981–1989 Live births to 1 year of age Population-based, multiple ascertainment 906,646 births Rate (per 10,000)	Atlanta, USA 1995–1997 Live births through 1 year, stillbirths, TOP >20 WGA Population-based, multiple ascertainment 937,195 births Rate (per 1,000)	Trondhein, Norway 1991–2001 Fetuses from 18 weeks GA to at least 2 years of age Area served by one major hospital 29,460 pregnancies Total Rate (per 1,000)
Heterotaxy, L-TGA	1.4	1.6	1
Conotruncal defects			
Tetralogy of Fallot	3.3	4.7	2.4
d-Transposition of the great arteries	2.3	2.4	4.8
Double-outlet right ventricle	0.7	2.2	1
Truncus	0.5	0.6	0.3
Atrioventricular septal defect			
with Down syndrome	2.3	2.4	4.8
without Down syndrome	1	1	3.4
Total anomalous pulmonary venous return	0.7	0.6	0.7
Ebstein's anomaly	0.6	0.6	0.3
Right heart defects			0.0
Tricuspid atresia	0.4	0.3	0.7
Pulmonic atresia, intact septum	0.6	0.6	0.0
Pulmonic stenosis, atresia	5.4	5.9	7.8
Peripheral pulmonic stenosis		7	1.7
Left heart defects			
Hypoplastic left heart	1.8	2.1	3.4
Coarctation of the aorta	1.4	3.5	4.1
Aortic arch atresia/hypoplasia		0.6	0.3
Aortic valve stenosis	0.8	0.8	4.4
Septal defects			0.0
Ventricular septal defects	11.2	24.9	83.8
Atrial septal defects	3.2	10	19
Patent ductus arteriosus	0.9	8.1	0.0
Other major CHD		9.7	2
Total	48.4	90.2	146
Major	17	23.2	27.2

BWIS, Baltimore-Washington Infant Study; TOP, termination of pregnancy; GA, gestational age; WGA, weeks gestational age; L-TGA, L-transposition of the great arteries; CHD, congenital heart disease.

conditions (23), and 9 per 1,000 to 15 to 20 per 1,000 when further including smaller septal defects and milder valvar stenoses (39,42). Estimates for specific conditions need to be interpreted in light of ascertainment and reporting methods, although rates for clinically severe conditions are likely to be relatively reliable compared with milder conditions.

Generalizing these findings from relatively small study areas to countries or continents should be done with caution. Assuming an average prevalence of 9 per 1,000 for heart defects in the aggregate, and 3 per 1,000 for serious heart defects, it can be estimated that 1.2 million affected babies are born worldwide every year (36,000 in the United States), of whom at least 400,000 babies are severely affected (12,000 in the United States).

These are probably minimum estimates, because they assume that rates in developed countries apply to developing countries, where most births occur but few reliable data are available (23,40). However, such estimates may be optimistic, because of the considerable challenges of nutrition, preconception care, and environmental exposures in many developing countries, which may increase the risk for heart defects. These considerations underscore the need for good data on

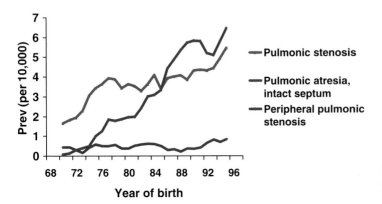

FIGURE 25.2 Trends of selected right heart defects, by severity, Atlanta 1968–1997. (Modified from *Pediatrics* 2001;107(3): E32, with permission.)

occurrence and burden of disease in much of the world (23,46,47). As the health profile of heart defects increases internationally, it will require a concerted effort to build and sustain a data infrastructure allowing for internal data gathering and international sharing.

Prevalence among children and adults is less known. The American Heart Association estimates that approximately one million adults (or approximately 1 in 300 people) live in the United States with a congenital heart defect. Such figures have been difficult to obtain directly and are usually estimated as a function of birth prevalence of specific conditions combined with their estimated survival rates (24,44). Although such figures are helpful, more detailed data and additional validation are urgently needed (2,3).

Also needed are epidemiologic data on the evolution of heart defects through the lifespan and their changing population impact. For example, many septal defects may become smaller or will have closed. In some cases, anatomy and function will have changed following surgery. In other cases, asymptomatic conditions such as bicuspid aortic valve may have evolved into significant, even life-threatening lesions requiring surgery (43,48,49). Developing and strengthening national, high-quality registries and networks will be extremely valuable in filling these data gaps.

Occurrence: The Future

Changes in diagnostic technology, parental choices, population structure, and environmental risk factors create new challenges for epidemiologic studies. A few examples are discussed by way of illustration.

A major challenge for current and future studies is capturing not only affected live births but also stillbirths, fetal deaths, and pregnancy terminations, which in some cases represent a considerable proportion of cases. Pregnancy terminations, in particular, currently account for as many as half or more of all cases of hypoplastic left heart syndrome in some countries (50,51) and a significant fraction in parts of the United States (38). Studies that do not include pregnancy terminations and fetal deaths will likely underestimate the impact of heart defects and may produce biased etiologic findings. Also, rates of pregnancy terminations may change as treatment options improve (e.g., for hypoplastic left heart syndrome), possibly leading to an apparent increase in birth prevalence that would otherwise be difficult to explain and leading to potentially unwarranted community concern.

Changing population structure could also affect the occurrence of some heart defects. For example, a shift toward older

maternal age in some populations may lead to more pregnancies with heart defects associated with chromosomal trisomies. The extent to which such increased occurrence translates into increased birth prevalence will depend on concurrent rates of fetal diagnosis and pregnancy termination.

Finally, the rising frequency of risk factors for heart defects (e.g., untreated diabetes) in many countries is also concerning. Monitoring and intervening to reduce such risk factors should be a clinical and public health priority in pediatric cardiology.

Detecting the Next Epidemic of Heart Defects

As the experience from retinoic acid and rubella has shown, teratogens can and have caused clusters of heart defects. Monitoring for the next unknown teratogen-induced 'epidemic' of birth defects is a stated goal for many monitoring programs. Yet, shifting background rates and the challenges of ascertainment for many heart defects make such a difficult activity even harder. For example, reliably detecting small increases in ventricular septal defects against a backdrop of already increasing rates can be extremely difficult.

Rising to these challenges requires innovative approaches and increased resources. Approaches can include improving clinical description and cardiology expertise available to the monitoring program, incorporating spatial analysis (to look for geographic clustering), concurrently monitoring risk factor prevalence, developing a rapid response capacity to alarms, connecting clinical and public health networks (regionally and nationally), and expanding the capacity for genetic and biomarker assessment. An increasingly important component of monitoring will likely be the astute clinician. By noting clusters of heart defects or clues to unusual associations of exposures and malformations, the astute clinician can provide a launching point for epidemiologic investigations into new or emerging causes of heart defects.

An effective system will have to balance the ability to detect true changes in occurrence (high sensitivity, low false-negative rates) with the risk and costs of reacting to too many false alarms (false-positive rates). This challenge will require close collaboration between epidemiologists and clinician to help discriminate among the multitude of signals those that have the greatest epidemiologic and biologic plausibility.

Outcomes: Mortality

Congenital heart defects are the leading cause of infant deaths owing to congenital anomalies, and this seems to be true worldwide (46,52). According to one estimate, in North America congenital heart defects contribute to one third of infant deaths because of congenital anomalies, and, overall, to approximately one tenth of all infant deaths (46,52). In developing countries, where most births occur, the impact is particularly severe because of high morbidity and mortality. One study estimated that the infant mortality owing to birth defects was roughly in inverse proportion to a country's per capita gross domestic product (52). Although based on incomplete data, these findings underscore the global impact that low-cost, effective strategies of primary prevention may have worldwide.

Surgical series document improving survival for many heart defects in the last decades in developed countries. Nationwide, population-based improvements in survival are less well documented (53,54). One such study in the United States, based on national death certificate data, reported that mortality from congenital heart defects declined by 40% from 1979 through 1997. Still, in 1995 to 1997 (the last years covered by the study), congenital heart defects were responsible for approximately 6,000 deaths per year. Mortality declined for many, but not all, heart defects. In particular, mortality for hypoplastic left heart syndrome has shown relatively little improvement compared with other conditions such as d-transposition of the great arteries, for which mortality has declined considerably. For this reason, hypoplastic left heart syndrome, on a population basis, is currently the leading cause of infant deaths owing to congenital heart defects (53). The U.S. study also identified a possible health disparity, in that mortality among black children was 20% higher than that among white children (53).

Although valuable, data from death certificates have limitations. Integrating these data with surgical and clinical cardiology networks and population-based registries would be very helpful in improving population-based assessment of mortality and other clinical outcomes. Such assessments can then guide interventions and help reduce disparities.

Outcomes: Neurodevelopmental Disabilities

With improving survival, interest is increasingly focusing on quality of life and long-term outcomes, particularly neurodevelopmental outcomes (55–58). Neurodevelopmental outcomes are a major concern for clinicians and parents. In one study, both clinicians and parents rated neurologic disability more concerning than cardiac disability when assessing quality of life for children with congenital heart defects (59).

Neurodevelopmental outcomes and related clinical issues are discussed in detail elsewhere in this volume (see Chapter 80). From an epidemiologic perspective, which is the focus here, the frequency, range, and causes of neurodevelopmental outcomes associated with heart defects are still incompletely known. Unsurprisingly, neurodevelopmental challenges are common in children with a congenital heart defect who also have an identifiable genetic condition or multiple congenital anomalies. However, increasing data suggest that also children without such obvious extracardiac involvement may be at risk for adverse neurologic outcomes, possibly because of subtle brain anomalies, altered hemodynamics, cyanosis, or the stress and complications of surgery (57). For example, microcephaly, neuronal migration defects and Chiari I malformation have been identified in children with apparently isolated heart defects (60). Altered hemodynamics, particularly in ductal-dependent lesions, may pose a risk for seizures, intraventricular hemorrhage, and periventricular leukomalacia (55,61,62). The stress and complications of surgery have been cited as a particular concern for children with functional single ventricle who undergo the Norwood operation or heart transplantation (55). Finally, neuropsychiatric conditions, including attention deficit and hyperactivity disorders, anxiety, and depression, are being increasingly diagnosed in older children and adults with congenital heart defects.

Information on neurodevelopmental outcomes evaluated today in adolescents and adults with heart defects is useful in planning management and identifying underrecognized issues. However, because of changes in surgical and medical treatment, timing, and management, it is unclear that long-term outcomes that are observed in older children today, who were born and treated years or decades ago, will necessarily be applicable to today's newborn. For this reason, epidemiologically sound studies of long-term outcomes are urgently needed. In particular, longitudinal, population-based studies will be very valuable as a basis for evaluating and improving neurodevelopmental outcomes.

Outcomes: Long-Term Studies and Quality of Life

Health-related quality of life is an evolving area of research in pediatric cardiology. One strength of the quality of life perspective is that it incorporates the view of the person with a heart defect. This is also a major challenge for researchers, because such a personal view is not captured by most traditional data sources such as vital statistics, hospital records, or administrative databases. Hence the need for novel tools and methods, further tailored to the patient's condition and age, and, in the case of children, inclusive of both a parental and child component (63–66). Because of the challenges and relative novelty of quality of life studies, one review suggested that published studies are not uniformly rigorous conceptually and methodologically (67). A further recognized data gap relates to specific studies on long-term quality of life outcomes (58,68), including school functioning, social functioning, independent living, and social integration, whose findings would be very helpful for counseling, early treatment, and anticipatory guidance (56).

Findings from such studies are not always consistent. Differences among studies may be related to many factors, both personal and societal, that can influence quality of life, including the condition's severity, surgery, health care support, family support, insurance coverage, income, and societal attitudes toward chronic illness (58,69–73).

Selected issues can be illustrated by examples. In Finland, researchers evaluated a population-based cohort of people in Finland with congenital heart defects ≤45 years after diagnosis. They found that, as a group, surviving patients appeared to cope well, and compared with the general population, had similar education, employment level, and tendency to live in a steady relationship (74). Although not directly addressing quality of life, the findings underscore the potentially good outcome for affected people (most of whom had relatively simple heart defects) living in a socially advanced society with a universal, comprehensive health care system.

By contrast, several studies in North America and Europe have also reported that patients with heart defects, after surgery, report worse health-related quality of life compared with reference groups (75–77). Quality of life may vary by anatomic lesion and type of surgery. For example, among children with transposition of the great arteries, better scores were noted among people with simpler lesions and arterial switch repair (71), although quality of life scores were also good after atrial switch operation (78). Family income may also affect quality of life, as noted in one study of survivors of the Fontan operation, in which lower family income negatively affected both physical and psychosocial aspects of quality of life (69). Compared with those of younger children, psychosocial components of quality of life tend to be particularly evident among adolescents and adults (79–81).

Factors beyond individual and family may also affect quality of life. For example, living with a heart defect in a rural area may be especially challenging because of stigma and difficulties in obtaining employment or health insurance (82). Difficulties in obtaining life insurance or a mortgage may, in fact, be a more general issue, even among people with mild or minor congenital heart defects (83).

In summary, current findings point to deficits in health status and quality of life among many patients with heart defects, as well as in parents of affected children. In addition to issues directly related to medical and surgical treatment, an increasing body of literature underscores the importance of extracardiac, psychosocial, and economic aspects in the lives of people with heart defects. From an epidemiologic perspective, quality of life studies are an area of growth. Studies of representative cohorts of patients, ideally population based, with appropriate stratification by clinical phenotype, are especially desirable.

Outcomes: Disparities

Health disparities include differences in the occurrence, mortality, and burden of disease among specific population groups. Disparities may be due to related factors such as the distribution of risk factors, access to care, environment, socioeconomic status, mechanisms of disease, or genetic variation. Understanding and responding to health disparities is a crucial step in ensuring that a community's health is equitable and just (84).

Disparities in survival between developed and developing countries are well known and were briefly discussed. Health disparities within countries are especially troubling, because they should be more easily preventable. In the United States, the 20% higher heart defect–associated mortality among

black children compared with white children remained nearly unchanged throughout the two decades examined by the already cited national death certificate study (53,54). Another United States study, using a large inpatient database, reported a higher risk of death among black and Hispanic children (74% and 34% higher, respectively) compared with white children (85). Such ongoing gaps are concerning and call for urgent investigations and decisive interventions (84).

Outcomes: Cost

Substantial resources are used yearly to care for people with congenital heart defects. Yet, comprehensive and recent estimates of the economic costs of birth defects are largely unavailable. Valid cost data are needed for cost–benefit and cost–effectiveness analyses and are crucial components of a rational approach to planning and prioritizing intervention and prevention. In 1995, a landmark study estimated that the lifetime cost of illness for babies born each year in the United States with a few selected heart defects (Table 25.5) exceeded 500 million dollars in medical costs and 1.2 billion dollars in total costs (in 1992 dollars) (86,87). This figure was largely based on the profile of services received by infants and children with these conditions in California during the late 1980s and early 1990s. The figure included estimates of direct costs (medical, developmental, and special education services) and some indirect costs (costs of lost work and household productivity). Most of the costs were driven by the expenses of early surgical interventions in infancy and childhood, as well as by lost productivity owing to death in infancy.

There are several reasons to suggest that this estimate, while large, may represent only a fraction of the overall economic cost of congenital heart defects. First, whereas the heart defects used in the estimate are severe and associated with considerable costs, there are many more heart defects than those examined. The five conditions combined have a yearly birth prevalence of approximately 1.5 per 1,000, compared with 3 to 6 per 1,000 for all severe or moderately severe conditions and 9 per 1,000

TABLE 25.5

LIFETIME COSTS FOR SELECTED BIRTH DEFECTS FOR BABIES BORN IN ONE YEAR IN THE UNITED STATES

	Medical costs	Total cost	Cost/case
Congenital heart defect			
Single ventricle	$ 61,659,000	$ 172,631,000	$ 344,000
Truncus arteriosus	107,578,000	209,676,000	505,000
Tetralogy of Fallot	185,122,000	360,486,000	262,000
Transposition of great arteries	166,334,000	514,529,000	267,000
Total	520,693,000	1,257,322,000	
Other congenital anomalies			
Spina bifida	204,512,000	489,289,000	294,000
Down syndrome	278,696,000	1,847,752,000	451,000
Cerebral palsy	851,809,000	2,425,781,000	503,000

Rate: cases per 1,000 live births (for cerebral palsy, rate per 1,000 3-year-olds).

All cost estimates are in 1992 U.S. dollars.
From Centers for Disease Control and Prevention, Waitzman NJ, Romano PS, et al. Economic costs of birth defects and cerebral palsy–United States, 1992. *MMWR Morb Mortal Wkly Rep* 1995;44:694–699; and Waitzman NJ, Romano PS, Scheffler RM. The cost of birth defects. University Press of America, 1996, with permission.

TABLE 25.6

DISTRIBUTION OF CONGENITAL HEART DEFECTS (CHD) AND ASSOCIATED DEFECTS,[a] REPORTED BY SELECTED STUDIES WITH A BIRTH POPULATION OF 1,000 OR MORE

Author, year	Isolated CHD (%)[a]	Multiple: CHD plus ≥1 major noncardiac defect[a]		
		Total (%)	Syndrome (%)	Unclassified multiple (%)
Greenwood et al., 1975	75	25	8	17
Wallgren et al., 1978[b]	56	44	Not specified	Not specified
Kramer et al., 1987	83	17[b]	13	8
Stoll et al., 1989	74	26	11.5	14.5
Ferencz et al., 1993[c]	77	23	17	6
Hanna et al., 1994	76	24	5	18
Bosi et al., 2003	76	24	13	[10]
Eskedal et al., 2004	80	20	[16]	[4]
Tegnander et al., 2006[d]				
– Prenatal diagnosis	[43]	67	Data on chromosome abnormality only	
– Postnatal diagnosis	[57]	43	Data on chromosome abnormality only	

[a]Figures in brackets were calculated from the data in the papers. Percentages are rounded. Total of syndrome and unclassified multiple may not equal the total of the multiple.
[b]Autopsy series.
[c]From Table 13.4 in Ferencz C, Loffredo CA, Correa-Villasenor A, et al. *Genetic and Environmental Risk Factors of Major Congenital Heart Disease: The Baltimore-Washington Infant Study 1981–1989.* Mount Kisco, NY: Futura Publishing, 1997, restricted to "pure" diagnoses, with permission.
[d]Data relative to major heart defects.
From References 15, 28, 39, and 88 to 94, with permission.

overall. Second, some common mild conditions may develop into serious conditions in the adult, requiring costly interventions. For example, bicuspid aortic valve may evolve into severe aortic valve disease in the adult, and the associated long-term medical care costs were not captured by the study. Third, technological advances over the past decade have led to reduction in mortality but may have increased the cost of surgical interventions and ongoing medical care. Fourth, other cost components merit consideration, including time spent and loss of productivity by family members for provision of care, and the residual psychosocial costs of illness not reflected in the estimates of care, which may exceed traditional cost components (86). Finally, costs related to education and developmental intervention were probably underestimated because, as discussed above, at the time, the frequency of adverse neurodevelopmental outcomes among children with congenital heart defects were less known than they are now.

Such emerging information on occurrence and outcomes highlights the need for a revised comprehensive assessment of the economic cost of congenital heart defects. Revised cost information can provide further impetus toward research focused on better interventions and primary prevention. For example, fully understanding that preventing one case of d-transposition of the great arteries through strict preconceptional treatment of a diabetic woman saves at least 277,000 U.S. dollars (in 1992 dollars) may strengthen public policy commitment to preventive services (86,87).

Patterns and Causes: Epidemiologic Findings

To gain insight into possible genetic causes and provide epidemiologic groupings, congenital heart defects can be classified as *isolated* or *multiple*, with further categorization into *syndromic* and *unknown* patterns. Several relevant studies have been published in the last 30 years, some of which are listed in Table 25.6 (15,28,39,88–94). In many of these studies approximately 75% to 80% of congenital heart defects were isolated, that is, without major extracardiac malformations. The higher proportion of nonisolated defects in a recent Norwegian study (39) could be due in part to the study design, which emphasized systematic fetal ascertainment.

Less consistent are the data on the proportion of heart defects associated with a recognizable chromosome or mendelian gene syndrome, or with a multiple anomaly complex of unknown cause. Two relatively large, population-based studies suggest that approximately 15% of people with a congenital heart defect plus extracardiac defects have a syndrome (15,88). Although chromosome analysis, gene testing, and clinical delineation of malformation syndromes are rapidly improving, the lack of a more dramatic proportional increase in known syndromes may be offset by the increased echocardiographic imaging detection of mild defects (notably, small atrial and ventricular septal defects and mild pulmonic stenosis), most of which are likely to be isolated and nonsyndromic. In this setting, describing the distribution of syndromic conditions as rates among births, rather than proportions among cases of heart defects, may better reflect the progress in syndrome identification.

Summarizing the distribution of specific extracardiac defects is likewise challenging, because some studies may list only major malformations or broadly defined categories of ICD-9 codes, or may fail to specify whether syndromic associations have been excluded. In general, the extracardiac anomalies more commonly associated with heart defects include urinary, central nervous system, alimentary tract, and skeletal defects (1,15,89,95).

Table 25.7 summarizes selected primary data on chromosomal and genetic causes. Over a 20-year period, the number of systematic epidemiologic studies is small. In the Baltimore-Washington Infant Study (1,15), 12% of newborns were

TABLE 25.7

CAUSES OF CONGENITAL HEART DEFECTS

Source	Chromosome abnormality (%)[a]	Mendelian gene defect (%)[b]	Microdeletion (%)	Maternal exposure (%)	Total (%)[c]	Comment
Kramer et al., 1987	5	5	Not specified	3	13	—
Stoll et al., 1989	9	"Non-chromosomal"	2.5		11.5	—
Boughman et al., Correa et al., in Ferencz et al., Table 9.1, 1993	12	7	Not specified	1–2	~20	—
Nora, 1994	~10	~10	Included in chromosome analysis	NS	~20	Meta-analysis
Correa and Botto, 2003	10	<5	5	1	~15	Meta-analysis includes data on deletion 22q11
Bosi et al., 2003	9	5	Not specified	NS	14	—
Botto et al., 2005	17	1	Included in chromosome abnormality	0.4	21	Major CHDs studied; ASD, VSD, and PDA excluded

NS, not specified; CHDs, congenital heart diseases; ASD, atrial septal defect; VSD, ventricular septal defect; PDA, patent ductus arteriosus.
[a,b]Refer to Chapter 26 on Genetics of Congenital Heart Defects for details about specific syndromes and conditions.
[c]Figures rounded.

reported to have a chromosome abnormality, slightly higher than the 9% estimate reported by studies in France (28) and Italy (88). One recent study in the United States reported chromosomal anomalies in 15% of births with heart defects (including stillbirths), including cases of deletion 22q11. Another study, also population based, reported chromosomal anomalies in 17% of serious major heart defects (i.e., excluding septal heart defects and patent ductus arteriosus), suggesting a higher contribution to the more serious group of heart defects (96). A more detailed description of associated syndromes and conditions can be found in Chapter 26.

RISK FACTORS: AN EPIDEMIOLOGIC ASSESSMENT

This section focuses on epidemiologic evidence for environmental risk factors of heart defects. Genetic risk factors are examined in a separate chapter and in recent reviews (97–99).

Two epidemiologic studies in particular, one in the Baltimore-Washington area and one in Finland, have systematically evaluated a wide range of environmental risk factors, using a case-control design. The main findings of the Baltimore-Washington infant study (BWIS), a population-based etiologic study of heart defects conducted in the 1980s, are summarized in two monographs (1,15). The findings from the Finnish study, which included all cases born in the country in 1982 to 1983 and a sample of controls, have also been extensively reported (100–106). Studies from the Centers for Disease Control and Prevention (CDC) (14,107–113) and from the California Birth Defects Monitoring Program (114–117) have also generated considerable information on specific phenotypes and a range of maternal exposures.

Much of the epidemiologic evidence on risk factors of heart defects has been presented and discussed in some detail in a recent review (118). Selected data are summarized here, but additional findings, tables, and references are available in the extended report (118). Additional resources for the clinician include online databases, such as REPROTOX and TERIS (119,120), which are regularly updated, and teratogen information services, such as those that are part of the OTIS (121) or ENTIS (122) networks, whose staff can be especially helpful.

Interpreting Epidemiologic Findings

Because much epidemiologic evidence derives from case-control studies, a discussion of their main strengths and limitation may be helpful to the clinician (118). Case-control studies compare genotypes or patterns of exposures with certain factors in affected and unaffected people and use these patterns to estimate the association between such factors and the heart defects. Environmental exposures are typically investigated through interviews with mothers of affected and unaffected pregnancies at variable times after the delivery of the pregnancy, although biomarkers are increasingly being developed and used.

The magnitude of the association between exposure and outcome is expressed as an odds ratio (OR) and, under certain conditions, estimates the relative risk of disease given the exposure. Because causality is a complex concept (123) and difficult to infer from these data alone, epidemiologic studies may be said, conservatively, to identify risk factors rather than establish causation.

Good epidemiologists go to considerable lengths to ensure that a study is rigorously designed and implemented. At stake are validity and precision. In assessing validity, major concerns are bias and confounding and their effects in generating or distorting associations (chance is also a concern, but generally a much more treatable one). For example, a study may find that smoking is associated with a certain heart defect. This finding by itself does not prove or imply that smoking is a cause or even a risk factor. Such association may be due to a confounder (e.g., alcohol use, if alcohol causes heart defects and is more common among smokers compared with nonsmokers); or it may be due to bias (e.g., recall bias, if mothers of affected babies are more likely than mothers of controls to remember or report smoking during pregnancy). Chance may also generate a spurious finding, if, for example, the predominance of smokers among case mothers in a case-control study is due to sampling alone.

Avoiding spurious associations is not trivial and requires investigators to carefully plan, implement, and analyze the study. Statistical analyses cannot fix a poorly planned or executed study. Moreover, even good studies can generate spurious findings, if only by chance. Thus, a reasonable indicator of a finding's validity is its reproducibility across several well-designed studies in different settings.

Studying environmental exposures currently has many limitations that may explain in part the slow progress and the often inconsistent findings. A major limitation has been the paucity of biomarkers of exposures, particularly during early pregnancy. Thus, exposure assessment is usually based on maternal recall (e.g., of fever, chronic illnesses, medication use), proxies of exposures (e.g., job title), or group-level data (e.g., use of pesticides in the community), often with little or no independent validation. Another limitation is the lack of information on susceptibility genotypes. Some environmental factors may become risk factors only or mainly in the presence of such genotypes, and without these data, epidemiologic assessment of environmental factors may miss or underestimate important health effects.

When examining risk estimates, it is helpful to consider several aspects of the association. These include the magnitude of the risk (e.g., the size of the odds ratio), the specific type(s) of heart defects associated with the exposure, potential interactions (the changes in effects by gender, race, age, or other factors), and the frequency of the risk factor in the population. As a group, these findings are helpful in evaluating the clinical and public health relevance of risk factors. For example, risk factors that are frequent in the population and that are associated with severe heart defects potentially have a considerable clinical and public health impact, as they may cause many cases and significant morbidity even if the magnitude of the risk (the relative risk) is not particularly high (123). In other words, the magnitude of the relative risk is not the only factor that plays into determining the impact of a risk factor (the attributable fraction) in a population.

Finally, most studies present risk estimates as point estimates with their confidence intervals. The confidence interval expresses the uncertainty, owing to the sample size of the study, regarding the true value of the point estimate. However, this does not mean that the true value is equally likely to be anywhere in the confidence interval. The best estimate remains the point estimate, and the likelihood of other values decreases the closer one gets to the limits of the interval (123). Because of this situation, confidence intervals can be chosen by the investigator, and there is nothing a priori special about the frequently seen 95% confidence interval and the associated p value of 0.05 (123). For this reason, it is reasonable and recommended (123) to consider point estimates and confidence intervals in a broader context of patterns of findings and sets of studies, rather than using the p value (or the inclusion of the null value

in the interval) as a dichotomous decision rule to assess whether a finding is present, relevant, or important.

The following section, rather than providing an exhaustive discussion, will focus on selected exposures (Table 25.8), chosen either because they are established risk factors for heart defects (e.g., diabetes, retinoic acid) or because they are common enough (e.g., smoking, obesity) that they may be of concern even if associated with mildly increased risks for heart defects. In addition to risk factors, there is a discussion on vitamin supplements as potential preventive measures.

Selected Risk Factors

Diabetes

Maternal pregestational diabetes is an established teratogen, which affects not only the developing heart but also numerous extracardiac organs (1,109,112,124–128). Many studies do not distinguish risks associated with type 1 and type 2 diabetes (see Table 25.8). Heart defects consistently associated with maternal diabetes include laterality defects (situs inversus, heterotaxy), several conotruncal defects, and, less consistently, some left ventricular outflow obstructive defects and septal defects (1,109,112,124,127,129). Among conotruncal defects, the risk appears to be strong for outflow defects with normally related great arteries and, to a lesser extent, d-transposition of the great arteries (usually complex rather than simple d-transposition) (1,109,124,127,129). Obstructive hypertrophic cardiomyopathy occurs with maternal diabetes but typically resolves. For heart defects in the aggregate, studies have estimated relative risks of approximately 4 to 5, with higher estimates for some heart defects and for heart defects associated with extracardiac anomalies (1,109,124,126,127) (Table 25.9). Some studies suggest that gestational diabetes may be a risk factor for heart defects, but it is unclear to what extent such association, when identified, may be driven by pregestational diabetes uncovered by or diagnosed during pregnancy (130–132).

The risk for diabetic embryopathy can be considerably reduced by strict glycemic control before conception, thus providing an important opportunity for primary prevention (84,133). In practice, however, prevention has been a challenge, and many affected pregnancies continue to occur (84,126,134). Estimates of the prevalence of diabetes among women of childbearing age vary. One recent report estimates that diabetes affects approximately 2% or 1.85 million women of childbearing age in the United States, such that preconceptional diabetes management could decrease the risk for pregnancy loss and congenital malformation for approximately 113,000 births per year (84). The high and rising rates of diabetes and diabetes-related risk factors (135,136) underscores the need for a renewed call to action for health providers to help prevent diabetes-related heart defects.

Obesity

The findings relating maternal obesity with heart defects in the offspring continue to be inconsistent across studies. Two studies identified an increased risk for heart defects in the aggregate (113,137), and one study did not (1). Findings are also discordant for conotruncal anomalies, with studies reporting no clear increase in risk (1,138) or an increased risk (139). Studies of obesity are challenging because of the potential for reporting bias, variations in body mass index categorization, and confounding by unrecognized diabetes or other factors associated with obesity. Also, the biology of obesity is likely to

TABLE 25.8

COMMON EXPOSURES ASSOCIATED WITH INCREASED RISK FOR CONGENITAL HEART DEFECTS: ESTIMATED EFFECTS, RISK, AND PREVENTION

Factor	Congenital heart defect	Estimated risk	Exposure type and frequency	Comments
Diabetes	Early developmental CHDs, i.e., laterality defects, looping, conotruncal defects, AV septal defects	OR usually 3 to 10, higher for some phenotypes	Pregestational diabetes:	1%–2% of women of childbearing age in United States; increasing in many countries
Febrile illness, influenza	LVOTO, including coarctation of the aorta; tricuspid atresia, dTGA and other conotruncal malformations, VSD, possibly others.	For febrile illness, relative risk between 1.5 and 3 (generally ~2), thought possibly higher for tricuspid atresia. For influenza, similar risk estimates	First trimester febrile illness reported in approximately 6%–8% of pregnancies. Generally associated with respiratory or influenzalike symptoms.	Relative contribution of hyperthermia and underlying infection unclear. Risk may be higher when influenzalike illness is associated with high fever.
Maternal phenylketonuria	Tetralogy of Fallot, VSD, PDA, LVOTO	Relative risk up to 6	Frequency of PKU is approximately 1 in 10,000 among whites	Known teratogen. Relatively rare, but effects preventable with strict dietary compliance from before conception
Retinoic acid	Conotruncal defects	High absolute risk	Isotretinoin, etretinate by mouth are teratogenic, topical tretinoin probably not	Retinoic acid use is subject to rigorous controls in some countries but not others. Exposure is a concern because many users are young women
Obesity	Several heart defects, including conotruncal defects, unclear if specific	Relative risk between 1 and 3, but some studies are negative. Causality not clear	Risks typically associated with BMI >29, but some studies show risks at BMI 25 to 29	Causality not clear. Association possibly owing in part to unrecognized diabetes. Important individual and public health concern, as obesity is increasing in many countries
Smoking	Septal defects, others	Relative risk between 1 and 3, but some studies are negative. Causality not clear	In individual studies, risk present if both parents smoke and if father alone smokes (secondhand smoking)	Causality not clear, but preventable. Smoking can cause other adverse pregnancy outcomes
Caffeine	No clear association with structural CHDs	No clear association has been demonstrated	No clear increased risk, no trend for increased risk with increasing amount of caffeine	Caffeine crosses the placenta and can have cardiovascular effects. However, several large studies failed to identify increased risk for heart defects or other malformations
Alcohol	Possibly several heart defects, including conotruncal defects	Inconsistent findings; some studies do not find association	Possible higher risk with high exposure, but not consistent finding	Known teratogen, major effects on central nervous system, association with specific heart defects still being investigated

AV, atrioventricular; OR, odds ratio; LVOTO, left ventricular outflow tract obstruction; dTGA, d-transposition of the great arteries; VSD, ventricular septal defect; PDA, patent ductus arteriosus; BMI, body mass index; CHDs, congenital heart diseases.

TABLE 25.9

PERICONCEPTIONAL USE OF VITAMINS AND OCCURRENCE OF CONGENITAL HEART DEFECTS

Type of study	Authors and year	Population-based	Study participants	Exposure	Relative risk (95% confidence interval)		
					Heart defects (overall)	Outflow tract defects (OTD)	Ventricular septal defect (VSD)
Randomized clinical trial	Czeizel et al., 1998	—	2,471 women on MV supplements; 2,391 on trace elements	MV pill with 0.8 mg folic acid	0.42 (0.19–0.98)	0.48 (0.04–5.34)	0.24 (0.05–1.14)
Case-control	Shaw et al., 1995	Yes	207 with OTD, 481 controls	MV supplements	—	0.7 (0.46–1.1)	—
Case-control	Scanlon et al., 1997	Yes	126 with OTD, 679 controls	MV supplements with folic acid	—	0.97 (0.6–1.6)	—
Case-control	Botto et al., 1996 & 2000	Yes	958 with heart defects, 3,029 controls	MV supplements	0.76 (0.6–0.97)	0.46 (0.24–0.86)	0.61 (0.38–0.99)
Case-control	Werler et al., 1999	No	157 with OTD, 186 with VSD, 521 controls	MV supplements	—	1 (0.7–1.5)	1.2 (0.8–1.8)

MV, multivitamin.

be complex and heterogeneous. Yet, because of the high and rising frequency of obesity in the United States and other countries, identifying even small increases in risk is important because of the potentially large number of pregnancies that such risk would affect (136).

Rubella

Gregg's description of the teratogenicity of rubella infection in 1941 and the subsequent understanding of its wide-ranging effects on cardiac development were key steps in the process that has led to widespread immunization of prepubertal girls (140). Heart defects in congenital rubella syndrome include most commonly pulmonic stenosis (valvar, supravalvar, or peripheral) and patent ductus arteriosus but infrequently include others, such as tetralogy of Fallot (141).

Through sustained immunization campaigns, congenital rubella syndrome has been nearly eliminated in the United States, but continued vigilance is necessary (141,142). Worldwide, rubella infection and congenital rubella syndrome remain a significant problem, highlighting the importance of global eradication of this preventable condition (143).

Fever and Flu

Although the evidence in animal models is convincing (144–146), characterizing the cardiac teratogenicity of other febrile illnesses in humans remains a challenge. For example, validating reports of febrile illness in pregnancy is difficult in retrospective studies, as is disentangling the potential interactions between underlying infection, fever, and medications. Nevertheless, several studies indicate that first-trimester febrile or flulike illnesses (the terms flu and influenza are often used in the literature interchangeably) may be associated with an approximately twofold increased risk for congenital heart defects in the aggregate and possibly higher risks for specific lesions such as tricuspid atresia, coarctation of the aorta, aortic stenosis, and ventricular septal defects (101,110,115,124,145,147).

The number of exposed pregnancies is unknown but may be considerable, since in several studies, approximately 6% to 8% of women in the control groups reported at least one respiratory infection or febrile illness during the first trimester of pregnancy (101,110,115,147). Thus, among the estimated 4 million newborns born yearly in the United States, approximately ≥250,000 may have been exposed to some form of febrile or flulike illness in early pregnancy.

If febrile illnesses cause an increased risk for heart defects, avoidance of ill contacts, and possibly preconceptional immunization before flu season, may be effective. Also of potential relevance are reports that periconceptional use of multivitamin supplements may be associated with a reduced risk of congenital heart defects associated with febrile illnesses (110,115).

Maternal Phenylketonuria

Women with maternal phenylketonuria (PKU) who have high levels of phenylalanine when pregnant have a high likelihood of having children with microcephaly and mental retardation, a presentation that exemplifies maternal PKU syndrome (148–150). Except for the brain, the heart is the major organ affected by maternal PKU, in the form of increased risk mainly for left-sided defects (coarctation of the aorta to hypoplastic left heart syndrome), tetralogy of Fallot, septal defects, and possibly patent ductus arteriosus (148–150). Estimates of relative risk have been high (6 to 15) in various studies and for different heart defects. In one major study, the absolute risk for heart defects was 14% among pregnancies exposed to high

levels of phenylalanine (34 of 235 pregnancies) compared with pregnancies with good biochemical control (148).

The number of women of childbearing age with PKU is unknown. Based on the birth prevalence of PKU (1 in 10,000 births), an estimated 200 girls with PKU are born yearly in the United States and will eventually be at risk for having an affected pregnancy if untreated. Although maternal PKU may be relatively rare, because it is preventable, every effort should be made to identify and treat women at risk before conception to reduce the risk for cardiac and developmental disability in their pregnancies.

Seizure Disorders and Seizure Medications

The issue of teratogenicity of seizure disorder and anticonvulsant medications is especially complex because of heterogeneity of seizure disorders, the number of available medications, the range of dosages, the frequency of polytherapy, and ongoing marketing of new medications. Most women with seizure disorders have uneventful pregnancies, and seizure medications, rather than seizure disorders per se, are currently the main concern for teratogenicity (151). Exposure to phenytoin, hydantoin, and valproic acid has been associated with increased risk for malformations (152–157), although reliable estimates of risk for specific types of heart defects are unavailable.

In the United States, seizure medications are prescribed for an estimated 1 million women (19 per 1,000), potentially affecting an estimated 75,000 pregnancies every year (84). Preconceptional counseling of women with a seizure disorder is particularly important, in particular to evaluate the benefits and risks of lowering dosage, switching to less teratogenic medications, and ensuring that women understand and follow recommendations for a healthy pregnancy, including the use of folic acid supplements (84,155–157).

Thalidomide and Retinoic Acid Congeners

Thalidomide and retinoic acid congeners have some features in common. These medications are potent teratogens for which there is no known safe dose, and they can cause severe and complex heart defects, including conotruncal anomalies, in addition to other major birth defects (158–160).

Retinoic acid and its congeners, which include isotretinoin and etretinate, are a particular concern because of their use among young women for the treatment of acne, and possibly other less-specific indications (161). Although strict regulatory guidelines have been issues in some countries, health care providers should be alert to improper use (84,161,162).

Vitamin A

Vitamin A occurs in one of two forms, beta-carotene and retinol. Both forms are widely available alone or in combination in supplements, which include some high-dose formulations. Both forms are liposoluble, and therefore may accumulate in the body. The chemical similarities of these compounds with retinoids have long raised concerns for teratogenicity.

Beta-carotene has not been associated with increased risks for congenital heart defects; however, findings for retinol have been less consistent. In some studies, use of supplements containing retinol at high doses (>10,000 IU) was associated with an increased risk for heart defects, and in particular d-transposition of the great arteries (20,163,164). Other studies did not find an increased risk with high retinol intake (165–168). Because of such uncertainties, except in cases where vitamin A is especially beneficial (i.e., among vitamin A–deficient people), it seems prudent to avoid high-dose retinol supplements in the periconceptional period and to favor vitamin A preparations containing beta-carotene.

Sulfa Antibiotics

Some commonly used antibiotics such as dihydrofolate reductase inhibitors are folic acid antagonists. Specifically, trimethoprim-sulfonamide and sulfasalazine have been associated with a mild to moderate increase in risk for heart defects (169,170). In one study, the use of folic acid supplements decreased the excess risk associated with these compounds (170).

Ampicillin, Corticosteroids, Oral Contraceptives

There is no evidence that these commonly used medications increase materially the risk for congenital heart defects, as discussed in a recent review (118). In many cases, initial reports suggestive of teratogenicity were followed by larger studies that failed to confirm such findings (118).

Lithium

After initial reports suggesting that lithium was a strong risk factor for heart defects, and particularly for Ebstein's anomaly, more recent data have prompted a reassessment of such estimates (171–173). Recent estimates suggest that the risk associated with lithium is smaller than previously thought, although small to moderate increases in risk for Ebstein's anomaly cannot be excluded (171–173). More generally, women with manic-depressive conditions may be at risk for adverse pregnancy outcomes and may benefit from careful preconceptional and prenatal care (171–174).

Dietary, Lifestyle, and Demographic Factors

Caffeine. Because of frequent consumption and known effects on cardiovascular physiology, reproductive risks of caffeine intake have been extensively investigated. To date, several studies (175–177), including the BWIS (1) and Finnish (100,103) cardiac studies, have failed to detect evidence of cardiac teratogenicity related to consumption of coffee and other caffeine-containing beverages, including soft drinks.

Alcohol. Alcohol is an established human teratogen and causes a wide range of structural malformations and neurologic abnormalities (178,179). Methodologic issues, including the challenge of documenting exposure reliably and precisely, make studies of alcohol effects in humans especially difficult. In the BWIS, significant association with alcohol exposure was limited to small ventricular septal defects and was noted only in women who reported heavy consumption (1). In the Finnish cardiac study, the authors reported possible associations with ventricular septal defects (102), atrial septal defects (100,104), and possibly conotruncal defects (103), although dose-response patterns were unimpressive. In the Atlanta population-based study, no associations with conotruncal anomalies were identified (108).

Nevertheless, the general teratogenic effects of alcohol use make prevention of alcohol effects in pregnancy an important public health priority (84,180). According to recent estimates, approximately 7 million women of childbearing age in the United States are frequent drinkers, and without preconception interventions, alcohol misuse might affect approximately 577,000 births per year (84).

Smoking. Smoking increases the risk for low birth weight, preterm birth, and other adverse outcomes, but findings relative to heart defects are inconsistent. Most recent data seem to support such association, with generally low but statistically significant findings. Such studies include two cohort studies, one from Sweden (odds ratio for all heart defects, 1.1; for conotruncal anomalies, 1.2) (181) and one from the United States (odds ratio for all heart defects, 1.56) (182). Among case-control studies, the BWIS reported an increased risk for d-transposition of the great arteries (odds ratio, 2.1) (1), and a study from California reported an increased risk for conotruncal anomalies (odds ratio, 2.2.) among women who did not use vitamin supplements in the periconceptional period (115). Even small increases in risk are of concern because of the frequency of smoking in women. In 2003, an estimated 11% of pregnant women in the United States smoked during pregnancy (84). Also of concern is the increasing rate of smoking among women in many countries (183).

Race/Ethnicity. Racial variations in the occurrence of congenital heart defects have been consistently reported. In the United States, for example, findings from the BWIS (41) and a CDC study (13) suggest that white infants, compared with black infants, have higher rates of several heart defects, including left-sided defects (aortic stenosis, coarctation of the aorta, hypoplastic left heart); some, but not all, conotruncal defects (d-transposition of the great arteries, truncus arteriosus); and Ebstein's anomaly. In the same studies, compared with black infants, white infants tended to have lower rates of pulmonic stenosis and atrial septal defect. Other racial and ethnic groups have been less studied.

International surveys of heart defect occurrence show differences by country and race/ethnicity (23,40,44). However, interpreting these findings in terms of effects of ethnic background is complicated by the concurrent variations in ascertainment and reporting across countries.

Potential Protective Factors: Folic Acid and Multivitamin Supplements

The notion that vitamin supplementation may reduce the risk for some heart defects is receiving increasing attention (184–187). Confirming such preventive effects would be a major breakthrough for primary prevention of heart defects, for several reasons. Based on initial data, the fraction of preventable heart defects may be large, many women of childbearing age may benefit, and many vitamins, including folic acid, are inexpensive and easily transportable. Thus the potential worldwide impact of vitamin-based prevention is considerable.

The data that most directly assess the relation between vitamin supplementation and risk for heart defects derive from one randomized clinical trial and several observational studies. Most data, although not all, are consistent with a reduced risk for selected heart defects among women who take multivitamin supplements from before conception (Table 25.9). In the randomized clinical trial of folic acid and multivitamin supplements for the prevention of birth defects, the overall risk for congenital heart defects was reduced by 52% in children of women taking the multivitamin supplement with 0.8 mg of folic acid, compared with the reference group (women taking a supplement with trace elements only) (188,189). Such reduction was driven largely by lower rates of conotruncal and ventricular septal defects (Table 25.9).

Among the population-based case-control studies, findings include a decreased risk for congenital heart defects in the aggregate (14), for conotruncal anomalies (14,117), for ventricular septal defects (14), and possibly coarctation of the aorta (14). However, one study showed no decrease in risk of ventricular septal defects (190), and in another study on conotruncal anomalies, the results were mixed, with a trend of reduced risk for tetralogy of Fallot but not other conotruncal anomalies (191). Some of the risk estimates are associated with relatively wide confidence intervals. Although the best estimate of risk (the point estimate) is consistent with a reduced risk associated with multivitamin use, larger studies with more precise estimates would be very helpful.

Other studies also report that multivitamin supplement use was associated with a decrease in the teratogenic risk from other exposures. For example, multivitamin supplements appeared to reduce the risk for heart defects among pregnancies of women whose risk was increased because of first-trimester use of certain medications (mainly certain antibiotics with antifolate effects) (170). In two other studies, the risk for heart defects associated with first-trimester febrile illness was decreased among women who also took multivitamin supplements from before conception (110,115). As in previous studies, some of these findings are associated with wide confidence intervals and would be important to replicate in larger studies.

To examine plausibility and potential mechanism, human and experimental studies are also evaluating the relation between micronutrient (vitamin) intake, genotype, and cardiac phenotype, with particular attention to the network of genes involved in the metabolism of folate and other factors of one-carbon metabolism. Initial data, which relate mainly to the folate-related gene MTHFR (methylenetetrahydrofolate reductase) and its 677C->T variant, are inconsistent. Some studies found no evidence of an association of such MTHFR variant with conotruncal or other heart defects (18,192–194), whereas others found an association (195–197). Case selection, choice of controls, analytic methods, and other methodologic issues may have contributed to the discrepant findings. Large, well-designed population-based studies with good clinical and laboratory data would be very helpful in elucidating the relation between heart defects and the set of folate genes. One study examined the reduced folate carrier gene RFC1 and reported an increased risk for heart defects with the variant genotype, which increased further among women who did not use folic acid supplementation (198).

In mice, the combination of mild MTHFR deficiency and low dietary folate caused increased rates of heart malformations, which were not seen among mice on a folate-sufficient diet (199). In a similar experimental setup, these researchers then showed that proliferation of embryonic myocardium is sensitive to maternal dietary folate and concluded that folate supplementation during pregnancy is important for normal heart development (200). Also, in mice, impaired folic acid transport (owing to knockout of the folic acid–binding protein one Folbp1) resulted in extensive apoptosis-mediated cell death, concentrated in the interventricular septum and conotruncal region. The authors concluded that altered folate transport could mediate susceptibility to heart defects, in particular in the conotruncal area (201).

Following implementation of flour fortification in the United States in 1998, researchers have begun monitoring for concurrent changes in birth defect prevalence rates. Fortification in the United States can be viewed as equivalent to increasing, by a small amount, the average intake of folic acid in most of the population. Except for perhaps a small decrease in tetralogy of Fallot, to date there does not seem to have been a decrease in occurrence rates of heart defects (or of newborn hospitalizations for heart defects). This suggests that small doses of folic acid are probably not effective in preventing a significant fraction of heart defects (fortification seems to have

decreased the occurrence of neural tube defects, albeit by a smaller amount than achieved in the randomized trials of supplements).

How can one reconcile the mostly negative findings from the fortification experience with the mostly positive findings from the Hungarian randomized trial and some observational studies? One possibility is that a relatively large amount of folic acid is needed for a measurable effect on heart defects (as suggested also for cleft lip and palate). Another possibility is that a multivitamin combination (found in supplements) may be more effective than folic acid alone (used in fortification).

In summary, these accumulating findings are encouraging but not conclusive. Because of the importance of conclusively establishing the preventive potential of vitamin supplements, a large randomized trial of vitamin supplementation (versus the recommended dose of folic acid alone) would be very helpful. The cost of heart defects is such that such a randomized trial would easily be cost effective.

From a practical perspective, pediatric cardiologists need not wait for such a trial. Because of the established protective effect against neural tube defects, daily periconceptional use of folic acid is recommended for all women of childbearing age. By promoting periconceptional use of a multivitamin supplement containing folic acid (400 μg), pediatric cardiologists would provide all women with the benefits of a reduced risk for a neural tube defect–affected pregnancy and, at the same time, possibly a lower risk for heart defects.

APPROACH TO PREVENTION

Although current knowledge on risk factors is incomplete, some guidelines can be proposed for the primary prevention of heart defects (118). One may attempt to separate strategies to prevent heart defects from strategies to prevent other congenital anomalies and adverse pregnancy outcomes (e.g., preterm birth, intrauterine growth retardation). However, guidelines to prevent heart defects in the broader context of child health is likely more desirable and practical (84). A set of suggested prevention guidelines is presented in Table 25.10.

At the basis of many specific recommendations is the emphasis on preconception care (84). This is a crucial time to identify and treat potentially risky exposures and behaviors. A helpful guiding concept is that of the 12-month pregnancy, that is, a time period that includes also the trimester *before* conception. This preconceptional period, together with at least the first 2 months of pregnancy, provides a crucial opportunity for promoting healthy cardiac development. Most cardiac structures develop in the first 7 weeks postconception (9 weeks following last menstrual period), during which time many women may be unaware of the pregnancy, potentially exposed to teratogens, and with limited or no prenatal care.

For the individual, preconceptional health includes some key actions: Identifying and managing chronic illnesses or exposures; avoiding exposures to acute illnesses, alcohol, and smoking; and taking a daily multivitamin containing folic acid. For population-based interventions, crucial areas of improvement include increasing health care access, improving health behaviors, and refocusing health professionals on common preventable risk factors for heart defects, from maternal diabetes, to supplement use, to medication use. Specific to population-based interventions are monitoring and interventions to reduce health disparities.

Specifically, all women of childbearing age should be encouraged to take a daily vitamin supplement containing folic acid, to reduce the occurrence of neural tube defects and

TABLE 25.10

SUGGESTED GUIDELINES FOR PRIMARY PREVENTION OF CONGENITAL HEART DEFECTS

Step	Comments
Take a daily multivitamin containing folic acid.	Start using before conception. Prevents neural tube defects and may prevent some congenital heart diseases. Recommended daily dose of folic acid is 0.4 mg. Consider higher dose of folic acid if there was a previously affected pregnancy.
Get preconceptional assessment of risk factors and maternal conditions.	Target diabetes, chronic illness, and medication use, maternal phenylketonuria, smoking, alcohol, rubella immunization.
Stop common exposures, including smoking and alcohol use, from before conception.	Also avoid secondhand smoke; encourage smoking cessation by other members of the household.
Reassess medication use.	Target medications with known teratogenic effect, (e.g., modify seizure medications), be aware of others that have not been evaluated sufficiently for their safety. Contact Organization of Teratogen Informations Services for resources. Reassess over-the-counter medications use.
Avoid exposures to heavy metals, herbicides, pesticides, and organic solvents.	Assess exposure associated with household activities, work-related (self and partner), or environmental.
Avoid close contact with ill individuals, especially those with febrile illnesses.	Discuss safe ways to decrease high fever if it occurs. It is unclear to what extent risk associated with febrile illness is related to fever or illness.

possibly also some congenital heart defects. Health providers, in concert with their clients, should reevaluate and treat chronic conditions from before conception, especially diabetes (the increased prevalence of birth defects among infants of women with type 1 or type 2 diabetes is substantially reduced through proper management of diabetes from before conception throughout the pregnancy). Women diagnosed with PKU as infants should be targeted for interventions aimed at ensuring adherence to a low phenylalanine diet before conception and continue it throughout their pregnancy.

Before conception, women who are on a regimen of teratogenic medications (e.g., valproic acid) and who are contemplating pregnancy should be prescribed a lower dosage of these drugs. Among women with childbearing potential who use isotretinoins (e.g., Accutane), effective pregnancy prevention should be implemented to avoid unintended pregnancies while on this medication. Rubella vaccination provides protective seropositivity and prevents congenital rubella syndrome.

Because only 20% of women successfully control tobacco dependence during pregnancy, cessation of smoking is recommended before pregnancy (84). In addition to the evidence on risk for congenital heart defects, preterm birth, low birth weight, and other adverse perinatal outcomes associated with maternal smoking in pregnancy can be prevented if women stop smoking before or during early pregnancy. Alcohol misuse is a significant concern. As previously discussed, although the evidence for specific cardiac teratogenicity is mixed, fetal alcohol syndrome and alcohol-related birth defects can be prevented if women cease intake of alcohol before conception.

With respect to obesity, the risk associated with cardiovascular anomalies is not convincingly established. However, obesity is associated with several adverse perinatal outcomes, including neural tube defects, preterm delivery, diabetes, and hypertensive and thromboembolic disease. Appropriate weight loss and improving nutritional health before pregnancy reduces these risks. Additional recommendations for preconception care include vaccination for hepatitis B, identification and treatment of HIV/AIDS and sexually transmitted diseases, treatment of hypothyroidism, and reassessment of oral anticoagulant therapy for warfarin users (84,118).

These general guidelines can reasonably apply to all women of childbearing age to prevent the occurrence of heart defects and other congenital anomalies. Pediatric cardiologists, perhaps more than other specialists, will also see and be called to counsel women who have a heart defect or a previously affected child and who are contemplating (or not actively excluding) another pregnancy. In this group, the search for modifiable risk factors should be especially rigorous. Also, evaluation for underlying genetic conditions (e.g., deletion 22q11), including referral to an experienced medical geneticist, may be extremely helpful in defining and managing recurrence risk. In the setting of prevention of recurrence of neural tube defects, data from a randomized trial have shown the efficacy of a high dose (4 mg) of folic acid, with no adverse effect. No comparable data are available for heart defects.

CONCLUSION

Epidemiology can contribute significantly to finding risk factors, assessing outcomes, and evaluating interventions. Data gaps are significant in all three areas, and filling these gaps requires a concerted effort by the clinical, research, and public health community. In particular, large population-based studies are needed.

Two examples can illustrate the potential of these studies as well as the challenges. In the United States, the National Birth Defect Prevention Study (NBDPS) is an example of an ongoing large multicenter case-control study focused on the etiologic factors of heart defects and other congenital anomalies (202,203). The NBDPS includes rigorous phenotyping, collection of biologic samples from children and parents, and parental interviews. The large scale is critical to reach the statistical power necessary to investigate the role of genotype, environment, and gene–environment interactions.

The National Children's Study (NCS) represents a complementary, powerful approach. Also a population-based study, the NCS strives to identify and follow a cohort of 100,000 babies from pregnancy (or even preconception) through at least 18 years of age (204). Concurrent collection of comprehensive environmental, biologic, and clinical data will provide an unprecedented opportunity to assess risk factors for many common health conditions (204), including the more common heart defects, and to study their natural and modified longitudinal history. Studies such as these represent significant opportunities but require sustained public support as well as multidisciplinary collaboration, including that between epidemiologists and pediatric cardiologists.

With respect to prevention, conclusive evidence on the potential preventive effect of vitamin supplements will be extremely helpful as a basis for national and international action to reduce the occurrence of heart defects. A randomized clinical trial targeted specifically at heart defects, although challenging, would provide the best evidence. Such effort would be justifiable, given the significant health impact of heart defects worldwide and the benefits of finding an effective, inexpensive strategy of primary prevention.

Finally, in addition to seeking risk factors and preventive factors, epidemiologic studies need to keep expanding their scope to keep pace with the needs of people with heart defects, in particular as it relates to mortality, morbidity, cost, and broadly, quality of life. Population-based studies, in particular, can help identify priority areas for interventions, including health disparities, so as to benefit both the person with a heart defect and the community.

References

1. Ferencz C, Loffredo CA, Correa-Villasenor A, et al. *Genetic and Environmental Risk Factors of Major Congenital Heart Disease: The Baltimore-Washington Infant Study 1981–1989.* Mount Kisco, NY Futura Publishing, 1997.
2. Warnes CA, Liberthson R, Danielson GK, et al. Task force 1: The changing profile of congenital heart disease in adult life. *J Am Coll Cardiol* 2001; 37:1170–1175.
3. Williams RG, Pearson GD, Barst RJ, et al. Report of the National Heart, Lung, and Blood Institute Working Group on research in adult congenital heart disease. *J Am Coll Cardiol* 2006;47:701–707.
4. Mavroudis C, Gevitz M, Elliott MJ, et al. Virtues of a worldwide congenital heart surgery database. *Semin Thorac Cardiovasc Surg Pediatr Card Surg Annu* 2002;5:126–131.
5. Jacobs JP, Jacobs ML, Maruszewski B, et al. Current status of the European Association for Cardio-Thoracic Surgery and the Society of Thoracic Surgeons Congenital Heart Surgery Database. *Ann Thorac Surg* 2005;80: 2278–2283; discussion 2283–2274.
6. Jacobs JP, Lacour-Gayet FG, Jacobs ML, et al. Initial application in the STS congenital database of complexity adjustment to evaluate surgical case mix and results. *Ann Thorac Surg* 2005;79:1635–1649; discussion 1635–1649.
7. Jacobs JP, Maruszewski B, Tchervenkov CI, et al. The current status and future directions of efforts to create a global database for the outcomes of therapy for congenital heart disease. *Cardiol Young* 2005;15(suppl 1): 190–197.
8. Jacobs JP, Mavroudis C, Jacobs ML, et al. Lessons learned from the data analysis of the second harvest (1998–2001) of the Society of Thoracic Surgeons (STS) Congenital Heart Surgery Database. *Eur J Cardiothorac Surg* 2004;26:18–37.
9. Jacobs JP. Software development, nomenclature schemes, and mapping strategies for an international pediatric cardiac surgery database system. *Semin Thorac Cardiovasc Surg Pediatr Card Surg Annu* 2002;5:153–162.
10. Clark EB. Pathogenetic mechanisms of congenital cardiovascular malformations revisited. *Semin Perinatol* 1996;20:465–472.
11. Clark EB. Etiology of congenital cardiovascular malformations: Epidemiology and genetics. In: Allen HD, Gutgesell HP, Clark EB, et al., eds. *Moss and Adams' Heart Disease in Infants, Children, and Adolescents.* 6th ed. Philadelphia: Lippincott Williams & Wilkins, 2001:64–79.
12. Khoury MJ, Moore CA, James LM, et al. The interaction between dysmorphology and epidemiology: Methodologic issues of lumping and splitting. *Teratology* 1992;45:133–138.
13. Botto LD, Correa A, Erickson JD. Racial and temporal variations in the prevalence of heart defects. *Pediatrics* 2001;107:E32.
14. Botto LD, Mulinare J, Erickson JD. Occurrence of congenital heart defects in relation to maternal multivitamin use. *Am J Epidemiol* 2000;151: 878–884.
15. Ferencz C, Loffredo CA, Rubin JD, et al. *Epidemiology of Congenital Heart Disease: The Baltimore-Washington Infant Study 1981–1989.* Mount Kisco, NY: Futura Publishing, 1993.
16. Lewin MB, McBride KL, Pignatelli R, et al. Echocardiographic evaluation of asymptomatic parental and sibling cardiovascular anomalies associated with congenital left ventricular outflow tract lesions. *Pediatrics* 2004;114:691–696.
17. Loffredo CA, Chokkalingam A, Sill AM, et al. Prevalence of congenital cardiovascular malformations among relatives of infants with hypoplastic left heart, coarctation of the aorta, and d-transposition of the great arteries. *Am J Med Genet A* 2004;124:225–230.
18. McBride KL, Fernbach S, Menesses A, et al. A family-based association study of congenital left-sided heart malformations and 5,10 methylenetetrahydrofolate reductase. *Birth Defects Res A Clin Mol Teratol* 2004;70: 825–830.
19. McBride KL, Marengo L, Canfield M, et al. Epidemiology of noncomplex left ventricular outflow tract obstruction malformations (aortic valve stenosis, coarctation of the aorta, hypoplastic left heart syndrome) in Texas, 1999–2001. *Birth Defects Res A Clin Mol Teratol* 2005;73:555–561.
20. Botto LD, Loffredo C, Scanlon KS, et al. Vitamin A and cardiac outflow tract defects. *Epidemiology* 2001;12:491–496.
21. Harris JA, Francannet C, Pradat P, et al. The epidemiology of cardiovascular defects, part 2: A study based on data from three large registries of congenital malformations. *Pediatr Cardiol* 2003;24:222–235.
22. Mason CA, Kirby RS, Sever LE, et al. Prevalence is the preferred measure of frequency of birth defects. *Birth Defects Res A Clin Mol Teratol* 2005; 73:690–692.
23. Hoffman JI, Kaplan S. The incidence of congenital heart disease. *J Am Coll Cardiol* 2002;39:1890–1900.
24. McCrindle BW. The prevalence of congenital cardiac lesions. In: Freedom RM, Yoo S-J, Mikailian H, et al., eds. *The Natural and Modified History of Congenital Heart Disease.* New York: Futura, Blackwell Publishing, 2004.
25. Rosenthal GR. Prevalence of congenital heart disease. In: Garson AJ, Bricker JT, Fisher DJ, et al., eds. *The Science and Practice of Pediatric Cardiology.* Baltimore: Williams & Wilkins, 1998:1098.
26. Ursell PC, Byrne JM, Strobino BA. Significance of cardiac defects in the developing fetus: A study of spontaneous abortuses. *Circulation* 1985;72: 1232–1236.
27. Chinn A, Fitzsimmons J, Shepard TH, et al. Congenital heart disease among spontaneous abortuses and stillborn fetuses: Prevalence and associations. *Teratology* 1989;40:475–482.
28. Stoll C, Alembik Y, Roth MP, et al. Risk factors in congenital heart disease. *Eur J Epidemiol* 1989;5:382–391.
29. Fyler DC, Buckley LP, Hellenbrand WE, et al. Report of the New England Regional Infant Cardiac Program. *Pediatrics* 1980;65(suppl):376.
30. Grabitz RG, Joffres MR, Collins-Nakai RL. Congenital heart disease: Incidence in the first year of life. The Alberta Heritage Pediatric Cardiology Program. *Am J Epidemiol* 1988;128:381–388.
31. Fixler DE, Pastor P, Chamberlin M, et al. Trends in congenital heart disease in Dallas County births, 1971–1984. *Circulation* 1990;81:137–142.
32. Kidd SA, Lancaster PA, McCredie RM. The incidence of congenital heart defects in the first year of life. *J Paediatr Child Health* 1993;29:344–349.
33. Samanek M. Boy:girl ratio in children born with different forms of cardiac malformation: A population-based study. *Pediatr Cardiol* 1994;15:53–57.
34. Abu-Harb M, Hey E, Wren C. Death in infancy from unrecognised congenital heart disease. *Arch Dis Child* 1994;71:3–7.
35. Tanner K, Sabrine N, Wren C. Cardiovascular malformations among preterm infants. *Pediatrics* 2005;116:e833–838.
36. Roy DL, McIntyre L, Human DG, et al. Trends in the prevalence of congenital heart disease: Comprehensive observations over a 24-year period in a defined region of Canada. *Can J Cardiol* 1994;10:821–826.
37. Eichhorn P, Sutsch G, Jenni R. Congenital heart defects and abnormalities newly detected with echocardiography in adolescents and adults [in German]. *Schweiz Med Wochenschr* 1990;120:1697–1700.
38. Lin AE, Herring AH, Amstutz KS, et al. Cardiovascular malformations: Changes in prevalence and birth status, 1972–1990. *Am J Med Genet* 1999;84:102–110.

39. Tegnander E, Williams W, Johansen OJ, et al. Prenatal detection of heart defects in a non-selected population of 30,149 fetuses—detection rates and outcome. *Ultrasound Obstet Gynecol* 2006;27:252–265.

40. Hoffman JI. Incidence of congenital heart disease: I. Postnatal incidence. *Pediatr Cardiol* 1995;16:103–113.

41. Correa-Villasenor A, McCarter R, Downing J, et al. White-black differences in cardiovascular malformations in infancy and socioeconomic factors. The Baltimore-Washington Infant Study Group. *Am J Epidemiol* 1991;134:393–402.

42. Hiraishi S, Agata Y, Nowatari M, et al. Incidence and natural course of trabecular ventricular septal defect: Two-dimensional echocardiography and color Doppler flow imaging study. *J Pediatr* 1992;120:409–415.

43. Ward C. Clinical significance of the bicuspid aortic valve. *Heart* 2000; 83:81–85.

44. Hoffman JI, Kaplan S, Liberthson RR. Prevalence of congenital heart disease. *Am Heart J* 2004;147:425–439.

45. Wren C, Richmond S, Donaldson L. Temporal variability in birth prevalence of cardiovascular malformations. *Heart* 2000;83:414–419.

46. Lopez AD, Mathers CD. Measuring the global burden of disease and epidemiological transitions: 2002–2030. *Ann Trop Med Parasitol* 2006;100: 481–499.

47. Murray CJL, Lopez AD. *Health Dimensions of Sex and Reproduction: The Global Burden of Sexually Transmitted Diseases, HIV, Maternal Conditions, Perinatal Disorders, and Congenital Anomalies.* Boston: Harvard University Press, 1998.

48. Chambers J. Aortic stenosis. *BMJ* 2005;330:801–802.

49. Cecconi M, Nistri S, Quarti A, et al. Aortic dilatation in patients with bicuspid aortic valve. *J Cardiovas Med (Hagerstown)* 2006;7:11–20.

50. Garne E, Loane M, Dolk H, et al. Prenatal diagnosis of severe structural congenital malformations in Europe. *Ultrasound Obstet Gynecol* 2005;25:6–11.

51. Khoshnood B, De Vigan C, Vodovar V, et al. Trends in prenatal diagnosis, pregnancy termination, and perinatal mortality of newborns with congenital heart disease in France, 1983–2000: A population-based evaluation. *Pediatrics* 2005;115:95–101.

52. Rosano A, Botto LD, Botting B, et al. Infant mortality and congenital anomalies from 1950 to 1994: An international perspective. *J Epidemiol Community Health* 2000;54:660–666.

53. Boneva RS, Botto LD, Moore CA, et al. Mortality associated with congenital heart defects in the United States: Trends and racial disparities, 1979–1997. *Circulation* 2001;103:2376–2381.

54. Gillum RF. Epidemiology of congenital heart disease in the United States. *Am Heart J* 1994;127:919–927.

55. Mahle W. Spectrum of heart disease. In: Rubin I, Crocker A, eds. *Medical Care for Children and Adults with Developmental Disabilities.* Baltimore: Paul H Brooks Publishing, 2006:379–386.

56. Brown MD, Wernovsky G, Mussatto KA, et al. Long-term and developmental outcomes of children with complex congenital heart disease. *Clin Perinatol* 2005;32:1043–1057, xi.

57. Wernovsky G. Outcomes regarding the central nervous system in children with complex congenital cardiac malformations. *Cardiol Young* 2005; 15(suppl 1):132–133.

58. Williams WG. Surgical outcomes in congenital heart disease: Expectations and realities. *Eur J Cardiothorac Surg* 2005;27:937–944.

59. Knowles RL, Griebsch I, Bull C, et al. Quality-of-life and congenital heart defects: Comparing parent and professional values. *Arch Dis Child* 2006. (Epub ahead of print.)

60. Limperopoulos C, Majnemer A, Shevell MI, et al. Neurodevelopmental status of newborns and infants with congenital heart defects before and after open heart surgery. *J Pediatr* 2000;137:638–645.

61. Limperopoulos C, Majnemer A, Shevell MI, et al. Predictors of developmental disabilities after open heart surgery in young children with congenital heart defects. *J Pediatr* 2002;141:51–58.

62. Mahle WT, Clancy RR, Moss EM, et al. Neurodevelopmental outcome and lifestyle assessment in school-aged and adolescent children with hypoplastic left heart syndrome. *Pediatrics* 2000;105:1082–1089.

63. Eiser C, Morse R. Can parents rate their child's health-related quality of life? Results of a systematic review. *Qual Life Res* 2001;10:347–357.

64. Eiser C, Morse R. The measurement of quality of life in children: Past and future perspectives. *J Dev Behav Pediatr* 2001;22:248–256.

65. Eiser C, Morse R. A review of measures of quality of life for children with chronic illness. *Arch Dis Child* 2001;84:205–211.

66. Goldbeck L, Melches J. Quality of life in families of children with congenital heart disease. *Qual Life Res* 2005;14:1915–1924.

67. Moons P, Van Deyk K, Budts W, et al. Caliber of quality-of-life assessments in congenital heart disease: A plea for more conceptual and methodological rigor. *Arch Pediatr Adolesc Med* 2004;158:1062–1069.

68. Schultz AH, Wernovsky G. Late outcomes in patients with surgically treated congenital heart disease. *Semin Thorac Cardiovasc Surg Pediatr Card Surg Annu* 2005;145–156.

69. McCrindle BW, Williams RV, Mitchell PD, et al. Relationship of patient and medical characteristics to health status in children and adolescents after the Fontan procedure. *Circulation* 2006;113:1123–1129.

70. Goldbeck L, Melches J. The impact of the severity of disease and social disadvantage on quality of life in families with congenital cardiac disease. *Cardiol Young* 2006;16:67–75.

71. Culbert EL, Ashburn DA, Cullen-Dean G, et al. Quality of life of children after repair of transposition of the great arteries. *Circulation* 2003;108: 857–862.

72. Moons P, Van Deyk K, De Geest S, et al. Is the severity of congenital heart disease associated with the quality of life and perceived health of adult patients? *Heart* 2005;91:1193–1198.

73. Rose M, Kohler K, Kohler F, et al. Determinants of the quality of life of patients with congenital heart disease. *Qual Life Res* 2005;14:35–43.

74. Sairanen HI, Nieminen HP, Jokinen EV. Late results and quality of life after pediatric cardiac surgery in Finland: A population-based study of 6,461 patients with follow-up extending up to 45 years. *Semin Thorac Cardiovasc Surg Pediatr Card Surg Annu* 2005:168–172.

75. Spijkerboer AW, Utens EM, De Koning WB, et al. Health-related quality of life in children and adolescents after invasive treatment for congenital heart disease. *Qual Life Res* 2006;15:663–673.

76. Lane DA, Lip GY, Millane TA. Quality of life in adults with congenital heart disease. *Heart* 2002;88:71–75.

77. Green A. Outcomes of congenital heart disease: A review. *Pediatr Nurs* 2004;30:280–284.

78. Moons P, De Bleser L, Budts W, et al. Health status, functional abilities, and quality of life after the Mustard or Senning operation. *Ann Thorac Surg* 2004;77:1359–1365; discussion 1365.

79. Rietveld S, Mulder BJ, van Beest I, et al. Negative thoughts in adults with congenital heart disease. *Int J Cardiol* 2002;86:19–26.

80. Lip GY, Lane DA, Millane TA, et al. Psychological interventions for depression in adolescent and adult congenital heart disease. *Cochrane Database Syst Rev* 2003;(3):CD004394.

81. Claessens P, Moons P, de Casterle BD, et al. What does it mean to live with a congenital heart disease? A qualitative study on the lived experiences of adult patients. *Eur J Cardiovasc Nurs* 2005;4:3–10.

82. Jefferies JL, Noonan JA, Keller BB, et al. Quality of life and social outcomes in adults with congenital heart disease living in rural areas of Kentucky. *Am J Cardiol* 2004;94:263–266.

83. Crossland DS, Jackson SP, Lyall R, et al. Life insurance and mortgage application in adults with congenital heart disease. *Eur J Cardiothorac Surg* 2004;25:931–934.

84. Johnson K, Posner SF, Biermann J, et al. Recommendations to Improve Preconception Health and Health Care—United States. *MMWR Recomm Rep* 2006:1–23.

85. Benavidez OJ, Gauvreau K, Jenkins KJ. Racial and ethnic disparities in mortality following congenital heart surgery. *Pediatr Cardiol* 2006;27:321–328.

86. Centers for Disease Control and Prevention, Waitzman NJ, Romano PS, et al. Economic costs of birth defects and cerebral palsy—United States, 1992. *MMWR Morb Mortal Wkly Rep* 1995;44:694–699.

87. Waitzman NJ, Romano PS, Scheffler RM. *The Cost of Birth Defects.* Lanham, MD: University Press of America, 1996.

88. Bosi G, Garani G, Scorrano M, et al. Temporal variability in birth prevalence of congenital heart defects as recorded by a general birth defects registry. *J Pediatr* 2003;142:690–698.

89. Eskedal L, Hagemo P, Eskild A, et al. A population-based study of extracardiac anomalies in children with congenital cardiac malformations. *Cardiol Young* 2004;14:600–607.

90. Greenwood RD, Rosenthal A, Parisi L, et al. Extracardiac abnormalities in infants with congenital heart disease. *Pediatrics* 1975;55:485–492.

91. Hanna EJ, Nevin NC, Nelson J. Genetic study of congenital heart defects in Northern Ireland (1974–1978). *J Med Genet* 1994;31(11):858–863.

92. Kramer HH, Majewski F, Trampisch HJ, et al. Malformation patterns in children with congenital heart disease. *Am J Dis Child (1960)* 1987;141: 789–795.

93. Nora JJ. Causes of congenital heart diseases: Old and new modes, mechanisms, and models. *Am Heart J* 1993;125:1409–1419.

94. Wallgren EI, Landtman B, Rapola J. Extracardiac malformations associated with congenital heart disease. *Eur J Cardiol* 1978;7:15–24.

95. Pradat P. A case-control study of major congenital heart defects in Sweden—1981–1986. *Eur J Epidemiol* 1992;8:789–796.

96. Botto LD, Feldkamp M, Carey JC. Actual causes of congenital heart defects: A population based study, Utah 1999–2003. Paper presented at the American Society of Human Genetics, Salt Lake City, UT, 2005.

97. Pierpont ME, Basson CT, Benson WD, et al. The genetic basis for congenital heart defects: Current knowledge. *Circulation.* In press.

98. Garg V. Insights into the genetic basis of congenital heart disease. *Cell Mol Life Sci* 2006;63:1141–1148.

99. Gruber PJ. Cardiac development: New concepts. *Clin Perinatol* 2005;32:845–855, vii.

100. Tikkanen J, Heinonen OP. Risk factors for cardiovascular malformations in Finland. *Eur J Epidemiol* 1990;6:348–356.

101. Tikkanen J, Heinonen OP. Maternal hyperthermia during pregnancy and cardiovascular malformations in the offspring. *Eur J Epidemiol* 1991;7: 628–635.

102. Tikkanen J, Heinonen OP. Risk factors for ventricular septal defect in Finland. *Public Health* 1991;105:99–112.
103. Tikkanen J, Heinonen OP. Risk factors for conal malformations of the heart. *Eur J Epidemiol* 1992;8:48–57.
104. Tikkanen J, Heinonen OP. Risk factors for atrial septal defect. *Eur J Epidemiol* 1992;8:509–515.
105. Tikkanen J, Heinonen OP. Risk factors for coarctation of the aorta. *Teratology* 1993;47:565–572.
106. Tikkanen J, Heinonen OP. Risk factors for hypoplastic left heart syndrome. *Teratology* 1994;50:112–117.
107. Erickson JD. Risk factors for birth defects: Data from the Atlanta Birth Defects Case-Control Study. *Teratology* 1991;43:41–51.
108. Adams MM, Mulinare J, Dooley K. Risk factors for conotruncal cardiac defects in Atlanta. *J Am Coll Cardiol* 1989;14:432–442.
109. Becerra JE, Khoury MJ, Cordero JF, et al. Diabetes mellitus during pregnancy and the risks for specific birth defects: A population-based case-control study. *Pediatrics* 1990;85:1–9.
110. Botto LD, Erickson JD, Mulinare J, et al. Maternal fever, multivitamin use, and selected birth defects: Evidence of interaction? *Epidemiology* 2002;13:485–488.
111. Botto LD, Mulinare J, Erickson JD. Do multivitamin or folic acid supplements reduce the risk for congenital heart defects? Evidence and gaps. *Am J Med Genet A* 2003;121:95–101.
112. Correa A, Botto L, Liu Y, et al. Do multivitamin supplements attenuate the risk for diabetes-associated birth defects? *Pediatrics* 2003;111:1146–1151.
113. Watkins ML, Botto LD. Maternal prepregnancy weight and congenital heart defects in offspring. *Epidemiology* 2001;12:439–446.
114. Carmichael SL, Shaw GM, Yang W, et al. Maternal periconceptional alcohol consumption and risk for conotrunal heart defects. *Birth Defects Res A Clin Mol Teratol* 2003;67:875–878.
115. Shaw GM, Nelson V, Carmichael SL, et al. Maternal periconceptional vitamins: Interactions with selected factors and congenital anomalies? *Epidemiology* 2002;13:625–630.
116. Shaw GM, Nelson V, Iovannisci DM, et al. Maternal occupational chemical exposures and biotransformation genotypes as risk factors for selected congenital anomalies. *Am J Epidemiol* 2003;157:475–484.
117. Shaw GM, O'Malley CD, Wasserman CR, et al. Maternal periconceptional use of multivitamins and reduced risk for conotruncal heart defects and limb deficiencies among offspring. *Am J Med Genet* 1995;59:536–545.
118. Jenkins KJ, Correa A, Feinstein JA, et al. Non-inherited risk factors and congenital cardiovascular defects: Current knowledge. *Circulation* 2006.
119. TERIS - Teratogen information service and online version of *Shepard's Catalog of Teratogenic Agents*, University of Washington, 2006.
120. REPROTOX - information system on environmental hazards to human reproduction and development. Available at www.reprotox.org. Accessed February 6, 2007.
121. Organization of Teratology Information Specialists. Available at www.otispregnancy.org. Accessed February 6, 2007.
122. European Network Teratology Information Services. Available at www.entis-org.com. Accessed February 6, 2007.
123. Rothman KJ. *What Is Causation? Epidemiology: An Introduction*. New York: Oxford University Press, 2002.
124. Loffredo CA. Epidemiology of cardiovascular malformations: Prevalence and risk factors. *Am J Med Genet* 2000;97:319–325.
125. Moore LL, Singer MR, Bradlee ML, et al. A prospective study of the risk of congenital defects associated with maternal obesity and diabetes mellitus. *Epidemiology* 2000;11:689–694.
126. Ray JG, O'Brien TE, Chan WS. Preconception care and the risk of congenital anomalies in the offspring of women with diabetes mellitus: A meta-analysis. *QJM* 2001;94:435–444.
127. Wren C, Birrell G, Hawthorne G. Cardiovascular malformations in infants of diabetic mothers. *Heart* 2003;89:1217–1220.
128. Kousseff BG. Diabetic embryopathy. *Curr Opin Pediatr* 1999;11:348–352.
129. Rowland TW, Hubbell JP Jr, Nadas AS. Congenital heart disease in infants of diabetic mothers. *J Pediatr* 1973;83:815–820.
130. Aberg A, Westbom L, Kallen B. Congenital malformations among infants whose mothers had gestational diabetes or preexisting diabetes. *Early Hum Dev* 2001;61:85–95.
131. Martinez-Frias ML, Bermejo E, Rodriguez-Pinilla E, et al. Epidemiological analysis of outcomes of pregnancy in gestational diabetic mothers. *Am J Med Genet* 1998;78:140–145.
132. Sheffield JS, Butler-Koster EL, Casey BM, et al. Maternal diabetes mellitus and infant malformations. *Obstet Gynecol* 2002;100:925–930.
133. Cousins L. Etiology and prevention of congenital anomalies among infants of overt diabetic women. *Clin Obstet Gynecol* 1991;34:481–493.
134. Holing EV, Beyer CS, Brown ZA, et al. Why don't women with diabetes plan their pregnancies? *Diabetes Care* 1998;21:889–895.
135. Harris MI, Flegal KM, Cowie CC, et al. Prevalence of diabetes, impaired fasting glucose, and impaired glucose tolerance in U.S. adults. The Third National Health and Nutrition Examination Survey, 1988–1994. *Diabetes Care* 1998;21:518–524.
136. Mokdad AH, Ford ES, Bowman BA, et al. Prevalence of obesity, diabetes, and obesity-related health risk factors, 2001. *JAMA* 2003;289:76–79.
137. Mikhail LN, Walker CK, Mittendorf R. Association between maternal obesity and fetal cardiac malformations in African Americans. *JAMA* 2002;94:695–700.
138. Shaw GM, Todoroff K, Schaffer DM, et al. Maternal height and prepregnancy body mass index as risk factors for selected congenital anomalies. *Paediatr Perinat Epidemiol* 2000;14:234–239.
139. Waller DK, Mills JL, Simpson JL, et al. Are obese women at higher risk for producing malformed offspring? *Am J Obstet Gynecol* 1994;170:541–548.
140. Forrest JM, Turnbull FM, Sholler GF, et al. Gregg's congenital rubella patients 60 years later. *Med J Aust* 2002;177:664–667.
141. Reef SE, Plotkin S, Cordero JF, et al. Preparing for elimination of congenital rubella syndrome (CRS): Summary of a workshop on CRS elimination in the United States. *Clin Infect Dis* 2000;31:85–95.
142. Reef SE, Redd SB, Abernathy E, et al. The epidemiological profile of rubella and congenital rubella syndrome in the United States, 1998–2004: The evidence for absence of endemic transmission. *Clin Infect Dis* 2006; 43(suppl 3):S126–132.
143. Robertson SE, Featherstone DA, Gacic-Dobo M, et al. Rubella and congenital rubella syndrome: Global update. *Rev Panam Salud Publica* 2003; 14:306–315.
144. Edwards MJ, Shiota K, Smith MS, et al. Hyperthermia and birth defects. *Reprod Toxicol* 1995;9:411–425.
145. Graham JM, Jr., Edwards MJ. Teratogen update: Gestational effects of maternal hyperthermia due to febrile illnesses and resultant patterns of defects in humans. *Teratology* 1998;58:209–221.
146. Roulston A, Marcellus RC, Branton PE. Viruses and apoptosis. *Annu Rev Microbiol* 1999;53:577–628.
147. Zhang J, Cai WW. Association of the common cold in the first trimester of pregnancy with birth defects. *Pediatrics* 1993;92:559–563.
148. Levy HL, Guldberg P, Guttler F, et al. Congenital heart disease in maternal phenylketonuria: Report from the Maternal PKU Collaborative Study. *Pediatr Res* 2001;49:636–642.
149. Matalon KM, Acosta PB, Azen C. Role of nutrition in pregnancy with phenylketonuria and birth defects. *Pediatrics* 2003;112:1534–1536.
150. Rouse B, Azen C. Effect of high maternal blood phenylalanine on offspring congenital anomalies and developmental outcome at ages 4 and 6 years: The importance of strict dietary control preconception and throughout pregnancy. *J Pediatr* 2004;144:235–239.
151. Holmes LB, Harvey EA, Coull BA, et al. The teratogenicity of anticonvulsant drugs. *N Engl J Med* 2001;344:1132–1138.
152. Barrett C, Richens A. Epilepsy and pregnancy: Report of an Epilepsy Research Foundation Workshop. *Epilepsy Res* 2003;52:147–187.
153. Samren EB, van Duijn CM, Christiaens GC, et al. Antiepileptic drug regimens and major congenital abnormalities in the offspring. *Ann Neurol* 1999;46:739–746.
154. Samren EB, van Duijn CM, Koch S, et al. Maternal use of antiepileptic drugs and the risk of major congenital malformations: A joint European prospective study of human teratogenesis associated with maternal epilepsy. *Epilepsia* 1997;38:981–990.
155. American College of Obstetricians and Gynecologists. Seizure disorders in pregnancy. Number 231, December 1996. Committee on Educational Bulletins of the American College of Obstetricians and Gynecologists. *Int J Gynaecol Obstet* 1997;56:279–286.
156. Crawford P. Best practice guidelines for the management of women with epilepsy. *Epilepsia* 2005;46(suppl 9):117–124.
157. Pschirrer ER. Seizure disorders in pregnancy. *Obstet Gynecol Clin North Am* 2004;31:373–384, vii.
158. Smithells RW, Newman CG. Recognition of thalidomide defects. *J Med Genet* 1992;29:716–723.
159. Coberly S, Lammer E, Alashari M. Retinoic acid embryopathy: Case report and review of literature. *Pediatr Pathol Lab Med* 1996;16:823–836.
160. Lammer EJ, Chen DT, Hoar RM, et al. Retinoic acid embryopathy. *N Engl J Med* 1985;313:837–841.
161. Honein MA, Paulozzi LJ, Erickson JD. Continued occurrence of Accutane-exposed pregnancies. *Teratology* 2001;64:142–147.
162. Perlman SE, Rudy SJ, Pinto C, et al. Caring for women with childbearing potential taking teratogenic dermatologic drugs. Guidelines for practice. *J Reprod Med* 2001;46:153–161.
163. Rothman KJ, Moore LL, Singer MR, et al. Teratogenicity of high vitamin A intake. *N Engl J Med* 1995;333:1369–1373.
164. Werler MM, Lammer EJ, Rosenberg L, et al. Maternal vitamin A supplementation in relation to selected birth defects. *Teratology* 1990;42:497–503.
165. Khoury MJ, Moore CA, Mulinare J. Vitamin A and birth defects. *Lancet* 1996;347:322.
166. Mastroiacovo P, Mazzone T, Addis A, et al. High vitamin A intake in early pregnancy and major malformations: A multicenter prospective controlled study. *Teratology* 1999;59:7–11.
167. Mills JL, Simpson JL, Cunningham GC, et al. Vitamin A and birth defects. *Am J Obstet Gynecol* 1997;177:31–36.

168. Shaw GM, Wasserman CR, Block G, et al. High maternal vitamin A intake and risk of anomalies of structures with a cranial neural crest cell contribution. *Lancet* 1996;347:899–900.

169. Czeizel AE, Rockenbauer M, Sorensen HT, et al. The teratogenic risk of trimethoprim-sulfonamides: A population based case-control study. *Reprod Toxicol* 2001;15:637–646.

170. Hernandez-Diaz S, Werler MM, Walker AM, et al. Folic acid antagonists during pregnancy and the risk of birth defects. *N Engl J Med* 2000;343: 1608–1614.

171. Cohen LS, Friedman JM, Jefferson JW, et al. A reevaluation of risk of in utero exposure to lithium. *JAMA* 1994;271:146–150.

172. Jacobson SJ, Jones K, Johnson K, et al. Prospective multicentre study of pregnancy outcome after lithium exposure during first trimester. *Lancet* 1992;339:530–533.

173. Warner JP. Evidence-based psychopharmacology 3. Assessing evidence of harm: What are the teratogenic effects of lithium carbonate? *J Psychopharmacol* 2000;14:77–80.

174. Kallen B, Tandberg A. Lithium and pregnancy. A cohort study on manic-depressive women. *Acta Psychiatr Scand* 1983;68:134–139.

175. Linn S, Schoenbaum SC, Monson RR, et al. No association between coffee consumption and adverse outcomes of pregnancy. *N Engl J Med* 1982;306:141–145.

176. Olsen J, Overvad K, Frische G. Coffee consumption, birthweight, and reproductive failures. *Epidemiology* 1991;2:370–374.

177. Rosenberg L, Mitchell AA, Shapiro S, et al. Selected birth defects in relation to caffeine-containing beverages. *JAMA* 1982;247:1429–1432.

178. Hoyme HE, May PA, Kalberg WO, et al. A practical clinical approach to diagnosis of fetal alcohol spectrum disorders: Clarification of the 1996 institute of medicine criteria. *Pediatrics* 2005;115:39–47.

179. Jones KL. *Smith's Recognizable Patterns of Human Malformation.* Philadelphia: WB Saunders, 2005.

180. Institute of Medicine Ed. Committee to Study Fetal Alcohol Syndrome, *Fetal Alcohol Syndrome—Diagnosis, Epidemiology, Prevention and Treatment.* Washington, DC: National Academy Press, 1996.

181. Kallen K. Maternal smoking and congenital heart defects. *Eur J Epidemiol* 1999;15:731–737.

182. Woods SE, Raju U. Maternal smoking and the risk of congenital birth defects: A cohort study. *J Am Board Fam Pract* 2001;14:330–334.

183. Amos A, Haglund M. From social taboo to "torch of freedom": The marketing of cigarettes to women. *Tob Control* 2000;9:3–8.

184. Bailey LB, Berry RJ. Folic acid supplementation and the occurrence of congenital heart defects, orofacial clefts, multiple births, and miscarriage. *Am J Clin Nutr* 2005;81:1213S–1217S.

185. Daly S, Cotter A, Molloy AE, et al. Homocysteine and folic acid: Implications for pregnancy. *Semin Vasc Med* 2005;5:190–200.

186. Huhta JC, Hernandez-Robles JA. Homocysteine, folate, and congenital heart defects. *Fetal Pediatr Pathol* 2005;24:71–79.

187. Botto LD, Olney RS, Erickson JD. Vitamin supplements and the risk for congenital anomalies other than neural tube defects. *Am J Med Genet C Semin Med Genet* 2004;125:12–21.

188. Czeizel AE. Periconceptional folic acid containing multivitamin supplementation. *Eur J Obstet Gynecol Reprod Biol* 1998;78:151–161.

189. Czeizel AE, Dudas I. Prevention of the first occurrence of neural-tube defects by periconceptional vitamin supplementation *N Engl J Med* 1992; 327:1832–1835.

190. Werler MM, Hayes C, Louik C, et al. Multivitamin supplementation and risk of birth defects. *Am J Epidemiol* 1999;150:675–682.

191. Scanlon KS, Ferencz C, Loffredo CA, et al. Preconceptional folate intake and malformations of the cardiac outflow tract. Baltimore-Washington Infant Study Group. *Epidemiology* 1998;9:95–98.

192. Shaw GM, Iovannisci DM, Yang W, et al. Risks of human conotruncal heart defects associated with 32 single nucleotide polymorphisms of selected cardiovascular disease-related genes. *Am J Med Genet A* 2005; 138:21–26.

193. Hobbs CA, James SJ, Jernigan S, et al. Congenital heart defects, maternal homocysteine, smoking, and the 677 C>T polymorphism in the methylenetetrahydrofolate reductase gene: Evaluating gene-environment interactions. *Am J Obstet Gynecol* 2006;194:218–224.

194. Pereira AC, Xavier-Neto J, Mesquita SM, et al. Lack of evidence of association between MTHFR C677T polymorphism and congenital heart disease in a TDT study design. *Int J Cardiol* 2005;105:15–18.

195. van Beynum IM, Kapusta L, den Heijer M, et al. Maternal MTHFR 677C>T is a risk factor for congenital heart defects: Effect modification by periconceptional folate supplementation. *Eur Heart J* 2006;27:981–987.

196. Junker R, Kotthoff S, Vielhaber H, et al. Infant methylenetetrahydrofolate reductase 677TT genotype is a risk factor for congenital heart disease. *Cardiovasc Res* 2001;51:251–254.

197. Wenstrom KD, Johanning GL, Johnston KE, et al. Association of the C677T methylenetetrahydrofolate reductase mutation and elevated homocysteine levels with congenital cardiac malformations. *Am J Obstet Gynecol* 2001;184:806–812; discussion 812–807.

198. Pei L, Zhu H, Zhu J, et al. Genetic variation of infant reduced folate carrier (A80G) and risk of orofacial defects and congenital heart defects in China. *Ann Epidemiol* 2006;16:352–356.

199. Li D, Pickell L, Liu Y, et al. Maternal methylenetetrahydrofolate reductase deficiency and low dietary folate lead to adverse reproductive outcomes and congenital heart defects in mice. *Am J Clin Nutr* 2005;82:188–195.

200. Li D, Rozen R. Maternal folate deficiency affects proliferation, but not apoptosis, in embryonic mouse heart. *J Nutr* 2006;136:1774–1778.

201. Tang LS, Wlodarczyk BJ, Santillano DR, et al. Developmental consequences of abnormal folate transport during murine heart morphogenesis. *Birth Defects Res A Clin Mol Teratol* 2004;70:449–458.

202. Rasmussen SA, Olney RS, Holmes LB, et al. Guidelines for case classification for the National Birth Defects Prevention Study. *Birth Defects Res A Clin Mol Teratol* 2003;67:193–201.

203. Yoon PW, Rasmussen SA, Lynberg MC, et al. The National Birth Defects Prevention Study. *Public Health Rep* 2001;116(suppl 1):32–40.

204. Branum AM, Collman GW, Correa A, et al. The National Children's Study of environmental effects on child health and development. *Environ Health Perspect* 2003;111:642–646.

CHAPTER 26 ■ GENETICS OF CONGENITAL HEART DEFECTS

ELIZABETH GOLDMUNTZ, MD, AND ANGELA E. LIN, MD

Enormous progress has been made in the medical and surgical management of children born with congenital heart defects (CHDs). Patients with significant heart disease now routinely survive well into adulthood. With these advances come new questions about variability in clinical outcome, long-term survival, fetal intervention, and recurrence risk. Although differences in clinical management affect clinical outcome and survival, evidence suggests that the etiologic basis of these malformations contributes to outcome as well (1–4). These observations highlight the importance of understanding the causes of CHDs.

Both environmental and genetic factors contribute to the cause of CHDs (Table 26.1). The environmental impact is discussed in Chapter 25. Evidence for a genetic contribution

TABLE 26.1

CAUSES OF CONGENITAL HEART DEFECTS

Etiology	Example: Patient with Tetralogy of Fallot (TOF)
Chromosomal change	
Change in chromosome number	Trisomy 18 or 21
Translocation between chromosomes	Translocation 1p36 and other autosome
Deletion of chromosome segment	Deletion 5p or 22q11
Duplication of chromosome segment	Partial trisomy 8q
Single gene or gene pair abnormality	
Isolated congenital heart defect	Newborn with TOF, whose mother also had TOF repaired in childhood, sister has malalignment-type VSD (probable autosomal dominant inheritance)
Associated with syndrome	*JAG1* mutation in Alagille syndrome
Mitochondrial defect	None known
Environmental exposure	Fetus found to have TOF, mother known to have maternal phenylketonuria
Multifactorial causation (gene/environmental interaction)	TOF in a child with ectopia cordis
Stochastic events	Isolated TOF

VSD, ventricular septal defect.

comes from several observations. First, specific types of CHDs are commonly seen in conjunction with specific chromosomal abnormalities. For example, atrioventricular septal defects are most commonly diagnosed in patients with trisomy 21, and patients with trisomy 21 are commonly diagnosed with atrioventricular septal defects. Second, CHDs can occur in multiple members of a family, suggesting a genetic basis. Recent studies have demonstrated particularly high heritability in certain subsets of CHDs such as left-sided lesions (5–7). Third, epidemiologic studies demonstrate an increased precurrence and recurrence risk for CHDs in families with one affected member (8–11).

These observations also suggest that many CHDs result from complex genetic and environmental interactions rather than simple mendelian inheritance. For example, although the vast majority of patients with Down syndrome have a complete third copy of chromosome 21, only 40% to 50% of patients have CHD. This observation is consistent with incomplete penetrance (as opposed to full penetrance of mental retardation) and suggests that other genetic and/or environmental factors contribute to the risk of CHDs even in the presence of a major chromosomal alteration. Similarly, the likelihood that parents with one affected child will have a second affected child is increased as compared with the initial risk in the general population, but the recurrence risk is significantly lower than simple mendelian inheritance would predict.

The heterogeneous etiologic factors of CHDs also make it more complicated to understand the basis of these disorders. For example, several different genetic alterations are now known to be associated with tetralogy of Fallot including trisomy 21, the 22q11 deletion, and *JAG1* mutations (Table 26.1 and see below: Genetics of Specific CHDs). Tetralogy of Fallot is also found in many other genetic syndromes and can be associated with maternal exposure to retinoic acid and maternal phenylketonuria. Therefore, defining the genetic

alterations that contribute to the cause of specific CHDs and identifying those that affect clinical outcome is challenging.

Nonetheless, notable advances have begun to unravel the genetic basis of these disorders. The first edition of this text published in 1968 cited 15 genetic syndromes and conditions, including storage diseases (personal correspondence from Dr. George Emmanouilides, Harbor-UCLA Medical Center). In contrast, this chapter lists nearly 50 malformation syndromes characterized in part by CHDs, and many more are known. Specific genetic causes for some of these syndromes are now defined. This change represents a threefold increase in the number of recognized syndromes in almost 40 years and a marked increase in the number of specific genetic causes known for CHDs. As discoveries are made, the number of children with defined genetic causes of their CHD will increase. The information should help the physician counsel families more accurately about recurrence risks and clinical outcome and, it is hoped, lead to novel medical therapeutics to improve clinical outcomes. Since rapid progress is likely to continue, the medical caregiver will need a firm understanding of this area to anticipate its impact on clinical medicine.

This chapter reviews the genetic basis of CHDs. The term CHDs refers to developmental changes of the intracardiac structures and major vessels and is interchangeable with the terms cardiovascular malformation or congenital heart disease. The genetic basis of cardiomyopathies and arrhythmias, both of which may be associated with a CHD, are discussed in other chapters. Instead of listing all possible genetic syndromes associated with each CHD (which can be found in multiple on-line and textbook resources listed below), this chapter will present an alternative approach for considering the genetic causes of CHD: the chapter is ordered by genetic mechanism to help the reader understand and anticipate future developments in this field. In addition, Tables 26.2 through 26.4 summarize the growing number of syndromes that are either common conditions

TABLE 26.2

CHROMOSOME ABNORMALITY SYNDROMES ASSOCIATED WITH CONGENITAL HEART DEFECTS

Syndrome	Reference	Gene(s)[b]	OMIM no.	Frequency of CHD[a] All (%)	Frequency of CHD[a] Distinctive or common	Distinctive features[c]
Changes in chromosome number						
Trisomy 13	(A,B)			50–80	Conotruncal CHDs: DORV, TOF VSD, ASD, PDA AVC Polyvalvar dysplasia	Polydactyly Cleft lip and palate CNS anomalies (holoprosencephaly) Renal, GU anomalies Scalp cutis aplasia Microphthalmia
Trisomy 18	(C)			95	Polyvalvar dysplasia Conoventricular VSD TOF, DORV AVC	Overlapping fingers CNS anomalies (posterior fossas) Small facial features Rocker bottom feet Renal, GU anomalies
Down syndrome (trisomy 21 most common)	(D–F)		190685	40	AVC defects: Complete AVSD Primum ASD VSD, all types Secundum ASD PDA TOF	GI anomalies Endocrine anomalies Fifth finger clinodactyly Leukemoid reaction Microbrachycephaly
Turner syndrome (45,X most common)	(G–L)			25	LVOTO CHDs: BAV +/− AS(V) Coarctation MV anomalies, MVP PAPVC, LSVC Aortic dilation, dissection Hypertension	Horseshoe kidney Short fourth metacarpal Neck webbing Lymphedema Infertility Short stature Nevi, keloids
Chromosome deletion or duplication						
Deletion 1p36	(M,N)		607872	35	Assorted CHD TOF/PA PDA Ebstein DCM	Obesity Cleft lip/palate Epilepsy Hearing loss Brachydactyly
Deletion 3p25	(O, P)			25	Primum ASD Assorted CHDs	Ptosis Abnormal ears Postaxial polydactyly
Duplication 3q	(Q)			75	Assorted CHDs	Craniosynostosis Short neck GU anomalies Cleft palate Fifth finger clinodactyly
Deletion 4p16	(R)	WHSC1 WHSC2	194190	30–50	Secundum ASD PS(V) VSD	Abnormal ears Cleft lip/palate GU anomalies

(*continued*)

TABLE 26.2

CHROMOSOME ABNORMALITY SYNDROMES ASSOCIATED WITH CONGENITAL HEART DEFECTS (CONTINUED)

Syndrome	Reference	Gene(s)[b]	OMIM no.	Frequency of CHD[a]		Distinctive features[c]
				All (%)	Distinctive or common	
Deletion 4qter	(S)			40	RVOTO PS	Abnormal pinnae Cleft palate Pierre-Robin sequence Fifth fingernail tapered, pointed/duplicated
Deletion 5p15	(T)		123450	20	Assorted CHDs VSD PDA TOF	Catlike cry Cleft lip/palate Abnormal ears Preauricular tags
Williams syndrome Deletion 7p13	(U)	ELN1	194050	75[d]	SVAS +/− AS(V) PS PPS Coarctation Coronary artery stenosis	Abnormal calcium levels Hypodontia Characteristic behavior and personality
Deletion 8p23	(V–Y)			65–80	PS Secundum ASD AVSD VSD	GU anomalies Abnormal ears Minor hand anomalies
Duplication 8q (recombinant 8)	(Z)		179613	45	Conotruncal CHDs: TOF, DORV, truncus	Short fifth finger
Deletion 9p	(AA)		158170	35	Assorted CHDs	Trigonocephaly Extra flexion creases
Deleteion 10p	(BB)		601362	50	VSD +/− ASD PDA	Minor hand/foot anomalies Renal anomalies DiGeorge phenotype
Deletion 11q23 Jacobsen Syndrome	(CC)		147791	55	VSD LVOTO: HLHS	Thrombocytopenia or abnormal platelets Undescended testes Renal anomalies
Deletion 17p11.2 Smith–Magenis syndrome	(DD,EE)	RAI1	182290	10	Assorted CHDs	Brachycephaly Aggressive, self-injurious behavior Sleep disturbances Eye, ear anomalies
Deletion 18q	(FF,GG)		601808	15–30	PS ASD VSD	Wide-spaced nipples Cleft palate GU anomalies
Tetrasomy 22p Cat-eye syndrome	(HH)		115470	50	TAVPC PAPVC Assorted CHDs	Rectoanal anomalies Coloboma Preauricular tag/pit GU anomalies
Derivative 11;22	(II,JJ)		609029	60	ASD, VSD, PDA LSVC	Preauricular tag/pit Cleft palate Genital anomalies

(continued)

TABLE 26.2

CHROMOSOME ABNORMALITY SYNDROMES ASSOCIATED WITH CONGENITAL HEART DEFECTS (CONTINUED)

Syndrome	Reference	Gene(s)[b]	OMIM no.	Frequency of CHD[a]		Distinctive features[c]
				All (%)	Distinctive or common	
Deletion 22q11 DiGeorge sequence Velocardiofacial syndrome Conotruncal anomaly face syndrome	(KK–OO)	*TBX1*	192430 602054	75–85	IAA type B Truncus TOF VSD Aortic arch anomalies	Cleft palate Hypocalcemia T-cell dysfunction Feeding and speech disorders Psychiatric disorders

ASCA, aberrant subclavian artery; ASD, atrial septal defect; AS(V), aortic stenosis (valvar specified); AVC, atrioventricular canal; AVSD, atrioventricular septal defect; BAV, bicuspid aortic valve; CHDs, congenital heart defects; CNS, central nervous system; DCM, dilated cardiomyopathy; DORV, double-outlet right ventricle; FAVS, facioauriculovertebral spectrum; GI, gastrointestinal; GU, genitourinary; HCM, hypertrophic cardiomyopathy; HLHS, hypoplastic left heart syndrome; IAA, A/B, interrupted aortic arch, type A or B; LSVC, left superior vena cava; LVOTO, left ventricular outflow tract obstruction; MS, mitral stenosis; MVP, mitral valve prolapse; OMIM, on line Mendelian inheritance of man; PA, pulmonary atresia; PAPVC, partial anomalous pulmonary venous connection; PDA, patent ductus arteriosus; (P)PS, (peripheral) pulmonic stenosis; PS(V), pulmonary stenosis (valvar specified); RVOTO, right ventricular outflow tract obstruction; TAVPC, total anomalous pulmonary venous connection; TOF, tetralogy of Fallot; VSD, ventricular septal defect.

[a] Frequency figures rounded. When not specified in an article, data were calculated independently. Congenital heart "defects" excluded valve regurgitation, patent foramen ovale, and unspecified murmur, cyanosis, or heart disease. Some syndrome-specific nonstructural anomalies were included.

[b] Genes listed map to the disease locus and are specifically associated with the cardiovascular features of the syndrome, though other genes in the chromosomal region may also be related to the syndrome.

[c] Most syndromes have growth delay, some degree of developmental delay/mental retardation, and dysmorphic facial features, which can be reviewed in general genetics references (20,23).

[d] Frequency reflects cases with molecular confirmation.

References

A. Musewe NN, Alexander DJ, Teshima I, et al. Echocardiographic evaluation of the spectrum of cardiac anomalies associated with trisomy 13 and trisomy 18. *J Am Coll Cardiol* 1990;15(3):673–677.

B. Lehman CD, Nyberg DA, Winter TC 3rd, et al. Trisomy 13 syndrome: Prenatal US findings in a review of 33 cases. *Radiology* 1995;194(1):217–222.

C. Van Praagh S, Truman T, Firpo A, et al. Cardiac malformations in trisomy-18: A study of 41 postmortem cases. *J Am Coll Cardiol* 1989;13(7):1586–1597.

D. Ferencz C, Loffredo CA, Corea-Villasenor A, et al. *Genetic and Environmental Risk Factors of Major Congenital Heart Defects: The Baltimore-Washington Infant Study: 1981–1989.* Armonk, NY: Futura Publishing, 1997.

E. Freeman SB, Taft LF, Dooley KJ, et al. Population-based study of congenital heart defects in Down syndrome. *Am J Med Genet* 1998;80(3):213–217.

F. McElhinney DB, Straka M, Goldmuntz E, et al. Correlation between abnormal cardiac physical examination and echocardiographic findings in neonates with Down syndrome. *Am J Med Genet* 2002, 113(3):238–241.

G. Mazzanti L, Cacciari E. Congenital heart disease in patients with Turner syndrome. Italian Study Group for Turner Syndrome (ISGTS). *J Pediatr* 1998;133(5):688–692.

H. Ho VB, Bakalov VK, Cooley M, et al. Major vascular anomalies in Turner syndrome: Prevalence and magnetic resonance angiographic features. *Circulation* 2004;110(12):1694–1700.

I. Loscalzo ML, Van PL, Ho VB, et al. Association between fetal lymphedema and congenital cardiovascular defects in Turner syndrome. *Pediatrics* 2005;115(3):732–735.

J. Gravholt CH, Landin-Wilhelmsen K, Stochholm K, et al. Clinical and epidemiological description of aortic dissection in Turner's syndrome. *Cardiol Young* 2006;16(5):430–436.

K. Bondy CA. The Turner Syndrome Consensus Study Group: Guidelines for the Care of Girls and Women with Turner Syndrome. *J Clin Endocrinol Metab* 2006.

L. Bondy CA, Van PL, Bakalov VK, et al. Growth hormone treatment and aortic dimensions in Turner syndrome. *J Clin Endocrinol Metab* 2006;91(5):1785–1788.

M. Slavotinek A, Shaffer LG, Shapira SK. Monosomy 1p36. *J Med Genet* 1999;36(9):657–663.

N. Heilstedt HA, Ballif BC, Howard LA, et al. Physical map of 1p36, placement of breakpoints in monosomy 1p36, and clinical characterization of the syndrome. *Am J Hum Genet* 2003;72(5):1200–1212.

O. Green EK, Priestley MD, Waters J, et al. Detailed mapping of a congenital heart disease gene in chromosome 3p25. *J Med Genet* 2000;37(8):581–587.

P. Robinson SW, Morris CD, Goldmuntz E, et al. Missense mutations in CRELD1 are associated with cardiac atrioventricular septal defects. *Am J Hum Genet* 2003;72(4):1047–1052.

Q. Faas BH, De Vries BB, Van Es-Van Gaal J, et al. A new case of dup(3q) syndrome due to a pure duplication of 3qter. *Clin Genet* 2002;62(4):315–320.

R. Battaglia A, Carey JC, Wright TJ. Wolf-Hirschhorn (4p-) syndrome. *Adv Pediatr* 2001;48:75–113.

S. Huang T, Lin AE, Cox GF, et al. Cardiac phenotypes in chromosome 4q- syndrome with and without a deletion of the dHAND gene. *Genet Med* 2002;4(6):464–467.

T. Hills C, Moller JH, Finkelstein M, et al. Cri du chat syndrome and congenital heart disease: A review of previously reported cases and presentation of an additional 21 cases from the Pediatric Cardiac Care Consortium. *Pediatrics* 2006;117(5):e924–927.

U. Smoot L, Zhang H, Klaiman C, et al. Medical Overview and genetics of Williams-Beuren syndrome. *Progr Pediatr Cardiol* 2005;20:195–205.

(continued)

TABLE 26.2

CHROMOSOME ABNORMALITY SYNDROMES ASSOCIATED WITH CONGENITAL HEART DEFECTS (CONTINUED)

V. Digilio MC, Marino B, Guccione P, et al. Deletion 8p syndrome. *Am J Med Genet* 1998;75(5):534–536.
X. Pehlivan T, Pober BR, Brueckner M, et al. GATA4 haploinsufficiency in patients with interstitial deletion of chromosome region 8p23.1 and congenital heart disease. *Am J Med Genet* 1999;83(3):201–206.
Y. Devriendt K, Matthijs G, Van Dael R, et al. Delineation of the critical deletion region for congenital heart defects, on chromosome 8p23.1. *Am J Hum Genet* 1999;64(4):1119–1126.
Z. Digilio MC, Angioni A, Giannotti A, et al. Truncus arteriosus and duplication 8q. *Am J Med Genet A* 2003;121(1):79–81.
AA. Huret JL, Leonard C, Forestier B, et al. Eleven new cases of del(9p) and features from 80 cases. *J Med Genet* 1988;25(11):741–749.
BB. Van Esch H, Groenen P, Fryns JP, et al. The phenotypic spectrum of the 10p deletion syndrome versus the classical DiGeorge syndrome. *Genet Couns* 1999;10(1):59–65.
CC. Grossfeld PD, Mattina T, Lai Z, et al. The 11q terminal deletion disorder: a prospective study of 110 cases. *Am J Med Genet A* 2004;129(1):51–61.
DD. Potocki L, Shaw CJ, Stankiewicz P, et al. Variability in clinical phenotype despite common chromosomal deletion in Smith-Magenis syndrome [del(17)(p11.2p11.2)]. *Genet Med* 2003;5(6):430–434.
EE. Girirajan S, Vlangos CN, Szomju BB, et al. Genotype-phenotype correlation in Smith-Magenis syndrome: Evidence that multiple genes in 17p11.2 contribute to the clinical spectrum. *Genet Med* 2006;8(7):417–427.
FF. Cody JD, Ghidoni PD, DuPont BR, et al. Congenital anomalies and anthropometry of 42 individuals with deletions of chromosome 18q. *Am J Med Genet* 1999;85(5):455–462.
GG. Linnankivi T, Tienari P, Somer M, et al. 18q deletions: Clinical, molecular, and brain MRI findings of 14 individuals. *Am J Med Genet A* 2006;140(4):331–339.
HH. Berends MJ, Tan-Sindhunata G, Leegte B, et al. Phenotypic variability of cat-eye syndrome. *Genet Couns* 2001;12(1):23–34.
II. Lin AE, Bernar J, Chin AJ, et al. Congenital heart disease in supernumerary der(22),t(11;22) syndrome. *Clin Genet* 1986;29(4):269–275.
JJ. McDermid HE, Morrow BE. Genomic disorders on 22q11. *Am J Hum Genet* 2002;70(5):1077–1088.
KK. McDonald-McGinn DM, LaRossa D, Goldmuntz E, et al. The 22q11.2 deletion: Screening, diagnostic workup, and outcome of results; report on 181 patients. *Genet Test* 1997;1(2):99–108.
LL. Ryan AK, Goodship JA, Wilson DI, et al. Spectrum of clinical features associated with interstitial chromosome 22q11 deletions: A European collaborative study. *J Med Genet* 1997;34(10):798–804.
MM. Baldini A. DiGeorge syndrome: The use of model organisms to dissect complex genetics. *Hum Mol Genet* 2002;11(20):2363–2369.
NN. Goldmuntz E. DiGeorge syndrome: New insights. *Clin Perinatol* 2005;32(4):963–978, ix–x.
OO. Goldmuntz E, Clark BJ, Mitchell LE, et al. Frequency of 22q11 deletions in patients with conotruncal defects. *J Am Coll Cardiol* 1998;32(2):492–498.

Adapted from Lin AE, Ardinger HH. Genetic epidemiology and an overview of the genetics of congenital heart defects. *Progr Pediatr Cardiol.* 2005;20:113–126; and Lin AE, Belmont J, Ghaffar S. The heart. In: Stevenson RE, Hall JG, eds. *Human Malformations and Related Anomalies.* 2nd ed. New York: Oxford University Press, 2006:85–120.

frequently associated with any type of CHD, or uncommon syndromes associated with a distinctive pattern of CHD. The chapter will conclude with suggested guidelines for the genetic evaluation of a child with a CHD.

METHODS AND MECHANISMS

In large part, the identification of novel genetic abnormalities associated with disease has been driven by increasingly sensitive methods to detect genetic alterations. In the first era of chromosome analysis, the *karyotype* displayed the 23 pairs of human chromosomes and detected changes in chromosome number (such as trisomy 21) or large changes in chromosome architecture such as translocations (the exchange of pieces between two chromosomes). Smaller changes such as visible *deletions* or *duplications* of chromosomal segments were subsequently detected by new "banding" methods, such as Giemsa staining, which resulted in characteristic dark and light bands for each chromosome. More recently, *fluorescence in situ hybridization* (FISH) has been used to detect small deletions and duplications of chromosome segments that could not otherwise be seen on a standard or even high-resolution karyotype. Identification of disease-related *mutations* or alterations in the genetic code for a single gene can be detected using various techniques.

Accordingly, changes in chromosome number such as trisomy 21 or Turner syndrome were among the first identified genetic causes of CHDs. Deletion syndromes such as the 22q11 deletion or William syndromes were subsequently recognized with the advent of new banding techniques and then FISH. Increasingly automated mutation detection and gene

sequencing techniques now identify disease-related mutations in single-gene disorders such as Holt–Oram or Alagille syndromes. The growing ability to identify disease-related mutations in gene sequence has allowed additional clinical genetic testing in individual patients or families.

Investigators have used two main approaches to identify the genetic cause of CHDs to date. First, the identification of a consistent chromosomal alteration on a karyotype has pinpointed where investigators might look for the genetic basis of that disease. For example, 5% to 10% of patients with Alagille syndrome were originally noted to have a chromosomal deletion involving the "p" (short) arm of chromosome 20 (see Alagille syndrome). This observation suggested that other patients might have submicroscopic alterations of that region or a mutation in a gene in that region. Further investigations found disease-causing mutations in a gene called *JAG1* that mapped into the region of 20p, thereby establishing *JAG1* as the disease gene for Alagille syndrome.

Alternatively, if a large kindred with multiple affected members is identified, then a parametric linkage analysis can be performed that maps a chromosomal position or locus of the disease gene. Parametric linkage analyses have been very informative and are responsible for identifying the disease gene in Marfan, Holt–Oram and Noonan syndromes as well as familial cases of atrial septal defect with atrioventricular conduction blockade, to name a few (see in Single Gene Disorders). The Human Genome Project has greatly simplified and accelerated the identification of disease genes once a disease locus is defined.

These investigative strategies are limited by the relative rarity of large kindred or consistent chromosomal changes associated

TABLE 26.3

SINGLE-GENE DISORDERS ASSOCIATED WITH CONGENITAL HEART DEFECTS

Syndrome	Reference	Gene(s)	OMIM no.	Frequency of CHD[a]		Distinctive features[b]
				All (%)	Distinctive or most common	
Autosomal dominant						
Alagille syndrome	(A)	*JAG1* *NOTCH2*	118450	90[c]	PPS TOF+/− PA ASD, VSD Coarctation	Bile duct paucity Chronic cholestasis Butterfly vertebrae Posterior embryotoxon
Cardiofaciocutaneous syndrome	(B,C)	*BRAF* *MEK1* *MEK2* *KRAS*	*115150*	75[c]	PS(V) Secundum ASD Other valve dysplasia HCM	Sparse, curly hair Low, rotated ears Hyperkeratosis
Char syndrome	(D,E)	*TFAP2β*	169100	20–70	PDA Muscular VSD	Anomalies of fifth finger Supernumerary nipple
CHARGE syndrome Hall-Hittner syndrome	(F)	*CHD7* *SEMA3E*	214800	90[c]	Conotruncal CHDs: TOF, DORV+/−AVSD Aortic arch anomalies Assorted CHD	Coloboma Choanal atresia Genital anomalies Ear anomalies Facial asymmetry Cleft lip/palate
Cornelia de Lange syndrome	(G)	*NIPBL*	122470	25	VSD, ASD PS	Upper limb deficiency GI anomalies
Costello syndrome	(H–J)	*HRAS*	218040	75[c]	PS(V), other valve dysplasia HCM Atrial tachycardia	Skin/joint laxity Fine/curly hair Ulnar deviation Papillomata
Holt–Oram syndrome	(K,L)	*TBX5*	142900	75[c]	ASD, VSD PAPVR Assorted CHDs Conduction defect	Upper limb anomalies
LEOPARD syndrome	(M–O)	*PTPN11*	163950	70–100	PS(V) HCM Conduction defect	Café au lait macules Lentigines Deafness, ear anomalies
Neurofibromatosis	(P,Q)	*NF1*	162200	2	PS(V) ASV, Coarctation HCM	Café au lait macules Optic glioma Scoliosis Pseudarthrosis Neurofibromas
Noonan syndrome	(M, R–W)	*PTPN11* *KRAS* *SOS1*	163950	85[c]	PS(V) ASD AVSD, partial Coarctation HCM	Short, webbed neck Pectus deformity Cryptorchidism
Rubenstein-Taybi syndrome	(X)	*CREBBP*	180849	30	PDA, ASD, VSD Coarctation, HLHS	Broad thumbs, great toes
Townes-Brocks syndrome	(Y)	*SALL1*	107480	25[c]	Truncus, TOF ASD, VSD	Thumb malformations Ear anomalies Imperforate anus

(continued)

TABLE 26.3

SINGLE-GENE DISORDERS ASSOCIATED WITH CONGENITAL HEART DEFECTS (CONTINUED)

| Syndrome | Reference | Gene(s) | OMIM no. | Frequency of CHD[a] | | Distinctive features[b] |
				All (%)	Distinctive or most common	
Autosomal recessive						
Ellis–van Creveld syndrome	(Z)	EVC	225500	60	AVC defects: Common atrium Primum ASD, Complete AVSD Secundum ASD	Short limbs Polydactyly Hypoplastic nails Dental anomalies
Keutel syndrome	(AA)	MGP	245150	70	PS, peripheral	Short digits Mixed hearing loss Cartilage calcification
McKusick–Kaufman syndrome	(BB,CC)	MKKS	604896	15–50	AVSD defects: Complete AVSD Primum ASD, common atrium	Hydrometrocolpos Postaxial polydactyly
Smith–Lemli–Opitz syndrome	(DD)	DHCR7	270400	45	Secundum ASD, VSD Complete AVSD TAPVR	2–3 toe syndactyly Cleft palate Lung anomalies Genital anomalies
Simpson–Golabi–Behmel syndrome	(EE)	GPC3	312870	25	Secundum ASD, VSD Rare, variable cardiomyopathy	Macrosomia Cleft palate Supernumerary nipples Hypospadias Polysyndactyly

See Table 26.2 for definition of abbreviations. PAPVR, partial anomalous pulmonary venous return; TAPVR, total anomalous pulmonary venous return.
[a] Frequency figures rounded. When not specified in an article, data were calculated independently. Congenital heart "defects" excluded valve regurgitation, patent foramen ovale and unspecified murmur, cyanosis, or heart disease. Some syndrome-specific nonstructural anomalies were included.
[b] Most syndromes have growth delay, some degree of developmental delay or mental retardation, and dysmorphic facial features, which can be reviewed in general genetics references (20,23).
[c] Frequency reflects cases with molecular confirmation.

References

A. Spinner NB, Colliton RP, Crosnier C, et al. Jagged1 mutations in Alagille syndrome. *Hum Mutat* 2001;17(1):18–33.
B. Rodriguez-Viciana P, Tetsu O, Tidyman WE, et al. Germline mutations in genes within the MAPK pathway cause cardio-facio-cutaneous syndrome. *Science* 2006:311:1287–1290.
C. Niihori T, Aoki Y, Narumi Y, et al. Germline KRAS and BRAF mutations in cardio-facio-cutaneous syndrome. *Nat Genet* 2006;38(3):294–296.
D. Sweeney E, Fryer A, Walters M. Char syndrome: A new family and review of the literature emphasising the presence of symphalangism and the variable phenotype. *Clin Dysmorphol* 2000;9(3):177–182.
E. Char syndrome (www.genetests.org) April 12, 2007.
F. Lalani SR, Safiullah AM, Fernbach SD, et al. Spectrum of CHD7 mutations in 110 individuals with CHARGE syndrome and genotype-phenotype correlation. *Am J Hum Genet* 2006;78(2):303–314.
G. Jackson L, Kline AD, Barr MA, et al. de Lange syndrome: A clinical review of 310 individuals. *Am J Med Genet* 1993;47(7):940–946.
H. Lin AE, Grossfeld PD, Hamilton RM, et al. Further delineation of cardiac abnormalities in Costello syndrome. *Am J Med Genet* 2002;111(2):115–129.
I. Gripp KW, Lin AE, Stabley DL, et al. HRAS mutation analysis in Costello syndrome: Genotype and phenotype correlation. *Am J Med Genet A* 2006;140(1):1–7.
J. Gripp KW, Stabley DL, Nicholson L, et al. Somatic mosaicism for an HRAS mutation causes Costello syndrome. *Am J Med Genet A* 2006;140(20):2163–2169.
K. Sletten LJ, Pierpont ME. Variation in severity of cardiac disease in Holt-Oram syndrome. *Am J Med Genet* 1996;65(2):128–132.
L. Holt-Oram syndrome (www.GeneTests.org)
M. Sarkozy A, Conti E, Seripa D, et al. Correlation between PTPN11 gene mutations and congenital heart defects in Noonan and LEOPARD syndromes. *J Med Genet* 2003;40(9):704–708.
N. Keren B, Hadchouel A, Saba S, et al. PTPN11 mutations in patients with LEOPARD syndrome: A French multicentric experience. *J Med Genet* 2004;41(11):e117.
O. Digilio MC, Conti E, Sarkozy A, et al. Grouping of multiple-lentigines/LEOPARD and Noonan syndromes on the PTPN11 gene. *Am J Hum Genet* 2002;71(2):389–394.

(continued)

TABLE 26.3

SINGLE-GENE DISORDERS ASSOCIATED WITH CONGENITAL HEART DEFECTS (CONTINUED)

P. Lin AE, Birch PH, Korf BR, et al. Cardiovascular malformations and other cardiovascular abnormalities in neurofibromatosis 1. *Am J Med Genet* 2000;95(2):108–117.

Q. Friedman JM, Arbiser J, Epstein JA, et al. Cardiovascular disease in neurofibromatosis 1: Report of the NF1 Cardiovascular Task Force. *Genet Med* 2002;4(3):105–111.

R. Noonan JA. Noonan syndrome and related disorders. *Progr Pediatr Cardiol* 2005;20:177–185.

S. Zenker M, Lehmann K, Schulz AL, et al. Expansion of the genotypic and phenotypic spectrum in patients with KRAS germline mutations. *J Med Genet* 2007;44:131–135.

T. Sarkozy A, Obregon MG, Conti E, et al. A novel PTPN11 gene mutation bridges Noonan syndrome, multiple lentigines/LEOPARD syndrome and Noonan-like/multiple giant cell lesion syndrome. *Eur J Hum Genet* 2004;12(12):1069–1072.

U. Roberts AE, Araki T, Swanson KD, et al. Germline gain-of-function mutations in SOS1 cause Noonan syndrome. *Nat Genet* 2007;29:70–74.

V. Tartaglia M, Kalidas K, Shaw A, et al. PTPN11 mutations in Noonan syndrome: Molecular spectrum, genotype-phenotype correlation, and phenotypic heterogeneity. *Am J Hum Genet* 2002;70(6):1555–1563.

W. Tartaglia M, Mehler EL, Goldberg R, et al. Mutations in PTPN11, encoding the protein tyrosine phosphatase SHP-2, cause Noonan syndrome. *Nat Genet* 2001;29(4):465–468.

X. Stevens CA, Bhakta MG. Cardiac abnormalities in the Rubinstein-Taybi syndrome. *Am J Med Genet* 1995;59(3):346–348.

Y. Surka WS, Kohlhase J, Neunert CE, et al. Unique family with Townes-Brocks syndrome, SALL1 mutation, and cardiac defects. *Am J Med Genet* 2001;102(3):250–257.

Z. Digilio MC, Marino B, Ammirati A, et al. Cardiac malformations in patients with oral-facial-skeletal syndromes: Clinical similarities with heterotaxia. *Am J Med Genet* 1999;84(4):350–356.

AA. Teebi AS, Lambert DM, Kaye GM, et al. Keutel syndrome: Further characterization and review. *Am J Med Genet* 1998;78(2):182–187.

BB. Kumar D, Primhak RA, Kumar A. Variable phenotype in Kaufman-McKusick syndrome: Report of an inbred Muslim family and review of the literature. *Clin Dysmorphol* 1998;7(3):163–170.

CC. Slavotinek AM, Biesecker LG. Phenotypic overlap of McKusick-Kaufman syndrome with Bardet-Biedl syndrome: A literature review. *Am J Med Genet* 2000;95(3):208–215.

DD. Lin AE, Ardinger HH, Ardinger RH Jr, et al. Cardiovascular malformations in Smith-Lemli-Opitz syndrome. *Am J Med Genet* 1997;68(3):270–278.

EE. Lin AE, Neri G, Hughes-Benzie R, et al. Cardiac anomalies in the Simpson-Golabi-Behmel syndrome. *Am J Med Genet* 1999;83(5):378–381.

Adapted from Lin AE, Ardinger HH. Genetic epidemiology and an overview of the genetics of congenital heart defects. *Progr Pediatr Cardiol* 2005;20:113–126; and Lin AE, Belmont J, Ghaffar S. The heart. In: Stevenson RE, Hall JG, eds. *Human Malformations and Related Anomalies.* 2nd ed. New York: Oxford University Press, 2006:85–120.

with specific syndromes or CHDs. New technologies such as microarrays of single nucleotide polymorphisms (so-called SNPs) are likely to identify new submicroscopic chromosomal deletions or duplications and may lead to the identification of new disease loci or genes (12). In addition, it is increasingly apparent that a proportion of CHDs are complex in origin, resulting from a combination of genetic and environmental risk factors in any one patient or family (11). New approaches that consider this complexity are required to identify new genetic and environmental risk factors for CHDs. For example, genome-wide association studies that test for the association between common single nucleotide polymorphisms and CHDs may identify novel sequence changes that contribute to the risk for CHDs. If genetic risk factors are identified, then strategies to decrease the risk of occurrence or improve outcome may be possible.

PATTERNS OF INHERITANCE AND FAMILIAL RISKS

Assessing the risk of recurrence (the chance that an affected parent will have an affected child or that unaffected parents will have a second affected child) for a patient or their relative is an ongoing challenge. Historically, different study designs, variable classification schemes of CHDs, different modes of ascertainment, and evolving methods of diagnosis have made it difficult to compare studies and have complete confidence in the results. Most cases of CHD have been thought to be sporadic. Overall, low recurrence risks of 2% to 4% have been quoted for all types of CHDs with one affected sibling or parent (13–16). Studies suggest that the recurrence risk increases if more than

one sibling is affected (11) although it has been unclear if an affected mother confers a greater risk than an affected father (17,18). Recurrent CHDs within a family are usually concordant, or derive from the same class of defects (15).

Data from these studies are valuable but must be used with some caution. Earlier studies did not consider the more recently described Mendelian syndromes and chromosomal causes of CHDs, factors that affect the overall recurrence frequency. In addition, familial cases of almost every type of CHD have been observed as has every pattern of inheritance including autosomal dominant, autosomal recessive, X-linked, or complex nonmendelian patterns of inheritance. The observed pattern of inheritance greatly influences the risk of recurrence for any one family and must be considered for counseling purposes.

Instead of recurrence risk, investigators from the Baltimore-Washington Infant Study analyzed the rate of precurrence (the number of currently affected relatives at the time of birth) (8). These studies demonstrate substantial rates of familial disease and suggest that CHDs may not be as sporadic as once thought. Precurrence rates may vary substantially with the type of CHD under consideration (8).

Left-sided obstructive defects have been the subject of several recent large family studies. Echocardiography was performed on first-degree relatives of probands to complement extensive pedigree analysis and better assess the occurrence of CHD in each family. These reports found that 8% to 19% of first-degree relatives of patients with left-sided CHDs had predominantly concordant CHDs (5–7,19). These data suggest that left-sided CHDs commonly result from inherited genetic traits. Of note, CHDs were identified with higher frequency in first-degree relatives of probands with hypoplastic left heart syndrome (19.3%) and coarctation of the aorta (9.4%) than

TABLE 26.4

CONDITIONS WITH PRESUMED BUT UNKNOWN GENETIC CAUSE ASSOCIATED WITH CONGENITAL HEART DEFECTS

Syndrome	Reference	Gene(s)	OMIM no.	Frequency of CHD[a] All (%)	Frequency of CHD[a] Distinctive or most common	Distinctive features[b]
Autosomal dominant						
Adams-Oliver syndrome	(A,B)		100300	20	LVOTO CHDs: Coarctation, parachute MV TOF Pulmonary vascular malformations	Scalp cutis aplasia Terminal transverse limb defect
Kabuki syndrome	(C,D)		147920	45–55	ASD, VSD LVOTO CHDs: BAV, Coarctation Parachute MV, Shone's complex	Long palpebral fissures Cleft lip/palate Skeletal abnormalities Fetal fingerpads
Autosomal recessive						
Fryns syndrome	(E)		229850	50	Secundum ASD, VSD Conotruncal CHDs	Diaphragmatic hernia Distal digital hypoplasia GU, GI anomalies
Hydrolethalus syndrome	(F)		236680	60	AVSD defects: Complete AVSD, common atrium ASD	Hydrocephalus Keyhole occipital defect Polydactyly Cleft lip/palate
Oral-facial-digital syndrome, II	(G)		252100	50	Primum ASD Complete AVSD	Tongue hamartomas Median cleft lip, alveolus Complex polysyndactyly
Ritscher–Schinzel syndrome (3C)	(H)		220210	100	TOF, DORV Complete AVSD, primum ASD ASD, VSD	Dandy–Walker malformation Prominent forehead Cleft palate Coloboma
Etiologic heterogeneity with autosomal gene(s), in some cases						
PHACES syndrome	(I)		606519	90	Coarctation IAA type A Right, double, or cervical aortic arch	Posterior fossa malformation Hemangiomas Eye anomalies
Hemifacial microsomia, Goldenhar syndrome, oculoauricular vertebral spectrum	(J)		164210	30	VSD Conotruncal CHDs: TOF	Microtia, ear tags, pits Hypoplasia face Epibulbar dermoid Vertebral anomalies Radial deficiency GU anomalies
Heterotaxy	(K–M)	LEFTY2 ACVR2B CFC1 ZIC3	601877 602730 605376 306955	95	Dextrocardia D-transposition L-transposition AVSD defects TAPVR Interrupted IVC Left SVC	Visceral situs anomalies Lung lobation anomalies Cleft lip, palate GU, brain anomalies Biliary atresia Malrotation, bowel atresia Spleen anomalies

(continued)

TABLE 26.4

CONDITIONS WITH PRESUMED BUT UNKNOWN GENETIC CAUSE ASSOCIATED WITH CONGENITAL HEART DEFECTS (CONTINUED)

Syndrome	Reference	Gene(s)	OMIM no.	Frequency of CHD[a]		Distinctive features[b]
				All (%)	Distinctive or most common	
VATER association	(N)		192350	50	Assorted CHDs Single umbilical artery	Vertebral anomalies anorectal anomalies Renal anomalies Radial deficiency

See Table 26.2 for definitions of abbreviations. IVC, inferior vena cava; SVC, superior vena cava; TAPVR, total anomalous pulmonary venous return.

References

A. Lin AE, Westgate MN, van der Velde ME, et al. Adams-Oliver syndrome associated with cardiovascular malformations. *Clin Dysmorphol* 1998;7(4):235–241.
B. Maniscalco M, Zedda A, Faraone S, et al. Association of Adams-Oliver syndrome with pulmonary arterio-venous malformation in the same family: A further support to the vascular hypothesis. *Am J Med Genet A* 2005;136(3):269–274.
C. Armstrong L, Abd El Moneim A, Aleck K, et al. Further delineation of Kabuki syndrome in 48 well-defined new individuals. *Am J Med Genet A* 2005;132(3):265–272.
D. White SM, Thompson EM, Kidd A, et al. Growth, behavior, and clinical findings in 27 patients with Kabuki (Niikawa–Kuroki) syndrome. *Am J Med Genet A* 2004;127(2):118–127.
E. Lin AE, Pober BR, Mullen MP, et al. Cardiovascular malformations in Fryns syndrome: Is there a pathogenic role for neural crest cells? *Am J Med Genet A* 2005;139(3):186–193.
F. Visapaa I, Salonen R, Varilo T, et al. Assignment of the locus for hydrolethalus syndrome to a highly restricted region on 11q23-25. *Am J Hum Genet* 1999;65(4):1086–1095.
G. Digilio MC, Marino B, Giannotti A, et al. The atrioventricular canal defect is the congenital heart disease connecting short rib-polydactyly and oral-facial-digital syndromes. *Am J Med Genet* 1997;68(1):110–112.
H. Leonardi ML, Pai GS, Wilkes B, et al. Ritscher-Schinzel cranio-cerebello-cardiac (3C) syndrome: Report of four new cases and review. *Am J Med Genet* 2001;102(3):237–242.
I. Bronzetti G, Giardini A, Patrizi A, et al. Ipsilateral hemangioma and aortic arch anomalies in posterior fossa malformations, hemangiomas, arterial anomalies, coarctation of the aorta, and cardiac defects and eye abnormalities (PHACE) anomaly: Report and review. *Pediatrics* 2004;113(2):412–415.
J. Kumar A, Friedman JM, Taylor GP, et al. Pattern of cardiac malformation in oculoauriculovertebral spectrum. *Am J Med Genet* 1993;46(4):423–426.
K. Lin AE, Ticho BS, Houde K, et al. Heterotaxy: Associated conditions and hospital-based prevalence in newborns. *Genet Med* 2000;2(3):157–172.
L. Ticho BS, Goldstein AM, Van Praagh R, Extracardiac anomalies in the heterotaxy syndromes with focus on anomalies of midline-associated structures. *Am J Cardiol* 2000;85(6):729–734.
M. Ware SM, Peng J, Zhu L, et al. Identification and functional analysis of ZIC3 mutations in heterotaxy and related congenital heart defects. *Am J Hum Genet* 2004;74(1):93–105.
N. Botto LD, Khoury MJ, Mastroiacovo P, et al. The spectrum of congenital anomalies of the VATER association: an international study. *Am J Med Genet* 1997;71(1):8–15.

in first-degree relatives of probands with d-transposition of the great arteries (2.7%) (7). Similar studies detailing the heritability of other types or classes of CHDs have not yet been performed to provide similar data.

Collectively, these findings suggest that precurrence and recurrence rates are likely to vary between specific types of CHD and within different kindred. Therefore, instead of using population-based empiric data alone, counseling for recurrence risk for an individual family requires that multiple factors are considered including the specific type of CHD, the presence of additional affected family members, and the presence of known genetic or syndromic risk factors.

GENETIC SYNDROMES

Genetic syndromes are defined as a consistent pattern of malformation caused by a genetic alteration. A malformation syndrome consists of multiple structural defects that are thought to be due to a single cause, even if the suspected cause has not

yet been identified (20). The cause can include genetic alterations such as changes in chromosome number, translocations between chromosomes, deletions or duplications of specific chromosomal regions, or single gene defects, or can involve a teratogen (Table 26.1). The most common genetic syndromes will be described in the following sections organized by the type of associated genetic alteration. For each syndrome the genetic basis, clinical and cardiac phenotype, diagnostic testing, natural history, and population frequency are described. A more extensive table of syndromes is provided for reference (Tables 26.2–26.4). In addition to the common conditions summarized in this chapter, comprehensive listings of chromosome defects associated with a cardiac defect (21,22) may be useful and serve as sources for potential pathogenic gene loci. Genetic textbooks, chapters, and on-line services also provide extensive descriptions of each syndrome (20,23–25). An alternative listing of syndromes by cardiac subclasses may be more practical for the cardiologist searching for information based on the specific type of heart defect, especially when a dysmorphic child lacks a specific syndromic diagnosis (26).

Syndromes Associated with Chromosome Abnormalities

In population-based studies, a chromosome abnormality was detected in approximately 13% of children in the first year (27,28), and in 19% to 36% of miscarriages and stillborn fetuses with a cardiac defect (29). This material is reviewed in greater detail in Chapter 25 of this text. Chromosome abnormalities can be classified according to an increase or decrease in whole chromosome number (aneuploidy), an increase or decrease of part of a chromosome (duplication or deletion, partial trisomy, or partial monosomy), or a more complex rearrangement.

Change in Chromosome Number (Aneuploidy)

Down Syndrome. Down syndrome is the most familiar syndrome to cardiologists. Most patients with Down syndrome have complete trisomy 21 (94%) with a complete extra copy of chromosome 21 (Table 26.2). In rare cases (6% overall), partial trisomy of chromosome 21 is present owing to a chromosomal translocation or mosaicism.

The well-known facial appearance changes with age and varies with ethnic background (Fig. 26.1). Most newborns have hypotonia, followed by global developmental delays and moderate mental retardation. Other characteristic features include microbrachycephaly, small facial features, including small ears, protruding tongue, short upslanting eyes with epicanthal folds, transverse palmar creases, and sparse hair. Skeletal anomalies include fifth finger clinodactyly, brachydactyly, a gap between first and second toes, atlantoaxial

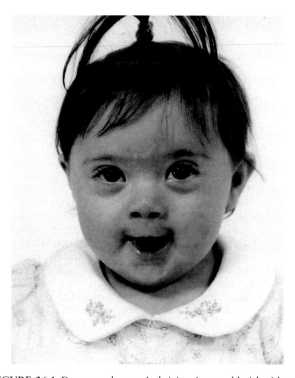

FIGURE 26.1 Down syndrome. A thriving 1-year-old girl with epicanthal folds, small nose, small mouth, small ears, and atrioventricular canal. (Courtesy of Sara S. Halbach, MS, CGC; Donna McDonald-McGinn, MS, CGC; Terri Anderson, MD; and Elaine Zackai, MD, The Children's Hospital of Philadelphia).

instability, hypoplastic pelvis, and joint laxity. Additional problems involve the visual, auditory, endocrine, hematologic, reproductive, and gastrointestinal systems.

Approximately half of liveborn Down syndrome individuals have CHD, of which approximately 40% have a complete atrioventricular septal defect (atrioventricular canal defect or endocardial cushion defect). When primum-type atrial septal defect, canal-type ventricular septal defect, and transitional atrioventricular septal defect are included, the frequency of the atrioventricular family of septal defects increases to almost 60% (27,30,31). The association of Down syndrome and atrioventricular septal defects is underscored by the fact that approximately 75% of patients with a complete atrioventricular septal defect have Down syndrome. Other common CHDs include secundum atrial septal defect, perimembranous and muscular ventricular septal defect, tetralogy of Fallot (with and without atrioventricular septal defect), and hemodynamically significant patent ductus arteriosus.

Mothers older than age 35 years have an increased risk of conceiving a child with an extra chromosome, including Down syndrome. The most recent national livebirth prevalence estimate for Down syndrome (1999 to 2001), adjusted for maternal age, is 1.36 per 1,000 (about 5,500 cases per year) (32). Overall survival has improved, although prenatally diagnosed CHDs and/or growth retardation may predict a poorer outcome (33). Population-based data from the United States notes that the median age at death increased from 25 to 49 years in the interval from 1983 to 1997 (34). Equivalent if not better surgical results for atrioventricular septal defect repair with similar postoperative residual cardiovascular defects have been reported in Down as compared with non-Down syndrome individuals (35,36). The frequency and severity of CHDs in patients with Down syndrome mosaicism was decreased in a single survey of this uncommon Down syndrome karyotype (37).

The strong association of Down syndrome and atrioventricular septal defects prompted a search for a cardiac gene on chromosome 21. A Down syndrome critical region on chromosome 21 (21q22) and CHD candidate genes have been proposed, although causation for atrioventricular septal defects has not been demonstrated (38).

Trisomy 18. The distinctive phenotype of trisomy 18 includes the nonspecific features of short palpebral fissures, small mouth, micrognathia, and growth retardation; and the more specific features of a prominent occiput, clenched hands, disorganized or hypoplastic palmar creases, hyperconvex nails, short sternum, small nipples, and radial deficiency; and anomalies of almost every organ system.

CHDs are nearly ubiquitous and include perimembranous ventricular septal defect, tetralogy of Fallot, double-outlet right ventricle, and polyvalvar dysplasia in which valve leaflets are thickened, myxomatous, or dysplastic (39–41). A natural history study of trisomy 18 in the United Kingdom reported that the prevalence at 18 weeks' gestational age was about 1 in 4,000, which decreased to 1 in 8,000 at birth (42). Recent population-based analyses of trisomy 18 (and trisomy 13) born during 1968 to 1999 reaffirmed that the vast majority (91%) die in the first year of life, although CHDs did not seem to affect survival (43). Although the high lethality and obligatory severe mental retardation among survivors is well recognized, some parents of trisomy 18 infants advocate for cardiac surgery, among other procedures.

There is no single trisomy 18 critical region. Instead, analysis of individuals with duplication of distal 18q provides insights into chromosome regions that may contribute to the trisomy 18 phenotype (44).

Turner Syndrome. The liveborn prevalence of Turner syndrome is approximately 1 per 2,000 (45). The phenotype depends on whether the X chromosome is absent (45,X occurs in almost 50% of patients) or structurally abnormal as an isochromosome, short or long arm deletion, or ring (46). The most common presentation is a spontaneously aborted fetus with hydrops, often with a lymphatic malformation in the neck or mediastinum. Lymphedema in fetal life produces neck webbing, protruding ears, loose nuchal skin, low hairline, puffy hands and feet, deep-set nails and lower-extremity edema in later life (Fig. 26.2). Frequent skeletal features include short fourth metacarpals and metatarsals, cubitus valgus, Madelung deformity (abnormal growth of the end of the radius), knee anomalies, osteoporosis, kyphoscoliosis, and broad chest with apparently widely spaced nipples. Structural renal abnormalities (horseshoe kidney), nevi, and conductive hearing loss with progressive sensorineural hearing loss are common. Premature ovarian failure begins perinatally and results in infertility in most women. Autoimmune diseases are common, as well as deficits in visual-spatial/perceptual abilities, attention, and social skills. Of note, some women with Turner syndrome have imperceptible syndromic facial features.

Turner syndrome women with 45,X generally have more malformations as compared with those with only partial deletion of the X chromosome. Deletion Xp predicts short stature and skeletal features such as brachydactyly and Madelung deformity. Individuals with a small ring X chromosome appear more likely to have mental deficiency and an atypical facial appearance. Mosaicism involving 45,X/46,XX is usually associated with a milder phenotype. Individuals with 45,X/46,XY mosaicism are at risk for gonadoblastoma (46).

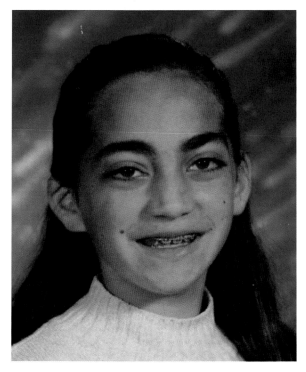

FIGURE 26.2 Turner syndrome. Eleven-year-old girl with hypertelorism, facial nevi, and dysplastic right pinnae. She has short stature, normal intelligence, thyroiditis, and no CHDs (Courtesy of Angela E. Lin, MD.)

Approximately 25% to 30% of Turner syndrome patients have a CHD, which usually involves obstruction of the left-sided cardiac structures (46–48). About 50% of adults have thoracic anomalies detected by MRI (49,50). The mildest CHD is an asymptomatic bicuspid aortic valve (15%), which may progress to aortic stenosis (10%). Coarctation of the aorta, isolated or with a bicuspid aortic valve, is present in 10% of Turner syndrome patients. These findings are significantly associated with the presence of neck webbing. Many investigators have hypothesized that the altered lymphatic drainage itself causes the associated left-sided obstructive lesions (48,51). However, it is unproven whether haploinsufficiency for genes on the X chromosome that may impair lymphatic and vascular development represent the underlying cause instead (52). Elongation of the transverse arch and/or pseudocoarctation has been reported in almost half of adults with Turner syndrome (50). Mitral valve anomalies occur in <5% of patients, and hypoplastic left heart syndrome is rare, but these illustrate the entire spectrum of left-sided obstructive lesions that can be seen in this population. Secundum atrial septal defect, perimembranous ventricular septal defect, partial anomalous pulmonary venous connection often involving the upper left pulmonary vein, and persistent left superior vena cava also occur, but complex CHDs are noticeably rare (47,48,50).

Turner syndrome women are at risk for aortic root dilation, dissection, and sudden death. Aortic dilation was originally thought to occur infrequently (approximately 10%) based on clinical series, but prospective MRI of older patients doubles the echocardiographic detection (33% vs. 16%) (49). Arterial dilation and arterial wall abnormalities suggest that there may be a more diffuse vasculopathy (53). A recent epidemiologic description of aortic dissection calculated a sixfold population-based risk (36 per 100,000 Turner syndrome years), or an approximate 1.4% risk (54). Aortic dissection in Turner syndrome is almost always associated with a risk factor such as bicuspid aortic valve, coarctation of the aorta or hypertension, and the few individuals without an underlying cause may reflect inadequate examination (55,56). Consensus guidelines (52) for monitoring and caring for the increasing number of older women with Turner syndrome include baseline imaging of the aorta at the time the condition is diagnosed and ongoing blood pressure monitoring. MRI may provide superior images to echocardiography depending on age, coexisting CHDs, previous surgery, and body habitus (49,50). Repeat imaging should be done every 5 to 10 years, when the clinical situation is appropriate (such as transitioning from pediatric to adult care), with the appearance of hypertension, or if pregnancy is contemplated (52,57). Several studies have begun to evaluate the impact of growth hormone on aortic dilation with conflicting results (58–60). A registry to identify individuals with Turner syndrome and aortic dissection may provide a sufficient cohort to yield further insight (61). A disturbing number of deaths owing to aortic dissection raise concern about the safety of pregnancy (57). For the increasing number of women who consider pregnancy using assisted reproductive technology, it seems prudent to plan the pregnancy with a cardiologist to monitor aortic size from a baseline study throughout the postpartum period, especially when risk factors are present (52).

Adult women with Turner syndrome require monitoring for postoperative recoarctation and hypertension, and aortic stenosis and regurgitation. Unrepaired bicuspid aortic valve should be monitored for the development of progressive stenosis and aortic dilation. Hypertension and coronary artery disease are more common than in the general population (56,62). Prospective ECG monitoring may also be indicated since recent data demonstrate conduction and repolarization abnormalities (including prolongation of the QTc interval) (63).

Studies correlating genotype with clinical phenotype suggest that haploinsufficiency of the short stature-homeobox (*SHOX*) gene on the short arm of the X chromosome leads to short stature and skeletal changes. Genes on both arms of the X chromosome are important for ovarian function. However, there is no known critical region on the X chromosome for CHDs.

Deletion–Duplication Syndromes

Increasingly sensitive cytogenetic techniques including FISH and array comparative genomic hybridization (CGH) have identified an increasing number of small chromosomal deletions and duplications that are not apparent on a high-resolution karyotype in patients with various clinical syndromes. A chromosomal *deletion* occurs when there is a missing segment of a chromosome on one of the two copies of the same chromosome resulting in one copy or haploinsufficiency of that region (partial monosomy). Conversely, a chromosomal duplication occurs when there is an extra copy of one segment of a chromosome resulting in three copies of that region (partial trisomy). Research has defined an expanding list of deletion and duplication syndromes over the last decade. Most of these syndromes are characterized by multiple congenital anomalies, presumably because of the number of genes involved in the deleted or duplicated segments. They also display marked clinical variability between individuals. Many of these syndromes are associated with CHDs and thus constitute an increasingly important group of syndromes with which a cardiologist should be familiar. Examples of the most common deletion syndromes with cardiovascular features are described below, and others are highlighted in Table 26.2.

The 22q11 Deletion Syndrome (DiGeorge, Velocardiofacial, or Conotruncal Anomaly Face Syndromes). DiGeorge syndrome was originally described as a rare developmental field defect characterized by aplasia or hypoplasia of the thymus, aplasia or hypoplasia of the parathyroid glands, conotruncal CHDs, and specific facial features (64,65). Infants presented with hypocalcemia, immunodeficiency, and severe CHDs (most commonly interrupted aortic arch type B, truncus arteriosus, or tetralogy of Fallot). The syndrome was observed to be etiologically heterogeneous, occurring in the context of maternal diabetes or alcohol use and in conjunction with various chromosomal abnormalities. Approximately 10% to 20% of patients with DiGeorge syndrome had chromosomal alterations resulting in the loss of the proximal long arm of one copy of chromosome 22. Further molecular studies demonstrated that nearly 90% of subjects with the DiGeorge phenotype had a deletion of chromosome 22 in the region of 22q11 (66,67). Subsequently, it was noted that patients with velocardiofacial (Shprintzen syndrome) (68) and conotruncal anomaly face syndrome (described in Japan) (69) shared similar clinical characteristics of patients with DiGeorge syndrome. Molecular studies demonstrated that the vast majority of patients with the clinical diagnosis of DiGeorge, velocardiofacial (Shprintzen syndrome), or conotruncal anomaly face syndromes shared a common genetic cause, namely a 22q11 deletion (70,71) (reviewed in [72]). Thus, patients with a 22q11 deletion represent a single disorder regardless of the associated clinical label. The 22q11 deletion syndrome is currently the most common deletion syndrome known and is estimated to occur in approximately 1 in 6,000 live births (28,73).

The clinical phenotype of the 22q11 deletion syndrome is highly variable among related and unrelated individuals (74).

The presentation can be severe and easily recognized at birth or subtle and detected late in life. Approximately 6% to 10% of cases are familial, implying that the affected child inherited the chromosomal deletion from a parent. Frequently the parent is recognized to carry a 22q11 deletion only after their more severely affected child is diagnosed. The most common features include CHDs, palate anomalies, feeding disorders, speech and learning disabilities, hypocalcemia, immunodeficiency, renal anomalies, behavioral and psychiatric disorders, and typical facial features (reviewed in [75]) (Fig. 26.3). However, the facial features can be difficult to identify in infants and may be underappreciated in certain populations such as African Americans (76).

Congenital heart defects are estimated to occur in 75% to 80% of patients with a 22q11 deletion (77,78). The prevalence of CHDs may be overestimated because of increased ascertainment in the pediatric population with CHDs as compared with adults with more subtle features (79). The most common CHDs associated with a 22q11 deletion include: tetralogy of Fallot, interrupted aortic arch type B, truncus arteriosus, perimembranous ventricular septal defect, and aortic arch anomalies. It should be noted that a wide range of CHDs has been reported in patients with a 22q11 deletion, including pulmonary valve stenosis, atrial septal defect, heterotaxy syndrome, and hypoplastic left heart syndrome.

Because CHDs are common in the 22q11 deletion syndrome, several studies have estimated the frequency with which a 22q11 deletion is found in patients with CHDs typical of DiGeorge or velocardiofacial syndromes. At least 50% of patients with an interrupted aortic arch type B, 35% with truncus arteriosus,

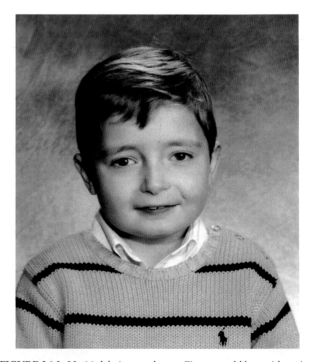

FIGURE 26.3 22q11 deletion syndrome. Five-year-old boy with typical facial features of the 22q11 deletion syndrome including malar flattening, small mouth, bulbous tipped nose with hypoplastic alae nasi, and micrognathia. He also had tetralogy of Fallot, developmental delay, mild immune suppression, and late emergence of speech. (Courtesy of Donna McDonald-McGinn, MS, CGC; Elaine Zackai, MD; and Elizabeth Goldmuntz, MD, The Children's Hospital of Philadelphia.)

24% with an isolated aortic arch anomaly, 15% with tetralogy of Fallot, and 10% with a perimembranous ventricular septal defect are found to have a 22q11 deletion (80–89). In contrast, <1% of patients with double-outlet right ventricle or d-transposition of the great arteries are found to have a 22q11 deletion. Several studies have demonstrated that patients with one of these intracardiac anomalies and a concurrent aortic arch anomaly (either abnormal sidedness, cervical location, or abnormal branching pattern) are more likely to have a 22q11 deletion. For example, only 3% of patients with a perimembranous ventricular septal defect and a normal left-sided aortic arch with normal branching pattern were diagnosed with the 22q11 deletion, whereas 45% with a perimembranous ventricular septal defect and concurrent aortic arch anomaly had a 22q11 deletion (82). Therefore, the presence of an aortic arch anomaly increases the risk of finding a 22q11 deletion regardless of the intracardiac anatomy. Studies also suggest that the subset of patients with tetralogy of Fallot associated with absent pulmonary valve syndrome or aortopulmonary collaterals are at higher risk of having a 22q11 deletion (84,90). Collectively, these findings demonstrate that a 22q11 deletion is commonly found in a significant subset of patients with congenital cardiovascular defects.

Identifying the cardiac patient with a 22q11 deletion early in life can provide substantial benefits to the child and family. Currently, it is recommended that infants with interrupted aortic arch, truncus arteriosus, tetralogy of Fallot, and isolated aortic arch anomalies undergo testing for a 22q11 deletion given the high frequency with which these patients are found to harbor a 22q11 deletion (91). Likewise, it is suggested that patients with a perimembranous ventricular septal defect and aortic arch anomaly, or any infant with noncardiac features of the 22q11 deletion syndrome (regardless of the CHD) undergo 22q11 deletion testing. Although somewhat controversial, current recommendations for testing seek to identify the deletion-bearing patient as early as possible to anticipate associated medical conditions and provide accurate family genetic counseling. Parents found to carry the deletion have a 50% chance of transmitting the deletion-bearing chromosome in subsequent pregnancies.

Although the evaluation must be tailored to each patient's needs, infants or children diagnosed with the 22q11 syndrome should be evaluated for associated noncardiac features including hypocalcemia, immunodeficiency, palate anomalies, feeding and speech disorders, renal and skeletal anomalies, cognitive deficiencies, and behavioral issues (75). Parents should be tested for a 22q11 deletion as well. A 22q11 deletion is now easily detected from a sample of whole blood using FISH. Results are usually available within 1 to 2 weeks. More rapid assays are currently under development.

Many children present with noncardiac symptoms and are diagnosed with a 22q11 deletion later in infancy or childhood. Although these patients are unlikely to have major intracardiac anomalies, aortic arch anomalies are commonly identified in this subset of patients. In particular, 38% of patients diagnosed with a 22q11 deletion after 9 months of age were found to have an aortic arch anomaly, of whom 27% had a symptomatic vascular ring (92). A remarkable variety of aortic arch anomalies has been found in the 22q11 deleted population including absent or isolated subclavian arteries where retrograde flow through the vertebral artery provides flow into the absent or isolated subclavian artery predisposing to a steal phenomenon (93). Since respiratory symptoms including asthma and airway anomalies are commonly diagnosed in the 22q11 deleted population, it is important to identify which children have concurrent vascular rings contributing to or

causing their respiratory symptoms and which should undergo surgical ligation.

Several laboratories have studied which gene or genes mapping to the deleted segment of chromosome 22 cause the malformations associated with the 22q11 deletion syndrome. Approximately 30 genes have been identified in the deleted segment and their role in the development of involved organs evaluated. *TBX1* is of particular interest because it maps into the deleted region and is expressed in regions of the mouse embryo critical to cardiovascular development. Several mouse models lacking partial or complete expression of this gene have been engineered and have demonstrated features consistent with but not completely reminiscent of the human 22q11 deletion syndrome (reviewed in [94–96]). In one report three human subjects with the clinical features of the 22q11 deletion syndrome but without a chromosomal 22q11 deletion were found to have presumably disease-causing mutations of *TBX1* (97). Thus, *TBX1* appears to play a critical role in the clinical phenotype. It is likely that other genetic and environmental factors modulate the expression of the deletion to result in the highly variable clinical features seen in this syndrome.

7q11 Deletion (Williams–Beuren Syndrome). Williams–Beuren syndrome is another familiar multisystem disorder that occurs in 1 per 20,000 livebirths. It is characterized in part by CHDs, hypercalcemia in infancy, skeletal and renal anomalies, cognitive deficits, social personality, and elfin facies (Fig. 26.4). As with other deletion syndromes, children with Williams syndrome can be diagnosed at different ages and present with a broad range of clinical features (reviewed in [98]). Early in life, feeding disorders and growth retardation are common. Hypercalcemia is seen in 15% of infants and usually resolves over time (99). The neurocognitive profile of Williams syndrome most commonly includes mild mental retardation, although the

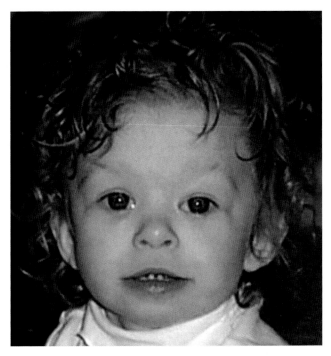

FIGURE 26.4 Williams syndrome. Seventeen-month-old girl with typical facial appearance including flared eyebrows, bright stellate irides, and wide mouth. She has mild supravalvar aortic stenosis. (Courtesy of Amy E. Roberts, MD, Children's Hospital, Boston.)

full-scale IQ ranges from low normal intelligence to severe mental retardation. Cognitive strengths and weaknesses relative to other patients with mental retardation include relatively good auditory rote memory but extreme difficulty with visuospatial construction tasks (100). The familiar high sociability and overly friendly demeanor seen in some patients with Williams syndrome may be accompanied by substantial behavioral disorders, including inattention and hyperactivity.

Approximately 55% to 80% of patients with Williams syndrome have CHDs, which typically include supravalvar aortic stenosis and/or supravalvar pulmonary stenosis (101,102). The degree of cardiovascular involvement and the relative involvement of the pulmonic or aortic vessels varies widely. Although supravalvar pulmonary stenosis usually improves with time, supravalvar aortic stenosis progresses in most cases (102–104). If significant supravalvar aortic stenosis is left untreated, cardiac hypertrophy followed by cardiac failure can result. Surgical and catheter interventions have met with success in some cases (105). Sudden cardiac death is another reported cardiovascular complication. Sudden death was described in ten young children with Williams syndrome, seven of whom had coronary artery stenosis along with severe biventricular outflow tract obstruction (106). Presumably, sudden cardiac death resulted from myocardial ischemia, decreased cardiac output, or arrhythmias. Finally, patients with Williams syndrome may commonly develop hypertension either because of renal artery stenosis or other undefined mechanisms (101). Because of the generally diffuse arteriopathy and potential for hypertension, lifelong cardiovascular monitoring is recommended for patients with Williams syndrome (98).

Approximately 90% of patients with the clinical diagnosis of Williams syndrome have a deletion at chromosome 7q11.23, which is not generally apparent on a routine karyotype but can be detected by FISH. Clinical testing is readily available in most standard cytogenetic clinical laboratories. Given the clinical variability of Williams syndrome, it is appropriate to consider testing all patients with supravalvar aortic or pulmonic stenosis for a 7q11.23 deletion.

Most patients with Williams syndrome have a 7q11.23 deletion of the same size. The genes mapping to this region have been defined and include the elastin gene, ELN. Mutations within the elastin gene have also been found in patients with isolated supravalvar aortic stenosis (107–109). Therefore, deletion of the elastin gene in patients with Williams syndrome is thought to account for the cardiovascular phenotype. Molecular studies of rare patients with smaller deletions implicate the gene LIMK1 in the impaired visuospatial constructive cognition (110). Additional genes mapping into the deleted region are thought to contribute to the neurocognitive features and are under further study. In contrast to the 22q11 deletion syndrome, these findings suggest that Williams syndrome is a true contiguous gene deletion syndrome in which the deletion of specific genes corresponds to distinct clinical features.

Studies further suggest that specific types of mutations in the elastin gene result in different clinical syndromes. As noted, a 7q11.23 deletion results in complete loss of one copy of the elastin gene (as well as other genes) and the diffuse arteriopathy seen in Williams syndrome. Disruption or mutation of the elastin gene alone can also result in isolated forms of supravalvar aortic and pulmonic stenosis. Both sporadic cases of supravalvar aortic stenosis and families with autosomal dominant inheritance have been found to have intragenic elastin gene mutations that result in functional hemizygosity (half of the functional gene dosage), similar to deletion of the entire gene (109). Recently, mutations in the elastin gene have been identified in some patients with the autosomal dominant form of cutis laxa, another connective tissue disorder characterized by loose, saggy, inelastic skin. Both autosomal recessive and dominant forms have been observed in this genetically heterogeneous disorder (111,112). Studies suggest that these elastin mutations are functionally distinct from those associated with the diffuse arteriopathy, acting instead as a dominant negative effect. Thus, the specific elastin gene mutation appears to correlate with a specific clinical phenotype. These findings serve to demonstrate the complexity and heterogeneity of even seemingly straightforward genetic syndromes.

Subtelomere Deletion Syndromes. The subtelomeric region of the chromosome contains a gene-rich segment located just before the end (or telomere) of each chromosome. The subtelomeric region has been a difficult area in which to identify chromosomal rearrangements (including deletions and duplications) using standard techniques. More recently, investigators have developed a unique set of probes that test specifically for deletions and alterations in the subtelomeric regions of each chromosome. Patients with moderate to severe mental retardation of unknown cause were the first population tested for subtelomeric chromosomal rearrangements that were not otherwise apparent on high-resolution karyotypes. The first studies identified subtelomeric deletions in approximately 7% of patients with severe or moderate mental retardation (113,114).

Many reported patients with mental retardation and a subtelomeric deletion have additional congenital anomalies (114–116). These observations have led many clinical geneticists to test patients with multiple congenital anomalies (particularly those with mental retardation) and a normal karyotype for subtelomeric deletions using these new techniques (117). An increasing number of patients with multiple congenital anomalies has been found to have subtelomeric deletions leading to the description of new clinical syndromes. For example, some patients with similar clinical phenotypes were found to have a 1p36 deletion, thereby defining a new deletion syndrome (118,119). Some of these new deletion syndromes are associated with CHDs, and it is likely that more will be described in the future. For example, patients with a 9q34 deletion have mental retardation, distinct facial features, and CHDs (120). Further evaluation of these new deletion syndromes will help define the cause of the disorder for a growing number of patients but may also identify novel disease loci and genes for CHDs.

Genetic Syndromes Caused by Mutations in Single Genes

An increasing number of malformation syndromes have been found to be caused by a mutation of a single gene in contrast to a larger chromosomal abnormality (see Table 26.3). These mutations can be inherited in a mendelian fashion and demonstrate an autosomal dominant pattern of inheritance in families, with a 50% risk of recurrence. As with larger chromosomal alterations, single-gene disorders are characterized by a variable phenotype between related and unrelated affected individuals, suggesting that additional genetic and environmental factors modify the clinical phenotype of any single mutation. The type of intragenic mutation may be variable (as in Alagille syndrome) or fairly consistent (as in achondroplasia) and may include nonsense, frameshift, missense, or splice site mutations. Specific mutations may result in different biologic consequences and may cause different clinical phenotypes. These observations have been well characterized in

Noonan and LEOPARD syndrome most recently (see Noonan Syndrome). It is important to note that even single-gene disorders can be genetically heterogeneous, implying that mutation of more than one gene can result in the same observed clinical phenotype, as illustrated by the discussions on Alagille and Noonan syndromes in the following sections. The most common genetic syndromes for which a specific disease gene has been defined are described below.

Alagille Syndrome (*JAG1 and Notch2*). Alagille syndrome was originally defined as the presence of bile duct paucity on liver biopsy in conjunction with three of the following five findings: cholestasis, CHDs, skeletal or ocular abnormalities, or typical facial features (121,122) (Fig. 26.5). An autosomal dominant disorder, it was noted that a subset of patients with clinical features of Alagille syndrome had deletions of chromosome 20p12 (123–125). The Notch ligand, *JAG1*, was subsequently mapped into the commonly deleted region (126). Two reports identified mutations of *JAG1* in patients with Alagille syndrome and therefore demonstrated that *JAG1* is a disease gene for this disorder (127,128). *JAG1* mutations were also identified in family members with milder presentations or microforms of Alagille syndrome, demonstrating that there is a broad spectrum of clinical phenotypes associated with *JAG1* mutations. Using the most sensitive techniques, mutations can be identified in 94% of patients with features of Alagille syndrome (129). Approximately 5% of patients will have a chromosomal deletion involving one copy of the entire gene, whereas most will have various intragenic mutations (129,130). Mutations introducing a shift in the reading frame of the genetic code (so-called frameshift mutations) are the most common type of mutation, but missense mutations that alter only a single amino acid have also been identified. As a result of most mutations, there is only one functional copy of the gene and presumably half the amount of functional protein. Therefore, the disease mechanism appears to be that of haploinsufficiency.

Alagille syndrome is characterized by right-sided CHDs including peripheral pulmonary stenosis (diffuse hypoplasia of the pulmonary arterial bed as well as discrete stenosis), pulmonary valve stenosis, and tetralogy of Fallot. Left-sided lesions and septal defects have also been reported (131). Examination of pedigrees of patients with Alagille syndrome and/or *JAG1* mutations suggested that some patients with CHDs without overt hepatic involvement would have *JAG1* mutations. Indeed, *JAG1* mutations have been identified in patients and kindred who do not have overt hepatic disease and therefore do not meet the classic criteria of Alagille syndrome but have CHDs typical of Alagille syndrome and other mild syndromic features (132,133). Therefore, the diagnosis of Alagille syndrome or *JAG1* mutation should be considered in families in which more than one member has a right-sided heart defect. Conversely, patients with right-sided CHDs should be carefully examined for subclinical features of Alagille syndrome and questioned for a relevant family history to identify the patient at risk for Alagille syndrome or a *JAG1* mutation. Patients suspected of having Alagille syndrome should undergo cytogenetic testing including a karyotype and FISH analysis for deletion of chromosomal region 20p12. Testing for intragenic *JAG1* mutations is not yet clinically available.

Several studies have reported additional vascular anomalies and complications in patients with Alagille syndrome, highlighting the fact that the observed arteriopathy can affect more than the pulmonary arterial bed. In particular, Kamath et al. (134) reported that 9% of their cohort with Alagille syndrome had noncardiac vascular anomalies or events including basilar,

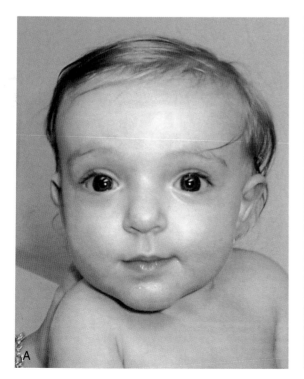
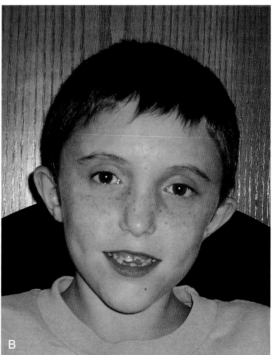

FIGURE 26.5 Alagille syndrome. Representative facial features of two boys with Alagille syndrome aged 7 months (**A**) and 9 years (**B**). Note the broad forehead, deep-set eyes, rounded tip and pearlike shape of the nose, and pointed chin. The features give the face an inverted triangle appearance. (Courtesy of the parents; David Piccoli, MD; and Elizabeth Goldmuntz, MD, The Children's Hospital of Philadelphia.)

internal carotid, and middle cerebral artery aneurysms. Other reported arterial anomalies include renal artery stenosis and moyamoya disease. Vascular events accounted for 34% of the mortality in this cohort. The true prevalence of such arterial anomalies is still unknown, and thus it is not yet clear whether routine screening for other vascular anomalies is clinically warranted. However, these observations point to a diffuse vasculopathy in Alagille syndrome and should heighten the clinician's awareness for these potentially devastating complications.

The encoded protein, Jagged1, is a cell surface protein that serves as a ligand for the Notch transmembrane receptor. The Notch signaling pathway is thought to regulate cell fate decisions. The mouse homozygous null for *JAG1* dies early in embryogenesis, and the heterozygote for *JAG1* does not recapitulate the Alagille phenotype (135). However, the double heterozygous mouse with only one functional copy of *JAG1* and one functional copy of *NOTCH2* has all of the classic features of Alagille syndrome (136). Because of this observation and because there remains a subset of patients for whom *JAG1* mutations cannot be identified, McDaniell et al. (137) evaluated the *JAG1* mutation-negative subset of patients for mutations in *NOTCH2*. They identified two unrelated kindred with *NOTCH2* mutations out of 11 *JAG1* mutation-negative patients with the clinical features of Alagille syndrome. Of note, all of the patients with *NOTCH2* mutations had renal manifestations, which are less commonly seen in the cohort of Alagille patients with *JAG1* mutations. This study demonstrates that Alagille syndrome is in fact a genetically heterogeneous disorder even though most patients have *JAG1* mutations. These results also further highlight the critical role of the *NOTCH* signaling pathway in cardiovascular development and disease.

Holt–Oram Syndrome (*TBX5*).

Holt–Oram syndrome is the most common "heart-hand" syndrome and is estimated to occur in 1 of 100,000 live births. An autosomal dominant disorder, it is characterized by skeletal anomalies of the upper limbs and CHDs (138,139). The skeletal anomalies involve the preaxial radial ray and are fully penetrant (i.e., everyone with the diagnosis of Holt–Oram syndrome must have a skeletal anomaly), although they range in severity. Some patients have subclinical skeletal changes with only radiographically evident abnormalities of the carpal bone whereas others have obvious severe manifestations such as phocomelia. The thumb is frequently affected and can be triphalangeal, hypoplastic, or absent. Skeletal anomalies can be seen in one or both upper limbs and may be symmetric or asymmetric.

Approximately 75% of patients diagnosed with Holt–Oram syndrome have CHD (140). Although atrial and ventricular septal defects are most commonly seen (58% and 28%, respectively), additional CHDs including atrioventricular septal defects, conotruncal anomalies, and left-sided defects are also reported. Atrioventricular conduction delay, which can begin as first-degree atrioventricular block and progress to complete heart block, is also an important cardiovascular feature.

Linkage analyses performed on families demonstrating autosomal dominant inheritance identified a disease locus at 12q24 (141,142). Subsequent investigations identified mutations in *TBX5* in patients with Holt–Oram syndrome (143,144). Since the initial discovery, nonsense, frameshift, and missense mutations have been identified in familial and sporadic cases. Mutations of *TBX5* are found in approximately 70% of patients with the clinical features of Holt–Oram syndrome. Presumably those with the correct diagnosis of Holt–Oram syndrome in whom a mutation cannot be readily identified have a mutation in a regulatory domain that is not routinely tested since the disorder is not thought to be genetically heterogeneous. Although in most cases the diagnosis of Holt–Oram syndrome can be reliably made by clinical examination, genetic testing for *TBX5* mutations is clinically available in several specialized laboratories and may be useful in specific situations where the diagnosis is ambiguous or needed for prenatal counseling.

The diagnosis of Holt–Oram syndrome should be considered in the patient with heart and upper limb anomalies. Given the variable phenotype, Holt–Oram syndrome should also be considered in the patient with an apparently isolated septal defect and family history of septal or upper limb anomalies. The patient suspected of having Holt–Oram syndrome should be evaluated for radial ray and cardiac and conduction abnormalities. Although most commonly a sporadic rather than familial disorder, selected family members of affected members should be examined for subtle features to allow for appropriate genetic counseling. Some reports have suggested a genotype/phenotype correlation (i.e., certain mutations may be associated with more severe cardiac or skeletal manifestations), but caution must be exercised for the individual when counseling about the implications of each mutation.

Noonan Syndrome (*PTPN11, KRAS, SOS1*).

Noonan syndrome occurs in 1 per 1,000 to 1 per 2,500 live births diagnosed clinically (145) and is characterized by hypertelorism, ptosis, short stature, and CHDs (146,147) (Fig. 26.6). Approximately 50% to 80% of clinically defined patients have CHD, most commonly pulmonary valve stenosis and hypertrophic cardiomyopathy. Additional cardiac manifestations include secundum-type atrial septal defect, ventricular septal defect, tetralogy of Fallot, pulmonary artery stenosis,

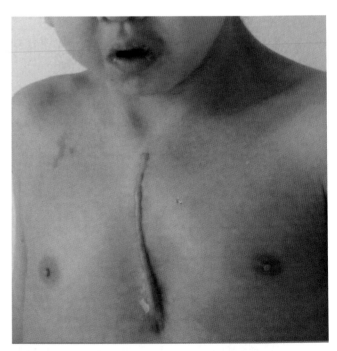

FIGURE 26.6 Noonan syndrome. Nine-year-old girl who had repair of stenotic bicuspid pulmonary valve. This thorax shows the classic combination-type pectus of Noonan syndrome, which protrudes superiorly (carinatum) and dips inferiorly (excavatum), accompanied by postoperative keloid. (Courtesy of Gurkan Cetin, MD; Mete Gursoy, MD; Alican Hatemi, MD; Aybala Tongut, MD; and Ulas Kumbasar, MD, Istanbul University Institute of Cardiology Department of Cardiac Surgery, Turkey.)

coarctation of the aorta, incomplete atrioventricular septal defect (primum-type atrial septal defect), and polyvalvulopathy (148,149). Other noncardiac anomalies include webbed neck, skeletal anomalies, bleeding diathesis, lymphatic disorders, mental retardation, and cryptochordism.

Most cases of Noonan syndrome are sporadic, although families with a pattern of autosomal dominant inheritance are well known. There is marked clinical variability among affected individuals; some parents have been diagnosed with this disorder only on the diagnosis of their more severely affected offspring.

Recent investigations have confirmed that Noonan syndrome is a genetically heterogeneous disorder. Linkage analyses and candidate gene studies first identified mutations in patients with Noonan syndrome in the gene *PTPN11*, a gene encoding the non–receptor-type protein tyrosine phosphatase SHP-2 (src homology region 2-domain phosphatase-2) that functions in the ras/MAPK pathway (150). Approximately half of patients with Noonan syndrome have a mutation in *PTPN11* (151–154). Studies correlating genotype with cardiac phenotype suggest that mutations of *PTPN11* are more common in Noonan syndrome patients with pulmonary valve stenosis (almost 80%) compared to those with hypertrophic cardiomyopathy (<10%). Yoshida et al. (152) observed that only those with *PTPN11* mutations had hematologic disorders such as bleeding diathesis or juvenile myelomonocytic leukemia. Otherwise, there did not appear to be any clinical difference between those Noonan patients with or without a *PTPN11* mutation (151,152). These and other studies (155) demonstrate that Noonan syndrome is a genetically heterogeneous disorder given that only half of Noonan patients have mutations in *PTPN11*.

Mutations of *PTPN11* have also been found in syndromes whose features overlap with those of Noonan syndrome, demonstrating that these are allelic disorders sharing a common genetic basis. Mutations of *PTPN11* have been identified in several patients with Noonan-like/multiple giant cell lesion syndrome, a syndrome characterized by features of Noonan syndrome and giant cell lesions of bone and soft tissue (cherubism) (132,151,156–158). A subset of patients with LEOPARD syndrome has also been found to have *PTPN11* mutations (159–162). LEOPARD syndrome is an autosomal dominant disorder characterized by multiple lentigines, electrocardiographic conduction abnormalities, ocular hypertelorism, pulmonary valve stenosis, hypertrophic cardiomyopathy, growth retardation, abnormal genitalia, and sensorineural deafness. LEOPARD syndrome itself appears to be genetically heterogeneous since not all patients with this clinical diagnosis have a *PTPN11* mutation (160,161). Although *PTPN11* mutations resulting in Noonan syndrome are thought to confer a gain in function of the encoded protein, SHP-2 (150), mutations found in LEOPARD syndrome appear to have a dominant negative effect (163), which may explain the distinct phenotype.

Recently, mutations in two additional genes in the ras/MAPK pathway, *SOS1* and *KRAS*, have been identified in a subset of patients with Noonan syndrome who do not have a *PTPN11* mutation. *SOS1* mutations have been reported in approximately 20% of *PTPN11* mutation-negative Noonan syndrome patients, or 10% of the Noonan syndrome population overall (164,165). *KRAS* mutations have been found in a few patients with *PTPN11* mutation-negative Noonan syndrome (166–169). These findings contribute to a complicated phenotype and novel story that is only now unfolding.

Ellis–van Creveld Syndrome (*EVC* and *EVC2*). Of the short rib–polydactyly syndromes which have similar phenotypes, Ellis–van Creveld syndrome can be distinguished by its frequent occurrence among the Old Order Amish of Pennsylvania and the combination of both skeletal and ectodermal dysplasia. Only half of patients with Ellis–van Creveld syndrome die in infancy because the short ribs and narrow thorax are not always severely restrictive. Short stature with short limbs, postaxial polydactyly, type A, hypoplastic nails, neonatal teeth, small teeth, and alveolar frenula complete the memorable appearance. More than 50% of patients with Ellis–van Creveld syndrome have a CHD, which is most commonly a large atrial septal defect (170). One hypothesis views Ellis–van Creveld syndrome as part of the spectrum of oral-facial-skeletal syndromes, which share a predisposition to atrioventricular septal defects and heterotaxy (171). This autosomal recessive disorder is caused by mutations in the *EVC* (172) and nonhomologous *EVC2* genes on chromosome 4p16 (173).

CHARGE Syndrome/Hall-Hittner Syndrome (*CHD7*). A long-standing discussion about whether the CHARGE malformation complex should be termed an association or syndrome (174) was resolved after the discovery of causative mutations in the chromodomain helicase DNA-binding gene (*CHD7*) on chromosome 8q12.1 (12). The cause of CHARGE syndrome is likely to be genetically heterogeneous given that *CHD7* mutations have been found in only approximately 65% of patients diagnosed clinically (12,175–178). The original diagnostic criteria specified coloboma (usually involving the retina or choroid coloboma), heart defects, choanal atresia (membranous or bony), retardation of postnatal growth and development (hypotonia), brain anomalies, genitourinary anomalies (more commonly recognized in males, including hypogonadotropic hypogonadism), and external ear anomalies (small, square, cupped) and/or deafness (all types) (Fig. 26.7). The mnemonic was updated to highlight the diagnostic value of cranial nerve weakness or palsy (especially facial asymmetry) and hypoplasia of the cochlea and semicircular canals. Oral clefts and neurogenic swallowing problems are now appreciated as supportive of the CHARGE syndrome (178,179). The developmental, behavioral, and personality profile is complex since visual and auditory sensory handicaps exaggerate cognitive limitations, and may include some features of autism (180).

CHDs have always been part of the core phenotype, and the availability of molecular testing provides more accurate analysis of a core phenotype. A CHD was present in 92% of *CHD7* mutation-positive and 71% *CHD7* mutation-negative individuals (176). Assorted CHDs have been reported, with conotruncal and aortic arch anomalies consistently overrepresented in clinical series. The clinical features of the DiGeorge phenotype have been observed concurrently in patients with CHARGE syndrome (179).

The frequency of the CHARGE syndrome has been reported to range from 1 per 10,000 to 1 per 15,000 live births, although one population-based study estimated a frequency of 1 in 8,500 live births (181). Most cases of the CHARGE syndrome are sporadic in occurrence, but autosomal dominant inheritance and germline mosaicism, long clinically suspected, have now been confirmed by molecular testing (176).

Common Conditions with a Presumed But Unknown Genetic Cause

Table 26.4 lists syndromes that are presumed to be due to mendelian genes based on observed family inheritance (e.g., affected siblings with Fryns syndrome suggest autosomal

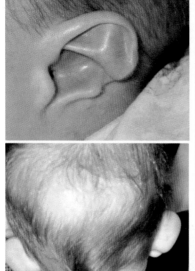

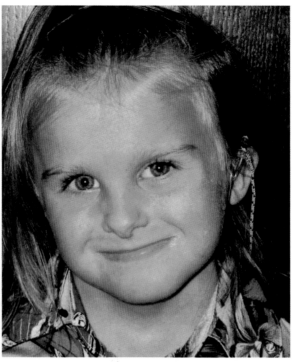

FIGURE 26.7 CHARGE syndrome. The characteristic ear anomalies include pinnae that are severely malformed (**A**), protruding (**B**), or small (**C**), as in this 5-year-old girl with very mild facial features and laryngotracheomalacia. She carries the *CHD7* mutation and had a more severely affected brother, presumably representing gonadal mosaicism. (Courtesy of the parents; Margaret A. Hefner, MS, CGS; and the CHARGE Syndrome Foundation, Inc.)

recessive inheritance). Familiar disorders that are etiologically heterogeneous are also listed and discussed in more detail below.

Heterotaxy

Heterotaxy is neither a genetic syndrome in the typical sense nor a straightforward CHD, but a familiar malformation complex involving right-left axis determination with a birth prevalence of 1 of 10,000 (182,183). Heterotaxy implies that the laterality of thoracoabdominal viscera is neither situs solitus (normal position) nor situs inversus (mirror image). Cardiac, pulmonary, renal, and gastrointestinal defects may also be accompanied by midline defects of the brain and face (184); hence the description of heterotaxy as a developmental field defect or laterality sequence.

Family studies have been invaluable in delineating the genetic basis of heterotaxy. Kindred in which some members had situs inversus and others had heterotaxy suggested that laterality defects represent a spectrum of disease. The phenotypic spectrum of heterotaxy may include certain types of isolated CHD given pedigrees where some members have overt heterotaxy "syndrome" and others have an isolated CHD such as transposition of the great arteries or double-outlet right ventricle.

Recognized risk factors for heterotaxy syndrome include maternal insulin-dependent diabetes, but assorted chromosome abnormalities have also been identified (27,182,185). The first genetic basis of a laterality disorder was observed in Kartagener syndrome in which situs inversus is accompanied by bronchiectasis, chronic sinusitis, nasal polyps, and infertility owing to immotile sperm from impaired ciliary function. Autosomal recessive inheritance, and less commonly autosomal dominant and X-linked recessive inheritance, have been described in Kartagener syndrome. Genetic heterogeneity is supported by the discovery of mutations in the gene encoding axonemal dynein intermediate chain on chromosome 9p21, with additional loci on 7p21 and 5p14 (186–188).

Pedigrees with X-linked patterns of inheritance for heterotaxy led to the discovery of the first heterotaxy gene, *ZIC3*, which maps to Xq24-27.1 (189,190). Many genes have also been found in animal models to participate in the establishment of asymmetry and laterality in the embryo. Several of these genes were tested for mutations in patients with heterotaxy and are implicated as potential disease-related genes including *LEFTY A, CRYPTIC/CFC1, ACVR2β, NKX2.5,* and *CRELD1* (191–197). However, such studies were limited and additional research is needed to define the contribution of these candidate genes to the disease spectrum.

VATER/VATERR/VACTERL Association

The VATER association is usually a sporadic occurrence of unknown cause. In rare cases as an association, it can occur in a child with an underlying syndrome, such as trisomy 18 (198). The original acronym was VATER to include *v*ertebral anomalies, *a*nal atresia (with or without fistula), *t*racheoesophageal fistula, and *r*enal dysplasia. Later, radial defects including radial or thumb absence or hypoplasia, and preaxial polydactyly expanded the *R*. The presence of CHDs, a single umbilical artery, and lower spine anomalies were also included. A general diagnostic guideline required three or more defects to establish the diagnosis (199).

Various types of CHDs have been reported. Traditional clinical analysis of relatively small series has progressed to epidemiologic analyses of registries. An international study with careful phenotyping found CHDs to be significantly associated with VATER defects (199). In contrast, a smaller collaboration suggested that CHDs were not part of the VATER core cluster (200). VATER is generally a sporadic occurrence. However, when VATER occurs with hydrocephalus (especially owing to aqueductal stenosis) and/or is associated with a family history of hydrocephalus, it is viewed as a distinct mendelian disorder (201). Autosomal dominant, X-linked recessive and autosomal recessive inheritance have been described. Because the VATER association is not thought to have a single pathogenetic pathway, it would not be suspected of having a single causative gene. When sonic hedgehog (Shh) signaling is defective in mice, the pattern of defects resembles VATER (202), which may provide insights into the human condition.

Goldenhar Syndrome, First and Second Branchial Arch Syndrome, Hemifacial Microsomia, Facioauriculovertebral Spectrum, and Oculoauriculovertebral Spectrum

Although Goldenhar syndrome is the most familiar eponym, it is perhaps the least accurate description of what is considered a spectrum of craniofacial anomalies (20). Referring to the complex as suspected errors in morphogenesis of the first and second branchial arches is cumbersome though accurate. A practical approach using the acronym OMENS is favored by many craniofacial specialists and builds on the fundamental hemifacial microsomia; the additional defects of eye, mandible, ear, nerve, and soft tissue involvement are added (203). Dysmorphologists prefer the literal terms facioauriculovertebral spectrum (FAVS) and oculoauriculovertebral spectrum (OAVD). A few cases are familial, and autosomal dominant inheritance has been reported. Maternal diabetes is a familiar association (204). Other risk factors that have been studied include vasoactive medications and vascular events (205).

Involvement is usually unilateral with variable hypoplasia of facial structures (including bone, soft tissue, ears, eyes, or mouth). Ear tags or ear pits, epibulbar dermoids (characteristic of Goldenhar syndrome), and deafness are also characteristic. Oral clefts may involve the lip, palate, and corner of the mouth, creating macrostomia. There can be associated vertebral, radial, or rib defects, as well as renal anomalies and midline brain defects (especially agenesis of the corpus callosum, encephalocele, and lipoma). The breadth of associated anomalies has prompted many descriptions of overlapping complexes (206,207).

The largest single-center review noted CHDs in almost 20% of the 32 patients who were defined as having oculoauriculovertebral spectrum (208). The authors acknowledged the wide range of previously reported frequencies (5% to 58%) and attributed this to the selection bias (clinical series, population-based ascertainment) and the variability in case definition. They reported tetralogy of Fallot and ventricular septal defect in about two thirds of those with a CHD, but many other CHDs were noted. The increased frequency of conotruncal CHDs has led many investigators to suspect a role for neural crest cell migration in producing the head and neck anomalies.

Genetics Of Isolated Congenital Heart Defects: *NKX2.5, GATA4, NOTCH1*

Little is known about the genetic basis of isolated, nonsyndromic CHDs although they constitute the vast majority of clinical cases. The evaluation of kindred with multiple affected members has begun to identify specific disease genes for isolated CHDs in recent years. In particular, the transcription factors *NKX2.5* and *GATA4*, and the regulator of cell fate, *NOTCH1*, have been identified as disease genes for a small subset of patients with specific types of nonsyndromic CHDs. These findings and the remaining questions are described below.

NKX2.5

Schott et al. (209) identified four families whose affected members most commonly had atrial septal defects and atri-

oventricular conduction disorders. An informative parametric linkage analysis identified a disease locus on chromosome 5q. The gene, *NKX2.5,* mapped into this locus and was already known to participate in cardiovascular development from animal models. Mutations of *NKX2.5* specific to each family were found in the affected members and were not found in any normal control subjects. Each mutation was predicted to alter the encoded protein function, and most mutations disrupted the highly conserved DNA binding domain. Subsequent reports identified *NKX2.5* mutations in other sporadic and familial cases with atrioventricular conduction abnormalities with or without ASDs (210,211). These studies not only identified the first disease gene for isolated CHD but also made the surprising discovery that *NKX2.5* was critical to atrioventricular (AV) nodal development and function over time.

Because some family members in the original kindred had other types of CHDS, several investigators tested patients with other CHDs and normal AV nodal conduction for mutations of *NKX2.5*. These studies identified primarily missense mutations in a few patients with different lesions including tetralogy of Fallot, double-outlet right ventricle, coarctation of the aorta, and hypoplastic left heart syndrome (212–214). The mutations were not identified in control populations. Unlike patients with AV conduction anomalies, the mutations in these patients were mostly outside the DNA binding domain and only occasionally mapped into other highly conserved domains. Given the type and location of these mutations, it is more difficult to demonstrate that they alter the function of the encoded protein. However, these studies suggest that *NKX2.5* plays an important role in a range of CHDs.

Though investigations continue, it is clear that patients with atrial septal defects and atrioventricular conduction abnormalities are at risk for having a mutation of *NKX2.5*. It is also clear that those patients with *NKX2.5* mutations who present with first-degree AV block can progress to complete heart block over time and even sudden cardiac death if the conduction abnormality goes undiagnosed (212). These data suggest that patients with an atrial septal defect warrant assessment by ECG for AV prolongation. If first-degree AV block is diagnosed, then periodic evaluation for progression to higher grades of AV block seems warranted, even after surgical repair. It would also seem prudent to obtain a detailed family history for signs and symptoms of complete heart block and potentially to screen immediate family members (first-degree relatives) by ECG for subclinical AV conduction abnormalities to identify underlying familial disease. Likewise, the immediate family members of a patient with AV conduction abnormalities with or without other CHDs might warrant similar screening. Mutation studies of *NKX2.5* are not currently clinically available but might help identify the subset of patients with an atrial septal defect at risk for conduction abnormalities.

GATA4

Following the novel studies on *NKX.2.5*, Garg et al. (215) identified mutations in the transcription factor, *GATA4*, in two kindred with septal defects. These findings were of particular interest given that *GATA4*, which maps to chromosome 8p22-p23.1, is a molecular partner with *NKX2.5* and is deleted in some patients with CHDs and chromosome 8p23 deletions. Garg et al. (215) reported a *GATA4* mutation in one kindred in which multiple members had an atrial septal defect, and a second mutation in a different kindred with atrial septal defects, ventricular septal defects, and pulmonary valve stenosis. Subsequent investigators have reported *GATA4* mutations in familial cases of septal defects (210,211). Additional investigations are required to determine the frequency with which *GATA4* mutations are found in sporadic cases with septal or other CHDs. This work, in conjunction with that on *NKX2.5*, highlights the significance of this molecular pathway in cardiovascular development and disease.

NOTCH1

Studies of kindred with multiple affected members continue to identify novel molecular developmental pathways that contribute to cardiovascular disease and development. Most recently, Garg et al. (216) identified mutations in *NOTCH1* in two small families with bicuspid aortic valve and aortic valve stenosis. Of particular interest was that some patients did not have congenital bicuspid aortic valves but developed aortic valve calcification in later decades of life. Experiments confirmed that *NOTCH1* was expressed in the developing aortic valve. Experiments also suggested that *NOTCH1* mutations play a role in aortic valve calcification. Additional studies are required to estimate the frequency with which *NOTCH1* mutations are found in other familial and sporadic cases of aortic valve disease or related left-sided cardiac defects to assess its role in a broader population, but these studies have clearly opened up new avenues of investigation.

GENETICS OF SPECIFIC CARDIAC LESIONS

The growing body of genetic information now allows the clinician to consider whether a patient with a specific type of CHD has an associated genetic alteration (Table 26.5). The clinician needs to consider whether additional genetic consultation or genetic testing is warranted. For example, mutations in *NKX2.5*, *GATA4*, *MYH6*, and *TBX5* have been identified

TABLE 26.5

DISEASE LOCI OR GENES ASSOCIATED WITH SPECIFIC CONGENITAL HEART DEFECTS KNOWN TO DATE

Congenital heart defect	Associated genetic loci or disease genes[a]
Atrial septal defect (with or without atrioventricular conduction blockade)	*TBX5* (Holt–Oram syndrome) *NKX2.5*
Atrial septal defect (without atrioventricular conduction blockade)	*GATA4* *MYH6*
Perimembranous ventricular septal defect	*TBX5* (Holt–Oram syndrome) *GATA4* 22q11 deletion Many syndromes including trisomy 21
Tetralogy of Fallot	*NKX2.5* *JAG1* (Alagille syndrome) *PTPN11* (Noonan syndrome) 22q11 deletion Many syndromes including trisomy 21
Truncus arteriosus	22q11 deletion
Interrupted aortic arch	22q11 deletion
Patent ductus arteriosus	*TFAP2β* (Char syndrome)
Atrioventricular septal defect	*CRELD1* 1p 8p23 Trisomy 21 (21q22)
Heterotaxy syndrome	*ZIC3* *CFC1* Activan Lefty A
Valvar pulmonary stenosis	*JAG1* (Alagille syndrome) *PTPN11 KRAS SOS1* (Noonan syndrome) *HRAS* (Costello syndrome) *BRAF, MEK1/2* (Cardiofaciocutaneous syndrome)
Supravalvar aortic stenosis	Elastin (*ELN*)
Aortic valve stenosis/BAV	*NOTCH1*

BAV, bicuspid aortic valve.
[a]See text for relevant references.

in patients with atrial septal defects (144,209,215,217). Therefore, one can now consider whether a patient with an atrial septal defect has an associated syndrome (such as Holt–Oram syndrome) or mutation in one of these genes. Although clinical testing for mutations in these genes is not currently available, considering these possibilities should at least remind the clinician to review the family history for associated features such as atrioventricular block seen with *NKX2.5* and *TBX5* mutations, or skeletal anomalies seen in Holt–Oram syndrome. Similarly, patients with tetralogy of Fallot may be either syndromic or nonsyndromic and are at risk for different genetic alterations accordingly (Tables 26.1 and 26.5). Therefore, the patient with tetralogy of Fallot should be carefully evaluated for features of one of the known associated syndromes including trisomy 21, 22q11 deletions, and *JAG1* mutations. The family history should be carefully reviewed for CHDs or associated syndromic features that might suggest a 22q11 deletion or *JAG1* mutation, for example. Table 26.5 lists known genetic alterations associated with specific CHDs to help the clinician move from the cardiac to a concurrent genetic diagnosis. Since all of these CHDs are genetically heterogeneous, this table can list only the currently known associated disease genes. As new diagnostic tests and clinical discoveries are made, this list is likely to become more extensive and clinically relevant. Of course, many other genetic syndromes associated with each CHD are known; only those with recognized specific genetic alterations are listed here.

GENETIC EVALUATION AND COUNSELING

Although most of the care for a patient with CHD focuses on the diagnosis and treatment of the heart itself, it is critical for the referring primary care provider and the cardiologist to consider whether genetic consultation and counseling is warranted both at the time of diagnosis of the CHD and in later years. The chances of finding additional congenital anomalies or syndromic features in a patient with a CHD are high. Approximately 20% to 25% of infants ≤1 year of age have a noncardiac malformation, and approximately 5% to 17% have a genetic syndrome (9,27,218–221). The diagnosis of a genetic syndrome is more likely when growth and developmental delay are also present. Therefore, clinicians must examine the patient with a CHD with a critical eye for dysmorphic features, changes in body habitus, other congenital anomalies, neurocognitive deficits, or a family history of these same findings. Even in the apparent absence of dysmorphic features or other congenital anomalies, patients with certain CHDs should be suspect for genetic syndromes based on the known frequency of such associations. For example, the patient with interrupted aortic arch type B is so commonly found to have a 22q11 deletion that referral for genetic consultation and testing should be considered even in the absence of overt dysmorphic features. Finally, given the highly variable and often subtle presentation of many genetic syndromes, a concurrent genetic diagnosis can be easily overlooked or delayed if a high level of suspicion and willingness to seek genetic consultation is not maintained.

Importance of Identifying a Genetic Syndrome or Alteration

Identifying the underlying genetic syndrome or alteration in a patient with a CHD is of growing clinical importance. First, diagnosing the patient with a genetic syndrome allows the early identification and treatment of associated *noncardiac* features. For example, the patient found to carry a 22q11 deletion can be evaluated and treated for commonly associated noncardiac features such as feeding disorders, palate anomalies, speech disturbances, hypocalcemia, and others. Knowing that a patient with a CHD has a 22q11 deletion is important to define the cause of subsequent feeding disorders and failure to thrive, which might otherwise be accredited to heart failure alone. Second, establishing a specific genetic cause allows for appropriate family counseling regarding risks of recurrence (222). For example, parents of a patient with Alagille syndrome should be tested to determine if one of the parents is a potential carrier of a *JAG1* mutation since the parent with only subtle syndromic manifestations carrying the mutation has a 50% chance of having a second affected child. Depending on the age of the individual and circumstances, the geneticist may provide information about prenatal diagnosis including options for imaging the fetal heart and obtaining appropriate genetic tests. Third, establishing a genetic diagnosis in the future will most likely allow more accurate counseling regarding cardiac and noncardiac clinical outcome. Several studies suggest that specific genetic syndromes are associated with a worse clinical cardiac prognosis (1–4). Finally, for many patients and their families, knowing whether a CHD is associated with an identifiable cause such as a chromosome abnormality, gene mutation, or genetic risk factor can be important. Ultimately, determining the patient genetic phenotype is essential to provide more accurate clinical care, estimation of prognosis, and assessment of risk (Table I in [223]). In the future, genotype may in part influence management strategy.

When to Refer the Cardiac Patient for a Genetics Evaluation

The increasing number of possible genetic diagnoses and the rapid development of new genetic tests necessitates a close collaboration between the referring primary physician, cardiologist, and clinical geneticist. Much depends on the cardiologist's diagnostic ability, interest, and time to determine if a CHD is isolated, part of a familial CHD syndrome, or associated with other defects of a known syndrome or as of yet uncharacterized complex (25). Consultation from a clinical geneticist should be sought for the cardiac patient with the following: Dysmorphic features, multiple congenital anomalies, neurocognitive deficits, or a family history of CHD, congenital anomalies, or neurocognitive deficits. Although, historically, learning disabilities or developmental delay have been attributed to the cardiac defect and surgical intervention, instead these observations may prove to be independent problems that may indicate the presence of a genetic syndrome or chromosomal alteration. Families may also benefit from a genetic consultation for counseling purposes, particularly with respect to risks of recurrence. Early referral to a clinical geneticist allows the early diagnosis of associated noncardiac features, as well as early intervention and timely counseling. Finally, sometimes the primary care taker or cardiologist orders the basic genetic tests to screen for abnormalities with the intention of consulting genetics if an abnormality is discovered. However, this practice may greatly underserve the patient with no detectable chromosomal alteration who nonetheless may have a genetic syndrome or the patient who could benefit from more specialized genetic testing. Thus, genetic consultation should be considered in the suspicious patient to allow for specialized assessment and direction of genetic testing.

The Genetic Evaluation

The goal of the genetic evaluation is to establish a diagnosis and provide information to the patient and family about recurrence risk and expected outcomes that are known (222). The evaluation therefore considers both the patient under evaluation and the family medical history in detail. Geneticists will first consider the specific type of CHD and associated congenital anomalies present in the patient. The geneticist (or genetic counselor) then obtains a complete family history of malformations and genetic conditions, including malformation syndromes (222). Information is also sought about recurrent miscarriages, sudden death in childhood, developmental delays, and mental retardation.

The geneticist's physical exam begins with an overall appraisal of habitus, facial appearance, and movements. Occasionally when an immediate general impression based on characteristic dysmorphic features provides rapid diagnosis, restraint and confirmation is needed. In addition to height, weight, and head circumference, measurements may be made of facial landmarks and distances, or other body parts to quantify the qualitative sense of hypertelorism, small pinnae, or long fingers. Most geneticists do not perform complete neurodevelopmental examinations, substituting modified office screening tests, reports from family members, previous formal testing, or functional appraisal of the individual's interactions and performance in the office setting.

Depending on whether the consultation is performed during an admission to the hospital or as an out-patient visit, emergently or as a scheduled visit, and whether the location is the tertiary care center or a small satellite clinic, diagnostic testing can be performed at the same time as the initial evaluation or requested to be obtained under the direction of the primary care giver and/or cardiologist. Radiographic and ultrasonographic tests may be ordered to define internal organ structure and function. Medical, educational, and therapeutic specialists may be requested to characterize multisystem involvement, and to begin treatment.

Genetic Testing

The most commonly requested genetics tests include a cytogenetic examination ordered as a karyotype of lymphocytes in fresh whole blood. A FISH analysis is complementary to a standard chromosome analysis, which can be useful for rapid diagnosis (e.g., amniocentesis diagnosis of trisomy) and to detect small telomeric deletions. The most recent technique for detecting an alteration of DNA quantity in an individual is called comparative genomic hybridization (CGH).

When a Mendelian gene disorder is suspected, geneticists determine if molecular testing is available and whether the testing is being done at a research or clinical lab. Details are sought from the referral laboratory and literature. Before testing can be done, the genetics team needs to know if the laboratory is approved to report clinical results, how specimens are shipped, the cost and potential for reimbursement by insurance, the length of time it takes to complete the test, and how results are communicated. This process can consume as much time as the genetics examination itself.

Practically speaking, the timing and location of having these tests completed may be determined more by medical insurance coverage and less by referring physician or patient preference. Likewise, whether the individual will be permitted to return for a follow-up genetics visit is highly dependent on health care coverage. Regardless of whether the genetics evaluation was conducted on a critically ill neonate on an emergent basis, or during an extensive consultation with the extended family of multiply affected individuals, communication and collaboration with the cardiologist is essential. Of course, the primary care physician and the individual (and family) should be included in all discussions.

A Partnership

Since approximately 75% of CHDs currently have no identifiable cause (9,24,27,218–221) or underlying condition, the notion of a formal genetic evaluation may appear to be unnecessary in many cases. However, the list of genetic causes of CHDs is expanding rapidly and is ever more difficult to understand, and many syndromes are now recognized to present with subtle and often unrecognized features. As the list of genetic causes for CHDs continues to expand in length and complexity, and the list of genetic syndromes associated with CHDs grows as well, there is clearly a need for clinical partnership between primary caretakers, cardiologists, and geneticists. In many cases, the primary care taker and cardiologist will call on the geneticist for consultation as described in the previous sections. For example, when coarctation is confirmed in a young girl who is noted subsequently to have short stature, redundant neck skin, and low-set ears, the geneticist can confirm the suspected diagnosis of Turner syndrome and provide long-term counseling to the patient and family. In other cases, the geneticist may call on the cardiologist to define the associated CHD in a patient under consideration for a particular genetic syndrome to assist with the diagnosis. For example, a geneticist may consider the diagnosis of Holt–Oram syndrome in a three-generation family with absent and unusual thumbs. Although *TBX5* mutation studies would be confirmatory, speedier diagnostic support would be provided by two-dimensional echocardiographic detection of a secundum ASD in mother and son.

It can be difficult to coordinate the cardiology and genetics consultations (223). Instead of being evaluated at different times, some patients are seen in cardiovascular genetics clinics with genetics and cardiology specialists working in tandem. With the assistance of supplemental imaging of other organs; confirmatory cytogenetic, molecular, or metabolic blood tests; and the proven test of time, clinicians may make a unifying diagnosis to enhance each case.

CONCLUSIONS

In concert with the field of human genetics, our understanding of the genetic contribution to CHDs has advanced dramatically over the last 10 years. The field has moved from detailing genetic syndromes to the definition of specific genetic alterations causing those clinical phenotypes. Specific genetic causes of isolated CHDs have also begun to be identified. The remarkable and rapid advancements in human genetics and developmental biology are likely to lead to new discoveries in the field of cardiovascular genetics in the near future. Given these discoveries, an increasing number of patients with a CHD could be given a concurrent genetic diagnosis. It will be of increasing importance for the cardiologist caring for patients with CHDs to have a working knowledge of these discoveries and available genetic testing. It will also be increasingly important for the general pediatrician and cardiologist to work in concert with the clinical geneticists and genetic counselors to identify concurrent genetic diagnoses. The clinical implications of the associated genetic diagnosis, such as associated noncardiac features, will be increasingly important to recognize and address. In the future, genotype-specific management strategies and outcomes may result from these discoveries. Most important, understanding the genetic basis of these disorders, in conjunction with advances in developmental biology, will improve our understanding of cardiovascular development and disease and allow for novel, improved management strategies.

References

1. Gaynor JW, Mahle WT, Cohen MI, et al. Risk factors for mortality after the Norwood procedure. *Eur J Cardiothorac Surg* 2002;22(1):82–89.
2. Mahle WT, Crisalli J, Coleman K, et al. Deletion of chromosome 22q11.2 and outcome in patients with pulmonary atresia and ventricular septal defect. *Ann Thorac Surg* 2003;76(2):567–571.
3. Michielon G, Marino B, Formigari R, et al. Genetic syndromes and outcome after surgical correction of tetralogy of Fallot. *Ann Thorac Surg* 2006;81(3):968–975.
4. Anaclerio S, Di Ciommo V, Michielon G, et al. Conotruncal heart defects: Impact of genetic syndromes on immediate operative mortality. *Ital Heart J* 2004;5(8):624–628.
5. Cripe L, Andelfinger G, Martin LJ, et al. Bicuspid aortic valve is heritable. *J Am Coll Cardiol* 2004;44(1):138–143.
6. Lewin MB, McBride KL, Pignatelli R, et al. Echocardiographic evaluation of asymptomatic parental and sibling cardiovascular anomalies associated with congenital left ventricular outflow tract lesions. *Pediatrics* 2004;114(3):691–696.
7. Loffredo CA, Chokkalingam A, Sill AM, et al. Prevalence of congenital cardiovascular malformations among relatives of infants with hypoplastic left heart, coarctation of the aorta, and d-transposition of the great arteries. *Am J Med Genet A* 2004;124(3):225–230.
8. Boughman JA, Berg KA, Astemborski JA, et al. Familial risks of congenital heart defect assessed in a population-based epidemiologic study. *Am J Med Genet* 1987;26(4):839–849.
9. Hanna EJ, Nevin NC, Nelson J. Genetic study of congenital heart defects in Northern Ireland (1974–1978). *J Med Genet* 1994;31(11):858–863.
10. Calzolari E, Garani G, Cocchi G, et al. Congenital heart defects: 15 years of experience of the Emilia-Romagna Registry (Italy). *Eur J Epidemiol* 2003;18(8):773–780.
11. Nora JJ, Nora AH. Update on counseling the family with a first-degree relative with a congenital heart defect. *Am J Med Genet* 1988;29(1):137–142.
12. Vissers LE, van Ravenswaaij CM, Admiraal R, et al. Mutations in a new member of the chromodomain gene family cause CHARGE syndrome. *Nat Genet* 2004;36(9):955–957.
13. Nora JJ, Nora AH. Genetic and environmental factors in the etiology of congenital heart diseases. *South Med J* 1976;69(7):919–926.
14. Burn J, Brennan P, Little J, et al. Recurrence risks in offspring of adults with major heart defects: Results from first cohort of British collaborative study. *Lancet* 1998;351:311–316.
15. Gill HK, Splitt M, Sharland GK, et al. Patterns of recurrence of congenital heart disease: An analysis of 6,640 consecutive pregnancies evaluated by detailed fetal echocardiography. *J Am Coll Cardiol* 2003;42(5):923–929.
16. Pradat P. Recurrence risk for major congenital heart defects in Sweden: A registry study. *Genet Epidemiol* 1994;11(2):131–140.
17. Nora JJ, Nora AH. Maternal transmission of congenital heart diseases: New recurrence risk figures and the questions of cytoplasmic inheritance and vulnerability to teratogens. *Am J Cardiol* 1987;59(5):459–463.
18. Whittemore R, Wells JA, Castellsague X. A second-generation study of 427 probands with congenital heart defects and their 837 children. *J Am Coll Cardiol* 1994;23(6):1459–1467.
19. McBride KL, Pignatelli R, Lewin M, et al. Inheritance analysis of congenital left ventricular outflow tract obstruction malformations: Segregation, multiplex relative risk, and heritability. *Am J Med Genet A* 2005;134(2):180–186.
20. Jones K. *Smith's Recognizable Patterns of Human Malformation*. 6th ed. Philadelphia: Elsevier Sanders, 2005.
21. Brewer C, Holloway S, Zawalnyski P, et al. A chromosomal deletion map of human malformations. *Am J Hum Genet* 1998;63(4):1153–1159.
22. van Karnebeek CD, Hennekam RC. Associations between chromosomal anomalies and congenital heart defects: A database search. *Am J Med Genet* 1999;84(2):158–166.
23. Gorlin R, Cohen MM, Hennekam RCM. *Syndromes of the Head and Neck*. Oxford: Oxford University Press; 2001.
24. Burn J, Goodship J. Congenital Heart Disease. In: Rimoin D, Connor J, Pyeritz R, et al., eds. *Emery and Rimoin's Principles and Practice of Medical Genetics*. London: Churchill Livingstone, 2002:1239–1326.
25. Lacro R. Dysmorphology. In: Keane JF, Lock LJ, Fyler DC, ed. *Nadas' Pediatric Cardiology*. Boston: WB Saunders; 2006.
26. Lin AE, Belmont J, Ghaffar S. The Heart. In: Stevenson RE, Hall JG, eds. *Human Malformations and Related Anomalies*. 2nd ed. New York: Oxford University Press; 2006:85–120.
27. Ferencz C, Loffredo CA, Corea-Villasenor A, et al. *Genetic and Environmental Risk Factors of Major Congenital Heart Defects: The Baltimore-Washington Infant Study: 1981–1989*. Armonk, NY: Futura Publishing, 1997.
28. Botto LD, May K, Fernhoff PM, et al. A population-based study of the 22q11.2 deletion: Phenotype, incidence, and contribution to major birth defects in the population. *Pediatrics* 2003;112(1 pt 1):101–107.
29. Chinn A, Fitzsimmons J, Shepard TH, et al. Congenital heart disease among spontaneous abortuses and stillborn fetuses: Prevalence and associations. *Teratology* 1989;40(5):475–482.
30. Freeman SB, Taft LF, Dooley KJ, et al. Population-based study of congenital heart defects in Down syndrome. *Am J Med Genet* 1998;80(3):213–217.
31. McElhinney DB, Straka M, Goldmuntz E, et al. Correlation between abnormal cardiac physical examination and echocardiographic findings in neonates with Down syndrome. *Am J Med Genet* 2002;113(3):238–241.
32. Centers for Disease Control and Prevention (CDC). Improved national prevalence estimates for 18 selected major birth defects—United States, 1999–2001. *MMWR Morb Mort Wkly Rep* 2005;54:1301–1305.
33. Wessels MW, Los FJ, Frohn-Mulder IM, et al. Poor outcome in Down syndrome fetuses with cardiac anomalies or growth retardation. *Am J Med Genet A* 2003;116(2):147–151.
34. Yang Q, Rasmussen SA, Friedman JM. Mortality associated with Down syndrome in the USA from 1983 to 1997: A population-based study. *Lancet* 2002;359:1019–1025.
35. Reller MD, Morris CD. Is Down syndrome a risk factor for poor outcome after repair of congenital heart defects? *J Pediatr* 1998;132(4):738–741.
36. Marino B, Diociaiuti L, Calcagni G, et al. Outcome in Down syndrome fetuses with cardiac anomalies. *Am J Med Genet A* 2004;128(1):101–102; author reply 103.
37. Marino B, de Zorzi A. Congenital heart disease in trisomy 21 mosaicism. *J Pediatr* 1993;122(3):500–501.
38. Barlow GM, Chen XN, Shi ZY, et al. Down syndrome congenital heart disease: A narrowed region and a candidate gene. *Genet Med* 2001;3(2):91–101.
39. Van Praagh S, Truman T, Firpo A, et al. Cardiac malformations in trisomy-18: A study of 41 postmortem cases. *J Am Coll Cardiol* 1989;13(7): 1586–1597.
40. Balderston SM, Shaffer EM, Washington RL, et al. Congenital polyvalvular disease in trisomy 18: Echocardiographic diagnosis. *Pediatr Cardiol* 1990;11(3):138–142.
41. Musewe NN, Alexander DJ, Teshima I, et al. Echocardiographic evaluation of the spectrum of cardiac anomalies associated with trisomy 13 and trisomy 18. *J Am Coll Cardiol* 1990;15(3):673–677.
42. Embleton ND, Wyllie JP, Wright MJ, et al. Natural history of trisomy 18. *Arch Dis Child Fetal Neonatal Ed* 1996;75(1):F38–41.
43. Rasmussen SA, Wong LY, Yang Q, et al. Population-based analyses of mortality in trisomy 13 and trisomy 18. *Pediatrics* 2003;111(4 pt 1):777–784.
44. Boghosian-Sell L, Mewar R, Harrison W, et al. Molecular mapping of the Edwards syndrome phenotype to two noncontiguous regions on chromosome 18. *Am J Hum Genet* 1994;55(3):476–483.
45. Nielsen J, Wohlert M. Sex chromosome abnormalities found among 34,910 newborn children: Results from a 13-year incidence study in Arhus, Denmark. *Birth Defects Orig Artic Ser* 1990;26(4):209–223.
46. Sybert VP, McCauley E. Turner's syndrome. *N Engl J Med* 2004;351Z: 1227–1238.
47. Mazzanti L, Cacciari E. Congenital heart disease in patients with Turner's syndrome. Italian Study Group for Turner Syndrome (ISGTS). *J Pediatr* 1998;133(5):688–692.
48. Loscalzo ML, Van PL, Ho VB, et al. Association between fetal lymphedema and congenital cardiovascular defects in Turner syndrome. *Pediatrics* 2005;115(3):732–735.
49. Ostberg JE, Brookes JA, McCarthy C, et al. A comparison of echocardiography and magnetic resonance imaging in cardiovascular screening of adults with Turner syndrome. *J Clin Endocrinol Metab* 2004;89(12):5966–5971.
50. Ho VB, Bakalov VK, Cooley M, et al. Major vascular anomalies in Turner syndrome: Prevalence and magnetic resonance angiographic features. *Circulation* 2004;110(12):1694–1700.
51. Lacro RV, Jones KL, Benirschke K. Coarctation of the aorta in Turner syndrome: A pathologic study of fetuses with nuchal cystic hygromas, hydrops fetalis, and female genitalia. *Pediatrics* 1988;81(3):445–451.

52. Bondy CA. Turner Syndrome Study Group. Care of Girls and Women with Turner syndrome: A guideline of the Turner Syndrome Study Group. *J Clin Endocrinol Metab* 2007; 92:10–25.

53. Ostberg JE, Donald AE, Halcox JP, et al. Vasculopathy in Turner syndrome: Arterial dilatation and intimal thickening without endothelial dysfunction. *J Clin Endocrinol Metab* 2005;90(9):5161–5166.

54. Gravholt CH, Landin-Wilhelmsen K, Stochholm K, et al. Clinical and epidemiological description of aortic dissection in Turner's syndrome. *Cardiol Young* 2006;16(5):430–436.

55. Lin AE, Lippe B, Rosenfeld RG. Further delineation of aortic dilation, dissection, and rupture in patients with Turner syndrome. *Pediatrics* 1998;102(1):e12.

56. Gravholt CH, Hansen KW, Erlandsen M, et al. Nocturnal hypertension and impaired sympathovagal tone in Turner syndrome. *J Hypertens* 2006;24(2):353–360.

57. Karnis MF, Zimon AE, Lalwani SI, et al. Risk of death in pregnancy achieved through oocyte donation in patients with Turner syndrome: A national survey. *Fertil Steril* 2003;80(3):498–501.

58. Bondy CA, Van PL, Bakalov VK, et al. Growth hormone treatment and aortic dimensions in Turner syndrome. *J Clin Endocrinol Metab* 2006;91(5):1785–1788.

59. van den Berg J, Bannink EM, Wielopolski PA, et al. Aortic distensibility and dimensions and the effects of growth hormone treatment in the Turner syndrome. *Am J Cardiol* 2006;97(11):1644–1649.

60. Lopez L, Boukas K, Carey H, et al. 45,X karyotype and bicuspid aortic valve are independent risk factors for aortic root enlargement in Turner Syndrome [abstract]. *Circulation* 2004;110:III–389.

61. https://www.ohsu.edu/pedscardturner/TSform-test.htm accessed 4/23/07.

62. Elsheikh M, Dunger DB, Conway GS, et al. Turner's syndrome in adulthood. *Endocr Rev* 2002;23(1):120–140.

63. Bondy CA, Ceniceros I, Van PL, et al. Prolonged rate-corrected QT interval and other electrocardiogram abnormalities in girls with Turner syndrome. *Pediatrics* 2006;118(4):e1220–1225.

64. Kirkpatrick JA Jr, DiGeorge AM. Congenital absence of the thymus. *Am J Roentgenol Radium Ther Nucl Med* 1968;103(1):32–37.

65. Conley ME, Beckwith JB, Mancer JF, et al. The spectrum of the DiGeorge syndrome. *J Pediatr* 1979;94(6):883–890.

66. Scambler PJ, Carey AH, Wyse RK, et al. Microdeletions within 22q11 associated with sporadic and familial DiGeorge syndrome. *Genomics* 1991;10(1):201–206.

67. Driscoll DA, Budarf ML, Emanuel BS. A genetic etiology for DiGeorge syndrome: Consistent deletions and microdeletions of 22q11. *Am J Hum Genet* 1992;50(5):924–933.

68. Shprintzen RJ, Goldberg RB, Lewin ML, et al. A new syndrome involving cleft palate, cardiac anomalies, typical facies, and learning disabilities: Velo-cardio-facial syndrome. *Cleft Palate J* 1978;15(1):56–62.

69. Kinouchi A, Mori K, Ando M, et al. Facial appearance of patients with conotruncal abnormalities. *Pediat Jpn* 1976;17:84.

70. Driscoll DA, Spinner NB, Budarf ML, et al. Deletions and microdeletions of 22q11.2 in velo-cardio-facial syndrome. *Am J Med Genet* 1992;44(2):261–268.

71. Burn J, Takao A, Wilson D, et al. Conotruncal anomaly face syndrome is associated with a deletion within chromosome 22q11. *J Med Genet* 1993;30(10):822–824.

72. Greenberg F. DiGeorge syndrome: An historical review of clinical and cytogenetic features. *J Med Genet* 1993;30(10):803–806.

73. Oskarsdottir S, Vujic M, Fasth A. Incidence and prevalence of the 22q11 deletion syndrome: A population-based study in Western Sweden. *Arch Dis Child* 2004;89(2):148–151.

74. Digilio MC, Angioni A, De Santis M, et al. Spectrum of clinical variability in familial deletion 22q11.2: From full manifestation to extremely mild clinical anomalies. *Clin Genet* 2003;63(4):308–313.

75. Goldmuntz E. DiGeorge syndrome: New insights. *Clin Perinatol* 2005;32(4):963–978, ix–x.

76. McDonald-McGinn DM, Minugh-Purvis N, Kirschner RE, et al. The 22q11.2 deletion in African-American patients: An underdiagnosed population? *Am J Med Genet* 2005;134(3):242–246.

77. McDonald-McGinn DM, LaRossa D, Goldmuntz E, et al. The 22q11.2 deletion: Screening, diagnostic workup, and outcome of results; report on 181 patients. *Genet Test* 1997;1(2):99–108.

78. Ryan AK, Goodship JA, Wilson DI, et al. Spectrum of clinical features associated with interstitial chromosome 22q11 deletions: A European collaborative study. *J Med Genet* 1997;34(10):798–804.

79. Shooner KA, Rope AF, Hopkin RJ, et al. Genetic analyses in two extended families with deletion 22q11 syndrome: Importance of extracardiac manifestations. *J Pediatr* 2005;146(3):382–387.

80. Goldmuntz E, Clark BJ, Mitchell LE, et al. Frequency of 22q11 deletions in patients with conotruncal defects. *J Am Coll Cardiol* 1998;32(2):492–498.

81. McElhinney DB, Clark BJ 3rd, Weinberg PM, et al. Association of chromosome 22q11 deletion with isolated anomalies of aortic arch laterality and branching. *J Am Coll Cardiol* 2001;37(8):2114–2119.

82. McElhinney DB, Driscoll DA, Levin ER, et al. Chromosome 22q11 deletion in patients with ventricular septal defect: Frequency and associated cardiovascular anomalies. *Pediatrics* 2003;112(6 pt 1):e472.

83. Momma K, Ando M, Matsuoka R. Truncus arteriosus communis associated with chromosome 22q11 deletion. *J Am Coll Cardiol* 1997;30(4):1067–1071.

84. Momma K, Kondo C, Matsuoka R. Tetralogy of Fallot with pulmonary atresia associated with chromosome 22q11 deletion. *J Am Coll Cardiol* 1996;27(1):198–202.

85. Frohn-Mulder IM, Wesby Swaay E, Bouwhuis C, et al. Chromosome 22q11 deletions in patients with selected outflow tract malformations. *Genet Couns* 1999;10(1):35–41.

86. Lewin MB, Lindsay EA, Jurecic V, et al. A genetic etiology for interruption of the aortic arch type B. *Am J Cardiol* 1997;80(4):493–497.

87. Takahashi K, Kido S, Hoshino K, et al. Frequency of a 22q11 deletion in patients with conotruncal cardiac malformations: A prospective study. *Eur J Pediatr* 1995;154(11):878–881.

88. Iserin L, de Lonlay P, Viot G, et al. Prevalence of the microdeletion 22q11 in newborn infants with congenital conotruncal cardiac anomalies. *Eur J Pediatr* 1998;157(11):881–884.

89. Amati F, Mari A, Digilio MC, et al. 22q11 deletions in isolated and syndromic patients with tetralogy of Fallot. *Hum Genet* 1995;95(5):479–482.

90. Johnson MC, Strauss AW, Dowton SB, et al. Deletion within chromosome 22 is common in patients with absent pulmonary valve syndrome. *Am J Cardiol* 1995;76(1):66–69.

91. Pierpont ME, Basson CT, Benson DW, et al. The genetic basis for congenital heart defects: Current knowledge. *Circulation.* In press.

92. McElhinney DB, McDonald-McGinn D, Zackai EH, et al. Cardiovascular anomalies in patients diagnosed with a chromosome 22q11 deletion beyond 6 months of age. *Pediatrics* 2001;108(6):E104.

93. Johnson TR, Goldmuntz E, McDonald-McGinn DM, et al. Cardiac magnetic resonance imaging for accurate diagnosis of aortic arch anomalies in patients with 22q11.2 deletion. *Am J Cardiol* 2005;96(12):1726–1730.

94. Baldini A. DiGeorge syndrome: The use of model organisms to dissect complex genetics. *Hum Mol Genet* 2002;11(20):2363–2369.

95. Baldini A. Dissecting contiguous gene defects: TBX1. *Curr Opin Genet Dev* 2005;15(3):279–284.

96. Yamagishi H, Srivastava D. Unraveling the genetic and developmental mysteries of 22q11 deletion syndrome. *Trends Mol Med* 2003;9(9):383–389.

97. Yagi H, Furutani Y, Hamada H, et al. Role of TBX1 in human del22q11.2 syndrome. *Lancet* 2003;362:1366–1373.

98. Morris CA, Mervis CB. Williams syndrome and related disorders. *Annu Rev Genomics Hum Genet* 2000;1:461–484.

99. Kruse K, Pankau R, Gosch A, et al. Calcium metabolism in Williams-Beuren syndrome. *J Pediatr* 1992;121(6):902–907.

100. Mervis CB, Robinson BF, Bertrand J, et al. The Williams syndrome cognitive profile. *Brain Cogn* 2000;44(3):604–628.

101. Kececioglu D, Kotthoff S, Vogt J. Williams-Beuren syndrome: A 30-year follow-up of natural and postoperative course. *Eur Heart J* 1993;14(11):1458–1464.

102. Eronen M, Peippo M, Hiippala A, et al. Cardiovascular manifestations in 75 patients with Williams syndrome. *J Med Genet* 2002;39(8):554–558.

103. Kim YM, Yoo SJ, Choi JY, et al. Natural course of supravalvar aortic stenosis and peripheral pulmonary arterial stenosis in Williams' syndrome. *Cardiol Young* 1999;9(1):37–41.

104. Wessel A, Pankau R, Kececioglu D, et al. Three decades of follow-up of aortic and pulmonary vascular lesions in the Williams-Beuren syndrome. *Am J Med Genet* 1994;52(3):297–301.

105. Cherniske EM, Carpenter TO, Klaiman C, et al. Multisystem study of 20 older adults with Williams syndrome. *Am J Med Genet A* 2004;131(3):255–264.

106. Bird LM, Billman GF, Lacro RV, et al. Sudden death in Williams syndrome: Report of ten cases. *J Pediatr* 1996;129(6):926–931.

107. Curran ME, Atkinson DL, Ewart AK, et al. The elastin gene is disrupted by a translocation associated with supravalvular aortic stenosis. *Cell* 1993;73(1):159–168.

108. Li DY, Toland AE, Boak BB, et al. Elastin point mutations cause an obstructive vascular disease, supravalvular aortic stenosis. *Hum Mol Genet* 1997;6(7):1021–1028.

109. Metcalfe K, Rucka AK, Smoot L, et al. Elastin: Mutational spectrum in supravalvular aortic stenosis. *Eur J Hum Genet* 2000;8(12):955–963.

110. Frangiskakis JM, Ewart AK, Morris CA, et al. LIM-kinase1 hemizygosity implicated in impaired visuospatial constructive cognition. *Cell* 1996;86(1):59–69.

111. Tassabehji M, Metcalfe K, Hurst J, et al. An elastin gene mutation producing abnormal tropoelastin and abnormal elastic fibres in a patient with autosomal dominant cutis laxa. *Hum Mol Genet* 1998;7(6):1021–1028.

112. Zhang MC, He L, Giro M, et al. Cutis laxa arising from frameshift mutations in exon 30 of the elastin gene (ELN). *J Biol Chem* 1999;274(2):981–986.

113. Flint J, Wilkie AO, Buckle VJ, et al. The detection of subtelomeric chromosomal rearrangements in idiopathic mental retardation. *Nat Genet* 1995;9(2):132–140.

114. Knight SJ, Regan R, Nicod A, et al. Subtle chromosomal rearrangements in children with unexplained mental retardation. *Lancet* 1999;354:1676–1681.

115. de Vries BB, White SM, Knight SJ, et al. Clinical studies on submicroscopic subtelomeric rearrangements: A checklist. *J Med Genet* 2001;38(3):145–150.

116. De Vries BB, Winter R, Schinzel A, et al. Telomeres: A diagnosis at the end of the chromosomes. *J Med Genet* 2003;40(6):385–398.

117. Ravnan JB, Tepperberg JH, Papenhausen P, et al. Subtelomere FISH analysis of 11 688 cases: An evaluation of the frequency and pattern of subtelomere rearrangements in individuals with developmental disabilities. *J Med Genet* 2006;43(6):478–489.

118. Slavotinek A, Shaffer LG, Shapira SK. Monosomy 1p36. *J Med Genet* 1999;36(9):657–663.

119. Heilstedt HA, Ballif BC, Howard LA, et al. Physical map of 1p36, placement of breakpoints in monosomy 1p36, and clinical characterization of the syndrome. *Am J Hum Genet* 2003;72(5):1200–1212.

120. Stewart DR, Huang A, Faravelli F, et al. Subtelomeric deletions of chromosome 9q: A novel microdeletion syndrome. *Am J Med Genet A* 2004;128(4):340–351.

121. Watson GH, Miller V. Arteriohepatic dysplasia: Familial pulmonary arterial stenosis with neonatal liver disease. *Arch Dis Child* 1973;48(6):459–466.

122. Alagille D, Odievre M, Gautier M, et al. Hepatic ductular hypoplasia associated with characteristic facies, vertebral malformations, retarded physical, mental, and sexual development, and cardiac murmur. *J Pediatr* 1975;86(1):63–71.

123. Spinner NB, Rand EB, Fortina P, et al. Cytologically balanced t(2;20) in a two-generation family with Alagille syndrome: Cytogenetic and molecular studies. *Am J Hum Genet* 1994;55(2):238–243.

124. Krantz ID, Rand EB, Genin A, et al. Deletions of 20p12 in Alagille syndrome: Frequency and molecular characterization. *Am J Med Genet* 1997;70(1):80–86.

125. Byrne JL, Harrod MJ, Friedman JM, et al. del(20p) with manifestations of arteriohepatic dysplasia. *Am J Med Genet* 1986;24(4):673–678.

126. Pollet N, Boccaccio C, Dhorne-Pollet S, et al. Construction of an integrated physical and gene map of human chromosome 20p12 providing candidate genes for Alagille syndrome. *Genomics* 1997;42(3):489–498.

127. Li L, Krantz ID, Deng Y, et al. Alagille syndrome is caused by mutations in human Jagged1, which encodes a ligand for Notch1. *Nat Genet* 1997;16(3):243–251.

128. Oda T, Elkahloun AG, Pike BL, et al. Mutations in the human Jagged1 gene are responsible for Alagille syndrome. *Nat Genet* 1997;16(3):235–242.

129. Warthen DM, Moore EC, Kamath BM, et al. Jagged1 (JAG1) mutations in Alagille syndrome: Increasing the mutation detection rate. *Hum Mutat* 2006;27(5):436–443.

130. Spinner NB, Colliton RP, Crosnier C, et al. Jagged1 mutations in Alagille syndrome. *Hum Mutat* 2001;17(1):18–33.

131. McElhinney DB, Krantz ID, Bason L, et al. Analysis of cardiovascular phenotype and genotype-phenotype correlation in individuals with a JAG1 mutation and/or Alagille syndrome. *Circulation* 2002;106(20):2567–2574.

132. Krantz ID, Smith R, Colliton RP, et al. Jagged1 mutations in patients ascertained with isolated congenital heart defects. *Am J Med Genet* 1999;84(1):56–60.

133. Eldadah ZA, Hamosh A, Biery NJ, et al. Familial tetralogy of Fallot caused by mutation in the jagged1 gene. *Hum Mol Genet* 2001;10(2):163–169.

134. Kamath BM, Spinner NB, Emerick KM, et al. Vascular anomalies in Alagille syndrome: A significant cause of morbidity and mortality. *Circulation* 2004;109(11):1354–1358.

135. Xue Y, Gao X, Lindsell CE, et al. Embryonic lethality and vascular defects in mice lacking the Notch ligand Jagged1. *Hum Mol Genet* 1999;8(5):723–730.

136. McCright B, Lozier J, Gridley T. A mouse model of Alagille syndrome: Notch2 as a genetic modifier of Jag1 haploinsufficiency. *Development* 2002;129(4):1075–1082.

137. McDaniell R, Warthen DM, Sanchez-Lara PA, et al. NOTCH2 mutations cause Alagille syndrome, a heterogeneous disorder of the notch signaling pathway. *Am J Hum Genet* 2006;79(1):169–173.

138. Basson CT, Cowley GS, Solomon SD, et al. The clinical and genetic spectrum of the Holt-Oram syndrome (heart-hand syndrome). *N Engl J Med* 1994;330:885–891.

139. Newbury-Ecob RA, Leanage R, Raeburn JA, et al. Holt-Oram syndrome: A clinical genetic study. *J Med Genet* 1996;33(4):300–307.

140. Bruneau BG, Logan M, Davis N, et al. Chamber-specific cardiac expression of Tbx5 and heart defects in Holt-Oram syndrome. *Dev Biol* 1999;211(1):100–108.

141. Bonnet D, Pelet A, Legeai-Mallet L, et al. A gene for Holt-Oram syndrome maps to the distal long arm of chromosome 12. *Nat Genet* 1994;6(4):405–408.

142. Terrett JA, Newbury-Ecob R, Cross GS, et al. Holt-Oram syndrome is a genetically heterogeneous disease with one locus mapping to human chromosome 12q. *Nat Genet* 1994;6(4):401–404.

143. Li QY, Newbury-Ecob RA, Terrett JA, et al. Holt-Oram syndrome is caused by mutations in TBX5, a member of the Brachyury (T) gene family. *Nat Genet* 1997;15(1):21–29.

144. Basson CT, Bachinsky DR, Lin RC, et al. Mutations in human TBX5 (corrected) cause limb and cardiac malformation in Holt-Oram syndrome. *Nat Genet* 1997;15(1):30–35.

145. Nora JJ, Nora AH, Sinha AK, et al. The Ullrich-Noonan syndrome (Turner phenotype). *Am J Dis Child* 1974;127(1):48–55.

146. Noonan JA. Hypertelorism with Turner phenotype. A new syndrome with associated congenital heart disease. *Am J Dis Child* 1968;116(4):373–380.

147. Allanson JE. Noonan Syndrome. In: Cassidy SB, Allanson JE, eds. *Management of Genetic Syndromes.* 2nd ed. Hoboken, NJ: Wiley-Liss; 2005:385.

148. Marino B, Digilio MC, Toscano A, et al. Congenital heart diseases in children with Noonan syndrome: An expanded cardiac spectrum with high prevalence of atrioventricular canal. *J Pediatr* 1999;135(6):703–706.

149. Bertola DR, Kim CA, Sugayama SM, et al. Cardiac findings in 31 patients with Noonan's syndrome. *Arq Bras Cardiol* 2000;75(5):409–412.

150. Tartaglia M, Mehler EL, Goldberg R, et al. Mutations in PTPN11, encoding the protein tyrosine phosphatase SHP-2, cause Noonan syndrome. *Nat Genet* 2001;29(4):465–468.

151. Tartaglia M, Kalidas K, Shaw A, et al. PTPN11 mutations in Noonan syndrome: Molecular spectrum, genotype-phenotype correlation, and phenotypic heterogeneity. *Am J Hum Genet* 2002;70(6):1555–1563.

152. Yoshida R, Hasegawa T, Hasegawa Y, et al. Protein-tyrosine phosphatase, nonreceptor type 11 mutation analysis and clinical assessment in 45 patients with Noonan syndrome. *J Clin Endocrinol Metab* 2004;89(7):3359–3364.

153. Jongmans M, Otten B, Noordam K, et al. Genetics and variation in phenotype in Noonan syndrome. *Horm Res* 2004;62(suppl 3):56–59.

154. Musante L, Kehl HG, Majewski F, et al. Spectrum of mutations in PTPN11 and genotype-phenotype correlation in 96 patients with Noonan syndrome and five patients with cardio-facio-cutaneous syndrome. *Eur J Hum Genet* 2003;11(2):201–206.

155. Jamieson CR, van der Burgt I, Brady AF, et al. Mapping a gene for Noonan syndrome to the long arm of chromosome 12. *Nat Genet* 1994;8(4):357–360.

156. Lee JS, Tartaglia M, Gelb BD, et al. Phenotypic and genotypic characterisation of Noonan-like/multiple giant cell lesion syndrome. *J Med Genet* 2005;42(2):e11.

157. Lee SM, Cooper JC. Noonan syndrome with giant cell lesions. *Int J Paediatr Dent* 2005;15(2):140–145.

158. Sarkozy A, Obregon MG, Conti E, et al. A novel PTPN11 gene mutation bridges Noonan syndrome, multiple lentigines/LEOPARD syndrome and Noonan-like/multiple giant cell lesion syndrome. *Eur J Hum Genet* 2004;12(12):1069–1072.

159. Legius E, Schrander-Stumpel C, Schollen E, et al. PTPN11 mutations in LEOPARD syndrome. *J Med Genet* 2002;39(8):571–574.

160. Digilio MC, Conti E, Sarkozy A, et al. Grouping of multiple-lentigines/LEOPARD and Noonan syndromes on the PTPN11 gene. *Am J Hum Genet* 2002;71(2):389–394.

161. Kalidas K, Shaw AC, Crosby AH, et al. Genetic heterogeneity in LEOPARD syndrome: Two families with no mutations in PTPN11. *J Hum Genet* 2005;50(1):21–25.

162. Digilio MC, Sarkozy A, Pacileo G, et al. PTPN11 gene mutations: Linking the Gln510Glu mutation to the "LEOPARD syndrome phenotype". *Eur J Pediatr* 2006;165(11):803–805.

163. Kontaridis MI, Swanson KD, David FS, et al. PTPN11 (Shp2) mutations in LEOPARD syndrome have dominant negative, not activating, effects. *J Biol Chem* 2006;281(10):6785–6792.

164. Roberts AE, Araki T, Swanson KD, et al. Germline gain-of-function mutations in SOS1 cause Noonan syndrome. *Nat Genet* 2006.

165. Tartaglia M, Pennacchio LA, Zhao C, et al. Gain-of-function SOS1 mutations cause a distinctive form of Noonan syndrome. *Nat Genet* 2006.

166. Schubbert S, Zenker M, Rowe SL, et al. Germline KRAS mutations cause Noonan syndrome. *Nat Genet* 2006;38(3):331–336.

167. Carta C, Pantaleoni F, Bocchinfuso G, et al. Germline missense mutations affecting KRAS Isoform B are associated with a severe Noonan syndrome phenotype. *Am J Hum Genet* 2006;79(1):129–135.

168. Zenker M, Lehmann K, Schulz AL, et al. Expansion of the genotypic and phenotypic spectrum in patients with KRAS germline mutations. *J Med Genet* 2006.

169. Niihori T, Aoki Y, Narumi Y, et al. Germline KRAS and BRAF mutations in cardio-facio-cutaneous syndrome. *Nat Genet* 2006;38(3):294–296.

170. Digilio MC, Marino B, Giannotti A, et al. The atrioventricular canal defect is the congenital heart disease connecting short rib-polydactyly and oral-facial-digital syndromes. *Am J Med Genet* 1997;68(1):110–112.

171. Digilio MC, Marino B, Ammirati A, et al. Cardiac malformations in patients with oral-facial-skeletal syndromes: Clinical similarities with heterotaxia. *Am J Med Genet* 1999;84(4):350–356.

172. Ruiz-Perez VL, Ide SE, Strom TM, et al. Mutations in a new gene in Ellis-van Creveld syndrome and Weyers acrodental dysostosis. *Nat Genet* 2000;24(3):283–286.
173. Ruiz-Perez VL, Tompson SW, Blair HJ, et al. Mutations in two nonhomologous genes in a head-to-head configuration cause Ellis-van Creveld syndrome. *Am J Hum Genet* 2003;72(3):728–732.
174. Graham JM Jr. A recognizable syndrome within CHARGE association: Hall-Hittner syndrome. *Am J Med Genet* 2001;99(2):120–123.
175. Jongmans MC, Admiraal RJ, van der Donk KP, et al. CHARGE syndrome: The phenotypic spectrum of mutations in the CHD7 gene. *J Med Genet* 2006;43(4):306–314.
176. Lalani SR, Safiullah AM, Fernbach SD, et al. Spectrum of CHD7 Mutations in 110 Individuals with CHARGE Syndrome and Genotype-Phenotype Correlation. *Am J Hum Genet* 2006;78(2):303–314.
177. Aramaki M, Udaka T, Kosaki R, et al. Phenotypic spectrum of CHARGE syndrome with CHD7 mutations. *J Pediatr* 2006;148(3):410–414.
178. Verloes A. Updated diagnostic criteria for CHARGE syndrome: A proposal. *Am J Med Genet A* 2005;133(3):306–308.
179. Blake KD, Davenport SL, Hall BD, et al. CHARGE association: An update and review for the primary pediatrician. *Clin Pediatr (Phila)* 1998;37(3):159–173.
180. Graham JM Jr, Rosner B, Dykens E, et al. Behavioral features of CHARGE syndrome (Hall-Hittner syndrome) comparison with Down syndrome, Prader-Willi syndrome, and Williams syndrome. *Am J Med Genet A* 2005;133(3):240–247.
181. Issekutz KA, Graham JM Jr, Prasad C, et al. An epidemiological analysis of CHARGE syndrome: Preliminary results from a Canadian study. *Am J Med Genet A* 2005;133(3):309–317.
182. Lin AE, Ticho BS, Houde K, et al. Heterotaxy: Associated conditions and hospital-based prevalence in newborns. *Genet Med* 2000;2(3):157–172.
183. Lim JS, McCrindle BW, Smallhorn JF, et al. Clinical features, management, and outcome of children with fetal and postnatal diagnoses of isomerism syndromes. *Circulation* 2005;112(16):2454–2461.
184. Ticho BS, Goldstein AM, Van Praagh R. Extracardiac anomalies in the heterotaxy syndromes with focus on anomalies of midline-associated structures. *Am J Cardiol* 2000;85(6):729–734.
185. Aylsworth AS. Clinical aspects of defects in the determination of laterality. *Am J Med Genet* 2001;101(4):345–355.
186. Witt M, Wang Y, Wang S, et al. Exclusion of chromosome 7 for Kartagener syndrome but suggestion of linkage in families with other forms of primary ciliary dyskinesia. *Am J Hum Genet* 1999;64(1):313–318.
187. Guichard C, Harricane MC, Lafitte JJ, et al. Axonemal dynein intermediate-chain gene (DNAI1) mutations result in situs inversus and primary ciliary dyskinesia (Kartagener syndrome). *Am J Hum Genet* 2001;68(4):1030–1035.
188. Olbrich H, Haffner K, Kispert A, et al. Mutations in DNAH5 cause primary ciliary dyskinesia and randomization of left-right asymmetry. *Nat Genet* 2002;30(2):143–144.
189. Casey B, Devoto M, Jones KL, et al. Mapping a gene for familial situs abnormalities to human chromosome Xq24-q27.1. *Nat Genet* 1993;5(4):403–407.
190. Gebbia M, Ferrero GB, Pilia G, et al. X-linked situs abnormalities result from mutations in ZIC3. *Nat Genet* 1997;17(3):305–308.
191. Kosaki K, Bassi MT, Kosaki R, et al. Characterization and mutation analysis of human LEFTY A and LEFTY B, homologues of murine genes implicated in left-right axis development. *Am J Hum Genet* 1999;64(3):712–721.
192. Bamford RN, Roessler E, Burdine RD, et al. Loss-of-function mutations in the EGF-CFC gene CFC1 are associated with human left-right laterality defects. *Nat Genet* 2000;26(3):365–369.
193. Kosaki R, Gebbia M, Kosaki K, et al. Left-right axis malformations associated with mutations in ACVR2B, the gene for human activin receptor type IIB. *Am J Med Genet* 1999;82(1):70–76.
194. Watanabe Y, Benson DW, Yano S, et al. Two novel frameshift mutations in NKX2.5 result in novel features including visceral inversus and sinus venosus type ASD. *J Med Genet* 2002;39(11):807–811.
195. Robinson SW, Morris CD, Goldmuntz E, et al. Missense mutations in CRELD1 are associated with cardiac atrioventricular septal defects. *Am J Hum Genet* 2003;72(4):1047–1052.
196. Ozcelik C, Bit-Avragim N, Panek A, et al. Mutations in the EGF-CFC gene cryptic are an infrequent cause of congenital heart disease. *Pediatr Cardiol* 2006;27(6):695–698.
197. Belmont JW, Mohapatra B, Towbin JA, et al. Molecular genetics of heterotaxy syndromes. *Curr Opin Cardiol* 2004;19(3):216–220.
198. Weaver DD, Mapstone CL, Yu PL. The VATER association. Analysis of 46 patients. *Am J Dis Child* 1986;140(3):225–229.
199. Botto LD, Khoury MJ, Mastroiacovo P, et al. The spectrum of congenital anomalies of the VATER association: An international study. *Am J Med Genet* 1997;71(1):8–15.
200. Kallen K, Mastroiacovo P, Castilla EE, et al. VATER non-random association of congenital malformations: Study based on data from four malformation registers. *Am J Med Genet* 2001;101(1):26–32.
201. Evans JA, Stranc LC, Kaplan P, et al. VACTERL with hydrocephalus: Further delineation of the syndrome(s). *Am J Med Genet* 1989;34(2):177–182.
202. Kim J, Kim P, Hui CC. The VACTERL association: Lessons from the Sonic hedgehog pathway. *Clin Genet* 2001;59(5):306–315.
203. Vento AR, LaBrie RA, Mulliken JB. The O.M.E.N.S. classification of hemifacial microsomia. *Cleft Palate Craniofac J* 1991;28(1):68–76; discussion 77.
204. Wang R, Martinez-Frias ML, Graham JM Jr. Infants of diabetic mothers are at increased risk for the oculo-auriculo-vertebral sequence: A case-based and case-control approach. *J Pediatr* 2002;141(5):611–617.
205. Werler MM, Sheehan JE, Hayes C, et al. Vasoactive exposures, vascular events, and hemifacial microsomia. *Birth Defects Res A Clin Mol Teratol* 2004;70(6):389–395.
206. Bergmann C, Zerres K, Peschgens T, et al. Overlap between VACTERL and hemifacial microsomia illustrating a spectrum of malformations seen in axial mesodermal dysplasia complex (AMDC). *Am J Med Genet A* 2003;121(2):151–155.
207. Kallen K, Robert E, Castilla EE, et al. Relation between oculo-auriculo-vertebral (OAV) dysplasia and three other non-random associations of malformations (VATER, CHARGE, and OEIS). *Am J Med Genet A* 2004;127(1):26–34.
208. Kumar A, Friedman JM, Taylor GP, et al. Pattern of cardiac malformation in oculoauriculovertebral spectrum. *Am J Med Genet* 1993;46(4):423–426.
209. Schott JJ, Benson DW, Basson CT, et al. Congenital heart disease caused by mutations in the transcription factor NKX2-5. *Science* 1998;281:108–111.
210. Sarkozy A, Conti E, Neri C, et al. Spectrum of atrial septal defects associated with mutations of NKX2.5 and GATA4 transcription factors. *J Med Genet* 2005;42(2):e16.
211. Hirayama-Yamada K, Kamisago M, Akimoto K, et al. Phenotypes with GATA4 or NKX2.5 mutations in familial atrial septal defect. *Am J Med Genet A* 2005;135(1):47–52.
212. Benson DW, Silberbach GM, Kavanaugh-McHugh A, et al. Mutations in the cardiac transcription factor NKX2.5 affect diverse cardiac developmental pathways. *J Clin Invest* 1999;104(11):1567–1573.
213. McElhinney DB, Geiger E, Blinder J, et al. NKX2.5 mutations in patients with congenital heart disease. *J Am Coll Cardiol* 2003;42(9):1650–1655.
214. Harvey RP, Lai D, Elliott D, et al. Homeodomain factor Nkx2-5 in heart development and disease. *Cold Spring Harb Symp Quant Biol* 2002;67:107–114.
215. Garg V, Kathiriya IS, Barnes R, et al. GATA4 mutations cause human congenital heart defects and reveal an interaction with TBX5. *Nature* 2003;424:443–447.
216. Garg V, Muth AN, Ransom JF, et al. Mutations in NOTCH1 cause aortic valve disease. *Nature* 2005;437:270–274.
217. Ching YH, Ghosh TK, Cross SJ, et al. Mutation in myosin heavy chain 6 causes atrial septal defect. *Nat Genet* 2005;37(4):423–428.
218. Kramer HH, Majewski F, Trampisch HJ, et al. Malformation patterns in children with congenital heart disease. *Am J Dis Child* 1987;141(7):789–795.
219. Stoll C, Alembik Y, Roth MP, et al. Risk factors in congenital heart disease. *Eur J Epidemiol* 1989;5(3):382–391.
220. Bosi G, Garani G, Scorrano M, et al. Temporal variability in birth prevalence of congenital heart defects as recorded by a general birth defects registry. *J Pediatr* 2003;142(6):690–698.
221. Eskedal L, Hagemo P, Eskild A, et al. A population-based study of extracardiac anomalies in children with congenital cardiac malformations. *Cardiol Young* 2004;14(6):600–607.
222. Hoess K, Goldmuntz E, Pyeritz RE. Genetic counseling for congenital heart disease: New approaches for a new decade. *Curr Cardiol Rep* 2002;4(1):68–75.
223. Lin AE, Salbert BA, Belmont J, et al. Total is more than the sum of the parts: Phenotyping the heart in cardiovascular genetics clinics. *Am J Med Genet A* 2004;131(2):111–114.

CHAPTER 27 ■ DEVELOPMENT OF MYOCARDIAL STRUCTURE AND FUNCTION

LYNN MAHONY, MD

Myocardial contraction and relaxation change throughout fetal life and during maturation from neonate to adult. A thorough understanding of these processes should provide the foundation for developing age-appropriate therapeutic strategies for fetuses, neonates and children with heart disease. This chapter reviews developmental changes in the physiologic, cellular, and molecular processes that determine myocardial performance. Developmental changes in the structure and function of cellular and subcellular elements of the myocyte are summarized. The effects of these changes on myocardial performance are then discussed. Many important concepts have been omitted or greatly simplified because of space limitations. The interested reader is referred to several excellent sources (1–6).

STRUCTURE

Maturation of the myocardium is marked by profound changes in myocyte composition and in the arrangement and appearance of intracellular organelles. Variation in the timing of these changes among different species complicates interpretation of experimental studies. Myocytes from rabbits (7,8), rats (9), dogs (10), and cats (11) are immature at birth, whereas myocytes from sheep (12) and guinea pigs (13) are relatively mature. Although differing rates of maturation explain some variation, morphometric differences among species are reflected in functional differences among adult hearts of different species.

Myocyte

Myocyte number and size increase during maturation (7,8,11,12,14). Myocyte division (hyperplasia) occurs mainly during fetal and early newborn life. After this time, increases in cell size (hypertrophy) account for most increases in ventricular mass (14); the mechanisms responsible for the switch from hyperplastic to hypertrophic growth are the subject of intense study. The cell shape changes from smooth and rounded in the immature heart to rodlike in the mature heart, and the surface area-to-volume ratio of the individual myocytes decreases steadily. The cell contour becomes irregular, and specialized cell–cell junctions (intercalated discs) are located on the plateau of steplike projections of the plasma membrane (15).

In mature myocytes, contractile proteins are organized into myofibrils that are arranged in rows parallel to the long axis of the cell. These rows are distributed across the cell and alternate with rows of mitochondria. In the immature myocyte, the proportion of the cell volume containing myofibrils is less than that of mature cells (8,12,16,17). In addition, the myofibrils are much less organized and may not be oriented parallel to the long axis of the cell (7,11,12). With further maturation, the myofibrils are properly oriented but are located only near the periphery of the cell. The nuclei and mitochondria are clumped in the center. Eventually, the myofibrils are distributed across the entire cell, as in the mature myocyte. Increases in cell size and in the relative volume of the myofibrils likely contribute to the observed developmental changes in myocardial force generation (16).

Sarcolemma

The sarcolemma or plasma membrane contains ion channels, ion pumps, and ion exchangers that contribute to maintenance of the chemical and charge differences between the intracellular and extracellular spaces (Fig. 27.1). Ion flow across this membrane controls membrane depolarization and repolarization. The sarcolemma also contains receptors for hormones (e.g., β-adrenergic receptors) and enzymes such as adenylate cyclase. An external glycocalyx to which calcium and sodium bind surrounds the sarcolemma.

The sodium-potassium pump is an enzyme that uses energy derived from adenosine triphosphate (ATP) hydrolysis to maintain the sodium gradient across the sarcolemmal membrane. The enzyme consists of three subunits. The intracellular domain of the α subunit contains an ATPase site that provides energy for active transport of ions. The binding site for cardiac glycosides, which inhibit the pump, is on the extracellular side of this subunit. The β and γ subunits are essential for normal transport activity. Developmental changes in isoform expression of the α subunit occur in rats (18,19). Activity of the sodium-potassium pump is less in sarcolemmal membranes isolated from immature hearts than that measured in membranes from mature hearts (20,21). The functional consequences of these changes are not known.

The inward sodium current enters myocardial cells through sarcolemmal sodium channels and results in depolarization. In human beings the channel is encoded by SCN5A. Mutations in this gene cause one form of the long QT syndrome (22–24) and some types of the Brugada syndrome (25). Developmental changes in the function of sodium channels are present in hearts from rats, rabbits, and chicks (26–29). However, fewer age-related differences are found in human atrial myocytes (30).

Multiple potassium channels present in the sarcolemma generate at least nine different potassium currents (1,31). The channels (and their currents and subunits) are named in a rather enigmatic fashion, and a full description is beyond the scope of this chapter. In general, potassium channels can be divided into two classes. Inward rectifier channels generate current that

573

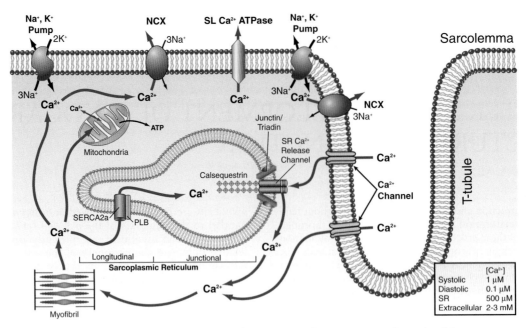

FIGURE 27.1 Diagrammatic representation of myocyte membrane systems and associated ion pumps and channels. After depolarization, calcium enters the myocytes through the calcium channels in the sarcolemma (plasma membrane). This triggers release of calcium to the myofibrils through the calcium release channels in the sarcoplasmic reticulum. After activation of muscle contraction, most of the calcium is taken up into the sarcoplasmic reticulum by the calcium pump (SERCA2a), but some is removed from the myoplasm by the Na^+-Ca^{2+} exchanger and the sarcolemmal calcium pump. SR, sarcoplasmic reticulum; SL, sarcolemma; PLB, phospholamban, NCX, Na^+-Ca^{2+} exchanger.

determines resting potential (phase 4 of the action potential). Outward rectifier channels generate currents that cause rapid repolarization after the upstroke of the action potential or cause the more sustained delayed rectifier currents that initiate phase 3 of the action potential. Mutations in potassium channel subunits cause some forms of the long QT syndrome (22–24).

Changes in the structure and function of potassium channels occur during maturation of the heart (32–37). These findings are often difficult to interpret because of methodologic, species, and age differences. Changes in various potassium currents during maturation of the heart likely contribute to age-related changes in the action potential and resting membrane potential.

Calcium enters the myocyte during the action potential through voltage-gated L-type calcium channels (also known as dihydropyridine receptors). These channels are integral membrane proteins and are composed of large α and α_1 subunits that surround an ion-selective pore. All three classes of calcium channel antagonists (dihydropyridines, phenylalkylamines, and benzothiazepines) bind to the α_1 subunit. The channels are gated by membrane potential and by the intracellular calcium concentration. Flow into the cell is passive because concentration of calcium in the extracellular space (1 mM) is greater than that in the cytosol of the resting myocyte (2×10^{-4} mM). In the mature heart, calcium influx through these channels provides the major source of activator calcium (discussed below in the excitation–contraction section).

Age-related changes in channel density and in the properties of the calcium current through these channels occur, but findings vary among species. For example, although voltage-dependent activation properties do not differ, peak calcium current density increases by twofold to threefold during maturation of rabbit heart (38–40). Tissue obtained from human

beings has been studied, but interpretation of the data is complicated by the fact that the tissue studied is almost always obtained from ill patients. In one study, decreased calcium current density measured in atria from 3-day-old to 4-year-old children was compared with published data from adult atria (41). In contrast, atrial calcium current density, steady-state inactivation, and kinetics of recovery from inactivation did not differ in tissue from infants <1 month of age compared with that from patients >1 year of age (42). However, calcium current measured in cells isolated from atria of children 3 days to 17 months of age inactivated about twofold more rapidly than that in cells isolated from adult atria. This may contribute to the relatively shortened action potential duration observed in immature compared with adult human atria.

The sarcolemmal Na^+-Ca^{2+} exchanger is an important component of the sarcolemmal membrane (43–47). Three sodium ions are exchanged for one calcium ion; thus, charge moves across the membrane. The cytosolic portion of the exchanger contains phosphorylation and other regulatory sites that alter the function of the exchanger in response to changing concentrations of sodium, calcium, and ATP, and to protein kinase–mediated phosphorylation. The direction of net calcium movement is determined by the calcium and sodium gradients, and by the membrane potential.

The exchanger primarily functions to extrude calcium from the myocyte after each contraction to maintain appropriate intracellular calcium content. Thus, one calcium ion leaves and three sodium ions enter the myocyte. The driving force for this calcium efflux is the sodium gradient between the intracellular and extracellular spaces. This gradient is maintained by the ATP-dependent sodium pump. Therefore, ATP hydrolysis is the ultimate energy source for transporting calcium out of the cell.

Calcium also enters the myocyte via the Na^+-Ca^{2+} exchanger. For example, during the plateau phase of the action potential, the large sodium entry raises subsarcolemmal sodium concentrations and thus the inside of the myocyte becomes positively charged. This favors reversal of the exchanger and results in calcium influx and sodium efflux. This phenomenon is likely more important in larger mammals who have relatively long action potentials. The possible role of this so-called reverse sodium–calcium exchange in excitation–contraction coupling is discussed below.

The inotropic effects of cardiac glycosides are mediated by the Na^+-Ca^{2+} exchanger. Inhibition of the sodium pump by cardiac glycosides increases cytosolic sodium concentration. This sodium is extruded from the cell by the exchanger, thus increasing intracellular calcium concentration, an important determinant of contractility.

Important differences in the activity of the Na^+-Ca^{2+} exchanger are noted in myocytes from various mammals (48). Inward Na^+-Ca^{2+} exchange currents elicited by caffeine-induced calcium release by the sarcoplasmic reticulum are largest in hamsters, smallest in rats, and intermediate in guinea pig and human myocytes. These differences may reflect differences in exchanger density, regulation, and spatial relationship to sarcoplasmic reticulum calcium release channels.

Striking changes in exchanger function occur during maturation of the heart. Exchanger mRNA, protein levels, and current are twofold to threefold higher in immature hearts and then decline to adult levels after birth in rabbits and rats (49–53). Consistent with the higher exchanger density, the velocity of calcium extrusion by the exchanger is higher in myocytes from neonatal rabbits than that from adults (54). The increased activity of the exchanger in immature hearts likely impacts processes controlling excitation–contraction coupling and relaxation in the developing heart (discussed below).

An ATP-dependent calcium pump in the sarcolemma also removes calcium from the myocytes (55). Binding of calcium and the calcium-binding protein, calmodulin, stimulate the pump by increasing both calcium sensitivity and maximal velocity. Thus, increased intracellular calcium stimulates pump activity. Although calcium efflux occurs by way of the sarcolemmal calcium pump, the rapid, high-capacity exchanger likely controls steady-state intracellular calcium concentration. Little information is available regarding changes in the structure or regulation of the sarcolemmal calcium pump during development.

The sarcolemma also contains a sodium–hydrogen exchanger (56). This exchanger uses the energy of the sodium gradient to transport protons out of the myocardial cell. The cardiac exchanger is located preferentially in the t-tubules and intercalated discs near the sarcoplasmic reticulum calcium channels. Numerous substances including protons and ATP tightly regulate the exchanger. Recent data attest to the importance of this exchanger in cell growth and death. Sodium–hydrogen exchange activity is higher in newborn hearts than that measured in adult hearts (57,58). This may contribute to the greater resistance of immature hearts to extracellular acidosis (59).

Transverse Tubule System

The t-tubule system is a continuation of the sarcolemma that extends transversely into the central regions of the cell and runs longitudinally between adjacent sarcomeres. T-tubules envelop the myofibril at the level of the Z-discs and form couplings with the sarcoplasmic reticulum. This arrangement allows transmission of the action potential to the interior of the myocardial cell, facilitating rapid activation of the entire cell.

Development of t-tubules is associated with maturation of the myocardial cell and is correlated with the large increase in cell volume that occurs during development (7,13,60–63). As myocytes enlarge, development of t-tubules facilitates communication between the extracellular space and the interior of the cell. At birth, considerable variation is observed in the degree of development of the t-tubule system. Myocytes from animals that are relatively mature at birth, such as guinea pigs and lambs, have well-developed t-tubules, but those from immature newborns, such as rabbits and rats, do not. T-tubules are first noted at about 30 weeks gestation in human beings (64). Variations in the degree of development of the t-tubule system contribute to species-related differences in the cellular processes regulating excitation–contraction coupling in immature animals.

Mitochondria

The size and relative volume of mitochondria increase during development (8,10,12,65–67). In addition, the inner mitochondrial membranes, the mitochondrial cristae, lengthen and become more densely packed. In several species, striking maturation of the mitochondria occurs immediately after birth (8,12,66).

These ultrastructural changes in the mitochondria parallel changes in substrate metabolism. Long-chain free fatty acids are the most important myocardial energy substrate in adult hearts. Activated free fatty acids are transported into the mitochondria and then are metabolized by β-oxidation, producing ATP. The enzyme carnitine palmityl coenzyme A transferase transports activated free fatty acids from the cytosol into the mitochondria. In immature hearts, the activity of this enzyme is decreased. As a result of these and other factors, the primary energy substrates in the immature heart are lactate and carbohydrates (68,69). Thus, age-related increases in mitochondrial-dependent aerobic metabolism may be explained in part by increases in mitochondrial volume and in the density of the inner cristal system.

Sarcoplasmic Reticulum

The sarcoplasmic reticulum is a tubular membrane network that surrounds the myofibrils and regulates cytosolic calcium concentration. The sarcoplasmic reticulum has two components: the junctional sarcoplasmic reticulum (subsarcolemmal cisternae) and the longitudinal or free sarcoplasmic reticulum (sarcotubular network) (Fig. 27.1). The longitudinal sarcoplasmic reticulum is responsible for calcium uptake, and the junctional sarcoplasmic reticulum is primarily responsible for calcium storage and release.

The junctional sarcoplasmic reticulum membranes in mammalian myocardium form tight associations with sarcolemmal (peripheral couplings or couplons) and t-tubule membranes (dyads) (70). The cytosolic surfaces of the junctional membrane contain the sarcoplasmic reticulum calcium release channel, which is also known as the ryanodine receptor because it binds the plant alkaloid ryanodine. Calcium flows through this channel to the myofilaments to initiate contraction. The corbular sarcoplasmic reticulum is a form of junctional sarcoplasmic reticulum located at the Z line of the sarcomere, which contains calcium release channels but does not form junctions with the sarcolemmal or t-tubule membranes.

Sarcoplasmic reticulum calcium release channels and the sarcolemmal L-type calcium channels are grouped together into functional clusters (calcium release units) with various other proteins including calsequestrin, triadin, and junctin

(71). Calsequestrin is a low-affinity calcium-binding protein that stores large amounts of releasable calcium within the sarcoplasmic reticulum. Mutations in calsequestrin are linked to catecholamine-induced polymorphic ventricular tachycardia in some patients (72). Triadin and junctin are small transmembrane proteins that facilitate anchoring of calsequestrin to the release channel at the junctional face membrane and likely contribute to regulation of these channels (73,74).

The sarcoplasmic reticulum calcium release channel is a large protein containing four subunits that functions as a scaffolding for a considerable number of regulatory proteins (67). These bulky macromolecular complexes are the junctional "feet" seen between the sarcoplasmic reticulum and sarcolemmal membranes on electron micrographs (70). The release channel is tightly regulated, and numerous proteins interact with the cytoplasmic domain of the release channels including calmodulin, protein kinase A, phosphatases 1 and 2A, and calstabin2 (FK-506 binding protein) (71,75). Calstabin2 binds to immunosuppressive drugs such as cyclosporine and regulates interactions of the channel subunits. Sympathetic stimulation results in channel phosphorylation by protein kinase A that increases calcium release. Mutations in the release channel are also linked to several types of ventricular tachycardia in relatively young patients (76).

The various parts of the junctional sarcoplasmic reticulum are connected by anastomosing strands of longitudinal sarcoplasmic reticulum. This portion of the sarcoplasmic reticulum is rich in ATP-dependent calcium pumps, which are encoded by the sarco(endo)plasmic reticulum calcium ATPase (SERCA) 2a gene. Active transport of calcium into the sarcoplasmic reticulum by calcium pumps results in muscle relaxation. Regulation of sarcoplasmic reticulum calcium pump activity is mediated by an intrinsic sarcoplasmic reticulum protein called phospholamban (77). This protein is an important regulator of baseline calcium cycling and of contractility, and is a critical determinant of the cardiac response to sympathetic stimulation. Dephosphorylated phospholamban inhibits calcium pump activity by decreasing the affinity of the pump for calcium. Phosphorylation of phospholamban by protein kinase A dissociates phospholamban from the calcium pump. The resulting increased affinity for calcium of the pump facilitates removal of calcium from troponin, thereby accelerating relaxation, which is an important element of the cardiovascular response to sympathetic stimulation. Additionally, the amount of calcium taken up by the sarcoplasmic reticulum is increased; thus, more calcium is available for release, which increases contractility.

In the mature heart, the sarcoplasmic reticulum regulates intracellular calcium concentration and is the most important source of activator calcium for binding to troponin C. Age-related changes in sarcoplasmic reticulum structure or function therefore likely affect myocardial function. The content of sarcoplasmic reticulum is decreased, and this membrane is less organized in the immature heart (7,17,78). In particular, separation of the junctional and free regions is less well defined (7). Dyads develop in parallel with t-tubule development (79).

Calcium uptake, calcium pump activity, the number of calcium pumps, calcium pump efficiency, and the amount of phospholamban are decreased in the immature heart compared with the mature heart in mice (80–82), rabbits (83–85), guinea pigs (86), and sheep (21,87). Administration of thyroid hormone increases expression of the calcium pump protein and mRNA in adult rabbits, mice, and baboons (88–92). Thus, the perinatal increase in thyroid hormone that occurs in most species (93) may contribute to the perinatal increase in sarcoplasmic reticulum calcium pump expression.

Contractile Proteins

The sarcomere, which is defined at both ends by Z-discs, is the fundamental contractile unit of striated muscle (Fig. 27.2). Sarcomeres are composed of proteins organized into strands called filaments. The I band is composed of thin (actin) filaments as well as the troponin complex and tropomyosin. The very dark Z-disc bisects the I band. Thick filaments are polymers of myosin and a very large protein called titin. The A band is composed of overlapping thin and thick filaments. The dark M band in the center of the A band consists of thick filaments cross-linked to titin by myosin-binding protein C, myomesin, and obscurin. Mutations in various contractile proteins cause some forms of familial hypertrophic cardiomyopathy (94,95).

Each of these contractile proteins is expressed in related but distinct forms (isoforms) that differ in amino acid sequence and functional properties. Isoform production is determined by cell type (skeletal vs. cardiac muscle, atrial vs. ventricular) and is regulated by physiologic stimuli. Complex and precise alterations in isoform expression occur for most of the contractile proteins during muscle development (96–99). These changes in isoforms result in changes in the functional properties of the sarcomere; therefore, they likely contribute to the changes in myocardial function known to occur during normal development.

Myosin

Myosin, the most abundant contractile protein, has two heavy chains and four light chains. The tails of the two heavy chains are woven together to form the thick filament (Fig. 27.2). The globular head projects up from hinge points on the long axis of the thick filament to form the cross-bridges. The myosin head contains adenosine triphosphatase (ATPase) activity that contributes to fiber shortening during contraction.

A multigene family encodes myosin heavy chains (MHC). Cardiac myosin contains two heavy chain isoforms, α-MHC and β-MHC. Myosin containing two α chains (V1) has the highest ATPase activity. V2 contains an α and a β chain. Myosin containing two β chains (V3) has the lowest ATPase activity. The ATPase activity of the heavy chain is correlated with the unloaded maximum velocity of shortening of the myofibril. Thus, changes in myosin isoforms have important functional implications (100).

Developmental changes in expression of myosin heavy chain isoforms vary among species (101). For example, in rats, the V3 isoform is most abundant in the ventricle during fetal life and is replaced by V1 in the adult heart. However, in the human ventricle, the V3 isoform predominates during fetal, neonatal, and adult life. The amount of α-MHC is <5% of the total myosin in the fetal ventricle. This increases to 5% to 10% in the adult ventricle and decreases to 0% to 2% in failing ventricles (102). Despite the relatively small amounts of the α-MHC isoform present in human ventricles, this isoform appears to play an important role in ventricular function because mutations in the α-MHC gene cause a spectrum of cardiomyopathies including ventricular hypertrophy and dilation (103).

Myosin light chains are located near the head portion of the myosin molecule. Myosin light chain 1 (MLC1) is called the essential light chain, and MCL2 is the regulatory light chain. Although the regulatory light chain has a well-defined role in regulating smooth muscle contraction, the physiologic role of the light chains in cardiac muscle is much less clear. Two isoforms of the MLC1 gene occur. The MLC1a gene is expressed in human fetal and adult atria and in fetal ventricle. As the ventricle matures, MLC1a is replaced by the ventricular isoform, MLC1v (104–106). The physiologic significance of this shift is

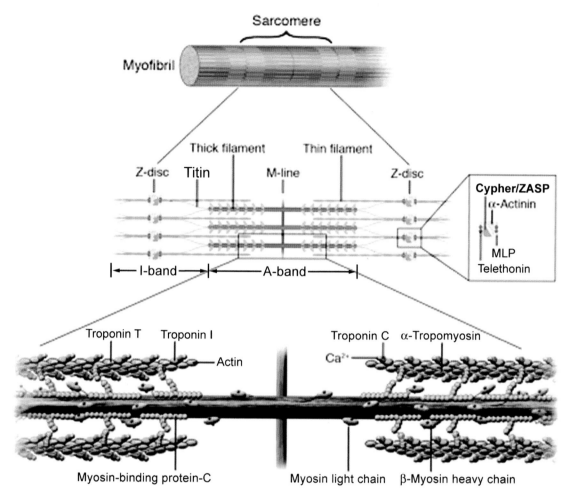

FIGURE 27.2 Schematic diagram of a sarcomere showing arrangement of thick and thin filaments. Thick filaments contain myosin, myosin-binding protein C, and titin. The tails of the myosin heavy chains are woven together to form the thick filament. The globular myosin head projects outward to form cross-bridges. The thin filaments include actin and the various troponins. Actin forms the backbone of the thin filament. Tropomyosin binds to troponin T at multiple sites along the major groove of the actin filament and inhibits actin–myosin interaction. Troponin T binds the troponin complex to tropomyosin, troponin I inhibits interactions between actin and myosin, and troponin C binds calcium. The sarcomere, which lies between two Z-discs, is anchored by interactions between titin and actin with Z-disc proteins including cypher/ZASP, α-actinin, muscle-specific LIM protein (MLP), and telethonin. (Modified from Morita H, Seidman J, Seidman C. Genetic causes of human heart failure. *J Clin Invest* 2005;115:518–526, with permission.)

unknown. There are also two isoforms of the MLC2 gene, MLC2a and MLC2v, which are expressed in human atria and ventricle. No known isoform shifts occur during development.

Actin

A polymer consisting of two strands of actin monomers forms the backbone of the thin filament. Actin is a small globular protein that is encoded by a multigene family. Two isoforms, skeletal α-actin and cardiac α-actin, are present in striated muscle. These isoforms differ by only four amino acids, two of which are in the myosin-binding region.

During development, both actin isoforms are expressed in the human ventricle (107). In fetal and neonatal hearts, skeletal α-actin mRNA constitutes >80% of the total actin. Cardiac α-actin mRNA constitutes >60% of the total actin in the mature heart. The impact of this isoform shift on contractile function of the human heart is unknown.

Tropomyosin

Tropomyosin consists of two helical peptide chains and exists as a homodimer or heterodimer of two isoforms, α and β, wound around each other to form a coil. Tropomyosin binds to troponin T at multiple sites along the major groove of the actin filament and modulates the interaction between actin and myosin (Fig. 27.3). The cooperative activation that is an important component of thin filament function is likely mediated in part by the overlap of adjacent tropomyosin molecules (108).

Troponin Complex

The troponin complex consists of three separate proteins (Fig. 27.3). Troponin T binds the complex to tropomyosin, troponin I inhibits interactions between actin and myosin, and troponin C binds calcium. Together with tropomyosin, the troponin complex confers calcium sensitivity to the process of cross-bridge formation. Calcium-induced changes in the actin-binding

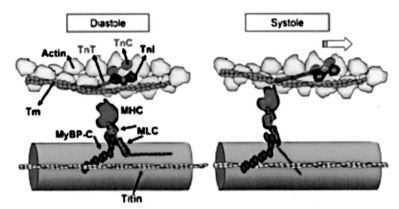

FIGURE 27.3 Movement of contractile proteins during activation of contraction. In diastole, Tm (tropomyosin) is held in place by protein interactions with troponin I (TnI) and troponin T (TnT) and blocks cross-bridge formation between actin and myosin heavy chain (MHC). In systole, calcium initiates contraction by binding to troponin C (TnC). Troponin I moves from being tightly bound to actin in diastole to being tightly bound to troponin C. As troponin I moves away from actin, troponin T shifts tropomyosin toward the middle of the groove between the actin strand. This alters actin–myosin interaction and allows formation of tightly bound cross-bridges. Cross-bridge formation is also regulated by interactions with myosin light chains (MLC), myosin-binding protein C (MyBP-C), and titin. (From Kass DA, Solaro RJ. Mechanisms and use of calcium-sensitizing agents in the failing heart. *Circulation* 2006:113:305–315, with permission.)

affinity of troponin I provide a molecular switch that identifies an increase in intracellular calcium as a signal that initiates contraction (108). Multiple isoforms of each troponin are expressed in a tissue- and developmental stage–specific manner (99).

Troponin T. Four isoforms of cardiac troponin T (cTnT1, cTnT2, cTnT3, cTnT4) are expressed in the human heart as a result of alternative splicing of a single gene (109). The relative expression of these isoforms, which differ in length and charge, changes significantly with development (110). All isoforms are expressed in fetal hearts, but only one isoform (cTnT3) is expressed in mature human hearts. The isoforms cTnT1 and cTnT4 are up-regulated in failing human hearts harvested from transplant patients (110) and in hearts from children with congestive heart failure secondary to congenital heart defects (111). Expression of cTnT4 is correlated with the severity of heart failure before surgery and with the duration of recovery. These isoform shifts modify the calcium sensitivity of force development and therefore likely affect contractility (112,113).

Troponin I. Troponin I has a relatively elongated structure with a rounded head on each end. Linking the ends of the molecule is the so-called inhibitory peptide, which binds to troponin C during systole and to actin during diastole. Troponin I acts as a strong inhibitor of actin–myosin interactions. Only the cardiac isoform of troponin I is found in normal and failing adult human hearts. Both the cardiac and slow skeletal isoforms are expressed in immature hearts (114–116). In fetal hearts the predominant (>70%) troponin I is the slow skeletal isoform, but this is not detected in a normal 9-month-old human heart (115). These isoform changes likely affect myocardial function (108,117).

These age-related alterations in troponin I expression may contribute to changes in cardiac function. An extended amino-terminal sequence containing serine residues is present in the cardiac isoform but not in the slow skeletal isoform. These serine residues are phosphorylated in response to β-adrenergic stimulation of the heart. Phosphorylation of troponin I at this site shifts cooperative interactions within the troponin complex. This decreases not only the sensitivity of troponin C and

myofilament activation for calcium but also the affinity of troponin I for troponin C, thus altering contractile performance (118,119). In addition, the slow skeletal troponin I isoform may contribute to the relative resistance of neonatal myofilament activity to deactivation by acidic pH (118,120–123).

Troponin C. Binding of calcium to troponin C changes the tertiary structure of troponin C, which results in changes in the structure of the other troponin subunits and tropomyosin. This causes tropomyosin to move into a position that allows strong myosin binding to actin, ultimately leading to muscle cell contraction. Fast skeletal and slow cardiac isoforms of troponin C have been identified (124). However, in contrast to other myofilament proteins, cardiac muscle expresses only the single cardiac isoform (125).

Cytoskeleton and Extracellular Matrix

The cytoskeleton functions as a scaffold for the cell on which various subcellular components are arranged such that efficient communication occurs between internal and external environments of the cell. The structural proteins in this framework organize the intracellular components and proteins that participate in cell signaling. The cytoskeleton determines cell size and organization and allows the tension developed by the contractile proteins to be transmitted to the myocyte, to adjacent cells, and to the extracellular matrix (126,127). Mutations in a number of the cytoskeletal proteins are linked to inherited forms of familial dilated and hypertrophic cardiomyopathies and to arrhythmias. The reader is referred to Chapters 56 and 57 in this book and to other sources (94,95,128).

The cytoskeleton is a dynamic structure and is critical to transduction of mechanical signals. This is facilitated by the juxtaposition of ion channels, signaling molecules, and messengers to the various cytoskeletal structures. Tremendous changes in cytoskeletal structure occur during normal cell growth. Additionally, cytoskeletal structure is remodeled in the mature cell in response to pathophysiologic signals such as systolic stress or diastolic stretch; these processes can be associated with ventricular hypertrophy or dilation (remodeling) (129).

Development of the heart and blood vessels is critically dependent on proteins within the cytoskeleton and extracellular matrix (130–133). Developmental changes in the organization of the intracellular organelles (7) likely reflect changes in the composition and organization of the cytoskeleton (134–137). Additionally, the developmental changes in the composition and organization of the cytoskeleton and extracellular matrix are integral to maturational changes in the active and passive properties of the myocardium.

Cytoskeletal Proteins Associated with the Thick Filaments

The most important function of the cytoskeletal proteins associated with the thick filaments is to link these filaments within the sarcomere. Titin, the largest protein known in human beings, spans half the sarcomere from the Z-disc at the end of the sarcomere to the M-line at the center of the sarcomere (138) (Fig. 27.2). The N-terminal ends of titin overlap within the Z-disc, and the C-terminal ends overlap at the M-line; this creates a continuous filament system that aligns the thick filaments within the myofibril. Functionally distinct motifs are present within titin at the Z-disc, I-band, A-band, and M-line; the segment of the protein at the I-band contains serial spring elements that determine passive tension of the myocardium, which is an important determinant of late diastolic filling and operating sarcomere length. In addition, this extensible region extends in the opposite direction of sarcomere stretch, thus developing restoring force. This restoring force contributes to the elastic recoil that drives early diastolic filling. Thus, titin is important in maintaining the structural integrity of the sarcomere, setting sarcomere length and influencing diastolic filling. As a continuous elastic element within the myofibrils, titin has multiple protein interactions with functionally diverse proteins known to be involved in force transmission and stretch sensing (138,139). Mutations in titin have been identified in some patients with dilated cardiomyopathy, confirming that defects in force transmission can cause dilated cardiomyopathy (95).

Differential splicing of a single titin gene creates titin isoforms with various extensibilities (140). Hearts from large mammals (including human beings) express both the stiffer N2B isoform and the more compliant N2BA isoform, but hearts from small mammals contain mostly the stiffer N2B isoform. The intrinsic heart rate is higher and the diastolic filling time is shorter in the relatively stiff rodent heart.

Titin isoforms are developmentally regulated; fetal hearts express even more compliant titin isoforms, which are replaced by stiffer isoforms in mature hearts with a time course that varies among species (141,142). This isoform change correlates with changes in passive stiffness measured in myofibrils and skinned fibers; myocardium is less stiff (more compliant) in the immature heart than in the adult. These data contrast with several early studies that suggest that the fetal heart is less compliant than the adult heart (16,143). The conflicting results may reflect differences in experimental preparations and technique.

Myosin-binding protein C stabilizes the thick filament by binding to myosin and titin, forming transverse fibers that connect adjacent myosin filaments near the center of the sarcomere (144) (Figs. 27.2 and 27.3). Along with myosin-binding protein C, other proteins found at the M-line including myomesin, M-protein, and obscurin facilitate force transmission along the thick filaments.

Z-Discs

The Z-disc, which defines the ends of the sarcomeres, is a complex array of proteins that links the myofilaments from opposing sarcomeres into a highly ordered lattice (Figs. 27.2 and 27.4) (128). Proteins located at the Z-disc include α-actinin, telethonin (T-cap), nebulette, muscle LIM protein, filamin, and myotilin. Z-discs are responsible for transmitting tension generated by individual sarcomeres along the length of the myofibril, allowing efficient contractile activity. Additionally, proteins of the Z-disc also serve as docking sites for transcription factors, calcium-signaling proteins, and for kinases and phosphatases. Increasing evidence implicates the Z-disc and its associated components as a sensor of cell stress and strain and as a mediator of signaling responsible for cell development, growth, and remodeling in response to altered hemodynamics. The recently demonstrated linking of the Z-discs to

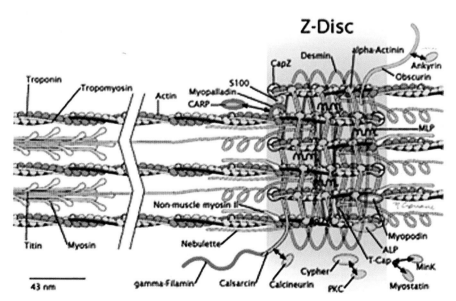

FIGURE 27.4 Schematic of the network of proteins constituting the Z-disc. Titin is shown with the PEVK region illustrated as a spring and capped by telethonin (T-cap). CARP, cardiac-restricted ankyrin repeated protein; MLP, muscle specific LIM protein; ALP, actinin-associated LIM protein. (From Pyle WG, Solaro WR. At the crossroads of myocardial signaling: the role of Z-discs in intracellular signaling and cardiac function. *Circ Res* 2004;94:296–305, with permission.)

the transverse tubules by a regulatory subunit of the sarcolemmal potassium channel (minK) suggests that Z-discs may also play a role in mechanoelectric feedback.

Extramyofibrillar Cytoskeleton

The cytoskeleton consists of myofibrillar and extramyofibrillar components. The contractile proteins described previously and titin constitute the myofibrillar cytoskeleton. The extramyofibrillar cytoskeleton is composed of three different filament systems: (i) microfilaments, (ii) intermediate filaments, and (iii) microtubules.

■ Microfilaments contain actin and are found in two places within the myocyte: Sarcomeric actin in the thin filaments of the sarcomere and nonsarcomeric or cortical actin that form a subsarcolemmal network. Microfilaments containing nonsarcomeric or cytoplasmic actin (F-actin) are critical to linking the intracellular cytoskeleton with adjoining cells and with the extracellular matrix (Fig. 27.5).

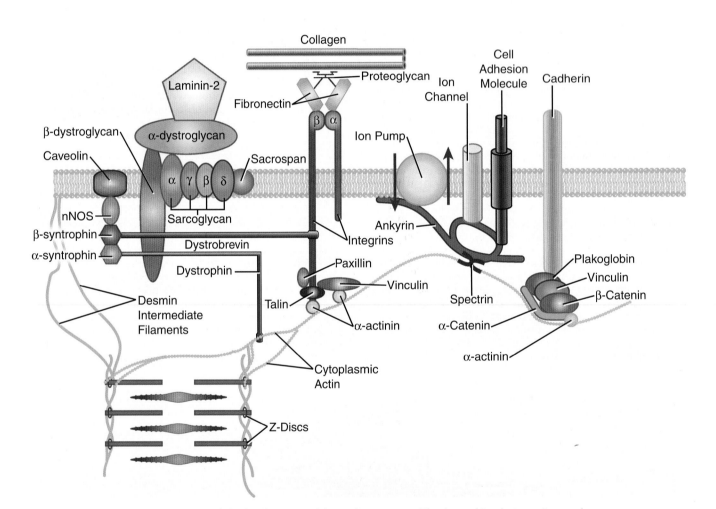

FIGURE 27.5 Cytoskeletal architecture of the cardiac myocyte. The dystrophin–glycoprotein complex links the plasma membrane to cytoplasmic actin filaments. Integrins bind the cell to the extracellular matrix and are composed of α and β subunits that attach through various proteins (fibronectin, laminin, proteoglycans) to collagen. The intracellular part of the β subunit binds to cytoplasmic actin filaments through another protein complex that includes α-actinin, talin, vinculin, and paxillin. Ankyrin links membrane proteins such as ion pumps and channels together, thereby organizing interactions among proteins with related functions. Spectrin links ankyrin to the cytoplasmic actin filaments and is also associated with both costameres and intercalated discs at the sarcolemmal membrane. Cadherins mediate connection of cell-to-cell contacts in both desmosomes and fascia adherens. In the fascia adherens, cadherins link the cytoplasmic actin filaments of adjacent cells through vinculin, catenins, plakoglobin, and α-actinin. In addition to contributing to the structural integrity of the cell, many of these proteins are critically involved in cell signaling as described in the text. (Adapted from Towbin JA, Bowles NE. The failing heart. *Nature* 2002;415:227–233; Katz AM. The cytoskeleton. In: *Physiology of the Heart*. Philadelphia: Lippincott Williams & Wilkins, 2006:127–139; and Liew CC, Dzau VJ. Molecular genetics and genomics of heart failure. *Nat Rev Genet* 2004;5:811–825, with permission.)

■ Intermediate fibers are composed primarily of desmin polymers in muscle and form a network that maintains the structural integrity of the myocytes (145). In addition to participating in the intercalated discs, the desmin filaments link Z-discs of adjacent myofilaments bundles to each other and link Z-discs to costameres (described below) and to the sarcoplasmic reticulum and sarcolemmal and nuclear membranes (Fig. 27.5). Stress-induced alteration of the spatial arrangement of this network may mediate alterations in gene expression. Mutations in desmin cause desmin-related myopathies that are characterized by abnormal intrasarcoplasmic desmin aggregation and accumulation.

■ Microtubules contain polymerized subunits of α and β tubulin that undergo continuous depolymerization and repolymerization within the cell. The total amount of tubulin and the proportion of the polymerized form likely affect the stiffness of the cytoskeleton (146). Microtubules surround the nucleus and spread longitudinally throughout the cell. They stabilize cell structure by anchoring subcellular organelles, and they transmit mechanical and chemical signals within and between cells.

Cytoskeletal Components of Cell-to-Cell Junctions

Intercalated discs are specialized cell-to-cell junctions that join myocytes at each end to adjacent myocytes; these junctions are important sites of force transmission between myocytes (Fig. 27.6) (147). The intercalated discs consist of fascia adherens (analogous to adherens junctions in nonmuscle cells), desmosomes, and gap junctions. Transmembrane proteins called cadherins mediate connection of cell–cell contacts in both the desmosomes and fascia adherens. The fascia adherens connects microfilaments to sarcomeric actin (thin filaments). The cadherins in the fascia adherens complex bind to the microfilaments (nonsarcomeric actin) via subsarcolemmal proteins called catenins that are then connected to sarcomeric

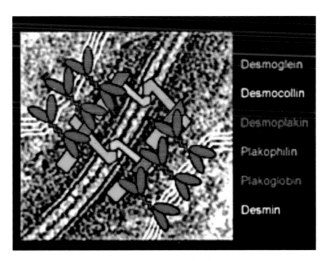

FIGURE 27.7 An electron micrograph of a desmosome with a superimposed model of the molecular constituents that make up the desmosome and connect it to the intermediate filaments of the cytoskeleton. (From Saffitz JE. Adhesion molecules: why they are important to the electrophysiologist. *J Cardiovasc Electrophysiol* 2006;17:225–229, with permission.)

actin via α-actinin and vinculin (Fig. 27.5). The desmosomes connect the intermediate (desmin) filaments of adjacent cells. Cadherins within the desmosome called desmoglein and desmocollin bind to the intermediate filaments through a protein complex containing plakoglobin (catenin γ), desmoglein, and desmoplakin (Fig. 27.7) (148).

Connections to the Extracellular Matrix

The many protein complexes that link the myofibrils and membrane systems of the myocyte to the extracellular matrix are essential for stabilizing cell structure during the stresses of contraction and relaxation. Additionally, these linking protein complexes are involved in organizing and coordinating membrane signaling systems with the contractile systems.

The various cytoskeletal networks within the myocyte, the sarcolemma, and the extracellular matrix are linked through highly complex protein networks called costameres (analogous to focal adhesions in nonmuscle cells and in cultured cardiomyocytes) (149,150). These structures, which contain proteins including vinculin, talin, tensin, paxillin, and zyxin, encircle the lateral aspects of the myocyte perpendicular to its long axis, forming a transmembrane physical attachment between the peripheral Z-discs and the extracellular matrix (Fig. 27.8). Costameres thus anchor the myofibrils to the sarcolemma and transmit lateral contractile force from the sarcomere to the extracellular matrix and ultimately to neighboring myocytes. Recent evidence suggests that costameric proteins likely play a role in converting mechanical stimuli to alterations in cell signaling and gene expression, which can result in cell growth or hypertrophy.

Integrins are also essential components of the protein network responsible for transmission of force between the myocytes and the extracellular matrix (150). These cell-adhesion molecules are heterodimers of various α and β subunits and are embedded within the sarcolemmal membrane adjacent to costameres. The intracellular domain of the β subunits binds to actin microfilaments through costamere proteins including α-actinin, talin filamin, tensin, and vinculin (see Fig. 27.5). The extracellular portion of integrin interacts with various

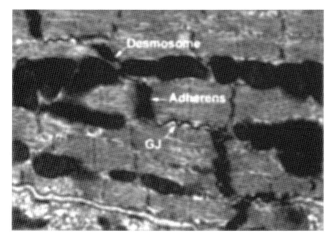

FIGURE 27.6 An intercalated disk connecting two ventricular myocytes as seen by transmission electron microscopy. There is an intimate spatial juxtaposition between gap junctions and adhesion junctions within the intercalated disk. Gap junctions (GJ) are typically located between rows of sarcomeres in offset regions of the disk situated between adherens junctions. Gap junctions also occur in close proximity to desmosomes. (From Saffitz JE. Adhesion molecules: Why they are important to the electrophysiologist. *J Cardiovasc Electrophysiol* 2006;17:225–229, with permission.)

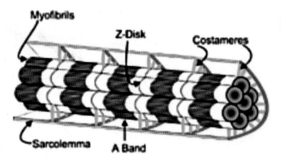

FIGURE 27.8 Schematic diagram depicting cellular location of costameres in striated muscle. Costameres are aligned circumferentially with the Z-disc to physically couple force-generating sarcomeres with the sarcolemmal membrane. (From Ervasti JM. Costameres: The Achilles' heel of Herculean muscle. *J Biol Chem* 2003;278:13591–13594, with permission.)

extracellular matrix proteins, including laminin, collagen, fibronectin, and vitronectin. Integrins also participate in a number of signaling pathways mediated by several G-proteins and protein kinases that modify interactions between the integrins and the extracellular matrix. These pathways are involved in both cell growth and apoptosis in response to stimuli such as passive stretch and active tension.

The dystrophin glycoprotein complex also plays an important role in linking the intracellular cytoskeleton and the extracellular matrix (151). This complex (composed of α- and β-dystroglycans, α-, β-, γ- and δ-sarcoglycans, caveolin-3, syntrophin, and dystrobrevin) binds the actin microfilaments to the extracellular matrix, thereby transmitting force to the extracellular matrix (Fig. 27.5). The N-terminal of dystrophin binds to the microfilaments. The C-terminal binds to a transmembrane protein called dystroglycan via a protein complex that includes α and β syntrophins and dystrobrevin. This latter complex functions as an intracellular protein signaling system. Sarcoglycans, a six-member family of membrane-spanning glycoproteins, bind dystroglycan to the plasma membrane. The extracellular portion of dystroglycan binds to laminin in the extracellular matrix. Mutations in dystrophin cause muscular dystrophy, and mutations in the components of the dystrophin glycoprotein complex are present in patients with dilated cardiomyopathy (151).

Spectrin is an actin-binding cytoskeletal protein that plays an important role in coordinating membrane signaling systems with the contractile filaments within the myocytes (152,153). Spectrin is associated with costameres and intercalated discs at the sarcolemmal membrane and is also a component of protein complexes related to the sarcoplasmic reticulum at the Z-discs. Ankyrins are adaptor proteins that bind to spectrin and also to a structurally diverse group of membrane proteins such as ion channels and pumps, calcium release channels, and cell-adhesion molecules (154) (Fig. 27.5). In this way, various proteins are linked together, thereby organizing interactions among proteins with related functions. For example, ankyrins localize the calcium release channels of the sarcoplasmic reticulum to the sarcolemmal calcium release channels thus facilitating excitation–contraction coupling. Additionally, ankyrins also link the sarcoplasminic reticulum membrane to proteins at the Z-disk region of titin, thus ensuring that the sarcoplasmic reticulum moves with the Z-disc. Mutations in ankyrins result in cell dysfunction because interactions such as these are disrupted. Mutations in ankyrins are known to cause cardiac arrhythmias in human beings and in mouse models (155).

The extracellular matrix is a supporting network that surrounds myocardial cells that serve both structural and cell regulatory functions (156–159). It is composed of (a) connective tissue, mainly various collagen types and elastin; (b) a gel-like ground substance consisting of proteoglycans; (c) basement membrane proteins such as collagen, laminin, and fibronectin; and (d) other molecules such as cytokines, growth factors, and proteases. Synthesis of these components is mediated by mechanical stretch and various growth factors. Once considered merely scaffolding to support and to align cells, this complex interstitium also mediates processes such as cell migration, proliferation, adhesion, and cell-to-cell signaling. The extracellular matrix plays a critical role in normal growth and development (130,133) as well as in the progression of pathologic remodeling of the ventricle (160,161).

FUNCTION

Overview of Contractile Function

Before considering developmental changes in myocardial function, it is useful to review the events involved in normal contraction and relaxation. Contraction of the heart begins when an action potential depolarizes the sarcolemma. Depolarization is caused by sequential inward currents of sodium and calcium ions. The slow inward calcium current enters through voltage-gated L-type channels in the sarcolemma and triggers release of a large amount of calcium from the sarcoplasmic reticulum, thus amplifying the inward calcium current.

The calcium released by the sarcoplasmic reticulum initiates contraction by binding to the amino terminal end of troponin C. This causes a conformational change in troponin C that increases its affinity to troponin I. Troponin I moves from being tightly bound to actin (diastole) to being tightly bound to troponin C (Fig. 27.3). This results in movement of the inhibitory portion of troponin I away from actin. In addition, tropomyosin shifts within the groove between the actin strands, which alters actin–myosin interaction and eventually allows formation of tightly bound cross-bridges. ATP binding causes conformational changes in the actin–myosin interface, ultimately resulting in displacement of actin toward the center of the sarcomere and contractile element shortening. The amount of force developed by the contracting myocyte depends, in part, on the number of cross-bridges formed. The number of cross-bridges formed depends on the amount of calcium released by the sarcoplasmic reticulum and on the intrinsic properties of the myofilaments (e.g., calcium sensitivity) (108). At a given intracellular calcium concentration, an increase in calcium sensitivity results in greater force, and a reduction in calcium sensitivity decreases force. Thin filament isoform expression, phosphorylation, and intracellular acidosis modulate the calcium sensitivity of the myofilaments.

Relaxation begins with removal of calcium from the myofilaments, mediated primarily by the sarcoplasmic reticulum calcium pump but also by the Na^+-Ca^{2+} exchanger. Removal of calcium from the myofilaments results in breaking of the cross-bridge and return to the resting state.

Excitation–Contraction Coupling

Excitation–contraction coupling is the sequence of steps that begins with an electrical signal resulting from the action potential and ends with binding of calcium to troponin C.

A large increase in intracellular calcium concentration is critical for binding of sufficient calcium to troponin C. Although calcium enters the myocyte across the sarcolemma during the plateau phase of the action potential, the absolute calcium flux is not more than a tenth of that required for maximal contraction (162). Similarly, calcium stored and released by mitochondria is quantitatively unimportant (163). Instead, the source of this activator calcium is the sarcoplasmic reticulum, and an intact sarcoplasmic reticulum is required for normal excitation–contraction coupling in mammalian myocytes.

The exact process by which calcium release from the sarcoplasmic reticulum is activated and then terminated has been the subject of intensive study (4,164,165). In skeletal muscle, the L-type channel (dihydropyridine receptor) behaves as a voltage sensor that provides the signal for release of calcium from the sarcoplasmic reticulum. In contrast, as Ringer showed in 1883, the coupling of depolarization of a cardiac muscle to muscle contraction cannot occur in the absence of extracellular calcium. Depolarization of the sarcolemma opens the voltage-dependent L-type calcium channels. Calcium entering the myocyte after depolarization interacts with the release channel in the sarcoplasmic reticulum (ryanodine receptor), inducing release of calcium to the myofilaments (calcium-induced calcium release) (166). Sarcoplasmic reticulum calcium release contributes to calcium-calmodulin–dependent inactivation of calcium influx through the sarcolemmal L-type calcium channels.

Although colocalization of L-type calcium channels and sarcoplasmic reticulum calcium release channels at junctional microdomains between the sarcolemmal and sarcoplasmic reticulum membranes (discussed above) likely facilitates close interaction, precise details concerning how calcium release to the myofilaments is activated are incompletely defined. Calcium release channels in the sarcoplasmic reticulum are relatively insensitive to physiologic concentrations of calcium within the myocytes. Instead, these channels are efficiently activated by local trigger calcium. The so-called local control theory proposes that a calcium signal through an L-type sarcolemmal channel activates a cluster of calcium release channels in the sarcoplasmic reticulum that are located in a microdomain within the dyad or peripheral coupling. Calcium entering the cell via an L-type calcium channel has preferential access to the sarcoplasmic reticulum channels located in its release cluster and does not trigger calcium release from neighboring clusters.

Very small calcium release events can be imaged with a confocal microscope and are called calcium sparks (167–169). Calcium sparks likely reflect the nearly simultaneous activation of a cluster of about 6 to 20 calcium release channels at a single dyad or peripheral coupling. Calcium sparks occur spontaneously but at a low rate in quiescent cells. These are local events that travel relatively small distances within the cell. Depolarization of the cardiac cell and resulting entry of calcium through L-type channels evoke multiple sparks arising from independent release clusters that summate spatially and temporally such that sufficient calcium reaches the myofilaments to cause contraction; thus, excitation is linked to contraction.

It is not completely clear why calcium-induced calcium release is not regenerative and uncontrolled, that is, why the release channel in the sarcoplasmic reticulum does not continue to respond to the calcium passing through it and release all the stored calcium. Termination of calcium release may involve several mechanisms including calcium-dependent inactivation of the channels involving another protein such as calmodulin, stochastic attrition (inherent random closing of individual channels), a cooperative interaction among release channels within the cluster, and local depletion of calcium from the sarcoplasmic reticulum (170).

Although the importance of the L-type calcium current in triggering calcium release from the sarcoplasmic reticulum is widely accepted, the possibility that calcium influx through the exchanger also induces calcium release has been a subject of intensive research and considerable controversy. Interpretation of available data is complicated by differences in the exchanger activity and in the processes controlling excitation–contraction coupling among mammalian species and the nonphysiologic conditions that are often a part of various experimental models. The precise contribution of reverse sodium–calcium exchange in triggering calcium release from the sarcoplasmic reticulum remains to be defined (46,171). Nevertheless, Na^+-Ca^{2+} exchanger activity will significantly affect excitation–contraction coupling because both forward- and reverse-mode operation affect intracellular calcium content.

The activation of myocyte contraction in the immature heart likely depends more on calcium influx across the sarcolemma than on calcium release from the sarcoplasmic reticulum (63). Immature hearts are more sensitive than adult hearts to the negative inotropic effects of calcium channel antagonists (172–174). As discussed earlier, sarcoplasmic reticulum content and calcium sequestration are decreased in the immature heart. Furthermore, ryanodine, a plant alkaloid that interferes selectively with calcium release from the sarcoplasmic reticulum (175), produces a decreased negative inotropic response in immature rabbit hearts compared with that in mature hearts (176). The high surface-to-volume ratio and the subsarcolemmal location of the contractile proteins support the feasibility of transsarcolemmal calcium influx as the source of the calcium binding to troponin C in the immature heart. As the myocytes mature and increase in size, development of transverse tubules and tight coupling of calcium entry to sarcoplasmic reticulum calcium release allow efficient excitation–contraction coupling throughout the cell (63,177).

Whether this activator calcium enters the immature myocyte via the L-type calcium channels or via reverse-mode Na^+-Ca^{2+} exchange is controversial. One study showed that contractions in neonatal myocytes from rabbits are much more sensitive to nifedipine than contractions in adult myocytes (178). Others postulated that the increased density of Na^+-Ca^{2+} exchangers allows reverse-mode function to be an important source of calcium for excitation–contraction coupling (51,52,63,172). However, whether calcium influx through the exchanger supports physiologically relevant contractions remains to be defined and is likely species dependent (54,179). Interestingly, no difference is detected in exchange current density between newborn and adult guinea pigs (50). This likely reflects the fact that guinea pigs are much more mature at birth than rabbits (13,180) and may be relevant to the situation in human beings. The observation that infants respond adversely (compared with adults) to administration of calcium channel antagonists (181) suggests that the immature human myocardium is relatively reliant on calcium influx through L-type calcium channels.

Systolic Function

Determinants of Systolic Function

Determinants of systolic function include the preload or amount of blood distending the ventricle before contraction, the load encountered during shortening (afterload), the heart rate, and myocardial contractility (Fig. 27.9). Because the

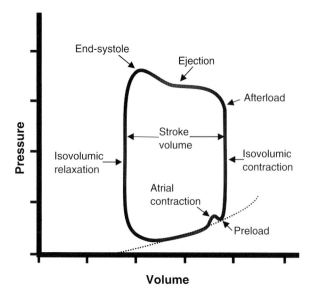

FIGURE 27.9 Left ventricular pressure–volume loop. Isovolumic contraction begins at a measurable end-diastolic pressure, which is defined as preload and proceeds until the ventricle reaches its afterload, at which point ejection occurs. When ejection ends, ventricular pressure and volume lie on the end-systolic pressure–volume relationship. Isovolumic relaxation then proceeds, at which time ventricular pressure decreases rapidly. When ventricular pressures falls below atrial pressure, ventricle filling begins and eventually ventricular pressure and volume lie on the end-diastolic pressure–volume relationship (*dotted line*). (Drawing courtesy of David Teitel, MD.)

ventricle consists of individual muscle fibers, investigators have characterized systolic function by examining individual determinants in isolated muscle strips as well as in the intact heart. However, these respective determinants are not mediated by separate cellular processes. Rather, they result from the interaction of several cellular processes; thus, none of these determinants is completely independent of another. Additionally, neurohumoral stimuli also affect almost all cellular processes in the intact circulation.

The force of contraction depends on initial sarcomere length (preload). Thus, in isolated muscle strips, tension varies with length and, in the intact heart, stroke volume varies with end-diastolic volume. This phenomenon is called the Frank–Starling relationship. The degree of overlap of the thick and thin filaments is determined by sarcomere length. At one time, the varying number of cross-bridges formed at different sarcomere lengths was thought to explain the Frank–Starling relationship. However, it is now known that the calcium sensitivity of the myofilaments is dependent on sarcomere length (182). As sarcomere length decreases from optimal (2.2 μm), developed tension is less than would be expected to result from the decrease in filament overlap. The mechanism by which this occurs is unknown but may involve interactions between titin and the thick and thin filaments (138).

The load or force encountered by the heart during contraction (afterload) includes inertia within the blood and ventricular mass, impedance of the central (elastic) vasculature, and resistance of the peripheral vascular bed. In general, increasing or decreasing afterload produces a reciprocal change in the volume of blood ejected if other determinants of systolic function remain constant. In the intact circulation, however, alterations in end-diastolic volume allow Starling's law to maintain stroke volume in the face of reasonable afterload changes.

Afterload is difficult to quantitate in the intact heart. Instantaneous wall stress and vascular impedance are reasonable estimates of afterload but are difficult to measure. Usually, systemic vascular resistance or even mean arterial pressure is used as a measure of afterload. However, these variables reflect only peripheral vascular resistance. Important changes in impedance and ventricular compliance could be missed.

Heart rate is another determinant of systolic function. If stroke volume is constant, cardiac output is a linear function of heart rate. In the intact mature heart, however, cardiac output is maintained over a broad range of heart rates because alterations in heart rate affect preload and therefore stroke volume according to the Frank–Starling relationship. For example, an increase in rate decreases diastolic filling (preload) and therefore decreases stroke volume. However, the increased heart rate offsets the decreased stroke volume, and cardiac output is maintained. At very high rates, diastolic filling is impaired to the extent that cardiac output decreases. Similarly, marked decreases in heart rate result in decreased cardiac output when increases in stroke volume are unable to compensate for the low rate.

Heart rate also affects systolic function by way of the force–frequency relationship. At any given frequency of stimulation, isolated cardiac muscle strips and intact hearts generate a certain force. An increase in the frequency of stimulation at low to moderate rates causes a stepwise increase in force until a new plateau is reached. Similarly, force decreases when the frequency of stimulation is decreased. This force–frequency relationship reflects alterations in the amount of calcium available to the myofilaments. As heart rate increases, more calcium enters the myocyte. Eventually, calcium influx and efflux equilibrate, but total intracellular calcium is increased. The exact mechanisms underlying the force–frequency relationship are incompletely understood. This relationship is abolished in the phospholamban knockout mouse, suggesting that heart rate–related alterations in the phosphorylation of phospholamban may play a role (183). Whether the additional calcium enters by way of the sarcolemmal calcium channels (use-dependent modulation of calcium current) or the Na^+-Ca^{2+} exchanger (184) remains to be determined.

Myocardial contractility is defined as the potential of cardiac muscle to do work independent of preload and afterload (1). This potential is determined by the interaction between myosin and actin, including (a) the number of cross-bridges formed, which is determined largely by the availability of calcium for binding to troponin C and by myofilament response to calcium binding; (b) the rate of cross-bridge cycling, which reflects myosin ATPase activity; and (c) the time course of cross-bridge activation and deactivation, which is determined by sarcoplasmic reticulum function, the calcium sensitivity of troponin C, and cooperative interactions between cross-bridges and the thin filament. Thus, preload, afterload, heart rate, and contractility are not independent determinants of systolic function. Heart rate affects the amount of activator calcium available to the myofilaments and, therefore, contractility. Preload also modulates contractility in that the initial sarcomere length affects the calcium sensitivity of the myofilaments. Certainly, experimental conditions can be constructed such that one of these determinants is relatively dominant. However, in the intact circulation, the effects of alterations in one determinant always depend on interaction with other determinants.

Developmental Aspects

Remarkably, despite the many morphologic changes that occur during maturation of the heart, myocardial mechanics are qualitatively similar in embryonic, fetal, neonatal, and mature hearts. For example, the arterial pressure and blood flow waveforms are nearly identical except for scale. Cardiac output is carefully regulated throughout development to match metabolic demands. In the early embryo, the heart is not innervated, so other mechanisms, including local modulation of contractile force, circulating vasoactive substances, and ventricular vascular coupling, maintain appropriate cardiac output (185).

In the fetus, ventricular function is evaluated in terms of combined ventricular output because the foramen ovale and ductus arteriosus provide communication between the right and left ventricles. The combined ventricular output in the fetus is high relative to the adult animal, and indices of ventricular performance are similar or higher (186). Limited increases in combined ventricular output occur in response to alterations in preload (187–189) and afterload (187,190). Although the combined ventricular output is sensitive to alterations in heart rate (191,192), the fetal heart is unable to maintain output in the presence of prolonged tachycardia. The relatively underdeveloped sarcoplasmic reticulum in the fetus likely precludes increases in the amount of activator calcium delivered to the myofilaments. Thus, hydrops often develops in human fetuses with poorly controlled tachycardia. The increased dependence on heart rate in fetal compared with mature hearts is related, in part, to decreased compliance and greater ventricular interaction in the fetus (discussed in a later section).

Force generated by isolated muscle strips and intact hearts during myocardial contraction increases during maturation (16,83,193–196). This can be explained, in part, by the previously discussed age-related increase in the relative amount of contractile protein and changes in contractile protein isoforms. However, because the number of cross-bridges formed is an important determinant of force generation, changes in the availability of activator calcium will have important functional consequences. Age-related changes in sarcoplasmic reticulum- and sarcolemmal-mediated influx of calcium most likely contribute to maturational changes in two indices of contractility: postextrasystolic potentiation and restitution. The contraction after an extrasystole is potentiated. Postextrasystolic potentiation reflects increased release of calcium from the sarcoplasmic reticulum and is present even in very immature hearts. However, the extent of the increase in the strength of the potentiated contraction increases during maturation of the heart (17,193,196). The relationship between the force resulting from an extrasystole and the interval between the previously normal beat and the extrasystole is called restitution and reflects the availability of activator calcium to the myofilaments. Maturational changes in the time course of restitution occur in cats (17) and rabbits (7).

At birth, when oxygen demands of respiratory and thermoregulatory work increase substantially, left ventricular output increases twofold to threefold (193,197,198). Immediately after birth, left ventricular preload increases and stroke volume increases via the Starling mechanism. Heart rate also increases. As a result, cardiac output increases greatly. Thus, despite myocyte immaturity, the newborn ventricle functions at a high level. In addition, filling and contraction of the left ventricle are not constrained by the right ventricle after birth. The increase in inotropic state that occurs immediately after birth also likely reflects increased β-adrenergic stimulation (197,199). Interestingly, cardiac output and heart rate do not increase normally at birth in fetal sheep subjected to thyroidectomy 2 to 3 weeks before delivery (200). Thyroid hormone may mediate the high level of β-adrenergic stimulation at birth because thyroid hormone increases the density of β-adrenergic receptors.

Contractile reserve increases as β-adrenergic tone decreases (193,197,201) and the myocyte matures.

The high resting cardiac output limits the ability of the newborn heart to respond to alterations in the determinants of ventricular function. Although the newborn myocardium does response to alterations in preload (202), the response is limited as compared to that of the mature myocardium (203). The normal heart rate in the newborn is near maximum. Decreasing the rate decreases cardiac output, but increasing the rate does not augment output (204). Atrial contraction contributes much more to ventricular output in the immature heart than it does in the mature heart (205). Thus, the newborn heart benefits from both a heart rate near the normal range and atrial-ventricular synchrony.

The newborn heart is also very sensitive to changes in afterload. Van Hare showed that limitations in the response to increased preload reflected increased afterload (206). The limited response to afterload persists even in older animals (207). Additionally, the ratio of contractility to afterload is already relatively high so that further increases in afterload will decrease output (193,201). This decreased contractile reserve likely reflects the high levels of β-adrenergic stimulation present at birth (208).

Relaxation and Diastole

Traditionally, diastole is defined as beginning with closure of the semilunar valves and is divided into four phases: (i) isovolumic relaxation (ends with opening of the atrioventricular valves), (ii) rapid filling, (iii) diastasis (passive filling), and (iv) atrial systole. However, from a physiologic perspective, relaxation is the process by which the ventricular myocardium returns to steady state after contraction. Relaxation is thus an active process and includes the phases of isovolumic relaxation and rapid filling. True diastole encompasses two phases: (i) diastasis and (ii) atrial systole.

Relaxation

Relaxation depends on rapid removal of calcium from troponin C. This is accomplished by four pathways including the calcium pump in the sarcoplasmic reticulum, the sarcolemmal Na^+-Ca^{2+} exchanger, the sarcolemma calcium pump, and mitochondrial uptake. The latter two processes contribute minimally and will not be discussed.

In mature hearts, the decline in cytosolic calcium is mediated primarily by active transport of calcium back into the sarcoplasmic reticulum. The sarcoplasmic reticulum calcium pump ATPase (SERCA2a) couples hydrolysis of ATP to active calcium transport. The rate of calcium uptake by the sarcoplasmic reticulum correlates well with the observed rate of myocardial relaxation. Transgenic mice overexpressing the cardiac or skeletal isoform of the pump show enhanced rates of contraction and relaxation, suggesting that calcium pump activity is an important determinant of contractility (209–211). The calcium taken up by the sarcoplasmic reticulum is stored in both the free, ionized form and bound to calsequestrin, and is available for release to initiate the next contraction. Calsequestrin and other proteins associated with the sarcoplasmic reticulum calcium may modulate intracellular calcium signaling (212).

As discussed in a previous section, dephosphorylated phospholamban inhibits calcium pump activity. Phospholamban is the principal protein phosphorylated in the heart in response to β-adrenergic stimulation. A direct correlation exists between isoproterenol-induced stimulation of the calcium pump and enhancement of isovolumic relaxation in isolated guinea pig hearts (213).

The role of phospholamban has been investigated by targeted ablation of the phospholamban gene in mice. The affinity of the calcium pump for calcium and basal contractility are greatly increased in phospholamban-deficient mice compared with wild-type mice (77,214). Experimental studies comparing wild-type with phospholamban-heterozygous and phospholamban-deficient mice show a close linear correlation between the relative amount of phospholamban in the heart and the affinity of the calcium pump for calcium as well as the rates of contraction and relaxation (215). The life span of these mice is normal. Interestingly, mutations in phospholamban are associated with dilated cardiomyopathy in a few human beings (216,217). In contrast to mice that function normally with little cardiac reserve, the heart rate is relatively low in human beings and the contractile reserve is relatively high. The impact of the decreased cardiac reserve caused by abnormal phospholamban is perhaps greater in human beings than in mice.

Calcium is also removed from the myofilaments by extrusion across the cell membrane. In the steady state, the amount of calcium removed from the myocyte equals the amount entering through the calcium channels (4,44). Most of the calcium removed is extruded by the Na^+-Ca^{2+} exchanger (43). This exchanger is sensitive to both membrane potential and the intracellular calcium concentration. As discussed earlier, the sarcolemmal calcium pump plays only a minor role in removing calcium from the myocyte in the mature heart.

The relative participation of the sarcoplasmic reticulum pump and the Na^+-Ca^{2+} exchanger in removing calcium from the cytosol during relaxation differs among species. Sequestration of calcium by the sarcoplasmic reticulum is dominant in rats and rabbits; however, a greater fraction of calcium is extruded by the exchanger in rabbits (28%) than in rats (7%) (218). These results are consistent with other studies showing species-related differences in exchanger activity (48). The relative role of the sarcoplasmic reticulum pump compared with that of the exchanger in human beings is similar to that of the rabbit and not like that of the mouse or rat (164).

Age-related changes in myocardial relaxation and in the relaxation response to various stimuli occur in the dog (195), rabbit (219,220), and guinea pig (86). For example, the percentage decrease in the time constant of isovolumic relaxation (tau) in response to isoproterenol is twice as high in adult as in newborn guinea pig hearts (86). Furthermore, in the same hearts, calcium uptake, calcium pump activity, and calcium pump density are all decreased in sarcoplasmic reticulum vesicles isolated from newborn hearts compared with values measured in vesicles from adult hearts. Thus, decreased calcium sequestration by the sarcoplasmic reticulum may contribute to limited augmentation of relaxation in response to β-adrenergic stimulation in the immature myocardium.

Infusion of ryanodine impairs relaxation, confirming the dependency of relaxation on calcium sequestration by the sarcoplasmic reticulum. Interestingly, ryanodine decreases isovolumic relaxation to a greater extent in adult than in newborn guinea pig hearts (86). The observations that Na^+-Ca^{2+} exchanger activity, protein content, and mRNA levels are all increased in immature compared with mature rabbit hearts support the hypothesis that removal of calcium from the myofilaments across the sarcolemma by way of the Na^+-Ca^{2+}

exchanger contributes substantially to relaxation in the immature heart (20,49,50,54). Further support for a compensatory role for the Na^+-Ca^{2+} exchanger in the presence of diminished sarcoplasmic reticulum function comes from studies of human hearts (221–223). Sarcoplasmic reticulum calcium pump protein and mRNA levels are decreased, but Na^+-Ca^{2+} exchanger protein and mRNA levels are increased in failing compared with nonfailing adult hearts.

Because relaxation requires removal of calcium from troponin C, the calcium affinity of troponin C may be another determinant of the rate and extent of relaxation. The calcium affinity of troponin C is modulated by phosphorylation of troponin I, isoform shifts involving troponin T, and sarcomere length (108,119). Information regarding the effects of changes in calcium affinity of troponin C on relaxation is limited. However, isoform shifts that occur in troponin I (98,114,115) and troponin T(110,113) during maturation of the heart may contribute to developmental changes in augmentation of relaxation in the immature myocardium.

At the end of systole, the ventricular muscle fibers are compressed to lengths shorter than equilibrium length. Energy is stored in muscle fibers and in the extracellular matrix as in a compressed spring. The subsequent recoil, sometimes called "restoring force," is a manifestation of the ventricle's elastic properties. As discussed previously, developmental changes in titin isoforms likely result in changes in elastic properties during maturation of the heart.

Diastole

The response of the ventricle to passive and active (atrial systole) filling is characterized by the end-diastolic pressure–volume curve (Fig. 27.9). This phenomenon is mediated by the passive mechanical properties of the myocardium, ventricular interaction, and the pericardium. The developmental changes in the cytoskeleton and extracellular matrix likely affect passive properties including compliance or distensibility, stress, and elasticity. In rats, chickens, and human beings the ratio of passive to active filling increases dramatically during gestation (224–227).

The function of the two ventricles is linked (myocardial cross talk or ventricular interdependence) in the normal heart and is amplified by physiologic or structural abnormalities in either ventricle (228,229). Although the relative contributions are somewhat controversial, the right and left ventricles interact especially in diastole, when pressures are low. The position of the ventricular septum depends on the transseptal pressure difference. An increase in right ventricular volume or pressure impedes left ventricular filling. In the fetus, high right ventricular pressures and decreased ventricular compliance likely contribute to limits in left ventricular filling. After birth, the decrease in pulmonary vascular resistance and increased pulmonary blood flow are associated with an increase in pulmonary venous return. Increased left atrial pressure and left ventricular filling likely contribute to the increase in left ventricular output that occurs after birth. In the newborn, a pathologic increase in right ventricular volume or pressure as a result of, for example, persistent pulmonary hypertension could impair left ventricular output.

Pericardial pressure affects ventricular interaction and may limit ventricular filling. The pericardium, lungs, and rib cage modulate pericardial pressure. Acute ventricular dilation or a large pericardial effusion (pericardial tamponade) increases pericardial pressure and therefore decreases ventricular filling.

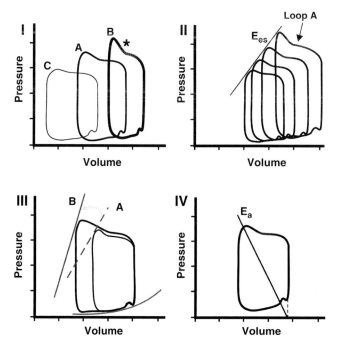

FIGURE 27.10 A: Pressure–volume (PV) loops showing alterations in afterload. Loop A represents a normal left ventricular curve. An increase in systemic vascular resistance (loop B) causes a decrease in stroke volume and a steeper and sharper late ejection contour (*asterisk*). In contrast, the late ejection curve is relatively flat when systemic vascular resistance is decreased (loop C). **B:** Loop A represents the resting PV loop. Decreasing preload by transient occlusion of the inferior vena cava allows generation of a series of PV loops; joining the end-systolic points creates a line. The slope of this line is end-systolic elastance (E_{es}), an index of ventricular contractility. **C:** Line A represents the resting PV loop with baseline E_{es}. An increase in contractility (E_{es}) (line B) results in increased end-systolic pressure and increased stroke volume. **D:** Vascular elastance is calculated as the slope of the line connecting the end-systolic point of the PV loop with the x-intercept of the end-diastolic volume. (Drawings courtesy of David Teitel, MD.)

Use of Pressure–Volume Loops to Evaluate Cardiovascular Function

The effects of alterations in contractility and relaxation as well as the relationship between cardiac function and the circulation are described efficiently by the pressure–volume loop (Fig. 27.9). This relationship describes the interaction of the pressure generated and the volume ejected from the ventricle causing pressure to increase as volume enters the circulation. Isovolumic contraction begins at a measurable end-diastolic pressure, which is defined as preload. The rate of pressure rise is determined by the ability of the myocytes to contract. When the ventricle reaches its afterload, the aortic valve opens and ejection occurs. The ventricle continues to contract, and the contour of this ejection phase is determined by the afterload against which the ventricle

contracts. This is primarily determined by the resistance of the peripheral arteries, but the elastic properties (impedance) of the large central arteries and inertial forces of the blood and within the ventricular wall also affect afterload. Changes in pressure–volume curves resulting from alterations in afterload are illustrated in Figure 27.10A. When ejection ends, the ventricle will be the stiffest or most resistant to stretch. Isovolumic relaxation then proceeds, at which time ventricular pressure decreases rapidly. When ventricular pressure falls below atrial pressure, the mitral valve opens and ventricle filling begins. Eventually ventricular pressure and volume lie on the end-diastolic pressure–volume relationship. This relationship reflects relaxation or lusitropy.

The end-systolic pressure–volume relationship characterizes contractility. A family of pressure–volume curves can be generated by sequentially decreasing preload (Fig. 27.10B). Joining the end-systolic points generates a line called the end-systolic pressure–volume relationship, the slope of which is end-systolic elastance (E_{es}), an index of contractility or inotropic state (230). As contractility increases, E_{es} increases because the increased number of actin-myosin cross-bridges that have formed makes the myocardium stiffer (Fig. 27.10C).

The profile of the pressure generated within the vascular bed as volume enters the circulation from the ventricle contributes to the physiologic effects of changes in contractility. Vascular elastance (E_a) can be calculated as the end-systolic pressure in the vessel (which is the same as that in the ventricle) divided by the stroke volume (Fig. 27.10D) (231,232). The concept of ventricular-arterial coupling (E_{es}/E_a) is used to describe how the arterial response determines the physiologic effect of changes in contractility (233). Coupling ratios of approximately one reflect optimal efficiency between ventricular work and oxygen consumption and are associated with the highest stroke work. However, stroke work varies minimally when E_{es}/E_a is between 0.3 and 1.3; decreases in stroke work are noted outside this range (234). Since the immature myocardium functions at a lower arterial elastance (afterload) and a higher ventricular elastance (contractility), the resting E_{es}/E_a is relatively high, which explains in part why newborns are very sensitive to increases in afterload (206).

CONCLUSION

The studies summarized in this chapter document important advances in our understanding of the cellular and molecular basis of developmental changes in myocardial function. Further investigation using the techniques of cellular and molecular biology will provide the means for characterizing the control systems that integrate developmental changes in various subcellular processes into global myocardial performance. Currently, many clinical decisions are based on empiric observation. In the future, diagnostic and therapeutic strategies will be based on a detailed understanding of the cellular and molecular bases of abnormal myocardial function resulting from acquired and congenital heart diseases.

References

1. Katz AM. *Physiology of the Heart*. Philadelphia: Lippincott Williams & Wilkins, 2006.
2. Artman M, Mahony L, Teitel DF. *Neonatal Cardiology*. McGraw-Hill, 2002.
3. Page E, Fozzard HA, Solaro RJ, eds. *Handbook of Physiology*, Section 2. The cardiovascular system. Vol I. *The Heart*. New York: Oxford, 2002.
4. Bers DM. Cardiac excitation-contraction coupling. *Nature* 2002;415:198–205.
5. Teitel DF. Physiologic development of the cardiovascular system in the fetus. In: Polin RA, Fox WW, eds. *Fetal and Neonatal Physiology*. Philadelphia: WB Saunders, 1998:827–836.

6. Anderson PAW. The heart and development. *Semin Perinatol* 1996;20:482–509.

7. Nassar R, Reedy MC, Anderson PAW. Developmental changes in the ultrastructure and sarcomere shortening of the isolated rabbit ventricular myocyte. *Circ Res* 1987;61:465–483.

8. Hoerter J, Mazet F, Vassort G. Perinatal growth of the rabbit cardiac cell. Possible implications for the mechanism of relaxation. *J Mol Cell Cardiol* 1981;13:725–740.

9. Olivetti G, Anversa P, Loud AV. Morphometric study of early postnatal development in the left and right ventricular myocardium of the rat: II. Tissue composition capillary growth and sarcoplasmic alterations. *Circ Res* 1980;46:503–512.

10. Legato MJ. Cellular mechanisms of normal growth in the mammalian heart: II. A quantitative and qualitative comparison between the right and left ventricular myocytes in the dog from birth to five months of age. *Circ Res* 1979;44:263–279.

11. Sheridan DJ, Cullen MJ, Tynan MJ. Qualitative and quantitative observations on ultrastructural changes during postnatal development in the cat myocardium. *J Mol Cell Cardiol* 1979;11:1173–1181.

12. Smolich JJ, Walker AM, Campbell GR et al. Left and right ventricular myocardial morphometry in fetal neonatal and adult sheep. *Am J Physiol* 1989;257:H1–H9.

13. Hirakow R, Gotoh T. Quantitative studies on the ultrastructural differentiation and growth of mammalian cardiac muscle cells: II. The atria and ventricles of the guinea pig. *Acta Anat* 1980;108:230–237.

14. Anversa P, Olivetti G, Loud AV. Morphometric study of early postnatal development in the left and right ventricular myocardium of the rat: I. Hypertrophy hyperplasia and binucleation of myocytes. *Circ Res* 1980;46:495–502.

15. Smolich JJ. Ultrastructural and functional features of the developing mammalian heart: A brief overview. *Reprod Fertil Dev* 1995;7:451–461.

16. Friedman WF. The intrinsic physiologic properties of the developing heart. *Prog Cardiovasc Dis* 1972;15:87–111.

17. Maylie JG. Excitation-contraction coupling in neonatal and adult myocardium of cat. *Am J Physiol* 1982;242:H834–H843.

18. Lucchesi PA, Sweadner KJ. Postnatal changes in Na K-ATPase isoform expression in rat cardiac ventricle. Conservation of biphasic ouabain activity. *J Biol Chem* 1991;266:9327–9331.

19. Orlowski J, Lingrel JB. Tissue-specific and developmental regulation of rat Na K-ATPase catalytic a isoform and b subunit mRNAs. *J Biol Chem* 1988;263:10436–10442.

20. Artman M. Sarcolemmal Na^+-Ca^{2+} exchange activity and exchanger immunoreactivity in developing rabbit hearts. *Am J Physiol* 1992;263:H1506–H1513.

21. Mahony L, Jones LR. Developmental changes in cardiac sarcoplasmic reticulum in sheep. *J Biol Chem* 1986;261:15257–15265.

22. Ackerman MJ. The long QT syndrome: Ion channel diseases of the heart. *Mayo Clin Proc* 1998;73:250–269.

23. Keating MT, Sanguinetti MC. Molecular and cellular mechanisms of cardiac arrhythmias. *Cell* 2001;104:569–580.

24. Shah M, Akar FG, Tomaselli GF. Molecular basis of arrhythmias. *Circulation* 2005;112:2517–2529.

25. Antzelevitch C, Brugada P, Borggrefe M, et al. Brugada syndrome: Report of the second consensus conference: Endorsed by the Heart Rhythm Society and the European Heart Rhythm Association. *Circulation* 2005;111:659–670.

26. Cheanvechai V, Hughes SF, Benson DW Jr. Relationship between cardiac cycle length and ventricular relaxation rate in the chick embryo. *Pediatr Res* 1992;31:480–482.

27. Fujii S, Ayer RK Jr, DeHaan RL. Development of the fast sodium current in early embryonic chick heart cells. *J Membrane Biol* 1988;101:209–223.

28. Xu Y-Q, Pickoff AS, Clarkson CW. Developmental changes in the effects of lidocaine on sodium channels in rat cardiac myocytes. *J Pharmacol Exp Ther* 1992;262:670–676.

29. Xu Y-Q, Pickoff AS, Clarkson CW. Evidence for developmental changes in sodium channel inactivation gating and sodium channel block by phenytoin in rat cardiac myocytes. *Circ Res* 1991;69:644–656.

30. Sakakibara Y, Wasserstrom JA, Furakawa T, et al. Characterization of the sodium current in single human atrial myocytes. *Circ Res* 1992;71:535–546.

31. Snyders DJ. Structure and function of cardiac potassium channels. *Cardiovasc Res* 1999;42:377–390.

32. Sánchez-Chapula J, Elizalde A, Navvaro-Polanco R, et al. Differences in outward currents between neonatal and adult rabbit ventricular cells. *Am J Physiol* 1994;266:H1184–H1194.

33. Crumb WJ Jr, Pigott JD, Clarkson CW. Comparison of Ito in young and adult human atrial myocytes: Evidence for developmental changes. *Am J Physiol* 1995;268:H1335–H1342.

34. Xie LH, Takano M, Noma A. Development of inwardly rectifying K+ channel family in rat ventricular myocytes. *Am J Physiol* 1997;272:H1741–H1750.

35. Wang L, Duff HJ. Developmental changes in transient outward current in mouse ventricle. *Am J Physiol* 1997;81:120–127.

36. Nakamura TY, Sturm E, Pountney DJ, et al. Developmental expression of NCS-1 (frequenin), a regulator of Kv4 K+ channels, in mouse heart. *Pediatr Res* 2003;53:554–557.

37. Morrissey A, Parachuru L, Leung M, et al. Expression of ATP-sensitive K^+ channel subunits during perinatal maturation in the mouse heart. *Pediatr Res* 2005;58:185–192.

38. Wetzel GT, Chen F, Klitzner TS. Ca2+channel kinetics in acute isolated fetal, neonatal and adult rabbit cardiac myocytes. *Circ Res* 1993;72:1065–1074.

39. Osaka T, Joyner RW. Developmental changes in calcium currents of rabbit ventricular cells. *Circ Res* 1991;68:788–796.

40. Huynh TV, Chen F, Wetzel GT, et al. Developmental changes in membrane Ca2+and K+ currents in fetal, neonatal, and adult rabbit ventricular myocytes. *Circ Res* 1992;70:508–515.

41. Hatem SN, Sweeten T, Vetter V, et al. Evidence for presence of Ca2+channel-gated Ca2+ stores in neonatal human atrial myocytes. *Am J Physiol* 1995;268:H1195–H1201.

42. Roca TP, Pigott JD, Clarkson CW, et al. L-type calcium current in pediatric and adult human atrial myocytes: Evidence for developmental changes in channel inactivation. *Pediatr Res* 1996;40:462–468.

43. Cannell MB. Contribution of sodium-calcium exchange to calcium regulation in cardiac muscle. *Ann N Y Acad Sci* 1991;639:428–443.

44. Barry WH, Bridge JHB. Intracellular calcium homeostasis in cardiac myocytes. *Circulation* 1993;87:1806–1815.

45. Egger M, Niggli E. Regulatory function of Na-Ca exchange in the heart: Milestones and outlook. *J Membrane Biol* 1999;168:107–130.

46. Philipson KD, Nicoll DA. Sodium-calcium exchange: A molecular perspective. *Annu Rev Physiol* 2000;62:111–133.

47. Hilgemann DW. New insights into the molecular and cellular workings of the cardiac Na^+/Ca^{2+} exchanger. *Am J Physiol Cell Physiol* 2004;287:C1167–C1172.

48. Sham JSK, Hatem SN, Morad M. Species differences in the activity of the Na^+-Ca^{2+} exchanger in mammalian cardiac myocytes. *J Physiol* 1995;488:623–631.

49. Boerth SR, Zimmer DB, Artman M. Steady-state mRNA levels of the sarcolemmal Na^+-Ca^{2+} exchanger peak near birth in developing rabbit and rat hearts. *Circ Res* 1994;74:354–359.

50. Artman M, Ichikawa H, Avkiran M, et al. Na^+-Ca^{2+} exchange current density in cardiac myocytes from rabbits and guinea pigs during postnatal development. *Am J Physiol* 1995;268:H1714–H1722.

51. Haddock PS, Coetzee WA, Artman M. Na^+/Ca^{2+} exchange current and contractions measured under Cl(-)-free conditions in developing rabbit hearts. *Am J Physiol* 1997;273:H837–H846.

52. Balaguru D, Haddock PS, Puglisi JL, et al. Role of the sarcoplasmic reticulum in contraction and relaxation of immature rabbit ventricular myocytes. *J Mol Cell Cardiol* 1997;29:2747–2757.

53. Koban MU, Moorman AF, Holtz J, et al. Expressional analysis of the cardiac Na-Ca exchanger in rat development and senescence. *Cardiovasc Res* 1998;37:405–423.

54. Huang J, Hove-Madsen L, Tibbits GF. Na^+/Ca^{2+} exchange activity in neonatal rabbit ventricular myocytes. *Am J Physiol Cell Physiol* 2005;288:C195–C203.

55. Katz AM. Excitation-contraction coupling. In: *Physiology of the Heart.* Philadelphia: Lippincott Williams & Wilkins, 2006:162–199.

56. Karmazyn M, Sawyer M, Fliegel L. The Na(+)/H(+) exchanger: A target for cardiac therapeutic intervention. *Curr Drug Targets Cardiovasc Haematol Disord* 2005;5:323–335.

57. Meno H, Jarmakani JM, Philipson KD. Developmental changes of sarcolemmal Na^+-Ca^{2+} exchange. *J Mol Cell Cardiol* 1989;21:1179–1185.

58. Haworth RS, Yasutake M, Brooks G, et al. Cardiac Na^+-H^+ exchanger during postnatal development in the rat: Changes in mRNA expression and sarcolemmal activity. *J Mol Cell Cardiol* 1997;29:321–332.

59. Chen F, Wetzel GT, Friedman WF, et al. Developmental changes in the effects of pH on contraction and Ca2+ current in rabbit heart. *J Mol Cell Cardiol* 1996;28:635–642.

60. Sheldon CA, Friedman WF, Sybers HD. Scanning electron microscopy of fetal and neonatal lamb cardiac cells. *J Mol Cell Cardiol* 1976;8:853–862.

61. Page E. Quantitative ultrastructural analysis in cardiac membrane physiology. *Am J Physiol* 1978;63:C147–C158.

62. Gotoh T. Quantitative studies on the ultrastructural differentiation and growth of mammalian cardiac muscle cells. The atria and ventricles of the cat. *Acta Anat* 1983;115:168–177.

63. Haddock PS, Coetzee WA, Cho E, et al. Subcellular [Ca2+]i gradients during excitation-contraction coupling in newborn rabbit ventricular myocytes. *Circ Res* 1999;85:415–427.

64. Kim H-D, Kim D-J, Lee I-J, et al. Human fetal heart development after mid-term: Morphometry and ultrastructural study. *J Mol Cell Cardiol* 1992;24:949–965.

65. Smith HE, Page E. Ultrastructural changes in rabbit heart mitochondria during the perinatal period. Neonatal transition to aerobic metabolism. *Dev Biol* 1977;57:109–117.

66. Rolph TP, Jones CT, Parry D. Ultrastructural and enzymatic development of fetal guinea pig heart. *Am J Physiol* 1982;243:H87–H93.

67. Barth E, Stammler G, Speiser B, et al. Ultrastructural quantitation of mitochondria and myofilaments in cardiac muscle from 10 different animal species including man. *J Mol Cell Cardiol* 1992;24:669–681.

68. Fisher DJ, Heymann MA, Rudolph AM. Myocardial oxygen and carbohydrate consumption in fetal lambs in utero and in adult sheep. *Am J Physiology* 1980;238:H399–H405.

69. Fisher DJ, Heymann MA, Rudolph AM. Myocardial consumption of oxygen and carbohydrates in newborn sheep. *Pediatr Res* 1981;15:843–846.

70. Franzini-Armstrong C, Protasi F, Ramesh V. Shape, size, and distribution of Ca(2+) release units and couplons in skeletal and cardiac muscles. *Biophys J* 1999;77:1528–1539.

71. Bers DM. Macromolecular complexes regulating cardiac ryanodine receptor function. *J Mol Cell Cardiol* 2004;37:417–429.

72. Viatchenko-Karpinski S, Terentyev D, Gyorke I, et al. Abnormal calcium signaling and sudden cardiac death associated with mutation of calsequestrin. *Circ Res* 2004;94:471–477.

73. Zhang L, Kelley J, Schmeisser G, et al. Complex formation between junctin, triadin, calsequestrin and the ryanodine receptor. *J Biol Chem* 1997;272:23389–23397.

74. Morad M, Cleemann L, Knollmann BC. Triadin: The new player on excitation-contraction coupling block. *Circ Res* 2005;96:607–609.

75. Fill M, Copello JA. Ryanodine receptor calcium release channels. *Physiol Rev* 2002;82:893–922.

76. Lehnart SE, Wehrens XH, Kushnir A, et al. Cardiac ryanodine receptor function and regulation in heart disease. *Ann N Y Acad Sci* 2004;1015:144–159.

77. MacLennan DH, Kranias EG. Phospholamban: A crucial regulator of cardiac contractility. *Nat Rev Mol Cell Biol* 2003;4:566–577.

78. Nakanishi T, Okuda H, Kamata K, et al. Development of the myocardial contractile system in the fetal rabbit. *Pediatr Res* 1987;22:201–207.

79. Wibo M, Bravo G, Godfraind T. Postnatal maturation of excitation-contraction coupling in rat ventricle in relation to the subcellular localization and surface density of 1,4-dihydropyridine and ryanodine receptors. *Circ Res* 1991;662–673.

80. Koss KL, Kranias EG. Phospholamban: A prominent regulator of myocardial contractility. *Circ Res* 1996;79:1059–1063.

81. Ganim J, Luo W, Ponniah S, et al. Mouse phospholamban gene expression during development in vivo and in vitro. *Circ Res* 1992;71:1021–1030.

82. Harrer JM, Haghighi K, Kim HW, et al. Coordinate regulation of SR Ca2+ -ATPase and phospholamban expression in developing murine heart. *Am J Physiol* 1997;272:H57–H66.

83. Nakanishi T, Jarmakani JM. Developmental changes in myocardial mechanical function and subcellular organelles. *Am J Physiol* 1984;246:H615–H625.

84. Fisher DJ, Tate CA, Phillips S. Developmental regulation of the sarcoplasmic reticulum calcium pump in the rabbit heart. *Pediatr Res* 1992;31:474–479.

85. Arai M, Otsu K, MacLennan DH, et al. Regulation of sarcoplasmic reticulum gene expression during cardiac and skeletal muscle development. *Am J Physiol* 1992;262:C614–C620.

86. Kaufman TM, Horton JW, White DJ, et al. Age-related changes in myocardial relaxation and sarcoplasmic reticulum function. *Am J Physiol* 1990;259:H309–H316.

87. Pegg W, Michalak M. Differentiation of sarcoplasmic reticulum during cardiac myogenesis. *Am J Physiol* 1987;252:H22–H31.

88. Rohrer D, Dillmann WH. Thyroid hormone markedly increases the mRNA coding for sarcoplasmic reticulum Ca2+-ATPase in the rat heart. *J Biol Chem* 1988;263:6941–6944.

89. Arai M, Otsu K, MacLennan DH, et al. Effect of thyroid hormone on the expression of mRNA encoding sarcoplasmic reticulum proteins. *Circ Res* 1991;69:266–276.

90. Ojamaa K, Samarel AM, Kupfer JM, et al. Thyroid hormone effects on cardiac gene expression independent of cardiac growth and protein synthesis. *Am J Physiol* 1992;263:E534–E540.

91. Khoury SF, Hoit BD, Vrushank D, et al. Effect of thyroid homone on left ventricular performance and regulation of contractile and Ca2+-cycling proteins in the baboon. *Circ Res* 1996;79:727–735.

92. Cernohorsky J, Kolar F, Pelouch V, et al. Thyroid control of sarcolemmal Na⁺/Ca²⁺ exchanger and SR Ca2+-ATPase in developing rat heart. *Am J Physiol* 1998;275:H264–H273.

93. Fisher DA. The unique endocrine milieu of the fetus. *J Clin Invest* 1986;78:603–611.

94. Towbin JA, Bowles NE. The failing heart. *Nature* 2002;415:227–233.

95. Morita H, Seidman J, Seidman CE. Genetic causes of human heart failure. *J Clin Invest* 2005;115:518–526.

96. Swynghedauw B. Developmental and functional adaptation of contractile proteins in cardiac and skeletal muscles. *Physiol Rev* 1986;66:710–771.

97. Wade R, Kedes L. Developmental regulation of contractile protein genes. *Annu Rev Physiol* 1989;51:179–188.

98. Murphy AM. Contractile protein phenotypic variation during development. *Cardiovasc Res* 1996;31:E25–E33.

99. Anderson PAW. Thin filament regulation in development. In: Solaro RJ, Moss RL, eds. *Molecular Control Mechanisms in Striated Muscle Contraction*. Boston: Kluwer Academic Publishers, 2002:329–377.

100. Barany M. ATPase activity of myosin correlated with speed of muscle shortening. *J Gen Physiol* 1967;50(suppl):197–218.

101. Lompre AM, Mercadier JJ, Wisnewsky C, et al. Species- and age-dependent changes in the relative amounts of cardiac myosin isoenzymes in mammals. *Dev Biol* 1981;84:286–290.

102. Reiser PJ, Portman MA, Ning XH, et al. Human cardiac myosin heavy chain isoforms in fetal and failing adult atria and ventricles. *Am J Physiol Heart Circ Physiol* 2001;280:H1814–H1820.

103. Carniel E, Taylor MR, Sinagra G, et al. Alpha-myosin heavy chain: A sarcomeric gene associated with dilated and hypertrophic phenotypes of cardiomyopathy. *Circulation* 2005;112:54–59.

104. Cummins P, Lambert SJ. Myosin transitions in the bovine and human heart. A developmental and anatomical study of heavy and light chain subunits in the atrium and ventricle. *Circ Res* 1986;58:846–858.

105. Barton PJ, Buckingham ME. The myosin alkali light chain proteins and their genes. *Biochem J* 1985;231:249–261.

106. Price KM, Littler WA, Cummins P. Human atrial and ventricular myosin light-chain subunits in the adult and during development. *Biochem J* 1980;191:571–580.

107. Boheler KR, Carrier L, de la Bastie D, et al. Skeletal actin mRNA increases in the human heart during ontogenic development and is the major isoform of control and failing adult hearts. *J Clin Invest* 1991;88:323–330.

108. Kobayashi T, Solaro RJ. Calcium, thin filaments, and the integrative biology of cardiac contractility. *Annu Rev Physiol* 2005;67:39–67.

109. Anderson PAW, Grieg A, Mark TM, et al. Molecular basis of human cardiac troponin T isoforms expressed in the developing, adult, and failing heart. *Circ Res* 1995;76:681–686.

110. Anderson PAW, Malouf NN, Oakeley AE, et al. Troponin T isoform expression in humans. *Circ Res* 1991;69:1226–1233.

111. Saba Z, Nassar R, Ungerleider RM, et al. Cardiac troponin T isoform expression correlates with pathophysiological descriptors in patients who underwent corrective surgery for congenital heart disease. *Circulation* 1996;94:472–476.

112. Gomes AV, Guzman G, Zhao J, et al. Cardiac troponin T isoforms affect the Ca2+ sensitivity and inhibition of force development. Insights into the role of troponin T isoforms in the heart. *J Biol Chem* 2002;277:35341–35349.

113. Nassar R, Malouf NN, Mao L, et al. cTnT1, a cardiac troponin T isoform, decreases myofilament tension and affects the left ventricular pressure waveform. *Am J Physiol Heart Circ Physiol* 2005;288:H1147–H1156.

114. Hunkeler NM, Kullman J, Murphy AM. Troponin I isoform expression in human heart. *Circ Res* 1991;69:1409–1414.

115. Sasse S, Brand NJ, Kyprianou P, et al. Troponin I gene expression during human cardiac development and in end-stage heart failure. *Circ Res* 1993;72:932–938.

116. Bodor GS, Oakeley AE, Allen PD, et al. Troponin I phosphorylation in the normal and failing human heart. *Circulation* 1997;96:1495–1500.

117. Siedner S, Kruger M, Schroeter M, et al. Developmental changes in contractility and sarcomeric proteins from the early embryonic to the adult stage in the mouse heart. *J Physiol* 2003;548:493–505.

118. Guo X, Wattanapermpool J, Palmiter KA, et al. Mutagensis of cardiac troponin I. Role of the unique NH2-terminal peptide in myofilament activation. *J Biol Chem* 1994;269:15210–15216.

119. Metzger JM, Westfall MV. Covalent and noncovalent modification of thin filament action: The essential role of troponin in cardiac muscle regulation. *Circ Res* 2004;94:146–158.

120. Solaro RJ, Kumar P, Blanchard EM, et al. Differential effects of pH on calcium activation of myofilaments of adult and perinatal dog hearts. *Circ Res* 1986;58:721–729.

121. Martin AF, Ball K, Gao L, et al. Identification and functional signficance of troponin I isoforms in neonatal rat heart myofibrils. *Circ Res* 1991;69:1244–1252.

122. Wolska BM, Vijayan K, Arteaga GM, et al. Expression of slow skeletal troponin I in adult transgenic mouse heart muscle reduces the force decline observed during acidic conditions. *J Physiol* 2001;536:863–870.

123. Day SM, Westfall MV, Fomicheva EV, et al. Histidine button engineered into cardiac troponin I protects the ischemic and failing heart. *Nat Med* 2006;12:181–189.

124. Parmacek MS, Leiden JM. Structure function and regulation of troponin C. *Circulation* 1989;80:219–233.

125. Toyota N, Shimada Y, Bader D. Molecular cloning and expression of chicken cardiac troponin C. *Circ Res* 1989;65:1241–1246.

126. Granzier HL, Irving TC. Passive tension in cardiac muscle: Contribution of collagen, titin, microtubules, and intermediate filaments. *Biophys J* 1995;68:1027–1044.

127. Stomer MH. The cytoskeleton in skeletal, cardiac and smooth muscle cells. *Histol Histopathol* 1998;13:283–291.

128. Pyle WG, Solaro RJ. At the crossroads of myocardial signaling: The role of Z-discs in intracellular signaling and cardiac function. *Circ Res* 2004;94:296–305.

129. Katz AM. The cytoskeleton. In: *Physiology of the Heart*. Philadelphia: Lippincott Williams & Wilkins, 2006:127–139.

130. Linask KK, Manisastry S, Han M. Cross talk between cell-cell and cell-matrix adhesion signaling pathways during heart organogenesis: Implications for cardiac birth defects. *Microsc Microanal* 2005;11:200–208.

131. Hagel M, George EL, Kim A, et al. The adaptor protein paxillin is essential for normal development in the mouse and is a critical transducer of fibronectin signaling. *Mol Cell Biol* 2002;22:901–915.

132. Wu JC, Sung HC, Chung TH, et al. Role of N-cadherin- and integrin-based costameres in the development of rat cardiomyocytes. *J Cell Biochem* 2002;84:717–724.

133. Corda S, Samuel JL, Rappaport L. Extracellular matrix and growth factors during heart growth. *Heart Fail Rev* 2000;5:119–130.

134. Small JVF, Furst DO, Thornell L-E. The cytoskeletal lattice of muscle cells. *Eur J Biochem* 1992;208:559–572.

135. Marijianowski MM, van der Loos CM, Mohrschladt MF, et al. The neonatal heart has a relatively high content of total collagen and type I collagen, a condition that may explain the less compliant state. *J Am Coll Cardiol* 1994;23:1204–1208.

136. van der Loop FT, Schaart G, Langmann H, et al. Rearrangement of intercellular junctions and cytoskeletal proteins during rabbit myocardium development. *Eur J Cell Biol* 1995;68:62–69.

137. van der Loop FT, Van Eys GJ, Schaart G, et al. Titin expression as an early indication of heart and skeletal muscle differentiation in vitro. Developmental re-organisation in relation to cytoskeletal constituents. *J Muscle Res Cell Motil* 1996;17:23–36.

138. Granzier HL, Labeit S. The giant protein titin: A major player in myocardial mechanics, signaling, and disease. *Circ Res* 2004;94:284–295.

139. Miller MK, Granzier H, Ehler E, et al. The sensitive giant: The role of titin-based stretch sensing complexes in the heart. *Trends Cell Biol* 2004;14:119–126.

140. Cazorla O, Freiburg A, Helmes M, et al. Differential expression of cardiac titin isoforms and modulation of cellular stiffness. *Circ Res* 2000;86:59–67.

141. Lahmers S, Wu Y, Call DR, et al. Developmental control of titin isoform expression and passive stiffness in fetal and neonatal myocardium. *Circ Res* 2004;94:505–513.

142. Opitz CA, Leake MC, Makarenko I, et al. Developmentally regulated switching of titin size alters myofibrillar stiffness in the perinatal heart. *Circ Res* 2004;94:967–975.

143. Romero T, Covell J, Friedman WF. A comparison of pressure-volume relations of the fetal, newborn, and adult heart. *Am J Physiol* 1972;222:1285–1290.

144. Flashman E, Redwood C, Moolman-Smook J, et al. Cardiac myosin binding protein C: Its role in physiology and disease. *Circ Res* 2004;94:1279–1289.

145. Capetanaki Y. Desmin cytoskeleton: A potential regulator of muscle mitochondrial behavior and function. *Trends Cardiovasc Med* 2002;12:339–348.

146. Ishibashi Y, Takahashi M, Isomatsu Y, et al. Role of microtubules versus myosin heavy chain isoforms in contractile dysfunction of hypertrophied murine cardiocytes. *Am J Physiol Heart Circ Physiol* 2003;285:H1270–H1285.

147. Perriard JC, Hirschy A, Ehler E. Dilated cardiomyopathy: A disease of the intercalated disc? *Trends Cardiovasc Med* 2003;13:30–38.

148. Huber O. Structure and function of desmosomal proteins and their role in development and disease. *Cell Mol Life Sci* 2003;60:1872–1890.

149. Ervasti JM. Costameres: The Achilles' heel of Herculean muscle. *J Biol Chem* 2003;278:13591–13594.

150. Samarel AM. Costameres, focal adhesions, and cardiomyocyte mechanotransduction. *Am J Physiol Heart Circ Physiol* 2005;289:H2291–H2301.

151. Lapidos KA, Kakkar R, McNally EM. The dystrophin glycoprotein complex: Signaling strength and integrity for the sarcolemma. *Circ Res* 2004;94:1023–1031.

152. Baines AJ, Pinder JC. The spectrin-associated cytoskeleton in mammalian heart. *Front Biosci* 2005;10:3020–3033.

153. Bennett PM, Baines AJ, Lecomte MC, et al. Not just a plasma membrane protein: In cardiac muscle cells alpha-II spectrin also shows a close association with myofibrils. *J Muscle Res Cell Motil* 2004;25:119–126.

154. Bennett V, Baines AJ. Spectrin and ankyrin-based pathways: Metazoan inventions for integrating cells into tissues. *Physiol Rev* 2001;81:1353–1392.

155. Mohler PJ, Bennett V. Ankyrin-based cardiac arrhythmias: A new class of channelopathies due to loss of cellular targeting. *Curr Opin Cardiol* 2005;20:189–193.

156. Weber KT. Cardiac interstitium in health and disease: The fibrillar collagen network. *J Am Coll Cardiol* 1989;13:1637–1652.

157. Sussman MA, McCulloch A, Borg TK. Dance band on the Titanic: Biomechanical signaling in cardiac hypertrophy. *Circ Res* 2002;91:888–898.

158. Camelliti P, Borg TK, Kohl P. Structural and functional characterisation of cardiac fibroblasts. *Cardiovasc Res* 2005;65:40–51.

159. Miner EC, Miller WL. A look between the cardiomyocytes: The extracellular matrix in heart failure. *Mayo Clin Proc* 2006;81:71–76.

160. Jane-Lise S, Corda S, Chassagne C, et al. The extracellular matrix and the cytoskeleton in heart hypertrophy and failure. *Heart Fail Rev* 2000;5:239–250.

161. Deschamps AM, Spinale FG. Disruptions and detours in the myocardial matrix highway and heart failure. *Curr Heart Fail Rep* 2005;2:10–17.

162. Fabiato A. Calcium-induced release of calcium from the cardiac sarcoplasmic reticulum. *Am J Physiol* 1983;245:C1–C88.

163. Crompton M. The role of Ca2+ in the function and dysfunction of heart mitochondria. In: Langer GA, ed. *Calcium and the Heart*. New York: Raven Press, 1990:167–198.

164. Bers DM. *Excitation-Contraction Coupling and Cardiac Contractile Force*. Dordrecht, Netherlands: Kluwer Academic Publishers, 2001.

165. Wang SQ, Wei C, Zhao G, et al. Imaging microdomain Ca2+ in muscle cells. *Circ Res* 2004;94:1011–1022.

166. Fabiato A. Appraisal of the physiological relevance of two hypotheses for the mechanism of calcium release from the mammalian cardiac sarcoplasmic reticulum: Calcium-induced release versus charge-coupled release. *Mol Cell Biochem* 1989;89:135–140.

167. Cheng H, Lederer WJ, Cannell MB. Calcium sparks: Elementary events underlying excitation-contraction coupling in heart muscle. *Science* 1993;262:740–744.

168. Wier WG, ter Keurs HEDJ, Marban E, et al. Ca2+ 'sparks' and waves in intact ventricular muscle resolved by confocal imaging. *Circ Res* 1997;81:462–469.

169. Cannell MB, Soeller C. Mechanisms underlying calcium sparks in cardiac muscle. *J Gen Physiol* 1999;113:373–376.

170. Stern MD, Cheng H. Putting out the fire: What terminates calcium-induced calcium release in cardiac muscle? *Cell Calcium* 2004;35:591–601.

171. Philipson KD. Na(+)-Ca(2+) exchange: Three new tools. *Circ Res* 2002;90:118–119.

172. Boucek RJ Jr, Shelton M, Artman M, et al. Comparative effects of verapamil, nifedipine, and diltiazem on contractile function in the isolated immature and adult rabbit heart. *Pediatr Res* 1984;18:948–952.

173. Artman M, Graham TP Jr, Boucek RJ Jr. Effects of postnatal maturation on myocardial contractile responses to calcium antagonists and changes in contraction frequency. *J Cardiovasc Pharmacol* 1985;7:850–855.

174. Seguchi M, Jarmakani JM, George BL, et al. Effect of Ca2+ antagonists on mechanical function in the neonatal heart. *Pediatr Res* 1986;20:838–842.

175. Bers DM, Bridge JH, MacLeod KT. The mechanism of ryanodine action in rabbit ventricular muscle evaluated with Ca2+-selective microelectrodes and rapid cooling contractures. *Can J Physiol Pharmacol* 1987;65:610–618.

176. Seguchi M, Harding JA, Jarmakani JM. Developmental change in the function of sarcoplasmic reticulum. *J Mol Cell Cardiol* 1986;18:189–195.

177. Artman M, Mahony L, Teitel DF. Regulation of myocyte contraction and relaxation. In: *Neonatal Cardiology*. McGraw-Hill, 2002:19–28.

178. Wetzel GT, Chen F, Klitzner TS. Na$^+$/Ca^{2+} exchange and cell contraction in isolated neonatal and adult rabbit cardiac myocytes. *Am J Physiol* 1995;268:H1723–H1733.

179. Chin TK, Christiansen GA, Caldwell JG, et al. Contribution of the sodium-calcium exchanger to contractions in immature rabbit ventricular myocytes. *Pediatr Res* 1997;41:480–485.

180. Goldstein MA, Traeger L. Ultrastructural changes in postnatal development of the cardiac myocyte. In: Legato ML, ed. *The Developing Heart*. Boston: Martinus Nijhoff Publishing, 1985:1–20.

181. Epstein ML, Kiel EA, Victorica BE. Cardiac decompensation following verapamil therapy in infants with supraventricular tachycardia. *Pediatrics* 1985;75:737–740.

182. Allen DG, Kentish JC. The cellular basis of the length-tension relation in cardiac muscle. *J Mol Cell Cardiol* 1985;17:821–840.

183. Bluhm WF, Kranias EG, Dillmann WH, et al. Phospholamban: A major determinant of the cardiac force-frequency relationship. *Am J Physiol Heart Circ Physiol* 2000;278:H249–H255.

184. Vila Petroff MG, Palomeque J, Mattiazzi AR. Na(+)-Ca2+ exchange function underlying contraction frequency inotropy in the cat myocardium. *J Physiol* 2003;550:801–817.

185. Keller BB. Overview: Functional maturation and coupling of the embryonic CV system. In: Clark EB, Markwald RR, Takao A, eds. *Developmental Mechanisms of Heart Disease.* Armonk, NY: Futura Publishing, 1995:367–385.
186. Rudolph AM, Heymann MA. The circulation of the fetus in utero. Methods for studying distribution of blood flow, cardiac output and organ blood flow. *Circ Res* 1967;21:163–184.
187. Thornburg KL, Morton MJ. Filling and arterial pressures as determinants of RV stroke volume in sheep fetus. *Am J Physiol* 1983;244:H656–H663.
188. Thornburg KL, Morton MJ. Filling and arterial pressures as determinants of left ventricular stroke volume in fetal lambs. *Am J Physiol* 1986;251:H961–H968.
189. Gilbert RD. Control of fetal cardiac output during changes in blood volume. *Am J Physiol* 1980;238:H80–H86.
190. Gilbert RD, Anderson PA, Glick KL, et al. Effects of afterload and baroreceptors on cardiac function in fetal sheep. The effect of heart rate on in utero left ventricular output in the fetal sheep. *J Dev Physiol* 1986;372:557–573.
191. Anderson PA, Glick KL, Killam AP, et al. The effect of heart rate on in utero left ventricular output in the fetal sheep. *J Physiol* 1986;372:557–573.
192. Anderson PA, Killam AP, Mainwaring RD, et al. In utero right ventricular output in the fetal lamb the effect of heart rate. *J Physiol* 1987;387:297–316.
193. Anderson PAW, Glick KL, Manring A, et al. Developmental changes in cardiac contractility in fetal and postnatal sheep: In vitro and in vivo. *Am J Physiol* 1984;247:H371–H379.
194. Nishioka K, Nakanishi T, George BL, et al. The effect of calcium on inotropy of catecholamine and paired electrical stimulation in the newborn and adult myocardium. *J Mol Cell Cardiol* 1981;13:511–520.
195. Park IS, Michael LH, Driscoll DJ. Comparative response of the developing canine myocardium to inotropic agents. *Am J Physiol* 1982;242:H13–H18.
196. Davies P, Dewar J, Tynan M, et al. Post-natal developmental changes in the length-tension relationship of cat papillary muscles. *J Physiol* 1975;253:95–102.
197. Teitel DF, Sidi D, Chin T, et al. Developmental changes in myocardial contractile reserve in the lamb. *Pediatr Res* 1985;19:948–955.
198. Teitel DF, Iwamoto HS, Rudolph AM. Effects of birth-related events on central blood flow patterns. *Pediatr Res* 1987;22:557–566.
199. Padbury JF, Roberman B, Oddie TH, et al. Fetal catecholamine release in response to labor and delivery. *Obstet Gynecol* 1982;60:607–611.
200. Breall JA, Rudolph AM, Heymann MA. Role of thyroid hormone in postnatal circulatory and metabolic adjustments. *J Clin Invest* 1984;73:1418–1424.
201. Teitel DF, Klautz R, Steendijk P, et al. The end-systolic pressure-volume relationship in the newborn lamb: Effects of loading and inotropic interventions. *Pediatr Res* 1991;29:473–482.
202. Berman W, Christensen D. Effects of acute preload and afterload stress of myocardial function in newborn and adult sheep. *Biol Neonate* 1983;43:61–66.
203. Klopfenstein HS, Rudolph AM. Postnatal changes in the circulation and responses to volume loading in sheep. *Circ Res* 1978;42:839–845.
204. Shaddy RE, Tyndall MR, Teitel DF, et al. Regulation of cardiac output with controlled heart rate in newborn lambs. *Pediatr Res* 1988;24:577–582.
205. Klautz RJ, Baan J, Teitel DF. Contribution of synchronized atrial systole to left ventricular contraction in the newborn pig heart. *Pediatr Res* 1998;43:331–337.
206. Van Hare GF, Hawkins JA, Schmidt KG, et al. The effects of increasing mean arterial pressure on left ventricular output in newborn lambs. *Circ Res* 1990;67:78–83.
207. Minoura S, Gilbert RD. Postnatal change of cardiac function in lambs: Effects of ganglionic block and afterload. *J Dev Physiol* 1987;9:123–135.
208. Smolich JJ, Cox HS, Berger PJ, et al. Left ventricular norepinephrine and epinephrine kinetics at birth in lambs. *Circ Res* 1997;81:438–447.
209. He H, Giordano FJ, Hilal-Dandan R, et al. Overexpression of the rat sarcoplasmic reticulum Ca2+ ATPase gene in the heart of transgenic mice accelerates calcium transients and cardiac relaxation. *J Clin Invest* 1997;100:380–389.
210. Loukianov E, Ji Y, Grupp IL, et al. Enhanced myocardial contractility and increased Ca2+ transport function in transgenic hearts expressing the fast-twitch skeletal muscle sarcoplasmic reticulum Ca2+-ATPase. *Circ Res* 1998;83:889–897.
211. Baker DL, Hashimoto K, Grupp IL, et al. Targeted overexpression of the sarcoplasmic reticulum Ca2+-ATPase increases cardiac contractility in transgenic mouse hearts. *Circ Res* 1998;83:1205–1214.
212. Beard NA, Casarotto MG, Wei L, et al. Regulation of ryanodine receptors by calsequestrin: Effect of high luminal Ca2+ and phosphorylation. *Biophys J* 2005;88:3444–3454.
213. Lindemann JP, Jones LR, Hathaway DR, et al. Beta-adrenergic stimulation of phospholamban phosphorylation and Ca2+-ATPase activity in guinea pig ventricles. *J Biol Chem* 1983;258:464–471.
214. Luo W, Grupp IL, Harrer J, et al. Targeted ablation of the phospholamban gene is associated with markedly enhanced myocardial contractility and loss of b-agonist stimulation. *Circ Res* 1994;75:401–409.
215. Luo W, Wolska BM, Grupp IL, et al. Phospholamban gene dosage effects in the mammalian heart. *Circ Res* 1996;78:839–847.
216. Schmitt JP, Kamisago M, Asahi M, et al. Dilated cardiomyopathy and heart failure caused by a mutation in phospholamban. *Science* 2003;299:1410–1413.
217. Haghighi K, Kolokathis F, Pater L, et al. Human phospholamban null results in lethal dilated cardiomyopathy revealing a critical difference between mouse and human. *J Clin Invest* 2003;111:869–876.
218. Bassani JWM, Bassani RA, Bers DM. Relaxation in rabbit and rat cardiac cells: Species-dependent differences in cellular mechanisms. *J Physiol* 1994;476:279–293.
219. Okuda H, Nakanishi T, Nakazawa M, et al. Effect of isoproterenol on myocardial mechanical function and cyclic AMP content in the fetal rabbit. *J Mol Cell Cardiol* 1987;19:151–157.
220. Szymanska G, Grupp IL, Slack JP, et al. Alterations in sarcoplasmic reticulum calcium uptake, relaxation parameters and their responses to b-adrenergic agonists in the developing rabbit heart. *J Mol Cell Cardiol* 1995;27:1819–1829.
221. Studer R, Reinecke H, Bilger J, et al. Gene expression of the cardiac Na+-Ca2+ exchanger in end-stage human heart failure. *Circ Res* 1994;75:443–453.
222. Flesch M, Schwinger RHG, Schiffer F, et al. Evidence for functional relevance of an enhanced expression of the Na+-Ca2+ exchanger in failing human myocardium. *Circulation* 1996;94:992–1002.
223. Wehrens XH, Lehnart SE, Marks AR. Intracellular calcium release and cardiac disease. *Annu Rev Physiol* 2005;67:69–98.
224. Reed KL, Sahn DJ, Scagnelli S, et al. Doppler echocardiographic studies of diastolic function in the human fetal heart: Changes during gestation. *J Am Coll Cardiol* 1986;8:391–395.
225. Nakazawa M, Miyagawa S, Ohno T, et al. Developmental hemodynamic changes in rat embryos at 11 to 15 days of gestation: Normal data of blood pressure and the effect of caffeine compared to data from chick embryo. *Pediatr Res* 1988;23:200–205.
226. Hu N, Connuck DM, Keller BB, et al. Diastolic filling characteristics in the stage 12 to 27 chick embryo ventricle. *Pediatr Res* 1991;29:334–337.
227. Wladimiroff JW, Huisman TW, Stewart PA, et al. Normal fetal Doppler inferior vena cava, transtricuspid and umbilical artery flow velocity waveforms between 11 and 16 weeks' gestation. *Am J Obstet Gynecol* 1992;166:921–924.
228. Bove AA, Santamore WP. Ventricular interdependence. *Prog Cardiovasc Dis* 1981;23:365–388.
229. Damiano RJ Jr, La FP Jr, Cox JL, et al. Significant left ventricular contribution to right ventricular systolic function. *Am J Physiol* 1991;261:H1514–H1524.
230. Sagawa K. The ventricular pressure-volume diagram revisited. *Circ Res* 1978;43:677–687.
231. Suga H. Left ventricular time-varying pressure-volume ratio in systole as an index of myocardial inotropism. *Jpn Heart J* 1971;12:153–160.
232. Sunagawa K, Sagawa K, Maughan WL. Ventricular interaction with the loading system. *Ann Biomed Eng* 1984;12:163–189.
233. Little WC, Cheng CP. Left ventricular-arterial coupling in conscious dogs. *Am J Physiol* 1991;261:H70–H76.
234. de Tombe PP, Jones S, Burkhoff D, et al. Ventricular stroke work and efficiency both remain nearly optimal despite altered vascular loading. *Am J Physiol* 1993;264:H1817–H1824.
235. Liew CC, Dzau VJ. Molecular genetics and genomics of heart failure. *Nat Rev Genet* 2004;5:811–825.

CHAPTER 28 ■ FETAL ECHOCARDIOGRAPHY AND FETAL CARDIOLOGY

CHARLES S. KLEINMAN, MD, JULIE S. GLICKSTEIN, MD, AND ROXANA SHAW, MD

HISTORICAL PERSPECTIVE

In the introduction to his epochal 1974 monograph, "Congenital Diseases of the Heart," Dr. Abraham M. Rudolph (1) emphasized the importance that characterization of the cardiovascular adaptation of the fetus during the months leading to delivery and the postnatal transition of the systemic and pulmonary circulatory system has in improving understanding of the clinical condition of the neonate, and in contributing to the formulation of logical and physiologically based management strategies for various forms of congenital heart disease. Toward this end Rudolph and associates developed techniques for the study of cardiovascular development, using chronically instrumented fetal lambs (2). Their studies included normal fetal animals, as well as fetuses in which pulmonary artery or ascending aortic banding was used to simulate pulmonary or aortic stenosis. Regional flow within the cardiovascular system was investigated through the use of radionuclide-labeled microspheres (3,4). These observations were extended to include the varied components of the transitional circulation, providing insights into the relative roles played by oxygenation, cord clamping, and the intrinsic fetal shunt pathways in the redistribution of blood flow in the fetus at the time of birth (5–8).

Rudolph's studies of the fetal lamb were postulated as a model for understanding the human fetal and transitional circulation, despite the recognition that the fetal lamb differed in substantial ways from the human fetus. These differences would be reflected in altered regional flow distribution to organs such as the brain, which constitutes a larger fraction of body mass in the primate and human than in the ovine fetus. In addition, the relative difference in the degree of "maturation" of the ovine neonate, compared with the human neonate, could also result in alterations in regional blood flow distribution between the two species.

In 1977, Rudolph's observations of the fetal lamb served as the foundation on which our understanding of the fetal and transitional circulation of the human fetus was based. In 1976 Dr. Frederick Morin completed a doctoral thesis toward his M.D. degree at the Yale University School of Medicine that was, in turn, based on the observations of a 1972 study (9) describing the use of M-mode echocardiographic recordings of fetal cardiac activity in the human fetus. This paper had speculated that fetal cardiac function in normal and abnormal pregnancies could be analyzed through the use of the measurement of left ventricular ejection fraction from M-mode recordings of cardiac wall motion against time. The same publication predicted that the small size, complex anatomy, and rapid heartbeat of the human fetus would not allow complex congenital cardiac malformations to be diagnosed prenatally.

This served as the intellectual underpinning for the initiation of a clinical research project at the Yale University School of Medicine aimed at applying fetal echocardiography to validate in the human fetus the observations that had been documented in the ovine fetal model. The first findings of significance related to paradoxic motion of the interventricular septum, reminiscent of the findings postnatally in patients with cardiac malformations associated with volume- and pressure-overloaded right ventricles. M-mode echocardiography in the human fetal heart thus provided noninvasive confirmation that the findings that had previously been made in the ovine fetus, where the fetal right ventricle functions as the dominant ventricle, ejecting a larger stroke volume than the left ventricle at systemic blood pressure, held, as well, for the fetal human.

Subsequent studies were undertaken to characterize the development of the human fetal cardiovascular system and were presented at the annual meetings of the Society for Gynecologic Investigation and the Society for Pediatric Research in the spring of 1978. At the latter, Dr. Helen Taussig commented on the importance of these findings, which offered the potential for the diagnosis of congenital heart disease in early gestation, and the potential for termination of such pregnancies, to decrease the individual and societal burden of congenital heart disease in these children.

Thereafter, our attention was turned toward establishing a clinical role for fetal echocardiography. Although we had speculated in 1978 that such studies could be useful for the diagnosis of congenital heart disease, it was not until a year had passed before we were able to prove this. Our first peer-reviewed publication on this topic appeared in 1980 (10). This paper suggested indications for detailed fetal echocardiographic study in pregnancies deemed to be at high risk for congenital heart disease. M-mode and two-dimensional echocardiography was used to document atrioventricular septal defect in a patient with left atrial isomerism and complete atrioventricular block, atrial flutter, and hydrops fetalis. M-mode echocardiography was used to document tricuspid atresia and hypoplastic right ventricle in a second fetus. M-mode echocardiography was used to demonstrate the presence of complete heart block in the fetus of a mother with systemic lupus erythematosus.

This article was reviewed by Dr. Alexander Nadas in the 1981 edition of the Yearbook of Pediatrics (10). Dr. Nadas noted the potential for the use of the technique for research purposes, but he doubted the potential for a clinical role for fetal echocardiography, owing to the improbability of establishing such diagnoses before the legal limits for termination of pregnancy.

During 1980, publications from San Diego (11) and from London (12,13) documented the potential for examination of the fetal heart using sequential, segmental analysis of cardiac structure. In 1981 deGeeter et al., from Strasbourg, hosted the first international meeting devoted to fetal echocardiography and clinical fetal cardiology.

In 1984, at the World Congress of Pediatric Cardiology, Fermont et al., from Paris, reported their experience with four-chamber screening of the fetal heart for the detection of congenital heart disease (13) This was followed by the description provided by Allan et al. (14) of a regional screening program in London. She went on to train ultrasonographers throughout Great Britain and the Continent to participate in similar screening programs throughout Europe.

INDICATIONS FOR FETAL ECHOCARDIOGRAPHY

While it must be recognized that most cases of congenital heart disease result from pregnancies in women who are not identified in advance to be at higher-than-average risk for congenital heart disease, most women referred for detailed fetal echocardiographic study have been judged to be at risk according to factors defined as fetal, maternal, or familial risks (Table 28.1).

TABLE 28.1

INDICATIONS FOR FETAL ECHOCARDIOGRAPHY

Familial risk factors
History of congenital heart disease
Previous sibling
Paternal
Mendelian syndromes that include congenital heart disease
Noonan
Tuberous sclerosis
Maternal risk factors
Congenital heart disease
Cardiac teratogen
Isotretinoin
Lithium carbonate
Ethanol
Phenytoin
Valproic acid
Trimethadione
Carbamazepine
Maternal metabolic disorders
Diabetes mellitus
Phenylketonuria
Fetal risk factors
Extracardiac anomalies
Chromosomal
Anatomic
Fetal cardiac arrhythmia
Irregular rhythm
Tachycardia (>180 bpm) in absence of amnionitis
Fixed bradycardia
Nonimmune hydrops fetalis
Abnormal fetal situs
Suspected fetal heart malformation on screening ultrasound
Lack of reassuring four-chamber view during basic obstetric scan

bpm, beats per minute.

SCREENING FOR CONGENITAL HEART DISEASE

As noted above, most infants with congenital heart disease are born to women without high-risk indications for congenital heart disease. Fermont et al. documented that the identification of fetuses with abnormal four-chamber views of the heart would improve case findings of major forms of congenital heart disease. The normal four-chamber view of the fetal heart may be obtained in approximately 95% of fetuses examined between the late second and early third trimesters of pregnancy. The fetal heart is normally a midline structure, with the apex pointing leftward toward the fetal stomach. The heart lies in a horizontal orientation, above the transverse liver. By orienting the ultrasound transducer approximately 30 degrees cephalad from the transverse plane where the fetal abdominal circumference is measured, a tomographic view of the fetal heart is obtained (Fig. 28.1) that demonstrates the four-chamber anatomy of the fetal heart. The central fibrous body of the normal fetal heart is intact, with the septal leaflet of the tricuspid valve inserting slightly closer to the cardiac apex than the insertion of the anterior leaflet of the mitral valve. The atrial cavities and the interposed atrial septum are visualized, with the foramen ovale representing the major source of blood flow into the left atrium from the inferior vena cava. The atrial septum primum undulates in the left atrial flow stream from the inferior vena cava and functions as a flap valve that functionally seals

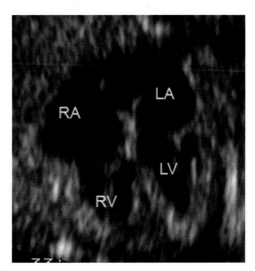

FIGURE 28.1 Normal four-chamber view of the fetal heart during midtrimester. Note the relatively equal transverse diameters of the right and left atria (RA, LA) and the right and left ventricles (RV, LV). The septal leaflet of the tricuspid valve is inserted into the central fibrous body of the heart in a position that is slightly offset toward the apex of the heart in comparison with the site of insertion of the anterior mitral leaflet to the central fibrous body. The moderator band is seen at the apex of the right ventricle. The posterior inflow portion of the ventricular septum is interposed between the two ventricular chambers. The foramen ovale represents an unrestricted flow orifice between the inferior vena cava and the left atrium. Relatively highly oxygenated umbilical venous return from the inferior vena cava is preferentially shunted into the left atrium through the left ventricle and into the descending aortic distribution. This provides the most highly oxygenated arterial blood to the fetal coronary arterial and cerebral circulation.

the foramen ovale following birth, owing to increased pulmonary venous return consequent to gaseous expansion of the lungs and postnatal decrease in pulmonary vascular resistance. The atrial chambers are normally symmetrical in appearance as are the ventricular chambers. The right ventricular chamber appears slightly foreshortened owing to the moderator band at the ventricular apex. The right ventricular surface of the ventricular septum is more coarsely trabeculated than the left ventricular septal surface. In the short-axis view, the two papillary muscles of the mitral valve are seen, and neither of these muscles is associated with the ventricular septum, whereas the tricuspid valve characteristically has a chordal insertion to the conal region of the right ventricular outflow tract.

Abnormalities of four-chamber anatomy may characterize certain forms of congenital heart disease. In many cases, the primary structural abnormality of the heart may be apparent in the view of the central fibrous body. Such defects may include complete atrioventricular septal (canal) defect, hypoplastic left heart syndrome, hypoplastic right heart syndrome, Ebstein malformation of the tricuspid valve, and various forms of single ventricle (Fig. 28.2). Disproportion of atrial or ventricular chambers may reflect altered flow patterns through the fetal cardiovascular system (15). In such

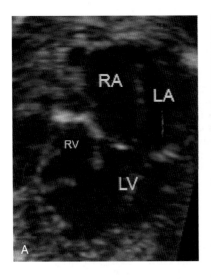
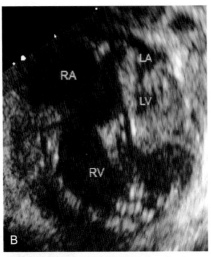
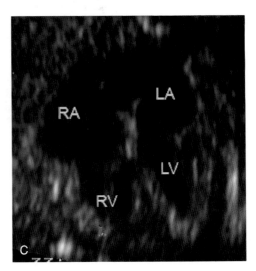
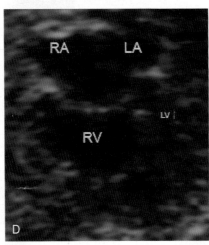
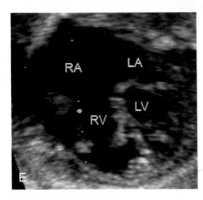
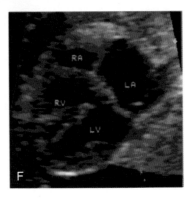

cases the four-chambers of the heart may change their volume and or wall thickness to reflect the volume and pressure of blood flow through them. Pulmonary valve stenosis, for example, may be associated with right ventricular wall hypertrophy, with decreased chamber volume secondary to increased right-to-left shunting across the foramen ovale, with right ventricular hypertrophy or with increased chamber volume if tricuspid regurgitation occurs (16). Similarly, disproportionate development of atria and ventricles may occur in the presence of discrete obstruction to left ventricular outflow (Fig. 28.3) (17–19). The latter findings have served as the foundation for the development of the first programs for fetal intervention.

The sensitivity and specificity of abnormal four-chamber screening for congenital heart disease has been discussed repeatedly in the literature during the past decade, with claims varying from a sensitivity of 0% to 10% (e.g., the RADIUS trial in the United States) (20–22) to a sensitivity of >80%, with most series suggesting a sensitivity in the range of approximately 40% (10,23–49) (Table 28.2).

Based on claims of the utility of four-chamber screening for congenital heart disease, bodies such as the American College of Radiology, The American College of Obstetrics and Gynecology, and the American Institute of Ultrasound in Medicine have recommended that four-chamber screening views of the heart be included in the evaluation of all fetuses undergoing ultrasound examination, regardless of indication.

Views of the ventricular outflow tracts may demonstrate ventriculoarterial connections and allow the integrity of the ventricular septum to be evaluated. The right ventricular outflow through the main pulmonary artery typically proceeds in a posterior sweep to the ductus arteriosus, the descending thoracic aorta, and the pulmonary arterial bifurcation, with the left pulmonary artery continuing posteriorly and the right pulmonary artery arising at a right angle where it passes under the aortic arch. The left ventricular outflow tract continues into the ascending aorta, which ascends vertically toward the head. The ascending aorta and main pulmonary artery crisscross one another after emerging from their respective outflow tracts. Tomographic imaging demonstrates the perpendicular courses of these great arteries by showing one vessel in a longitudinal view while the second vessel is seen as a circular cross section (Fig. 28.4). The presence of subvalvar, valvar, and/or supravalvar obstruction can be detected, and outflow tract abnormalities such as ventricular septal defect, conal septal malalignment, double-outlet ventricle, or arterial transposition may be documented (Fig. 28.5).

The sensitivity and specificity that is added to four-chamber screening of the fetal heart by the inclusion of long-axis views of the outflow tracts has resulted in revised standards for screening echocardiography by the American College of Radiology, the American College of Obstetrics and Gynecology, and the American Institute of Ultrasound in Medicine.

ECHOCARDIOGRAPHIC ASSESSMENT OF FETAL CARDIOVASCULAR PERFORMANCE

M-mode echocardiographic studies of the human fetus provide insight into the relative size and pressure of the fetal ventricles. The timing of mechanical events during various phases of the cardiac cycle as reflected by wall motion, and motion of the cardiac valves may be used to analyze cardiac rhythm (10) (Fig. 28.6).

Two-dimensional imaging may provide insight into relative chamber and blood vessel volume and pressure. The addition of color flow Doppler adds further information concerning the function of the atrioventricular and semilunar valves and flow within important fetal flow pathways such as the ductus venosus, foramen ovale, and ductus arteriosus (Fig. 28.7).

Feit et al. (50) used two-dimensional imaging of the fetal foramen ovale to estimate interatrial volume flow and demonstrated that fetuses with left heart obstruction had smaller transatrial flow volumes, whereas patients with right heart obstructive lesions had larger-volume right-to-left interatrial shunts. Berning et al. (51) emphasized the importance of color

FIGURE 28.2 Montage of six four-chamber views of the fetal heart (A–F). Five cases of congenital heart disease (A, B, D, E, F) involving the central fibrous body of the heart are contrasted with a normal four-chamber view (C). A: Four-chamber view of the heart of a fetus with tricuspid atresia and ventricular disproportion favoring a large left ventricle (LV). There is an absent right atrioventricular connection, with a solid bar of muscle interposed between the right atrium (RA) and the right ventricle (RV). The sole inflow to the right ventricle is through a small muscular ventricular septal defect, and the right ventricular cavity is hypoplastic. There is a large, single, mitral atrioventricular valve and a large left ventricle. B: Marked ventricular disproportion favoring the right ventricle in a patient with hypoplastic left heart. The left atrium (LA) is small and thick-walled. The mitral valve is miniscule, and the left ventricle is hypoplastic, with a hypertrophic, fibroelastotic, left ventricle. C: Normal four-chamber view of the fetal heart with proportionate ventricular and atrial cavites, normal atrioventricular valves, and intact central fibrous body. D: Unbalanced, right ventricular not dominant, atrioventricular septal defect in a fetus with trisomy 21. Although not visualized in this view, this fetus also had a hypoplastic aortic arch. E: Atrial and ventricular disproportion, with enlarged right-sided cardiac chambers in a fetus with the Ebstein malformation of the tricuspid valve. The tricuspid valve leaflets are redundant and thickened, with inferior displacement of the septal (visualized) and posterior (not seen in this view) leaflets. The anterior leaflet (visualized) is redundant and sail-like. A significant portion of the inflow tract of the right ventricle is "atrialized" owing to the apical displacement of the tricuspid valve. F: A balanced, complete, atrioventricular septal defect in a hydropic fetus with trisomy 21. The central fibrous portion of the heart is deficient, with a large ostium primum atrial septal defect, inflow ventricular septal defect, and a common atrioventricular valve.

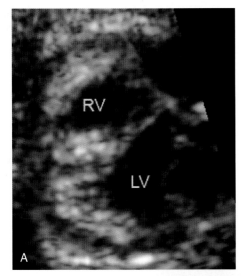

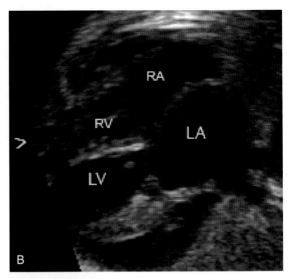

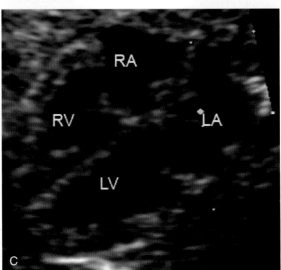

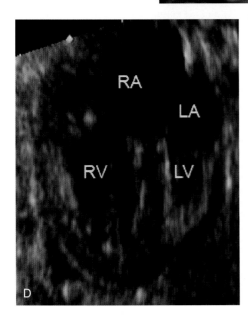

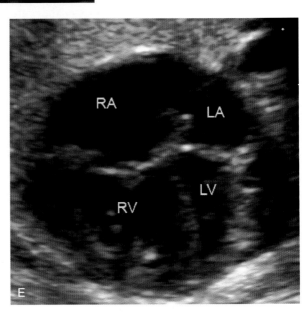

TABLE 28.2

PRENATAL SCREENING FOR CONGENITAL HEART DISEASE

Study	View	GA(Weeks)	Sensitivity
Wylie et al., 1994	4-Chamber View	18–20	18
Stoll et al., 1993	4-Chamber View	18–22	9.2
Sharland and Allan, 1992	4-Chamber View	—	69
Vergani et al., 1992	4-Chamber View	18–20	81
Buskens et al., 1996	4-Chamber View	16–24	5
Todros et al., 1997	4-Chamber View	18–22	15
Ott, 1995	4-Chamber View	—	14
Luck, 1992	4-Chamber + outflow	19	33.3
Tegnander et al., 1995	4-Chamber	16–22	10
Rustico et al., 1995	Full fetal echo	20–22	35.4
Hafner et al., 1998	Full fetal echo	16–22	43.8
Achiron et al., 1992	Extended fetal echo	18–24	78 (48 4-chamber)
Stümpflen et al., 1996	Extended fetal echo	18–28	88 (47 4-chamber)
Tegnander et al., 2006	4-Chamber + outflow	18	57

GA, gestational age.

flow in determining flow volume and direction across the fetal ductus arteriosus and foramen ovale in the diagnosis of left heart hypoplasia and /or obstruction to right ventricular outflow (Fig. 28.8).

Pulsed Doppler flow analysis has been used to estimate regional blood flow distribution within the human fetus during the third trimester of pregnancy. The radionuclide-labeled microsphere studies of Heymann and Rudolph had demonstrated that in the third trimester fetal lamb the fetal right ventricle ejects 67% of the combined output of the two ventricles, with only approximately 8% of the combined output traversing the high-resistance pulmonary vascular bed. This 8% of combined output enters the fetal left atrium as pulmonary venous return and combines with relatively oxygen-rich pulmonary venous return streaming through the ductus venosus and inferior vena cava, amounting to approximately 25% of combined ventricular output. Thus 33% of combined ventricular output crosses the mitral valve and is ejected as left ventricular output. This relatively oxygen-rich blood is preferentially distributed to the coronary arteries and cerebral circulation. In the 1970s Dr. Rudolph had estimated that the relatively larger brain in the primate and human would probably demand a larger volume of left ventricular output during fetal life. He estimated that the ratio of right-to-left ventricular combined output in the human would be in the range of 55%/45%. Doppler flow studies in the human fetus have confirmed that estimate (52,53).

Friedman et al. (54–56) described studies on isolated strips of myocardium as well as on whole heart preparations

FIGURE 28.3 Montage of five four-chamber views of the fetal heart (A–E), including one normal fetal heart (C) and five examples (A–C, E, F) of fetal four-chamber views that are abnormal, owing to perturbed flow distribution, in a setting of a normal central fibrous body. A: Four-chamber view of the heart of a fetus with pulmonary stenosis. The right ventricle (RV) is thick walled and has a slightly diminutive right ventricular cavity. In the presence of pulmonary valve stenosis and a competent tricuspid valve, the increased right ventricular afterload results in myocardial hypertrophy, whereas the decreased diastolic compliance of the hypertrophic myocardium results in increased right-to-left shunting at the level of the foramen ovale, with increased left ventricular (LV) diastolic filling volume and diminished right ventricular filling volume. B: Four-chamber view of the heart of a hydropic fetus with severe aortic stenosis, left ventricular dilation and fibroelastosis, with decreased systolic contraction. Severe mitral regurgitation resulted in marked left ventricular (LV) and left atrial (LA) dilation and premature closure of the foramen ovale. C: Normal four-chamber view of fetal heart demonstrating symmetrical right and left atria (RA, LA) and ventricles (RV, LV). D: Four-chamber view of fetal heart of a fetus with coarctation of the aorta. The right ventricle is disproportionately enlarged, whereas the left ventricle is relatively volume depleted. This is due to the abnormal distribution of blood flow, favoring outflow from the right ventricle at the expense of outflow from the left ventricle in this fetus with aortic arch hypoplasia. E: Four-chamber view of fetal heart near term. This image demonstrates the finding that disproportionate right ventricular dilation, while characteristic of flow redistribution in fetuses with coarctation of the aorta, is sensitive but not specific for this malformation. In this case the disproportion between ventricular dimensions is not associated with aortic coarctation, but rather, with normal flow redistribution near term in a fetus with mild constriction of the ductus arteriosus, with resulting increased right ventricular afterload. This image was found in one of the patients in our series who was incorrectly suspected to have coarctation of the aorta, based on this finding.

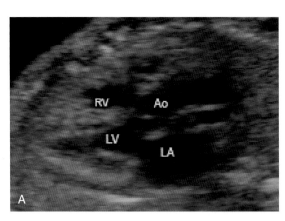

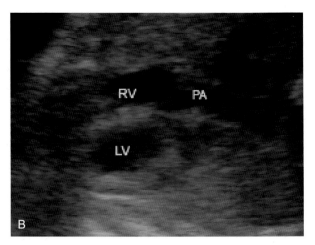

FIGURE 28.4 A: Long-axis view of the left ventricular outflow tract. The anterior right ventricle (RV) is separated from the posterior left ventricle (LV) by the ventricular septum. The integrity of the anterior ventricular septum can be evaluated. The membranous and conoventricular septa are intact and are in fibrous continuity with the anterior wall of the ascending aorta (Ao). The anterior mitral valve leaflet is in fibrous continuity with the posterior aortic wall, resulting in commitment of the left ventricle to the ascending aorta. The left atrium is posterior to the ascending aorta. The subaortic region is unobstructed. The right pulmonary passes beneath the aortic arch. **B:** Long-axis view of the right ventricular outflow tract. The right and left ventricles (RV, LV) are separated by the intact ventricular septum. The main pulmonary artery (PA) arises above the conus and dives posteriorly to continue into the ductal arch. The main pulmonary artery is perpendicular to the ascending aorta, which passes vertically until the branch point between the innominate artery and the aortic arch.

from mature and fetal sheep. These studies demonstrated that mature myocardium generates higher tension (pressure) at any end-diastolic length (volume) than does fetal myocardium. In addition, passive tension (pressure) is higher at any level of diastolic length (volume). These myocardial properties explain the findings of fetal animal studies, suggesting limited afterload and preload reserve. Possible explanations for the intrinsic differences between fetal and mature myocardium have been offered, including a paucity of contractile elements within immature myocytes, the increased amount of nuclear material within mature myocytes, the relatively haphazard orientation of contractile elements within immature myocardium versus the parallel orientation of the contractile elements of mature myocardium, and the relative deficiency of sarcomeres in fetal myocardium versus the rich distribution of sarcomeres and t-tubules that provide intracellular calcium stores to the contractile elements of mature myocardium.

Pulsed Doppler and Doppler tissue imaging studies of biventricular diastolic filling are suggestive of restrictive ventricular diastolic physiology throughout mid and late gestation (57–60) (Fig. 28.9). Recently, normative data have been presented for strain and strain rate analysis of the fetal myocardium (61,62). It is unclear at this point whether this technique will offer a reliable and reproducible means of analyzing fetal systolic and diastolic performance.

Rudolph (1) has summarized the known characteristics of fetal myocardium and the *in utero* environment to explain the proclivity of fetuses toward the development of interstitial edema and hydrops fetalis (Fig. 28.10). These findings explain the frequent development of hydrops fetalis among fetuses with pressure or volume overload, or sustained brady arrhythmias or tachyarrhythmias.

Huhta et al. (63,64) have proposed the use of a Cardiovascular Profile Score to determine the overall status of cardio-vascular compensation of given fetuses. They have suggested that this scoring system be used to predict the onset of cardiovascular decompensation in such fetuses (Fig. 28.11).

CONGENITAL HEART DISEASE AND ASSOCIATED ANOMALIES

The association of congenital heart disease with extracardiac malformations of the fetus and neonate is well recognized. In some cases the genetic basis for these associations has been defined (9,10,65–68).

Increased nuchal fold thickness during the first trimester of pregnancy may be associated with a high incidence of congenital heart disease. In some cases the increased nuchal thickness is related to karyotypic abnormalities such as Turner (XO) syndrome or trisomy 21 (69–74). In other cases karyotype may be normal, and increased nuchal thickness is thought to relate to elevated fetal venous pressure from congestive heart failure. Increased first trimester fetal nuchal thickness is another screening method that has been used as an indication for detailed fetal echocardiographic study (17,75–83).

Typical associations do exist between specific congenital heart malformations, extracardiac malformations, and karyotypic abnormalities. These associations include atrioventricular septal (canal) defects, increased nuchal thickness, macroglossia, hypoplastic fifth metacarpal, duodenal atresia, sandal foot, and trisomy 21; double-outlet right ventricle, intrauterine growth restriction, clinodactyly, rocker bottom feet, esophageal atresia, and trisomy 18; ventricular septal defect, holoprosencephaly, intrauterine growth restriction, cleft lip and palate, and trisomy 13; coarctation of the aorta, bicommissural aortic valve, cervical cystic hygroma, pedal

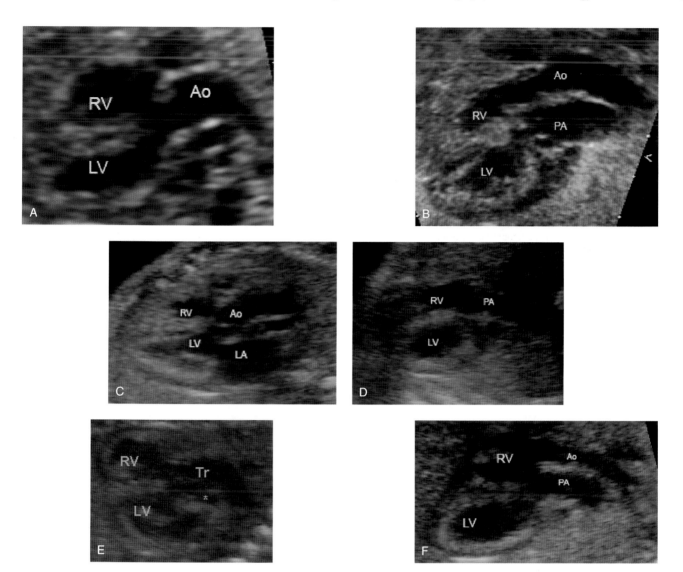

FIGURE 28.5 Montage of six long-axis views of the fetal heart. **A:** Long-axis view of the left ventricular outflow tract of a fetus with pulmonary atresia with ventricular septal defect. The ventricular septum is interposed between the left and right ventricles (LV, RV). The large ascending aorta (Ao) overrides a large, subaortic, conoventricular septal defect. The right ventricular outflow tract is not visualized in this view. **B:** Long-axis view of the left ventricular outflow tract in a fetus with d-transposition of the great arteries. The interventricular septum is intact. There is ventriculoarterial discordance, with the transposed ascending aorta (Ao) arising anteriorly from the right ventricle (RV) and the main pulmonary artery (PA) arising from the left ventricle. The parallel course of the great arteries is characteristic of transposition or malposition. **C and D:** Normal left (C) and right (D) ventricular outflow tracts. **E:** Long-axis view of the left ventricular outflow tract in a fetus with type I persistent truncus arteriosus. The common arterial trunk (Tr) overrides a large conoventricular septal defect. A common pulmonary artery (*asterisk*) arises from the left and posterior aspect of the common arterial trunk. **F:** Long-axis view of the left ventricular outflow tract of a fetus with Taussig-Bing double-outlet right ventricle. The parallel, d-malposed great arteries both arise from over the right ventricle, with the pulmonary artery overriding the subpulmonary ventricular septal defect. The anterior aorta is much smaller than the posterior pulmonary artery. Further investigation demonstrated a hypoplastic aortic arch.

edema, and Turner syndrome (XO). The association between conotruncal malformations and (del) 22q11.2, DiGeorge syndrome, and/or velocardiofacial syndrome has been well established (84–89).

We have found approximately 60% of fetuses presenting with complete, balanced, atrioventricular septal defect and previously undiagnosed karyotype to have trisomy 21.

Approximately 20% of patients with complete atrioventricular septal defect have abnormalities of situs and spleen formation. The association of interrupted inferior vena cava, azygous continuation to the superior vena cava, intestinal malrotation, complete heart block, and/or agenesis of the gall bladder and extrahepatic biliary atresia are strongly suggestive of left atrial isomerism and polysplenia.

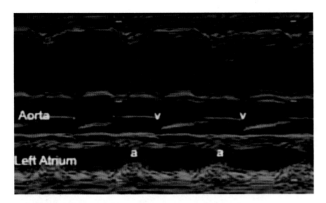

FIGURE 28.6 M-mode echocardiographic tracing recorded through aortic root of fetus with atrial ectopic tachycardia at 180 beats per minute. The aortic valve opening (v) corresponds to the mechanical response to electrical stimulation leading to ventricular myocardial contraction. Note that there is one atrial undulation (a) for each ventricular contraction.

On the other hand, the associated presence of double-outlet right ventricle, atrioventricular septal defect, pulmonary stenosis or atresia, totally anomalous pulmonary venous connection, and intestinal malrotation are strongly suggestive of right atrial isomerism with asplenia (90–96). Such fetuses represent some of the most difficult cases to manage postnatally.

The frequent association of karyotypic abnormalities with congenital heart disease diagnosed during the second trimester (30.5%) has led us to recommend genetic diagnosis whenever congenital heart disease is diagnosed in the human fetus (10,65,66,97,98). Although many patients have been reticent to submit to the risks involved with amniocentesis, chorion villus sampling, or fetal umbilical blood sampling, especially if they have no intention of terminating the pregnancy, even if a karyotypic abnormality is found, or if the pregnancy has already progressed past the legal limit for abortion, we have still recommended such testing in selected cases. Although termination of pregnancy is a compelling and common reason for genetic testing, the knowledge of an

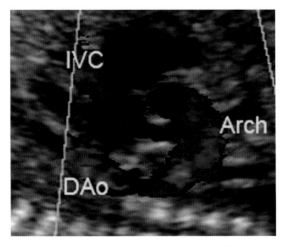

FIGURE 28.7 Color flow imaging demonstrating inferior vena caval (IVC) return to the fetal right atrium and aortic arch flow (Arch) into the descending thoracic aorta (DAo).

associated genetic abnormality may serve to change the aggressiveness of tocolytic therapy for the treatment of premature labor or the aggressiveness of fetal monitoring and the use of cesarean delivery for fetal distress during labor in the mothers of such fetuses.

The frequent association of congenital heart disease (C), especially conotruncal malformations and abnormalities of the vertebrae (V), anus (A), trachea (T), esophagus (E), kidneys (R), and limbs (L) (VACTERL) should raise suspicions when congenital heart disease is diagnosed in fetuses with polyhydramnios (e.g., impeded fetal swallowing), oligohydramnios (impeded urine production), scoliosis, or limb reduction (99,100).

Another, increasingly common, indication for targeted echocardiographic imaging is the presence of intensely echogenic foci within the left ventricular cavity (Fig. 28.12). This finding is thought to relate to increased mineralization of the tips of the papillary muscles within the left ventricle and, in and of itself, does not appear to have short- or long-term clinical consequences. Until recently there was some debate about whether these echogenic foci are clinical markers for the presence of trisomy 21. A recent meta-analysis concluded that such foci increase the odds that a given pregnancy is complicated by the Down syndrome by a factor of five to six. It is recommended, therefore, that this factor be included in the risk calculation (e.g., along with traditional serum markers and nuchal translucency evaluation) for consideration of invasive genetic diagnosis for affected fetuses (101–111).

WHAT IS IT THAT PARENTS WANT TO KNOW?

The value of prenatal diagnosis can best be assessed in light of what parents expect from these studies. It would be easier to cost account such studies if they had a clear-cut impact on neonatal survival or quality of survival. As we will see below, such an impact is difficult to demonstrate for many of these studies. On the other hand, there is little doubt that detailed prenatal diagnosis has an impact on prenatal counseling and on the process of obtaining informed consent from parents whose fetuses have complex congenital heart disease.

Our counseling process consists of a detailed description of the anatomic abnormalities in the fetus. This includes abnormalities of the heart and cardiovascular system, as well as extracardiac abnormalities that may have been diagnosed. The details of neonatal care, including the timing, location and mode of delivery; details of medical support, including the potential need for prostaglandin E₁ infusion for the maintenance of ductal patency, and the potential need for reparative or palliative surgery in the neonatal period are discussed. The details of neonatal and later surgical procedures are discussed, and the parents are given the opportunity to speak with the pediatric cardiac surgeons, pediatric surgeons, and neonatologists who are likely to be involved in neonatal management.

In large part, parents care little about the detailed name or anatomic description of their child's anomaly. They are, most often, interested in learning what the short-, mid-, and long-term prospects for survival are. These are often related to associated anomalies, genetic syndromes, or underlying anatomy. From a purely anatomic perspective, the breakpoint in the continuum of disease severity, from 1 (minimal) to 10 (most severe), occurs at 8. Eight to ten on this scale represents lesions that are not reparable into a two-ventricular physiology, and

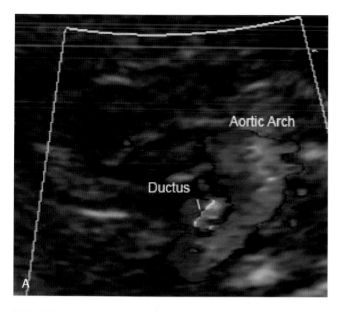

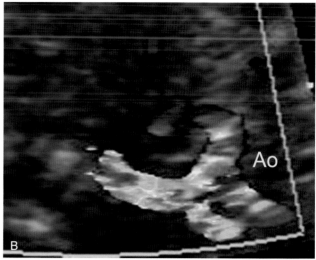

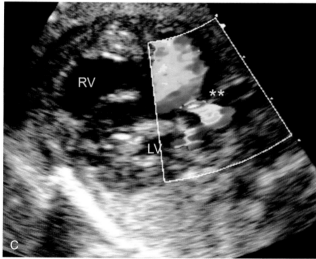

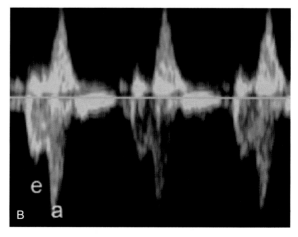

FIGURE 28.8 Series of figures demonstrating Doppler color flow analysis in fetuses with congenital heart disease. **A:** Retrograde flow in the ductus arteriosus (Ductus) of a fetus with complex congenital heart disease, including pulmonary atresia. **B:** Retrograde perfusion of the aortic arch (Ao) in a fetus with complex congenital heart disease including aortic arch hypoplasia. **C:** Left-to-right flow across the foramen ovale (*asterisks*) in a fetal patient with hypoplastic left heart syndrome. (LV, left ventricle; RV, right ventricle.)

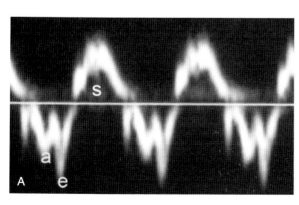

FIGURE 28.9 Doppler tissue imaging velocities from lateral tricuspid valve ring (**A**) and Doppler flow-velocity waveforms from right ventricular inflow of normal midtrimester fetus (**B**). Note dominant a′ and a waves. These waveforms are consistent with relatively restrictive fetal ventricular myocardium at this stage of development.

POSTNATAL
Tissue Pressure - 5 mm Hg
HP - 45 mm Hg
HP - 15 mm Hg
Arterial.
Venous.
COP - 25 mm Hg
COP - 25 mm Hg
15 mm Hg Out
Net Pressure
0 mm Hg
15 mm Hg In
FETAL
Tissue Pressure - 2 mm Hg
HP - 30 mm Hg
HP - 5 mm Hg
Arterial
Venous
COP - 15 mm Hg
COP - 15 mm Hg
13 mm Hg Out
Net Pressure
1 mm Hg out
12 mm Hg In

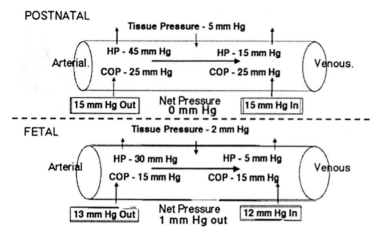

FIGURE 28.10 Schematic representation of idealized postnatal versus fetal capillary hemodynamics. The relationship between hydrostatic and plasma oncotic pressures and estimated interstitial tissue pressure result in a net outward pressure gradient of 1 mm Hg in the fetus, whereas in the postnatal cardiovascular system the net pressure gradient is 0. This explains the dependency of the fetal cardiovascular system on avid lymphatic drainage to prevent fetal edema and fluid third-spacing.

will, by definition, require Fontan's palliation and/or orthotopic transplantation.

The prospects for cardiac and neurodevelopmental outcome are discussed, and the parents are encouraged to ask questions of the physician management team and/or a team composed of parents of children with similar problems who have consented to be available, as requested.

DOES PRENATAL CARDIAC DIAGNOSIS MAKE A DIFFERENCE?

It has taken approximately a quarter-century of experience with prenatal cardiac diagnosis to demonstrate that such studies have a positive impact on survival (112–114). In fact, multiple studies that focused on the impact of prenatal diagnosis of hypoplastic left heart syndrome appeared to suggest that prenatal diagnosis had a negative influence on short-term survival (49,115–128). This is almost certainly related to a weighting toward prenatal diagnosis in a sicker subpopulation of fetuses. A study undertaken at Yale during the early 1990s failed to demonstrate a survival advantage related to the prenatal diagnosis of congenital heart disease with single-ventricle physiology, whereas fetuses with lesions reparable into two ventricular systems appeared to enjoy a significant enhancement of survival prospects (10). This study also demonstrated a common experience with several other series in which it was noted that prenatal cardiac diagnosis, by facilitating anticipatory use of prostaglandin E_1 to prevent closure of the ductus arteriosus in neonates with critical impairment of systemic or pulmonary blood flow, allows affected fetuses to avoid neonatal

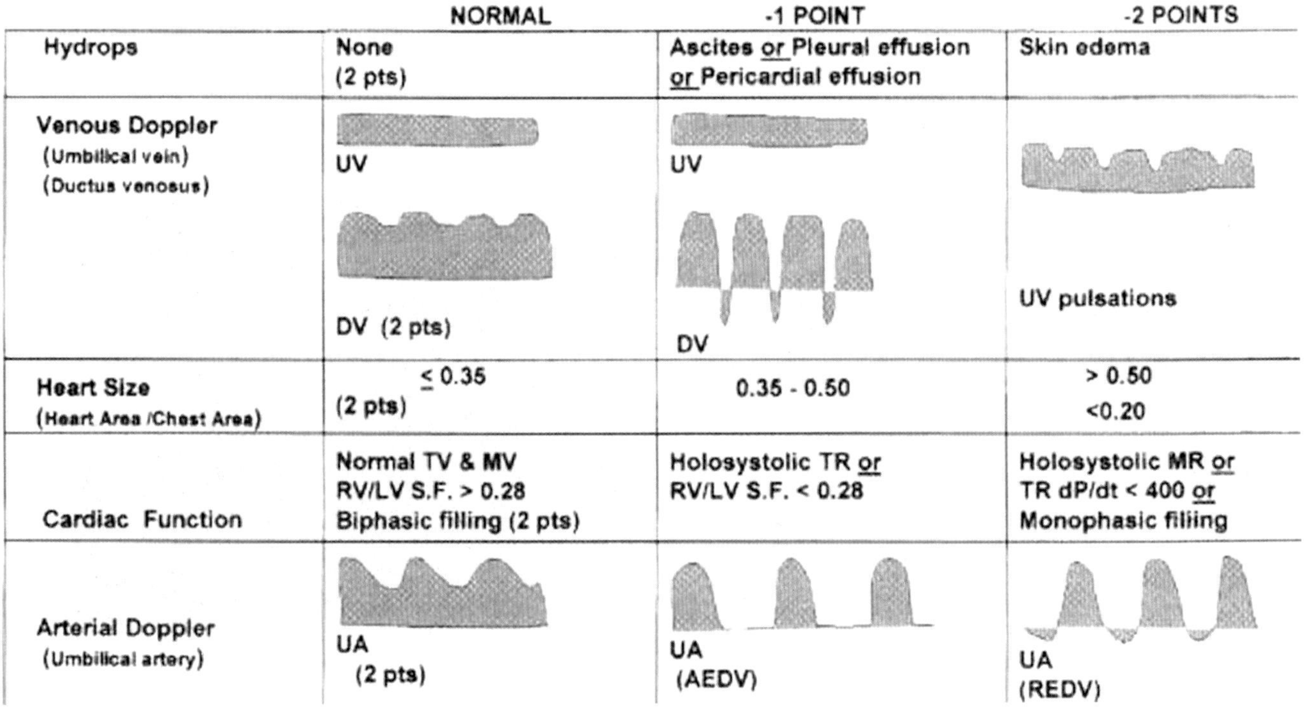

NORMAL
-1 POINT
-2 POINTS
Hydrops
None
(2 pts)
Ascites or Pleural effusion
or Pericardial effusion
Skin edema
Venous Doppler
(Umbilical vein)
(Ductus venosus)
UV
DV (2 pts)
UV
DV
UV pulsations
Heart Size
(Heart Area /Chest Area)
≤ 0.35
(2 pts)
0.35 - 0.50
> 0.50
<0.20
Cardiac Function
Normal TV & MV
RV/LV S.F. > 0.28
Biphasic filling (2 pts)
Holosystolic TR or
RV/LV S.F. < 0.28
Holosystolic MR or
TR dP/dt < 400 or
Monophasic filling
Arterial Doppler
(Umbilical artery)
UA
(2 pts)
UA
(AEDV)
UA
(REDV)

FIGURE 28.11 Huhta's proposed Cardiovascular Profile Score.

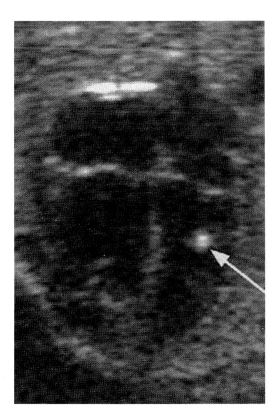

FIGURE 28.12 Intensely echogenic focus associated with the antero-lateral mitral papillary muscle. This does not represent a cardiac neo-plasm, nor does it represent a structural malformation of the fetal heart. There has been a suggestion that such foci are associated with an increased odds ratio of associated fetal Down syndrome.

acidemia (140,129,130). Although currently an unproven hypothesis, the potential neurodevelopmental advantage to be derived by the affected neonate who avoids acidemia may, in the long run, prove to be the most important long-term salutary effect of prenatal cardiac diagnosis (131). Among the individual cardiac lesions for which prenatal diagnosis has been suggested to impart a survival advantage are transposition of the great arteries, coarctation of the aorta, and hypoplastic left heart syndrome. A review of the experience in the latter series emphasizes the impact of prenatal diagnosis on the parental intention-to-treat decision-making process (10,49,122–124, 127,132).

The Impact of Prenatal Cardiac Diagnosis on Planning for Delivery

A relatively unique consideration of the impact of prenatal cardiac diagnosis on outcomes that is not readily appreciated in reviews of surgical outcome for individual lesions relates to the options for site of delivery of these patients. It has been demonstrated that surgical survival for neonates with hypoplastic left heart syndrome is directly related to the surgical volume of the individual surgical center (133). Prenatal diagnosis, by providing parents with the luxury of time to conduct research, may alter survival through alteration of the site of delivery and subsequent surgery. It is possible, if not likely, that the latter will exert a profound impact of prenatal cardiac diagnosis on postnatal survival.

With the possible exception of patients with associated extracardiac lesions (e.g., abdominal wall defects) that necessitate cesarean delivery (134), it is rare for the pediatric cardiologist to become involved in the decision making concerning mode of delivery. Possible exceptions include fetuses with cardiac rhythm disturbances that preclude effective intrapartum fetal heart rate monitoring. Such arrhythmias may include chaotic rhythms that confound the logic of external fetal heart rate monitors that calculate heart rate from instantaneous measurement of R-R intervals or regular tachyarrhythmias or bradyarrhythmias such as atrial flutter or complete heart block, where the heart rate may not vary with the alterations in sympathetic and parasympathetic tone that are associated with uterine contraction (10).

Cesarean delivery may be indicated in rare situations in which the coordinated care of the neonate requires the skills of multiple specialists who are assembled specifically at the time of delivery. During the past year at the Morgan Stanley Children's Hospital of New York–Presbyterian we have delivered four fetuses by cesarean section specifically for cardiac reasons. Two fetuses were delivered by cesarean section owing to prenatal identification of premature closure of the foramen ovale in fetuses with hypoplastic left heart syndrome with secondary pulmonary venous obstruction, whereas one fetus was delivered by cesarean section to undergo cardiac surgery because of obstructed totally anomalous pulmonary venous return in a setting of right atrial isomerism, atrioventricular septal defect, double-outlet right ventricle with d-malposition of the great arteries, and pulmonary atresia. One fetus, with d-transposition of the great arteries and congenital diaphragmatic hernia, was delivered by cesarean section and immediately placed on extracorporeal membrane oxygenation, pending surgical repair of diaphragmatic hernia and subsequent successful arterial switch repair of transposition of the great arteries.

It is unusual for neonates with congenital heart disease to require resuscitation in the delivery room. In such cases there is usually an associated problem that interferes with adequate lung inflation at the time of the first breath. Such issues may arise in fetuses with associated pleural effusions, in fetuses with associated congenital diaphragmatic hernia, or in fetuses in which marked cardiomegaly results in a mass effect and pulmonary hypoplasia (e.g., occasional cases of Ebstein malformation of the tricuspid valve or aortic stenosis with marked mitral regurgitation). In fetuses with severe pulmonary venous obstruction, such as those with totally anomalous pulmonary venous drainage with obstruction (particularly common among fetuses with visceral heterotaxy and right atrial isomerism), congenital atresia of the common pulmonary vein, or in fetuses with hypoplastic left heart syndrome and premature closure of the foramen ovale, gas exchange may be rendered inadequate by pulmonary edema. Doppler waveform analysis in the branch pulmonary veins may be predictive of critical pulmonary venous obstruction (Fig. 28.13). Fetuses with tetralogy of Fallot and absent pulmonary valve with aneurysmal pulmonary arteries may have inadequate ventilation owing to external airway compression with secondary tracheomalacia or bronchomalacia (Fig. 28.14).

REGIONAL BLOOD FLOW ANALYSIS AND FETAL CARDIOVASCULAR WELL-BEING

Techniques for the antenatal surveillance of the fetus are aimed at the detection of evidence of cardiovascular compromise secondary to hypoxemia and deterioration of acid-base balance

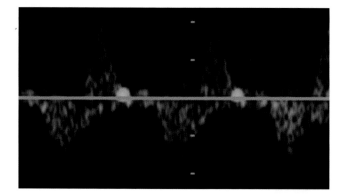

FIGURE 28.13 To-and-fro flow pattern in pulmonary vein in a fetal patient with obstructed left ventricular inflow and outflow. This pattern is highly suggestive of severe pulmonary venous obstruction. This fetus is likely to have critical pulmonary insufficiency in the neonatal period. Such fetuses may require emergent pulmonary vein decompression in the neonatal period and have been subjected to efforts at atrial septal fenestration *in utero*.

(69,135–143). Blood flow within the placental circulation is normally characterized by low placental vascular resistance with no evidence of autoregulation within the placental vascular bed, whereas regional arterial flow in the fetal organ beds is finely tuned through local autoregulation. Impaired forward arterial flow is almost invariably associated with altered preload and with abnormalities of flow within the fetal central venous system, including the inferior vena cava (IVC), ductus venosus (DV), and umbilical vein (UV). Abnormalities of flow in these three locations may be used to predict acid-base status in growth-retarded fetuses (Fig. 28.15). Progressive deterioration in cardiac pump function is associated with absent forward venous flow during atrial contraction or with atrial flow reversal in the central venous circulation. The finding of retrograde flow in the ductus venosus during atrial contraction is almost

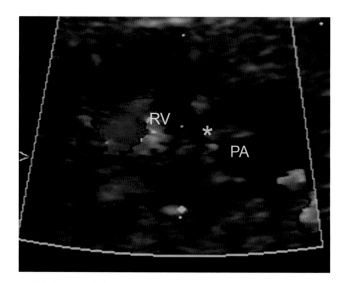

FIGURE 28.14 Pulmonary regurgitation (*asterisk*) through the rudimentary pulmonary valve structure in a fetus with tetralogy of Fallot with absent pulmonary valve results in dilation of the right ventricle (RV) and pulmonary artery (PA). Such fetuses are in danger of pulmonary insufficiency in the delivery room secondary to external compression of the major airways by the aneurysm-dilated main and proximal right pulmonary artery.

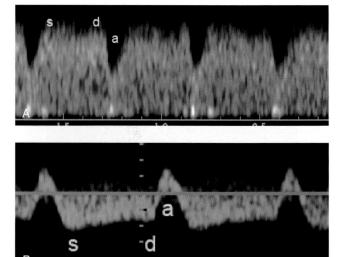

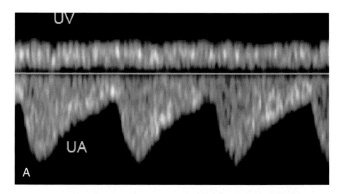

FIGURE 28.15 Ductus venosus flow waveforms. **A:** Normal ductus venosus flow demonstrates high continuous antegrade flow during systole (s) diastole (d) and during atrial contraction (a). **B:** Retrograde ductus venosus flow during atrial contraction. This is a finding that is associated with progressive ventricular dysfunction, with increased end-systolic volume, and increased end-diastolic pressure.

always associated with fetal acidemia, and diastolic notching of flow within the umbilical vein, especially with evidence of absent or reversed end-diastolic flow in the umbilical artery, is a finding that presages fetal death if delivery is not accomplished within the ensuing 72 hours (Fig. 28.16) (144–149).

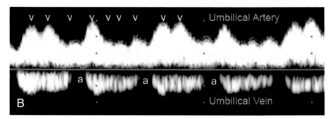

FIGURE 28.16 **A:** Simultaneous recording of umbilical artery (UA) and vein (UV) waveforms in normal fetus. Note the high end-diastolic velocity in the umbilical artery, characteristic of a low-resistance placental circulation. There is continuous antegrade flow in the umbilical vein. **B:** Umbilical arterial and venous flow in a fetus with paroxysmal polymorphic ventricular tachycardia and hydrops fetalis. Note chaotic, rapid, umbilical arterial undulations and marked umbilical venous notching associated with cannon a-waves. The latter are associated with elevated systemic venous pressure, hydrops fetalis, and fetal acidosis.

Ventricular-vascular coupling within a cardiovascular system based largely on massive blood flow through a low-resistance bed such as the placenta, with a propelling pump consisting of fetal myocardium, with limited preload and afterload reserve is markedly sensitive to alterations in placental resistance and/or to altered myocardial performance or intravascular volume (150). Elevation of placental vascular resistance is typically accompanied by an increase in umbilical arterial pulsatility (difference between peak arterial and end-diastolic flow velocity), whereas enhanced perfusion (organ-sparing) of fetal organs is associated with decreased local resistance and decreased arterial pulsatility. Brain-sparing has been demonstrated to be strongly predictive of perinatal morbidity in fetuses with intrauterine growth retardation and has been correlated with impaired cognitive outcome in children who were born as very preterm infants (151–153). It has been suggested that growth-restricted human fetuses with chronic cerebral hypoxemia and established brain-sparing centralization of blood flow may have limited capacity for further hyperperfusion in response to superimposed acute hypoxemia (154). Fouron et al. (155–157) have focused attention on the direction of blood flow in the aortic isthmus among patients with congenital heart disease. These workers have found that retrograde isthmus blood flow is correlated with impaired neurodevelopmental outcome, perhaps related to limited cerebral oxygen delivery. We have focused our attention on pulsed Doppler evidence of centralization of fetal blood flow as evidence of autoregulation of fetal cerebral blood flow in the presence of congenital cardiac malformations associated with impaired cerebral oxygen delivery owing to impaired cerebral arterial oxygen content or impaired cerebral blood flow volume (158). We have speculated that these alterations in blood flow may be associated with altered neurodevelopmental potential among these fetuses. Kaltman et al. (159) found similar cerebral flow redistribution among fetuses with right ventricular outflow obstruction, whereas Jouannic, et al. (160) found similar cerebral flow redistribution among fetuses with transposition of the great arteries.

THE PRENATAL EVOLUTION OF CONGENITAL HEART DISEASE

The principal underlying Rudolph's concept that understanding fetal cardiovascular adaptation to congenital heart disease will provide insight into the transitional and neonatal circulation is that in the fetal heart form follows function. It was postulated for many years prior to the availability of ultrasound for the observation of progressive cardiovascular development in the presence of congenital heart disease that certain congenital cardiac malformations evolve through the course of pregnancy, with a tendency toward progressive chamber and blood vessel disproportion (1).

It has been demonstrated, for example, that pulmonary outflow obstruction in fetuses with tetralogy of Fallot may progress in severity, even to the point of acquired pulmonary atresia, over the course of pregnancy (118,161,162). Aortic or pulmonary valvar stenosis may progress over the course of pregnancy into valvar atresia, and ventricular wall thickness may increase in concert with increased ventricular peak systolic pressure. Ventricular chamber development may be stunted by the development of endocardial fibroelastosis and diminished ventricular compliance through pregnancy (163).

On the other hand, the onset of atrioventricular valve regurgitation, related to papillary muscle dysfunction or chordal rupture, may result in marked progressive ventricular and atrial chamber enlargement.

PRENATAL TREATMENT OF CONGENITAL HEART DISEASE

In 1992, Tynan et al. reported an experience with a percutaneous technique for fetal aortic balloon valvuloplasty (127,164) involving needle puncture of the maternal abdomen, uterus, and fetal thorax, with direct catheterization of the fetal left ventricle by direct apical puncture and subsequent wire and catheter manipulation across the stenotic aortic valve. Four fetuses were subjected to this technique, with a single long-term survivor. That technique was devised against a background of appalling survival figures for neonates who were undergoing surgical treatment for that lesion at that time. Interestingly, between the announcement of that procedure in the popular press and the appearance of the publication in the scientific literature, that same group declared a moratorium on the procedure, related in part to improved surgical and interventional catheterization results with neonates with aortic stenosis (120). A subsequent publication described the world's experience with this technique and documented a 100% failure rate at several institutions (165), with the almost inexplicable conclusion that further investigation was merited to determine the potential role for the technique in the management of fetuses with congenital heart disease.

A decade later, the group from Boston Children's Hospital released to the press the results of a preliminary experience with the use of this same technique, which was being proposed as a means of preventing the evolution of severe fetal aortic stenosis with associated left ventricular fibroelastosis into hypoplastic left heart syndrome. This group has attempted to establish criteria for selection of candidates for this procedure and has preliminary data to suggest that in selected cases fetal balloon valvuloplasty may result in incremental aortic and left ventricular growth, and may result in adequate left heart development to obviate the need for Norwood-type palliation, with subsequent biventricular palliation of these patients. This group has suggested that retrograde perfusion of the aortic arch is one of the criteria that is predictive of hypoplastic left heart in patients who do not undergo palliation. Their experience suggests that successful aortic balloon valvuloplasty results in antegrade perfusion of the aortic arch and isthmus in these fetuses (112,166).

Tulzer et al. (167,168), from Austria, reported an experience with fetal percutaneous pulmonary balloon valvuloplasty, under ultrasound guidance, to alter the natural history of pulmonary atresia with intact ventricular septum. Their initial experience was undertaken to avoid the onset of hydrops fetalis. The potential for hydrops fetalis was assessed on the basis of the Cardiovascular Profile Score that was proposed by Huhta et al. (63). Subsequent experience has suggested that pulmonary outflow obstruction is almost invariably associated with atrial flow reversal in the inferior vena cava and ductus venosus that may affect the cardiovascular performance score and unduly increase the prediction of subsequent hydrops fetalis. Several centers have subsequently reported successful pulmonary valve dilation and biventricular management of fetuses who presented with pulmonary atresia and intact ventricular septum (169–171).

Rigorous evaluation of the selection criteria and outcome of such fetuses has not been reported at this point.

The Boston Children's Hospital group has also reported a preliminary experience with percutaneous balloon dilation of the atrial septum, in an effort to palliate fetuses with hypoplastic left heart syndrome and pulmonary venous obstruction secondary to premature stenosis or closure of the foramen ovale (112). This technique was devised to improve the results for the palliation of these fetuses, who may present with severe pulmonary hypertension and pulmonary lymphangiectasia. The experience reported to date suggests that needle perforation of the atrial septum, wire passage across the septum, and delivery of an angioplasty catheter with subsequent balloon septoplasty can be accomplished. This preliminary experience suggests that improvement in balloon technology will be required before the technique may be expected to result in a lasting fenestration of the atrial septum that is adequate to effect a positive impact on fetal physiology. This same group has recently reported successful coronary stent placement in the atrial septum of a fetus with hypoplastic left heart syndrome. This fetus survived and subsequently underwent successful Norwood stage I palliation. A recent report describes the use of fetoscopy to place an intracardiac ultrasound catheter into the esophagus of a human fetus with hypoplastic left heart syndrome to provide transesophageal imaging during an unsuccessful attempt to perform balloon septoplasty on a fetus with critical pulmonary venous obstruction (172).

Reports of the use of fetoscopy and laser fenestration of the atrial septum in such fetuses, and for the management of aortic stenosis, have emerged from Tampa (173). Ludomirsky et al., in St. Louis, are investigating the use of targeted ultrasound to create fenestrations of the fetal atrial septum. Scattered anecdotal reports of attempts to perform aortic and pulmonary balloon valvuloplasty procedures have surfaced at national and international cardiology meetings.

The overall results of these procedures ideally should be collected, analyzed, and reported in a critical fashion, lest the pediatric cardiology community repeat the hard lessons learned by the Maternal-Fetal Medicine community during the past 25 years. The latter have had a broad experience with fetal therapy, and have seen several promising techniques capture the imagination of the medical community and the popular press, only to be abandoned later after disappointing functional outcomes were found on follow-up of surviving infants. Such techniques were based on a seemingly sound understanding of physiology and on a genuine desire to be of help to these fetuses. These included procedures for fetal exteriorization for repair of diaphragmatic hernia and for palliation of urinary tract obstruction, and percutaneous cerebral ventriculoamniotic shunting for palliation of obstructive hydrocephalus (113,174–183).

THE CURRENT ROLE OF FETAL ECHOCARDIOGRAPHY

Although fetal echocardiography and fetal cardiology have been incorporated into many pediatric cardiology programs during the past two decades, the role of fetal cardiology varies considerably from location to location. In many cases the role of fetal cardiology is dependent on the relationship that exists between Maternal-Fetal Medicine and Pediatric Cardiology in the institution, and whether individual institutions have obstetric and neonatal services housed under the same roof.

We have reviewed the role that prenatal cardiac diagnosis has had during the last two calendar years (2004 and 2005) at the Morgan Stanley Children's Hospital of the Columbia University Medical Center campus of New York–Presbyterian Hospital. This service represents a highly evolved fetal cardiology service, with an extremely active Department of Obstetrics and Gynecology, with a Maternal-Fetal Medicine Division that has been actively involved in the performance of detailed fetal echocardiography for many years. Similarly, our Pediatric Echocardiography service has been extremely aggressive in its approach to fetal cardiology and the integration of these patients into the neonatal cardiology and cardiovascular surgery service.

Unlike the case at many centers, where the pediatric cardiology service provides screening services for fetal congenital heart disease, the service at our hospital is based on a model in which the pregnant woman is seen, almost exclusively, by the obstetric service, until a high-risk indication for a targeted fetal echocardiogram is identified. Although services that perform screening studies usually find evidence of fetal cardiovascular disease in approximately 10% of scans, with the predominant indication for scan being a previous family history of congenital heart disease, we have a very different experience (184,185).

In 2004 and 2005, our laboratory diagnosed 254 fetuses to have congenital cardiovascular abnormalities among only 878 fetuses (including 27 sets of twins) undergoing fetal echocardiography (yield 30%). These included seven false-positives (six cases of relative right heart enlargement and suspected coarctation of the aorta and one case of suspected pulmonary arterial hypoplasia). Three false-negative cases were documented, including one case of unappreciated partial anomalous pulmonary venous connection in a twin with a large cystic adenomatoid malformation of the lung with marked cardiac displacement; one fetus who presented at 2 weeks of age with evidence of coarctation of the aorta, which was successfully repaired; and one fetus with a congenital diaphragmatic hernia in which an aortic coarctation was missed (Table 28.3).

Six fetuses were found to have incomplete diagnoses, including one fetus with Down syndrome and complete atrioventricular septal defect who was diagnosed postnatally to also have type A aortic arch interruption. A second fetus, with trisomy 13 and double-outlet right ventricle with subaortic ventricular septal defect, was diagnosed postnatally to also have an aortopulmonary window. Aortic coarctations were unappreciated in three fetuses, one with atrioventricular septal defect, one with complete transposition of the great arteries, and one with tricuspid atresia and ventricular septal defect in whom transposition of the great arteries and the coarctation was overlooked. Dextrocardia and situs inversus were missed in a fetus in which the Shone complex was correctly diagnosed.

Of the 247 patients with congenital heart disease (excluding the 7 false-positives), follow-up is complete for 196. Fourteen patients have been lost to follow-up, and 37 are still awaiting delivery and postnatal evaluation as of the time of writing this chapter. Of the 247 cases of correctly identified congenital heart disease, the categories of abnormality, in descending order of frequency, consisted of conotruncal malformations (84), hypoplastic left heart variants (65), left-to-right shunt lesions (37) (including complete atrioventricular septal

TABLE 28.3

CONGENITAL CARDIAC MALFORMATIONS DIAGNOSED IN UTERO (2004–2005) ($n = 247$)

Diagnosis	No.
Conotruncal malformations	84
d-Transposition (+/− VSD)	19
Double-outlet RV (+/− malposition)	28
Tetralogy of Fallot	19
Pulmonary atresia/VSD	3
Tetralogy with absent PV syndrome	2
L-TGA (+/− VSD)	7
Truncus arteriosus	6
Hypoplastic left heart syndrome	55
HLHS (mitral/aortic atresia)	27
HLHS (Shone complex)	21
HLHS variant (not Shone)	4
Left-to-right shunt lesions	37
Atrioventricular septal defects	**29**
Complete Atrioventricular Septal Defect	28
Ostium Primum ASD	1
Ventricular Septal Defect	**7**
Atrial Septal Defect	**1**
Right Heart Obstructive Lesions	30
Tricuspid atresia (+/− d-TGA)	13
Pulmonary atresia + IVS	8
Critical PS	7
Tricuspid Stenosis	1
Pulmonary artery stenosis	1
Visceral heterotaxia	9
Double-inlet LV	6
Cardiac tumors	5
Aortic arch anomalies	5
Ascending aortic aneurysm	3
Interrupted aortic arch + VSD	2
Ebstein malformation of the TV	3
Single ventricle variants	2
Other (one of a kind)	11
TOTAL	247

defect (29), right heart obstructions (30), visceral heterotaxia (9), double-inlet left ventricle (6), aortic arch anomalies (5), cardiac tumors (5), Ebstein malformation of the tricuspid valve (3), single ventricle variants (2), and other one-of-a-kind anomalies (11).

Forty-five patients either underwent termination of pregnancy (40) or chose nonintervention (compassionate care) (5) for their offspring. The diagnoses of these fetuses are presented in Table 28.4, but were weighted toward severe anomalies such as hypoplastic left heart syndrome and visceral heterotaxia, with or without genetic abnormalities (e.g., trisomy 21, trisomy 13).

Fourteen patients suffered intrauterine fetal demise. These included five fetuses with trisomy 18, including one with double-outlet right ventricle with subaortic ventricular septal defect, one with double-outlet right ventricle with subpulmonary ventricular septal defect and d-malposition of the great arteries, one with atrioventricular septal defect, one with tetralogy of Fallot, and one with a large atrioventricular canal-type ventricular septal defect. Two additional fetuses that had fetal demise had persistent truncus arteriosus, one with interrupted aortic arch, the other with severe hydrops fetalis secondary to truncal valve stenosis and regurgitation. Both of these fetuses were chromosomally normal. One fetus with tetralogy of Fallot, absent pulmonary valve syndrome and severe ascites, was refused chromosomal study. A second fetus with tetralogy of Fallot and absent pulmonary valve with the unusual finding of hypoplastic pulmonary arteries was not karyotyped. The remaining fetuses with fetal demise did not have chromosomal study. They included the recipient twin of a twin-to-twin transfusion, a fetus with a massive atrial teratoma and hydrops fetalis (Table 28.5).

Of the 291 fetuses with suspected congenital cardiac malformations, arrhythmia, or cardiomyopathy, 97 underwent prenatal karyotyping. Twenty-five of these fetuses (26%) had identifiable genetic syndromes, including 13 cases of trisomy 21, 4 with trisomy 18, 3 with Turner syndrome, 2 with chromosome 22q11.2 microdeletion (1 fetus with interrupted aortic arch type B and ventricular septal defect and 1 with tricuspid atresia, ventricular septal defect, and persistent truncus arteriosus), and 1 with Klinefelter syndrome.

Sixteen fetuses were identified who had congenital cardiac malformations and associated extracardiac malformations. The latter included three fetuses with associated congenital

TABLE 28.4

TERMINATION OF PREGNANCY AND COMPASSIONATE CARE IN FETAL CONGENITAL HEART DISEASE (2004–2005) ($n = 46$)

Termination of pregnancy	
Diagnosis	No.
Hypoplastic left heart syndrome	11
Visceral heterotaxia	4
Double-outlet right ventricle	3
Pulmonary atresia/intact ventricular septum	5
Tetralogy of Fallot	3
Atrioventricular canal defect (trisomy 21)	2
Pulmonary atresia/ventricular septal defect	2
Tricuspid atresia (1 with trisomy 18)	2
d-Transposition of the great arteries	2
Left ventricular diverticulum	1
Aortic aneurysm	1
Ebstein malformation of the tricuspid valve	1
Double-inlet left ventricle	1
Multiple APCs/Dandy–Walker cyst	1
l-Transposition/VSD/pulmonary atresia	1

Compassionate care	
Diagnosis	No.
RV-dominant AV canal defect/ pulmonary atresia	1
Hypoplastic left heart variant/trisomy 21	1
Double-outlet right ventricle/ aortopulmonary window	1
Hypoplastic left heart/severe tricuspid regurgitation	1
Tricuspid atresia/VSD/d-transposition/ aortic atresia	1
Dilated cardiomyopathy	1

TABLE 28.5

CONGENITAL HEART DISEASE AND INTRAUTERINE FETAL DEMISE 2004–2005 ($n = 14$)

Pt. No.	Cardiac diagnosis	Other findings	Karyotype/22q11
1	Inflow VSD	Clinodactyly; choroid plexus cysts	Trisomy 18
2	Tetralogy of Fallot	Clinodactyly; IUGR; rocker bottom feet	Trisomy 18
3	Double-outlet RV	Twin pregnancy; IUGR; omphalocele	Trisomy 18
4	Pulmonary atresia/IVS coronary sinusoids	None	None
5	Tetralogy of Fallot; absent pulmonary valve; hypoplastic pulmonary arteries	None	None
6	L-TGA/VSD/pulmonary atresia	None	None
7	Truncus arteriosus; interrupted aortic arch	None	Normal
8	Pericardial tumor; pericardial effusion	Hydrops fetalis	None
9	Tetralogy of Fallot	Hydrops fetalis	None
10	Truncus arteriosus; truncal stenosis/regurgitation	Hydrops fetalis	Normal
11	Twin/twin transfusion; RV hypertrophy	Polyhydramnios	Normal
12	Double-outlet RV; d-malposition	Hydrops fetalis	Trisomy 18
13	AV septal defect	Hydrops fetalis	Trisomy 18
14	d-Transposition of the GAs	None	None

diaphragmatic hernia (one with d-transposition of the great arteries, one with complete atrioventricular septal defect, and one with tricuspid atresia ventricular septal defect and normally oriented great arteries).

Indications for detailed fetal echocardiographic study at New York–Presbyterian Hospital during 2004 and 2005 are presented in Table 28.6. Note the marked predominance of suspected congenital heart disease in this list and the relative infrequency of family history of congenital heart disease. We attribute this and the paucity of cases of associated chromosomal abnormalities to the maturity of the screening program within Maternal-Fetal Medicine at our hospital.

Of the 138 live-born fetuses with correctly identified congenital heart disease for which we have follow-up, and for which there was an intention to treat, 94 (68%) underwent surgery during the first month of life and 19 (14%) additional underwent surgery within the first 6 months of life.

FETAL CARDIAC ARRHYTHMIAS

Fetal cardiac arrhythmias have been recognized with increasing frequency during the past several years and in general have been associated with a greater degree of maternal and physician anxiety than they deserve. Most irregularities of fetal cardiac rhythm represent isolated extrasystoles, which frequently present as a perceived skipping of fetal heart beats. Extrasystoles are significant only because of the potential for an appropriately timed extrasystole to initiate sustained re-entry tachycardia in the presence of an appropriate anatomic substrate involving an accessory conduction pathway or a region of scar with unidirectional block and decremental conduction. The statistical likelihood of this occurring in the fetal or immediate neonatal period is in the range of 0.5% to 2%. The most common, important, sustained fetal arrhythmias are orthodromic reciprocating supraventricular tachycardia, atrial flutter with varying degrees of atrioventricular

block, or severe bradycardia associated with complete atrioventricular block (10).

Nineteen patients were found to have sustained fetal arrhythmias during 2004 and 2005. Nine fetuses had sustained atrial premature contractions. None of these fetuses went on to develop sustained supraventricular tachycardia, and none received prenatal therapy. Ten patients with sustained arrhythmias received in utero therapy and went on to live birth with normal neonatal cardiovascular function.

TABLE 28.6

INDICATIONS FOR FETAL ECHOCARDIOGRAPHY AT THE MORGAN STANLEY CHILDREN'S HOSPITAL OF NEW YORK–PRESBYTERIAN COLUMBIA UNIVERSITY MEDICAL CENTER CALENDAR 2005 ($n = 403$)

Indication	No. of referrals	% of total
Maternal	46	11
Diabetes mellitus	27	7
Drug ingestion	1	
Systemic disease	16	4
In vitro fertilization	2	
Fetal	309	77
Suspected CHD (includes inadequate visualization)	171	42
Extracardiac anomalies (includes abnormal karyotype, IUGR)	101	25
Fetal arrhythmia	18	5
Twins	19	5
Family History	48	12
TOTAL	403	

CHD, congenital heart disease; IUGR, intrauterine growth restriction.

TABLE 28.7

CLINICALLY IMPORTANT FETAL ARRHYTHMIAS ENCOUNTERED DURING 2004–2005 ($n = 13$)

Pt. no.	Arrhythmia	Cardiac structure	Cardiac function	Medication(s)	Comments	Outcome
1	ORT	Normal	Normal	Digoxin		NSR (A/W)
2	PJRT	Normal	Decreased (hydrops fetalis)	Digoxin; flecainide; propranolol		NSR Function normalized; hydrops resolved (A/W)
3	ORT (intermittent)	Normal	Normal	Propranolol		NSR (A/W)
4	ORT	Normal	Normal	Digoxin		NSR (A/W)
5	Atrial flutter	Normal	Decreased (hydrops fetalis)	Digoxin; sotalol		NSR function normalized; hydrops resolved (A/W)
6	EAT	Normal	Decreased	Digoxin; propranolol	In utero control	Neonatal recurrence resolved with amiodarone/ propranolol (A/W)
7	ORT	Normal	Decreased (hydrops fetalis)	Digoxin; sotalol		NSR function normalized; hydrops resolved (A/W)
8	ORT	Normal	Normal	Digoxin; flecainide	Therapy started elsewhere	NSR (A/W)
9	ORT	HLHS	Decreased RV function			Termination of pregnancy
10	Complete AV block	LA isomerism complex AVSD	Decreased hydrops fetalis			Termination of pregnancy
11	Complete AV block	LA isomerism complex AVSD	Decreased hydrops fetalis			Termination of pregnancy
12	Complete AV block	Normal	Decreased	Dexamethasone	Maternal lupus	Epicardial VVI pacemaker (A/W)
13	Primary AV block	Normal	Normal	Dexamethasone	Maternal anti-SS-A; anti-SS-B	NSR (A/W)

These included two fetuses with prolonged atrioventricular conduction (1) or complete heart block (1) in the presence of positive maternal titers against Ro or La antibodies. The first fetus received dexamethasone as part of a multicenter study and was born with normal atrioventricular conduction. The second of these fetuses required cardiac pacing in the neonatal period, owing to recalcitrant complete heart block. Two fetuses, with left atrial isomerism, complete atrioventricular septal defect, hydrops fetalis, and complete heart block were classified as heterotaxy syndrome and were not included in the group presenting with sustained arrhythmia as the chief complaint. One patient with hypoplastic left heart syndrome and intermittent supraventricular tachycardia was classified among fetuses with congenital heart disease as the primary diagnosis.

The other eight fetuses had sustained supraventricular tachyarrhythmias, including atrial flutter (1), ectopic atrial tachycardia (2), and orthodromic reciprocating tachycardia

(5). They responded to antiarrhythmic therapy protocols that contained digoxin, alone or in combination with propranolol, sotalol, or flecainide (Table 28.7).

In the presence of sustained fetal tachyarrhythmia, it is common for the fetus to develop hydrops fetalis (10). The latter arises because of the development of venous hypertension in the presence of significant atrial backflow into the inferior vena caval circulation. The increase in hydrostatic pressure results in a net increase in extravasation of fluid into the interstitial space that is not adequately compensated by fetal lymphatic drainage. It is not uncommon, therefore, for hydrops fetalis to develop despite maintenance of normal or nearly normal systolic ventricular shortening. Sustained fetal tachycardia and hydrops fetalis has been associated with neonatal hypoalbuminemia and hyperbilirubinemia, even weeks following resolution of the tachycardia and fetal anasarca (186). This is probably attributable to high inferior vena caval pressure and associated hepatic dysfunction, with decreased albumin production and biliary stasis. The decreased albumin production, resulting in decreased fetal and neonatal serum oncotic pressure, contributes both to the production of fetal edema and anasarca and to the considerable delay that is often encountered between arrhythmia control and resolution of hydrops fetalis.

Bradycardia associated with complete atrioventricular block may result from autoimmune damage to the atrioventricular conduction system, related to transplacental passage of anti-Ro (SS-A) or La (SS-B) antibodies. Such mothers may have clinical symptoms of systemic lupus erythematosus or Sjögren syndrome, although in many young women, the detection of fetal heart block may be the first evidence of an elevated antibody titer in an otherwise asymptomatic mother (187–194).

Bradycardia owing to complete atrioventricular block may be diagnosed in fetuses with negative maternal antibody titers. Many of these fetuses have complex congenital cardiac disease with malformations involving the development of the central fibrous portion of the heart (e.g., atrioventricular discordant connections in corrected l-transposition of the great arteries or left atrial isomerism with ambiguous atrioventricular connections). Complete heart block must be distinguished from sinus bradycardia, which may be associated with fetal hypoxemia, or from blocked atrial bigeminy, in which every second atrial contraction is so premature that the atrioventricular node is still refractory because of the previous sinus beat and therefore unable to conduct the premature contraction (95,195).

These three forms of bradycardia can be distinguished from one another through careful evaluation of atrial rhythm. In sinus bradycardia, there is a one-to-one relationship between the slow atrial rate and the equal ventricular response rate. In complete heart block, the atrial rate is regular and exceeds the slower, regular, idioventricular rhythm. In blocked atrial bigeminy, the atrial rate is regularly irregular, with paired beating between the conducted beat and the blocked premature atrial beat, which is not conducted. Magnetocardiographic studies of fetal patients with recurrent episodes of supraventricular tachycardia have suggested that many of the premature atrial beats that occur in these fetuses are echo beats that re-enter the atrium via accessory pathways but are not conducted back into the ventricle through the atrioventricular node (196).

Analysis and Treatment of Fetal Cardiac Arrhythmias

In the absence of reliable electrocardiographic recordings of fetal atrial and ventricular electrical activity, M-mode, pulsed Doppler, and color-encoded M-mode echocardiographic recordings of mechanical and flow events are used to time and sequence the electrical activation underlying these events (Fig. 28.17) (10,52,197–217). Rein et al. (218) described the use of Doppler tissue imaging to time the mechanical activation sequence of the atria and ventricles to analyze cardiac rhythm using a ladder diagram or kinetocardiogram to provide similar information. Recent reports have demonstrated that magnetocardiography may provide important information regarding fetal atrial activation and the morphology of fetal QRS complexes, QT intervals, and T-wave morphology. This procedure is laborious, requires special equipment and magnetic shielding, and is not widely available, but may well emerge as the preferable means of analyzing clinically significant fetal arrhythmias (196,219–223).

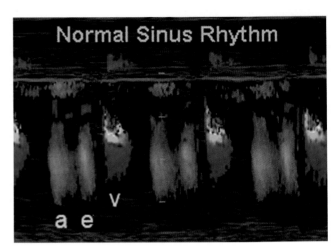

FIGURE 28.17 Color-encoded M-mode echocardiogram. The M-mode tracing imparts temporal resolution to the color flow recording. In this orientation diastolic filling of the fetal ventricle is toward the transducer, resulting in the biphasic e and a waves, whereas the ejection into the aorta is away from the transducer and is inscribed as the aliased blue/cyan image.

Fetal Antiarrhythmic Therapy

The existence of techniques for the analysis and treatment of fetal cardiac arrhythmias is insufficient justification to expose a mother and fetus to the potential hazards of antiarrhythmic therapy. Fetal therapy offers the potential for dramatic success, but also has the potential for catastrophic consequences for two patients at once. The management schema for such patients should be predicated on an understanding of the natural history of the arrhythmia, a precise knowledge of the electrophysiologic basis for the arrhythmia, and a detailed appreciation of the pharmacokinetics and pharmacology of antiarrhythmic agents in the fetus, mother, and placenta. These must be factored in a commonsense risk/benefit analysis. Neonatal risk increases proportionately with the degree of prematurity and lung immaturity at the time of the initial diagnosis. This must be balanced against the degree of cardiovascular compromise accompanying the arrhythmia. In the absence of extreme prematurity, or without evidence of severe fetal hemodynamic compromise (e.g., hydrops fetalis), fetal intervention is difficult to justify.

Analysis of Fetal Tachyarrhythmias

Figure 28.18 presents a suggested algorithm for the analysis and treatment of fetal tachyarrhythmias. If tachycardia is associated with atrioventricular (AV) dissociation or is sustained in the presence of varying degrees of AV block, AV re-entry tachycardia (AVRT) (either orthodromic or antidromic) or AV nodal re-entry tachycardia (AVNRT) cannot be the underlying electrophysiologic mechanism of the tachycardia, since those tachycardias are characterized by a 1:1 atrioventricular contraction sequence, driven by a circus movement of electrical energy at the atrioventricular junction.

If there is AV dissociation, with a ventricular rate in excess of atrial rate (A:V ratio <1:1), one may assume that the tachycardia arises below the bundle of His and does not depolarize the atrium in a retrograde direction with a 1:1 ratio. The latter is characteristic of ventricular tachycardia (VT) or junctional ectopic tachycardia (JET). When there is some degree of AV block with an A:V ratio of >1:1, one may be dealing with intra-atrial re-entry tachycardia (IART), ectopic atrial tachycardia

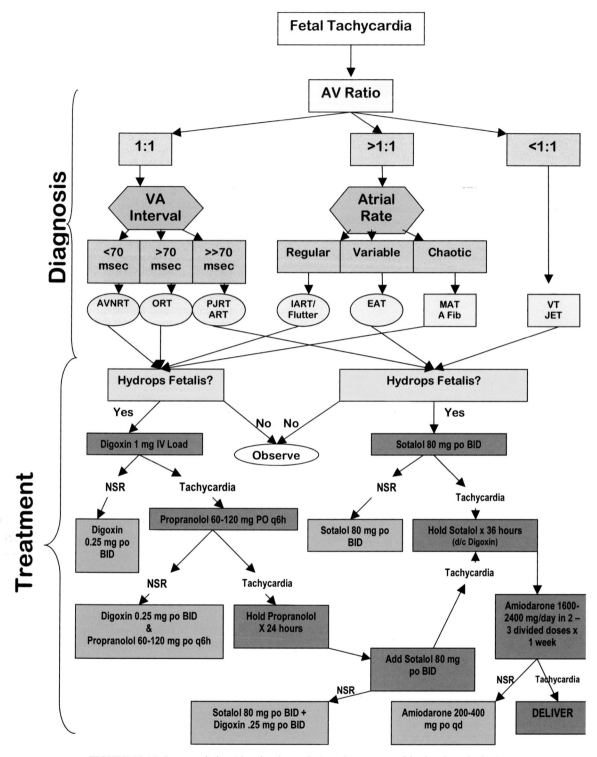

FIGURE 28.18 Suggested algorithm for the analysis and treatment of fetal tachyarrhythmias.

(EAT), multifocal atrial tachycardia (MAT), atrial flutter (AF), or atrial fibrillation. In the presence of these arrhythmias, the atrial rate exceeds that of the ventricles, with the relationship dictated by the degree of AV block.

In the presence of a strict 1:1 A:V ratio, we evaluate the ventriculoatrial (VA) interval. Using simultaneous recordings of central venous and arterial pulsed Doppler flow waveforms, the time sequence of atrial and ventricular electrical activation can be discerned. Such recordings can be obtained by placement of the Doppler sample volume to overlap the fetal superior vena cava and ascending aorta (224) or fetal right pulmonary artery and right pulmonary vein (Fig. 28.19) (225).

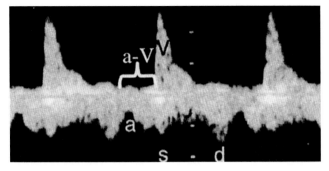

FIGURE 28.19 Simultaneous inscription of flow waveforms from the right upper pulmonary artery (above the baseline) and right upper pulmonary vein (below the baseline). The undulations of the pulmonary vein representing atrial contraction (a) are related to the timing of the upstroke of the systolic ejection into the branch pulmonary artery (v). The atrioventricular (a-V) and ventriculoatrial (V-a) conduction times may be measured, and related to the electrical events underlying the mechanical responses that result in the flow events recorded in this image.

The atrioventricular mechanical interval may be used as a surrogate of electrocardiographic PR interval, and the ventriculoatrial (VA) time interval may also be calculated.

In the presence of a very short VA interval or one slightly >70 ms, the most likely electrophysiologic mechanism of the tachycardia is orthodromic AVRT or AVNRT. If the A:V ratio is >1:1 with a regular atrial tachycardia, the likely diagnosis is AF or IART. Depending on gestational age, the likelihood of pulmonary maturity, and the presence or absence of hydrops fetalis, we may or may not consider the use of *in utero* antiarrhythmic treatment to the fetus. A fetus with unsustained tachycardia or without hydrops fetalis is not in immediate danger and is not likely to be offered prenatal therapy. On the other hand, in the presence of sustained tachyarrhythmia, with hydrops fetalis, the risk/benefit analysis tips in the direction of *in utero* therapy.

Intrauterine Antitachyarrhythmic Therapy

In the face of severe prematurity, immediate delivery for postnatal treatment may not be a logical option. The frequent association of hydrops fetalis with sustained supraventricular tachycardia (SVT) and the dismal prognosis for such fetuses and neonates in a setting of extreme prematurity may justify vigorous efforts at in utero therapy, if such treatment can be offered at a tolerably low risk to the mother. Even a moderate risk to the fetus could be justified in this setting, in light of the poor prognosis for the neonate if the arrhythmia and hydrops fetalis are unremitting. The decision regarding the institution of fetal treatment should consider the following: (a) the fetal hemodynamic state (Is there hydrops fetalis?), (b) the potential risks to mother and fetus inherent in fetal treatment, (c) availability of facilities for monitoring of mother and fetus, and (d) willingness of the mother to submit to such treatment and monitoring.

Many antiarrhythmic drugs have a narrow therapeutic margin and may be associated with significant toxicity, including proarrhythmic potential. Only the Vaughn-Williams class II (β-blocker) agents appear to lack the potential for late proarrhythmic mortality. Type IA or type III agents, alone or in combination with medications that interfere with drug metabolism through the cytochrome P-450 pathway, may precipitate polymorphic ventricular tachycardia (torsades de pointes). Type IC agents such as flecainide may cause QRS prolongation and ventricular tachycardia recalcitrant to treatment. The absence of a readily available technique to monitor fetal QTc or QRS duration during antiarrhythmic therapy constitutes a fundamental hazard associated with fetal antiarrhythmic therapy.

Prior to the initiation of antiarrhythmic therapy, the therapeutic goal should be established. In some circumstances rate control may provide an adequate opportunity to recover fetal cardiovascular function, whereas in many cases complete control of the arrhythmia is necessary to allow resolution of hydrops fetalis.

The literature is filled with many reports touting the virtues of different antiarrhythmic agents for the control of fetal tachyarrhythmias (10,226–242). Few of these reports discussed medication choices based on a detailed analysis of the electrophysiologic mechanism of the arrhythmia. The algorithm that we present is based on a sequential analysis of arrhythmia mechanism modeled after the framework suggested by Walsh et al. (243). The suggested sequence of drug administration has evolved considerably over the past several years and has been influenced by personal experience and the literature. This is offered as a step-off point for consideration by the reader when fetal antitachycardia treatment is anticipated. Just as different cardiac centers use differing medical regimens for the same arrhythmia in infants and children, it is expected that fetal antiarrhythmic treatment protocols will be individualized, based on local experience with specific antiarrhythmic medications. A rational approach to the treatment of these patients should consider the nature of the arrhythmia, the hemodynamic impact of the rhythm disturbance, and the pharmacology and pharmacokinetics of the maternal-placental-fetal unit. We have settled on a simplified treatment protocol, focusing on the administration of digoxin, propranolol, sotalol, and amiodarone. We have had limited experience with the use of flecainide in the fetus, although some centers have found the latter to be a safe and effective agent for the treatment of some fetal arrhythmias. We have made a team approach to the administration of antiarrhythmic treatment to the pregnant woman. This team includes maternal-fetal medicine, pediatric cardiology, and adult cardiology specialists to focus on the care of these complex patients. Such teams should devise their own treatment plans, which may differ at individual medical centers or for individual patients.

Treatment of the Fetus with Bradycardia

The most important sustained fetal bradyarrhythmia is congenital complete heart block. These fetuses may develop hydrops fetalis. The latter may occur in the subgroup of fetuses with associated congenital heart disease. The association of fetal heart failure with congenital heart block, with or without congenital heart disease, represents an absolute indication for electrical pacemaker therapy in the neonate. In the fetus, the association of complete heart block and hydrops fetalis is dire. When associated with congenital heart disease, the outcome is almost invariably fatal, with or without fetal therapy (195).

The initial report of the use of electrical pacemaker therapy for the treatment of fetal congenital heart block involved a fetus presenting with heart block in the absence of congenital heart disease (244). This fetus presumably incurred immune complex–mediated damage to the fetal conduction system and myocardium. There was severe bradycardia and hydrops fetalis. In desperation, the treating physicians placed a pacing catheter within the fetal heart via percutaneous puncture of the maternal abdomen, uterus, fetal thorax, and ventricular wall. Fetal ventricular capture was demonstrated, without clinical improvement. Subsequent attempts to use similar pacing systems have been, likewise, unsuccessful.

Laboratory models of complete heart block have been created in fetal lambs, with subsequent resolution of hydrops fetalis following fetal exteriorization and surgical implantation of permanent pacemakers connected to epicardial pacing leads (245). An attempt to implant a pacemaker in this fashion in a human fetus was unsuccessful. Although it may well be that some human fetuses with heart block and hydrops fetalis have deteriorated solely because of bradycardia, we are concerned that some neonates do not respond to pacing alone. This subgroup of patients may have immune-mediated damage to the contractile elements of the heart from the same mechanism that damaged the fetal conduction system (246–250). Although it has been demonstrated that the administration of β-mimetic agents to the pregnant woman may increase the intrinsic ventricular rate of the fetus by 50%, there has been no consistent evidence that such treatment ameliorates hydrops fetalis in affected fetuses (251–254).

A preliminary experience in our laboratory with the administration of absorbable corticosteroid to pregnant women whose fetuses had developed high-grade second-degree or recent-onset third-degree heart block in the presence of high titers of anti–SS-A or SS-B antibodies suggested that such treatment might halt the progression or even reverse the damage to the conduction tissue (10). This study spawned a multicenter investigation designed to evaluate the impact of maternally administered corticosteroid on echocardiographically estimated fetal AV conduction intervals (255–262). Some centers have adopted steroid therapy for the routine treatment of fetuses with antibody-mediated congenital complete heart block, based on improved mortality statistics in the current era compared with historical controls (263–266). The results of the multicenter study noted above are likely to provide an important insight into the appropriateness of such therapy (267).

References

1. Rudolph AM. *Congenital Diseases of the Heart*. Chicago: Yearbook, 1974.
1a. Rudolph AM. *Congenital Diseases of the Heart*. 2nd ed. Armonk, NY: Futura, 2001.
2. Rudolph AM, Heymann MA. The circulation of the fetus in utero. Methods for studying distribution of blood flow, cardiac output and organ blood flow. *Circ Res* 1967;21(2):163–184.
3. Heymann MA, et al. Blood flow measurements with radionuclide-labeled particles. *Prog Cardiovasc Dis* 1977;20(1):55–79.
4. Rudolph AM, Heymann MA. Measurement of flow in perfused organs, using microsphere techniques. *Acta Endocrinol Suppl (Copenh)* 1972; 158:112–217.
5. Rudolph AM, Iwamoto HS, Teitel DF. Circulatory changes at birth. *J Perinat Med* 1988;16(suppl 1):9–21.
6. Teitel DF, Iwamoto HS, Rudolph AM. Effects of birth-related events on central blood flow patterns. *Pediatr Res* 1987;22(5):557–566.
7. Iwamoto HS, Teitel D, Rudolph AM. Effects of birth-related events on blood flow distribution. *Pediatr Res* 1987;22(6):634–640.
8. Iwamoto HS, Teitel DF, Rudolph AM. Effect of birth-related events on metabolism in fetal sheep. *Pediatr Res* 1991;30(2):158–164.
9. Winsberg F. Echocardiography of the fetal and newborn heart. *Invest Radiol* 1972;7(3):152–158.
10. Kleinman CS, Copel JA. Fetal cardiovascular physiology and therapy. *Fetal Diagn Ther* 1992;7(2):147–157.
11. Lange LW, et al. Qualitative real-time cross-sectional echocardiographic imaging of the human fetus during the second half of pregnancy. *Circulation* 1980;62(4):799–806.
12. Allan LD, et al. Echocardiographic and anatomical correlates in the fetus. *Br Heart J* 1980;44(4):444–451.
13. Kachaner J, Fermont L. Prenatal cardiology [in French]. *Presse Med* 1985;14(9):517–519.
14. Allan LD, et al. Prenatal screening for congenital heart disease. *Br Med J (Clin Res Ed)* 1986;292:1717–1719.
15. Brown DL, Durfee SM, Hornberger LK. Ventricular discrepancy as a sonographic sign of coarctation of the fetal aorta: How reliable is it? *J Ultrasound Med* 1997;16(2):95–99.
16. Hornberger LK, Need L, Benacerraf BR. Development of significant left and right ventricular hypoplasia in the second and third trimester fetus. *J Ultrasound Med* 1996;15(9):655–659.
17. Hornberger LK, et al. Echocardiographic study of the morphology and growth of the aortic arch in the human fetus. Observations related to the prenatal diagnosis of coarctation. *Circulation* 1992;86(3):741–747.
18. Hornberger LK, et al. Antenatal diagnosis of coarctation of the aorta: A multicenter experience. *J Am Coll Cardiol* 1994;23(2):417–423.
19. Hornberger LK, et al. Left heart obstructive lesions and left ventricular growth in the midtrimester fetus. A longitudinal study. *Circulation* 1995;92(6):1531–1538.
20. Crane JP, et al. A randomized trial of prenatal ultrasonographic screening: Impact on the detection, management, and outcome of anomalous fetuses. The RADIUS Study Group. *Am J Obstet Gynecol* 1994;171(2):392–399.
21. Ewigman BG, et al. Effect of prenatal ultrasound screening on perinatal outcome. RADIUS Study Group. *N Engl J Med* 1993;329:821–827.
22. LeFevre ML, et al. A randomized trial of prenatal ultrasonographic screening: Impact on maternal management and outcome. RADIUS (Routine Antenatal Diagnostic Imaging with Ultrasound) Study Group. *Am J Obstet Gynecol* 1993;169(3):483–489.
23. Presbitero P, et al. Fetal echocardiography: Diagnosis of congenital cardiomyopathies in a population at risk [in Italian]. *G Ital Cardiol* 1985;15(6):590–596.
24. Sharland GK, Allan LD. Screening for congenital heart disease prenatally. Results of a 2 1/2-year study in the South East Thames Region. *Br J Obstet Gynaecol* 1992;99(3):220–225.
25. Achiron R, et al. Extended fetal echocardiographic examination for detecting cardiac malformations in low risk pregnancies. *Bmj* 1992;304(6828):671–674.
26. Vergani P, et al. Screening for congenital heart disease with the four-chamber view of the fetal heart. *Am J Obstet Gynecol* 1992;167(4 Pt 1):1000–1003.
27. Stoll C, et al. Evaluation of prenatal diagnosis of congenital heart disease. *Prenat Diagn* 1993;13(6):453–461.
28. Hofbeck M, et al. Prenatal findings in patients with prolonged QT interval in the neonatal period. *Heart* 1997;77(3):198–204.
29. Giancotti A, et al. Prenatal evaluation of congenital heart disease in high-risk pregnancies. *Clin Exp Obstet Gynecol* 1995;22(3):225–229.
30. Buskens E, et al. Efficacy of fetal echocardiography and yield by risk category. *Obstet Gynecol* 1996;87(3):423–428.
31. Sinclair BG, Sandor GG, Farquharson DF. Effectiveness of primary level antenatal screening for severe congenital heart disease: A population-based assessment. *J Perinatol* 1996;16(5):336–340.
32. Kleinert S. Routine prenatal screening for congenital heart disease. *Lancet* 1996;348:836.
33. Stumpflen I, et al. Effect of detailed fetal echocardiography as part of routine prenatal ultrasonographic screening on detection of congenital heart disease. *Lancet* 1996;348:854–857.
34. Alembik Y, Stoll C. Routine fetal echocardiography and detection of congenital heart disease. *Lancet* 1996;348:1732.
35. Buskens E, et al. Routine prenatal screening for congenital heart disease: What can be expected? A decision-analytic approach. *Am J Public Health* 1997;87(6):962–967.
36. Crane JM, et al. Abnormal fetal cardiac axis in the detection of intrathoracic anomalies and congenital heart disease. *Ultrasound Obstet Gynecol* 1997;10(2):90–93.
37. Todros T, et al. Accuracy of routine ultrasonography in screening heart disease prenatally. Gruppo Piemontese for Prenatal Screening of Congenital Heart Disease. *Prenat Diagn* 1997;17(10):901–906.
38. Hess DB, et al. Obtaining the four-chamber view to diagnose fetal cardiac anomalies. *Obstet Gynecol Clin North Am* 1998;25(3):499–515.
39. Stoll C, et al. Evaluation of prenatal diagnosis of congenital heart disease. *Prenat Diagn* 1998;18(8):801–807.
40. Hafner E, et al. Detection of fetal congenital heart disease in a low-risk population. *Prenat Diagn* 1998;18(8):808–815.
41. Kirk JS, et al. Fetal cardiac asymmetry: A marker for congenital heart disease. *Obstet Gynecol* 1999;93(2):189–192.
42. Tometzki AJ, et al. Accuracy of prenatal echocardiographic diagnosis and prognosis of fetuses with conotruncal anomalies. *J Am Coll Cardiol* 1999;33(6):1696–1701.
43. Paladini D. Prenatal screening of congenital heart disease between ethics and cost-effectiveness. Time for a change in current prenatal ultrasound screening policies? *Ultrasound Obstet Gynecol* 1999;14(4):225–228.
44. Cohen EH, Rein AJ. Antenatal diagnosis of cardiac malformation: A structural study. *Fetal Diagn Ther* 2000;15(1):54–60.

45. Saxena A, Soni NR. Fetal echocardiography: Where are we? *Indian J Pediatr* 2005;72(7):603–608.

46. Simpsom JM, et al. Accuracy and limitations of transabdominal fetal echocardiography at 12–15 weeks of gestation in a population at high risk for congenital heart disease. *Bjog* 2000;107(12):1492–1497.

47. Fesslova V, Villa L, Kustermann A. Long-term experience with the prenatal diagnosis of cardiac anomalies in high-risk pregnancies in a tertiary center. *Ital Heart J* 2003;4(12):855–864.

48. Sharland G. Routine fetal cardiac screening: What are we doing and what should we do? *Prenat Diagn* 2004;24(13):1123–1129.

49. Sklansky M, et al. Prenatal screening for congenital heart disease using real-time three-dimensional echocardiography and a novel 'sweep volume' acquisition technique. *Ultrasound Obstet Gynecol* 2005;25(5):435–443.

50. Feit LR, Copel JA, Kleinman CS. Foramen ovale size in the normal and abnormal human fetal heart: An indicator of transatrial flow physiology. *Ultrasound Obstet Gynecol* 1991;1(5):313–319.

51. Berning RA, et al. Reversed shunting across the ductus arteriosus or atrial septum in utero heralds severe congenital heart disease. *J Am Coll Cardiol* 1996;27(2):481–486.

52. Reed KL, et al. Cardiac Doppler flow velocities in human fetuses. *Circulation* 1986;73(1):41–46.

53. Kenny JF, et al. Changes in intracardiac blood flow velocities and right and left ventricular stroke volumes with gestational age in the normal human fetus: A prospective Doppler echocardiographic study. *Circulation* 1986;74(6):1208–1216.

54. Friedman WF. The intrinsic physiologic properties of the developing heart. *Prog Cardiovasc Dis* 1972;15(1):87–111.

55. Friedman WF, Kirkpatrick SE. In situ physiological study of the developing heart. *Recent Adv Stud Cardiac Struct Metab* 1975;5:497–504.

56. Sheldon CA, Friedman WF, Sybers HD. Scanning electron microscopy of fetal and neonatal lamb cardiac cells. *J Mol Cell Cardiol* 1976;8(11):853–862.

57. Harada K, et al. Tissue Doppler imaging in the normal fetus. *Int J Cardiol* 1999;71(3):227–234.

58. Paladini D, et al. Prenatal diagnosis of congenital heart disease in the Naples area during the years 1994–1999—the experience of a joint fetal-pediatric cardiology unit. *Prenat Diagn* 2002;22(7):545–552.

59. Paladini D, et al. The association between congenital heart disease and Down syndrome in prenatal life. *Ultrasound Obstet Gynecol* 2000;15(2):104–108.

60. Jamjureeruk V. Evaluation of ventricular myocardial velocities and heart motion of the fetal heart by tissue Doppler image. *J Med Assoc Thai* 2001;84(8):1158–1163.

61. Larsen LU, et al. Strain rate derived from color Doppler myocardial imaging for assessment of fetal cardiac function. *Ultrasound Obstet Gynecol* 2006;27(2):210–213.

62. Di Salvo G, et al. Quantification of regional left and right ventricular longitudinal function in 75 normal fetuses using ultrasound-based strain rate and strain imaging. *Ultrasound Med Biol* 2005;31(9):1159–1162.

63. Huhta JC. Fetal congestive heart failure. *Semin Fetal Neonatal Med* 2005;10(6):542–552.

64. Huhta JC. Right ventricular function in the human fetus. *J Perinat Med* 2001;29(5):381–389.

65. Paladini D, et al. Prenatal diagnosis of congenital heart disease and fetal karyotyping. *Obstet Gynecol* 1993;81(5 (pt 1)):679–682.

66. Fogel M, et al. Congenital heart disease and fetal thoracoabdominal anomalies: Associations in utero and the importance of cytogenetic analysis. *Am J Perinatol* 1991;8(6):411–416.

67. Fasnacht MS, Jaeggi ET. Fetal and genetic aspects of congenital heart disease [in German]. *Ther Umsch* 2001;58(2):70–75.

68. Moyano D, Huggon IC, Allan LD. Fetal echocardiography in trisomy 18. *Arch Dis Child Fetal Neonatal Ed* 2005;90(6):F520–522.

69. Ghi T, et al. Incidence of major structural cardiac defects associated with increased nuchal translucency but normal karyotype. *Ultrasound Obstet Gynecol* 2001;18(6):610–614.

70. Hyett JA, et al. Intrauterine lethality of trisomy 21 fetuses with increased nuchal translucency thickness. *Ultrasound Obstet Gynecol* 1996;7(2):101–103.

71. Cheng PJ, et al. First-trimester nuchal translucency measurement and echocardiography at 16 to 18 weeks of gestation in prenatal detection for trisomy 18. *Prenat Diagn* 2003;23(3):248–251.

72. Surerus E, Huggon IC, Allan LD. Turner's syndrome in fetal life. *Ultrasound Obstet Gynecol* 2003;22(3):264–267.

73. Hyett J. Does nuchal translucency have a role in fetal cardiac screening? *Prenat Diagn* 2004;24(13):1130–1135.

74. Sciarrone A, et al. First-trimester fetal heart block and increased nuchal translucency: An indication for early fetal echocardiography. *Prenat Diagn* 2005;25(12):1129–1132.

75. Ducarme G, et al. Increased nuchal translucency and cystic hygroma in the first trimester: Prenatal diagnosis and neonatal outcome [in French]. *Gynecol Obstet Fertil* 2005;33(10):750–754.

76. Hyett J, Moscoso G, Nicolaides K. Increased nuchal translucency in trisomy 21 fetuses: Relationship to narrowing of the aortic isthmus. *Hum Reprod* 1995;10:3049–3051.

77. Kagan KO, et al. Relation between increased fetal nuchal translucency thickness and chromosomal defects. *Obstet Gynecol* 2006;107(1):6–10.

78. D'Alton M, Cleary-Goldman J. First and second trimester evaluation of risk for fetal aneuploidy: The secondary outcomes of the FASTER Trial. *Semin Perinatol* 2005;29(4):240–246.

79. Malone FD, et al. First-trimester or second-trimester screening, or both, for Down's syndrome. *N Engl J Med* 2005;353:2001–2011.

80. Carvalho JS. Nuchal translucency, ductus venosus and congenital heart disease: An important association—a cautious analysis. *Ultrasound Obstet Gynecol* 1999;14(5):302–306.

81. Devine PC, Simpson LL. Nuchal translucency and its relationship to congenital heart disease. *Semin Perinatol* 2000;24(5):343–351.

82. Mavrides E, et al. Limitations of using first-trimester nuchal translucency measurement in routine screening for major congenital heart defects. *Ultrasound Obstet Gynecol* 2001;17(2):106–110.

83. Huggon IC, et al. Fetal cardiac abnormalities identified prior to 14 weeks' gestation. *Ultrasound Obstet Gynecol* 2002;20(1):22–29.

84. Driscoll DA, et al. Deletions and microdeletions of 22q11.2 in velo-cardio-facial syndrome. *Am J Med Genet* 1992;44(2):261–268.

85. Kelly D, et al. Confirmation that the velo-cardio-facial syndrome is associated with haplo-insufficiency of genes at chromosome 22q11. *Am J Med Genet* 1993;45(3):308–312.

86. Goldmuntz E, et al. Microdeletions of chromosomal region 22q11 in patients with congenital conotruncal cardiac defects. *J Med Genet* 1993;30(10):807–812.

87. Driscoll DA, et al. Prevalence of 22q11 microdeletions in DiGeorge and velocardiofacial syndromes: Implications for genetic counselling and prenatal diagnosis. *J Med Genet* 1993;30(10):813–817.

88. Shprintzen RJ. Velocardiofacial syndrome and DiGeorge sequence. *J Med Genet* 1994;31(5):423–424.

89. Johnson MC, et al. The genetic basis of paediatric heart disease. *Ann Med* 1995;27(3):289–300.

90. Phoon CK, et al. Left atrial isomerism detected in fetal life. *Am J Cardiol* 1996;77(12):1083–1088.

91. Atkinson DE, Drant S. Diagnosis of heterotaxy syndrome by fetal echocardiography. *Am J Cardiol* 1998;82(9):1147–1149, A10.

92. Berg C, et al. Prenatal diagnosis of cardiosplenic syndromes: A 10-year experience. *Ultrasound Obstet Gynecol* 2003;22(5):451–459.

93. Pasquini L, et al. The implications for fetal outcome of an abnormal arrangement of the abdominal vessels. *Cardiol Young* 2005;15(1):35–42.

94. Tongsong T, et al. Prenatal diagnosis of transposition-like double-outlet right ventricle with mitral valve atresia in heterotaxy syndrome. *J Clin Ultrasound* 2005;33(4):197–200.

95. Schneider C, et al. Development of Z-scores for fetal cardiac dimensions from echocardiography. *Ultrasound Obstet Gynecol* 2005;26(6):599–605.

96. Bernasconi A, et al. Fetal dextrocardia: Diagnosis and outcome in two tertiary centres. *Heart* 2005;91(12):1590–1594.

97. Wladimiroff JW, et al. Prenatal diagnosis and management of congenital heart defect: Significance of associated fetal anomalies and prenatal chromosome studies. *Am J Med Genet* 1985;21(2):285–290.

98. Hyett JA, Moscoso G, Nicolaides KH. Cardiac defects in 1st-trimester fetuses with trisomy 18. *Fetal Diagn Ther* 1995;10(6):381–386.

99. Brons JT, et al. Prenatal ultrasonographic diagnosis of radial-ray reduction malformations. *Prenat Diagn* 1990;10(5):279–288.

100. Geggel RL. Conditions leading to pediatric cardiology consultation in a tertiary academic hospital. *Pediatrics* 2004;114(4):e409–417.

101. Koklanaris N, et al. Isolated echogenic intracardiac foci in patients with low-risk triple screen results: assessing the risk of trisomy 21. *J Perinat Med* 2005;33(6):539–542.

102. Borgida AF, et al. Frequency of echogenic intracardiac focus by race/ethnicity in euploid fetuses. *J Matern Fetal Neonatal Med* 2005;18(1):65–66.

103. Finberg HJ. An isolated echogenic heart focus is a low-level risk marker for Down syndrome. *J Ultrasound Med* 2004;23(7):1008–1009; author reply 1009.

104. Coco C, Jeanty P, Jeanty C. An isolated echogenic heart focus is not an indication for amniocentesis in 12,672 unselected patients. *J Ultrasound Med* 2004;23(4):489–496.

105. Sotiriadis A, Makrydimas G, Ioannidis JP. Diagnostic performance of intracardiac echogenic foci for Down syndrome: A meta-analysis. *Obstet Gynecol* 2003;101(5 pt 1):1009–1016.

106. Souter VL, et al. Correlation of ultrasound findings and biochemical markers in the second trimester of pregnancy in fetuses with trisomy 21. *Prenat Diagn* 2002;22(3):175–182.

107. Caughey AB, et al. The impact of the use of the isolated echogenic intracardiac focus as a screen for Down syndrome in women under the age of 35 years. *Am J Obstet Gynecol* 2001;185(5):1021–1027.

108. Huggon IC, et al. Isolated echogenic foci in the fetal heart as marker of chromosomal abnormality. *Ultrasound Obstet Gynecol* 2001;17(1):11–16.

109. Wax JR, et al. A preliminary study of sonographic grading of fetal intracardiac echogenic foci: Feasibility, reliability and association with aneuploidy. *Ultrasound Obstet Gynecol* 2000;16(2):123–127.

110. Winter TC, et al. Echogenic intracardiac focus in 2nd-trimester fetuses with trisomy 21: Usefulness as a US marker. *Radiology* 2000;216(2):450–456.

111. Bromley B, et al. Significance of an echogenic intracardiac focus in fetuses at high and low risk for aneuploidy. *J Ultrasound Med* 1998;17(2):127–131.

112. Tworetzky W, et al. Usefulness of magnetic resonance imaging of left ventricular endocardial fibroelastosis in infants after fetal intervention for aortic valve stenosis. *Am J Cardiol* 2005;96(11):1568–1570.

113. Franklin O, et al. Prenatal diagnosis of coarctation of the aorta improves survival and reduces morbidity. *Heart* 2002;87(1):67–69.

114. Bonnet D. [Plasticity of the myocardium in pediatric cardiology]. *Arch Pediatr* 1996;3(12):1273–1275.

115. Munn MB, et al. Prenatally diagnosed hypoplastic left heart syndrome—outcomes after postnatal surgery. *J Matern Fetal Med* 1999;8(4):147–150.

116. Eapen RS, Rowland DG, Franklin WH. Effect of prenatal diagnosis of critical left heart obstruction on perinatal morbidity and mortality. *Am J Perinatol* 1998;15(4):237–242.

117. Sharland GK, et al. Factors influencing the outcome of congenital heart disease detected prenatally. *Arch Dis Child* 1991;66(3):284–287.

118. Smythe JF, Copel JA, Kleinman CS. Outcome of prenatally detected cardiac malformations. *Am J Cardiol* 1992;69(17):1471–1474.

119. Magnier S, et al. Outcome of 77 live born children with cardiac or rhythmic anomalies diagnosed in the prenatal period. Apropos of 77 cases [in French]. *Arch Mal Coeur Viass* 1995;88(5):747–752.

120. Simpson JM, Sharland GK. Natural history and outcome of aortic stenosis diagnosed prenatally. *Heart* 1997;77(3):205–210.

121. Eronen M. Outcome of fetuses with heart disease diagnosed in utero. *Arch Dis Child Fetal Neonatal Ed* 1997;77(1):F41–46.

122. Allan LD, Apfel HD, Printz BF. Outcome after prenatal diagnosis of the hypoplastic left heart syndrome. *Heart* 1998;79(4):371–373.

123. Boldt T, Andersson S, Eronen M. Outcome of structural heart disease diagnosed in utero. *Scand Cardiovasc J* 2002;36(2):73–79.

124. Brick DH, Allan LD. Outcome of prenatally diagnosed congenital heart disease: An update. *Pediatr Cardiol* 2002;23(4):449–453.

125. Verheijen PM, et al. Prenatal diagnosis of the fetus with hypoplastic left heart syndrome management and outcome. *Herz* 2003;28(3):250–256.

126. Fountain-Dommer RR, et al. Outcome following, and impact of, prenatal identification of the candidates for the Norwood procedure. *Cardiol Young* 2004;14(1):32–38.

127. Simpson JM, et al. Outcome of intermittent tachyarrhythmias in the fetus. *Pediatr Cardiol* 1997;18(2):78–82.

128. Mellander M. Perinatal management, counselling and outcome of fetuses with congenital heart disease. *Semin Fetal Neonatal Med* 2005;10(6):586–593.

129. Jouannic JM, et al. Sensitivity and specificity of prenatal features of physiological shunts to predict neonatal clinical status in transposition of the great arteries. *Circulation* 2004;110(13):1743–1746.

130. Verheijen PM, et al. Prenatal diagnosis of congenital heart disease affects preoperative acidosis in the newborn patient. *J Thorac Cardiovasc Surg* 2001;121(4):798–803.

131. Lavrijsen SW, et al. Severe umbilical cord acidemia and neurological outcome in preterm and full-term neonates. *Biol Neonate* 2005;88(1):27–34.

132. Kadar K. [Prognosis for the fetus with congenital heart defects in the era of modern diagnostics and therapeutics]. *Orv Hetil* 2004; 145(16):849–853.

133. Checchia PA, et al. The effect of surgical case volume on outcome after the Norwood procedure. *J Thorac Cardiovasc Surg* 2005;129(4):754–759.

134. Hagberg S, et al. Prenatally diagnosed gastroschisis—a preliminary report advocating the use of elective caesarean section. *Z Kinderchir* 1988;43(6):419–421.

135. Wood C. Fetal scalp sampling: Its place in management. *Semin Perinatol* 1978;2(2):169–179.

136. Woods JR Jr. Birth asphyxia: Pathophysiologic events and fetal adaptive changes. *Clin Perinatol* 1983;10(2):473–486.

137. Low JA. The role of blood gas and acid-base assessment in the diagnosis of intrapartum fetal asphyxia. *Am J Obstet Gynecol* 1988;159(5):1235–1240.

138. Weiner CP. The relationship between the umbilical artery systolic/diastolic ratio and umbilical blood gas measurements in specimens obtained by cordocentesis. *Am J Obstet Gynecol* 1990;162(5):1198–1202.

139. Favre R, et al. Standard curves of cerebral Doppler flow velocity waveforms and predictive values for intrauterine growth retardation and fetal acidosis. *Fetal Diagn Ther* 1991;6(3–4):113–119.

140. Pattinson RC, et al. Obstetric and neonatal outcome in fetuses with absent end-diastolic velocities of the umbilical artery: A case-controlled study. *Am J Perinatol* 1993;10(2):135–138.

141. Hata T, et al. Real-time 3-D echocardiographic evaluation of the fetal heart using instantaneous volume-rendered display. *J Obstet Gynaecol Res* 2006;32(1):42–46.

142. Seelbach-Gobel B, et al. The prediction of fetal acidosis by means of intrapartum fetal pulse oximetry. *Am J Obstet Gynecol* 1999;180(1 pt 1):73–81.

143. Baz E, et al. Abnormal ductus venosus blood flow: A clue to umbilical cord complication. *Ultrasound Obstet Gynecol* 1999;13(3):204–206.

144. Arduini D, Rizzo G, Romanini C. Changes of pulsatility index from fetal vessels preceding the onset of late decelerations in growth-retarded fetuses. *Obstet Gynecol* 1992;79(4):605–610.

145. Rizzo G, et al. The value of fetal arterial, cardiac and venous flows in predicting pH and blood gases measured in umbilical blood at cordocentesis in growth retarded fetuses. *Br J Obstet Gynaecol* 1995;102(12):963–969.

146. Reuwer PJ, et al. Feto-placental circulatory competence. *Eur J Obstet Gynecol Reprod Biol* 1986;21(1):15–26.

147. Carvalho FH, et al. Ductus venosus Doppler velocimetry to predict acidemia at birth in pregnancies with placental insufficiency [in Portuguese]. *Rev Assoc Med Bras* 2005;51(4):221–227.

148. Kaukola T, et al. Suboptimal neurodevelopment in very preterm infants is related to fetal cardiovascular compromise in placental insufficiency. *Am J Obstet Gynecol* 2005;193(2):414–420.

149. Baschat AA, et al. Venous Doppler in the prediction of acid-base status of growth-restricted fetuses with elevated placental blood flow resistance. *Am J Obstet Gynecol* 2004;191(1):277–284.

150. Gardiner HM. Successes and shortcomings of fetal echocardiography. *Hosp Med* 2001;62(10):634–639.

151. Baschat AA, et al. Doppler and biophysical assessment in growth restricted fetuses: Distribution of test results. *Ultrasound Obstet Gynecol* 2006;27(1):41–47.

152. Harman CR, Baschat AA. Comprehensive assessment of fetal wellbeing: Which Doppler tests should be performed? *Curr Opin Obstet Gynecol* 2003;15(2):147–157.

153. Sterne G, Shields LE, Dubinsky TJ. Abnormal fetal cerebral and umbilical Doppler measurements in fetuses with intrauterine growth restriction predicts the severity of perinatal morbidity. *J Clin Ultrasound* 2001;29(3):146–151.

154. Fu J, Olofsson P. Restrained cerebral hyperperfusion in response to superimposed acute hypoxemia in growth-restricted human fetuses with established brain-sparing blood flow. *Early Hum Dev* 2006;82(3):211–216. Epub 2005 Dec 2.

155. Fouron JC. The unrecognized physiological and clinical significance of the fetal aortic isthmus. *Ultrasound Obstet Gynecol* 2003;22(5):441–447.

156. Fouron JC, et al. Correlation between prenatal velocity waveforms in the aortic isthmus and neurodevelopmental outcome between the ages of 2 and 4 years. *Am J Obstet Gynecol* 2001;184(4):630–636.

157. Sonesson SE, Fouron JC. Doppler velocimetry of the aortic isthmus in human fetuses with abnormal velocity waveforms in the umbilical artery. *Ultrasound Obstet Gynecol* 1997;10(2):107–111.

158. Donofrio MT, et al. Autoregulation of cerebral blood flow in fetuses with congenital heart disease: The brain sparing effect. *Pediatr Cardiol* 2003;24(5):436–443.

159. Kaltman JR, et al. Impact of congenital heart disease on cerebrovascular blood flow dynamics in the fetus. *Ultrasound Obstet Gynecol* 2005;25(1):32–36.

160. Jouannic JM, et al. Middle cerebral artery Doppler in fetuses with transposition of the great arteries. *Ultrasound Obstet Gynecol* 2002;20(2):122–124.

161. Fesslova V, Nava S, Villa L. Evolution and long term outcome in cases with fetal diagnosis of congenital heart disease: Italian multicentre study. Fetal Cardiology Study Group of the Italian Society of Pediatric Cardiology. *Heart* 1999;82(5):594–599.

162. Trines J, Hornberger LK. Evolution of heart disease in utero. *Pediatr Cardiol* 2004;25(3):287–298.

163. Sharland GK, et al. Left ventricular dysfunction in the fetus: Relation to aortic valve anomalies and endocardial fibroelastosis. *Br Heart J* 1991;66(6):419–424.

164. Allan LD, et al. Survival after fetal aortic balloon valvoplasty. *Ultrasound Obstet Gynecol* 1995;5(2):90–91.

165. Kohl T, et al. World experience of percutaneous ultrasound-guided balloon valvuloplasty in human fetuses with severe aortic valve obstruction. *Am J Cardiol* 2000;85(10):1230–1233.

166. Wilkins-Haug LE, et al. In-utero intervention for hypoplastic left heart syndrome—a perinatologist's perspective. *Ultrasound Obstet Gynecol* 2005;26(5):481–486.

167. Arzt W, et al. Invasive intrauterine treatment of pulmonary atresia/intact ventricular septum with heart failure. *Ultrasound Obstet Gynecol* 2003;21(2):186–188.

168. Tulzer G, et al. Fetal pulmonary valvuloplasty for critical pulmonary stenosis or atresia with intact septum. *Lancet* 2002;360:1567–1568.

169. Galindo A, et al. Pulmonary balloon valvuloplasty in a fetus with critical pulmonary stenosis/atresia with intact ventricular septum and heart failure. *Fetal Diagn Ther* 2006;21(1):100–104.

170. Satomi G, et al. Interventional treatment for fetus and newborn infant with congenital heart disease. *Pediatr Int* 2001;43(5):553–557.

171. Huhta J, et al. Advances in fetal cardiac intervention. *Curr Opin Pediatr* 2004;16(5):487–493.

172. Kohl T, et al. Fetal transesophageal echocardiography: Clinical introduction as a monitoring tool during cardiac intervention in a human fetus. *Ultrasound Obstet Gynecol* 2005;26(7):780–785.

173. Suh E, et al. How to grow a heart: Fibreoptic guided fetal aortic valvotomy. *Cardiol Young* 2006;(16 suppl 1):43–46.

174. Harrison MR, et al. Fetal surgical treatment. *Pediatr Ann* 1982;11(11):896–899, 901–903.

175. Harrison MR, et al. Successful repair in utero of a fetal diaphragmatic hernia after removal of herniated viscera from the left thorax. *N Engl J Med* 1990;322:1582–1584.

176. Lorenz HP, Adzick NS, Harrison MR. Open human fetal surgery. *Adv Surg* 1993;26:259–273.

177. Harrison MR, et al. Correction of congenital diaphragmatic hernia in utero VIII: Response of the hypoplastic lung to tracheal occlusion. *J Pediatr Surg* 1996;31(10):1339–1348.

178. Harrison MR, et al. Correction of congenital diaphragmatic hernia in utero IX: Fetuses with poor prognosis (liver herniation and low lung-to-head ratio) can be saved by fetoscopic temporary tracheal occlusion. *J Pediatr Surg* 1998;33(7):1017–1022; discussion 1022–1023.

179. Harrison MR, et al. Fetoscopic temporary tracheal occlusion by means of detachable balloon for congenital diaphragmatic hernia. *Am J Obstet Gynecol* 2001;185(3):730–733.

180. Cortes RA, et al. Survival of severe congenital diaphragmatic hernia has morbid consequences. *J Pediatr Surg* 2005;40(1):36–45; discussion 45–46.

181. Harrison MR, et al. A randomized trial of fetal endoscopic tracheal occlusion for severe fetal congenital diaphragmatic hernia. *N Engl J Med* 2003;349:1916–1924.

182. Clewell WH, et al. Placement of ventriculo-amniotic shunt for hydrocephalus in a fetus. *N Engl J Med* 1981;305:955.

183. Clewell WH. Congenital hydrocephalus: Treatment in utero. *Fetal Ther* 1988;3(1–2):89–97.

184. Hamar BD, et al. Trends in fetal echocardiography and implications for clinical practice: 1985 to 2003. *J Ultrasound Med* 2006;25(2):197–202.

185. Mohan UR, Kleinman CS, Kern JH. Fetal echocardiography and its evolving impact 1992 to 2002. *Am J Cardiol* 2005;96(1):134–136.

186. Vanderhal AL, et al. Conjugated hyperbilirubinemia in a newborn infant after maternal (transplacental) treatment with flecainide acetate for fetal tachycardia and fetal hydrops. *J Pediatr* 1995;126(6):988–990.

187. Vetter VL, Rashkind WJ. Congenital complete heart block and connective-tissue disease. *N Engl J Med* 1983;309:236–238.

188. Scott JS, et al. Connective-tissue disease, antibodies to ribonucleoprotein, and congenital heart block. *N Engl J Med* 1983;309:209–212.

189. McCue CM, et al. Congenital heart block in newborns of mothers with connective tissue disease. *Circulation* 1977;56(1):82–90.

190. Veille JC, Sunderland C, Bennett RM. Complete heart block in a fetus associated with maternal Sjogren's syndrome. *Am J Obstet Gynecol* 1985;151(5):660–661.

191. McCormack GD, Barth WF. Congenital complete heart block with maternal primary Sjogren's syndrome. *South Med J* 1985;78(4):471–473.

192. Sholler GF, Whight CM, Celermajer JM. Fetal echocardiography: Experience and reason. *Med J Aust* 1986;144(5):250–252.

193. Taylor PV, et al. Maternal antibodies against fetal cardiac antigens in congenital complete heart block. *N Engl J Med* 1986;315:667–672.

194. Horsfall AC, et al. Ro and La antigens and maternal anti-La idiotype on the surface of myocardial fibres in congenital heart block. *J Autoimmun* 1991;4(1):165–176.

195. Schmidt KG, et al. Perinatal outcome of fetal complete atrioventricular block: A multicenter experience. *J Am Coll Cardiol* 1991;17(6):1360–1366.

196. Van Leeuwen P. Fetal magnetocardiography: Time intervals and heart rate variability. *Neurol Clin Neurophysiol* 2004;2004:46.

197. Herruzo A, et al. Bigeminal fetal rhythm [in Spanish]. *Acta Obstet Ginecol Hisp Lusit* 1979;27(9):593–600.

198. Martinez J, et al. Ventricular fetal extrasystole [in Spanish]. *Acta Obstet Ginecol Hisp Lusit* 1979;27(9):579–590.

199. Madison JP, et al. Echocardiography and fetal heart sounds in the diagnosis of fetal heart block. *Am Heart J* 1979;98(4):505–509.

200. Baumgarten K, Frohlich H. Fetal rhythm disorders during pregnancy and birth [in Geerman]. *Z Geburtshilfe Perinatol* 1972;176(4):249–265.

201. Chitkara U, et al. Persistent supraventricular tachycardia in utero. *Diagn Gynecol Obstet* 1980;2(4):291–298.

202. Hawrylyshyn PA, et al. The role of echocardiography in fetal cardiac arrhythmias. *Am J Obstet Gynecol* 1981;141(2):223–225.

203. DeVore GR, Siassi B, Platt LD. Fetal echocardiography. III. The diagnosis of cardiac arrhythmias using real-time-directed M-mode ultrasound. *Am J Obstet Gynecol* 1983;146(7):792–799.

204. Stewart PA, Tonge HM, Wladimiroff JW. Arrhythmia and structural abnormalities of the fetal heart. *Br Heart J* 1983;50(6):550–554.

205. Allan LD, et al. Evaluation of fetal arrhythmias by echocardiography. *Br Heart J* 1983;50(3):240–245.

206. Wester HA, Grimm G, Lehmann F. Echocardiographic diagnosis of fetal heart insufficiency caused by supraventricular tachycardia [in German]. *Z Kardiol* 1984;73(6):405–408.

207. Shapiro I, Sharf M, Abinader EG. Prenatal diagnosis of fetal arrhythmias: A new echocardiographic technique. *J Clin Ultrasound* 1984;12(6):369–372.

208. Crowley DC, et al. Two-dimensional and M-mode echocardiographic evaluation of fetal arrhythmia. *Clin Cardiol* 1985;8(1):1–10.

209. Silverman NH, et al. Recognition of fetal arrhythmias by echocardiography. *J Clin Ultrasound* 1985;13(4):255–263.

210. Wladimiroff JW, Stewart PA. Treatment of fetal cardiac arrhythmias. *Br J Hosp Med* 1985;34(3):134–140.

211. Truccone NJ, Mariona FG. Prenatal diagnosis and outcome of congenital complete heart block: The role of fetal echocardiography. *Fetal Ther* 1986;1(4):210–216.

212. Castillo R, et al. Fetal echocardiography: diagnosis and management of fetal arrhythmias. *J Med Assoc Ga* 1986;75(12):730–733.

213. Lingman G, Marsal K. Fetal cardiac arrhythmias: Doppler assessment. *Semin Perinatol* 1987;11(4):357–361.

214. Cameron A, et al. Evaluation of fetal cardiac dysrhythmias with two-dimensional, M–mode, and pulsed Doppler ultrasonography. *Am J Obstet Gynecol* 1988;158(2):286–290.

215. Gembruch U, Bald R, Hansmann M. Color-coded M-mode Doppler echocardiography in the diagnosis of fetal arrhythmia [in German]. *Geburtshilfe Frauenheilkd* 1990;50(4):286–290.

216. Chaoui R, et al. Fetal echocardiography: Part III. Fetal arrhythmia [in German]. *Zentralbl Gynakol* 1991;113(24):1335–1350.

217. Maeno Y. Fetal arrhythmias; intrauterine diagnosis and treatment. *Kurume Med J* 1991;38(4):327–336.

218. Rein AJ, et al. Use of tissue velocity imaging in the diagnosis of fetal cardiac arrhythmias. *Circulation* 2002;106(14):1827–1833.

219. Wakai RT, et al. Magnetocardiographic rhythm patterns at initiation and termination of fetal supraventricular tachycardia. *Circulation* 2003;107(2):307–312.

220. Comani S, et al. Characterization of fetal arrhythmias by means of fetal magnetocardiography in three cases of difficult ultrasonographic imaging. *Pacing Clin Electrophysiol* 2004;27(12):1647–1655.

221. Hosono T, et al. Prenatal diagnosis of fetal complete atrioventricular block with QT prolongation and alternating ventricular pacemakers using multi-channel magnetocardiography and current-arrow maps. *Fetal Diagn Ther* 2002;17(3):173–176.

222. Menendez T, et al. Prenatal diagnosis of QT prolongation by magnetocardiography. *Pacing Clin Electrophysiol* 2000;23(8):1305–1307.

223. Hamada H, et al. Prenatal diagnosis of long QT syndrome using fetal magnetocardiography. *Prenat Diagn* 1999;19(7):677–680.

224. Fouron JC, et al. Management of fetal tachyarrhythmia based on superior vena cava/aorta Doppler flow recordings. *Heart* 2003;89(10):1211–1216.

225. DeVore GR, Horenstein J. Simultaneous Doppler recording of the pulmonary artery and vein: A new technique for the evaluation of a fetal arrhythmia. *J Ultrasound Med* 1993;12(11):669–671.

226. Lingman G, Ohrlander S, Ohlin P. Intrauterine digoxin treatment of fetal paroxysmal tachycardia. Case report. *Br J Obstet Gynaecol* 1980;87(4):340–342.

227. Kerenyi TD, et al. Transplacental cardioversion of intrauterine supraventricular tachycardia with digitalis. *Lancet* 1980;2:393–394.

228. Dumesic DA, et al. Transplacental cardioversion of fetal supraventricular tachycardia with procainamide. *N Engl J Med* 1982;307(18):1128–1131.

229. King CR, et al. Successful treatment of fetal supraventricular tachycardia with maternal digoxin therapy. *Chest* 1984;85(4):573–575.

230. Allan LD, et al. Evaluation and treatment of fetal arrhythmias. *Clin Cardiol* 1984;7(9):467–473.

.31. Truccone N, Mariona F. Intrauterine conversion of fetal supraventricular tachycardia with combination of digoxin and verapamil. *Pediatr Pharmacol (New York)* 1985;5(2):149–153.

232. Lingman G, et al. Fetal cardiac arrhythmia. Clinical outcome in 113 cases. *Acta Obstet Gynecol Scand* 1986;65(3):263–267.

233. Killeen AA, Bowers LD. Fetal supraventricular tachycardia treated with high-dose quinidine: Toxicity associated with marked elevation of the metabolite, 3(S)–3-hydroxyquinidine. *Obstet Gynecol* 1987;70(3 pt 2):445–449.

234. Allan LD, et al. Flecainide in the treatment of fetal tachycardias. *Br Heart J* 1991;65(1):46–48.

235. Perry JC, Ayres NA, Carpenter RJ Jr. Fetal supraventricular tachycardia treated with flecainide acetate. *J Pediatr* 1991;118(2):303–305.

236. Pinsky WW, Rayburn WF, Evans MI. Pharmacologic therapy for fetal arrhythmias. *Clin Obstet Gynecol* 1991;34(2):304–309.

237. Azancot-Benisty A, et al. Clinical and pharmacologic study of fetal supraventricular tachyarrhythmias. *J Pediatr* 1992;121(4):608–613.

238. Parilla BV, Strasburger JF, Socol ML. Fetal supraventricular tachycardia complicated by hydrops fetalis: A role for direct fetal intramuscular therapy. *Am J Perinatol* 1996;13(8):483–486.

239. Amano K, et al. Successful treatment of supraventricular tachycardia with flecainide acetate: A case report. *Fetal Diagn Ther* 1997;12(6):328–331.

240. Mangione R, et al. Successful treatment of refractory supraventricular tachycardia by repeat intravascular injection of amiodarone in a fetus with hydrops. *Eur J Obstet Gynecol Reprod Biol* 1999;86(1):105–107.

241. Schmolling J, et al. Digoxin, flecainide, and amiodarone transfer across the placenta and the effects of an elevated umbilical venous pressure on the transfer rate. *Ther Drug Monit* 2000;22(5):582–588.

242. Nakata M, et al. Successful treatment of supraventricular tachycardia exhibiting hydrops fetalis with flecainide acetate. A case report. *Fetal Diagn Ther* 2003;18(2):83–86.
243. Walsh EP, Saul JP, Triedman JK. *Cardiac Arrhythmias in Children and Young Adults with Congenital Heart Disease.* Philadelphia: Lippincott Williams & Wilkins, Philadelphia, 2001.
244. Carpenter RJ Jr, et al. Fetal ventricular pacing for hydrops secondary to complete atrioventricular block. *J Am Coll Cardiol* 1986;8(6):1434–1436.
245. Crombleholme TM, et al. Complete heart block in fetal lambs. I. Technique and acute physiological response. *J Pediatr Surg* 1990;25(6):587–593.
246. Herreman G, et al. Fetal death caused by myocarditis and isolated congenital auriculoventricular block [in French]. *Presse Med* 1985;14(29):1547–1550.
247. Buyon JP, et al. Intrauterine therapy for presumptive fetal myocarditis with acquired heart block due to systemic lupus erythematosus. Experience in a mother with a predominance of SS-B (La) antibodies. *Arthritis Rheum* 1987;30(1):44–49.
248. Buyon JP, Winchester R. Congenital complete heart block. A human model of passively acquired autoimmune injury. *Arthritis Rheum* 1990;33(5):609–614.
249. Arroyave CM, et al. Myocardiopathy diagnosed in utero in a mother with SS-A antibodies treated with plasmapheresis [in Spanish]. *Ginecol Obstet Mex* 1995;63:134–137.
250. Udink ten Cate FE, et al. Dilated cardiomyopathy in isolated congenital complete atrioventricular block: Early and long-term risk in children. *J Am Coll Cardiol* 2001;37(4):1129–1134.
251. Matsushita H, et al. Successful prenatal treatment of congenital heart block with ritodrine administered transplacentally. *Arch Gynecol Obstet* 2002;267(1):51–53.
252. Huang HW, et al. Prenatal diagnosis of persistent fetal bradycardia: Report of four cases. *Chang Gung Med J* 2001;24(1):57–61.
253. Comas C, et al. Complete congenital atrioventricular block. Prenatal diagnosis and perinatal management. *Rev Esp Cardiol* 1997;50(7):498–506.
254. Koike T, et al. Fetal ventricular rate in case of congenital complete heart block is increased by ritodrine. Case report. *J Perinat Med* 1997;25(2):216–218.
255. Friedman DM, Buyon JP. Complete atrioventricular block diagnosed prenatally: Anything new on the block? *Ultrasound Obstet Gynecol* 2005;26(1):2–3.
256. Buyon JP, et al. Identifying an early marker for congenital heart block: When is a long PR interval too long? Comment on the article by Sonesson et al. *Arthritis Rheum* 2005;52(4):1341–1342.
257. Glickstein J, et al. The fetal Doppler mechanical PR interval: A validation study. *Fetal Diagn Ther* 2004;19(1):31–34.
258. Buyon JP, Friedman DM. Autoantibody-associated congenital heart block: The clinical perspective. *Curr Rheumatol Rep* 2003;5(5):374–378.
259. Brucato A, et al. Proposal for a new definition of congenital complete atrioventricular block. *Lupus* 2003;12(6):427–435.
260. Rosenthal D, et al. Validation of the Doppler PR interval in the fetus. *J Am Soc Echocardiogr* 2002;15(9):1029–1030.
261. Friedman DM, et al. Congenital heart block in neonatal lupus: The pediatric cardiologist's perspective. *Indian J Pediatr* 2002;69(6):517–522.
262. Saleeb S, et al. Comparison of treatment with fluorinated glucocorticoids to the natural history of autoantibody-associated congenital heart block: Retrospective review of the research registry for neonatal lupus. *Arthritis Rheum* 1999;42(11):2335–2345.
263. Raboisson MJ, et al. Fetal Doppler echocardiographic diagnosis and successful steroid therapy of Luciani-Wenckebach phenomenon and endocardial fibroelastosis related to maternal anti-Ro and anti-La antibodies. *J Am Soc Echocardiogr* 2005;18(4):375–380.
264. Jaeggi ET, et al. Is immune-mediated complete fetal atrioventricular block reversible by transplacental dexamethasone therapy? *Ultrasound Obstet Gynecol* 2004;23(6):602–605.
265. Jaeggi ET, et al. Transplacental fetal treatment improves the outcome of prenatally diagnosed complete atrioventricular block without structural heart disease. *Circulation* 2004;110(12):1542–1548.
266. Jaeggi ET, et al. Outcome of children with fetal, neonatal or childhood diagnosis of isolated congenital atrioventricular block. A single institution's experience of 30 years. *J Am Coll Cardiol* 2002;39(1):130–137.
267. Carvalho JS, Shinebourne EA, Kyle P. Efficacy unproved of maternal dexamethasone for fetal heart block. *Am J Obstet Gynecol* 1996;175(2):502–503.

CHAPTER 29 ■ CIRCULATION PHYSIOLOGY

DAVID F. TEITEL, MD, STEVEN C. CASSIDY, MD, AND JEFFREY R. FINEMAN, MD

The circulation can be divided into its central components, consisting of the central arteries, veins, and, in the fetus, central shunts; and its peripheral components, consisting of the various regional vascular beds. Each component undergoes significant changes throughout fetal and postnatal development. General physiologic principles of blood flow will be presented first, followed by specific considerations pertaining to blood flow through the central and peripheral circulations, including developmental changes.

PHYSIOLOGY

General Physiology

Physical Determinants of Flow

Physical factors that regulate flow through a vascular bed exert their effects through the hydraulic equivalent of Ohm's law (resistance equation) and the Poiseuille–Hagen relationship. In vascular terms, Ohm's law states that resistance to flow between two points along a tube equals the pressure difference between the two points divided by flow. With vascular resistance R and blood flow Q, the mean pressure decrease that occurs from the artery (P_a) to the vein (P_v) can be derived from the formula

$$R = \frac{P_a - P_v}{Q}$$

To assess changes in arterial blood pressure in response to changes in flow and resistance, the formula can be rearranged as

$$P_a = Q \cdot R + P_v$$

Thus, elevation of arterial blood pressure may occur with an increase in vascular resistance or blood flow. These factors are not independent, and arterial blood pressure may remain constant with increased blood flow because the increased flow has caused vascular resistance to decrease by dilating or recruiting arteries—if the product $Q \cdot R$ does not increase, arterial pressure does not.

Further factors that affect the resistance to flow can be approximated by the Poiseuille–Hagen relationship, which describes the relationship of pressure and flow of a Newtonian fluid flowing through a straight, round glass tube:

$$R = \frac{8l\eta}{\pi r^4}$$

where l is the length of the tube, r is its internal radius, and η is the fluid viscosity. Blood is not Newtonian; however, at normal hematocrits, this probably is of little consequence. The walls of the small arteries are not smooth, and the arteries branch, curve, and taper. Blood flow is pulsatile, so that additional energy (and therefore a higher pressure) is needed to overcome inertia and to accelerate the blood at each ejection. Because of short distances between arterial branch points, laminar flow is unlikely in peripheral vascular beds, and viscous pressure losses would be greater than in a physical model. Arteries are also distensible, and continuously changing transvascular pressure alters their radii; therefore, pressure–flow relationships are not linear. Last, vascular beds are composed of many blood vessels in parallel. These vessels are not all open all the time, and they may differ in radii in different zones.

Despite these differences, the general principles of changes in physical factors such as viscosity and radius apply. Vascular resistance is directly related to the viscosity of blood perfusing the vascular bed and inversely related to its cross-sectional area (r^4). Increasing viscosity or decreasing vessel radius therefore leads to an elevation of both arterial pressure and vascular resistance (1).

CENTRAL CIRCULATION

The central circulation is structured very differently in the fetus, primarily to accommodate the different site of oxygen uptake. In the postnatal state, oxygen uptake occurs in the pulmonary vascular bed, which is perfused independently by the right ventricle; the left ventricle separately supplies the regional systemic vascular beds with fully oxygenated blood. In the fetal state, oxygen uptake occurs in the placenta, which is perfused in parallel with the systemic vascular beds. To deliver relatively highly oxygenated blood to the metabolically active tissues (such as the heart and brain) and to deliver less oxygenated blood to the placenta for oxygen uptake, central shunts and preferential blood flow patterns exist. Shunts are present in the venous system (ductus venosus), the heart (foramen ovale), and the arterial system (ductus arteriosus) and are remarkably efficient at achieving this goal. At birth, these shunts are abolished over a very short period of time, and the mature postnatal central circulation is established within the first few days of life.

Fetal Circulation

The presence of central shunts allows the fetal circulation to be remarkably efficient at distributing oxygen and substrate. Figure 29.1 demonstrates that the fetal ventricles primarily perform their postnatal functions: The fetal right ventricle supplies most of its blood via the ductus arteriosus and descending aorta to the placenta for oxygen uptake, and the left ventricle supplies most of its blood via the ascending aorta

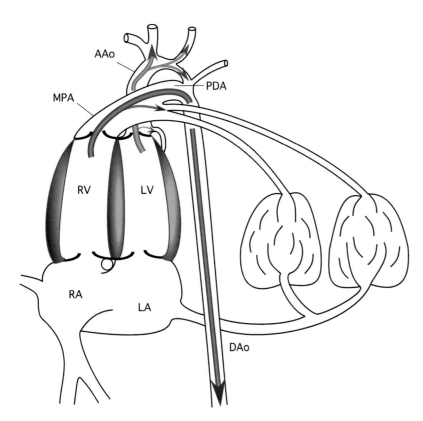

FIGURE 29.1 Preferential pattern of ventricular output. The left ventricle (LV) directs most of its highly saturated blood (*red arrow*) via the ascending aorta (AAo) to the highly metabolic heart and upper body. The right ventricle (RV) primarily ejects less oxygenated blood (*purple arrow*) via the main pulmonary artery (MPA) primarily down the ductus arteriosus (PDA) and via the descending aorta (DAo) to the placenta for oxygen uptake. RA, right atrium; LA, left atrium.

to the heart and brain for oxygen delivery. For the central venous circulation to facilitate the efficient performance of these tasks, the least saturated venous blood should be directed to the right ventricle and the most saturated should be directed to the left. To appreciate how this is achieved, it is best to divide the central venous circulation into five components: The venous return from the upper body, the myocardium, the lungs, the lower body, and the placenta.

The least saturated blood returns from the upper body, via the superior vena cava, and from the myocardium, via the coronary sinus. This blood is directed appropriately, through the tricuspid valve to the right ventricle. The leftward and superior course of the eustachian valve directs >95% of the blood flowing caudally from the superior vena cava away from the foramen ovale and toward the tricuspid valve. In addition, the location of the coronary sinus caudad to the foramen causes venous blood from the myocardium to flow through the tricuspid valve to the right ventricle (Fig. 29.1). Blood returning from the lungs is not well saturated, but by the nature of the normal drainage of the pulmonary veins to the left atrium, preferential flow to the right ventricle is not possible. However, pulmonary blood flow represents no more than 8% of combined ventricular output, so it does not have an appreciable effect on oxygen delivery (2).

Inferior vena caval return comes from the remaining two sources, the lower body and the placenta. Most lower body flow, except that from the liver, ascends the distal inferior vena cava. This stream of relatively desaturated blood enters the lateral margin of the right atrium and is directed primarily through the tricuspid valve. Placental (umbilical venous) and liver venous return is more complicated (Fig. 29.2). Under normal conditions in the fetal sheep, about 55% of the highly saturated umbilical venous return ascends via the ductus venosus to the inferior vena cava–right atrium junction, where it preferentially crosses the foramen ovale (2). Slightly less than half of the remaining umbilical venous return enters the left lobe of the liver, from which it reaches the left hepatic vein (3). The left hepatic vein joins the ductus venosus near the inferior vena cava, so that this highly saturated blood is also directed to the foramen ovale. The limbus of the foramen ovale helps to direct this blood into the left atrium. The remainder of the umbilical venous blood, along with >95% of the poorly saturated portal venous blood, is directed to the right lobe of the liver. From the right lobe, this much less saturated blood enters the right hepatic vein and tends to stream with the blood of the distal inferior vena cava to the tricuspid valve. The hepatic artery, which carries blood that is moderately well saturated, constitutes <10% of hepatic blood flow in the fetus, so it does not significantly contribute to oxygen supply. Hepatic arterial blood is distributed to both lobes of the liver, with the right lobe receiving somewhat more (3).

Thus, preferential streaming patterns among the different sources of venous return allow most of the poorly saturated blood from the upper body, myocardium, and lower body to reach the right ventricle, and the more highly saturated umbilical venous return to reach the left ventricle. Although the separation of fetal ventricular outputs is not as efficient as the postnatal separation, it is quite remarkable in its ability to allow the right and left ventricles to perform their normal postnatal functions of delivery of blood for oxygen uptake and oxygen supply, respectively.

Postnatal Circulation

The changes in the central circulation at birth are primarily caused by external events rather than by primary changes in the circulation itself. Most important of these external events

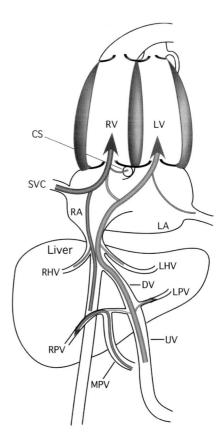

FIGURE 29.2 Preferential pattern of venous return to the right (RV) and left (LV) ventricles. More highly saturated blood (*red arrow*) from the umbilical vein (UV) passes via the ductus venosus (DV) and left hepatic vein (LHV) to the left atrium (LA) and LV. Less saturated blood (*blue arrows*) from the lower body via the inferior vena cava (IVC, not shown), from the main and right portal veins (MPV and RPV) via the right hepatic vein (RHV), from the coronary sinus (CS), and from the superior vena cava (SVC) passes to the right atrium (RA) and RV.

are the rapid and large decrease in pulmonary vascular resistance and the disruption of the umbilical-placental circulation. The various mechanisms responsible for the decrease in pulmonary vascular resistance are discussed later in this chapter. This decrease has profound effects on the central shunts in the systemic circulation. Abruptly at birth, the ductus arteriosus changes from a right-to-left conduit of blood to the descending aorta, to a left-to-right conduit of blood to the lungs, until it closes in the first hours or days of life. This shunt may be prolonged in the premature infant, causing a steal of blood from the regional vascular beds of greatest resistance. The physiologic basis of normal closure of the ductus arteriosus and problems associated with delayed closure are discussed elsewhere (see Chapter 33).

As previously mentioned, the ductus venosus carries umbilical venous return primarily to the left heart. Although the amount of umbilical venous blood that enters the ductus venosus is variable and is greatly affected by stresses such as hypoxemia, changes in flow do not appear to be caused by active vasoconstriction of the ductus venosus, but rather, occur passively in accordance with changes in umbilical blood flow. At birth, the umbilical-placental circulation is abolished, causing a marked reduction in ductus venosus flow and in flow to the left lobe of the liver. However, portal venous flow through the ductus venosus increases from <5%

to >50% by 1 hour of age so that, despite an increase in portal venous flow at birth, hepatic flow actually decreases substantially (4). This shunt of portal venous blood through the ductus venosus is transient, generally lasting for 1 day to 2 weeks. The functional closure of the ductus venosus is probably a passive phenomenon, although it has been demonstrated that the isolated ductus venosus can respond to adrenergic stimulation and prostanoids. In the intact newborn lamb, it can dilate in response to prostaglandin E_1 (5). Thus, its closure may be partly induced by the same hormonal changes that are implicated in the closure of the ductus arteriosus.

Although vasoactive processes are involved in the closure of the ductus arteriosus, and may be involved in closure of the ductus venosus, closure of the foramen ovale at birth is entirely passive, secondary to alterations in the relative return of blood to the right and left atria. Prior to birth, direct left atrial return via the pulmonary veins is only about 8% of combined venous return. Thus, the pressure gradient from right to left maintains a large flow of blood through the foramen ovale, which appears as a wind sock bulging into the left atrium. With the onset of oxygen ventilation, the proportion of combined venous return that directly enters the left atrium via the pulmonary veins increases dramatically, to >50% (2), because of the marked increase in pulmonary blood flow, which includes a transient left-to-right shunt through the ductus arteriosus. Left atrial pressure thus exceeds right, and the redundant flap of tissue of the foramen ovale that previously bowed into the left atrium is now pressed against the septum. Small left-to-right shunts may be visualized in the newborn by color Doppler ultrasonography, but these shunts are not hemodynamically significant. Although patency of the foramen ovale may be present for several years, shunts of any significance occur only when the primum septum is deficient, thus forming a secundum atrial septal defect. (See chapter 30.)

PULMONARY CIRCULATION

Although considerable information is available regarding the complex physiologic regulation of pulmonary vascular resistance, the exact mechanisms involved in intrinsic relaxation and constriction of the pulmonary vascular smooth muscle are not completely understood. The important functional role of the vascular endothelium and its interactions with smooth muscle are only now being brought to light. The pulmonary vessels not only produce many vasoactive substances, but also actively metabolize many. Changes in pulmonary vascular resistance can occur at different levels within the circulation, and vasoactive substances and their properties may change during passage through the pulmonary vascular bed. Accurate physiologic characterization of the pulmonary circulation varies with the gender, age, and species of the model used and the exact compartment of the pulmonary circulation evaluated. Whether all the principles that apply to general vascular smooth muscle also apply to the pulmonary circulation is not yet clear; however, the final common pathway by which vascular smooth muscle constricts is by Ca^{2+}-mediated stimulation of excitation–contraction coupling; relaxation occurs mainly either through a cyclic guanosine monophosphate (cGMP)- or cyclic adenosine monophosphate (cAMP)-mediated mechanism. Many interacting factors are responsible for the physiologic and physical control of pulmonary vascular resistance in the fetus and for its normal decrease after birth.

MORPHOLOGIC DEVELOPMENT

The stage of morphologic development of the pulmonary circulation affects the vascular responses in the perinatal period. In the fetus and newborn, all small pulmonary arteries have a thicker medial smooth muscle layer in relation to diameter than similar arteries in adults. This increased muscularity is partly responsible for the increased vasoreactivity and pulmonary vascular resistance in the fetus, particularly near term. In fetal lamb lungs, when perfusion is fixed at pressures equivalent to those in utero, the muscle is most prominent in the smallest resistance arteries (identified as fifth- and sixth-generation arteries; external diameter 20 to 50 mm), and over the latter half of gestation, the thickness remains constant in relation to diameter.

Similar observations using slightly different techniques have been made in human lungs. In these, the small pulmonary arteries are identified by their relationship to airways. Preacinar arteries course proximal to or along with terminal bronchioli; intra-acinar arteries course along with respiratory bronchioli or alveolar ducts, or within the alveolar walls. In arteries traced along the airways toward the alveoli, a point is reached at which the completely encircling medial smooth muscle coat gives way to a region of incomplete muscularization; in these partially muscularized arteries, the smooth muscle is arranged in a spiral or helix. The muscle then disappears from the arteries that are still larger than capillaries (nonmuscularized small pulmonary arteries). In these arteries, an incomplete pericyte layer is found within the endothelial basement membrane; in the nonmuscular portions of the partially muscular small pulmonary arteries are intermediate cells (i.e., cells intermediate in position and structure between pericytes and mature smooth muscle cells). These cells are precursor smooth muscle cells; under certain conditions, such as hypoxia, they may rapidly differentiate into mature smooth muscle cells.

In the near-term fetus, only about half the precapillary arteries (those associated with respiratory bronchioli) are muscularized or partially muscularized, and the alveoli are free of muscular arteries. In the first 4 to 6 weeks after birth, there is progressive involution of the circumferential medial smooth muscle with overall reduction in medial muscular thickness of the walls of the small pulmonary arteries. In adults, circumferential muscularization extends peripherally along the intraacinar arteries so that most are completely muscularized, although with only a very thin layer of smooth muscle; this adultlike pattern is reached at about puberty.

During fetal growth, the number of small arteries increases greatly. In humans the main preacinar pulmonary arterial branches that accompany the larger airways are developed by 16 weeks' gestation; however, the intraacinar circulation follows alveolar development late in gestation and after birth, and arteries multiply as alveoli develop, a process generally complete by about 10 years of age (6,7).

Fetal Circulation

In the fetus, gas exchange occurs in the placenta and pulmonary blood flow is low, supplying nutritional requirements for lung growth and allowing the lung to serve a metabolic or paraendocrine function. Pulmonary blood flow in near-term fetal lambs (term being 145 days of gestation) is about 100 mL/100 g wet lung weight (8% to 10% of combined ventricular output). Pulmonary blood flow is low despite the dominance of the right ventricle, which in the fetus ejects 55% to 60% of total cardiac output. Most of the right ventricular output is diverted away from the lungs through the widely patent ductus arteriosus to the descending thoracic aorta and the placenta for oxygenation (Fig. 29.1). In young fetuses at about 0.5 gestation, 3% to 4% of total cardiac output perfuses the lungs; this increases to about 6% at 0.8 gestation, corresponding temporally with the onset of the release of surface active material into lung fluid. There is a further progressive slow increase thereafter to 8% to 10% near term. Fetal pulmonary arterial mean blood pressure increases progressively with gestation and at term is about 50 mm Hg, exceeding mean aortic blood pressure by 1 to 2 mm Hg. Total pulmonary vascular resistance early in gestation is extremely high relative to that in the infant or adult, probably owing to the small number of small arteries present. Total pulmonary vascular resistance decreases progressively over the last half of gestation, with growth of new arteries and an overall increase in cross section. However, when lung growth is accounted for, the pulmonary vascular resistance per unit of lung tends to increase over late gestation (8,9).

Transitional Circulation

At birth, with initiation of pulmonary ventilation, pulmonary vascular resistance decreases rapidly and is associated with an eightfold to tenfold increase in pulmonary blood flow. In normal full-term lambs, pulmonary arterial blood pressure decreases to near adult levels within 2 to 3 hours. In humans this takes longer, and by 24 hours of age, mean pulmonary arterial blood pressure may be only half systemic. After the initial rapid decrease in pulmonary vascular resistance and pulmonary arterial blood pressure, there is a slow, progressive decrease, with adult levels reached after 2 to 6 weeks (Fig. 29.3). This is due to vascular remodeling, muscular involution, and rheologic changes.

Physiologic Regulation of Pulmonary Vascular Resistance

As previously discussed, pulmonary vascular resistance in the fetal lung is initially high and decreases slightly throughout the final third of gestation. Many factors, including mechanical effects, state of oxygenation, and the production of vasoactive substances, regulate the tone of the fetal pulmonary circulation. The most prominent factor associated with high fetal pulmonary vascular resistance is the normally low blood O_2 tension (pulmonary arterial blood pO_2 = 17 to 20 torr). In the fetal lamb, resistance is further increased by hypoxemia and lowered by increasing oxygen tension, a vasoactive response that becomes active in the latter third of gestation. The exact mechanism and site of hypoxic pulmonary vasoconstriction in the fetal pulmonary circulation remains unclear. In isolated fetal pulmonary arteries, oxygen modulates the production of both prostacyclin and endothelium-derived nitric oxide (EDNO); two potent vasoactive substances that may in part underlie the responses of the developing pulmonary circulation to changes in oxygenation. In addition to the low oxygen environment, many substances constrict the pulmonary circulation of the fetus, such as α agonists, thromboxane, and the leukotrienes. However, their role, if any, in the maintenance of the high fetal pulmonary vascular resistance does not appear prominent (10–12). In addition to the production of vasoconstrictors, the fetal pulmonary circulation actively and

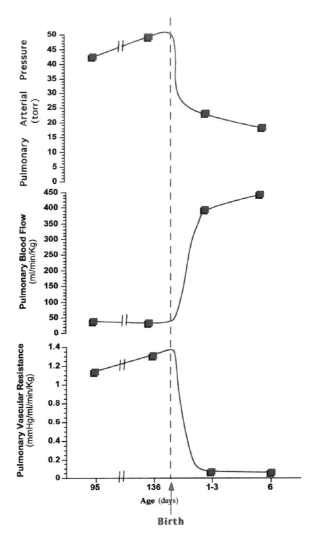

FIGURE 29.3 The changes in pulmonary arterial pressure, blood flow, and vascular resistance that occur around birth. (Data from Morin FC III, Egan E. Pulmonary hemodynamics in fetal lambs during development at normal and increased oxygen tension. *J Appl Physiol* 1992;73:213–218; and Soifer SJ, Morin FC III, Kaslow DC, et al. The developmental effects of prostaglandin D2 on the pulmonary and systemic circulation in the newborn lamb. *J Dev Physiol* 1983;5:237–250.)

continuously produces vasodilating substances that modulate the degree of vasoconstriction under normal conditions and may play a more active role during periods of fetal stress. These substances are mainly endothelially derived and include EDNO and prostacyclin (PGI$_2$). EDNO is synthesized by the oxidation of the guanidino nitrogen moiety of L-arginine. After certain stimuli, such as shear stress or the receptor binding of specific vasodilators (endothelium-dependent vasodilators), nitric oxide (NO) is synthesized by the activation of NO synthase, and NO is then released from the endothelial cells. Once released from endothelial cells, NO diffuses into vascular smooth muscle cells and activates soluble guanylate cyclase, the enzyme that catalyzes the production of guanosine-3′-5′-cyclic monophosphate (cGMP) from guanosine-5′-triphosphate. Activation of guanylate cyclase increases the concentrations of cGMP, thus initiating a cascade that results in smooth muscle relaxation (Fig. 29.4). Endothelial production of NO and

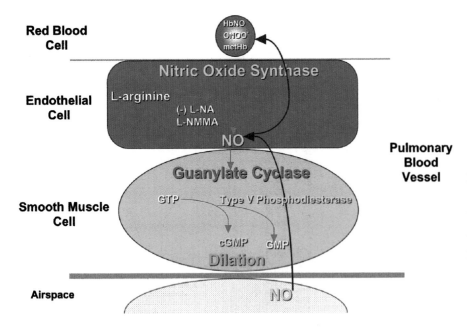

FIGURE 29.4 Schematic of the nitric oxide (NO)-cGMP pathway. Endogenous NO is produced from L-arginine within the pulmonary vascular endothelial cell. After diffusing into the smooth muscle cell, NO activates guanylate cyclase. The resulting increase in cGMP concentration induces relaxation. Exogenous NO (inhaled NO) diffuses from the airspace into the smooth muscle cell, where it activates guanylate cyclase. When it diffuses into the bloodstream, NO binds to hemoglobin to form methemoglobin and is inactivated.

cGMP has been demonstrated in the fetal, newborn, and adult pulmonary vasculature. In fetal lambs, inhibition of EDNO synthesis produces marked increases in resting fetal pulmonary vascular resistance and inhibits the oxygen-induced decrease in pulmonary vascular resistance. In addition, studies of intrapulmonary arteries and isolated lung preparations of the sheep reveal maturational increases in NO-mediated relaxation during the late fetal and early postnatal period. These data suggest that basal EDNO production is an important mediator of both normal fetal pulmonary vascular tone and the dramatic decrease in resistance that occurs with the onset of oxygen ventilation at birth (13–15). Prostacyclin is synthesized primarily in vascular endothelial cells and produces vasodilation by activating adenylate cyclase via receptor G protein–coupled mechanisms. Activation of adenylate cyclase results in increased adenosine 3′,5′-cyclic monophosphate (cAMP) concentrations, thus initiating a cascade that results in smooth muscle relaxation. Although there is a maturational increase in PGI_2 production throughout gestation, basal PGI_2 activity does not appear to be an important mediator of resting fetal pulmonary vascular tone. Interestingly, endothelin-1 (ET-1) is another potent endothelially derived vasoactive factor with both vasodilating and vasoconstricting effects. The hemodynamic effects of ET-1 are mediated by at least two distinct receptor populations, ET_A and ET_B. ET_A receptors are located on vascular smooth muscle cells and are likely responsible for the vasoconstricting effects of ET-1, whereas most ET_B receptors are located on endothelial cells and are likely responsible for the vasodilating effects of ET-1. The predominant effect of exogenous ET-1 in the fetal and newborn pulmonary circulation is vasodilation, mediated via ET_B receptor activation and EDNO release. However, the predominant effect in the juvenile and adult pulmonary circulation is vasoconstriction, mediated via ET_A receptor activation. In fetal lambs, selective ET_A receptor blockade produces small decreases in resting fetal pulmonary resistance, suggesting a potential, minor role for basal ET-1–induced vasoconstriction in maintaining the high fetal pulmonary vascular resistance. Although plasma concentrations of ET-1 are increased at birth, animal data suggest that basal ET-1 activity does not

play an important role in mediating the transitional or resting postnatal pulmonary circulation (16).

The decrease in pulmonary vascular resistance and increase in pulmonary blood flow with ventilation were, for a long time, thought mainly to be due to the increase in alveolar oxygen tension with a contribution from the physical expansion of the lung; the role of oxygen was supported by increased pulmonary flow with hyperbaric oxygenation without ventilation. Some pulmonary vasodilation occurs by inflating the lungs with a low oxygen-containing gas mixture that does not change arterial blood gas composition. Adding oxygen completes the vasodilator process. The exact mechanisms of oxygen-induced pulmonary vasodilation during the transitional circulation remain unclear. The increase in alveolar or arterial oxygen tension may decrease pulmonary vascular resistance either directly via potassium channel activation or indirectly by stimulating the production of vasodilator substances such as PGI_2, bradykinin, adenosine, adenosine-5′-triphosphate, or EDNO. Inflating the lung with a low-oxygen gas mixture may lower pulmonary vascular resistance by either physical or chemical mechanisms. One mechanism operates through changes in alveolar surface tension. Another more important mechanism is the production and release of prostaglandins (predominantly PGI_2), which occurs either with mechanical stimulation of the lung or with rhythmic lung expansion (17,18).

Exogenous prostaglandins, particularly PGI_2, lower pulmonary vascular resistance in the fetus. In addition, inhibiting prostaglandin production with indomethacin before fetal lung ventilation attenuates the subsequent decrease in pulmonary vascular resistance that occurs after the initial (approximately first 30 seconds) rapid decrease in resistance. However, exogenous PGE_2 and PGI_2 also produce systemic vasodilation in fetal animals, whereas systemic vascular resistance normally rises when ventilation begins. Therefore, other prostaglandins, such as PGD_2, could be involved in pulmonary vasodilation. In newborn animals, PGD_2 produces greater pulmonary than systemic vasodilation; this differential effect is lost by about 12 to 15 days of age, when PGD_2 produces pulmonary vasoconstriction. This is similar to the effects of histamine, a modest pulmonary vasodilator in the immediate perinatal period and later a pulmonary vasoconstrictor. Both PGD_2 and histamine are released from mast cells, which increase in number in the lungs over the last portion of gestation; after birth, they decrease markedly. Thus, the stimulus of lung expansion may cause mast cells to degranulate, release PGD_2 and histamine, and contribute to the initial postnatal pulmonary vasodilation.

Adenosine and adenosine triphosphate also produce potent pulmonary vasodilation in the fetus via purine receptor activation. Preliminary animal studies suggest that their release at birth has a significant role in oxygen-induced pulmonary vasodilation. Bradykinin, another vasoactive agent, also is a potent pulmonary vasodilator in the fetus. However, bradykinin receptor blockade does not attenuate the decrease in pulmonary vascular resistance at birth in the lamb, casting doubt over the importance of bradykinin in postnatal pulmonary vasodilation.

Endothelium-derived NO has been implicated as an important mediator of the decrease in pulmonary vascular resistance at birth associated with increased oxygenation. For example, inhibition of NO synthesis attenuates the increase in pulmonary blood flow owing to oxygenation of fetal lambs induced by either maternal hyperbaric oxygen exposure or in utero ventilation with oxygen. In utero ventilation without changing fetal blood gases increases epithelial nitric oxide synthase (eNOS) gene expression in lung parenchyma of fetal lambs; this is further increased by ventilation with 100% oxygen. In vitro data reveal a maturational increase in EDNO production from late gestation to the early postnatal period that is modulated, in part, by oxygen. Moreover, both acute and chronic inhibition of NO synthesis prior to delivery significantly attenuate the normal increase in pulmonary blood flow at birth. These data suggest an important role for EDNO activity during the transitional circulation. However, the immediate decrease in pulmonary vascular resistance minutes after birth is not attenuated by NO inhibition. Therefore, there appear to be at least two components to the decrease in pulmonary vascular resistance with the initiation of ventilation and oxygenation. First, pulmonary vasodilation is caused by physical expansion of the lung and the production of prostaglandins (PGI_2 and PGD_2). This probably is independent of fetal oxygenation and results in a modest increase in pulmonary blood flow and decrease in pulmonary vascular resistance. Second, there is a further maximal pulmonary vasodilation associated with fetal oxygenation that is independent of prostaglandin production; it is most likely caused by the synthesis of EDNO, although the exact stimuli for EDNO production have not yet been defined. Both components are necessary for the successful transition to extrauterine life.

Control of the perinatal pulmonary circulation, therefore, probably reflects a balance between factors producing active pulmonary vasoconstriction (leukotrienes, low oxygen, and possibly even ET-1 acting through the ET_A receptor) and those leading to pulmonary vasodilation (EDNO, ET-1 acting through the ET_B receptor, bradykinin, and prostaglandins). The dramatic increase in pulmonary blood flow after birth most likely reflects a shift from active pulmonary vasoconstriction to active pulmonary vasodilation. It is possible that arachidonic acid metabolism shifts from lipoxygenase products in the fetus toward cyclo-oxygenase products owing either to mechanical stimulation with lung expansion or to the higher oxygen environment after birth.

After the immediate postnatal period, the more important factors affecting pulmonary vascular tone and resistance are oxygen concentration, pH, the basal production of EDNO,

the effects of alveolar distention, and perhaps the production of other vasoactive agents such as histamine, 5-hydroxytryptamine, ET-1, prostanoids, thromboxanes, and the leukotrienes. The interaction of oxygen and pH is particularly important. Decreasing oxygen tension and decreases in pH elicit pulmonary vasoconstriction of the resting pulmonary circulation. The mechanisms of acute hypoxic pulmonary vasoconstriction remain unclear and are the subject of several extensive reviews. Acidosis potentiates hypoxic pulmonary vasoconstriction, and alkalosis reduces it. The exact mechanism of pH-mediated pulmonary vasoactive responses also remains incompletely understood, but appears to be independent of $paCO_2$ (6,15). Recent data suggest that potassium channels play an important role in mediating these responses (19,20).

POSTNATAL PERIPHERAL CIRCULATION

The peripheral circulation is composed of a wide variety of regional vascular beds, each with its own characteristics. Several mechanisms regulate blood flow to these beds and affect each bed to a varying degree. These include central regulatory mechanisms such as neural activity and hormonal levels, and local mechanisms including local metabolic and pressure–flow (autoregulation) control. These mechanisms will first be presented, and then the individual vascular beds will be discussed according to the control mechanisms.

Controls over the Peripheral Circulation

Neural Control

Neural control of the systemic circulation allows rapid regulation of the circulation and provides simultaneous control of different parts of the peripheral circulation. Neural regulation consists of feedback (afferent limb) information provided by baroreceptors and cardiac stretch receptors, and neurologic control (efferent limb) through the autonomic nervous system, composed of the sympathetic and parasympathetic systems. Nearly all blood vessels in the body are innervated by the autonomic system; the effect of this control varies from one vascular bed to another.

The afferent limb of the neural control mechanisms consists of baroreceptors in arterial walls and stretch receptors within heart muscle. Baroreceptors are found in each carotid sinus and in the aortic arch. Two types of baroreceptors have been identified. Type 1 receptors control dynamic changes in blood pressure; type 2 receptors are responsible for control of resting blood pressure (21). These receptors respond to stretch of the arterial wall and send nerve impulses to the cardioinhibitory and vasomotor centers of the medulla. Stimulation of carotid sinus receptors results in slowing of heart rate, vasodilation, and a decrease in arterial blood pressure. Smooth muscle in the walls of these baroreceptor regions is innervated by vasoconstrictor efferent fibers, suggesting that sympathetic activity may modify baroreceptor responses.

Stretch receptors are also found in the walls of the atria and ventricles. Atrial stretch receptors are located in the walls of both atria at the venoatrial junctions (22). Two kinds of atrial receptors have been described. Type A receptors fire during atrial contraction and respond to changes in atrial pressure, and type B receptors fire during ventricular systole and respond to changes in atrial volume (23). Type A receptors stimulate and type B receptors inhibit sympathetic activity.

These stretch receptors provide feedback to the hypothalamus and inhibit secretion of antidiuretic hormone (vasopressin) (23). Atrial stretch causes secretion of atrial natriuretic factor (ANF), which is discussed in more detail later. Atrial receptors also alter sympathetic stimulation of the renal circulation (21). By these mechanisms, atrial stretch receptors play an important role in regulation of intravascular volume. They are also responsible for stimulation of increased heart rate by the Bainbridge reflex (22).

Two different types of stretch receptors are found in ventricular myocardium. The first fire in a pulsatile manner in time with cardiac rhythm and are small in number. The second respond to mechanical stimulation and to various drugs and chemicals through nonmyelinated afferent nerves known as C fibers (22). Stimulation of C fibers, primarily located in the left ventricle, causes hypotension and bradycardia by parasympathetic stimulation and sympathetic inhibition (22). There is evidence to suggest that carotid baroreceptors are more important for control of sympathetic regulation of muscle blood flow, whereas cardiac receptors are more important in control of sympathetic regulation of kidney blood flow.

The efferent limb of neural control of the circulation, the autonomic nervous system, is divided into the sympathetic and parasympathetic systems. There are two different types of sympathetic nerve fibers: Vasoconstrictor and vasodilator. Sympathetic stimulation of the arterioles by vasoconstrictor fibers increases vascular resistance; these vessels are called resistance vessels. The nerve endings of these sympathetic vasoconstrictor fibers contain the vasoconstrictor norepinephrine, which is released on nerve stimulation. Other substances present at the neurovascular junction, including monoamines, polypeptides, purines, and amino acids, can influence the release and the effects of norepinephrine (21). Impulses carried through vasoconstrictor fibers contribute the normal vascular tone or baseline constriction that is present at rest in most vascular beds. These vasoconstrictor fibers are more prevalent in skeletal muscles, where intrinsic tone is fairly high under resting conditions. They are much less prevalent in the cerebral and coronary beds. Sympathetic vasoconstriction of larger arteries and of veins changes their volume and therefore changes the circulating volume; these vessels are known as capacitance vessels.

Sympathetic stimulation by vasodilator fibers increases blood flow to a vascular bed. These fibers are primarily found in the vascular beds of skeletal muscle. The transmitter in vasodilator fibers is thought to be acetylcholine, although in primates it may be epinephrine. These vasodilator fibers may cause a small anticipatory increase of blood flow to the skeletal muscle; however, once muscle exercise begins, local vasodilation probably plays a more important role.

The parasympathetic system primarily controls heart function and rate and has a very limited role in control of the peripheral circulation. The transmitter stored in nerve endings of the parasympathetic system is acetylcholine. Parasympathetic vasodilator fibers are found in the cerebral circulation and in the bladder, rectum, and external genitalia.

Hormonal Control

Hormonal control of the peripheral circulation can best be described as vascular constriction or dilation in response to circulating hormones. The vasculature in the peripheral circulation is responsive to various hormones, including catecholamines, angiotensin II, vasopressin, eicosanoids, nitric oxide (NO), and peptide hormones.

Catecholamines are the hormones of the adrenergic system. Adrenergic receptors to catecholamines are present in the smooth muscle throughout the peripheral vascular system and can be categorized as α and β receptors. Stimulation of α receptors causes vascular smooth muscle to contract, causing vasoconstriction; stimulation of β receptors causes vascular smooth muscle to relax, causing vasodilation. These receptors are responsive to both endogenous catecholamines and sympathomimetic drugs. Norepinephrine, β-adrenergic agonist, is secreted by the adrenal medulla and is carried by the bloodstream to receptors in the peripheral vasculature. Preganglionic sympathetic fibers innervate the adrenal medulla and stimulate norepinephrine secretion. There is, therefore, central control of this hormonal regulation. Epinephrine is also secreted by the adrenal medulla, but it is a much weaker vascular stimulant and tends to exert a β-agonistic effect at physiologic concentrations.

Angiotensin II, a powerful vasoconstrictor, is produced by activation of the renin–angiotensin–aldosterone system. The juxtaglomerular apparatus in the kidney secretes renin in response to decreased renal arterial pressure or a decrease in extracellular fluid volume. Renin, in turn, cleaves angiotensinogen to angiotensin I, which is then converted to angiotensin II by a converting enzyme found in lung and vascular endothelium. Angiotensin II has direct vasoconstrictor properties, acts centrally to stimulate the vasoconstrictor centers of the brain, and stimulates the secretion of antidiuretic hormone (vasopressin). Antidiuretic hormone is synthesized in the hypothalamus and secreted by the posterior pituitary. It is a very potent vasoconstrictor but plays a minimal role in regulation of the circulation under resting conditions.

Prostaglandins and other eicosanoids play a small role in regulation of flow in the systemic circulation and have been discussed in detail above. Another hormone that participates in regulation of the systemic circulation is atrial natriuretic factor (ANF). This peptide hormone is released from atrial myocytes of both atria and in smaller amounts from the ventricular myocytes. Ventricular production of ANF decreases with maturation; large amounts of ANF are produced in fetal ventricular myocardium, and only small amounts are produced by adult ventricles (24). ANF is released in response to stretch of either atrium; increased circulating levels of ANF are detected when left atrial pressure is elevated even when the right atrial pressure is normal. In the kidney, ANF decreases tubular reabsorption of sodium. In the circulatory system, ANF has vasodilator and cardioinhibitory effects (24). Circulating levels of ANF are increased in certain pathophysiologic conditions, such as congenital heart disease associated with elevated atrial pressures, congestive heart failure, valve disease, hypertension, coronary artery occlusion, and atrial arrhythmias (24).

Endothelial Function

The vascular endothelium plays an important role in regulating vascular tone, platelet adhesion, and inflammation. Receptors are present on the endothelial cell membrane for a number of locally produced and remotely secreted hormones and substances, including peptides, kinins, amines, nucleotides, and eicosanoids. The endothelium responds to changes in blood flow and stretch and generally promotes vasodilation (24). The endothelium produces vasoactive substances in response to different stimuli.

Endothelial cells produce a number of vasoactive hormones. Vasodilator substances produced by the endothelium include PGI_2, EDNO, adenosine, and endothelium-derived hyperpolarizing factor (EDHF) (25). PGI_2 and EDNO have been discussed above. The identity of EDHF has yet to be determined. It produces hyperpolarization of vascular smooth muscle cells (25) by activating K^+ channels, thereby inhibiting voltage-gated calcium channels, lowering cytosolic calcium, and promoting relaxation (26). Vasoconstrictor substances produced by the endothelium include ET-1, a locally acting peptide hormone also discussed earlier in this chapter. Angiotensin II is also produced in the endothelium by angiotensin-converting enzyme, found in vascular endothelial cells. Other vasoconstrictor factors are postulated to be produced by the endothelium, but are yet to be identified (25).

Local Metabolic Control

Tissues have the ability to regulate their own blood flow in response to changes in metabolic demands. The local chemical environment of arterioles can cause vasodilation or, to a lesser extent, vasoconstriction. For example, a decrease in pO_2, an increase in pCO_2, or an increase in H^+ or K^+ concentration each causes arteriolar vasodilation. Many tissues will release adenosine, a potent vasodilator, in response to increased metabolism or decreased oxygen tension.

Autoregulation

Blood flow to tissues remains relatively constant over a wide range of arterial blood pressure owing to autoregulation. The mechanisms of this phenomenon are largely unknown. Several hypothetical mechanisms exist, including local metabolic control, myogenic activity of vascular smooth muscle, tubuloglomerular feedback in the kidney, and tissue pressure. These mechanisms may act alone or in combination. The metabolic hypothesis suggests that blood flow is closely linked to tissue metabolism. Reduction of inflow of blood would cause an accumulation of vasodilator substances, which would in turn cause vasodilation and increased blood flow. In organs with high oxygen consumption, autoregulation of blood flow is dependent on tissue oxygenation. A second proposed mechanism of autoregulation is myogenic control (27). According to this theory, increased intravascular pressure stimulates vasoconstriction of vascular smooth muscle. A venous-arterial reflex has been described in which an increase in venous pressure causes arteriolar constriction, probably by a neurally mediated mechanism (27). A tubuloglomerular feedback mechanism may help to autoregulate renal blood flow. According to this hypothesis, increased renal blood pressure and flow increase the concentration of solutes in the tubular fluid; this increase is sensed in the macula densa, causing vasoconstriction by an unknown mechanism. Tissue pressure is another possible mechanism for autoregulation. By this proposed mechanism, increased tissue pressure in areas in encapsulated organs or in the brain leads to decreased blood flow to those areas. Autoregulation seems to play a more significant role in control of resting blood flow in vital organs such as the brain and heart and becomes significant in other areas during times of increased metabolic demand.

Specific Regional Vascular Beds

The different regional vascular beds in the fetus and child are controlled to varying extents by the different mechanisms discussed above. Generally, the highly metabolically active organs such as the brain and heart are primarily regulated by local mechanisms, whereas the less active beds are under central neural and hormonal controls. Specialized beds such as the renal and hepatic circulations, which receive blood for unique activities such as metabolic degradation and excretion, hematopoiesis, and blood pressure control, have unique combinations of control mechanisms. The myocardium will not be discussed in this section because it is considered elsewhere (see Chapter 27).

Cerebral Circulation

The cerebral circulation of the fetus and neonate has been the most extensively studied and characterized. It is unique in four main respects. First, there is a blood–brain barrier created by a continuous lining of endothelial cells linked by tight junctions and by degradative enzymes; thus, changes in circulating concentrations of various constituents such as H^+ and catecholamines may have a limited effect. Second, the large arteries form a significant component of the resistance circuit, having been shown to respond in a similar fashion to the arterioles in response to stresses such as hypoxia (28). Third, the cerebral circulation is encased in a closed box, the skull, so that perfusion pressure is particularly important to blood flow characteristics. And fourth, there is great heterogeneity in blood flow patterns to the different regions of the brain; they have very different resting blood flows and are controlled to different extents by different mechanisms. For example, in the fetus, the greatest blood flow occurs in the oldest regions phylogenetically: The brain stem receives the most, then the cerebellum, and last, the cortex. In the newborn, the pattern is immediately reversed, with the cortex receiving the greatest blood flow, then the cerebellum, and last, the brain stem (29). These differences are thought to exist because of differences in sensitivity to hypoxia and hyperoxia.

Autoregulation is an essential component in the control of cerebral blood flow. To limit the risk of hemorrhage and inadequate blood supply to the brain in the face of acute increases and decreases in blood pressure, it is important that flow remains constant over a wide range of perfusion pressures. In the brain, it appears that alterations in local adenosine concentrations mediate the autoregulatory response: Interstitial levels of adenosine increase during hypotension, an adenosine analogue increases blood flow in the autoregulatory range, and autoregulation is abolished by blocking the adenosine receptor (30). Prostanoids are another group of vasoactive substances that have been implicated in the control of autoregulation. Dilator prostanoids such as prostacyclin increase in response to hemorrhage, and cyclooxygenase inhibition decreases cerebral blood flow and the response to hypotension. Autoregulation has been demonstrated in young fetal sheep as early as 93 days' gestation (approximately 0.67 gestation) and exists over a wide range of mean cerebral arterial pressures (30). However, the lower limit of this range is close to the normal mean perfusion pressure, putting the fetus at relatively high risk for hypotension-associated problems. This is particularly important in the subependymal germinal matrix, which exists until about 36 weeks' gestation in the human fetus, and in the choroid plexus, which are the primary sites of intraventricular hemorrhage in the premature infant. In addition, autoregulation does not appear to exist in the white matter of the immature fetus, and this also might contribute to the risk of hypotensive damage to the immature brain. At birth, studies are conflicting as to whether the autoregulatory range increases significantly. However, the lower limit of the autoregulatory range is much further below the normal mean perfusion pressure than in the premature infant.

Another major regulating factor of cerebral blood flow is blood oxygen concentration. Because of the critical importance of oxygen delivery to the brain, this is not surprising. However, although it had been assumed that pCO_2 is a more important determinant of cerebral blood flow, recent studies have shown that the fetus and newborn are relatively insensitive to pCO_2 changes but can change blood flow twofold to threefold in response to changes in arterial pO_2 (30). In the immature brain, oxygen sensitivity follows the same hierarchy as flow patterns: The brain stem is most sensitive and the cortex least sensitive to changes in pO_2. This is perhaps a protective mechanism to permit the maintenance of basic autonomic function during profound hypoxia. The mechanisms behind oxygen sensitivity are not certain, although local factors produced by the endothelium probably play a considerable role. In addition to vasoactive substances, oxygen may have a direct effect on various ATP-mediated reactions (28).

Carbon dioxide also has a significant effect on cerebral blood flow, although less than in the mature brain, and, like oxygen, has its greatest effects on the brain stem (29). Moreover, this effect has been demonstrated in all regions of the brain as early as 0.4 gestation in the fetal sheep (31). Because of the blood–brain barrier, this effect is specific to a change in pCO_2; cerebral blood flow does not change in the face of metabolic acidosis or alkalosis. The effect of pCO_2 appears to be exerted by changing extracellular brain H^+, but how this change in H^+ then affects the production or release of endothelium-derived vasoactive substances is not known. It is apparent, however, that prostanoids are significantly involved in this response (32).

Other factors also can modulate cerebral blood flow, including sympathetic innervation, circulating hormones such as vasopressin and catecholamines, and blood hematocrit level, but it is clear that this highly metabolically active organ is under exquisite control from very early in gestation by a host of local regulatory mechanisms.

Peripheral Tissues

In contrast to the cerebral circulation, the peripheral circulation (skin, muscle, and bone) is primarily under central control. The vasoactivity of each component of the peripheral tissues is controlled somewhat differently. For example, the skin is predominantly under α-adrenergic tone with no significant autoregulation, whereas the muscle has a higher proportion of β-adrenergic control and has intact autoregulation. This group of vascular beds is presented together because the primary control of vascular tone of these beds and the responses to major stresses such as hypotension and hypoxemia are similar and are predominantly mediated by the autonomic nervous system and circulating hormones. Because peripheral blood flow is needed primarily for growth and thermoregulation in the developing organism and essential oxygen demands are small, central controls that limit flow during stress can be invoked with few sequelae. Thus, from early fetal life, a large variety of vascular receptors ($\alpha2$-adrenergic, $\beta1$- and $\beta2$-adrenergic, dopaminergic A1 and A2, vasopressinergic V1, muscarinic, etc.) develop. They transduce alterations in levels of circulating and synaptic compounds via various intracellular second messengers, into alterations of peripheral vascular smooth muscle tone.

Early in gestation, the peripheral circulation is predominantly under α-adrenergic influences, with little cholinergic tone. Changes in basal tone can be demonstrated with the administration of α-adrenergic agonists and not by β-agonists or cholinergic agents. Similarly, blocking of α-adrenergic

activity invokes a large decrease in peripheral vascular resistance, whereas the dominant effect of β-adrenergic blockade is to slow heart rate. Although parasympathetic tone is limited in early gestation, receptors are present and can be stimulated. Late in gestation, resting activity increases rapidly toward the high levels normally seen after birth. Very early in fetal life, response of autonomic receptors requires that circulating catecholamines be secreted by the adrenal medulla and nonadrenal chromaffin tissue; innervation is a significantly later event than receptor development. As innervation proceeds rapidly in early fetal life, neural mechanisms can be invoked to alter peripheral blood flow. The primary neural mechanisms invoked are the central vasomotor controls, which are primarily medullary, peripheral baroreceptors located in the carotid sinus and peripheral chemoreceptors located in the carotid and aortic bodies. Activity of both the baroreceptor and chemoreceptor mechanisms has been documented early in gestation, and although the manifestations may be blunted by the existence of central shunts and the umbilical-placental circulation, peripheral vasoconstriction is evident. The critical importance of baroreceptor control of the peripheral circulation is demonstrated by the marked fluctuations in arterial blood pressure induced by sinoaortic denervation in immature fetal sheep (33).

In addition to circulating catecholamines and the autonomic nervous system, other circulating hormones exert significant effects on the peripheral circulation throughout fetal and postnatal life. The renin–angiotensin system probably plays a major role in controlling peripheral vascular tone even in the young fetus; infusion of angiotensin II significantly increases peripheral vascular resistance (34). Plasma vasopressin increases during hypotension in the fetus and the newborn (35). Although atrial natriuretic peptide has been demonstrated as early as 21 weeks in the human fetus and does appear to have a small effect on blood volume, there is no evidence of a peripheral vascular effect (36).

Last, circulating hormones can affect the peripheral circulation indirectly via their effects on the central nervous system as well as in peripheral autonomic ganglia and the adrenal medulla. The roles of vasopressin and angiotensin II in the central control of the peripheral circulation are not clear, but these agents, along with various neurotransmitters, apparently exert significant controls via stimulation and inhibition of various central regions. Endogenous opioids are intimately involved in the cardiovascular response to shock by exerting both central and adrenal medullary effects in the adult. Endogenous opioids at concentrations higher than those seen in the mother have been demonstrated throughout gestation, and fetal plasma β-endorphin levels have been shown to increase in response to maternal hypoxemia (37).

Renal Circulation

Aspects unique to the renal circulation are its exceptionally high blood flow because of the requirements of glomerular ultrafiltration, the presence of two distinct capillary beds to allow for filtration and reabsorption, and the delayed maturational processes in regional blood flow and its controls as compared with other systemic vascular beds.

Blood flow to the adult kidney represents up to 25% of cardiac output. Most of this flow courses via the afferent arterioles in the renal cortex to the glomerular capillary bed. This capillary bed is under relatively high pressure to allow for a large production of ultrafiltrate into the renal collecting system. Distal to an efferent arteriolar system that significantly decreases hydrostatic pressure, significantly less blood passes to the medullary capillary bed. This low pressure in addition to osmotic forces favors the reuptake of the reabsorbate. Within the two regions, the cortex and medulla, there is preferential distribution of blood as well. The outer cortex receives a relatively small proportion of cortical blood and is composed of small glomeruli with low single-nephron glomerular filtration. The inner or juxtaglomerular cortex receives far more blood flow per weight and is composed of very large glomeruli with high filtration rates. The medulla is composed of the outer medulla (the descending and thick ascending limbs of the loops of Henle and collecting duct segments) and the inner medulla (thin segments of the loops of Henle and the terminal portions of the collecting system). The inner medulla is perfused by the vasa recta and receives the least blood per weight and at very slow transit times. This is critical to the reuptake of ultrafiltrate and thus concentration of urine: There is an inverse relationship between inner medullary blood flow and urine osmolality.

Under normal conditions, the primary mechanism for control of renal cortical blood flow is autoregulation, which matures quite late. It is present in the newborn of most species but of reduced efficiency. Because the immature kidney excretes far more prostanoids than the mature kidney, it is possible that impaired autoregulation is caused not so much by an immaturity of the mechanisms controlling autoregulation as by an overabundance of prostanoid production. In normal conditions, however, there is no evidence that prostanoids play a role in the control of renal blood flow. A mechanism unique to the kidney that contributes to autoregulatory control of renal blood flow is tubuloglomerular feedback. This mechanism is a single-nephron phenomenon and is initiated by alterations in filtrate and solute flow from the proximal to distal tubule. An alteration in either distal tubule reabsorption or fluid delivery alters the blood flow and glomerular filtration, probably by constriction or dilation of the afferent arteriole. The renin–angiotensin system mediates afferent arteriolar vasoconstriction so that glomerulotubular feedback depends on an intact and mature juxtaglomerular apparatus and renin–angiotensin system. The immature kidney does not show tubuloglomerular feedback until after birth, probably because of an immature renin–angiotensin system. In addition to the elevated renal prostanoids already discussed, basal levels of angiotensin II are elevated so that the ability of the juxtaglomerular apparatus to further activate the system is greatly limited; moreover, the immature renal vasculature is relatively insensitive to the constrictor effects of angiotensin II. Thus, unlike in the cerebral circulation, fine control of renal blood flow in resting conditions is significantly impaired in the fetus and newborn.

During stress, however, autonomic rather than autoregulatory mechanisms predominate and act primarily to limit renal blood flow. Both α1- and α2-adrenergic receptors are present in the kidney throughout fetal and postnatal life, and stimulation of both by neural discharge or circulating catecholamines causes renal vasoconstriction, redistributing blood away from the kidney as blood is distributed away from the peripheral circulation. Dopaminergic and β-adrenergic receptors are also present across development, although dopamine-2 receptor density decreases with age (38). Stimulation of both causes vasodilation but their physiologic significance is uncertain in the immature kidney; there is no evidence of resting β-adrenergic tone, and β-adrenergic blockade does not enhance α-adrenergically mediated vasoconstriction in the fetal sheep. However, the adult is more sensitive to stimulation of both β-adrenergic and dopaminergic receptors, developing significantly more vasodilation.

The role of other circulating factors in the control of cortical blood flow in the young is less significant and often less clear. The renin–angiotensin system has been discussed in regard to autoregulation. Although it is very important to the autoregulatory ability of the adult kidney, the renin-angiotensin system has significantly limited effects on autoregulation in the very young. Although captopril increases renal blood flow in the newborn lamb (39), this may be caused by its inhibition of kininase II in the kallikrein–kinin system, rather than by inhibition of angiotensin-converting enzyme. Similar to angiotensin, vasopressin is not known to have effects on resting renal blood flow in the young (40), despite the presence of V1 receptors.

Control over medullary flow in the adult kidney is primarily by vasopressin, with no evidence of autoregulation. As medullary flow decreases in response to release of vasopressin, the osmotic gradient increases and reuptake of the resorbate increases. As mentioned, the medulla consists of two distinct zones with complex vasculature to allow for the countercurrent multiplication and exchange critical to the reuptake of the vast majority of the ultrafiltrate. It is in the inner medulla that the extreme concentration of the urine occurs and the greatest sensitivity to vasopressin exists.

In addition to regional and developmental differences in the control of cortical and medullary blood flow, there are significant developmental differences in intrarenal regional blood flows and flow distribution, as suggested above. Up to 25% of cardiac output is distributed to the kidney in the adult, with about 90% of that flow being cortical. Most of that cortical flow is distributed to the larger juxtamedullary nephrons, yielding a very high glomerular filtration rate. Conversely, the immature kidney receives far less blood, and the distribution of that blood is less specific. The very low cortical flow is associated with a markedly reduced glomerular filtration rate in the fetus and newborn, and the relatively high medullary flow with limited vasopressin sensitivity is associated with poor concentrating ability. The lesser renal blood flow is caused only in small part by fewer nephrons. Glomerulogenesis is complete in the human by 36 weeks' gestation, yet the kidneys still account for only about 5% of cardiac output at birth. Over the first weeks of life, both renal blood flow and glomerular filtration rate double as afferent arteriolar resistance decreases. The ultimate increase in renal blood flow and ultrafiltration is related to further alterations in the renal vasculature, particularly in conjunction with the large increase in the size of glomeruli, which is not complete until late adolescence.

In summary, the renal vascular and glomerular beds are very immature at birth, so that renal function and control over renal blood flow and its distribution are limited. Throughout much of childhood, maturation proceeds, although most is accomplished in the first few months of life. The control mechanisms of renal flow are centered on three requirements: Maintenance of adequate ultrafiltration in the cortex, maintenance of filtrate concentration in the medulla, and redistribution of blood away from the kidney in periods of stress. The three functions are primarily controlled by different mechanisms that mature at different rates.

Splanchnic Circulation

The splanchnic circulation consists of the vascular beds of the spleen, gastrointestinal tract, and liver. Similar to the renal circulation, the splanchnic circulation receives about 25% of cardiac output in the adult, but it is also a large reservoir of blood, containing about 20% to 25% of total blood volume. Thus, response to stresses such as hemorrhage leads not only to redistribution of blood flow away from the splanchnic circulation but also to mobilization of blood volume from that vascular bed to the central vessels and other organs. Control over the splanchnic bed in response to stress is primarily central rather than local, with neurohumoral catecholamine stimulation being the major mechanism controlling vasoconstriction. Stimulation of both carotid and aortic baroreceptors causes sympathetic neural stimulation of splanchnic resistance and capacitance vessels and large decreases in splanchnic blood flow and volume. Also, secondary to the active vasoconstriction of the resistance (arterial) component of the splanchnic circulation are decreases in the venous capacitance size. It appears that approximately half the decrease in splanchnic blood volume is secondary to active vasoconstriction of the capacitance (venous) system and half secondary to its passive decrease in volume. Specific to the splanchnic bed is the property that exercise and thermal stresses also induce large decreases in flow and volume with redistribution to the skeletal muscle and skin, respectively. The afferent limbs of these responses are uncertain because, unlike with hemorrhage, stimulation of baroreceptors does not occur. Responses specific to the individual components of the splanchnic vascular bed will be discussed next.

The spleen has significant sympathetic adrenergic innervation and responds to stimulation with vasoconstriction. Although there are β-adrenergic receptors as well as α-adrenergic receptors, the former are less active. In addition to sensitivity to adrenergic stimulation, human splenic arterioles respond to vasopressin and angiotensin with vasoconstriction. There is no evidence of autoregulatory or other local controls over splenic blood flow. Thus, in response to stress, central mechanisms direct blood flow away from the spleen. Unlike other mammals, humans do not show significant reduction in splenic venous capacitance with stimulation, so it does not contribute significantly to the blood reservoir when mobilized with stress. It is the other components of the splanchnic circulation that contribute to increasing blood volume during hypovolemic stresses.

The gastrointestinal tract has a more complex vascular bed, controlled by a greater variety of mechanisms. Like the splenic vessels, the mesenteric vessels are richly innervated with sympathetic nerves, which respond to stimulation with vasoconstriction, although there are some vasodilatory β-adrenergic receptors as well. Constriction of the venous effluent vessels in addition to the passive decrease in venous capacitance causes mobilization of blood volume from this large reservoir. The intestinal circulation also responds similarly to the splenic circulation during hemorrhage, with marked vasoconstriction in response to increases in angiotensin II and vasopressin. However, unlike the splenic circulation, the intestinal circulation escapes from vasoconstriction as vascular resistance decreases and flow increases secondary to autoregulatory escape. This escape phenomenon is not well defined, but it is probably secondary to sensitivity of the arteriolar bed to vasodilator metabolites such as adenosine, in much the same way that adenosine is involved in local regulation of other vascular beds, such as the cerebral and myocardial circulations. This metabolic mechanism may explain why the fed adult dog, which has a greater oxygen extraction under normal pressure, exhibits better autoregulation than the fasted dog. This greater local regulatory response during conditions of greater oxygen extraction is also evident in the young (35 days) pig during hypoxic and ischemic stresses (41). However, similar to but not as pronounced as the case in the renal vascular bed, autoregulatory mechanisms are immature in the newborn, both at rest and in hypoxic and ischemic conditions.

The response of the intestinal circulation to feeding is also of interest. In anticipation of food, the response is central in origin and largely sympathetic, causing vasoconstriction. Once food has been ingested, there are major local vascular responses related to the type of food, the products of digestion in different parts of the intestine, and the secondary effects of various gastrointestinal hormones. The hydrolytic products of carbohydrates and fat are particularly potent local vasodilators and appear to act on a metabolic basis similar to that of autoregulation by increasing local oxygen consumption. Local hormones that may play a role in vasodilation include cholecystokinin, secretin, gastrin, glucagon, and vasoactive intestinal polypeptide. The overall response to feeding yields increases in local blood flow of $\leq 300\%$ within 60 to 90 minutes (42). Because of the large increase in oxygen consumption, however, these increases are not enough to meet the increased metabolic demand, so that oxygen extraction also increases.

The hepatic circulation is even more complex, receiving both highly oxygenated blood from the hepatic arteries and blood of lesser saturation but greater substrate concentrations from the portal vein. The incorporation of umbilical venous blood in the fetal circulation was discussed earlier. A review by Lautt and Greenway (43) clearly describes the hepatic circulation and its control. The portal vein terminates in the hepatic sinusoids, and the hepatic arterioles split into a complex capillary network that also drains into the sinusoids. These vessels, along with the biliary ductules and lymph vessels and nerves, occupy the portal triad. In these sinusoids, which allow free contact with the hepatic cells, the blood passes radially away from the center of the hepatic glomus to the periphery, where it passes into the hepatic venules on its way to the hepatic veins and inferior vena cava. As the blood passes from the center (zone 1) to the periphery (zone 3), near the hepatic venules, different metabolic activities predominate.

As with the kidney, blood flow to the liver is large (about 25% of cardiac output in the adult) and far exceeds its metabolic demand for oxygen. As with the intestinal circulation, hepatic blood volume is large (about 10% of total blood volume) and is mobilized during periods of stress. Conversely, as hepatic venous pressure increases, hepatic blood volume increases greatly because of the large compliance of these capacitance vessels. There are also sphincters described in the hepatic venules that may regulate hepatic blood volume by varying sinusoidal volume and portal resistance. These sphincters respond to norepinephrine and angiotensin.

Portal venous blood contributes about 75% of hepatic blood flow, and this flow is determined primarily by mechanisms that regulate splenic and intestinal flow, although presinusoidal sphincters exist as well. Alterations in hepatic venous pressure affect neither portal flow nor its intrahepatic distribution. The hepatic arterial circulation is innervated in a similar fashion as the mesenteric arterial circulation and responds prominently to α-adrenergic stimulation during stress, as well as to other stress hormones such as angiotensin II and vasopressin. Similarly, there are vasodilatory $\beta2$-adrenergic receptors and there is some responsiveness to vasodilatory gastrointestinal hormones such as glucagon, secretin, and pentagastrin. An additional regulatory mechanism of hepatic arterial flow exists that is somewhat analogous to intestinal autoregulation. Although there is no autoregulation within the arterial circulation, as portal venous flow decreases, there is a reciprocal increase in hepatic arterial flow. The mechanism is thought to be adenosine regulated: Adenosine is released into the central sinusoids and comes in contact with the hepatic arterioles; as portal flow decreases, the washout of adenosine from this region is decreased, and thus more is present to dilate the hepatic arterioles (42).

Perhaps the largest changes in regional blood flow in the perinatal period occur in the liver, but this is not because of maturation of the hepatic circulation but rather because of loss of the umbilical-placental circulation. Prior to birth, the primary source of hepatic blood flow is the umbilical vein, which joins the portal venous blood in the portal sinus. About 45% of umbilical venous return passes to the liver, with the right lobe receiving somewhat more than the left (3). Portal venous blood is distributed much more unequally, with almost all of it passing to the right lobe, which therefore is perfused with blood of much lower hemoglobin oxygen saturation compared with the left. Hepatic arterial blood flow is very limited in the fetus and is distributed approximately equally to the two lobes. At birth, the loss of the umbilical-placental circulation is not associated with immediate closure of the ductus venosus, which can remain patent for several days (23). Some portal venous blood is shunted away from the liver to the inferior vena cava via the ductus venosus. This, along with the absence of an immediate increase in hepatic arterial flow, causes a marked reduction in hepatic blood flow at birth and a halving of oxygen consumption (2). By 1 week of age, hepatic blood flow increases and oxygen consumption returns to fetal levels, although hepatic arterial blood flow remains at the very low fetal levels, contributing only 5% of total hepatic blood flow. The mechanisms that underlie the increase in hepatic flow and oxygen consumption in early postnatal life and the subsequent increase in hepatic arterial flow are uncertain, as are the implications of these changes on liver function and maturation.

References

1. Roos A. Poiseuille's law and its limitations in vascular systems. *Med Thorac* 1962;19:224–238.
2. Teitel DF, Iwamoto HS, Rudolph AM. Effects of birth-related events on central blood flow patterns. *Pediatr Res* 1987;22:557–566.
3. Edelstone DI, Rudolph AM, Heymann MA. Liver and ductus venosus blood flows in fetal lambs in utero. *Circ Res* 1978;42:426–433.
4. Townsend SF, Rudolph CD, Rudolph AM. Changes in ovine hepatic circulation and oxygen consumption at birth. *Pediatr Res* 1989;25:300–304.
5. Adeagbo AS, Coceani F, Olley PM. The response of the lamb ductus venosus to prostaglandins and inhibitors of prostaglandin and thromboxane synthesis. *Circ Res* 1982;51:580–586.
6. Levin DL, Rudolph AM, Heymann MA, et al. Morphological development of the pulmonary vascular bed in fetal lambs. *Circulation* 1976;53:144–151.
7. Reid L. The pulmonary circulation: Remodeling in growth and disease. *Am Rev Respir Dis* 1979;119:531–546.
8. Rudolph AM, Heymann MA. Circulatory changes during growth in the fetal lamb. *Circ Res* 1970;26:289–299.
9. Lewis AB, Heymann MA, Rudolph AM. Gestational changes in pulmonary vascular responses in fetal lambs in utero. *Circ Res* 1976;39:536–541.
10. Rudolph AM, Yuan S. Response of the pulmonary vasculature to hypoxia and H$^+$ ion concentration changes. *J Clin Invest* 1966;45:399–411.
11. Cassin S. Role of prostaglandins and thromboxanes in the control of the pulmonary circulation in the fetus and newborn. *Semin Perinatol* 1980;4:101–107.
12. Fineman JR, Soifer SJ, Heymann MA. Regulation of pulmonary vascular tone in the perinatal period. *Annu Rev Physiol* 1995;57:115–134.
13. Furchgott RF. Role of endothelium in responses of vascular smooth muscle. *Circ Res* 1983;53:557–573.
14. Ignarro LJ. Biological actions and properties of endothelium-derived nitric oxide formed and released from artery and vein. *Circ Res* 1989;65:1–21.
15. Shaul PW. Nitric oxide in the developing lung. *Adv Pediatr* 1995;42:367–414.
16. Yanagisawa M, Kurihara H, Kimura S, et al. A novel potent vasoconstrictor peptide produced by vascular endothelial cells. *Nature* 1988;332:411–415.
17. Leffler CW, Hessler JR, Green RS. The onset of breathing at birth stimulates pulmonary vascular prostacyclin synthesis. *Pediatr Res* 1984;18:938–942.
18. Soifer SJ, Fineman JR, Heymann MA. The pulmonary circulation. In: Gluckman PA, Heymann MA, eds. *Pediatrics and Perinatology. The Scientific Basis.* Kent, England: Edward Arnold, 1996:749–755.
19. Cornfield DN, Resnik ER, Herron JM, et al. Pulmonary vascular K$^+$ channel expression and vasoreactivity in a model of congenital heart disease. *Am J Physiol Lung Cell Mol Physiol* 2002;283:L1210–1219.
20. Vander Heyden MA, Halla TR, Madden JA, et al. Multiple Ca$^{(2+)}$-dependent modulators mediate alkalosis-induced vasodilation in newborn piglet lungs. *Am J Physiol Lung Cell Mol Physiol* 2001;280:L519–526.
21. Ebert TJ, Stowe DF. Neural and endothelial control of the peripheral circulation—implications for anesthesia, Part I. Neural control of the peripheral vasculature. *J Cardiothorac Vasc Anesth* 1996;10:147–158.
22. Linden RJ. Function of cardiac receptors. *Circulation* 1973;48:463–480.
23. Little RC, Little WC. The output of the heart and its control. In: *Physiology of the Heart and Circulation.* Chicago: Year Book Medical, 1989:165–198.
24. Athanassopoulos G, Cokkinos DV. Atrial natriuretic factor. *Prog Cardiovasc Dis* 1991;33:313–328.
25. Stowe DF, Ebert TJ. Neural and endothelial control of the peripheral circulation—implications for anesthesia. Part II. Endothelium-mediated effects in the normal and diseased circulation. *J Cardiothorac Vasc Anesth* 1996;10:159–171.
26. Archer SL, Gragasin FS, Wu X, et al. Endothelium-derived hyperpolarizing factor in human internal mammary artery is 11,12-epoxyeicosatrienoic acid and causes relaxation by activating smooth muscle BK(Ca) channels. *Circulation* 2003;107:769–776.
27. Johnson PC. Autoregulation of blood flow. *Circ Res* 1986;59:483–495.
28. Longo LD, Pearce WJ. Fetal and newborn cerebral vascular responses and adaptations to hypoxia. *Semin Perinatol* 1991;15:49–57.
29. Szymonowicz W, Walker AM, Cussen L, et al. Developmental changes in regional cerebral blood flow in fetal and newborn lambs. *Am J Physiol* 1988;254:H52–H58.
30. Laudignon N, Beharry K, Farri E, et al. The role of adenosine in the vascular adaptation of neonatal cerebral blood flow during hypotension. *J Cereb Blood Flow Metab* 1991;11:424–431.
31. Habgood MD, Jones SE, Maroni JM, et al. Cerebral blood flow in the anaesthetized immature sheep fetus and the response to hypercapnia. *Exp Physiol* 1991;76:495–505.
32. Wagerle LC, Mishra OP. Mechanism of CO_2 response in cerebral arteries of the newborn pig: Role of phospholipase, cyclooxygenase, and lipoxygenase pathways. *Circ Res* 1988;62:1019–1026.
33. Itskovitz J, LaGamma EF, Rudolph AM. Baroreflex control of the circulation in chronically instrumented fetal lambs. *Circ Res* 1983;52:589–596.
34. Iwamoto HS, Rudolph AM. Effects of angiotensin II on the blood flow and its distribution in fetal lambs. *Circ Res* 1981;48:183–189.
35. Zubrow AB, Daniel SS, Stark RI, et al. Plasma vasopressin, renin and catecholamines during nitroprusside-induced hypotension in the newborn lamb. *J Perinat Med* 1989;17:271–277.
36. Hargrave BY, Iwamoto HS, Rudolph AM. Renal and cardiovascular effects of atrial natriuretic peptide in fetal sheep. *Pediatr Res* 1989;26:1–5.
37. Wardlaw SL, Stark RI, Daniel S, et al. Effects of hypoxia on beta-endorphin and beta-lipotropin release in fetal, newborn, and maternal sheep. *Endocrinology* 1981;108:1710–1715.
38. Felder RA, Nakamura KT, Robillard JE, et al. Dopamine receptors in the developing sheep kidney. *Pediatr Nephrol* 1988;2:156–162.
39. Robillard JE, Nakamura KT. Neurohormonal regulation of renal function during development. *Am J Physiol* 1988;254:F771–F779.
40. Robillard JE, Weitzman RE. Developmental aspects of the fetal renal response to exogenous arginine vasopressin. *Am J Physiol* 1980;238:F407–F414.
41. Nowicki PT, Miller CE, Edwards RC. Effects of hypoxia and ischemia on autoregulation in postnatal intestine. *Am J Physiol* 1991;261:G152–G157.
42. Vatner SF, Franklin D, Van CR. Mesenteric vasoactivity associated with eating and digestion in the conscious dog. *Am J Physiol* 1970;219:170–174.
43. Lautt WW, Greenway CV. Conceptual review of the hepatic vascular bed. *Hepatology* 1987;7:952–963.

PART VII ■ CONGENITAL CARDIOVASCULAR MALFORMATIONS

CHAPTER 30 ■ ATRIAL SEPTAL DEFECTS

CO-BURN J. PORTER, MD, AND WILLIAM D. EDWARDS, MD

Any opening in the atrial septum, other than a competent foramen ovale, is an atrial septal defect (ASD). Defects that result from abnormal formation of the endocardial cushions are discussed in the chapter on atrioventricular septal defects (see Chapter 31).

SECUNDUM ATRIAL SEPTAL DEFECTS

Secundum ASDs represent 6% to 10% of all cardiac anomalies and are more frequent in females than males by about 2:1 (1). ASDs occur in 1 child per 1,500 live births (2). Most ASDs occur sporadically; however, a few families have the defect as a genetic abnormality. In 1960, Holt and Oram (3) noted the association between ASDs and anomalies of the upper extremities. In 1997, Li et al. (4) reported that Holt–Oram syndrome is caused by mutations in *TBX5*, a member of the Brachyury (T) gene family. Further understanding of genetic abnormalities causing ASDs is still in its early stages. To date, heterozygous mutations in two genes, *NKX2.5* and *GATA4*, have been identified to be causative for a subset of familial ASD through genetic linkage analysis of pedigrees with nonsyndromic congenital cardiovascular diseases (5). These two mutations also cause various other congenital heart diseases, especially isolated ASD (6). Most recently, a missense mutation in myosin heavy chain 6 (on chromosome 14q12) has been found to cause familial ASD (7).

Anatomy, Embryology, and Pathology

Atrial septal defects are classified according to their location relative to the fossa ovalis (Fig. 30.1) and their proposed embryogenesis. Interatrial communications in the region of the fossa ovalis may represent either a true secundum ASD or a valvular incompetent patent foramen ovale. Defects anterior to the fossa ovalis (primum defects) often are associated with a cleft in the anterior leaflet of the mitral valve. Those posterior and superior to the fossa ovalis, the sinus venosus defects, usually occur in conjunction with anomalous connection of the right pulmonary veins. Finally, interatrial communications at the expected site of the coronary sinus ostium are often associated with an unroofed coronary sinus and left atrial connection of a persistent left superior vena cava.

Throughout cardiac embryogenesis, an avenue for interatrial blood flow is maintained, despite the development of two separate septal structures. The sequence of atrial septation (Fig. 30.2) was well described several years ago by Van Mierop (8).

The septum primum, which is the first septum to develop, is an incomplete thin-walled partition in which the anteroinfe-

rior free edge is above the atrioventricular canal and becomes lined by tissue derived from the superior and inferior endocardial cushions. Before the resultant interatrial opening (ostium primum) becomes sealed by endocardial cushion tissue, programmed cell death in an area near the anterosuperior aspect of the septum primum creates small cribriform perforations. These perforations coalesce to form a large, second interatrial communication (ostium secundum) maintaining interatrial blood flow.

At this time, to the right of the first septum, an anterosuperior infolding of the atrial roof occurs and forms a second septal structure (septum secundum). It expands posteroinferiorly as a thick-walled muscular ridge to form an incomplete partition that overlies the ostium secundum. As atrial septation is accomplished, septum secundum forms the limbus of the fossa ovalis and septum primum forms the valve of the fossa ovalis. The channel for interatrial blood flow through the ostium secundum is known as the foramen ovale.

Concurrently with atrial septation, the left horn of the sinus venosus forms the coronary sinus, and the right sinus horn becomes a part of the right atrium. Infolding at the sinoatrial junction forms the right and left venous valves. Whereas the right venous valve is maintained and forms the rudimentary valves of the inferior vena cava (eustachian valve) and the coronary sinus (thebesian valve), the left venous valve becomes fused to the superior, posterior, and inferior margins of the fossa ovalis.

Patent Foramen Ovale

The foramen ovale represents a normal interatrial communication that is present throughout fetal life (Fig. 30.3A, B). Functional closure of the foramen ovale occurs postnatally as pressure in the left atrium exceeds that in the right atrium. As a result, the valve of the fossa ovalis is pressed against the limbus and forms a competent seal. During the first year of life, fibrous adhesions may develop between the limbus and valve and thereby produce a permanent anatomic seal and an imperforate atrial septum. In 25% to 30% of people, however, anatomic closure does not occur, and a potential interatrial channel persists through which blood or air may shunt whenever pressure in the right atrium exceeds that in the left atrium (9).

If atrial dilation occurs among individuals with a patent foramen ovale, the limbus may become so stretched that the ostium secundum (valve of the fossa ovalis) may no longer be covered by the limbic ledge. The result is a valvular incompetent patent foramen ovale that allows interatrial shunting throughout the cardiac cycle and thus constitutes an acquired ASD (Fig. 30.3C).

Atrial Septum

Defects at the level of the fossa ovalis presumably result from deficiency, perforation, or absence of the septum primum (the

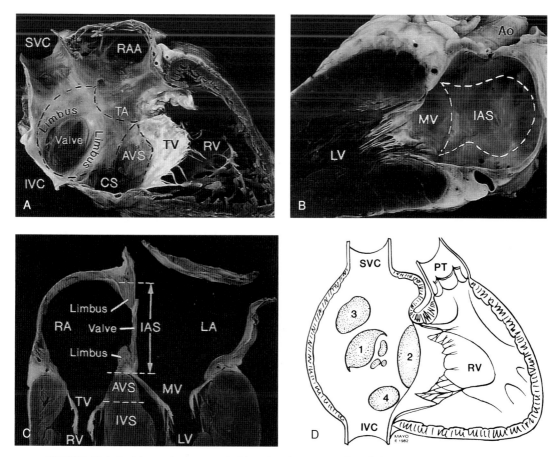

FIGURE 30.1 Atrial septal anatomy. **A:** Two-chamber view, right-sided. **B:** Two-chamber view, left-sided. The interatrial septum (IAS, outlined by *dotted lines*) is relatively small and is associated primarily with the limbus and valve of the fossa ovalis. Anterosuperiorly, the aortic root indents the right atrial free wall as the torus aorticus (TA). **C:** Four-chamber view. The IAS lies between the right and left atria (RA, LA), whereas the atrioventricular septum (AVS) lies between the RA and left ventricle (LV) **D:** Schematic diagram showing the location of atrial septal defects, numbered in decreasing order of frequency: 1, secundum; 2, primum; 3, sinus venosus; 4, coronary sinus (CS) type. IVC, inferior vena cava; IVS, interventricular septum; MV, mitral valve; PT, pulmonary trunk; RAA, right atrial appendage; RV, right ventricle; SVC, superior vena cava; TV, tricuspid valve. (Reprinted by permission of the Mayo Foundation.)

valve of the fossa ovalis) (Fig. 30.4A, B). Because the ostium secundum appears enlarged or unguarded, these defects are labeled as secundum type. In patients with a relatively small solitary defect that can be closed with sutures instead of a patch, it is likely that the interatrial communication represents a valvular incompetent patent foramen ovale rather than a true congenital secundum ASD. More recently, these have been closed in the catheterization suite.

Secondary Effects on the Heart

In the setting of a large interatrial communication, a chronic left-to-right shunt imposes a volume overload on the right-sided cardiac structures and results in dilation of the right atrium and right ventricle (Fig. 30.4C). Although volume enlargement of the right atrium and right ventricle produces capacious chambers, mural thrombus formation is distinctly uncommon.

In some cases, right ventricular dilation is so marked that the cardiac apex is formed entirely by the right ventricle. As the right ventricle dilates, the ventricular septum begins to straighten, such that the two ventricular chambers become D

shaped when viewed in the echocardiographic short-axis plane. In extreme cases, leftward bowing of the septum results in reversal of the cross-sectional shapes, with a circular right ventricle and a crescentic left ventricle.

The tricuspid and pulmonary annuli can become dilated, and the valves can be incompetent and mildly thickened. Dilation of the central pulmonary arteries also may occur. Dilation of the left atrium usually is mild. The wall thickness and mass of the left ventricle tend to be normal in patients with isolated secundum ASD.

Secondary Effects on the Lungs

The chronic volume overload causes dilation of the entire pulmonary vascular bed. Microscopically, the arteries, capillaries, and veins are engorged. Medial hypertrophy is evident in the muscular pulmonary arteries and the pulmonary veins, although its extent is usually masked by vascular dilation. Muscularization of arterioles also may occur (10).

In a few patients with a secundum ASD, severe and irreversible hypertensive pulmonary vascular disease develops, and there is a striking female preponderance for this association

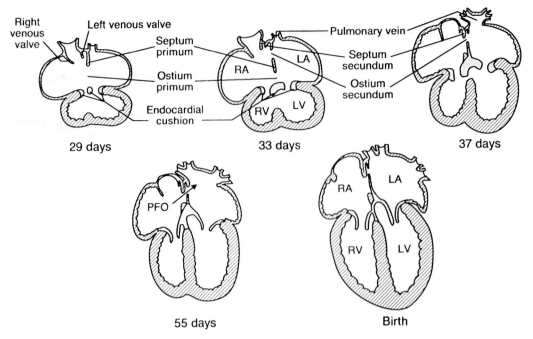

FIGURE 30.2 Schematic diagram showing the embryologic sequence of atrial septation. LA, left atrium; LV, left ventricle; PFO, patent foramen ovale; RA, right atrium; RV, right ventricle. (Modified from Van Mierop LHS. Embryology of the atrioventricular canal region and pathogenesis of endocardial cushion defects. In: Feldt RH, McGoon DC, Ongley PA, et al., eds. *Atrioventricular Canal Defects*. Philadelphia: WB Saunders, 1976:1–12, with permission.)

(Fig. 30.4D) (11). Obstructive lesions include not only plexiform lesions but also thrombotic lesions (12). In older patients, the coexistence of chronic pulmonary venous hypertension (owing to left ventricular hypertrophy or failure) or chronic hypoxic pulmonary hypertension (owing to chronic obstructive or interstitial pulmonary disease) may contribute to the pulmonary vascular disease associated with the interatrial communication and thereby add to risk of closure.

Physiology

The direction in which blood flows through the defect primarily is related to the relative compliances of the ventricles. Generally, the right ventricle is more compliant than the left, resulting in less resistance to filling from the right atrium. In most situations, shunting is left to right.

In infancy, the right ventricle is thick, stiff, and not very compliant. Therefore, there is a minimal amount of left-to-right shunting. In the first few weeks of life, the pulmonary vascular resistance decreases, the right ventricle becomes more compliant, and the amount of left-to-right shunting increases. Most infants with isolated ASDs are asymptomatic. However, there have been reports of infants with ASDs who present with heart failure. The hemodynamic findings at cardiac catheterization in these infants have been no different from those in children who do not have heart failure. Thus, the pathophysiology for heart failure in these infants is not fully understood. These infants tend to have a high incidence of extracardiac anomalies, developmental delay, and growth failure, which does not totally reverse after closure of the defect (13).

Generally, there is increased pulmonary blood flow; often three to four times normal. However, the pulmonary artery pressure is only slightly increased, and in most patients, pulmonary resistance remains in the normal range. A wide spectrum of hemodynamic findings in ASDs has been reported, including pulmonary vascular obstructive disease occurring in patients as young as 3 months of age (10). Steele et al. (11) reported their results for 702 patients found to have isolated ASDs of the ostium secundum or sinus venosus type at cardiac catheterization. Of these 702 patients, 40 (6%) had pulmonary vascular obstructive disease, defined as a total pulmonary resistance of ≥ 7 U/m²; there were 34 women (85%) and 6 men. Interestingly, no patient younger than 19 years of age presented with an ASD and pulmonary vascular obstructive disease. Haworth (10) reported on 10 patients with ASDs and pulmonary vascular obstructive disease (pulmonary arteriolar resistance of 4 to 16 U/m²). Four of the patients were younger than 6 months of age at the time of catheterization and presented with congestive heart failure and failure to grow. Five patients were evaluated at 2 to 9 years of age, and two had severe pulmonary vascular disease (pulmonary resistance of 16.5 and 15.5 U/m²).

Although encountered infrequently, patients with isolated secundum ASDs may have severe cyanosis owing to pulmonary vascular obstructive disease. Another cause of cyanosis in patients with secundum ASDs is a large sinus venosus valve, eustachian valve, or thebesian valve, which may divert blood from the inferior vena cava across the ASD. These abnormal valves can be identified by echocardiography, and this is an important diagnosis to establish because closure of the ASD is curative.

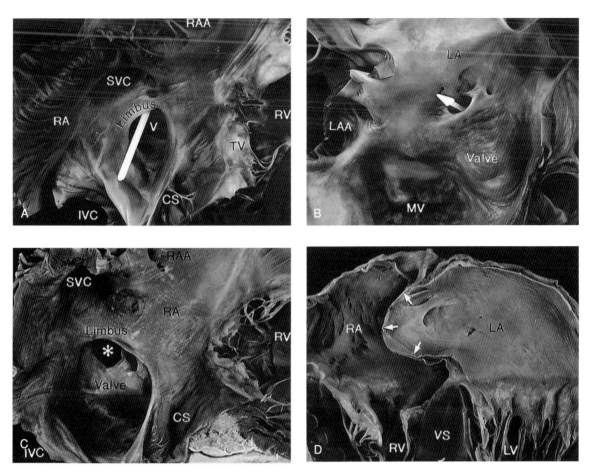

FIGURE 30.3 Patent foramen ovale. **A:** Right atrial view. **B:** Left atrial view. A white probe passes between the limbus and valve (V) of the fossa ovalis and enters the left atrium (LA) through the ostium secundum (*white arrow*), a normally prominent fenestration in the valve. **C:** Right atrial view. In this patient, atrial dilation has produced a valvular-incompetent patent foramen ovale, that is, an acquired atrial septal defect, indicated by the *asterisk*. **D:** Four-chamber view. An aneurysm of the fossa ovalis (*arrows*) bulges rightward in this patient, who also had a patent foramen ovale. (See Fig. 30.1 for abbreviations.) LAA, left atrial appendage; VS, ventricular septum.

Clinical Features

Most infants with ASDs are asymptomatic, and the condition goes undetected. They may present at 6 to 8 weeks of age with a soft systolic ejection murmur and possibly a fixed and widely split S_2. More recently, infants with heart murmurs have been referred earlier for echocardiographic evaluation so that the average age at which ASDs are being detected is about 6 months old. Older children with a moderate left-to-right shunt often are asymptomatic. Children with large left-to-right shunts are likely to complain of some fatigue and dyspnea. Growth failure is very uncommon. Rarely, ASDs in infants are associated with poor growth, recurrent lower respiratory tract infection, and heart failure.

Inspection of the chest may reveal a precordial bulge and a hyperdynamic cardiac impulse, especially in the older child and when the left-to-right shunt is large. Palpation of the precordium reveals a prominent systolic impulse. There are three important auscultatory features: (a) a typical wide and fixed splitting of the second heart sound, (b) a soft systolic ejection murmur at the second left intercostal space, and (c) an early to middiastolic murmur at the lower left sternal border. The term "fixed" refers to the constant time interval between A_2 and P_2 throughout the respiratory cycle. A delay in P_2 is due, in part, to prolonged emptying of the right ventricle because of increased volume of blood to be ejected; additionally, considerable vasodilation of the pulmonary vasculature delays intra-arterial pulmonary tension necessary to close the pulmonary valve.

The increased flow of blood across the pulmonary valve produces a crescendo–decrescendo (ejection-type) systolic murmur, heard maximally over the upper left sternal border and transmitted into both lung fields. The increased volume of blood shunted and flowing across the tricuspid valve results in the early to middiastolic murmur, maximal along the lower left sternal border.

When significant pulmonary hypertension develops, the above characteristic findings change because of a smaller or absent left-to-right shunt. The widely split S_2 can disappear, P_2 becomes louder, the systolic murmur becomes shorter, and the diastolic murmur disappears.

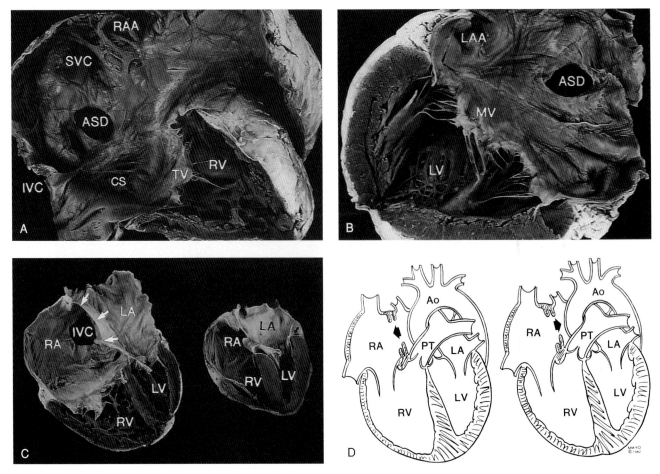

FIGURE 30.4 Secundum atrial septal defect (ASD). **A:** Right atrial view. **B:** Left atrial view. The defect involves the region of the fossa ovalis. **C:** Four-chamber view, with normal heart at right for comparison. The right ventricle exhibits volume enlargement and both atria are dilated. The ASD (*arrows*) is large. **D:** ASDs are shown schematically in a patient without pulmonary hypertension (with a left-to-right shunt). (See Fig 30.1 for abbreviations.) Ao, aorta; LAA, left atrial appendage. (Reprinted by permission of the Mayo Foundation.)

Radiologic Features

The heart is usually enlarged, with a cardiothoracic ratio >0.5 (Fig. 30.5). Pulmonary vascular markings are increased because of engorged pulmonary arteries, and this finding becomes more prominent with age and the larger the left-to-right shunt. If pulmonary vascular obstructive disease develops, the main pulmonary artery becomes quite large and the peripheral lung fields become clear or oligemic.

Electrocardiographic and Electrophysiologic Features

Usually, normal sinus rhythm is present (Fig. 30.6); however, in a few patients, usually older, junctional rhythm or supraventricular tachyarrhythmia, such as atrial flutter, can occur (14). In most patients, the mean frontal plane QRS axis is from +95 to +170 degrees. The P-R interval may be pro-

longed, especially in older patients, because of intra-atrial and sometimes H-V conduction delay, resulting in first-degree atrioventricular block (15). In about half the cases, tall P waves reflect right atrial enlargement. There is usually some variant of the rsR′ or RSR′ pattern (incomplete right bundle branch block pattern) in lead V1, consistent with right ventricular volume overload. The duration of the QRS complex is less ≤0.10 second, and R′ in lead V1 is somewhat prolonged.

Intracardiac electrophysiology studies (16–18) of patients with ASDs before repair have documented abnormalities of uncertain clinical significance. Apparent sinus node dysfunction has been reported (abnormal corrected sinus node recovery times and sinoatrial conduction times). However, only rarely do patients have abnormal findings on resting ECGs or 24-hour ambulatory monitoring. A few patients have atrioventricular node dysfunction diagnosed based on a prolonged A-H interval or an atrioventricular node Wenckebach periodicity at low atrial pacing rates. Again, abnormalities have not been demonstrated clinically. Perhaps

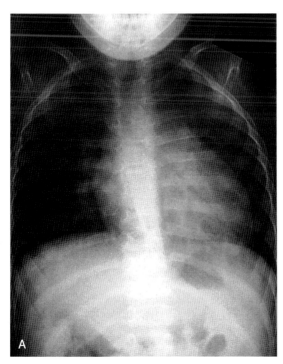
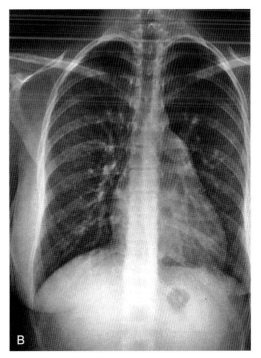

FIGURE 30.5 Chest radiographs. **A:** Two-year-old patient with secundum atrial septal defect (ASD). The radiograph shows cardiomegaly, right atrial prominence, upturned apex, and increased pulmonary vascular markings. **B:** Twenty-one-year-old patient with secundum ASD. The radiograph shows a nearly normal heart size, prominence of the left heart border with lifting of the apex, prominence of the main pulmonary artery, and increased pulmonary vascular markings.

these abnormal electrophysiologic findings are due to an imbalance of the autonomic nervous system control of the sinoatrial and atrioventricular nodes (19). Intra-atrial conduction time is prolonged in the older patient, and right atrial effective refractory periods are increased in some patients. Patients with these findings may be predisposed to atrial arrhythmias.

Echocardiographic/Doppler Features

Echocardiography shows increased right atrial and right ventricular dimensions and the defect in the atrial septum. The subcostal examination is the most effective for diagnosis because it places the ultrasound beam nearly perpendicular to

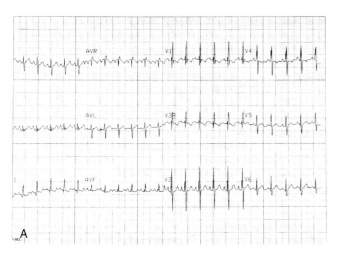
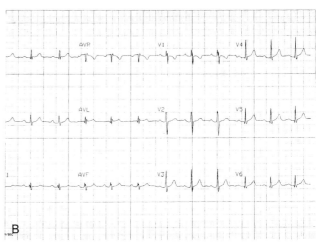

FIGURE 30.6 Electrocardiograms. **A:** Two-year-old patient with a secundum atrial septal defect (ASD). There is normal sinus rhythm with a prominent P wave in lead II, indicating right atrial enlargement. The frontal plane QRS axis is to the right, and right ventricular volume overload is manifested by rsR′ in lead V1 and terminal widening of the S wave in lead V6. **B:** Twenty-one-year-old patient with a secundum ASD. There is normal sinus rhythm with first-degree atrioventricular block. The frontal plane QRS axis is +20 degrees. The QRS complexes in the chest leads appear normal except for subtle widening of the S wave in lead V6.

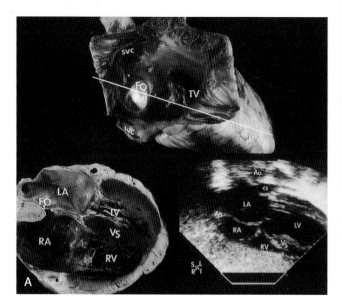

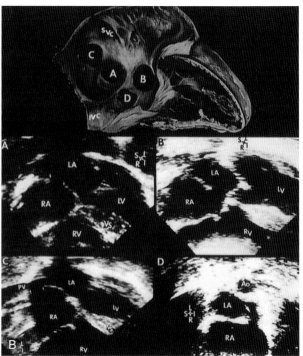

FIGURE 30.7 A: Two-dimensional echocardiography. Subcostal two-dimensional echocardiographic examination is the best view for diagnosis. This transducer orientation places the ultrasound beam nearly perpendicular to the plane of the atrial septum. **Top:** Anatomic specimen with the free wall of the right atrium removed. The line indicates the plane of section used to view the atrial septum from the subcostal transducer position. This line transects the middle portion of the atrial septum, including the fossa ovalis (FO). **Bottom left:** Anatomic specimen in the four-chamber plane of section. The right atrium (RA), left atrium (LA), and atrial septum are clearly delineated. Superior and inferior tilt of the transducer permits imaging of related portions of the atrial septum. **B:** Echocardiographic findings for various types of atrial septal defects (ASD). **Top:** Anatomic locations of various types of ASDs. **Lower panels** show the corresponding two-dimensional echocardiographic features of each defect. **A:** Secundum ASD. Defect is located in the middle portion of the atrial septum (*small arrows*). **B:** Primum valve. The septal portion of the mitral valve is displaced inferiorly, placing both atrioventricular valves at the same insertion level at the crest of the ventricular septum. **C:** Sinus venosus ASD. The defect is located in the posterosuperior atrial septum (*small arrows*), usually just beneath the orifice of the superior vena cava. This defect is commonly associated with partial anomalous connection of the right upper pulmonary veins (PV). **D:** Coronary sinus ASD. The defect is located at the expected position of the orifice of the coronary sinus (*arrow*) and is located just above the orifice of the IVC. (See Fig.30.1 for abbreviations.) Ao, aorta; VS, ventricular septum. (From Feldt RH, Porter CJ, Edwards WD, et al. Defects of the atrial septum and the atrioventricular canal. In: Adams FH, Emmanouilides GC, Riemenschneider TA, eds. *Moss's Heart Disease in Infants, Children, and Adolescents*. 4th ed. Baltimore: Williams & Wilkins 1989:170–179, by permission of the Mayo Foundation.)

the plane of the atrial septum (Fig. 30.7A). Each type of ASD has been characterized by tomographic two-dimensional echocardiographic examination (Fig. 30.7B). The secundum ASD is characterized by dropout of the midatrial septum; the primum ASD by a defect in the lower atrial septum; the sinus venosus ASD by a deficiency in the posterosuperior atrial septum; and the coronary sinus ASD by a communication at the level of the orifice of the coronary sinus (20).

In the pediatric patient, the presence of an ASD usually is apparent using surface echocardiography. However, in older patients transesophageal echocardiography (TEE) has become the most accepted diagnostic examination (Fig. 30.8). Associated partial anomalous pulmonary venous connection also can be diagnosed and characterized confidently using TEE (Fig. 30.9).

Peripheral contrast-enhanced echocardiography, in certain circumstances, can clarify the type and relative degree of left-to-right and right-to-left shunting (20). This examination best delineates the presence of right-to-left shunting by visualiza-

tion of agitated saline contrast bubbles in the left atrium or left ventricle. Left-to-right shunts also can be appreciated by a negative contrast effect (undyed blood visualized within the opacified right atrium).

Left-to-right shunting at the atrial level has a characteristic flow pattern that can be demonstrated by pulsed Doppler echocardiography (Fig. 30.10, top) (20). Blood shunting from left to right across the atrial septum typically begins in midsystole. The velocity and volume of blood progressively decrease until early diastole, when atrial contraction again accentuates the left-to-right shunt. Early in ventricular systole, there may be a transient right-to-left shunt. The Doppler flow pattern characteristic of an interatrial shunt is confirmatory of an ASD. Doppler examination has greatly increased the sensitivity of the echocardiographic examination.

Using Doppler technology, one can reasonably determine the ratio of pulmonary (Q_p) to systemic (Q_s) blood flow ($Q_p:Q_s$). However, most echocardiographers more commonly use a combination of direct visualization of the size of

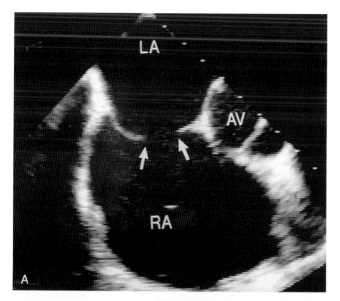

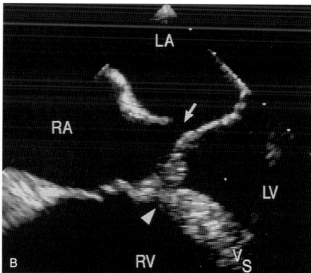

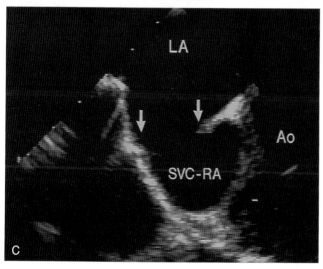

FIGURE 30.8 Atrial septal defect (ASD) diagnosis by transesophageal echocardiography. **A:** Secundum ASD. The transducer is posterior, adjacent to the left atrium (LA). In the midportion of the atrial septum there is an ASD (*arrows*). **B:** Primum ASD. The atrioventricular valves insert into the crest of the ventricular septum (VS) at the same level (*arrowhead*). A primum ASD (*arrow*) is visualized in the inferior atrial septum. **C:** Sinus venosus ASD. High in the atrial septum at the superior vena caval–right atrial junction (SVC-RA), there is a typical sinus venosus defect (*arrows*) communicating with the LA (see Fig. 30.1 for abbreviations). AV, aortic valve.

the defect and the visible features of volume overload as a means of assessing the significance of shunting. Using Doppler echocardiography, one can estimate right ventricular systolic pressure and pulmonary artery pressure from the tricuspid and pulmonary valve regurgitation Doppler velocity waveforms.

Color-flow imaging permits visualization of volumes of blood moving within the cardiac chamber and allows the blood traversing an ASD to be demonstrated (Fig. 30.10, bottom). These images are comparable to the angiographic visualization of intracardiac shunting. The unique contribution of color-flow imaging to the assessment of ASDs is its ability to show associated defects such as partial anomalous pulmonary venous connection.

Cardiac Catheterization

Cardiac catheterization is unnecessary for the diagnosis of secundum ASD. Occasionally, questions about pulmonary vascular obstructive disease or associated cardiac defects arise that require catheterization. However, for most patients clinical assessment in conjunction with noninvasive testing provides the correct diagnosis.

An ASD is suspected when the oxygen saturation in the right atrium is greater than that in the superior and inferior venae cavae. An increase in oxygen saturation of ≥10% from the superior vena cava to the right atrium in one series of blood samples or an increase of 5% in two series of samples usually indicates an interatrial communication. However, a ventricular septal defect with tricuspid insufficiency, a left ventricular to right atrial shunt, or partial or complete atrioventricular septal defect may produce similar findings. Anomalous pulmonary venous connection to the right atrium or vena cava or systemic arteriovenous fistula also will produce increased oxygen saturation in the right atrium and may be mistaken for an ASD.

Phasic and mean pressures in the right and left atria are equal with large defects. Generally, the right ventricular systolic pressures are slightly increased to 25 to 35 mm Hg. A few patients have modest increases in the right ventricular pressure and, in some patients, systolic pressure differences of

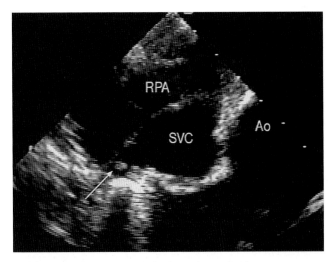

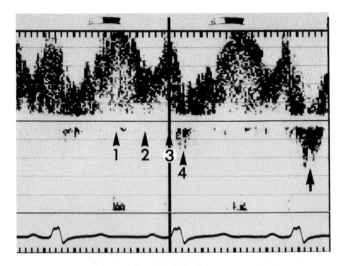

FIGURE 30.9 Transesophageal echocardiography demonstrates partial anomalous pulmonary venous connection in a patient (same as in Fig. 30.8C) with a sinus venosus atrial septal defect. The right upper pulmonary vein (*arrow*) enters the superior vena cava (SVC). This form of partial anomalous pulmonary vena cava is visualized by withdrawing the transesophageal echocardiogram scope to the level of the right pulmonary artery (RPA). Ao, aorta.

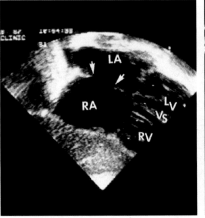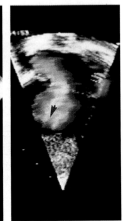

FIGURE 30.10 Pulsed Doppler echocardiographic findings in an atrial septal defect (ASD). The pulsed Doppler echocardiographic signal is consistent with a left-to-right shunt at the atrial level (recorded from a subcostal transducer position). The Doppler signal has a characteristic phasic change. **Top:** 1, left-to-right shunt (positive Doppler signal) begins in late systole; 2, diminishes through middiastole; 3, is enhanced by atrial contraction; and 4, reverses in early systole, consistent with a transient right-to-left shunt. The early systolic right-to-left shunt is enhanced with inspiration (*arrow*) and diminishes with expiration. **Bottom:** Secundum ASD. Photograph of a color-flow Doppler echocardiographic image of a left-to-right shunt through a secundum ASD. **Left:** Subcostal four-chamber two-dimensional echocardiographic examination shows a large secundum ASD (*arrows*). **Right:** Left-to-right shunt at the atrial level is characterized as a velocity volume moving across the plane of the atrial septum and is displayed as an orange-red signal moving toward the transducer (*arrow*). (See Fig. 30.1 for abbreviations.) VS, ventricular septum.

≤15 to 30 mm Hg are noted between the right ventricle and the pulmonary artery. Peak systolic gradients as high as 40 mm Hg across a normal pulmonic valve have been reported. Pulmonary artery pressure usually is normal to slightly increased; however, a small but significant number of patients may have moderate increases in the pulmonary artery pressure. In the usual situation, the pulmonary arteriolar resistance is <4.0 U/m².

Angiography almost never is necessary for the diagnosis of ASDs because echocardiography and, if necessary, cardiac catheterization to ascertain hemodynamic variables are satisfactory diagnostic procedures.

Natural History

The natural course of ASDs is relatively benign except for the largest openings and those associated with other cardiac defects. Typically, patients with ASDs remain active and asymptomatic through early childhood, and many patients have lived into their fourth, fifth, sixth, and even seventh decades with ASDs of moderate size before symptoms developed (21,22).

Secundum ASDs can close spontaneously, remain open, or enlarge. Spontaneous closure of isolated ASDs has been reported with some frequency. Prior to the advent of echocardiography, cardiac catheterization was necessary to confirm the diagnosis of secundum ASDs. In 1983 Cocherham et al. (23) reported results of 87 children who underwent cardiac catheterization at <4 years old because of significant secundum ASD. At follow-up they found that 15 of 87 (17%) had spontaneous closure. For those whose first study was done at <1 year old, spontaneous closure occurred in 22%. If the study was done between 1 and 2 years old, spontaneous closure occurred in 33%. If the first study was done between 2 and 4 years, the spontaneous closure rate was down to 3%. Their recommendation was to wait until after age 4 years for elective closure.

Using echocardiography, one has been able to evaluate more accurately the size and hemodynamic effects of an ASD. A prospective echocardiographic study suggested that as many as 24% of newborns have evidence of an opening (3 to 8 mm) in the atrial septum in the first week of life (24). However, by a little more than 1 year of age, 92% of the patients were found to have spontaneous closure of the opening, and in most patients, there was evidence of a valve-like opening of the atrial septum that was believed to contribute to closure. It appears that spontaneous closure, or a decrease in size, is most likely to occur in ASDs <7 to 8 mm and with younger age at diagnosis. Radzik et al. (25) reviewed the results in 101 infants diagnosed at a mean age of 26 days with an average follow-up of 9 months. Spontaneous closure occurred in all 32 ASDs <3 mm in diameter, 87% of 3- to 5-mm ASDs, 80% of 5- to 8-mm ASDs, and in none of 4 infants with defects >8 mm. These authors concluded that no follow-up is necessary if a defect is <3 mm in diameter, but for those with a defect 3 to 5 mm or 5 to 8 mm, they should be evaluated by the end of the 12th and 15th month, respectively, by which time >80% of the defects will be closed.

Helgason and Jonsdottir (26) reviewed the medical records of all patients in Iceland with a diagnosis of ASD born between 1984 and 1993. ASD was confirmed by 2-D echocardiogram, and data only from patients with secundum ASDs were analyzed. A total of 84 children diagnosed at a mean age of 12 months were followed for 4 years. Spontaneous closure or decreased size was observed in 89% with a 4-mm ASD, 79% with a 5- to 6-mm defect, and only 7% with a defect >6 mm. Even infants with congestive heart failure can have spontaneous closure or a reduction in the size of the ASD years after the diagnosis (27). Occasionally, spontaneous closure will occur as late as 16 years (27). One should be careful about proceeding too rapidly to close an ASD in an asymptomatic young patient.

Unfortunately, some ASDs can enlarge enough over time to require closure. McMahon et al. (28) evaluated 104 children who were diagnosed with their ASDs at a much older mean age of 4.5 years and followed for a mean of about 3 years. The defects were defined as small (3 to <6 mm), moderate (6 to <12 mm), or large (>12 mm). Among the 34 patients with a small ASD, 7 increased to moderate size and 3 increased to large size. Among 40 patients with a moderate ASD, 8 became large, and for the 30 patients with large defects, all remained large. Overall the defects enlarged in 65% of patients, and some to the extent (>20 mm) that they could not be closed by transcatheter techniques.

The presence and severity of functional limitation among patients with ASDs seem to increase with age. Congestive heart failure rarely is found in the first decades of life, but it can become common once the patient is older than 40 years of age (29). The onset of atrial fibrillation or, less commonly, atrial flutter can be a hallmark in the course of patients with ASDs. The incidence of atrial arrhythmias increases with advancing age (29) to as high as 13% in patients older than 40 years of age (30) and 52% in those older than 60 years of age (21).

Pulmonary vascular disease can occur in 5% to 10% of patients with untreated ASDs, predominantly in females (11). Usually it occurs after 20 years of age, although rare cases in early childhood have been recorded (10). Debate continues about what causes pulmonary vascular obstructive disease, which patients are at risk, and at what age it occurs It does not appear simply to be the magnitude of the shunt persisting for several decades.

Treatment

Surgery

Prior to the advent of interventional catheter procedures for major ASDs (Qp:Qs ratio >1.5:1) in children and young adults, surgical repair was the treatment of choice. Since most ASDs are well tolerated in infancy and may spontaneously close, elective repair frequently has been deferred

until the child is at least 4 years of age. Is some patients with very large ASDs, closure is done at younger ages. There is no advantage in delaying repair much beyond this age, and there may be harm in delaying repair to the teenage years and beyond (29). Long-standing volume overload of the right atrium and ventricle causes certain irreversible changes in the right atrium and right and left ventricles that possibly contribute to atrial arrhythmias and premature death. Early operation has been recommended for those infants and young children who have unremitting heart failure or associated pulmonary hypertension.

Indications for closure of an ASD in adults have been controversial. In 1970, Campbell (22) reported that adults with ASDs appeared to die at an earlier age than normal adults of the same age and gender. It is possible that asymptomatic individuals without complex ASDs could have been missed in this study. In 1994, Shah et al. (31) reported on a selected group of 82 adults with uncomplicated secundum or sinus venosus ASDs and no pulmonary hypertension, only some of whom had undergone repair. All patients were older than 25 years of age at presentation and were older than 45 years of age at the time of study. The investigators found no difference in survival or symptoms between the medically and surgically treated groups. There were no differences in incidence of new supraventricular arrhythmia (including atrial fibrillation), stroke, embolic phenomenon, or cardiac failure. Limitations of this study included nonrandom assignment of medical versus surgical therapy, exclusion of patients with pulmonary hypertension, and the proportion of patients lost to follow-up (22%). Long-term follow-up data from Murphy et al. (29) suggested that adults older than 41 years of age derived minimal benefit from operative closure.

Elective surgical repair of ASDs has been a safe and simple operation in the hands of an experienced surgical team. In 1998, the Pediatric Cardiac Care Consortium (32) reported its results from 1984 to 1995. Nine deaths occurred among 2,471 patients (0.4%) undergoing intracardiac repair of secundum or sinus venosus ASDs. Six of the nine deaths occurred in infants, and one of these was found to have Werdnig-Hoffman disease after surgical repair. Only one of 208 adult patients died. There was a slight trend toward relatively more infant operations in the years 1990 to 1993 (51% of the total number of operations), compared with 1989 to 1989 (31% of operations). In 1985 to 1986, 73% of patients stayed in the hospital 6 days or longer, whereas in 1992 to 1993, only 41% of patients stayed in the hospital 6 days or more. One reason for shorter hospital stay may have been earlier extubation and minimal ventilator care.

The usual approach is through a median sternotomy; however, recent reports have advocated a partial sternal split and a limited skin incision, providing adequate surgical exposure (33). For large defects, closure requires the use of a pericardial or prosthetic patch.

Catheter Device Closure

Transcatheter techniques for closure of ASDs have been available for several years. In 1976, King et al. (34) reported the first transcatheter closure of a secundum ASD in humans with a double-umbrella device. It was successful in five of ten patients. Since then, devices have undergone several evolutionary changes in an attempt to improve the design and the technique of delivering the devices. Early models included the Rashkind Atrial Septal Defect Occluder, Lock-USCI

Clamshell Occluder, CardioSEAL device, the Sideris Buttoned device, Atrial Septal Defect Occlusion System (ASDOS), Das-Angel Wings occlusion device, and Amplatzer Septal Occluder (35). Problems encountered using these devices included residual shunt, fractures of the hardware, embolization of the device, large delivery systems, and defects too large to close.

In December 2001, the Amplatzer septal occluder (ASO) device became the only FDA-approved device for transcatheter closure of ASDs. Recently there have been reports of long-term outcomes of transcatheter ASD closure using the ASO. Masura et al. (36) reported 4.7- to 9-year (median 6 years) follow-up of 151 patients (average age 12 years; average weight 36 kg.) who had transcatheter closure of ASDs from September 1995 to January 2000 . Complete closure was seen at 3-year follow-up, and there were no deaths or significant complications. Butera et al. (37) reported a single-center comparison of ASO (153 patients) to third-generation CardioSEAL/STARFlex devices (CS/SF) (121 patients). Procedure and fluoroscopy times were shorter in the ASO group, and residual shunts at procedure and discharge were significantly more frequent in the CS/SF group. There was no difference in complication rates, but late residual shunt was significantly more frequent in CS/SF group (4% at 24 months versus none in ASO group). Erosion and thrombus formation have occurred with use of septal occluder devices. The incidence of ASO device erosion in the United States was reported at 0.1%. Most occur in the first 72 hours, but one case occurred 3 years after implant (38). In a single-center report of 407 patients where 9 different atrial septal occluder devices were used, thrombus formation in the right or left atrium was found in 1.2% of patients. The CS/SF device had the highest incidence of thrombus, and the ASO device had no thrombus formation (39). Temporary atrioventricular block (first, second, and third) has been reported in a few patients, all resolving by 6 months after the procedure.

Late Outcomes of Surgically Treated Atrial Septal Defects

In 1990, Murphy et al. (29) reported the follow-up results (27 to 32 years or until death) for the first 123 consecutive patients who had closure of an ASD at the Mayo Clinic between 1956 and 1960. The perioperative mortality rate was 3.3% (four deaths). All four patients who died were 46 to 50 years of age, and all had pulmonary hypertension. Kaplan–Meier estimates of survival in the 119 patients included in the survival analysis were 97% 5 years after operation, 90% at 10 years, 83% at 20 years, and 74% at 30 years compared with 99%, 98%, 94%, and 85%, respectively, in an age- and sex-matched control population. The survival rate of patients under 25 years of age at operation was not different from that in a comparable control group (Fig. 30.11). The actuarial survival rate was 40% for patients who underwent surgery after the age of 41 years (at 27 years after surgery) compared with 59% in the control group. The presence of moderate or severe pulmonary hypertension (systolic pressure ≥40 mm Hg) had a markedly adverse effect on survival in patients over 24 years of age at the time of operation (Fig. 30.12). Age at operation and preoperative main pulmonary artery systolic pressure were significant predictors of long-term survival, according to univariate and multivariate analysis.

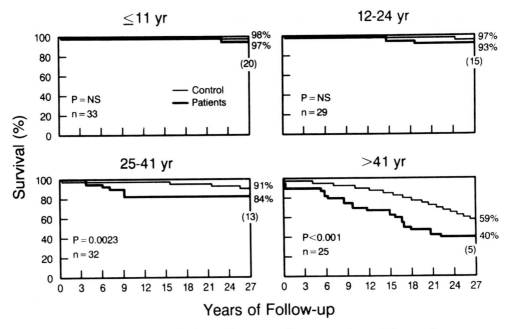

FIGURE 30.11 Long-term survival of patients surviving the perioperative period, according to age at operation. Expected survival in an age- and sex-matched control population is also shown. Probability values for the comparison of observed with expected survival were calculated using the log-rank test; values in parentheses denote the numbers of patients alive at the end of the follow-up periods. NS, not significant. (From Murphy JG, Gersh BJ, McGoon MD, et al. Long-term outcome after surgical repair of isolated atrial septal defect. *N Engl J Med* 1990;323:1645–1650, with permission.)

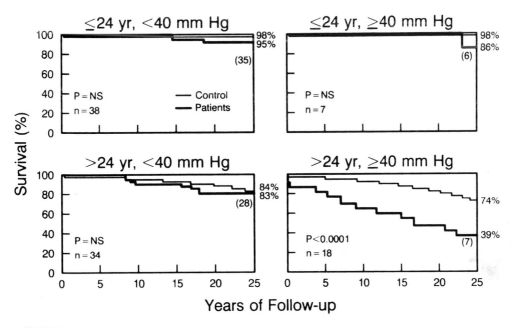

FIGURE 30.12 Long-term survival of patients surviving the perioperative period, according to age at operation and main pulmonary artery systolic pressure before operation. Probability values for the comparison of observed with expected survival were calculated using the log-rank test. NS, not significant. (From Murphy JG, Gersh BJ, McGoon MD, et al. Long-term outcome after surgical repair of isolated atrial septal defect. *N Engl J Med* 1990;323:1645–1650, with permission.)

There were 27 late deaths in the study by Murphy et al. (29). Of these, 18 (67%) were reported as cardiovascular deaths: 13 cardiac deaths and 5 deaths owing to stroke. All patients for whom stroke was listed as the cause of death had been in atrial fibrillation during follow-up.

Late fatal and nonfatal cardiovascular events occurred in 57% of the patients who were older than age 24 years at operation but in only 15% of those age 24 years or younger at operation. Both preoperative and atrial fibrillation or flutter became more frequent as the age at operation increased. Nineteen of the 123 patients were in atrial fibrillation or flutter before repair of their ASDs, and 13 of these 19 (68%) were still in atrial fibrillation or flutter at late follow-up. Of the 104 patients in sinus rhythm preoperatively, 80 (77%) remained in sinus rhythm during long-term follow-up.

SINUS VENOSUS ATRIAL SEPTAL DEFECTS

Sinus venosus ASDs account for 5% to 10% of ASDs and are located posterior and superior to the fossa ovalis (Fig. 30.13). Most often, the defect is rimmed by atrial septal tissue only anteroinferiorly. Its posterior aspect is the right atrial free wall, and its superior border is often absent because of an overriding superior vena cava. Infrequently, the defect may be directly posterior to the fossa ovalis or may be posteroinferior such that the inferior vena cava may join both atria.

The sinus venosus defect commonly is associated with anomalous connection of the right pulmonary veins to either the right atrium or the superior vena cava near the caval-atrial junction. Pulmonary veins from the right upper lobe or, less commonly, from the entire right lung connect anomalously, whereas the remaining veins join the left atrium normally. Indeed, the defect may result from "unroofing" of the pulmonary vein.

The preoperative electrocardiogram shows that about half of patients have a frontal plane P-wave axis of <30 degrees (40). In a patient with typical auscultatory findings of an ASD and a P-wave axis of <30 degrees on the electrocardiogram, one should think immediately of a sinus venosus defect.

Two-dimensional echocardiography permits direct examination of the atrial septum, and by the use of multiple tomography projections, in particular the subcostal approach, the sinus venosus ASD can be visualized (Fig. 30.7B, C). In some patients, it may be difficult to visualize a sinus venosus defect using transthoracic echocardiography. One should be suspicious of such a defect if one observes turbulent flow patterns in the superior vena cava or otherwise unexplained volume overload of the right atrium and ventricle. Also, in older patients, TEE may be necessary to make an accurate diagnosis (Figs. 30.8C and 30.9).

For the high sinus venous defects associated with partial anomalous pulmonary venous connection to the superior vena cava, repair must include the construction of a tunnel connecting the orifice of the anomalous vein with the ASD. This tunnel is best constructed with an autologous pericardial patch.

CORONARY SINUS ATRIAL SEPTAL DEFECT

The coronary sinus ASD is a rare anomaly. It is located inferior and anterior to the fossa ovalis, at the anticipated site of the coronary sinus ostium (Fig. 30.14) (41). It is usually part of a developmental complex that includes unroofing of the coronary sinus and a persistent left superior vena cava that joins the roof of the left atrium. This anomaly may be associated with complete atrioventricular septal defect, particularly in the asplenia syndrome, and the ASDs of both malformations then merge.

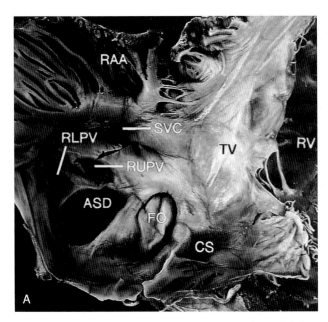
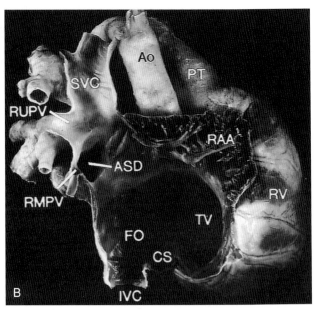

FIGURE 30.13 Sinus venosus atrial septal defect (ASD). **A:** Right atrial view. Right upper (RUPV) and lower (RLPV) pulmonary veins join the right atrium near the site of the defect, posterosuperior to the fossa ovalis (FO). **B:** Right atrial view. The sinus venosus defect is posterior to the FO, and the right upper and middle (RMPV) pulmonary veins anomalously join the superior vena cava (SVC). (See Fig. 30.1 for abbreviations.) Ao, aorta.

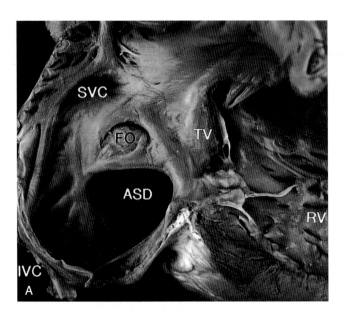
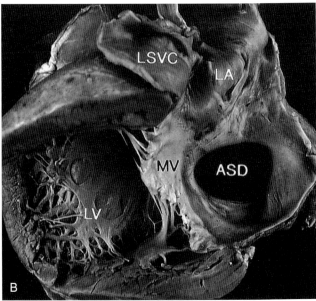

FIGURE 30.14 Coronary sinus atrial septal defect (ASD). **A:** Right atrial view. **B:** Left atrial view. The defect is at the expected site of the coronary sinus ostium, anteroinferior to the fossa ovalis (FO). A persistent left superior vena cava (LSVC) joins the left atrial wall (LA). (See Fig. 30.1 for abbreviations.)

References

1. Fyler DC. Atrial septal defect secundum. In: *Nadas' Pediatric Cardiology*. Philadelphia: Hanley & Belfus, 1992:513–524.
2. Sam'anek M. Children with congenital heart disease: Probability of natural survival. *Pediatr Cardiol* 1992;13:152–158.
3. Holt M, Oram S. Familial heart disease with skeletal malformations. *Br Heart J* 1960;22:236–242.
4. Li QY, Newbury-Ecob RA, Terrett JA, et al. Holt-Oram syndrome is caused by mutation in TBX5, a member of the Brachyury (T) gene family. *Nat Genet* 1997;15:21–29.
5. Srivastava D, Olson EN. A genetic blueprint for cardiac development. *Nature* 2000:407:221–225.
6. Schott JJ, Benson DW, Basson CT, et al. Congenital heart disease caused by mutations in the transcription factor *NKX2-5*. *Science* 1998;281:108–111.
7. Ching YH, Ghosh TK, Cross SJ, et al. Mutation in myosin heavy chain 6 causes atrial septal defect. *Nat Genet* 2005;37:423–428.
8. Van Mierop LHS. Embryology of the atrioventricular canal region and pathogenesis of endocardial cushion defects. In: Feldt RH, McGoon DC, Ongley PA, et al., eds. *Atrioventricular Canal Defects*. Philadelphia: WB Saunders, 1976:1–12.
9. Hagen PT, Scholz DG, Edward WD. Incidence and size of patent foramen ovale during the first 10 decades of life: An autopsy study of 965 normal hearts. *Mayo Clin Proc* 1984;59:17–20.
10. Haworth SG. Pulmonary vascular disease in secundum atrial septal defect in childhood. *Am J Cardiol* 1983;51:265–272.
11. Steele PM, Fuster V, Cohen M, et al. Isolated atrial septal defect with pulmonary vascular obstructive disease: Long-term follow-up and prediction of outcome after surgical correction. *Circulation* 1987;76:1037–1042.
12. Schamroth CL, Sareli P, Pocock WA, et al. Pulmonary arterial thrombosis in secundum atrial septal defect. *Am J Cardiol* 1987;60:1152–1156.
13. Mainwaring RD, Mirali-Akbar H, Lamberti JJ, et al. Secundum-type atrial septal defects with failure to thrive in the first year of life. *J Cardiol Surg* 1996;11:116–120.
14. Garson A Jr, Bink-Boelkens M, Hesslein PS, et al. Atrial flutter in the young: A collaborative study of 380 cases. *J Am Coll Cardiol* 1985;6:871–878.
15. Shiku DJ, Stijns M, Lintermans JP, et al. Influence of age on atrioventricular conduction intervals in children with and without atrial septal defect. *J Electrocardiol* 1982;15:9–14.
16. Clark EB, Kugler JD. Preoperative secundum atrial septal defect with coexisting sinus node and atrioventricular node dysfunction. *Circulation* 1982;65:976–980.
17. Karpawich PP, Antillon JR, Cappola PR, et al. Pre- and postoperative electrophysiologic assessment of children with secundum atrial septal defect. *Am J Cardiol* 1985;55:519–521.
18. Bink-Boelkens MTE, Bergstra A, Landsman MLJ. Functional abnormalities of the conduction system in children with an atrial septal defect. *Int J Cardiol* 1988;20:263–272.
19. Finley JP, Nugent ST, Hellenbrand W, et al. Sinus arrhythmia in children with atrial septal defect: An analysis of heart rate variability before and after surgical repair. *Br Heart J* 1989;61:280–284.
20. Seward JB, Tajik AJ, Edwards WD, et al. Congenital heart disease. In: *Two-dimensional Echocardiographic Atlas*. Vol. 1. New York: Springer-Verlag, 1987.
21. St. John Sutton MG, Tajik AJ, McGoon DC. Atrial septal defect in patients ages 60 years or older: Operative results and long-term postoperative follow-up. *Circulation* 1981;64:402–409.
22. Campbell M. Natural history of atrial septal defect. *Br Heart J* 1970;32:820–826.
23. Cockerham JT, Martin TC, Gutierrez FR, et al. Spontaneous closure of secundum atrial septal defect in infants and young children. *Am J Card* 1983;52:1267–1271.
24. Fukazawa M, Fukushige J, Ueda K. Atrial septal defects in neonates with reference to spontaneous closure. *Am Heart J* 1988;116:123–127.
25. Radzik D, Davignon A, Van Doesburg N, et al. Predictive factors for spontaneous closure of atrial septal defects diagnosed in the first 3 months of life. *J Am Coll Cardiol* 1993;22:851–853.
26. Helgason H, Jonsdottir G. Spontaneous closure of atrial septal defects. *Pediatr Cardiol* 1999;20:195–199.
27. Brassard M, Fouron JC, van Doesburg NH, et al. Outcome of children with atrial septal defect considered too small for surgical closure. *Am J Cardiol* 1999;83:1552–1555.
28. McMahon CJ, Feltes TF, Fraley JK, et al. Natural history of growth of secundum atrial septal defects and implications for transcatheter closure. *Heart* 2002;87:256–259.
29. Murphy JG, Gersh BJ, McGoon MD, et al. Long-term outcome after surgical repair of isolated atrial septal defect. *N Engl J Med* 1990;323:1645–1650.
30. Hamilton WT, Haffajee CI, Dalen JE, et al. Atrial septal defect secundum: Clinical profile with physiologic correlates. In: Roberts WC, ed. *Adult Congenital Heart Disease*. Philadelphia: FA Davis Co, 1987:395–407.
31. Shah D, Azhar M, Oakley CM, et al. Natural history of secundum atrial septal defect in adults after medical or surgical treatment: A historical prospective study. *Br Heart J* 1994;71:224–228.
32. Gessner IH. Atrial septal defect. In: Moller JH, ed. *Perspectives in Pediatric Cardiology*. Vol. 6. *Surgery of Congenital Heart Disease*. Pediatric Cardiac Care Consortium 1984–1995. Armonk, NY: Futura Publishing, 1998:31–44.
33. Black MD, Freedom RM. Minimally invasive repair of atria septal defects. *Ann Thorac Surg* 1998;65:765–767.
34. King TD, Thompson SL, Steiner C, et al. Secundum atrial septal defect: Nonoperative closure during cardiac catheterization. *JAMA* 1976;235:2506–2509.
35. O'Laughlin MP. Catheter closure of secundum atrial septal defects. *Tex Heart Inst J* 1997;24:287–292.
36. Masura J, Gavora P, Podnar T. Long-term outcome of transcatheter secundum-type atrial septal defect closure using Amplatzer septal occluders. *J Am Coll Cardiol* 2005;45:505–507.
37. Butera G, Carminati M, Chessa M, et al. CardioSEAL/STARflex versus Amplatzer devices for percutaneous closure of small to moderate (up to 18 mm) atrial septal defects. *Am Heart J* 2004;148:507–510.
38. Amin Z, Hijazi ZM, Bass JL, et al. Erosion of Amplatzer septal occluder device after closure of secundum atrial septal defects: Review of registry of complications and recommendations to minimize future risk. *Catheter Cardiovasc Interv* 2004;63:496–502.
39. Krumsdorf U, Ostermayer S, Billinger K, et al. Incidence and clinical course of thrombus formation on atrial septal defect and patient foramen ovale closure devices in 1,000 consecutive patients. *J Am Coll Cardiol* 2004;43:302–309.
40. Davia JE, Cheitlin MD, Bedynek JL. Sinus venosus atrial septal defect: Analysis of fifty cases. *Am Heart J* 1973;85:177–185.
41. Raghib G, Ruttenberg HD, Anderson RC, et al. Termination of left superior vena cava in left atrium, atrial septal defect, and absence of coronary sinus: A developmental complex. *Circulation* 1965;31:906–918.

CHAPTER 31 ■ ATRIOVENTRICULAR SEPTAL DEFECTS

FRANK CETTA, MD, L. LUANN MINICH, MD, WILLIAM D. EDWARDS, MD,
JOSEPH A. DEARANI, MD, AND FRANCISCO J. PUGA, MD

ACKNOWLEDGMENT

The authors would like to acknowledge the contributions of Robert H. Feldt, M.D. He was the lead author of this chapter in previous editions. Doctor Feldt died in 2004. He was a mentor and friend to many clinicians in this field. His dedication to improved care for patients with congenital heart disease and his contributions to advance the science of congenital cardiology are missed and remembered.

NOMENCLATURE

Atrioventricular septal defects (AVSD) are a group of anomalies that share a defect of the atrioventricular septum and abnormalities of the atrioventricular valves. The terms "atrioventricular canal defects" or "endocardial cushion defects" also describe these lesions but, for the purposes of this chapter, the term *atrioventricular septal defect* will be used. These lesions are divided into partial and complete forms. In partial AVSD, a primum atrial septal defect (ASD) is always present and there are two distinct mitral and tricuspid valve annuli. The mitral valve invariably is cleft. The complete form also includes a primum ASD, but it is contiguous with an inlet ventricular septal defect (VSD) and the common atrioventricular valve has a single annulus. Similarly, the clinical manifestations and management of these patients depend on the extent and severity of the lesions present.

Several classifications have been used to describe AVSDs. *Transitional AVSD* is a subtype of partial AVSD. This term is used when a partial AVSD also has a small inlet VSD that is partially occluded by dense chordal attachments to the ventricular septum. *Intermediate AVSD* is a subtype of complete AVSD that has distinct right and left atrioventricular valve orifices despite having only one common annulus. These separate orifices are referred to as right and left atrioventricular valve orifices rather than tricuspid and mitral. This also is true when describing the valves after repair of complete AVSD. Unfortunately, the terms "transitional" and "intermediate" have been confused in the literature. Rather than relying on the terminology of these subtypes, the clinician, echocardiographer, and surgeon should communicate by simply describing the anatomy and shunting observed (Fig. 31.1).

Surgical repair of AVSD has been one of the great successes of the last several decades of congenital cardiac surgery. Studer et al. (1) reported average operative mortality <2%. Long-term survival has been excellent. A cumulative 20-year survival of 95% has been reported (2). However, at least 25% of patients (3) await reoperation, most commonly because of progressive left atrioventricular valve regurgitation or relief of left ventricular outflow tract obstruction.

DEMOGRAPHICS

AVSDs account for 4% to 5% of congenital heart disease and an estimated occurrence of 0.19 in 1,000 live births (4,5). In a large fetal echocardiography experience, AVSD was the most common anomaly detected, constituting 18% of abnormal fetal hearts (6). *In utero* diagnosis of an AVSD is readily made on routine fetal four-chamber imaging. Gender distribution is approximately equal or may show a slight female preponderance (4).

About 40% to 45% of children with Down syndrome have congenital heart disease, and among these, approximately 40% have an AVSD, usually the complete form (4). Complete AVSDs also occur in patients with heterotaxy syndromes (more common with asplenia than with polysplenia). Common atrium has been associated with Ellis–van Creveld syndrome.

EMBRYOGENESIS

Faulty development of the endocardial cushions and of the atrioventricular septum is thought to be responsible for the broad range of AVSDs. In partial AVSDs, incomplete fusion of the superior and inferior endocardial cushions results in a cleft in the midportion of the anterior mitral leaflet, often associated with mitral regurgitation. In contrast, complete AVSD is associated with lack of fusion between the superior and inferior cushions and, consequently, with the formation of separate anterior and posterior bridging leaflets along the subjacent ventricular septum (Fig. 31.2).

Failure of the endocardial cushions to fuse creates a defect in the atrioventricular septum. The primum atrial septal component of this defect is usually large. This results in downward displacement of the anterior mitral leaflet to the level of the septal tricuspid leaflet (7). In AVSDs, the atrioventricular valves have the same septal insertion level in contrast to the leaflet arrangement in the normal heart (Fig. 31.3). The distance from the cardiac crux to the left ventricular apex is foreshortened, and the distance from the apex to the aortic valve is increased. This is in contrast to the normal heart, in which the two distances are roughly equal (Fig. 31.4). In AVSDs the disproportion between the two distances causes anterior displacement of the left ventricular outflow tract (LVOT). As a result, the LVOT is longer and narrower than normal and produces the "gooseneck" deformity. After surgical repair of the defect, progressive subaortic stenosis may develop (8).

Since the dextrodorsal conus cushion contributes to the development of the right atrioventricular valve and the outflow tracts lie adjacent to their respective inflow tracts, AVSDs

AVSD Summary

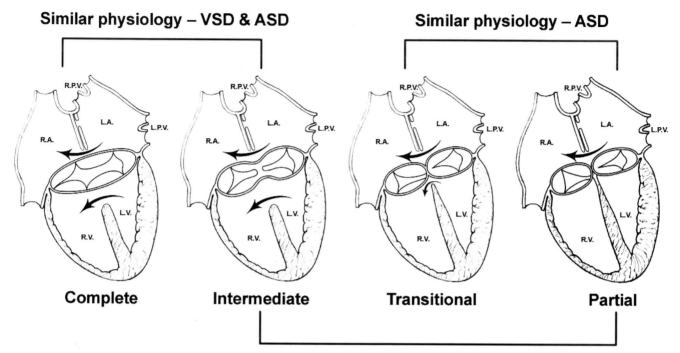

Similar physiology – VSD & ASD

Similar physiology – ASD

Complete   **Intermediate**   **Transitional**   **Partial**

Similar AV valve anatomy:
A tongue of tissue divides the common AV valve
into a right and left component by connecting the
anterior and posterior "bridging" leaflets centrally

FIGURE 31.1 Summary of AVSD. Anatomic and physiologic similarities between the different forms of atrioventricular septal defect (AVSD) are illustrated. Complete AVSDs have one annulus with large interatrial and interventricular communications. Intermediate defects (one annulus, two orifices) are a subtype of complete AVSD. Complete AVSDs have physiology of ventricular septal defects (VSD) and atrial septal defects (ASD). In contrast, partial AVSDs have physiology of ASDs. Transitional defects are a form of partial AVSD in which a small inlet VSD is also present. Partial defects and the intermediate form of complete AVSD share a similar anatomic feature: A tongue of tissue divides the common atrioventricular valve into distinct right and left orifices. LA, left atrium; LPV, left pulmonary vein; LV, left ventricle; RA, right atrium; RPV, right pulmonary vein; RV, right ventricle (with permission of Patrick W. O'Leary, MD).

may be associated with conotruncal anomalies, such as tetralogy of Fallot and double-outlet right ventricle. In addition, shift of the atrioventricular valve orifice may result in connection of the valve primarily to only one ventricle, creating disproportionate or unbalanced ventricles.

PARTIAL ATRIOVENTRICULAR SEPTAL DEFECT

Pathology

In partial AVSD, the mitral and tricuspid annuli are separate. The most frequent form of partial AVSD consists of a primum ASD and a cleft anterior mitral valve leaflet (Figs. 31.5 and 31.6). Most primum ASDs are large and located anteroinferiorly to the fossa ovalis. The defect is bordered by a crescentic rim of atrial septal tissue posterosuperiorly and by mitral-tricuspid

valvular continuity anteroinferiorly. These defects are not amenable to transcatheter device closure because of their proximity to the atrioventricular valves.

The mitral and tricuspid valves achieve the same septal insertion level because the mitral annulus is displaced toward the apex. As a result, the deficient atrioventricular septum is associated with an interatrial communication rather than an interventricular or right atrial to left ventricular communication. Nonetheless, the defect imparts a scooped-out appearance to the inlet ventricular septum, and the distance from mitral annulus to the left ventricular apex is less than the distance from the aortic annulus to the apex (Fig. 31.4).

The cleft in the anterior mitral leaflet is directed toward the midportion of the ventricular septum, along the anteroinferior rim of the septal defect (Fig. 31.7). In contrast, isolated mitral clefts (not otherwise associated with AVSD) are directed toward the aortic valve annulus (9). The mitral orifice is triangular rather than elliptical as in a normal heart and resembles a mirror-image tricuspid orifice. The cleft mitral valve usually

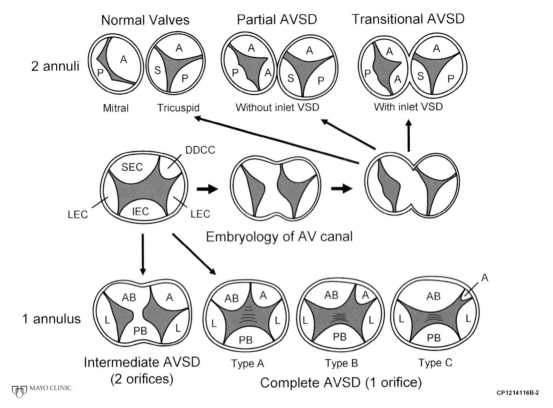

FIGURE 31.2 Diagram of the embryologic development of the atrioventricular canal region and the spectrum of AVSD, including partial, transitional, complete, and intermediate forms. A, anterior leaflet; AB, anterior bridging leaflet; DDCC, dextrodorsal conus cushion; IEC, inferior endocardial cushion; LEC, lateral endocardial cushion; P, posterior leaflet; PB, posterior bridging leaflet; S, septal leaflet; SEC, superior endocardial cushion; L, lateral leaflet.

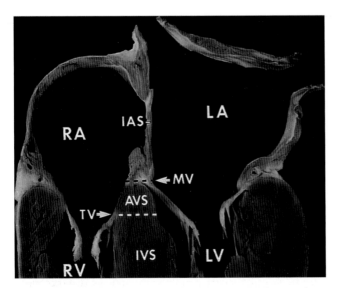

FIGURE 31.3 Atrioventricular septum in the normal heart (four-chamber view). The atrioventricular septum (AVS) lies between the right atrium (RA) and the left ventricle (LV) with the interatrial septum (IAS) above and the interventricular septum (IVS) below. The septal tricuspid leaflet (TV) normally inserts at a lower (more apical) level than the anterior mitral leaflet (MV). LA, left atrium; RV, right ventricle. (From Edwards WD. Applied anatomy of the heart. In: Brandenburg RO, Fuster V, Giuliani ER, et al., eds. *Cardiology: Fundamentals and Practice*. Vol. 1. Chicago: Year Book Medical, 1987:47–109; with permission of Mayo Foundation.)

is regurgitant and, with time, becomes thickened and exhibits secondary hemodynamic alterations in morphology that resemble mitral valve prolapse.

The most common associated anomalies with partial AVSD are a secundum ASD and persistence of a left superior vena cava connecting to the coronary sinus. Less frequently, pulmonary stenosis, tricuspid stenosis or atresia, cor triatriatum, coarctation of the aorta, patent ductus arteriosus, membranous VSD, pulmonary venous anomalies, and hypoplastic left ventricle have been reported (10–12).

Clinical Manifestations

Although patients with partial AVSD may be asymptomatic until adulthood, symptoms of excess pulmonary blood flow typically occur in childhood. Tachypnea and poor weight gain occur most commonly when the defect is associated with moderate or severe mitral valve regurgitation or with other hemodynamically significant cardiac anomalies. Patients with primum ASDs usually have earlier and more severe symptoms, including growth failure, than patients with secundum ASDs.

An uncomplicated primum ASD often is discovered in young children when echocardiography is performed to investigate a murmur. The murmur has typical systolic ejection qualities and is best heard over the upper left sternal border with radiation to the lung fields. The second heart sound is widely split and fixed during respiration. A holosystolic murmur owing to mitral regurgitation through the cleft may be

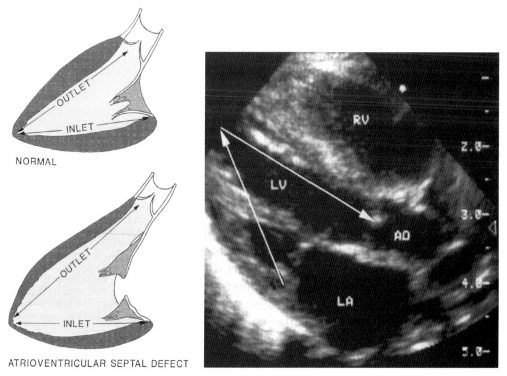

FIGURE 31.4 Elongate left ventricular outflow tract (LVOT) in atrioventricular septal defect (AVSD): Because of deficiency of the ventricular component of the atrioventricular septum and the "sprung" atrioventricular junction, the distance from the LV apex to the posterior left atrioventricular valve annulus is 20% to 25% shorter than the distance from the apex to the aortic annulus. Ao, aorta; LA, left atrium; LV, left ventricle; RV, right ventricle (with permission of Robert H. Anderson, MD).

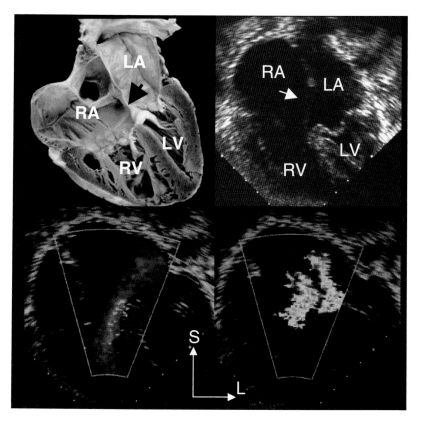

FIGURE 31.5 Top left: Four-chamber anatomic specimen demonstrating a large primum atrial septal defect (ASD) (*arrow*), severe right atrium (RA) and right ventricle (RV) dilation and connection of both atrioventricular valves to the septum at the same level. **Top right:** Corresponding apical four-chamber diastolic image demonstrating severe RA and RV dilation owing to a large primum ASD (*arrow*). **Bottom left:** Color Doppler scan from the apex, demonstrating a large left-to-right shunt crossing the primum ASD in diastole (red flow jet). **Bottom right:** Systolic color flow Doppler displaying moderate right and left atrioventricular valve regurgitation. LA, left atrium.

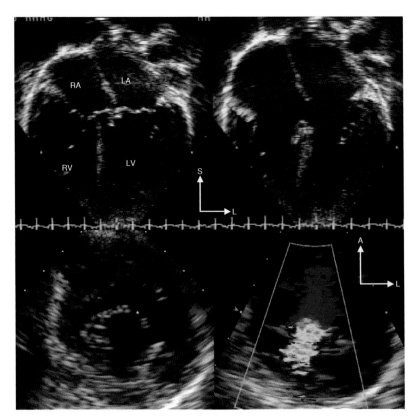

FIGURE 31.6 Partial AVSD: Atrioventricular valve anatomy. **Top left:** Systolic apical four-chamber image demonstrating that both right and left atrioventricular valves insert onto the crest of the ventricular septum at the same level. **Top right:** Corresponding diastolic frame revealing a large primum ASD. Systolic frames often understate the size of the interatrial communication. There is significant right atrium (RA) and right ventricle (RV) enlargement. **Bottom panels:** These are parasternal short-axis scans focused at the valve leaflet level in the left ventricular inflow. The left panel demonstrates the cleft in the anterior leaflet of the left atrioventricular valve (*asterisk*). The anterior leaflet is made of two separate components that move independently. This creates the diastolic gap in the leaflet (*asterisk*). Color Doppler on the right panel shows considerable regurgitation through the cleft. LA, left atrium; LV, left ventricle.

heard at the apex. A low-pitched middiastolic murmur heard at the left lower sternal border may be present if the shunt is large or if significant mitral regurgitation is present.

Echocardiography

Two-dimensional echocardiography is the primary imaging technique for diagnosing AVSDs (13–15). It is particularly useful for delineating the morphology of the atrioventricular valves. In larger patients or in patients with associated complex abnormalities, transesophageal echocardiography can provide incremental diagnostic information.

The internal cardiac crux is the most consistent echocardiographic imaging landmark. The apical four-chamber imaging plane clearly visualizes the internal crux. The primum ASD is seen as an absence of the lower atrial septum. The size of the primum ASD is made reliably from this imaging position (Fig. 31.8). Accurate visualization of the cardiac crux also permits assessment of the atrioventricular valves. Several two-dimensional echocardiographic features are shared by all forms of AVSD: Deficiency of a portion of the inlet ventricular

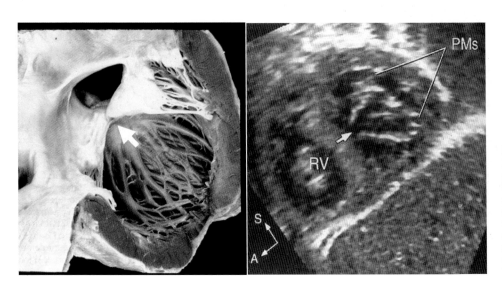

FIGURE 31.7 Cleft left atrioventricular valve: **Left:** In AVSD, the cleft in the anterior leaflet of the left atrioventricular valve is typically oriented toward the midportion of the ventricular septum (*arrow*) along the anterior-inferior rim of the septal defect. **Right:** Subcostal sagittal image demonstrating the septal orientation of the cleft. A, anterior; PMs, papillary muscles; RV, right ventricle; S, superior.

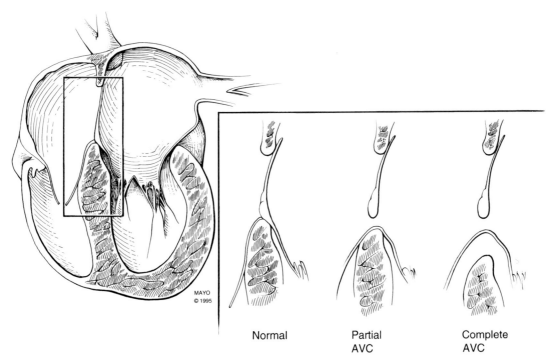

Normal   Partial   Complete
                AVC   AVC

FIGURE 31.8 AVSD and the internal cardiac crux. The internal cardiac crux is best visualized in the apical four-chamber imaging plane. Normally, the mitral insertion appears to be more superiorly fixed than the corresponding tricuspid septal leaflet. In all forms of AVSD, both right and left atrioventricular valve components insert at the same level on the crest of the inflow ventricular septum. A cleft in the mitral valve occurs in conjunction with the downward displacement of the anterior leaflet. In partial AVSD, there is a defect in the lower fatty portion of the atrial septum (i.e., within the atrial ventricular septum). In complete AVSD, there is a defect beneath the atrioventricular valves in the inflow ventricular septum. In general, these easily recognized anatomic features distinguish normal from partial and complete AVSD. AVC, atrioventricular canal.

septum, inferior displacement of the atrioventricular valves, and attachment of a portion of the left atrioventricular (mitral) valve to the septum. The atrioventricular valves are displaced toward the ventricles, with the septal portions inserting at the same level onto the crest of the ventricular septum. Therefore, in these defects, the two separate atrioventricular valve orifices are equidistant from the cardiac apex.

In the transitional form of partial AVSD, there is aneurysmal replacement of a portion of the inlet ventricular septum (16) (Fig. 31.9). Although small shunts may occur, this so-called tricuspid pouch usually obstructs any shunting at the ventricular level. Spectral and color flow Doppler hemodynamic assessment are useful to determine the severity of atrioventricular valve stenosis or insufficiency and to quantitate right ventricular systolic pressure. Doppler echocardiography often is not useful for evaluating the degree of mitral stenosis in the setting of a primum ASD that will decompress flow and pressure from the left atrium into the right atrium.

Other mitral valve abnormalities are typical with both the partial and complete forms of AVSD (Fig. 31.10). The most common abnormality, a cleft, is best visualized from the parasternal and subcostal short-axis imaging planes. Rarely, parachute mitral valve and double-orifice mitral valve also occur.

In the normal heart, the aortic valve is wedged between the mitral and tricuspid annuli. In AVSD the aortic valve is displaced or "sprung" anteriorly (Fig. 31.11). This anterior displacement creates an elongate, so-called gooseneck deformity of the LVOT. (Fig. 31.12) LVOT obstruction may occur in all forms of AVSD. It is more frequent when two atrioventricular valve orifices are present than when there is a common orifice. The superior bridging leaflet attaches to the crest of the ventricular septum, causing the outflow tract to become elongated and consequently narrowed. In addition, discrete subaortic fibromuscular ridges, septal hypertrophy, abnormal left atrioventricular valve chordal attachments, and abnormally oriented papillary muscles can exacerbate subaortic stenosis. LVOT obstruction may be subtle and therefore not appreciated during preoperative echocardiographic assessment. Obstruction may develop *de novo* after initial repair of the AVSD and closure of the mitral valve cleft (17) (Fig. 31.13). The LVOT obstruction often is progressive.

Detailed and comprehensive echocardiographic assessment is required to evaluate associated lesions and determine their significance. Tetralogy of Fallot, double-outlet right ventricle, pulmonary valve atresia, and anomalous pulmonary venous connections are associated with AVSDs but are less frequent with partial defects. In contrast, atrioventricular valve abnormalities and left ventricular hypoplasia are more frequent in two-orifice atrioventricular connections. Coarctation of the aorta occurs with equal frequency in partial and complete AVSD.

(text continues on page 654)

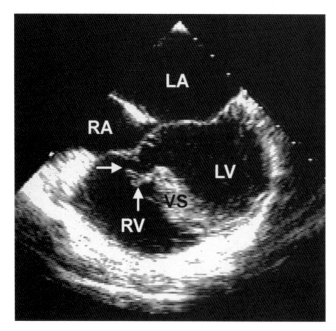

FIGURE 31.9 Transitional AVSD. Note the membranous aneurysm in the inflow ventricular septum (*arrows*). There is a primum atrial septal defect (ASD); thus, functionally, the entity presents as a partial AVSD. There can be restrictive ventricular septal defects (VSDs) in the inflow aneurysmal membrane. This patient did not have additional features that occur in this form of AVSD, such as a restrictive VSD, parachute mitral valve, or left ventricular outflow tract (LVOT) obstruction. LA, left atrium; LV, left ventricle; RA, right atrium; RV, right ventricle; VS, ventricular septum.

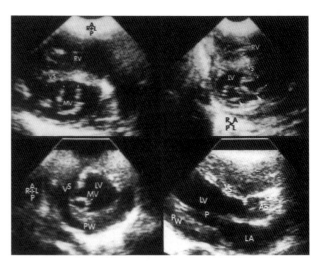

FIGURE 31.10 Echocardiographic features of associated anomalies with partial AVSDs. **Top left:** Cleft mitral valve. The anterior leaflet of the mitral valve (MV) has a characteristic break (*small arrows*) that represents a cleft in the anterior leaflet. This feature is common to both partial and complete forms of AVSDs. **Top right:** Double-orifice atrioventricular valve. Typically, a double-orifice mitral valve is encountered with partial AVSD. Each papillary muscle receives a separate atrioventricular valve orifice (*large arrows*). The anterolateral valve orifice is usually cleft (*small arrows*). **Bottom left:** Parachute valve. A single atrioventricular valve orifice inserts into a single or dominant papillary muscle. The mitral orifice (*arrow*) is often small and may result in stenosis. A, anterior; I, inferior; L, left; LA, left atrium; LV, left ventricle; P, posterior; PW, posterior wall; R, right; RV, right ventricle; S, superior; VS, ventricular septum. (Modified from Seward JB, Tajik AJ, Edwards WD, et al. *Two-Dimensional Echocardiographic Atlas.* Vol. 1. *Congenital Heart Disease.* New York: Springer-Verlag, 1987:270–292, with permission.)

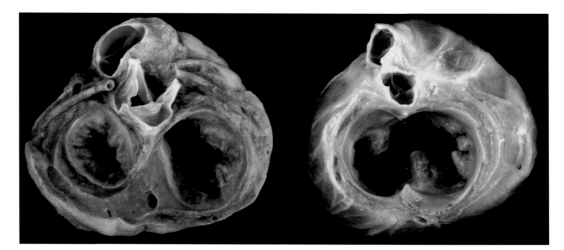

FIGURE 31.11 Sprung aortic valve: **Left:** Normal heart pathologic specimen cut in short axis at the base demonstrating where the atrioventricular junction has a figure-of-8 configuration. **Right:** Similar projection in an AVSD heart where the atrioventricular junction is "sprung." The aortic valve (instead of being wedged) between the atrioventricular valve annuli is anterior of the sprung atrioventricular junction.

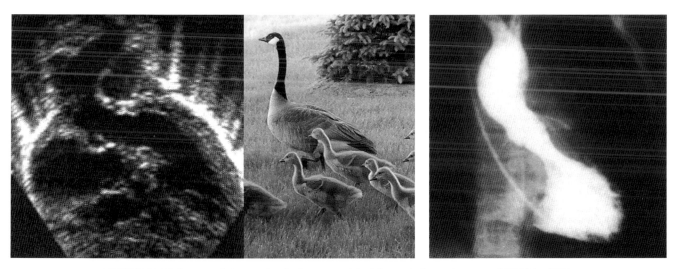

FIGURE 31.12 Because of the anterior displacement of the left ventricular outflow tract (LVOT) in AVSD, the elongate LVOT has been described as a "goose neck" with echocardiographic and angiographic imaging.

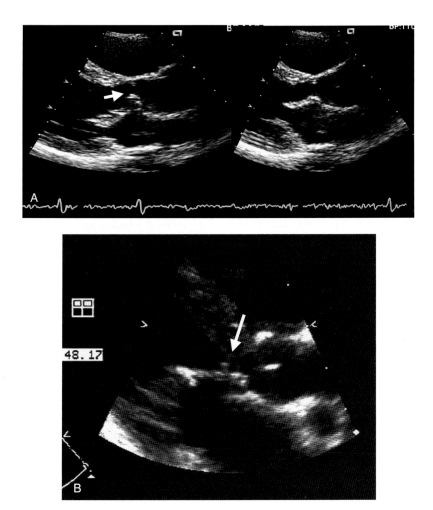

FIGURE 31.13 A: Left ventricular outflow tract (LVOT) obstruction: systolic (**left**) and diastolic (**right**) echocardiographics demonstrating LVOT obstruction in a 17-year-old who had repair of a partial AVSD at age 15 months. LVOT obstruction (*arrow*) is usually progressive and may be undetected at time of initial repair. **B:** LVOT obstruction: parasternal long-axis projection demonstrating left AV valve attachments (*arrow*) to the septum in a patient after repair of partial AVSD. Ten percent of patients with AVSD may require reoperation to relieve LVOT obstruction. Progressive LVOT obstruction is more common in partial than in complete AVSD. Mechanisms of LVOT obstruction include attachments of superior bridging leaflet to ventricular septum, extension of the anterolateral papillary muscle into the LVOT, discrete fibrous subaortic stenosis, tissue from an aneurysm of the membranous septum bowing into the LVOT.

653

Radiography

Typically, chest radiography demonstrates cardiomegaly and prominent pulmonary vascular markings. Because the jet of mitral regurgitation often is directed into the right atrium, right atrial enlargement rather than left atrial enlargement may be apparent.

Electrocardiography and Electrophysiology

The position of the AVSD dictates the position of the atrioventricular conduction tissues. Accordingly, the atrioventricular node is displaced posteriorly, near the orifice of the coronary sinus, and the His bundle is displaced inferiorly, along the inferior rim of the septal defect. The displacement of the atrioventricular conduction tissues, in conjunction with loss of ventricular septal myocardium, results in characteristic electrocardiographic (ECG) features (Fig. 31.14).

Sinus rhythm is present in most patients with a primum ASD. Prolongation of the P-R interval in relation to the patient's age and heart rate, seen in 18% to 70% of patients, is due primarily to increased intra-atrial conduction time from high right atrium to low septal right atrium (18). P-wave changes indicating right atrial, left atrial, or biatrial enlargement are seen in 54% of patients. The mean QRS axis in the frontal plane ranges from −30 degrees to −120 degrees, with most axes directed between −30 degrees and −90 degrees (Fig 31.15). Anatomic and electrophysiologic studies show that this abnormal vectorcardiographic pattern is associated with a specific anomaly of the conduction system (19,20). Right ventricular volume overload results in right ventricular hypertrophy and some variation of the rsR′ or RSR′ pattern in the right precordial leads in 84% of patients; 10% of patients have a qR pattern. Patients with significant mitral regurgitation may have evidence of left ventricular hypertrophy.

Except for prolonged intra-atrial conduction time, other intracardiac electrophysiologic measurements usually are normal, including sinus node and atrioventricular node function, His–Purkinje conduction time, and atrial and ventricular refractory periods (18).

Cardiac Catheterization and Angiography

Cardiac catheterization and angiography rarely are required for diagnosis or management of patients with a partial AVSD. Current echocardiographic techniques accurately define the anatomy and physiology of this lesion. In an older patient, cardiac catheterization may have a role in assessing the degree of pulmonary vascular obstructive disease or coronary artery disease.

A large left-to-right shunt can be demonstrated at the atrial level by a significantly higher oxygen saturation sampled from the right atrium compared with the blood in the inferior and superior vena cavae. Because of the anatomic position of the ASD, blood samples taken from the inflow portion of the right ventricle may have elevated oxygen saturation. The calculated left-to-right shunt often exceeds 50%. In most patients, right ventricular pressure is <60% of systemic pressure. A significant increase in calculated pulmonary vascular resistance is unusual in infants (1). Left ventricular angiography will demonstrate the elongate gooseneck deformation of the LVOT (Fig. 31.12).

Surgical Treatment of Partial Atrioventricular Septal Defect

The objectives of surgical repair include closure of the interatrial communication and restoration and preservation of left atrioventricular valve competence. These objectives can be accomplished by careful approximation of the edges of the valve cleft with interrupted nonabsorbable sutures. On occasion, it is necessary to add eccentric annuloplasty sutures to correct persistent central leaks. The repair is completed by closure of the interatrial communication (usually with an autologous pericardial patch), avoiding injury to the conduction tissue (21). This repair results in a two-leaflet valve (Fig. 31.16). Alternatively, if the left atrioventricular valve is to be considered a trileaflet valve, with the cleft viewed as a commissure, surgical repair demands that this commissure be left unsutured and that various annuloplastic sutures be placed to promote coaptation of the three leaflets. These morphologic concepts and surgical methods, favored by Carpentier (22) and Piccoli et al. (23), have not yet provided superior results.

The risk of hospital death for the surgical repair of partial AVSD is approximately 3%. Determinants of hospital mortality include congestive heart failure, cyanosis, failure to thrive, age at operation of <4 years, and moderate to severe left atrioventricular valve regurgitation. In a series of 334 patients from Mayo Clinic, 20- and 40-year survivals after repair of partial AVSD were 87% and 76%, respectively. Closure of the mitral cleft and age <20 years at time of operation were associated with better survival. Reoperation was performed for 11% of these patients. Repair of residual/recurrent mitral valve regurgitation or stenosis was the most common reason for reoperation (24). (See Reoperation after Repair of AVSD section.)

A low frequency of postoperative arrhythmias has been noted. Bradyarrhythmias, including severe sinus node dysfunction, may occur. The finding of surgical complete heart block has been rare. Permanent pacemaker implantation has been required for these patients. Late onset of atrial flutter has been rare.

Special Forms of Partial Atrioventricular Septal Defect

Malaligned Atrial Septum or Double-Outlet Right Atrium

Deviation of the atrial septum to the left of the atrioventricular junction has been reported rarely (25,26). When this occurs, both the right and left atrioventricular valves are visualized from the right atrium, which is connected to both ventricles through a large primum ASD. If deviation of the atrial septum to the left is extreme, the pulmonary veins may be isolated and obstructed, simulating cor triatriatum. Although the term "double-outlet" right atrium has been applied to this lesion (27), it is truly a form of AVSD.

Common Atrium

Common atrium is characterized by near absence of the atrial septum. In the presence of two ventricles, it always is associated with an AVSD (28). The pathologic spectrum of this lesion ranges from patients with coexistent primum and secundum ASDs to others who lack the entire septum except for a small muscular cord. Patients with asplenia syndrome

(text continues on page 657)

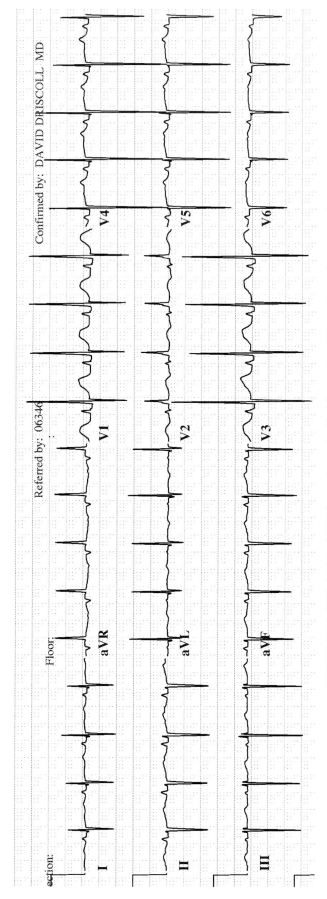

FIGURE 31.14 ECG: A 12-lead ECG from a 3-month-old with complete AVSD. Left axis deviation and right ventricular hypertrophy are present.

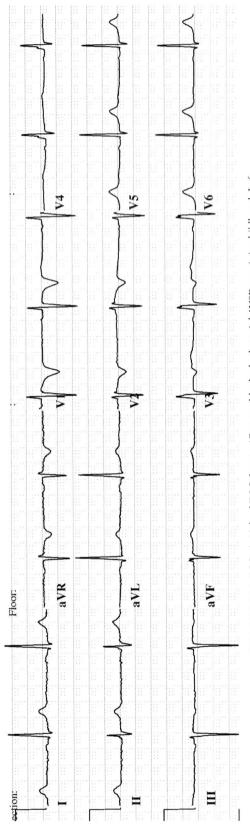

FIGURE 31.15 ECG: A 12-lead ECG from a 17-year-old who had partial AVSD repair in childhood. Left axis deviation and nonspecific T-wave changes are present.

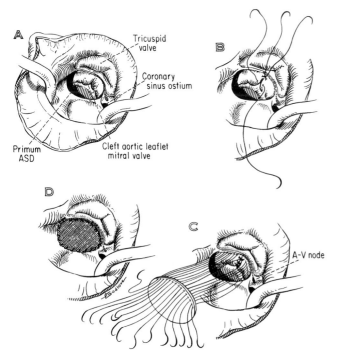

FIGURE 31.16 Repair of a partial AVSD. **A:** Surgical exposure. **B:** Closure of the mitral valve cleft. **C:** Prosthetic patch closure of an ostium primum defect. **D:** Repair completed. ASD, atrial septal defect; A-V, atrioventricular. (From Danielson GK. Endocardial cushion defects. In: Ravitch MM, Welch KJ, Benson CD, et al., eds. *Pediatric Surgery*. 3rd ed. Vol. 1. Chicago: Year Book Medical, 1979:720–726, with permission.)

with concomitant complex congenital heart disease compose the latter group. In these cases, transposition of the great arteries, double-outlet right ventricle, univentricular atrioventricular connection, and anomalous pulmonary venous connections frequently are encountered.

Clinical Manifestations. Most patients with common atrium present in infancy with symptoms of excess pulmonary blood flow, fatigue, tachypnea, and failure to thrive. However, if increased pulmonary vascular resistance develops, the left-to-right shunt decreases and the child will thrive. In general, these patients are symptomatic earlier in life than patients with only a primum ASD.

The precordium is hyperactive with a prominent right ventricular impulse. The second heart sound is widely split and fixed with respiration. The intensity of the pulmonary component of the second sound is proportionate to the severity of pulmonary hypertension. A crescendo–decrescendo systolic ejection murmur is present over the upper left sternal border and radiates to the axillae and to the back. A distinct holosystolic murmur of mitral valve regurgitation may be heard at the apex. A middiastolic murmur commonly is detected over the lower left sternal border resulting from an increase in right atrial to right ventricular blood flow. Patients with common atrium frequently have anomalies of cardiac and abdominal situs and asplenia.

The radiographic and electrocardiographic characteristics of patients with common atrium are indistinguishable from those with other forms of AVSD.

Echocardiography of Common Atrium. The subcostal four-chamber imaging plane is most suitable for accurate diagnosis. A muscle bundle or band coursing through the atrium should not be interpreted as an atrial septum.

Cardiac Catheterization and Angiography. The hemodynamic diagnosis of common atrium depends on the demonstration of complete mixing of systemic and pulmonary venous blood. The oxygen saturations of pulmonary and systemic arterial blood are nearly identical. Pulmonary blood flow exceeds systemic flow, except in patients with severe pulmonary vascular obstructive disease. Right ventricular pressure is increased more often than in secundum ASD or partial AVSD. If definitive repair is delayed, significant pulmonary vascular obstructive disease may develop more easily than in patients with secundum ASD or partial AVSD.

Treatment. Prior to surgical repair, medical therapy usually is instituted when signs and symptoms of excess pulmonary blood flow and failure to thrive are present. Digoxin and diuretic therapy are traditional forms of therapy. Common atrium requires surgical repair, which should be performed early in life because the patient usually has symptoms and is at risk for developing pulmonary vascular obstructive disease.

COMPLETE ATRIOVENTRICULAR SEPTAL DEFECT

Pathology

The complete form of AVSD is characterized by a large septal defect with interatrial and interventricular components and a common atrioventricular valve that spans the entire septal defect (28) (Fig. 31.17). The septal defect extends to the level of the membranous ventricular septum, which is usually deficient or absent.

The common atrioventricular valve has five leaflets. The posterior bridging leaflet drapes over the inlet ventricular septum and conceptually represents fusion of the septal tricuspid leaflet and the inferior half of the anterior mitral leaflet. Two lateral leaflets correspond to the posterior tricuspid and posterior mitral leaflets in a normal heart. The right-sided anterior leaflet, in essence, represents the normal anterior tricuspid leaflet, and the so-called anterior bridging leaflet corresponds to the superior half of the anterior mitral leaflet. The extent to which the anterior bridging leaflet actually straddles into the right ventricle varies considerably and has formed the basis for a classification system of complete AVSDs into types A, B, and C (see below). The common atrioventricular valve may be divided into distinct right and left orifices by a tongue of tissue that connects the two bridging leaflets, representing the intermediate form of AVSD.

Beneath the five commissures are five papillary muscles. The two left-sided papillary muscles are oriented closer together than in a normal heart, such that the lateral leaflet is smaller than a normal posterior mitral leaflet. In addition, the two papillary muscles often are rotated counterclockwise, such that the posterior muscle is farther from the septum than normal and the anterior muscle is closer to the septum. This papillary muscle arrangement, in conjunction with prominence of an anterolateral muscle bundle, may contribute to progressive LVOT obstruction. Moreover, the leaflets are prone to develop progressive regurgitation, and, with time, they become thickened and exhibit hemodynamic and

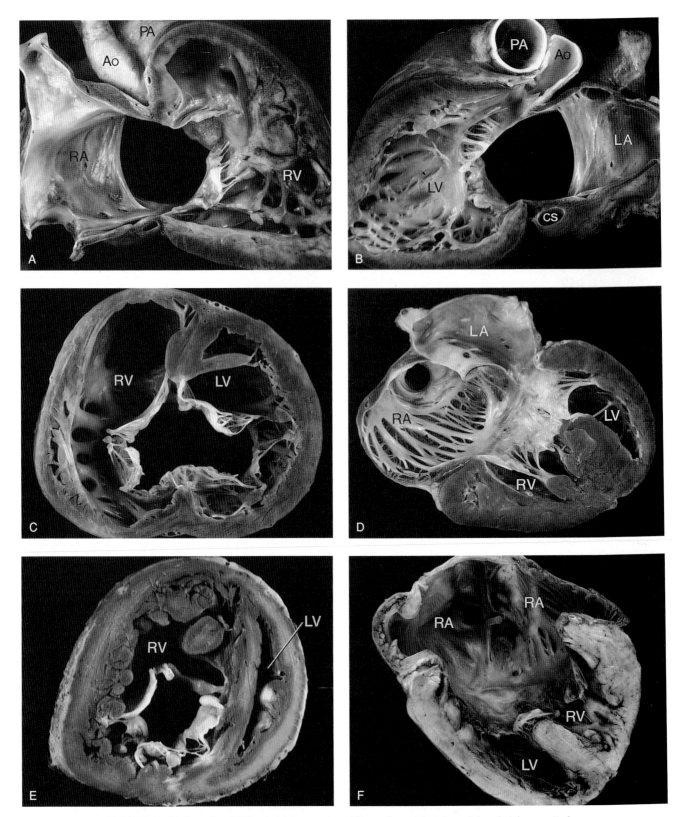

FIGURE 31.17 Complete AVSD. **A:** Right anterior oblique view with right atrial and right ventricular free walls removed, demonstrating a large septal defect. **B:** Left posterior oblique view (same specimens as in **A**) with left atrial and left ventricular free walls removed, showing the same septal defect. **C:** Short-axis view, illustrating a type A common atrioventricular valve with five leaflets. **D:** Four-chamber view, showing secondary right ventricular hypertrophy and right atrial dilation. **E:** Short-axis view of a biventricular specimen removed during cardiac transplantation, showing an unbalanced form of AVSD with dilation of a common inlet right ventricle, leftward septal bowing, and a hypoplastic left ventricle. **F:** Four-chamber view of a complete AVSD associated with right atrial isomerism, mirror-image ventricles (L-loop ventricular inversion), and asplenia. Ao, aorta; CS, coronary sinus; LA, left atrium; LV, left ventricle; PA, pulmonary artery; RA, right atrium; RV, right ventricle.

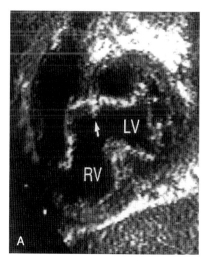
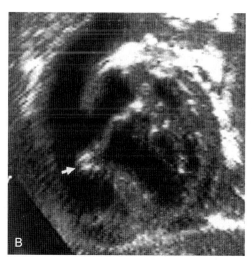
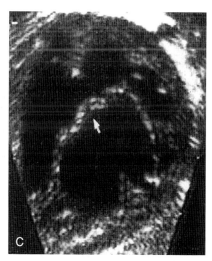

FIGURE 31.18 Echocardiographic findings in a complete AVSD. **A:** Type A complete AVSD. The defect is characterized by insertion of the atrioventricular valves to the crest of the ventricular septum (VS). **B:** Type B complete AVSD. The defect is characterized by dominant insertion of the anterior leaflets into papillary muscles in the right ventricle (RV). In this example, the anterior bridging leaflet inserts onto the crest of the ventricular septum, as well as onto a large ventricular papillary muscle (P). **C:** Type C AVSD. The anterior leaflet is unattached (*small arrows*) and overrides the crest of the ventricular septum. The free anterior leaflet does not insert onto the crest of the ventricular septum. I, inferior; L, left; LA, left atrium; LV, left ventricle; R, right; RA, right atrium; S, superior. (Modified from Seward JB, Tajik AJ, Edwards WD, et al. *Two-Dimensional Echocardiographic Atlas. Vol. 1. Congenital Heart Disease.* New York: Springer-Verlag, 1987:270–292, with permission.)

structural changes similar to that associated with mitral valve prolapse (29).

The potential for interventricular communication exists not only along the septal surface between the two bridging leaflets but also, in most cases, at the interchordal spaces beneath the leaflets. The posterior bridging leaflet characteristically overhangs the ventricular septum and has extensive septal chordal attachments; occasionally chordal fusion obliterates the interchordal spaces beneath this leaflet. The anatomic relationship between the anterior bridging leaflet and the ventricular septum is variable and forms the basis for a subclassification described by Rastelli et al. (30) (Fig. 31.18). For historical purposes this scheme is described below. In the modern era its clinical and surgical significance has become less important.

In type A (most common), the anterior bridging leaflet inserts entirely along the anterosuperior rim of the ventricular septum. It forms a true commissure with the right-sided anterior leaflet. Beneath this commissure is either a distinct medial papillary muscle or, more commonly, multiple direct chordal insertions along the septum. Interventricular communication beneath the anterior bridging leaflet may be minimal or absent in some cases owing to extensive interchordal fusion.

In type B (least common), the anterior bridging leaflet is larger and the right-sided anterior leaflet is smaller than in type A. As a result, the bridging leaflet straddles the septum and is associated with papillary muscle attachment along the septal or moderator band in the right ventricle. Because chordal anchors are not present between the anterior bridging leaflet and the underlying ventricular septum, free interventricular communication exists.

In type C, the anterior bridging leaflet is even larger than in type B, and its medial papillary muscle attachments have fused to the right-sided anterior papillary muscle. As a result, this leaflet is generally very small. Because the anterior bridging leaflet is not attached to the ventricular septum, free interventricular communication is possible, and the leaflet has been described as free floating.

The type of complete AVSD has some bearing on the likelihood of associated lesions. Type A usually is an isolated defect and is frequent in patients with Down syndrome. In contrast, type C is encountered with other complex anomalies, such as tetralogy of Fallot, double-outlet right ventricle, complete transposition of the great arteries, and heterotaxy syndromes (31,32). Coronary artery anomalies, when they occur, tend to be associated with coexistent conotruncal malformations rather than the AVSD. The combination of type C complete AVSD with tetralogy of Fallot is observed in patients with Down's syndrome, whereas double-outlet right ventricle is a feature of patients with asplenia.

Clinical Manifestations

Tachypnea and failure to thrive invariably occur early in infancy as a result of excessive pulmonary blood flow. Virtually all patients with complete AVSD have symptoms by 1 year of age. If these symptoms do not develop early on, the clinician should suspect premature development of pulmonary vascular obstructive disease. Atrioventricular valve regurgitation compounds these problems. After surgical repair, left atrioventricular valve regurgitation is the most common reason for reoperation. A recent study demonstrated that 19% of patients who have had repair developed severe left atrioventricular valve regurgitation (33). In that study preoperative atrioventricular valve regurgitation was an important risk factor for reoperation. Although spontaneous regression of postoperative left atrioventricular valve regurgitation does occur, many of these patients await reoperation.

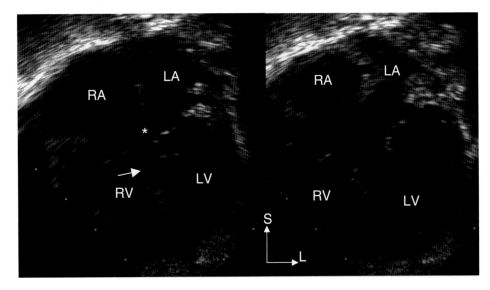

FIGURE 31.19 Complete AVSD: Apical four-chamber images in systole (**left**) and diastole (**right**) demonstrating a complete AVSD with large primum atrial septal defect (ASD) (*asterisk*), large inlet ventricular septal defect (VSD) (*arrow*), and common single-orifice atrioventricular valve. The **right panel** demonstrates the valve opening as a single unit with only lateral "hinge points" visible in this image. Biventricular volume overload and a small secundum ASD are present in this patient.

If severe pulmonary vascular obstructive disease is absent, there may be no systemic arterial oxygen desaturation. The physical examination demonstrates a hyperactive precordium, an accentuated first sound, and the second sound may move with respiration but it is quite variable. Because of elevated pulmonary artery pressures, the pulmonary closure sound is accentuated. A loud holosystolic murmur can be heard along the lower left sternal border and at the cardiac apex if left atrioventricular valve regurgitation is present. A separate crescendo–decrescendo systolic ejection murmur is heard over the upper left sternal border as a result of increased pulmonary blood flow. A middiastolic murmur can be heard along the lower left sternal border and frequently at the apex as a result of increased blood flow across the common atrioventricular valve. However, the physical examination findings of complete AVSD may be indistinguishable from those of an uncomplicated VSD or partial AVSD.

Echocardiography

Two-dimensional echocardiography is the primary diagnostic tool for evaluation of complete AVSDs (15,34). As described earlier, assessment of the internal cardiac crux from the apical and subcostal four-chamber projections provides excellent detail of the size and locations of defects in both the atrial and ventricular septa (Fig. 31.19). Additional secundum ASDs, a fairly common associated finding, can be detected from the subcostal four-chamber coronal view and with clockwise rotation of the transducer from the subcostal sagittal imaging plane (16). The VSD is located posteriorly in the inlet septum. Both right- and left-sided components of the common atrioventricular valve are displaced toward the ventricles and are associated with variable deficiency of the inflow ventricular septum. Spectral and color Doppler serve as adjuncts to assess the sites of shunting, severity of atrioventricular valve regurgitation, and connections of the pulmonary veins. Anomalous pulmonary venous connections are rarely associated with complete AVSDs and can be assessed with two-dimensional and Doppler echocardiography from multiple imaging planes. Fetal echocardiography readily detects complete AVSDs in a standard four-chamber view (Fig. 31.20).

When communicating with a surgeon, the echocardiographer must describe the morphology of the atrioventricular valve in precise detail. The surgeon needs to know the state of the atrioventricular valve orifices and whether a tongue of

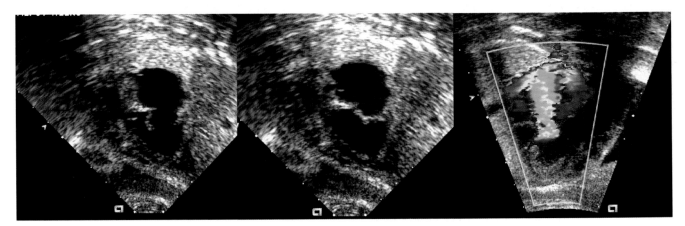

FIGURE 31.20 A 31-week gestation fetal echocardiograph with severe common atrioventricular valve regurgitation: four-chamber images in diastole (**left**), systole (**center**), and systole with color Doppler (**right**) demonstrating a common atrium, common atrioventricular valve, and common ventricle.

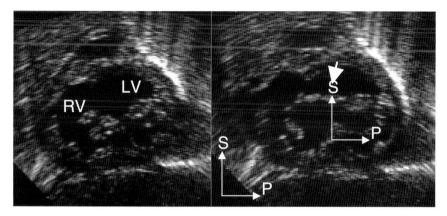

FIGURE 31.21 Subcostal sagittal imaging of common atrioventricular valve: Subcostal sagittal images in systole (**left**) and diastole (**right**) in a patient with complete AVSD. The right panel demonstrates the anterior bridging leaflet (*arrow*) of the common AV valve. This leaflet crosses (bridges) the ventricular septal defect (VSD) anteriorly and is shared by both ventricles. It is not divided into right and left components and has no attachments to the ventricular septum. This morphology is also called free floating or Rastelli's type C. During repair, unlike the naturally divided anterior bridging leaflet (type A), this leaflet must be incised into right and left components before attachment to the VSD patch.

tissue connects the superior and inferior bridging leaflets to form two distinct orifices. The subcostal *en face* view is essential for this determination. This view is obtained with counterclockwise rotation from the four-chamber coronal view until the atrioventricular valve leaflets appear en face (Fig. 31.21). Deliberate superior and inferior angulation of the probe will permit inspection of the cross section of all five valve leaflets. The valve is inspected from the inferior margin of the atrial septum to the superior margin of the ventricular septum (34,35). In the operating room, the transesophageal transgastric short-axis view will aid in this assessment.

Double-orifice left atrioventricular valve occurs rarely in AVSDs. This abnormality is more common when two distinct right and left atrioventricular valve orifices are present. The combined effective valve area of a double-orifice valve is always less than the valve area of a single-orifice valve. This predisposes the valve to postoperative stenosis. Standard subcostal and parasternal short-axis views usually demonstrate the double-orifice valve characteristics (Fig. 31.10).

Another rare association with complete AVSD is a single left ventricular papillary muscle. Similar to the double-orifice valve, a single papillary muscle will reduce the effective valve area. In patients with a single left ventricular papillary muscle, valve repair may be compromised owing to relative leaflet hypoplasia. Echocardiographic imaging techniques for this abnormality are similar to those for double-orifice left atrioventricular valves.

Two-dimensional echocardiography is essential for determining the relative sizes of the ventricular masses. In complete AVSDs that have a common or two distinct valve orifices, relative hypoplasia of one ventricle may occur. The clinical management of patients with unbalanced ventricles will be discussed later in this chapter. The echocardiographer needs to realize that when left ventricular hypoplasia and right ventricular dominance occur (the most frequent form of unbalanced AVSD), associated malformations such as aortic arch hypoplasia and coarctation are common. In contrast, if left ventricular dominance is present, pulmonary valve stenosis or atresia is a common associated defect. If unbalanced ventricles occur in the setting of a single atrioventricular valve orifice, the atrial

and ventricular septa often are malaligned. The subcostal *en face* view delineates the relative sizes of the atrioventricular valve orifices.

Several pitfalls make two-dimensional evaluation of an unbalanced AVSD difficult. First, the severity of valve malalignment may not correlate with the degree of ventricular hypoplasia. Second, a volume-overloaded right ventricle may cause the septum to bow toward the left ventricle, creating the false impression that it is hypoplastic. Third, a large ASD will allow preferential flow across the atrial septum and underfill the left ventricle (Fig. 31.22). Measurements of the relative right- and left-sided valve areas of the common atrioventricular valve have been used to determine the degree of hypoplasia and suitability for a two-ventricle repair (36) (Fig. 31.23). Similarly, van Son et al. (37) used a short-axis assessment of the ventricles with the presumption of normal septal configuration to predict the adequacy of the left ventricular volume after repair (Fig. 31.24).

Radiography

The heart is usually enlarged in patients with complete AVSD. Enlargement of the right atrium is suggested by increased convexity of the right heart border, and left atrial enlargement may give a characteristic flattening of the left heart border. The pulmonary artery is prominent, and the pulmonary vascular markings are increased.

Electrocardiography

Many patients have a prolonged P-R interval (18). Intracardiac studies have revealed increased intra-atrial conduction or prolonged atrioventricular node conduction as the cause of first-degree atrioventricular block. More than 50% of patients meet voltage criteria for atrial enlargement. A superior or northwest QRS axis is common (Fig. 31.15). The QRS axis in the frontal plane lies between −60 degrees and −135 degrees, with most patients having an axis between −90 degrees and

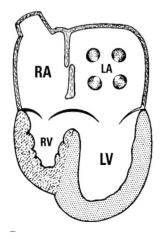
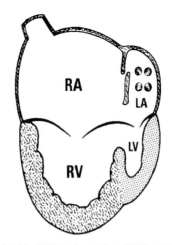

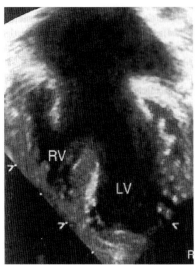
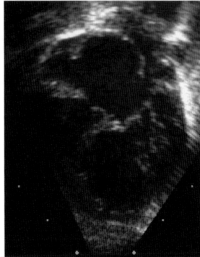

LV Dominant   RV Dominant

FIGURE 31.22 Right versus left ventricular dominance, based on a classification scheme from Bharati and Lev: Left ventricular dominance (**left panels**) and right ventricular dominance (**right panels**) are demonstrated. In the left ventricle–dominant case, the common atrioventricular valve opens predominantly into the left ventricle. Conversely, in the right ventricle–dominant case, the common atrioventricular valve opens predominantly into the right ventricle. LA, left atrium; LV, left ventricle; RA, right atrium; RV, right ventricle.

−120 degrees. Two thirds of the patients have some form of rsR, RSR′, or Rr′ in lead V1, and the rest have a qR or R pattern in the same chest lead, all indicating right ventricular hypertrophy. Left ventricular hypertrophy may also be present.

Cardiac Catheterization and Angiography

Cardiac catheterization and angiography rarely are needed for management of infants with complete AVSD. In an older child, when pulmonary vascular obstructive disease is suspected, there is a role for determining pulmonary vascular resistance. Severe pulmonary vascular obstructive disease (pulmonary vascular resistance of >10 U·m^2) has been reported in infants <1 year of age.

Cardiac catheterization reveals increased oxygen saturation at both the right atrial and the right ventricular levels. Pulmonary artery systolic pressure is invariably at or near systemic level, whereas in partial AVSDs, the pulmonary artery systolic pressure is usually $<60\%$ of systemic pressure. Pulmonary blood flow is increased as a result of left-to-right shunting at both atrial and ventricular sites, and the severity of shunting depends on the relationship of pulmonary to systemic vascular resistance. The hemodynamic abnormality in

complete AVSD may be complicated by severe common atrioventricular valve regurgitation, allowing blood to shunt freely among all four chambers. Left ventricular angiography rarely is required but reveals the typical LVOT gooseneck deformity and varying severity of left atrioventricular valve regurgitation.

Clinical Course

The timing of surgical intervention must take into account the propensity of pulmonary vascular disease to develop in these patients at an early age. The decision for operation is usually made in the first year of life. Children with complete AVSD frequently have surgical repair between 4 and 8 months of age.

Down Syndrome and Atrioventricular Septal Defect

Children with Down syndrome are more likely to have complete AVSD than children without Down syndrome. They are

RV dominant

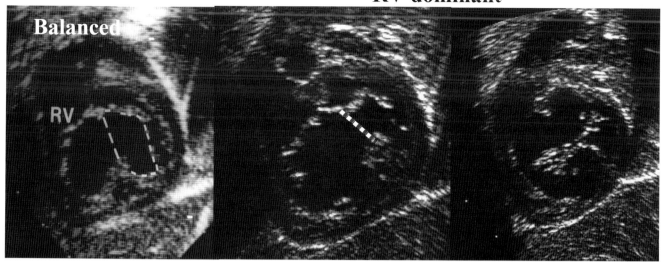

Balanced

RV

FIGURE 31.23 Echocardiographic assessment of ventricular dominance: Assessing unbalanced AVSDs using atrioventricular valve area measurements. **Left panel:** Diastolic frame from the subcostal sagittal plane demonstrating an en face view of the common atrioventricular valve. The planimetry demonstrates relative balance between the right and left portions of the common valve. **Center panel:** Diastolic frame demonstrating a right ventricle (RV)–dominant unbalanced AVSD with relative dominance of the right portion of the common atrioventricular valve. **Right panel:** Companion systolic frame of a right ventricle–dominant AVSD. (From Cohen M, Jacobs ML, Weinberg PM, et al. Morphometric analysis of unbalanced common atrioventricular canal using two-dimensional echocardiography. *J Am Coll Cardiol* 1996;28:1017, with permission.)

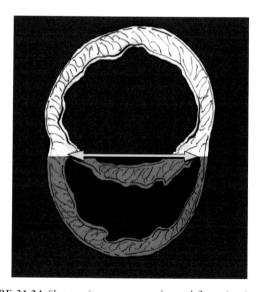

FIGURE 31.24 Short-axis assessment of septal flattening in unbalanced AVSD. Owing to right ventricular volume overload, the septum bows frequently toward the left ventricle. This may provide the misperception that the left ventricle is hypoplastic. However, if one assumes normalization of septal position, the potential volume of the left ventricle after repair may be predicted. From van Son, JAM, Phoon CK, Silverman NH, et al. Predicting feasibility of biventricular repair of right-dominant unbalanced atrioventricular canal. *Ann Thorac Surg* 1997;63:1657, with permission.)

also more likely to have associated tetralogy of Fallot (38,39). Sidedness (situs) and splenic anomalies are rare in patients with Down syndrome. Patients with Down syndrome usually do not have associated LVOT obstruction, left ventricular hypoplasia, coarctation of the aorta, or additional muscular VSDs (40,41).

The extent and progression of pulmonary vascular changes in children with Down syndrome and complete AVSD remain controversial. Histologic studies (42) have failed to reveal any differences in the extent of pulmonary vascular changes when patients with Down syndrome were compared with normal children who also had AVSD. Other studies (43) have suggested that children with Down syndrome have relative pulmonary parenchyma hypoplasia.

The hemodynamic assessment of children with Down syndrome must take into account that these patients may have chronic nasopharyngeal obstruction, relative hypoventilation, and sleep apnea. These factors contribute to carbon dioxide retention, relative hypoxia, and elevated pulmonary vascular resistance.

Patients with Down syndrome have a higher ratio of pulmonary to systemic resistance than patients without Down syndrome (44). This difference resolves with administration of 100% oxygen, suggesting that apparent hypoxia and hypoventilation are factors that can be corrected during hemodynamic study. Fixed and elevated pulmonary vascular resistance has been demonstrated in 11% of Down syndrome patients <1 year of age (44). Surgical results for patients with Down syndrome are similar to those of the general population (45).

Special Forms of Complete Atrioventricular Septal Defect

Unbalanced Defect

The term *unbalanced AVSD* has been applied when one ventricle and its corresponding atrioventricular valve are hypoplastic while the other ventricle receives the larger portion of the common atrioventricular valve. In this circumstance, the most common arrangement is a dominant right ventricle with a hypoplastic left ventricle (Fig. 31.22). The left-sided component of the common atrioventricular valve may be stenotic after two-ventricle repair has been performed.

In most examples of complete AVSD, the right atrium and pulmonary arteries are dilated and the right ventricular outflow tract bulges anteriorly. Often, the right ventricle is markedly hypertrophied, and the thickness of its free wall may equal or exceed that of the left ventricle. The left atrium is dilated, and the left ventricular outflow tract is long and narrow. Lateral displacement of the posteromedial left ventricular papillary muscle results in a small posterior left atrioventricular valve leaflet. Two-dimensional echocardiography provides valuable information regarding relative sizes and morphology of the atrioventricular valve(s) and the disproportionate sizes of the ventricles. The parasternal and subcostal short-axis views provide excellent imaging planes to determine relative ventricular sizes (Fig. 31.23).

Patients with severely unbalanced AVSD traditionally have had a modified Fontan operation. However, more recently, successful two-ventricle repair of unbalanced hearts has been possible when the atrioventricular valve index has exceeded 0.5 (46). In these patients, fenestration of the atrial septum may be required. Underfilling of the morphologic LV owing to a large shunt at the atrial level and bowing of the ventricular septum toward the LV may contribute to the perception that the LV is of inadequate size to sustain systemic circulation. In select patients with relative LV hypoplasia who have had successful two-ventricle repair, other associated cardiovascular features may have played an important role. In the small series described by van Son et al. (37), the interventricular communication was restrictive, there was antegrade flow into the ascending aorta from the LV, and the ductus arteriosus was closed or shunting only from left to right. Corresponding upper and lower extremity oxygen saturations were similar. Although successful operative results were reported, the long-term outcome of this surgical approach has not been determined.

Intermediate Defect

A rare subtype of complete AVSD occurs when the anterior and posterior bridging leaflets are fused atop the ventricular septum and the common atrioventricular valve is divided into distinct right and left orifices. This defect usually has a large primum ASD and a large inlet VSD. Patients present in the same manner as with other forms of complete AVSD. Surgical repair does not have to include division of separate right and left atrioventricular valve components (this has occurred naturally). The cleft in the left atrioventricular valve is closed, but the bridging leaflets often have insufficient tissue to reconstruct a competent anterior leaflet.

Surgical Treatment of Complete Atrioventricular Septal Defect

Surgical repair of complete forms of AVSD is indicated earlier in life than for the partial forms of AVSD. Repair of complete AVSD must be done prior to the development of irreversible pulmonary vascular obstructive disease. Repair should be done electively before 6 months of age. Earlier repair should be considered for infants with failure to thrive.

For the symptomatic infant, surgical options include palliative pulmonary artery banding and complete repair of the anomaly. Although in the modern age complete repair appears to be the procedure of choice for these infants, proponents of pulmonary banding have alluded to the relatively high risk of complete repair in infants <6 months of age (47). Silverman et al. (35) reported excellent results of pulmonary banding in 21 infants with complete AVSD who were <1 year of age. In that series, there was one surgical death (5%), and the remaining patients had excellent palliation. Williams et al. (48) recommended pulmonary artery banding for infants weighing <5 kg who were unresponsive to medical treatment or had significant associated anomalies. In the modern era, most centers perform complete repair in small infants who fail to thrive. This approach has largely obviated the need for pulmonary artery band placement.

The objectives of surgical repair include closure of interatrial and interventricular communications, construction of two separate and competent atrioventricular valves from available leaflet tissue, and repair of associated defects. Techniques for the surgical repair of complete AVSD have been standardized and are based on the use of a single patch or double patch (separate atrial and ventricular patches) to close the ASD and VSD and then reconstruction of the left atrioventricular valve as a bileaflet valve. Puga and McGoon (49) have described these techniques in detail.

Piccoli et al. (23) and Studer et al. (1) consider the cleft of the left atrioventricular valve a true commissure and envision this valve as a trileaflet valve. On the basis of these concepts, Carpentier (22) prefers the two-patch technique. The left atrioventricular valve remains a trileaflet structure (Fig. 31.25). The two-patch technique has become the method of choice.

In a series of 310 patients reported by Studer et al. (1), risk factors in the surgical repair of AVSDs were age at operation, severity of atrioventricular valve regurgitation, and preoperative functional class. Chin et al. (50) reported the results

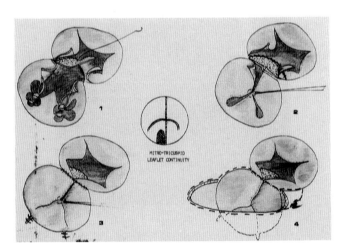

FIGURE 31.25 Carpentier technique for repair of complete AVSD with the double-patch technique. Concept of a trileaflet left atrioventricular valve. (From Carpentier A. Surgical anatomy and management of the mitral component of atrioventricular canal defects. In: Anderson RH, Shinebourne EA, eds. *Paediatric Cardiology*. Edinburgh: Churchill Livingstone, 1978: 477–490, with permission.)

obtained with complete repair in a group of patients whose mean age at operation was 10 months. Hospital mortality ranged from 62% in their early experience to 17% among 30 patients who underwent operation during the period 1978 to 1980. Bender et al. (51) reported 24 infants who had operation between 3 and 38 weeks of age (mean 18 weeks) and noted two operative deaths. Similar to repair of partial AVSD, postoperative sinus node dysfunction occurs. Complete heart block requiring permanent pacemaker placement is now rare.

Special Problems in Complete Atrioventricular Septal Defect Surgery

Parachute Deformity of the Mitral Valve. This problem has been addressed by David et al. (52). With such a deformity, closure of the mitral cleft at the time of repair may result in an obstructed mitral orifice. If the patient has significant atrioventricular valve regurgitation, valve replacement may be the only suitable option.

Double-Orifice Mitral Valve. The surgeon must resist the temptation of joining the two orifices by incising the intervening leaflet tissue. The combined opening of both orifices is satisfactory for adequate mitral valve function (53).

Right or Left Ventricular Hypoplasia. These anomalies may be severe enough to preclude septation. The only option for definitive surgical treatment is the modified Fontan's procedure preceded by adequate pulmonary artery banding in infancy.

Tetralogy of Fallot. In patients with this anomaly, all of whom have the complete form, the infundibular septum is displaced anteriorly, so that the typical inlet VSD extends anteriorly and superiorly toward the perimembranous area. In tetralogy of Fallot, there is obstruction of the right ventricular outflow tract. We prefer to treat these cyanotic infants initially with a systemic-to-pulmonary artery shunt and then by complete repair at 2 to 4 years of age. The intracardiac repair of these hearts is best accomplished through a combined right atrial and right ventricular approach (39).

Subaortic Stenosis. If discovered at the time of initial preoperative evaluation, subaortic stenosis tends to be of the fibromuscular membrane type and should be treated by appropriate resection during surgical repair. However, subaortic stenosis usually appears late after surgical repair of AVSD. The stenosis may be related to the uncorrected deficiency in the inlet septum. The obstruction usually is due to the formation of endocardial fibrous tags and fibromuscular ridges. Usually it can be treated by local resection, although in some patients a modified Konno procedure may be necessary.

REOPERATION AFTER REPAIR OF ATRIOVENTRICULAR SEPTAL DEFECTS

Partial Atrioventricular Septal Defect

Late reoperation following repair of partial AVSD may be required for regurgitation or stenosis of the left atrioventricular valve, subaortic stenosis, or residual recurrent ASD. Reoperation for mitral regurgitation occurs in 10% to 15% of survivors of primary repair of partial AVSD. Risk factors for reoperation include significant residual mitral regurgitation as assessed intraoperatively at the time of initial repair, the presence of a severely dysplastic mitral valve, and failure to close the cleft in the anterior (septal) mitral leaflet. Repeat repair is possible if valve dysplasia is not severe or when the mechanism of regurgitation is through an unsutured cleft. Eccentric commissural annuloplastic sutures often are needed to correct central regurgitation. Replacement of the mitral valve may be required in the presence of a severely dysplastic valve.

Reoperation for mitral stenosis may be necessary if the valve orifice is hypoplastic, or if the orifice is restricted owing to a parachute deformity of the subvalvular apparatus. Patient–prosthetic mismatch in patients who required mitral valve replacement during infancy or early childhood merits valve re-replacement. Relief of prosthetic mitral stenosis resulting from a small valve is technically challenging; the small valve requires replacement with a larger prosthesis, and there are no reliable techniques for mitral annular enlargement. Thorough debridement and excision of fibrous scar and old prosthetic material is necessary. In rare circumstances, the newer larger prosthesis is sewn into the left atrium above the original mitral annulus.

The late finding of the LVOT obstruction owing to subaortic stenosis is seen more frequently after correction of partial AVSD. This is likely due to the fact that during the conventional repair, the deficient portion of the inlet ventricular septum is not reconstructed so that the anterior (septal) leaflet of the mitral valve hinges on the line of fibrous fusion to the crest of the ventricular septum. Thus, the standard surgical repair does not modify the elongated and potentially narrowed LVOT. This is in contrast to complete AVSDs in which the deficient inlet septum is reconstructed with the subvalvular patch that effectively widens the outflow tract. Relief of LVOT obstruction can be accomplished in several ways, including transaortic resection of the fibrous or fibromuscular membrane and patch enlargement of the LVOT with a transaortic and right ventricular approach (modified Konno procedure). Others have described alternative approaches, including reconstruction of the deficient inlet septum, septal myectomy, and apicoaortic conduits (54–57). Reoperation for an isolated residual or recurrent ASD is rare after repair of partial AVSD.

Complete Atrioventricular Septal Defect

Late reoperation following repair of AVSD occurs in approximately 17% of patients during the first 20 years after surgical repair. Lesions requiring reoperation include left and right atrioventricular valve regurgitation, left atrioventricular valve stenosis (native and prosthetic), and residual/recurrent ASDs or VSDs.

Residual left atrioventricular valve regurgitation may result from inadequate surgical reconstruction. Intraoperative transesophageal echocardiography helps prevent patients from leaving the operating room with significant residual left atrioventricular valve regurgitation. Right atrioventricular valve regurgitation requiring reoperation is rare after repair of complete AVSD. It is more apparent with the presence of pulmonary hypertension or in association with tetralogy of Fallot with right ventricular dysfunction owing to persistent right ventricular outflow obstruction or pulmonary regurgitation. Residual shunts are rare causes for late reoperation.

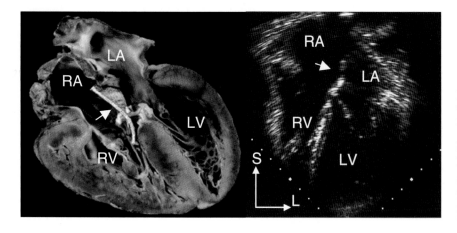

FIGURE 31.26 Left: Four-chamber anatomic specimen of a patient with partial AVSD after patch closure of a primum atrial septal defect (ASD) and repair of a cleft mitral valve. The patch (*arrow*) is attached to the right side of the atrial septum and the right atrioventricular valve to avoid damage to the conduction tissue and left atrioventricular valve. **Right:** corresponding apical four-chamber echocardiograph. L, left; LA, left atrium; LV, left ventricle; RA, right atrium; RV, right ventricle; S, superior.

POSTOPERATIVE ECHOCARDIOGRAPHIC ASSESSMENT

Echocardiographic assessment of the patient after repair of an AVSD includes a meticulous evaluation of the morphology of the atrioventricular valves (Fig. 31.26). Doppler interrogation for right and left atrioventricular valve stenosis or regurgitation is warranted. A search for residual shunts should be performed. Doppler evaluation of the velocity profiles across a ventricular level shunt and right atrioventricular valve regurgi-

tation can provide accurate determination of right ventricular systolic pressure. However, in the setting of a residual VSD, the VSD jet may contaminate the tricuspid regurgitation signal and preclude accurate quantification of right ventricular systolic pressure. In that setting, the echocardiographer should use indirect techniques such as assessment of ventricular septal flattening or bowing, right ventricular size and function, and Doppler interrogation of the pulmonary regurgitation velocity waveforms to assess pulmonary artery diastolic pressure. As stated frequently in this chapter, meticulous assessment of progressive left atrioventricular valve regurgitation/stenosis and development/progression of LVOT obstruction must be done during serial postoperative echocardiographic evaluations.

References

1. Studer M, Blackstone EH, Kirklin JW, et al. Determinants of early and late results of repair of atrioventricular septal (canal) defects. *J Thorac Cardiovasc Surg* 1982;84:523–542.
2. Aubert S, Henaine R, Raisky O, et al. Atypical forms of isolated partial atrioventricular septal defect increase the risk of initial valve replacement and reoperation. *Eur J Cardiothorac Surg* 2005;28:223–228.
3. McGrath LB, Gonzalez-Lavin L. Actuarial survival, freedom from reoperation, and other events after repair of atrioventricular septal defects. *J Thorac Cardiovasc Surg* 1987;94:582.
4. Fyler DC, Buckley LP, Hellenbrand WE, et al. Endocardial cushion defect. Report of the New England Regional Infant Cardiac Program. *J Pediatr* 1980;65(suppl):441–444.
5. Samanek M. Prevalence at birth, "natural" risk and survival with atrioventricular septal defect. *Cardiol Young* 1991;1:285–289.
6. Allan LD, Sharland GK, Milburn A, et al. Prospective diagnosis of 1006 consecutive cases of congenital heart disease in the fetus. *J Am Coll Cardiol* 1994;23:1452–1458.
7. Gutgesell HP, Huhta JC. Cardiac septation in atrioventricular canal defect. *J Am Coll Cardiol* 1986;8:1421–1424.
8. Taylor NC, Somerville J. Fixed subaortic stenosis after repair of ostium primum defects. *Br Heart J* 1981;45:689–697.
9. di Segni E, Edwards JE. Cleft anterior leaflet of the mitral valve with intact septa: A study of 20 cases. *Am J Cardiol* 1983;51:919–926.
10. Goel AK, Ganesan L, Edelstein M. Atrioventricular septal defect with cor triatriatum: Case report and review of the literature. *Pediatr Cardiol* 1998;19:243–245.
11. LaCorte MA, Cooper RS, Kauffman SL, et al. Atrioventricular canal ventricular septal defect with cleft mitral valve: Angiographic and echocardiographic features. *Pediatr Cardiol* 1982;2:289–295.
12. Silverman NH, Ho SY, Anderson RH, et al. Atrioventricular septal defect with intact atrial and ventricular septal structures. *Int J Cardiol* 1984;5:567–572.
13. Seward JB, Tajik AJ, Hagler DJ. Two-dimensional echocardiographic features of atrioventricular canal defect. In: Lundström N-R, ed. *Pediatric Echocardiography: Cross Sectional, M-mode and Doppler*. New York: Elsevier/North Holland, 1980:197–206.
14. Silverman NH, Ho SY, Anderson RH, et al. Atrioventricular septal defect with intact atrial and ventricular septal structures. *Int J Cardiol* 1984;5:567–572.
15. Snider RA, Serwer GA, Ritter SA. Defects in cardiac septation. In: *Echocardiography in Pediatric Heart Disease*. 2nd ed. St. Louis, MO: Mosby–Year Book. 1997:277–289.
16. Seward JB, Tajik AJ, Edwards WD, et al. Congenital heart disease. In: *Two-Dimensional Echocardiographic Atlas*. Vol. 1. New York: Springer-Verlag, 1987.
17. Reeder GS, Danielson GK, Seward JB, et al. Fixed subaortic stenosis in atrioventricular canal defect: A Doppler echocardiography study. *J Am Coll Cardiol* 1992;20:386–394.
18. Fournier A, Young M-L, Garcia OL, et al. Electrophysiologic cardiac function before and after surgery in children with atrioventricular canal. *Am J Cardiol* 1986;57:1137–1141.
19. Feldt RH, DuShane JW, Titus JL. The atrioventricular conduction system in persistent common atrioventricular canal defect: Correlations with electrocardiogram. *Circulation* 1970;42:437–444.
20. Boineau JP, Moore EN, Patterson DF. Relationship between the ECG, ventricular activation, and the ventricular conduction system in ostium primum ASD. *Circulation* 1973;48:556–564.
21. Thiene G, Wenink ACG, Frescura C, et al. Surgical anatomy and pathology of the conduction tissues in atrioventricular defects. *J Thorac Cardiovasc Surg* 1981;82:928–937.
22. Carpentier A. Surgical anatomy and management of the mitral component of atrioventricular canal defects. In: Anderson RH, Shinebourne EA, eds. *Paediatric Cardiology*. Edinburgh: Churchill Livingstone, 1978:477–490.
23. Piccoli GP, Wilkinson JL, Macartney FJ, et al. Morphology and classification of complete atrioventricular defects. *Br Heart J* 1979;42:633–639.
24. El-Najdawi E, Driscoll D, Puga F, et al. Operation for partial atrioventricular septal defect: A 40-year review. *J Thorac Cardiovasc Surg* 2000;119:880–889.
25. Alivizatos P, Anderson RH, Macartney FJ, et al. Atrioventricular septal defect with balanced ventricles and malaligned atrial septum: Double-outlet right atrium. *J Thorac Cardiovasc Surg* 1985;89:295–297.
26. Corwin RD, Singh AK, Karlson KE. Double-outlet right atrium. A rare endocardial cushion defect. *Am Heart J* 1983;106:1156–1157.
27. Horiuchi T, Saji K, Osuka Y, et al. Successful correction of double outlet left atrium associated with complete atrioventricular canal and l-loop double outlet right ventricle with stenosis of the pulmonary artery. *J Cardiovasc Surg (Torino)* 1976;17:157–161.

28. Titus JL, Rastelli GC. Anatomic features of persistent common atrioventricular canal. In: Feldt RH, McGoon DC, Ongley PA, et al., eds. *Atrioventricular Canal Defects*. Philadelphia: WB Saunders, 1976:13–35.

29. Fugelstad SJ, Danielson GK, Puga FJ, et al. Surgical pathology of the common atrioventricular valve: A study of 11 cases. *Am J Cardiovasc Pathol* 1988;2:49–55.

30. Rastelli GC, Kirklin JW, Titus JL. Anatomic observations on complete form of persistent common atrioventricular canal with special reference to atrioventricular valves. *Mayo Clin Proc* 1966;41:296–308.

31. Sridaromont S, Feldt RH, Ritter DG, et al. Double-outlet right ventricle associated with persistent common atrioventricular canal. *Circulation* 1975; 52:933–942.

32. Bharati S, Kirklin JW, McAllister HA Jr, et al. The surgical anatomy of common atrioventricular orifice associated with tetralogy of Fallot, double outlet right ventricle and complete regular transposition. *Circulation* 1980;61: 1142–1149.

33. Ten Harkel ADJ, Cromme-Dijkhuis AH, Heinerman BCC, et al. Development of left atrioventricular valve regurgitation after correction of atrioventricular septal defect. *Ann Thorac Surg* 2005;79:607–612.

34. Minich LL, Snider AR, Bove EL, et al. Echocardiographic evaluation of atrioventricular orifice anatomy in children with atrioventricular septal defect. *J Am Coll Cardiol* 1992;19:149–153.

35. Silverman N, Levitsky S, Fisher E, et al. Efficacy of pulmonary artery banding in infants with complete atrioventricular canal. *Circulation* 1983;68(suppl 2):II148–II153.

36. Cohen M, Jacobs ML, Weinberg PM, et al. Morphometric analysis of unbalanced common atrioventricular canal using two-dimensional echocardiography. *J Am Coll Cardiol* 1996;28:1017–1023.

37. van Son JAM, Phoon CK, Silverman NH, et al. Predicting feasibility of biventricular repair of right-dominant unbalanced atrioventricular canal. *Ann Thorac Surg* 1997;63:1657–1663.

38. Vet TW, Ottenkamp J. Correction of atrioventricular septal defect: Results influenced by Down syndrome? *Am J Dis Child* 1989;143:1361–1365.

39. Uretzky G, Puga FJ, Danielson GK, et al. Complete atrioventricular canal associated with tetralogy of Fallot: Morphologic and surgical considerations. *J Thorac Cardiovasc Surg* 1984;87:756–766.

40. De Biase L, Di Ciommo V, Ballerini L, et al. Prevalence of left-sided obstructive lesions in patients with atrioventricular canal without Down syndrome. *J Thorac Cardiovasc Surg* 1986;91:467–472.

41. Marino B. Atrioventricular septal defect – anatomic characteristics in patients with and without Down syndrome. *Cardiol Young* 1992;2:308–310.

42. Newfeld EA, Sher M, Paul MH, et al. Pulmonary vascular disease in complete atrioventricular canal defect. *Am J Cardiol* 1977;39:721–726.

43. Cooney TP, Thurlbeck WM. Pulmonary hypoplasia in Down syndrome. *N Engl J Med* 1982;307:1170–1173.

44. Hals J, Hagemo PS, Thaulow E, et al. Pulmonary vascular resistance in complete atrioventricular septal defect: A comparison between children with and without Down syndrome. *Acta Paediatr* 1993;82:595–598.

45. Rizzoli G, Mazzucco A, Maizza F, et al. Does Down syndrome affect prognosis of surgically managed atrioventricular canal defects? *J Thorac Cardiovasc Surg* 1992;104:945–953.

46. De Oliveira NC, Sittiwangkul R, McCrindle BW, et al. Biventricular repair in children with atrioventricular septal defects and a small right ventricle: Anatomic and surgical considerations. *J Thorac Cardiovasc Surg* 2005; 130:250–257.

47. Epstein ML, Moller JH, Amplatz K, et al. Pulmonary artery banding in infants with complete atrioventricular canal. *J Thorac Cardiovasc Surg* 1979;78:28–31.

48. Williams WH, Guyton RA, Michalik RE, et al. Individualized surgical management of complete atrioventricular canal. *J Thorac Cardiovasc Surg* 1983;86:838–844.

49. Puga FJ, McGoon DC. Surgical treatment of atrioventricular canal. *Mod Technics Surg* 1980;26:1–13.

50. Chin AJ, Keane JF, Norwood WI, et al. Repair of complete common atrioventricular canal in infancy. *J Thorac Cardiovasc Surg* 1982;84:437–445.

51. Bender HW Jr, Hammon JW Jr, Hubbard SG, et al. Repair of atrioventricular canal malformation in the first year of life. *J Thorac Cardiovasc Surg* 1982;84:515–522.

52. David I, Castaneda AR, van Praagh R. Potentially parachute mitral valve in common atrioventricular canal: Pathological anatomy and surgical importance. *J Thorac Cardiovasc Surg* 1982;84:178–186.

53. Lee C-N, Danielson GK, Schaff HV, et al. Surgical treatment of double-orifice mitral valve in atrioventricular canal defects: Experience in 25 patients. *J Thorac Cardiovasc Surg* 1985;90:700–705.

54. Mace L, Dervanian P, Folliguet T, et al. Atrioventricular septal defect with subaortic stenosis; extended valvular detachment and leaflet augmentation. *J Thorac Cardiovasc Surg* 1997;113:615–616.

55. van Son JA, Schneider P, Falk V. Repair of subaortic stenosis in atrioventricular canal with absent or restrictive interventricular communication patch augmentation of ventricular septum, resuspension of atrioventricular valves, and septal myectomy. *Mayo Clin Proc* 1997;72:220–224.

56. Van Ardsell GS, Williams WG, Boutin C, et al. Subaortic stenosis in the spectrum of atrioventricular septal defects. Solutions may be complex and palliative. *J Thorac Cardiovasc Surg* 1995;110:1534–1541.

57. DeLeon SY, Ilbawi MN, Wilson WR Jr, et al. Surgical opinions in subaortic stenosis associated with endocardial cushion defects. *Ann Thorac Surg* 1991;52:1082–1083.

CHAPTER 32 ■ VENTRICULAR SEPTAL DEFECTS

NANCY L. McDANIEL, MD, AND HOWARD P. GUTGESELL, MD

Ventricular septal defects (VSDs) are the most common form of congenital heart disease if bicuspid aortic valve is excluded. The defect can be in any portion of the ventricular septum, and the physiologic consequences can range from trivial to severe.

PREVALENCE

Approximately 20% of patients in congenital heart disease registries have VSD as a solitary lesion (1,2). Although historically the incidence of VSDs is cited as approximately 1.5 to 3.5 per 1,000 term infants (1–5) and 4.5 to 7 per 1,000 premature infants (3,5), recent echocardiographic studies demonstrated an incidence of VSD in newborns to be 5 to 50 per 1,000 (6–8). The lower prevalence in adults with congenital heart disease is

due to spontaneous closure of many defects. VSDs are slightly more common in females (3): Approximately 56% female, 44% male. VSDs are the most common lesion in many chromosomal syndromes, including trisomy 13, trisomy 18, and trisomy 21 groups, as well as in rarer syndromes (4). However, in most patients with VSDs (>95%), the defects are not associated with a chromosomal abnormality. A multifactorial cause has been proposed in which interaction between hereditary predisposition and environment results in the defect (4).

PATHOLOGY

The pathologic anatomy is depicted schematically in Figure 32.1. Although many classifications of VSD have been proposed, we prefer minor modifications of the system first

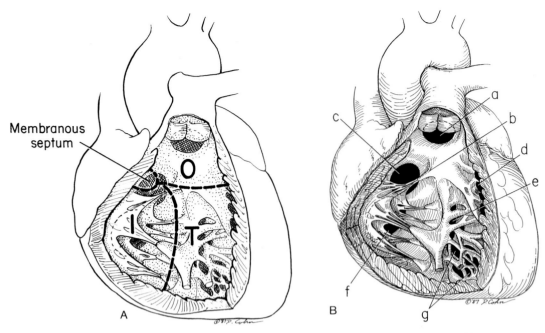

FIGURE 32.1 A: Ventricular septum viewed from right ventricular side is made up of four components: I, inlet component extends from tricuspid annulus to attachments of tricuspid valve; T, trabecular septum extends from inlet out to apex and up to smooth-walled outlet; O, outlet septum or infundibular septum, which extends up to pulmonary valve, and membranous septum. **B:** Anatomic position of defects: a, outlet defect; b, papillary muscle of the conus; c, perimembranous defect; d, marginal muscular defects; e, central muscular defects; f, inlet defect; g, apical muscular defects.

published by Soto et al. (9) (Table 32.1 and Fig. 32.1). In this classification, the ventricular septum is considered to have four components: An inlet septum separating the mitral and tricuspid valves; a trabecular septum, which extends from the attachments of the tricuspid leaflets outward to the apex and upward to the crista supraventricularis; the smooth-walled

TABLE 32.1

VSD CLASSIFICATION

1. Perimembranous: most common defect, 80% of surgical and autopsy series; usually extends into muscular, inlet, or outlet areas (synonyms: infracrystal, membranous)
2. Outlet: 5%–7% of autopsy and surgical series (29% in the Far East), situated just beneath the pulmonary value (synonyms: supracristal, conal, infundibular, subpulmonary, doubly committed subarterial)
3. Inlet: 5%–8%, posterior and inferior to perimembranous defect
4. Muscular: 5%–20%
   a. Central: mid-muscular, may have multiple apparent channels on RV side and coalesce to single defect on LV side
   b. Apical: multiple apparent channels on RV side may be single defect on LV side as with central defect
   c. Marginal: along RV septal junction
   d. "Swiss cheese" septum: large number of muscular defects

RV, right ventricular; LV, left ventricular

outlet or infundibular septum, which extends from the crista to the pulmonary valve; and the membranous septum, which is relatively small and is usually divided into two parts by the septal leaflet of the tricuspid valve (Fig. 32.1).

Defects involving the membranous septum with extension into the adjacent inlet, outlet, or muscular septum are termed perimembranous defects. A perimembranous defect lies in the outflow tract of the left ventricle immediately beneath the aortic valve. Synonyms include membranous defect and infracrystal defect. When viewed from the right side of the heart, the defect is beneath the crista supraventricularis and posterior to the papillary muscle of the conus (Fig. 32.1B). This is the location for approximately 80% of defects seen at surgery or at autopsy (10). These defects may involve varying amounts of muscular tissue adjacent to the membranous septum and have been variously subclassified as perimembranous inlet, perimembranous muscular, or perimembranous outlet VSD, depending on the extension of the defect. Minor anomalies of the tricuspid valve, which may be acquired secondary to left-to-right shunting, frequently are associated with perimembranous defects. These anomalies take the form of extra septal leaflet tissue or pouches that can partially or completely occlude the defect. These pouches have been called aneurysms of the ventricular septum and can be associated with spontaneous closure of the VSD. With the perimembranous defect, there can be a variable degree of anterior malalignment between the infundibular septum and the anterior ventricular septum such that the aortic valve appears to override the defect (9). Posterior or leftward malalignment also occurs, producing subaortic stenosis. When the septal commissure of the tricuspid valve is deficient at its attachment to the atrioventricular membranous septum, a left ventricular–to–right atrial shunt can occur (10). Such defects normally are associated with both left ventricular–to–right ventricular and left ventricular–to–right atrial shunting. Rarely, an isolated left ventricular–to–right atrial defect is found. Abnormalities of the tricuspid valve are common in this situation and include perforation, malformation, cleft, and widened commissure. Rarely, a defect can occur in the atrioventricular septum (Gerbode's defect) that produces an isolated left ventricular–to–right atrial shunt.

Defects in the outflow tract of the right ventricle beneath the pulmonary valve have been called supracristal, infundibular, conal, subpulmonary, or doubly committed subarterial defects (Fig. 32.1B). Outlet VSDs constitute approximately 5% to 7% of defects seen at surgery or autopsy, except in Japan and other Far Eastern countries, where the incidence is approximately 30% (9–11).

Inlet defects that are posterior and inferior to the membranous defect, beneath the septal leaflet of the tricuspid valve, and inferior to the papillary muscle of the conus have been called atrioventricular septal defects (Fig. 32.1B). This is a misnomer, because these defects usually are not associated with abnormalities of the mitral or tricuspid valves and the common atrioventricular bundle does not pass beneath the defect, as would be anticipated for a true atrioventricular septal defect (10). Inlet defects have been reported in 8% of 50 patients undergoing elective repair (10).

Defects in the muscular septum are frequently multiple and make up 5% to 20% of defects found at surgery or autopsy. There have been two recent attempts to classify muscular defects by location. Apical defects are the most common and frequently are difficult to visualize from the right ventricle because they are usually multiple with bordering and overlying trabeculae and tortuous channels (Fig. 32.1B). The left ventricular view shows fewer overlying trabeculae, and multiple defects frequently coalesce to form a single defect on the left side. Occasionally such apical defects are quite large (12,13).

Another type of muscular defect is the central defect (Fig. 32.1B), which is posterior to the trabecula septomarginalis (septal band of the crista) and in the midportion of the septum. Commonly, it is partially hidden by overlying trabeculae when viewed from the right ventricle and can give the impression of multiple defects. From the left ventricular view, this usually appears as a single rounded-off defect well away from the apex and the anterior and posterior left ventricular walls.

Small muscular defects near the septal–free wall margins have been termed marginal or anterior defects. These defects are usually multiple, small, tortuous, and distributed along the ventricular septal–free wall margins (Fig. 32.1B). Muscular defects can occur in combination with other muscular or nonmuscular defects, producing a Swiss cheese appearance of the septum.

Prolapse of one of the aortic valve cusps may occur with outlet or perimembranous VSDs. Patients with outlet defects usually have deficiency of muscular or fibrous support below the aortic valve with herniation of the right coronary leaflet through the VSD (14). The aortic commissures usually are normal. In contrast, patients with perimembranous VSDs and aortic insufficiency have herniation of the right or much less commonly the noncoronary cusp, have frequent abnormalities of aortic commissures (usually the right/noncoronary), and may have associated infundibular pulmonary stenosis. Echocardiography and angiography can show that the prolapsed aortic leaflet partially closes a moderate to large VSD and limits the left-to-right shunt. The prevalence of this complication is highest in patients with an outlet VSD but occurs with some perimembranous VSDs as well. The associated aortic valve insufficiency increases with age (15).

The relationship of the atrioventricular conduction pathways to the defect is important to surgical repair. In perimembranous defects, the bundle of His lies in a subendocardial position as it courses along the posterior-inferior margin of the defect. In inlet defects, the bundle of His passes anterosuperiorly to the defect (12). In muscular VSDs and outlet defects, there is little danger of heart block because the conduction tissue generally is far removed unless these defects extend into the perimembranous area.

PHYSIOLOGY

The primary anatomic variable that determines the physiologic state of the patient is defect size. In small or medium-sized VSD, the size of the defect limits the left-to-right shunt; however, in large defects (those approximately the size of the aortic orifice), there is essentially no resistance to flow across the VSD, and the relative resistances of the systemic and pulmonary circulations regulate flow across the defect.

Pulmonary vascular resistance determines the magnitude of the left-to-right shunt in infancy (16–20). Following birth, the small muscular pulmonary arteries normally change from the fetal state, with a small lumen and a thick medial muscle layer, to thin-walled structures with increased lumen size. The normal rate of decline in pulmonary vascular resistance that accompanies these changes is such that the right ventricular pressure is near adult levels within 7 to 10 days. In the presence of large VSDs, the rate of this process is delayed, and the increased pulmonary resistance prevents massive shunting of blood through the lungs. Elevation of left atrial pressure (pulmonary venous pressure) plays an important role in maintaining this phase of pulmonary vascular constriction (16).

Small VSDs, sometimes referred to as Roger's defect (21), are those less than one third the size of the aortic root and impose a high resistance to flow with a resultant large systolic pressure difference between the two ventricles. There is a small left-to-right shunt, normal right ventricular systolic pressure, and essentially normal work characteristics of the ventricles. The magnitude of the left-to-right shunt is related directly to the size of the defect, and there is no tendency for an increase in pulmonary vascular resistance. The pressure gradient across the defect favors the left ventricle throughout the cardiac cycle and can result in a continuous left-to-right shunt (22). The major gradient and left-to-right shunt occurs during ventricular ejection, with the direction of flow across perimembranous or outlet defects diverted into the outflow tract of the right ventricle and pulmonary artery. In some patients, the left-to-right shunt stops transiently at the end of isovolumic relaxation during a brief interval of early diastole when left ventricular pressure falls below that of the right. None of these patients has right-to-left shunting across the defect at this time.

Moderate-size VSDs are large enough to permit a moderate to large shunt, yet small enough to offer some resistance to flow. The VSD diameter is about equal to half that of the aortic orifice, and the peak systolic pressure difference is ≥20 mm Hg higher in the left than the right ventricle. It is extremely unusual for patients with moderate-sized VSDs to have marked elevation of pulmonary vascular resistance; most have moderate to large left-to-right shunts with volume overload of the left atrium and ventricle and left ventricular hypertrophy. Right ventricular systolic work and muscle mass are usually only mildly increased.

The intracardiac pressure flow events for moderate or large VSDs occur as described for small defects until right ventricular systolic pressures reach a level of 70% to 85% of systemic pressure (22). Patients with pressures at this level have a left-to-right gradient of 15 to 30 mm Hg throughout ventricular ejection. Left ventricular pressure increases more rapidly with the onset of systole than does right ventricular pressure, and this gradient is maintained throughout systole into the initial portion of isovolumic relaxation. The left ventricular pressure, however, decreases more rapidly than the right, with the development of a transient right-to-left gradient during relaxation. This is associated with a small right-to-left shunt across the defect into the outflow portion of the left ventricle. With the commencement of diastole, the pressure relationships across the defect favor the left ventricle, and flow again occurs from the left ventricle to the right ventricle. The small volume of blood that was shunted from the right ventricle into the left ventricle during isovolumic relaxation is returned to the right ventricle and thus does not enter the systemic circulation.

In many infants, large left-to-right shunts can be present with right ventricular pressures that are normal or only mildly to moderately elevated. In these patients, the size of the defect is restrictive, but the total amount of flow across the defect is relatively large. If the defect remains the same size and continues to restrict flow, the absolute amount of shunting will become less significant as the child becomes larger.

Defects are considered large when they are approximately the size of the aortic orifice. Because of the nonrestrictive character of the defect, the pulmonary circulation is subjected to the common ejectile force of both ventricles. Large left-to-right shunts ensue, with systemic pressure in both ventricles and frequently a small right-to-left shunt.

With large VSDs, a gradual decline of pulmonary vascular resistance usually occurs in the first few months of life, resulting in augmentation of the left-to-right shunt. The large blood volume handled by the left atrium results in left atrial and pulmonary venous hypertension. The increased return to the left side of the heart results in an enlarged left atrium and left ventricle as well as an increase in the left ventricular muscle mass (17). With the marked volume overload of the left ventricle, congestive heart failure is particularly likely to occur between the ages of 2 and 8 weeks. Compensatory mechanisms that allow the infant to adapt to this volume load include the Frank–Starling effect, increased sympathetic cardiac stimulation, and myocardial hypertrophy. The rapidity of the development of myocardial hypertrophy is one of the major factors in the ability of an infant to compensate adequately for a VSD with a large left-to-right shunt.

Excessive pulmonary blood flow can be associated with vessel injury. Chronic injury associated with a large unrepaired VSD can result in a thickened adventitia, medial hypertrophy, and intimal injury resulting in pulmonary vascular obstructive disease. Although the histology and progressive changes of pulmonary hypertension are documented (20,23,24), the basic mechanisms involved in this end stage of markedly sclerotic and damaged vessels remain to be clarified. A complex interaction between the vascular endothelium and the underlying smooth muscle cells, in the setting of increased flow and pressure, appears to trigger the pathologic vascular remodeling response (25).

Clinical Manifestations

History and Physical Examination

In infants with small VSDs, a murmur usually is detected at 1 to 6 weeks of age when the infant returns for the initial checkup after discharge from the newborn nursery. However, the murmur can be heard during the first days of life associated with a rapid decrease in pulmonary vascular resistance. With small defects, the clinical course is benign throughout infancy and childhood. There are normal patterns of feeding, growth, and development. The only risk is that of endocarditis, which is rare before the age of 2 years.

In accord with the mild hemodynamic changes associated with small defects, these children appear healthy. By palpation, the precordial activity is normal. A thrill may be palpable along the lower left sternal border and is associated with a grade IV to VI S-1 coincident holosystolic murmur that is plateau, crescendo, or crescendo–decrescendo (Fig. 32.2A). It frequently envelops the aortic component of the second sound and extends slightly past it. Because of the high-frequency components of the murmur, it is accentuated when auscultation is performed with the diaphragm. In some patients, the murmur can extend cephalad along the left parasternal region, owing to ejection across the outflow tract of the right ventricle. The murmur also can radiate to the right of the sternum. In children with an outlet defect, the murmur and thrill can be maximal at the second left intercostal space or suprasternal notch.

The holosystolic quality of the murmur correlates with the continuous systolic pressure gradient across the defect and provides indirect evidence that the right ventricular systolic pressure is significantly less than that of the left. The absence of a murmur during diastole, although flow continues across the defect, is related to the lack of turbulence owing to the small quantity of shunted blood. Infants with muscular defects can have softer short murmurs that cut off in midsystole, presumably because of closure of the defect owing to systolic contraction of septal musculature (Fig. 32.2B). This murmur can be differentiated from an innocent vibratory murmur by its starting with the first heart sound, its localization to the left sternal border, and its accentuation with the diaphragm because of its high-frequency components. This type of murmur is common in infancy and has a high likelihood of disappearance (approximately 80%) during the first year of life owing to spontaneous defect closure.

The valve closure sounds in small VSDs are usually normal. Some patients, however, have wide splitting of the second sound. If there is associated pulmonary stenosis or mitral insufficiency in a patient with VSD, these lesions may be suspected when the systolic murmur is transmitted to the upper left sternal border or apex, respectively.

Infants with moderate or large VSDs may develop symptoms as early as 2 weeks of age. The initial symptoms consist of tachypnea with increased respiratory effort, excessive sweating owing to increased sympathetic tone, and fatigue when feeding. The infant progressively tires with feeding; this symptom begins during the first month and increases in severity as pulmonary vascular resistance decreases. Symptoms occur earlier in the premature than in the full-term infant (3). It is not unusual for symptoms to be preceded by respiratory infection. This complication makes it difficult to clarify the degree to which the respiratory distress is due to heart failure from a large left-to-right shunt versus infection.

In the absence of infection, the cardiovascular basis for the respiratory symptoms probably is pulmonary edema of mild to moderate degree with elevated pulmonary venous pressure and decreased lung compliance. In infants with a large left-to-right shunt secondary to a VSD, dyspnea can occur with mean left atrial pressures slightly lower than 15 mm Hg (26).

In the presence of large shunts across the VSD, infants often have normal length and decreased weight. Precordial

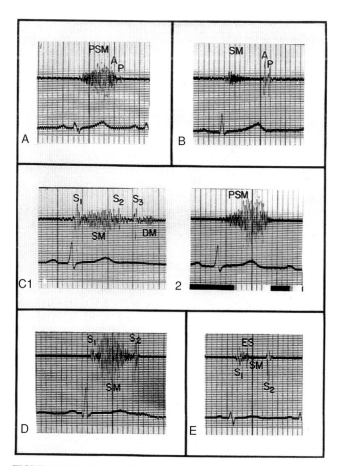

FIGURE 32.2 Phonocardiographic findings in ventricular septal defects with varying physiologic states. **A:** Small defect with normal right ventricular pressure and minimal left-to-right shunt. The murmur is harsh and pansystolic (PSM). Note the prominent splitting of S2, as commonly occurs in small defects. **B:** Small defect with non-holosystolic murmur. The murmur ends well before the second sound because of functional closure of the defect during ventricular contraction. **C:** Moderate-sized defect with mild elevation of right ventricular pressure and prominent left-to-right shunt. Phonocardiogram *(1)* at the apex illustrates the prominent S3 and diastolic rumble (DM) *(2)*. This tracing was recorded in the third interspace adjacent to the sternum. The murmur is most prominent in this area. **D:** Large defect with equal ventricular systolic pressures and large left-to-right shunt. This tracing was obtained from the left parasternal region in the third interspace. Notice the decrescendo nature of the murmur that shows marked diminution or termination before S2. **E:** Large defect with marked elevation of pulmonary vascular resistance and equal bidirectional shunting. This shows a predominant ejection sound (ES), a short ejection murmur (SM), and a single or closely split S2, with loud pulmonary component.

activity is accentuated and extends over both the right (parasternal) and left ventricular (apical) areas. The hyperdynamic precordium becomes more prominent as left ventricular volume increases owing to increased pulmonary blood flow and pulmonary venous return to the left side of the heart. In children with large shunts for ≥4 to 6 months, the left anterior thorax bulges outward.

The murmur with moderate-sized defects is usually associated with a thrill, is S1 coincident and holosystolic, and is harsh. Its duration and character suggest a significant pressure gradient across the defect. A prominent third sound with a short early middiastolic rumble (Fig. 32.2C) is frequently audible at the apex when pulmonary blood flow is twice systemic blood flow or greater. As in small defects, this murmur is most prominent over the right ventricular area along the lower left sternal border (Fig. 32.2C). The second sound usually is widely split with a slight variation with respiration. The intensity of the pulmonary component is normal or only slightly increased.

The S1 coincident murmur from a large VSD is maximal along the left sternal border, usually is decrescendo, and disappears during the latter third of systole before closure of the aortic valve (Fig. 32.2D). These characteristics differ from those in children maintaining a significant systolic pressure gradient across the defect throughout ventricular ejection. The pulmonary component of the second sound is usually loud, and splitting is narrow but detectable in most patients. Some patients have a murmur that extends into the upper left parasternal region generated by ejection of blood into the pulmonary artery. A few patients have an early faint diastolic decrescendo murmur in this region because of mild pulmonary valve insufficiency. The presence of an early diastolic decrescendo murmur, however, should alert one to the possibility of associated aortic insufficiency. In addition, there is usually a prominent third sound and a diastolic rumble in the apical area.

Some infants with large defects have very little decrease in pulmonary vascular resistance in the first few months of life and develop only mild to moderate left-to-right shunting. These infants do not pass through the phase of large left-to-right shunt (high-output cardiac failure). Their mild clinical course disguises the underlying physiologic abnormality because this group can develop pulmonary vascular obstructive disease with ultimate reversal of shunting.

A history of cyanosis not documented by physical examination is difficult to evaluate. In particular, cyanosis during the early weeks of life is often transient and frequently presents only with superimposed stress or illness. Persistent cyanosis from birth indicates a more complicated lesion than isolated VSD. However, the occurrence of cyanosis after infancy suggests reversal of the shunt to right to left because of progressive pulmonary vascular disease or the development of significant infundibular pulmonary stenosis.

Patients with large VSDs and marked elevation of pulmonary vascular resistance frequently appear well in childhood. Those with moderate to large right-to-left shunts will be cyanotic at rest. This is rare in infants, is occasionally seen by the age of 2 to 3 years, and is frequently seen in the adolescent and young adult. Palpation reveals a prominent right ventricular lift that is usually maximal in the xiphoid region. There may be a very short or no systolic murmur from the VSD (Fig. 32.2E). There may be a short pulmonary ejection murmur along the upper left parasternal region. A loud, harsh s1 coincident holosystolic murmur at the right lower sternal border indicates tricuspid valve insufficiency. Many patients have an early diastolic murmur of pulmonary valve insufficiency (27). The second sound is quite loud, palpable, and single or closely split. There is no diastolic rumble at the apex. However, a third sound of right ventricular origin may be present along the left sternal border. The eponym Eisenmenger's complex is now applied to the condition characterized by a VSD with marked elevation of pulmonary vascular resistance and a predominant right-to-left shunt (27,28).

In patients with Eisenmenger's complex, Wood (27) found that most had a history of cyanosis since infancy. It was his impression that the syndrome commonly was established at birth or developed during the first 2 years of life. Neither cyanosis nor breathlessness progressed markedly during childhood or adolescence, but deterioration occurred in young adults. Squatting was found in 15% of his patients, and hemoptysis occurred in 33% of patients (but never before 24 years of age). It occurred in 100% of patients by 40 years of age and was a contributing cause of death in 29%.

DIAGNOSTIC EVALUATION

Electrocardiography

The electrocardiogram (ECG) is usually normal with small VSDs. However, a few patients with small defects demonstrate an rsR′ in V1 or V4R. Left axis deviation is typical of atrioventricular septal defects but is occasionally seen in defects in other locations (29).

Patients with moderate-sized VSDs have moderate or large left-to-right shunts with volume overload of the left ventricle, and left ventricular hypertrophy is the rule (Fig. 32.3). Hypertrophy of both ventricles is common (30). In moderate-sized defects, there may be no right ventricular hypertrophy. However, mild or moderate elevation of right ventricular pressure can result in right ventricular hypertrophy, which is evident in lead V4R or V1 as an rsR′ pattern with the R′ increasing in amplitude with increasing right ventricular pressure.

In infants with large VSDs, the ECG features frequently are not as distinctive as in older children. In this age group, the presence of a counterclockwise QRS vector loop in the frontal vector plane can be helpful as an index of left ventricular hypertrophy. Some infants may show only increased biphasic voltages >4.5 mV over the midprecordium. Patients with

large VSDs and equal ventricular pressures demonstrate right ventricular hypertrophy (31). In patients with excessive pulmonary blood flow, left atrial enlargement is evidenced by biphasic P waves, which are usually most prominent in leads I, aVR, and V6. In addition, lead V1 frequently shows a biphasic P wave with a prominent negative deflection. In the presence of combined ventricular hypertrophy, the right ventricular hypertrophy pattern in lead V1 usually consists of a QRS complex of the rsR′ pattern or one with a prominent negative deflection on the upstroke of the R wave (rR′).

In patients with large VSDs and marked elevation of pulmonary resistance, left ventricular hypertrophy and left atrial enlargement are usually absent. Here, right ventricular hypertrophy produces a QRS pattern in lead V1 with slurring of the upstroke of the R wave and absent or minor S waves; V6 shows normal R waves and frequently a deep S wave.

Chest Radiography

The chest radiograph shows normal heart size and normal pulmonary vascularity in children with small VSDs. In contrast, chest radiographs in children with moderate VSDs show cardiac enlargement of varying severity and increased pulmonary vascular markings. There is downward and leftward elongation of the cardiac silhouette in the posterior-anterior view owing to left ventricular enlargement. The pulmonary vascular markings are increased in both the central and peripheral portions of the lung fields, and the main pulmonary artery segment is prominent. The left atrium is enlarged and can be appreciated on the lateral film, seen especially with a barium swallow;

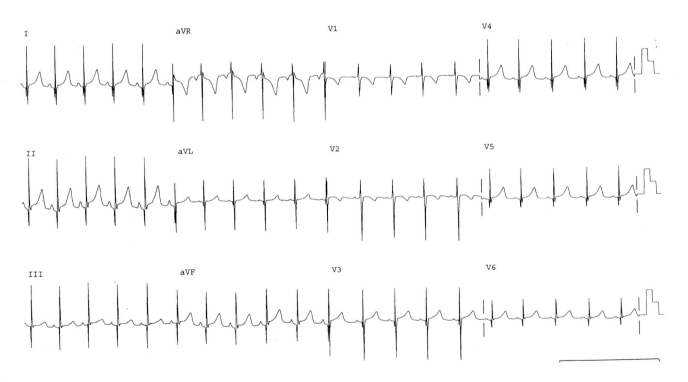

FIGURE 32.3 Electrocardiogram showing left ventricular hypertrophy in infant with large VSD. Note that precordial leads are at one-half standard.

in more severe degrees of left atrial enlargement, widening of the tracheal bifurcation with elevation of the left mainstem bronchus is obvious on the posterior-anterior film.

Similar to moderate VSDs, in those with large VSDs, moderately elevated pulmonary resistance and large left-to-right shunts, radiography demonstrates generalized cardiac enlargement, increased pulmonary vascular markings, and prominence of the main pulmonary artery. Hypertrophy and enlargement of the right ventricle frequently results in posterior displacement of the left ventricular apex.

Children with large VSDs and marked elevation of pulmonary vascular resistance have essentially normal-sized hearts. Characteristically with right ventricular hypertrophy, the cardiac apex will be rotated slightly upward to the left and posteriorly. There is also marked prominence of the main pulmonary artery and its adjacent vessels with decreased pulmonary vascular markings in the outer third of the lung fields. In patients who develop marked elevation of pulmonary vascular resistance after initially having a large shunt, the left ventricle and left atrium may remain somewhat enlarged for a period of time.

Echocardiography

Two-dimensional echocardiography, coupled with Doppler echocardiography and color flow mapping, can be used to determine the size and location of virtually all VSDs (32–36). Also, Doppler echocardiography can provide physiologic information regarding right ventricular and pulmonary artery systolic pressures and the interventricular pressure difference. Measurement of left atrial and left ventricular diameters provides semiquantitative information about shunt volume.

VSD sizes can be measured in absolute terms from the two-dimensional image (37). Not all defects are circular; thus,

dimensions of the defect may vary from one imaging plane to another. Defect size often is expressed in terms of the size of the aortic root. Lesions that approximate the size of the aorta are considered large; lesions one third to two thirds of the diameter of the aorta are moderate; and lesions less than one third the aortic root diameter are considered small. Pinhole lesions detected only by color flow mapping (<2 mm in diameter) might be termed very small or tiny.

VSD location s can be determined by analysis of the imaging planes from which the defect is visualized (Fig. 32.4). The left parasternal long-axis imaging plane transects the aortic root and the more anterior portions of the ventricular septum. Thus, this projection demonstrates some of the larger perimembranous VSDs, including those partially or totally closed by aneurysm tissue (38,39) (Fig. 32.5), subaortic defects seen in conditions such as tetralogy of Fallot, and defects in the anterior portion of the trabecular or muscular septum. Slight clockwise rotation of the transducer to a plane parallel to the right ventricular outflow tract allows visualization of subpulmonary defects in the outlet or infundibular septum.

On short-axis images obtained from projections near the semilunar valves, defects in the outlet septum appear at the 1 o'clock position of the aortic root–right ventricular outflow tract interface (Fig. 32.4). Aortic cusp prolapse may partially close the supracristal defect (Fig. 32.6). Defects in the subaortic septum appear at the 11 o'clock to 12 o'clock positions, and perimembranous defects appear at the 10 o'clock to 11 o'clock positions. From short-axis images obtained near the tips of the mitral valve leaflets, defects in the anterior portion of the trabecular septum appear at the 12 o'clock to 1 o'clock positions (Fig. 32.4), those in the midportion of the trabecular septum appear between the 9 o'clock and 12 o'clock positions, and defects of the inlet septum appear at the 7 o'clock to 9 o'clock positions.

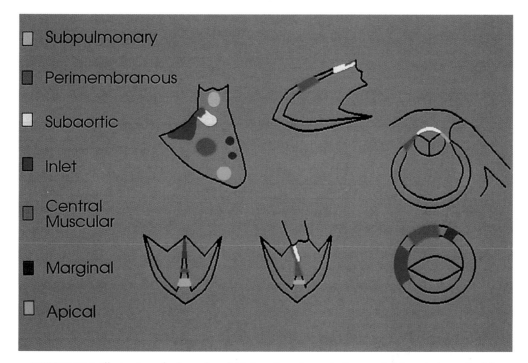

FIGURE 32.4 Illustration of scheme by which location of ventricular septal defects is determined by analysis of imaging planes in which the defect is visualized. The location of defects, as seen from the right side of the septum, is shown at upper left. Colors indicate where lesions are visualized on, proceeding clockwise, long-axis, short-axis, low short-axis, five-chamber, and four-chamber images.

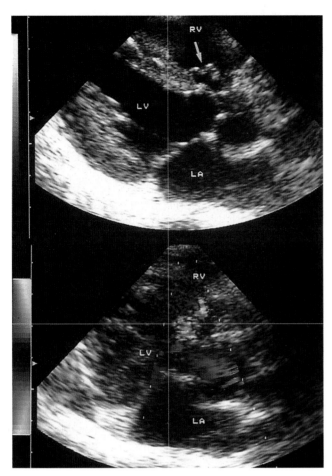

FIGURE 32.5 Two-dimensional (**top**) and color flow (**bottom**) images from left parasternal projection in 1-year-old infant with a perimembranous ventricular septal defect. Note the aneurysmal pouch formed by tricuspid valve tissue (*arrow*). Color flow image shows small left-to-right shunt through perforation in the aneurysm. LA, left atrium; LV, left ventricle; RV, right ventricle.

From four-chamber projections (either apical or subcostal), defects seen on the most posterior imaging planes, those passing through the atrioventricular valves, involve the inlet portion of the ventricular septum. Defects seen in more anterior (i.e., more shallow) imaging planes, especially those that pass through the aortic root, are in the perimembranous or subaortic portions of the ventricular septum. Defects in the outlet septum generally cannot be visualized from four-chamber projections but can be demonstrated by subcostal images in the sagittal plane, especially in small infants. Large defects often can be visualized in multiple imaging planes.

Virtually all moderate and large VSDs can be demonstrated by two-dimensional transthoracic echocardiography (TTE). Even very small defects are easily demonstrated by the use of color flow mapping (Fig. 32.4). Newer techniques such as three-dimensional (3-D) reconstruction imaging (Figs. 32.7 and 32.8) can be useful in defining VSD anatomy. This technique can be useful when standard echocardiographic evaluation of size does not match the clinical findings. Standard echocardiography also has been very useful in the detection of multiple defects, especially those in the middle and apical portions of the trabecular septum (40). Transesophageal echocardiography (TEE) is used occasionally in the child who is difficult to image or in whom there are additional anatomic issues

such as aortic insufficiency from cusp prolapse that need clarification (Fig. 32.9). TEE commonly is used to assess the adequacy of intraoperative repair or interventional catheterization closure of VSD (Fig. 32.8).

The interventricular pressure gradient may be estimated from the velocity of the flow jet as measured by Doppler echocardiography (41,42). The jet velocity is converted to pressure difference by the modified Bernoulli equation (gradient $= 4 \ V^2$, where V is velocity in meters per second). The technique is useful but has several limitations. If the ultrasound beam is not parallel to the VSD jet, the velocity of the jet will be underestimated and thus right ventricular pressure will be overestimated. Second, the velocity of the flow jet represents the maximal instantaneous difference between left and right ventricular pressure. Left ventricular pressure increases earlier in the cardiac cycle than right ventricular pressure, so the pressure difference in early systole may be somewhat greater than the ultimate peak-to-peak pressure difference. Despite these limitations, the Doppler method often provides a good estimate of right ventricular systolic pressure. When possible, this technique should be supplemented by estimation of right ventricular pressure from a tricuspid valve insufficiency jet (if present).

Echocardiography has provided insight into the mechanisms by which VSDs close spontaneously (43). Perimembranous defects often close by the development of a saccular pouch or aneurysm on the right ventricular septal surface, possibly derived from tissue from the septal leaflet of the tricuspid valve (Fig. 32.5). Muscular defects appear to close by progressive growth of tissue from the right ventricular side of the circumference of the defect (Fig. 32.10).

Doppler and color flow echocardiography have been used to demonstrate the shunting patterns in VSD (44,45). During isovolumetric contraction, flow is from the left ventricle to the right. During isovolumetric relaxation, flow is from the right to the left ventricle. In systole, flow is from left to right in people with isolated VSDs but is bidirectional in patients with extremely elevated pulmonary resistance or right ventricular outflow obstruction. In diastole, flow is initially from the right to the left ventricle but usually reverses in middiastole.

In addition to demonstration of the actual VSD, echocardiography is useful in identifying associated anomalies such as straddling or overriding atrioventricular valves, aortic cusp prolapse, aortic valve insufficiency, and ventricular outflow or inflow obstruction. Transesophageal studies can be extremely useful in patients with poor echocardiographic windows, particularly adolescents and adults. Intraoperative echocardiography, TEE and epicardial, have been used to assess the adequacy of repair and detect residual defects (46,47). Postoperative echocardiography is useful in determining the cause of residual murmurs and in confirming that pulmonary artery pressure has decreased following repair (47).

Magnetic Resonance Imaging

Magnetic resonance imaging (MRI) can be useful for imaging VSDs when ultrasonography is not feasible or when such studies are not diagnostic. However, transesophageal echocardiography should be used first.

Cardiac Catheterization

Cardiac catheterization is performed to document the number of defects, evaluate the magnitude of shunting, estimate

(text continues on page 677)

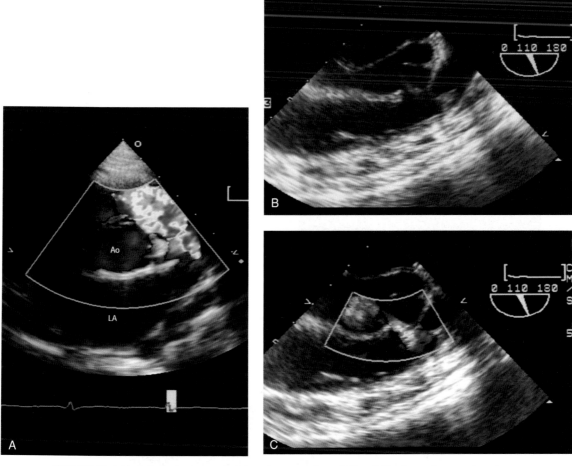

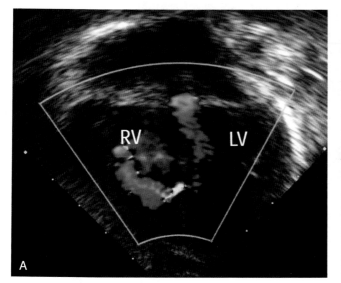

FIGURE 32.6 Transthoracic short axis (**A**) and transesophageal (**B** and **C**) echocardiograms in a 6-year-old with a supracristal VSD. Although the defect appeared small by color Doppler, it was >10 mm in diameter at surgery and was largely occluded by the prolapsing right aortic cusp (**B**). The location of the defect at 1 o'clock on the short-axis view of the aortic root (**A**) is characteristic of supracristal defects. Ao, aorta; LA, left atrium.

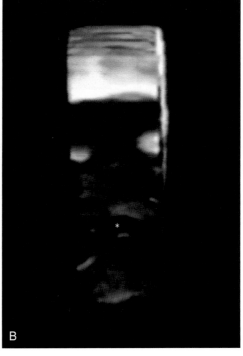

FIGURE 32.7 Apical four-chamber 2-D echocardiogram (**A**) and 3-D echocardiogram (**B**) in infant with large left-to-right shunt. Although the defect appeared quite small by color Doppler, the *en face* view of the septum seen on the 3-D echocardiogram reveals a banana-shaped defect (*asterisk*), which was 20 mm in its antero-posterior dimension. LV, left ventricle; RV, right ventricle.

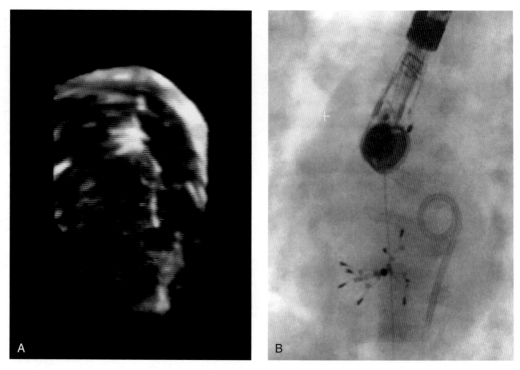

FIGURE 32.8 Three-dimensional echocardiogram (**A**) of a large defect in the lower portion of the ventricular septum. The defect was closed in the catheterization laboratory with a CardioSEAL device, which is visible by fluoroscopy (**B**).

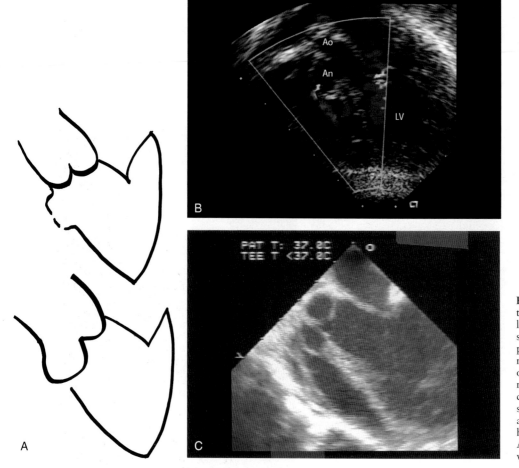

FIGURE 32.9 Diagram (**A**) illustrating the superficial similarity of a large aneurysm of the membranous septum (**top**) and an aortic cusp prolapsing through a perimembranous VSD. Doppler demonstration of left-to-right shunting through the middle of the protrusion (**B**) helps distinguish an aneurysm of the septum from a prolapsing cusp (**C**), as does careful attention to the hinge points of the aortic leaflets. Ao, aorta; An, aneurysm; LV, left ventricle.

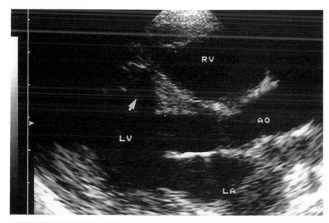

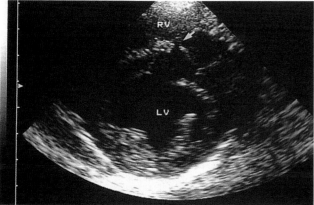

FIGURE 32.10 Long-axis (**top**) and short-axis images of a defect in the muscular septum of a 5-year-old, illustrating one mechanism by which defects close spontaneously. Despite the large defect on the left side of the septum (*arrow*, **top**), tissue growth on the upper right ventricular side has nearly closed the defect (*arrow*, **bottom**). Ao, aorta; LA left atrium; LV, left ventricle; RV, right ventricle.

pulmonary vascular resistance, estimate the workload of the two ventricles, document or exclude the presence or absence of associated defects, and provide the surgeon or interventional cardiologist with a clear anatomic picture of the location of the defect (or defects) in those patients needing intervention.

The procedure should be used for the procurement of information not apparent or available by other noninvasive means (48). Because conventional diagnostic techniques are sufficiently accurate to appraise the anatomic and physiologic state of the patient with a small defect, it is not necessary to catheterize such children.

Cardiac catheterization yields the maximum amount of useful information in two groups of patients: Infants with suspected VSDs with evidence of a large left-to-right shunt or heart failure, and patients with evidence of increased pulmonary vascular resistance with moderate or small left-to-right shunts. Improvements in echocardiographic/Doppler techniques now allow accurate diagnosis in many patients with isolated defects and can delay or obviate the need for catheterization in many patients.

We first perform a right-sided heart catheterization with measurement of the pressures and oxygen saturations in the pulmonary arteries, right side of the heart, and femoral artery for estimating pulmonary and systemic blood flows. Simultaneous pulmonary artery and aortic or peripheral arterial pressures are obtained, along with pulmonary wedge (or left

atrial) and right atrial pressures for estimation of pulmonary and systemic vascular resistances. Frequently, in infants the left side of the heart can be catheterized antegrade through a patent foramen ovale. In this situation, withdrawal of the catheter from the left ventricle to the left atrium to the right atrium and then rapid manipulation of the catheter into the right ventricle provides a means to assess the pressures in right and left ventricle to determine the magnitude of the shunt. In addition, the withdrawal from the left atrium to the right atrium provides a method to gauge the size of an associated atrial defect. In the presence of only a dilated foramen ovale, there is usually a mean pressure gradient from left atrium to right atrium of ≥3 mm Hg.

If a patent ductus arteriosus is not traversed in patients with pulmonary hypertension, left-sided heart catheterization is performed including retrograde aortography. Calculations of left ventricular end-diastolic volume (LVEDV), left ventricular ejection fraction (LVEF), left ventricular systolic output, left ventricular muscle mass, and left atrial maximal volume can be performed relatively easily and comparisons made with normal values (49). These data can be valuable in providing further information regarding pulmonary flow (20) and cardiac function. On the levogram phase of a right-sided heart injection, one can detect the presence or absence of a left-to-right shunt at the atrial level and anomalies of pulmonary venous return.

Left ventricular cineangiocardiography is used to document the location and number of VSDs. The long-axis oblique view is useful to visualize the ventricular septum, accurately delineate the size and number of defects, and evaluate the left ventricular outflow tract (50,51) (Fig. 32.11). If the long-axis view does not clearly delineate the defect(s), left ventricular injection with the four-chamber or hepatoclavicular view is performed. This view more clearly displays the posterior ventricular septum and is useful for demonstrating a left ventricular–to–right atrial communication.

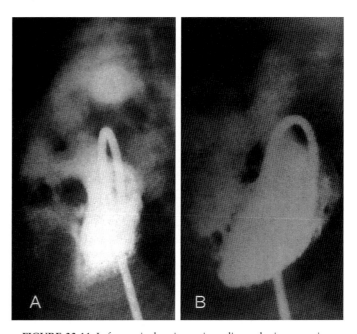

FIGURE 32.11 Left ventricular cineangiocardiography in a ventricular septal defect (VSD). Cranial left anterior-oblique view showing multiple VSDs in two patients. (Figures furnished by Dr. L. M. Bargeron, who developed this technique.)

In persons with a diastolic murmur suggesting semilunar valvular insufficiency, an aortogram is required for detection and estimation of the degree of aortic insufficiency. Additionally, documentation of coronary artery distribution is useful in situations in which a ventriculotomy is to be performed. Aortography also can demonstrate a left-to-right shunting patent ductus arteriosus, sidedness of the aortic arch, abnormalities of the branch vessels, and coarctation of the aorta, if present.

If pulmonary vascular resistance is elevated, the responsiveness of the pulmonary vascular bed should be tested by administration of 100% oxygen. Supplemental administration of nitric oxide may produce additional pulmonary vasodilation (52). Although the precise level of pulmonary vascular resistance that must be achieved to ensure safe surgical repair is uncertain, operation is generally advised if resistance decreases to a maximum of 6 to 8 $U \cdot m^2$ (53,54). Potentially correctable causes of pulmonary hypertension such as pulmonary vein obstruction and mitral stenosis should be excluded before the patient is deemed inoperable from pulmonary vascular disease.

DIFFERENTIAL DIAGNOSIS

In isolated VSD, the most common differential diagnostic problems arise in infants with large left-to-right shunts and in older children who have marked elevation of pulmonary vascular resistance. Cardiac catheterization is particularly helpful in infants to prove the presence of a ventricular defect or defects plus the presence or absence of associated defects in the unusual situation where echocardiographic data are equivocal.

Atrioventricular septal defects can be diagnosed from the ECG and echocardiogram. Occasionally, isolated VSDs may be associated with left-axis deviation and a counterclockwise loop in the frontal plane (29). If echocardiography is not diagnostic, left ventricular angiocardiography in the anterior-posterior view will demonstrate the characteristic gooseneck deformity of the atrioventricular septal defect.

Double-outlet right ventricle also can present with a large left-to-right shunt. Echocardiography is usually diagnostic, showing two arterial outlets arising from the right ventricle. Biplane cineangiocardiography usually will demonstrate the subaortic conus, and in the lateral view the separation of aortic and mitral valves leads one to this diagnosis.

By auscultation, pure infundibular pulmonary stenosis can sound very similar to a VSD. When the stenosis is severe, with greater than systemic systolic pressures in the right ventricle, the marked right ventricular hypertrophy evident on the ECG and prolongation of the murmur past aortic closure provide useful diagnostic clues to the diagnosis of infundibular pulmonary stenosis. It is common for these patients to have a VSD, although it may be small. Left ventricular cineangiocardiography is useful to demonstrate a VSD, which can be closed at the time that the stenosis is relieved surgically.

Double-chambered right ventricle also should be considered in situations with suspected VSD. Such patients also have significant right ventricular hypertrophy. Echocardiography and right ventricular angiography can clarify this diagnosis, which may be associated with a VSD.

Left ventricular–to–right atrial communications are suspected after finding a systolic murmur radiating to the right middle or upper sternal border, a diastolic rumble at the left sternal border, and right atrial enlargement on chest radiography or ECG. Pertinent catheterization findings include a large step-up in oxygen saturation at the right atrial level in the absence of an atrial septal defect and left ventricular angiography showing early right atrial opacification. These signs also can be present with VSD plus tricuspid insufficiency. Fortunately, preoperative diagnosis of left ventricular–to–right atrial communication is not essential for successful repair.

Occasionally, mild or moderate subaortic stenosis may be confused with a small VSD because of the overlap in the areas where the murmur is projected. The murmur in subaortic stenosis, however, usually radiates well to the upper right sternal border as well as toward the apex. In patients in whom the murmur suggests either a small VSD or subaortic stenosis, the presence of significant left ventricular hypertrophy on the ECG suggests subaortic stenosis. Echocardiographic/Doppler studies usually are diagnostic. Discrete subaortic stenosis can coexist with a VSD, and preoperative diagnosis is important.

Truncus arteriosus with increased pulmonary blood flow without visible cyanosis, aorticopulmonary window, and large patent ductus arteriosus can be mistaken for a VSD; however, accentuation of the arterial pulse pressure suggests a large aortic-pulmonary shunt. In addition, the chest film usually shows a concavity at the site of the main pulmonary artery in truncus arteriosus as well as rather high takeoffs for the right and left pulmonary artery. Retrograde aortography is essential in ruling out these defects in situations where echocardiographic studies are equivocal.

In the presence of a known VSD, associated lesions may present diagnostic problems. Associated aortic valve insufficiency (55) is indicated by a high-pitched, early diastolic decrescendo murmur in the second or third left interspace. It is unusual to detect the associated murmur of aortic valve insufficiency before 2 years of age. Once it becomes apparent, it may progress in severity.

In persons with corrected transposition of the great arteries with VSD and in those patients with common ventricle without pulmonary stenosis, the clinical picture may simulate isolated VSD. The ECG is useful for differentiating these patients, because Q waves in lead V1 or V4R occur commonly in the former two conditions. In addition, the echocardiogram usually is diagnostic.

Patients with transposition of the great arteries and large VSD can present with heart failure and minimal cyanosis. These patients are differentiated by the marked right ventricular hypertrophy on the ECG and by echocardiography.

TREATMENT: MEDICAL THERAPY

Children with small VSDs are asymptomatic and have excellent long-term prognosis. Neither medical therapy nor surgery is indicated.

If children with moderate or large VSDs develop symptomatic congestive heart failure (the clinical manifestation of pulmonary overcirculation and left-sided volume overload), a trial of medical therapy is indicated. Furosemide is used in a dosage of 1 to 3 mg/kg/day divided into two or three doses. Chronic furosemide can result in hypercalcemia and renal damage, as well as electrolyte disturbances. Addition of spironolactone can be helpful to minimize potassium loss. Potassium supplementation is difficult to achieve in most infants because of the unpalatable taste of the supplements. Additional initial therapy includes increasing the caloric density of the feedings. Systemic afterload reduction with enalapril (initial dosage of 0.1 mg/kg/24 hours divided into twice daily, gradually increasing to 0.5 mg/kg/24hours divided into twice daily dose, maximum of 40 mg/day) is also commonly prescribed. An acute trial has demonstrated efficacy in decreasing pulmonary flow and systemic resistance without decreasing pulmonary resistance (56). Symptomatic relief with a combination of diuretics and afterload reduction is common (57), although rigorous trials are lacking. The patient taking an angiotensin-converting enzyme inhibitor may experience a potassium-sparing effect, and spironolactone therapy should be discontinued.

A traditional approach has been to administer digoxin to infants with congestive heart failure associated with moderate or large VSD and increased pulmonary blood flow. Several studies have shown that the contractile function of the left ventricle is normal or increased, casting doubt on the usefulness of digoxin (58,59); however, symptomatic relief has been documented, and some experimental protocols have demonstrated acute benefit of digoxin on hemodynamic measurements (60). Digoxin may be indicated if diuresis and afterload reduction do not provide adequate symptom relief and surgery is not advisable. The usual dose of digoxin is 10 μg/kg/day that can be given once daily or in divided doses twice a day.

Many infants improve with medical therapy (61,62). Hypertrophy enables the left ventricle to handle a large volume and accounts for some of this improvement. Some patients show evidence of gradual decrease in the magnitude of the left-to-right shunt between 6 and 24 months of age. It is of paramount importance to assess accurately the cause of the decrease in left-to-right flow. It can result from an increase in pulmonary vascular resistance, a decrease in the relative size of the defect, or the development of hypertrophy of the outflow tract of the right ventricle with resultant functional or anatomic outflow obstruction. Although it may be difficult to determine how long to pursue medical management in the presence of continued symptomology and poor growth, improved surgical results have led many centers to recommend early surgery if symptoms do not respond to medical therapy.

Most children with VSD remain stable or improve following infancy. Heart failure rarely appears past infancy. Recurrence of symptoms may be due to respiratory infection, anemia, endocarditis, or development of an associated lesion such as aortic valve insufficiency.

A small group of patients will have developed severe pulmonary vascular obstructive disease with predominant right-to-left shunts by the time of referral (Eisenmenger's syndrome). Those inoperable patients will require symptomatic therapy and extensive counseling as their cyanosis increases and exercise capacity decreases. Red cell reduction by partial exchange transfusion may temporarily relieve symptoms of headache and extreme fatigue associated with extreme polycythemia. Relative iron deficiency anemia should be avoided. Selected patients may be candidates for lung or heart–lung transplantation (63) (see also Chapters 18 and 68, Heart–Lung Transplantation and Clinical Management of Patients with Pulmonary Hypertension, respectively). Some Eisenmenger's patients have acutely decompensated and died while at altitude. Supplemental oxygen should be available. This also applies to air travel where cabin pressurization may simulate an altitude of 5,000 to 7,000 feet.

SURGICAL THERAPY

Direct surgical repair has become the preferred operative therapy for VSD in most centers. Infants weighing as little as 2 kg can have operation. Current surgical mortality is <3% for single VSDs and VSDs with aortic valve insufficiency (AI), and about 5% for multiple VSD repair (64,65). Pulmonary artery banding, part of a two-stage repair strategy popular in the 1960s and 1970s, is largely reserved for critically ill infants with multiple VSDs or those with associated anomalies such as straddling atrioventricular valves or infants considered too small for complete repair.

Indications for surgical repair in infancy are uncontrolled congestive heart failure, including growth failure or recurrent respiratory infection. Large defects, even in the absence of symptoms, are repaired prior to 2 years of age (often prior to 1 year) if associated with elevated pulmonary artery pressure. Surgery generally is recommended for older, asymptomatic children with normal pulmonary pressure if the pulmonary-to-systemic flow ratio is >2:1. Defects associated with significant left ventricular dilation are often considered appropriate for repair.

There is a lower threshold for operation in patients with VSD and associated aortic insufficiency, especially if the latter is related to aortic cusp prolapse. Early repair may prevent progression of aortic valve insufficiency (66,67).

Most perimembranous and inlet defects are repaired using a transatrial surgical approach (the septal leaflet of the tricuspid valve may need to be detached to repair some inlet defects). Defects in the outlet septum can be repaired through the pulmonary valve. Multiple muscular defects, especially if near the apex, pose a difficult operative problem. Pulmonary banding may be preferred in small infants with severe heart failure. One approach to these lesions is to close the VSD with a single patch through an apical left ventriculotomy (68,69) (Fig. 32.12). Transcatheter therapy also has been successful (Fig. 32.8) but this technique is not yet in common use. Centers reporting results have shown good results with low complication rates in these difficult cases (70).

Postoperative Sequelae

A murmur of a residual VSD is frequent postoperatively. Echocardiography and color flow Doppler are useful in detecting residual shunt, but defect size may be difficult to determine (unless a large portion of the patch has split apart). Selective use of intraoperative TEE to assess VSD closure may be useful (46,47). Decisions regarding reoperation should be based on symptoms, left heart size, pulmonary pressure, and degree of shunting. In children with questionable indications for reoperation, catheterization is necessary.

Although patients who have required a left ventriculotomy for closure of a muscular VSD might show left ventricular dysfunction characterized by wall motion abnormalities, elevated end-diastolic pressure, or systolic dysfunction, a recent group of patients managed with this approach had normal indices of left ventricular function postoperatively (69). Longer follow-up of these patients at our institution has demonstrated no clinical symptoms or residual VSD. However, significant scarring of the LV apex on MRI has been observed (Fig. 32.13).

Right bundle branch block is common and may be due to ventriculotomy or direct injury to the right bundle itself. However, right bundle branch block occurs after a transatrial repair as well. Rarely, complete heart block can occur and is associated with late mortality. There is at least the theoretical possibility for a patient with right bundle branch block induced at surgery to develop complete heart block later in life if left bundle branch block is caused by acquired heart disease. Ventricular arrhythmias can be a late problem, particularly in persons with prior right or left ventriculotomies.

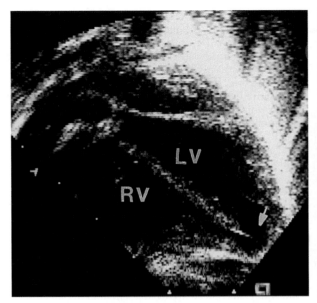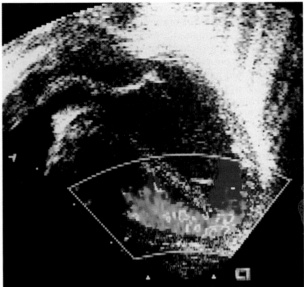

FIGURE 32.12 Apical four-chamber images of a large defect in the apical muscular septum of a 1-month-old infant. The color Doppler image on the **right** demonstrates left-to-right flow across the defect. The VSD was closed using a left ventricular apical incision. LV, left ventricle; RV, right ventricle.

CLINICAL COURSE AND PROGNOSIS

In general, long-term survival is good (71,72). Patients with small defects have an excellent prognosis, albeit with a small risk of endocarditis, aortic valve insufficiency, and late cardiac arrhythmia (73). A large number of these defects close spontaneously; this number approaches 75% to 80%, with most closing in the first 2 years of life. Those with perimembranous VSD will show an aneurysm of the ventricular septum or tricuspid valve pouch after spontaneous closure has occurred. These patients usually are followed indefinitely to detect spontaneous closure of the defect, to emphasize the importance of

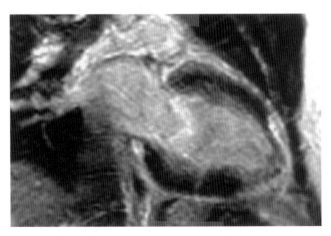

FIGURE 32.13 A late contrast-enhanced inversion recovery gradient echo magnetic resonance image (MRI) in a parasagittal two-chamber long-axis plane demonstrating enhancement of the left ventricular apex (*bright area*) consistent with chronic scar. (Courtesy of Dr. Christopher Kramer, University of Virginia, Departments of Internal Medicine, Cardiology, and Radiology.)

prophylactic antibiotics for endocarditis, and to observe for the occasional patient who develops a complication.

Patients with moderate-sized defects may develop large left-to-right shunts in infancy, and their main risk is heart failure between 1 and 6 months of age. Usually, this group can be managed medically without surgical intervention during infancy. If catheterization demonstrates that the right ventricular pressure is normal or only mildly elevated, most of these patients will have decreasing shunts over the first year of life and never require operative intervention (30,31). These patients, as well as those with large defects, occasionally develop significant infundibular pulmonary stenosis, which can progress in severity and require surgical intervention.

Approximately 15% to 20% of these patients continue to have large left-to-right shunts following infancy. If the clinical signs indicate that the shunt remains large, operation is recommended. However, in the Second Natural History of Congenital Heart Disease Study (73), 94.1% of patients with trivial, mild, or moderate VSDs managed medically were in New York State Heart Association Class I at follow-up 15 years after diagnosis.

Patients with large defects are the most difficult to manage because of the dangers of mortality in the first year of life owing to heart failure and associated pulmonary infections as well as the problem of development of elevated pulmonary vascular resistance. Patients who respond poorly to medical therapy and who continue to show signs of a large left-to-right shunt with growth failure and pulmonary infection undergo surgery within the first year of life.

The development of pulmonary vascular disease is uncommon in patients who undergo surgery before 2 years of age but may occur in as many as a quarter of patients with large defects who undergo surgery after 2 years of age (74). In addition, there was a progressively higher frequency of increased postoperative pulmonary resistance in the older patients. These data indicate that the pulmonary vascular obstructive changes can occur as early as 2 years of age. Generally, infants with VSD and increased pulmonary artery pressure should undergo repair between 3 and 12 months of age.

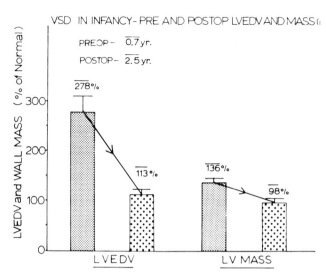

FIGURE 32.14 Normalization of left ventricular end-diastolic volume (LVEDV) and LV mass in infants undergoing repair of a ventricular septal defect in the first year of life.

There are at present limited data on long-term evaluation following operative correction of patients with moderate or large left-to-right shunts. Most patients have excellent results following operation, with normal growth, development, and activity. Longitudinal follow-up indicates that development of pulmonary hypertension is rare (4%) as is sinus node dysfunction (4%) but progressive aortic valve insufficiency is fairly common (16%) (75). Preoperative and postoperative left ventricular volume data in patients with large VSDs repaired at an average age of 5 years and restudied at an average of 1.6

years postsurgery demonstrated no significant residual shunts, LVEDV 118% of normal, left ventricular wall mass 134% of normal, and mildly depressed LVEF 85% of normal (76). Echocardiographic follow-up of children with surgically closed outlet VSD demonstrated that trivial or mild aortic valve insufficiency (AI) may develop in those without AI prior to surgery and that AI present before surgical closure improved in most cases (77).

It has been suggested that infants requiring surgery for VSDs early in life might show better postoperative left ventricular performance (78,79). Values for LVEDV and left ventricular mass are shown in Fig. 32.14 for seven infants who had closure of VSD at an average age of 12 months (78). The preoperative pulmonary-to-systemic flow ratio (Qp:Qs) averaged 2.1:1, right ventricular pressure averaged 96 mm Hg, and the ratio of right-to-left ventricular pressure was 1 in all patients. Repeat catheterization at an average of 1.5 years following operation showed that LVEDV had decreased from 278% to 113% of normal and left ventricular mass from 136% to 98% of normal. LVEF was normal postoperatively.

These data indicate that early closure of large VSDs in the first year of life is associated with a better result in terms of left ventricular function and regression of hypertrophy than surgery later in childhood. In evaluating early (<12 months) versus late operative results, multiple factors must be considered, including mortality, postoperative rhythm or conduction disturbances, pulmonary vascular resistance, ventricular function, and psychological impact. In children with large defects, there are no data to indicate a difference in mortality in infants versus older patients at surgical centers with a broad experience in infant cardiac surgery. Thus, repair in infancy is preferable in those symptomatic patients with large defects in whom a significant diminution in defect size during the first 18 months of life is unlikely.

References

1. Nadas AS, Fyler DC. *Pediatric Cardiology.* 3rd ed. Philadelphia: WB Saunders, 1972:348.
2. Keith JD, Rowe RD, Vlad P. *Heart Disease in Infancy and Childhood.* New York: Macmillan, 1967:3.
3. Hoffman JLE, Rudolph AM. The natural history of ventricular septal defects in infancy. *Am J Cardiol* 1965;16:634–653.
4. Nora JJ, Fraser FLC. *Medical Genetics.* Philadelphia: Lea & Febiger, 1974:334.
5. Moe DG, Guntheroth WG. Spontaneous closure of uncomplicated ventricular septal defect. *Am J Cardiol* 1987;60:674–678.
6. Tikanoja T. Effect of technical development on the apparent incidence of congenital heart disease. *Pediatr Cardiol* 1995;16:100–101.
7. Roguin N, Du Z-D, Barak M, et al. High prevalence of muscular ventricular septal defect in neonates. *J Am Coll Cardiol* 1995;26:1545–1548.
8. Ooshima A, Fukushige J, Ueda K. Incidence of structural cardiac disorders in neonates: An evaluation by color Doppler echocardiography and the results of a 1-year follow-up. *Cardiology* 1995;86:402–406.
9. Soto B, Becker AE, Moulaert AJ, et al. Classification of ventricular septal defects. *Br Heart J* 1980;43:332–343.
10. Lincoln C, Jamieson S, Shinebourne E, et al. Transatrial repair of ventricular septal defects with reference to their anatomic classification. *J Thorac Cardiovasc Surg* 1977;74:183–190.
11. Tatsuno K, Ando M, Takan A, et al. Diagnostic importance of aortography in conal ventricular-septal defect. *Am Heart J* 1975;89:171–177.
12. Anderson RH, Wilcox BR. The surgical anatomy of ventricular septal defect. *J Cardiac Surg* 1992;7:17–34.
13. Wennik ACG, Oppenheimer-Dekker A, Moulaert AJ. Muscular ventricular septal defects: A reappraisal of the anatomy. *Am J Cardiol* 1979;43:259–264.
14. Van Praagh R, McNamara JJ. Anatomic types of ventricular septal with aortic insufficiency. *Am Heart J* 1968;75:604–619.
15. Eroğlu AG, Öztunç F, Saltik L et al. Aortic valve prolapse and aortic regurgitation in patients with ventricular septal defect. *Pediatr Cardiol* 2003;24:36–39.
16. Rudolph AM. The effects of postnatal circulatory adjustments in congenital heart disease. *Pediatrics* 1965;36:763–772.
17. Jarmakani MM, Graham TP Jr, Canent RV Jr, et al. Effect of site of shunt on left heart volume characteristics with ventricular septal defect and patent ductus arteriosus. *Circulation* 1969;40:411–418.
18. Dammann JF Jr, Thompson WM Jr, Sosa O, et al. Anatomy, physiology and natural history of simple ventricular septal defects. *Am J Cardiol* 1960;5:136–166.
19. Ritter DG, Feldt RH, Weidman WH, et al. Ventricular septal defect. *Circulation* 1965;32(suppl 3):42–52.
20. Weidman WH, DuShane JW, Kirklin JW. Observations concerning progressive pulmonary vascular obstruction in children with ventricular septal defects. *Am Heart J* 1963;65:148–154.
21. Roger H. Recherches cliniques sur la communication congenitale des deux coeurs, par inocclusion du septum interventriculaire. *Bull Acad Nat Med (Paris)* 1879;8:1074.
22. Levin AE, Spach MS, Canent RV Jr, et al. Ventricular pressure-flow dynamics in ventricular septal defect. *Circulation* 1967;35:430–441.
23. Rabinovitch M, Keane JF, Norwood WI, et al. Vascular structure in lung tissue obtained at biopsy correlated with pulmonary hemodynamic findings after repair of congenital heart defects. *Circulation* 1984;69:655–667.
24. Haworth SG. Pulmonary vascular disease in ventricular septal defect: Structure and functional correlations in lung biopsies from 85 patients with outcome of intracardiac repair. *J Pathol* 1987;152:157–168.
25. Mecham RP. Conference summary: Biology and pathobiology of the lung circulation. *Chest* 1998;114(suppl):106–111.
26. Donald KE. Disturbances in pulmonary function in mitral stenosis and left heart failure. *Prog Cardiovasc Dis* 1958;1:298.
27. Wood P. The Eisenmenger syndrome or pulmonary hypertension with reversed central shunt. *BMJ* 1958;2:701–709, 755–762.
28. Abbott ME. Congenital heart disease. In: *Nelson's Loose-leaf Medicine.* Vol. 5. New York: Thomas Nelson & Sons, 1932:207.

29. Spach MS, Boineau JP, Long EC, et al. Genesis of the vectorcardiogram (electrocardiogram) in endocardial cushion defects. In: Hoffman I, Taymor RC, eds. *Vectorcardiography 1965*. New York: Elsevier/North Holland, 1966.

30. Van Hare GF, Soffer LJ, Sivakoff MC, et al. Twenty-five-year experience with ventricular septal defect in infants and children. *Am Heart J* 1987; 114:606–614.

31. van den Heuvel F, Timmers T, Hess J. Morphological, haemodynamic, and clinical variables as predictors for management of isolated ventricular septal defect. *Br Heart J* 1995;73:49–52.

32. Bierman FZ, Fellows K, Williams RG. Prospective identification of ventricular septal defects in infancy using subxyphoid two-dimensional echocardiography. *Circulation* 1980;62:807–817.

33. Cheatham JP, Latson LA, Gutgesell HP. Ventricular septal defect in infancy detection with two-dimensional echocardiography. *Am J Cardiol* 1981; 47:85–89.

34. Sutherland GR, Godman MJ, Smallhorn JF, et al. Ventricular septal defects: Two dimensional echocardiographic and morphological correlations. *Br Heart J* 1982;47:316–328.

35. Rein AJJT, Colan SD, Parness IA, et al. Regional and global left ventricular function in infants with anomalous origin of the left coronary artery from the pulmonary trunk: Preoperative and postoperative assessment. *Circulation* 1987;75:115–123.

36. Ortiz E, Robinson PJ, Deanfield JE, et al. Localization of ventricular septal defects by simultaneous display of superimposed colour Doppler and cross sectional echocardiographic images. *Br Heart J* 1985;54:53–60.

37. Sharef DS, Huhta JC, Marantz P, et al. Two-dimensional echocardiographic determination of ventricular septal defect size: Correlation with autopsy. *Am Heart J* 1989;117:1333–1336.

38. Canale JM, Sahn DJ, Valdes-Cruz LM, et al. Accuracy of two-dimensional echocardiography in the detection of aneurysms of the ventricular septum. *Am Heart J* 1981;101:255–259.

39. Sapire DW, Black IFS. Echocardiographic detection of aneurysms of the interventricular septum associated with ventricular septal defect: A method of noninvasive diagnosis and follow-up. *Am J Cardiol* 1975;36:797–801.

40. Ludomirsky A, Huhta JC, Vick GW III, et al. Color Doppler detection of multiple ventricular septal defects. *Circulation* 1986;74:1317–1322.

41. Houston AB, Lim MK, Doig WB, et al. Doppler assessment of the interventricular pressure drop in patients with ventricular septal defects. *Br Heart J* 1988;60:50–56.

42. Silbert DR, Brunson SC, Schiff R, et al. Determination of right ventricular pressure in the presence of a ventricular septal defect using continuous wave Doppler ultrasound. *J Am Coll Cardiol* 1986;8:379–384.

43. Eroğlu AG, Öztunç F, Saltik L, et al. Evolution of ventricular septal defect with special reference to spontaneous closure rate, subaortic ridge and aortic valve prolapse. *Pediatr Cardiol* 2003;24:31–35.

44. Pieroni DR, Nishimura RA, Bierman FZ, et al. Second natural study of congenital heart defects. Ventricular septal defect; echocardiography. *Circulation* 1993;87(suppl I):I80–I88.

45. Sommer RJ, Golinko RJ, Ritter SB. Intracardiac shunting in children with ventricular septal defect: Evaluation with Doppler color flow mapping. *J Am Coll Cardiol* 1990;16:1437–1444.

46. Muhiudeen IA, Roberson DA, Silverman NH, et al. Intraoperative echocardiography in infants and children with congenital cardiac shunt lesions: Transesophageal versus epicardial echocardiography. *J Am Coll Cardiol* 1990;16:1687–1695.

47. Rychik J, Norwood WI, Chin AJ. Doppler color flow mapping assessment of residual shunt after closure of large ventricular septal defects. *Circulation* 1991;84(suppl 3):III153–III161.

48. Carotti A, Marino B, Bevilacqua M, et al. Primary repair of isolated ventricular septal defect guided by echocardiography. *Am J Cardiol* 1997;79: 1498–1501.

49. Graham TP Jr, Jarmakani JM, Canent RV Jr, et al. Left heart volume estimations in infancy and childhood: Reevaluation of methodology and normal values. *Circulation* 1971;43:895–904.

50. Bargeron LM Jr, Elliott LP, Soto B, et al. Axial cineangiography in congenital heart disease. I: Concept, technical and anatomic consideration. *Circulation* 1977;56:1075–1083.

51. Elliott LP, Bargeron LM Jr, Bream PR, et al. Axial cineangiography in congenital heart disease. II: Specific lesions. *Circulation* 1977;56:1084–1094.

52. Atz AM, Adatia I, Lock JE, et al. Combined effects of nitric oxide and oxygen during acute pulmonary vasodilator testing. *J Am Coll Cardiol* 1999;33:813–819.

53. Day RW, Lynch JM, Shaddy RE, et al. Pulmonary vasodilatory effects of 12 and 60 parts per million inhaled nitric oxide in children with ventricular septal defect. *Am J Cardiol* 1995;75:196–198.

54. Neutze JM, Ishikawa T, Clarkson PM, et al. Assessment and follow-up of patients with ventricular septal defect and elevated pulmonary vascular resistance. *Am J Cardiol* 1989;63:327–331.

55. Halloran KH, Talner NS, Browne MJ. A study on ventricular septal defect associated with aortic insufficiency. *Am Heart J* 1965;69:320–326.

56. Webster MW, Neutze JM, Calder AL. Acute hemodynamic effects of converting enzyme inhibition in children with intracardiac shunts. *Pediatr Cardiol* 1992;13(3):129–135.

57. Montigny M, Davignon A, Fouron J-C, et al. Captopril in infants for congestive failure secondary to a large left to right shunt. *Am J Cardiol* 1989;63:631–633.

58. Berman W, Yabek SM, Dillon T, et al. Effects of digoxin in infants with a congested circulatory state due to a ventricular septa defect. *N Engl J Med* 1983;308:363–366.

59. Kimball TR, Daniels SR, Meyer RA, et al. Effect of digoxin on contractility and symptoms in infants with a large ventricular septal defect. *Am J Cardiol* 1991;68:1377–1382.

60. Stewart JM, Hintze TH, Woolf PK, et al. Nature of heart failure in patients with ventricular septal defect. *Am J Physiol* 1995;269:H1473–H1480.

61. Onat T, Ahunbay G, Batmaz G, et al. The natural course of isolated ventricular septal defect during adolescence. *Pediatr Cardiol* 1998;19: 230–234.

62. Krovetz JL. Spontaneous closure of ventricular septal defect. *Am J Cardiol* 1998;81:100–101.

63. Boucek MM, Faro A, Novick RJ, et al. The Registry of the International Society for Heart and Lung Transplantation: Fourth official pediatric report 2000. *J Heart Lung Transplant* 2001;20:39–52.

64. Arciniegas E, Farooki ZQ, Hakimi M, et al. Surgical closure of ventricular septal defect during the first twelve months of life. *J Thorac Cardiovasc Surg* 1980;80:921–928.

65. Hannan EL, Racz M, Kavey R-E, et al. Pediatric cardiac surgery: The effect of hospital and surgeon volume on in-hospital mortality. *Pediatrics* 1998;101:963–969.

66. Nadas AS, Thilenius OG, LaFarge CG, et al. Ventricular septal defect with aortic regurgitation: Medical and pathologic aspects. *Circulation* 1964;29: 862–873.

67. Yacoub MH, Khan H, Stavri G, et al. Anatomic correction of the syndrome of prolapsing right coronary aortic cusp, dilation of the sinus of Valsalva, and ventricular septal defect. *J Thorac Cardiovasc Surg* 1997;113:253–261.

68. McDaniel NL, Gutgesell HP, Nolan SP, et al. Repair of large muscular ventricular septal defects employing left ventriculotomy. *Ann Thorac Surg* 1989;47:593–594.

69. Hannan RL, McDaniel NL, Kron IL. Repair of large muscular ventricular septal defects in infants employing left ventriculotomy. *Ann Thorac Surg* 1997;63:288–289.

70. Knauth AL, Lock JE, Perry SB, et al. Transcatheter device closure of congenital and postoperative residual ventricular septal defects. *Circulation* 2004;110:501–507.

71. Moller JH, Patton C, Varco RL, et al. Late results (30 to 35 years) after operative closure of isolated ventricular septal defect from 1954 to 1960. *Am J Cardiol* 1991;68:1491–1497.

72. Ellis JH, Moodie DS, Sterba R, et al. Ventricular septal defect in the adult: Natural and unnatural history. *Am Heart J* 1987;114:115–120.

73. Kidd L, Driscoll DJ, Gersony WM, et al. Second natural history study of congenital heart defects: Results of treatment of patients with ventricular septal defects. *Circulation* 1993;87(suppl I):I38–I51.

74. DuShane JW, Krongrad E, Ritter DG, et al. The fate of raised pulmonary vascular resistance after surgery in ventricular septal defect. In: Rowe RD, Kidd BSL, eds. *The Child with Congenital Heart Disease after Surgery*. Mt. Kisco, NY: Futura Publishing, 1976.

75. Roos-Hesselin JW, Meijboom FJ, Spitaels SE, et al. Outcome of patients after surgical closure of ventricular septal defect at young age: Longitudinal follow-up of 22–34 years. *Eur Heart J* 2004;25:1057–1062.

76. Jarmakani JM, Graham TP Jr, Canent RV Jr, et al. The effect of corrective surgery on left heart volume and mass in children with ventricular septal defect. *Am J Cardiol* 1971;27:254–258.

77. Tomita H, Arakaki Y, Ono Y, et al. Evolution of aortic regurgitation following simple patch closure of doubly committed subarterial ventricular septal defect. *Am J Cardiol* 2000;86:540–542.

78. Cordell D, Graham TP Jr, Atwood GF, et al. Left heart volume characteristics following ventricular septal defect closure in infancy. *Circulation* 1976;54:294–298.

79. Graham TP Jr, Cordell GD, Bender HA Jr. Ventricular function following surgery. In: Rowe RD, Kidd BSL, eds. *The Child with Congenital Heart Disease after Surgery*. Mt. Kisco, NY: Futura Publishing, 1976:277–293.

CHAPTER 33 ■ PATENT DUCTUS ARTERIOSUS AND AORTOPULMONARY WINDOW

PHILLIP MOORE, MD, MBA, MICHAEL M. BROOK, MD, AND MICHAEL A. HEYMANN, MD

PATENT DUCTUS ARTERIOSUS

Anatomy

The ductus arteriosus, a large channel normally found in all mammalian fetuses, develops from the distal portion of the left sixth aortic arch and connects the main pulmonary trunk with the descending aorta, 5 to 10 mm distal to the origin of the left subclavian artery in a full-term infant. With a right aortic arch, the ductus arteriosus may be on the right, joining the right pulmonary artery and the right aortic arch just distal to the right subclavian artery; more commonly, it is on the left, joining the left pulmonary artery and the proximal portion of the left subclavian artery. Rarely, the ductus arteriosus may be bilateral. It varies in length and in the term fetus has a diameter of approximately 10 mm, similar to that of the descending aorta (1).

The microscopic structure of the ductus arteriosus differs from that of the adjacent pulmonary trunk or aorta. Although wall thicknesses are similar, the media of the latter are composed mainly of circumferentially arranged layers of elastic fibers, whereas the media of the ductus arteriosus consist largely of layers of smooth muscle arranged spirally in both leftward and rightward directions together with increased amounts of hyaluronic acid. The intimal layer of the ductus arteriosus is thicker than that of the adjoining arteries and contains an increased amount of mucoid substance. There are also small, thin-walled vessels in its subendothelial region (2,3).

Physiology

Role in the Fetus

By 6 weeks of gestation, the ductus arteriosus is developed sufficiently to carry most of the right ventricular output. The relative sizes of the great arteries and the ductus arteriosus reflect the proportions of cardiac output (combined ventricular output) carried by them (1). The right ventricle ejects about two thirds of combined ventricular output, and because lung flow is only 6% to 8%, the ductus arteriosus carries 55% to 60% of combined ventricular output (4). The ductus arteriosus permits flow to be diverted away from the high-resistance pulmonary circulation to the descending aorta and the low-resistance placental circulation. A large pulmonary blood flow during fetal life would represent wasted circulation, and the ductus arteriosus therefore reduces the total workload of the fetal ventricles (4).

Whether the ductus arteriosus plays an active physiologic role during fetal life is unknown. It had been considered a relatively passive structure until it was shown that prostaglandin E_2 (PGE_2) and prostacyclin (PGI_2) produce and maintain active relaxation (5–9).

Normal Postnatal Closure

Postnatal closure of the ductus arteriosus is effected in two phases. Immediately after birth, contraction and cellular migration of the medial smooth muscle in the wall of the ductus arteriosus produce shortening, increased wall thickness, and protrusion into the lumen of the thickened intima (intimal cushions or mounds), resulting in functional closure (3). This commonly occurs within 12 hours after birth in full-term human infants (10). The second stage usually is completed by 2 to 3 weeks in human infants, produced by infolding of the endothelium, disruption and fragmentation of the internal elastic lamina, proliferation of the subintimal layers, and hemorrhage and necrosis in the subintimal region. The mounds enlarge progressively, and there is connective tissue formation and replacement of muscle fibers with fibrosis and permanent sealing of the lumen to produce the ligamentum arteriosum (2).

The exact mechanisms responsible for the initial postnatal closure of the ductus arteriosus are not fully understood. During fetal life, the partial pressure of oxygen (pO_2) to which the ductus arteriosus is normally exposed is 18 to 28 mm Hg (4). An increase in pO_2, as occurs with ventilation after birth, constricts the ductus arteriosus in mature fetal animals (4,5,7,8,11); however, at about 0.6 gestation (term = 150 days), although capable of contracting, the ductus arteriosus is not constricted by increased oxygen even at high concentrations. With advancing gestation, the amount of constriction in response to increasing pO_2 is greater and the level of pO_2 required to initiate a response decreases (9,11). Other factors, such as the release of vasoactive substances (e.g., acetylcholine, bradykinin, or endogenous catecholamines), may contribute to postnatal closure of the ductus arteriosus under physiologic conditions (4,11).

Of greater importance is the role of prostaglandins, the cyclooxygenase-mediated products of arachidonic acid metabolism, in the ontogenic and overall physiology of the ductus arteriosus. Exogenous PGE_1, PGE_2, and PGI_2 dilate isolated ductus arteriosus strips or rings from term fetal lambs (5,6,8). Inhibitors of prostaglandin synthesis, either *in vitro* or when administered *in vivo* to pregnant animals near term, produce constriction of the ductus arteriosus (5,6,8), reversible by PGE_1 infusion (6), indicating that prostaglandins play an active role in maintaining the ductus arteriosus in a dilated state during normal fetal life. The exact sites of production of these prostaglandins *in vivo* are unclear. PGE_2 and PGI_2 are formed intramurally in the ductus arteriosus and may exert their action locally on muscle cells

(5–7). Endogenous PGI_2 production is about tenfold that of PGE_2; however, PGE_2 is three orders of magnitude more potent than PGI_2 as a relaxer of the ductus arteriosus (5,7). Prostaglandins are detectable only in very low concentrations in adult plasma, and most are not thought to act as circulating hormones because of their rapid catabolism in the lung (7). The fetus, however, has high circulating concentrations of prostaglandins, particularly PGE_2, probably owing to low fetal pulmonary blood flow and therefore decreased prostaglandin catabolism in the lungs, as well as to the fact that the placenta produces prostaglandins (5–7).

At birth, the placental source is removed, and the marked increase in pulmonary blood flow allows effective removal of circulating PGE_2. Thus, patency or closure of the ductus arteriosus represents a balance between the constricting effects of oxygen, and perhaps certain vasoconstrictive substances, and the relaxing effects of several prostaglandins (7,8).

The effects of prostaglandins, as well as of inhibitors of prostaglandin synthesis, vary at different gestational ages (5,7,9). Indomethacin constricts rings of ductus arteriosus from immature fetal lambs more than it does rings from close-to-term lambs. Both PGE_2 and PGI_2 relax the ductus arteriosus from immature lambs more than that from mature animals, reflecting the significantly greater sensitivity to PGE_2 and PGI_2 of the immature ductus arteriosus. This change in sensitivity is influenced by the increase in endogenous cortisol toward term.

The physiologic or pathophysiologic roles of other products of arachidonic acid metabolism by different pathways (e.g., cytochrome P450 monooxygenase) are not yet clearly established.

PERSISTENT PATENCY

Physiologic Considerations in Maintenance of Patency

Ontogenic differences in physiologic factors almost certainly account for the higher incidence of persistent patency of the ductus arteriosus (PDA) in preterm infants (9). Sensitivity of ductus arteriosus smooth muscle to PGE_2 is highest in immature animals and decreases with advancing gestation. In term infants, responsiveness is lost shortly after birth; this does not occur in the immature ductus. Pulmonary metabolism is important in reducing circulating concentrations of PGE_2; because this function is significantly reduced in immature lungs, increased circulating concentrations of PGE_2 as well as increased sensitivity are important contributors to persistent patency in preterm infants.

Physiologic Considerations of a Left-to-Right Shunt

General

As with all left-to-right shunts, with PDA three major, interrelated factors control the magnitude of shunting: The diameter and length of the ductus arteriosus, which governs the resistance offered to flow; the pressure difference between the aorta and the pulmonary artery; and the systemic and pulmonary vascular resistances.

Normally after birth, systemic vascular resistance (afterload) is high, whereas pulmonary vascular resistance decreases when ventilation begins. As a result, systemic arterial blood pressure becomes higher than that in the pulmonary artery. With a small PDA, a high resistance to flow is offered by the small cross-sectional opening of the ductus arteriosus, so that the left-to-right shunt will be small despite the large pressure difference. However, with a large communication, pressures tend to become equal, and the magnitude of shunting is then determined by the relationship of the systemic and pulmonary vascular resistances. For this reason left-to-right shunting through a PDA has been defined as dependent shunting (12). Because systemic vascular resistance does not change significantly after birth, changes in pulmonary vascular resistance are the major determinant in regulating the left-to-right shunting through a PDA. This is particularly important in the first 2 months after birth, when pulmonary vascular resistance normally is decreasing.

The physiologic features associated with left-to-right shunting through a PDA depend on the magnitude of the left-to-right shunt and the ability of the infant to handle the extra volume load (13). Left ventricular output, which normally is high in the immediate newborn period (14), is increased even further by the volume shunted left to right through the PDA (15). The resultant increase of pulmonary venous return to the left atrium and left ventricle increases ventricular diastolic volume (preload) and thereby left ventricular stroke volume (Frank–Starling's mechanism). Left ventricular dilation will result in an increased left ventricular end-diastolic pressure with secondary increase in left atrial pressure. This may lead to signs of overt left heart failure with left atrial dilation and pulmonary edema. Right ventricular failure may occur if there is a large PDA with pulmonary hypertension or pulmonary edema and an elevated left atrial pressure, in which case pulmonary vascular resistance may be increased. The net result of both these situations is an increased pressure load for the right ventricle. Left-to-right shunting through a stretched, incompetent foramen ovale secondary to left atrial dilation is a fairly common association (13).

Several compensatory physiologic mechanisms help to improve myocardial performance and thereby maintain a normal systemic output. In addition to the Frank–Starling mechanism, the sympathetic adrenal system is stimulated, as is the development of myocardial hypertrophy. Increased sympathetic stimulation leads to direct stimulation of nerve fibers within the myocardium, with local norepinephrine release as well as an increase in circulating catecholamines released from the adrenal glands. As a result, both the force of contraction and the heart rate are increased. These mechanisms are responsible for the rapid heart rate and the sweating often seen in infants with heart failure. If the increased volume load persists, hypertrophy of the ventricular myocardium will develop.

These compensatory mechanisms are ordinarily well developed in older children or adults; however, they are not as well developed in newborn infants and are even less so in prematurely born infants. It is most important, therefore, to consider the state of maturity (i.e., gestational age at time of birth) of an infant who has a PDA with left-to-right shunting. Many physiologic functions that are present in older children reach full maturation at different rates and periods of gestation. For example, sympathetic nervous innervation of the left ventricular myocardium may be completed only at term, or even after term (16), so that in an infant born prematurely, sympathetic stimulation of the left ventricular myocardium likely would be incomplete. Likewise, the myocardium in an immature animal responds less to stretch (Frank–Starling's mechanism) than does that in a more mature animal (17). The structure of the immature myocardium, too, is quite different from that at term in that there are far fewer contractile elements (17). Premature infants often have lower than normal serum Ca^{2+} concentrations, and this too may affect myocardial performance (18). Probably for one or all of these reasons, premature infants with left-to-right shunts through a PDA develop left ventricular failure earlier than their full-term counterparts and, in addition, with a smaller volume load. The altered myocardial structure also may be partly responsible for the poor response to digitalis of immature infants with left ventricular failure.

Of considerable importance as well is maintenance of myocardial perfusion. Because coronary arterial blood flow to the left ventricle occurs mainly during diastole and depends on the systemic arterial-intramyocardial diastolic pressure differences as well as the duration of diastole, alterations in either can affect coronary blood flow (19). A reduction in aortic diastolic pressure occurs in a large PDA, and with a significant shunt, left ventricular end-diastolic pressure may be increased and cause an increase in subendocardial intramyocardial pressure. The development of tachycardia will reduce the diastolic period. All three factors that affect adequate myocardial perfusion are therefore jeopardized in the presence of a large PDA.

Delivery of oxygen to the myocardium depends on not only the coronary blood flow, but also the oxygen content of arterial blood and the ability of arterial blood to deliver oxygen at the tissue sites. A low hemoglobin concentration caused by physiologic anemia in the newborn period, particularly in premature infants, or by repeated blood sampling as occurs with intensive neonatal care, jeopardizes oxygen delivery to the myocardium as well as to other organs. A further important factor, particularly in premature infants, is the amount of fetal hemoglobin present. Because fetal hemoglobin has a low affinity for the organic phosphates such as 2,3-diphosphoglycerate, the facilitation of oxygen delivery to peripheral tissues is reduced. This effect is greater with higher amounts of fetal hemoglobin (20).

Effects on the Pulmonary Circulation and Lungs

A small communication has little or no effect on the pulmonary arterial circulation. However, with a large communication, systemic and pulmonary arterial pressures will equalize, and because of the high flow and pressure, the small pulmonary arteries may not undergo their normal postnatal maturational changes. The medial smooth muscle does not regress as rapidly as normal or to the same extent, so that pulmonary vascular resistance falls more slowly and less completely than usual.

Initially the increase in pulmonary vascular resistance is associated only with an increased amount of medial smooth muscle. However, true pulmonary vascular disease (21) may occur subsequently, manifested by intimal damage with cellular proliferation, hyalinization, and finally thrombosis and fibrosis of the small pulmonary arteries. As more small pulmonary arteries become involved in this process, the pulmonary vascular resistance increases, the left-to-right shunt diminishes, and eventually a right-to-left shunt occurs. In severe pulmonary vascular obstructive disease, arteriovenous malformations may form with resultant hemoptysis.

Pulmonary edema occurs commonly in premature infants with only a moderate shunt and without severe heart failure.

Capillary permeability in newborn animals is greater than in adults, and may be even more pronounced in premature infants. A small elevation in pulmonary venous pressure therefore can produce significant pulmonary edema.

Delayed Closure in Term Infants

Although functional closure of the ductus arteriosus typically is completed on the first day after birth, it may be delayed for several days. Because pulmonary vascular resistance decreases normally, flow will occur from the aorta into the pulmonary artery throughout this period of functional patency. On careful auscultation, therefore, a murmur may be heard in the first few hours of life in many infants (22). Two particular murmurs have been described: A crescendo systolic murmur, and a continuous murmur with a crescendo systolic and diminuendo diastolic component. Neither murmur is very loud (grade 1 to 2 on a scale of 1 to 6), and both may be accentuated, or possibly only heard, during inspiration; the murmurs are heard best in the second to third left intercostal space and do not radiate widely. Because pulmonary arterial pressure is normal, the pulmonic component of the second sound is of normal intensity and the second sound is often well split (22). As the ductus arteriosus constricts, the diastolic component becomes inaudible and leaves only a crescendo systolic murmur that usually disappears by the second to third day of life. The electrocardiogram (ECG) and chest roentgenogram in these infants are normal. Real-time two-dimensional echocardiography shows normal intracardiac structures, and the ductus arteriosus generally is visualized directly. Doppler and color Doppler evaluation invariably detect and delineate the flow patterns of the shunt across the ductus arteriosus into the main pulmonary artery (23–25). Retrograde aortic flow is not seen in these infants. Hemodynamic studies performed in some of these infants in the past demonstrated small left-to-right shunts with essentially normal arterial pressures.

During the initial hours of constriction, any condition that lowers arterial blood pO_2 or increases circulating blood PGE_2 concentrations may delay normal closure (26). Likewise, before true anatomic closure occurs, the functionally closed ductus arteriosus may dilate with a reduced arterial blood pO_2 (27) or increased PGE_2 concentration. This may occur in asphyxial states and in the presence of any one of many different pulmonary diseases (e.g., meconium aspiration). Residing at a high-altitude location, a nonpulmonary cause of arterial hypoxemia, has been shown to produce delayed closure of the ductus arteriosus. The incidence of PDA is about 30 times greater at high altitude (4,500 to 5,000 m) than at sea level (28). With severe pulmonary disease or persistent pulmonary hypertension syndrome of the newborn, when there is an increase in pulmonary vascular resistance, no shunt or even a right-to-left shunt through the PDA may occur. This leads to a lower pO_2 in the lower extremities than in the upper. This difference in pO_2 may persist for many days, and with pulmonary disease the ductus arteriosus may remain patent for several weeks.

The initial constriction of the ductus arteriosus is most prominent at its pulmonary arterial end and extends progressively toward the aorta, thus accounting for the typical cone shape of the small PDA in which the diameter at the aortic end is considerably larger than at the pulmonary end. Even after the pulmonary arterial end has closed completely, the dilated aortic end of the ductus arteriosus may be apparent for many weeks. This ductus ampulla, or ductus bump, may be evident

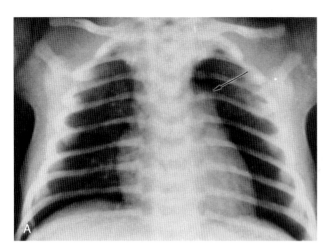
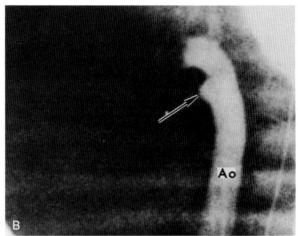

FIGURE 33.1 **A:** Posterior-anterior chest roentgenogram of a 2-day-old infant demonstrating the ductus bump (*arrow*). **B:** Angiogram in the lateral position of a 5-day-old infant demonstrating the ampulla of the ductus arteriosus (*arrow*). Ao, aorta.

on the chest roentgenogram (Fig. 33.1A) for several weeks (29). Persistence of the ductus ampulla (Fig. 33.1B) for many months or even years has been well demonstrated by angiograms in older children.

Persistent Patency in Premature Infants

Delayed closure of the ductus arteriosus in preterm infants is well recognized (10,30–34). With the advent of techniques for maintenance of ventilation in premature infants, survival, particularly of small premature infants, has improved dramatically. Improvement of lung function with surfactant replacement therapy, by decreasing pulmonary vascular resistance, has led to the clinical emergence of PDA earlier and more frequently in preterm infants (35). Because the constrictor response of the ductus arteriosus to oxygen and the dilator effect of PGE_2 are closely related to gestational age (5,7,11), it is not surprising that there is an extremely high incidence of PDA in low-birth-weight preterm infants, particularly the very low birth weight infant (<1,000 g) and those with pulmonary disease. Approximately 45% of infants <1,750 g birth weight have clinical evidence of PDA, and infants <1,200 g birth weight have a prevalence closer to 80%. Overall, the incidence of PDA in preterm infants is about 8 per 1,000 of all live births.

Manifestations

The clinical features depend on the magnitude of left-to-right shunt through the PDA and the ability of the infant to initiate compensatory mechanisms to handle the extra volume load. Because many premature infants have respiratory distress syndrome, the stage of development of this disease and the use of surfactant replacement therapy will determine the pulmonary vascular resistance and therefore the shunt. The maturity of the infant and the stage of myocardial development determine the ability to handle the shunt.

Three fairly distinct patterns of clinical presentation are recognized in these infants.

Patent Ductus Arteriosus with Little or No Lung Disease. In the first group, there is little or no underlying pulmonary

disease (usually infants whose birth weight exceeds 1,500 g). However, smaller infants are encountered, and in many instances their mothers have received steroid or other therapy prior to delivery, or the infants have received surfactant replacement therapy. A systolic murmur is first heard 24 to 72 hours after birth, and as the left-to-right shunt increases, this murmur becomes louder and more prolonged, extending to and often beyond the second heart sound into early diastole. The murmur commonly is heard best at the left sternal border in the second and third intercostal spaces. The classic continuous machinery murmur, described for older children with PDA, is not usual in premature infants, in whom the murmur generally has a high-frequency "rocky" quality. The pulmonic component of the second sound may become moderately accentuated. In the most mature infants in this group, a middiastolic flow rumble owing to increased diastolic flow across the normal mitral valve may be heard at the apex. If the shunt becomes large enough, a third heart sound due to rapid ventricular filling during diastole may be heard at the apex. The precordium becomes increasingly more hyperactive, the pulse pressure widens, and the peripheral pulses become more prominent and bounding as the left-to-right shunt increases. Increased peripheral pulses are best appreciated by the presence of palmar or forearm pulses.

If the shunt is allowed to become sufficiently large, clinical evidence of left ventricular failure may appear. This includes tachycardia, tachypnea, and rales on auscultation of the lung fields. Associated with the development of pulmonary edema, there may be a decrease in arterial blood pO_2. If left ventricular failure were allowed to progress, a significant number of these infants might develop episodes of apnea, often associated with severe bradycardia. Enlargement of the liver will occur, but usually quite late.

The ECG is not helpful early in the disease, but if a moderately large shunt persists for several weeks, left ventricular and left atrial hypertrophy may become evident. The chest roentgenogram may show enlargement of both the left atrium and left ventricle if there is a moderately large shunt, but heart size commonly is normal. Pulmonary vascularity is often increased. Dilation of the ascending aorta usually is not seen in premature infants, but may occur with a protracted moderately severe shunt.

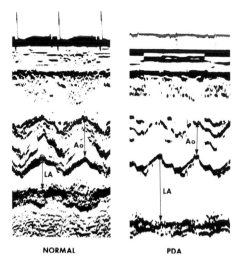

FIGURE 33.2 Echocardiograms from two premature infants, one without clinical evidence of a PDA (**left**) and the other (**right**) with a large left-to-right shunt through a PDA that was subsequently ligated. LA, left atrial diameter; Ao, aortic root diameter; PDA, with patent ductus arteriosus.

A full echocardiographic and Doppler evaluation has become essential in the clinical management of PDA and in assessing the magnitude of the shunt (23,24,36,37). This also will exclude congenital cardiac lesions with similar clinical findings as well as left ventricular failure owing to poor intrinsic myocardial function. Left atrial diameter varies with the size of the infant, so the ratio of the left atrial (LA) diameter to the aortic root (Ao) diameter can be used to determine LA enlargement (Fig. 33.2). The normal LA:Ao ratio in infants is between 0.8 and 1. A ratio >1.2 suggests left atrial enlargement, which, in the absence of left ventricular failure due to some other cause (such as aortic stenosis or volume overload),

most often indicates a significant left-to-right shunt. In the premature infant this is likely to be through a PDA. Two-dimensional echocardiography is now used to accurately assess left atrial and ventricular size directly. The dynamics of both left ventricular and descending aortic wall motion also indicate the magnitude of shunt. Direct visualization of the ductus arteriosus (Fig. 33.3) confirms the diagnosis. Doppler techniques (pulsed, continuous wave, and color) are applied to the evaluation of flow patterns in infants with PDA and are most helpful (24) (Fig. 33.4). Flow from the aorta into the pulmonary artery can be detected, and velocity profiles of flow in the main pulmonary artery, ductus arteriosus, and descending aorta in infants with PDA have been characterized. Doppler color flow mapping (25) also allows visualization of the extent of flow disturbance in the main pulmonary artery and the direction of the flow jet. Estimates of pulmonary arterial pressure also can be made if systemic arterial blood pressure is known (38).

Cardiac catheterization and angiography in these infants now is unnecessary because of the complete diagnostic information obtained by echocardiography. If performed, catheterization reveals moderate elevation of pulmonary arterial pressures and left-to-right shunting through the ductus arteriosus (30).

The use of biomarkers in the presence of PDA is currently being evaluated. As early as 1987, it was known that natriuretic peptide levels were abnormally elevated in the presence of a patent duct (39). More recently, B-type natriuretic peptide (BNP) has been studied in the presence of a duct in premature infants. BNP has been shown in adults to correlate to LV volume overload and LV failure (40). Small studies have showed that BNP levels are elevated in the presence of a large ductal shunt in premature infants (41,42). BNP levels decrease in both term and preterm infants rapidly after birth (43,44). In patients with a significant ductal shunt and elevated BNP levels, closure of the PDA results in a fall in BNP levels (45,46). BNP therefore, may be helpful in the screening and evaluation of newborn premature infants with a suspected ductal shunt, but its role in older infants (>2 weeks) or in asymptomatic patients has yet to be investigated.

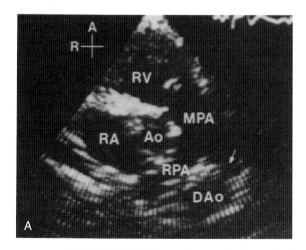
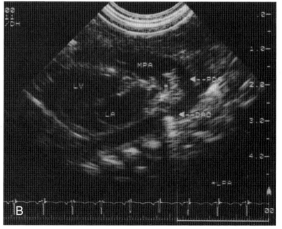

FIGURE 33.3 A: Echocardiogram in short-axis view demonstrating a patent ductus arteriosus (*arrow*). A, anterior; Ao, ascending aorta; DAo, descending aorta; MPA, main pulmonary artery; R, right; RA, right atrium; RPA, right pulmonary artery; RV, right ventricle. **B:** A high parasternal sagittal projection from the second left intercostal space parallel to the vertebral bodies (so-called ductus cut). The main pulmonary artery (MPA), patent ductus arteriosus (PDA), and descending aorta (DAO) are seen in a continuous arc. The origin of the left pulmonary artery (*LPA) is also seen. Posterior to the aorta, the vertebral bodies are seen behind the heart, showing the vertical orientation of the scan. LA, left atrium; LV, left ventricle.

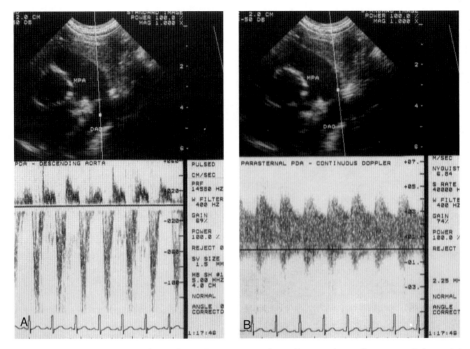

FIGURE 33.4 The **top** section of each figure demonstrates the real-time echocardiogram and the position of the Doppler sample volume and beam; the **bottom** section shows the resultant Doppler signal. **A:** This image evaluates blood flow in the descending aorta (DAO) just distal to the connection of the ductus arteriosus and the DAO. The pulsed Doppler signal shows systolic flow down the descending aorta (downward deflection, away from the transducer). During diastole there is reversal of flow into the main pulmonary artery (MPA) from the DAO (upward deflection above the baseline, toward the transducer). **B:** In this ductus cut, the Doppler beam is positioned through the MPA, ductus, and DAO. The continuous-wave Doppler signal shown represents the path determined by placing the transducer along this line of interrogation. Retrograde flow into the MPA occurs throughout. The continuous-wave signal samples the peak velocities through the ductus, which range from about 5 m/s in systole to about 3 m/s in diastole. These values, when used with systemic arterial blood pressure and the modified Bernoulli equation, allow for an estimation of pulmonary arterial pressures.

Many infants in this group do not develop severe left ventricular failure and ordinarily are easily managed with specific medical therapy to constrict the ductus arteriosus or conventional medical therapy of mild cardiac failure in preterm infants, fluid intake restriction, diuretics, and maintenance of hematocrit above 45%. Very rarely, intractable cardiac failure develops, and surgical closure may be required. More often existing premature lung disease, active or resolving, adds to respiratory and feeding difficulties, which prompt treatment as will be discussed in the next sections. If left alone, the ductus arteriosus closes spontaneously in most of these infants, commonly within 2 to 3 months after birth.

Patent Ductus Arteriosus in Infants Recovering from Lung Disease. The second and most common group of infants develops left-to-right shunting while recovering from severe or moderately severe respiratory distress syndrome. These infants usually weigh 1,000 to 1,500 g at birth. The idiopathic respiratory distress syndrome usually is evident within a few hours after birth, and if it follows the usual course, starts to improve after 3 to 4 days. As this improvement continues, early clinical evidence of a left-to-right shunt through a PDA appears. In addition, at about this age, fluid administration generally is increased to deliver adequate calories; this often aggravates the volume-loading effects of the left-to-right shunt on left ventricular function. Probably the ductus arteriosus has

been patent since birth and the pulmonary disease with a resultant increase in pulmonary vascular resistance has prevented a detectable left-to-right shunt. As the pulmonary disease improves, oxygenation increases and the ductus arteriosus should constrict. However, most of these infants are quite immature, so a good constrictor response may not occur. Many of these infants are still maintained on mechanical ventilators or continuous positive airway pressure (CPAP), so that careful clinical assessment is required to establish the presence of a shunt through the ductus arteriosus. In many instances the murmurs are not audible until the infant is briefly detached from the ventilator or CPAP system. Because recovery from the respiratory distress syndrome often is not continuously progressive but is interspersed with periods of deteriorating lung function, left-to-right shunting (and therefore the murmur) may be intermittent for several days. The murmur commonly disappears and reappears several times within short periods of time. Initially a systolic murmur alone is heard; however, as the shunt increases, the murmur extends into diastole. The murmur is similar in distribution and quality to that in the first group of premature infants with PDA. Because infants in the second group are usually more immature than those in the first, left ventricular failure may occur in them when clinically there seems to be less left-to-right shunting. A third sound often is heard, but a middiastolic flow rumble is uncommon. The pulmonic component of the second sound ordinarily is already accentuated because of the pulmonary disease but may become louder as the shunt increases. Increasing precordial activity is a good clinical indication of the magnitude of shunting in these infants, and increased heart rate, pulse pressure, and bounding pulses with a rapid upstroke are often detectable early. Palmar or forearm pulses are often palpable. Because most of these infants have indwelling umbilical arterial catheters, careful monitoring of the umbilical arterial blood pressure often shows a widening pulse pressure and a decrease in diastolic pressure as left-to-right shunting develops.

Rales are unreliable as an index of pulmonary edema and left ventricular failure because they may be suppressed by positive pressure ventilation used in these infants. However, in those extubated who have recovered sufficiently from their respiratory distress syndrome, rales may be heard. Apneic episodes are also common in this group and may be associated with short periods of bradycardia.

Deterioration in the ventilatory status of an infant recovering from respiratory distress syndrome is often a strong indication of a significant left-to-right shunt through a PDA. However, other causes, such as recurring lung disease and pneumothorax or sepsis, should be actively excluded. Deterioration of the ventilatory status is manifested by the requirement for an increasing concentration of inspired oxygen, alterations in ventilator rate or pressure settings, increased requirements of CPAP, and assisted ventilation and increasing arterial blood pCO_2. The ECG often shows increased right ventricular forces owing to the underlying pulmonary disease but generally is of little help. A chest roentgenogram will show the parenchymal changes of respiratory distress syndrome, and increased pulmonary vascularity therefore may be extremely difficult to assess. Cardiomegaly is variable, particularly if the infant is being artificially ventilated; however, increasing cardiomegaly may indicate an increasing shunt.

Because many of the changes described may be due to deterioration resulting from underlying pulmonary disease, it is important to be able to assess the contribution to the clinical picture of a PDA. For this purpose, the echocardiogram usually is very helpful. An increasing LA:Ao ratio will be produced by increasing left-to-right shunting, whereas a ratio that remains constant and within normal limits may indicate noncardiac causes of deterioration. Changes in the left ventricle, left atrium, and PDA size assessed reliably by two-dimensional Doppler echocardiography will determine the role of shunting through the PDA. It should be emphasized that very early diagnosis is possible with two-dimensional Doppler echocardiography, which is completely noninvasive and safe. In addition, BNP may become more useful in the coming years in the screening and evaluation of these patients. This, coupled with current, more aggressive management approaches, has altered the natural history of PDA so that infants rarely are allowed to develop many of the signs described above.

Patent Ductus Arteriosus Associated with Lung Disease. The third group consists of infants who have severe respiratory distress syndrome from birth. Because many of these are very low birth weight infants (<1,000 g), the likelihood of a PDA being present is very high (>80%). A few show no clinical signs even when carefully evaluated—the "silent" ductus arteriosus (47). Many do show clinical evidence of a left-to-right shunt through the PDA, or fail to show improved respiratory status at an age when they should start to recover from the primary pulmonary disease. They too are extremely sensitive to small increases in Na^+ and fluid administration. They require ventilatory assistance by mechanical respirators or CPAP. Deterioration commonly is manifested by the need for increasing ventilator pressure, rate, or oxygen, or CPAP support. Failure to improve is manifested by the inability to wean the infant from ventilatory support. An increase in arterial blood pCO_2 is common. Murmurs may be difficult to hear, and in some of these infants the ductus arteriosus may be so widely patent that a murmur is not produced (48). Changes in the ventilatory status may be due to progression of the primary pulmonary disease, and it is often even more difficult to separate left ventricular failure from increasing pulmonary problems than in the previous group. Increasing precordial activity, bounding pulses, and a widening arterial pulse pressure suggest the development of left-to-right shunting. When present, the murmur is usually only systolic, the pulmonic component of the second sound is accentuated, and a gallop rhythm is often heard. The ECG and chest radiograph usually are not helpful, but as outlined above, the two-dimensional Doppler echocardiographic evaluation is diagnostic even before clinical signs are apparent.

Management

Confirmation of Diagnosis. Infants with birth weights <1,500 g who have clinical evidence of significant left-to-right shunting are more likely to have a PDA. However, more severe forms of congenital heart disease should be considered. Clinical evaluation combined with a chest roentgenogram and ECG often cannot differentiate a PDA from such lesions as truncus arteriosus or aortopulmonary window unless an additional anomaly (e.g., a right aortic arch) is present. The two-dimensional echocardiogram Doppler study is diagnostic in distinguishing truncus arteriosus or aortopulmonary window from PDA.

Occasionally angiocardiographic confirmation is desired if there is a question of coarctation in association with the PDA. Because many infants with suspected PDA have an umbilical arterial catheter in place, it is ordinarily a simple procedure to replace this with an angiographic catheter and advance it to the thoracic aorta. Angiography gives a clear picture of the size of the PDA but only a rough estimate of the magnitude of shunting. Current practice in infants in whom the clinical and echocardiographic evidence indicates a PDA with left-to-right shunting is medical or surgical management without aortography to confirm the diagnosis. As noted above, BNP may become useful as a screening tool, decreasing the frequency of echocardiography in some infants.

Relationship to Systemic Organ Perfusion. Redistribution of systemic blood flow occurs even with moderate shunts (49). Retrograde aortic flow, decreased systemic blood flow, and moderate hypotension are common in premature infants with a PDA and may lead to decreased perfusion in many organs, with potential clinical consequences to each. Reduced cerebral blood flow or changes in cerebral blood flow velocity patterns have been implicated in the occurrence of intraventricular hemorrhage (50). Renal function may be compromised (51), and myocardial perfusion, particularly subendocardial blood flow, may be reduced (19).

A major factor involved in the development of necrotizing enterocolitis is bowel ischemia. A PDA with significant left-to-right shunting may be one of the contributing conditions in the production of bowel ischemia, but its role in the incidence of necrotizing enterocolitis is not proven. We therefore carefully monitor abdominal girth and residual gastric volumes prior to feeding and perform hematests on all stools and gastric aspirates in all premature infants with a PDA. We feel that when signs of necrotizing enterocolitis develop in an infant with significant left-to-right shunting through a PDA, early surgical closure of the ductus arteriosus has significantly reduced mortality. Therefore, if persistent abdominal distention, increasing residuals before feedings, blood in the stools or gastric aspirate, decreasing bowel sounds, and, particularly, intramural air occur in association with a significant left-to-right shunt through a PDA, immediate surgical closure is recommended.

Treatment

An important consideration in treating a premature infant with a PDA is maintenance of an adequate hematocrit and hemoglobin. A reduction in hemoglobin requires an increased cardiac output to maintain peripheral oxygenation, and with a left-to-right shunt and an already compromised myocardium, anemia may further impair cardiac function. In addition, because myocardial oxygen delivery depends on blood oxygen content, low hemoglobin exacerbates tissue ischemia, particularly in the abdomen and lower body where blood flow is reduced. Because arterial blood gas sampling is common, the hematocrit often decreases, and care must be taken to maintain it >45%. Because peripheral tissue oxygen delivery is retarded by fetal hemoglobin, exchange transfusion replacing fetal hemoglobin with adult hemoglobin may help to facilitate peripheral oxygenation (20). Because most premature infants require repeated blood sampling and blood transfusions, this is, in fact, usually accomplished. Electrolyte, glucose, and nutritional requirements must be carefully maintained. Caloric intake is often a major problem, and intravenous hyperalimentation may be required. Because volume overload may precipitate left ventricular failure, Na^+ and fluid administration commonly are restricted to low maintenance amounts. Previously, left ventricular failure was treated by digitalization and the use of diuretics, particularly furosemide. More recently it has become evident that in very small preterm infants, digitalis is relatively ineffective, and owing to potential toxic reactions, digitalis is rarely used now. All of the above are aimed at supportive treatment of a left-to-right shunt with myocardial failure. Optimally, treatment should be aimed directly at removing the shunt and its effects by closing the ductus arteriosus. The timing of such a maneuver and the method to be used remain open to debate.

Surgical closure before 10 days of age reduces the duration of ventilatory support and hospital stay and lowers morbidity (52). The use of oral or, preferably, intravenous (lyophilized) indomethacin to constrict the ductus arteriosus has led to successful nonsurgical closure in a large proportion of treated infants (53–55); the effects of indomethacin apparently are best when it is administered before 10 days of age and in less mature infants. Originally, indomethacin was administered only to infants in whom standard medical management had failed and surgery was contemplated (53); however, this is no longer the case. Dose schedules vary, but commonly a first dose of 0.2 mg/kg is given by nasogastric tube or intravenously. For intravenous indomethacin, subsequent doses depend on the age at initial treatment—if <48 hours, the subsequent two doses are 0.10 mg/kg; if 2 to 7 days, 0.20 mg/kg; and if >7 days, 0.25 mg/kg. A total of three doses usually is given 12 to 24 hours apart depending on urinary output; if urine flow decreases, fewer doses may be used or the time between doses may be extended. If clinical signs reappear after an initially successful course of therapy, a second course may be considered. Because signs of a shunt reappear in some infants, a more prolonged initial course of therapy has been suggested. Indomethacin should not be administered to infants with renal dysfunction (serum creatinine >1.6 mg/dL or blood urea nitrogen >20 mg/dL), overt bleeding, shock, necrotizing enterocolitis, or any suspicion thereof, or if there is electrocardiographic evidence of myocardial ischemia (56). The renal side effects of oliguria and hyponatremia do not always occur, and when they do they usually are transient; no obvious long-term adverse effects have been experienced (57). These renal side effects are more common, and often more severe, when significant fluid restriction precedes therapy. Administration to infants with PDA before they show obvious major hemodynamic complications has been used with good success, particularly in infants with birth weight <1,000 g (54). In this group of infants, the initiation of therapy is suggested immediately on diagnosis, which ordinarily is before 72 hours of age. True prophylactic therapy on the first day after birth appears to have no advantage, and because not all infants develop a PDA, a certain number would receive indomethacin unnecessarily.

Some studies have investigated combined treatment with indomethacin and inhibition of the nitric oxide pathway for very premature infants refractory to indomethacin alone (58). The combination of L-NMMA and indomethacin improved the closure rate, but the use adversely affected the creatinine and produced systemic hypertension, limiting its usefulness.

More recently, ibuprofen has also been evaluated as a possible alternative to indomethacin in preterm infants (59–64). In addition, meta-analysis of the available studies has shown a comparable rate of ductal closure after ibuprofen treatment (65–67). Some evidence exists that there may be less effect of ibuprofen on renal function and urine output (59,60). In addition, ibuprofen has less effect on cerebral vasculature and cerebral blood flow but has not shown a decreased risk for intraventricular hemorrhage (61,63,64). However, in trials using ibuprofen for prophylaxis, there has been an increased incidence of pulmonary hypertension (68) such that this trial was ended prematurely.

As with early surgical ligation, early treatment probably will reduce overall morbidity associated with a PDA. In premature baboons, ligation results in improved lung mechanics and ventilation at 14 days; however, there is no effect on histologic progression of chronic lung injury (69). Improved lung mechanics have been confirmed in premature infants 26 to 29 weeks' gestation after ligation showing an increase in dynamic compliance, tidal volume, and minute ventilation (70). The benefit of treatment in premature infants with lung disease has been confirmed in a retrospective study showing a fourfold mortality risk for infants <28 weeks with persistent PDA after medical treatment as compared with those without PDA or those successfully closed (71).

If after 48 to 72 hours of adequate medical management left ventricular failure is still uncontrolled, surgical closure is performed. Despite the small risk of recanalization, ligation rather than division of the ductus arteriosus has been recommended, although many surgeons still clip ligate to minimize the need for dissection and associated injury. Surgery now can be performed with minimal morbidity and mortality (72). Thorascopic surgery is used at some centers to minimize the effect on chest wall mechanics (73).

Prevention

Despite the efficacy of treatment of the patent duct in preterm infants, significant morbidity remains. Therefore, it would seem that early closure, before the development of clinical symptoms, may reduce associated morbidity. Indeed, prophylactic administration of indomethacin in preterm infants prior to 28 weeks decreases the incidence of serious pulmonary hypertension, grade III/IV intraventricular hemorrhage, and need for surgical closure, but has not been shown to alter mortality (74). Prophylactic ibuprofen also decreases the need for symptomatic treatment but has not yet been shown to alter the incidence of intraventricular hemorrhage (75). In addition, one trial reported an incidence of significant pulmonary hypertension after prophylactic ibuprofen administration (68).

Persistent Patency in Term Infants

The incidence of isolated PDA in full-term infants is about 1 in 2,000 live births (76), accounting for about 5% to 10% of all types of congenital heart disease. Unlike the ductus arteriosus in premature infants, in whom failure of closure is due to physiologic developmental retardation, the ductus arteriosus in full-term infants is abnormal, and failure to constrict is probably related to a significant structural abnormality.

Patency of the ductus arteriosus may occur in more than one member of a family, suggesting possible genetic factors in certain instances. Patent ductus arteriosus has been produced by genetic inbreeding in poodles (77). Recent gene linkage and chromosome analysis studies in humans have shown abnormalities on chromosome 12 in isolated PDA patients in Iran (78) and on chromosome 16 in association with aortic aneurysm (79).

Manifestations

In mature infants and older children, the factors determining the clinical features are the same as in premature infants, namely, the size of the communication, the relationship between pulmonary and systemic vascular resistances, and the ability of the myocardium to handle the extra volume load.

Small Ductus Arteriosus. With a small communication, pulmonary vascular resistance and therefore pulmonary arterial pressure normally decrease after birth. However, because the resistance to flow across the ductus arteriosus is high, only a small left-to-right shunt develops. Pulmonary blood flow is increased only minimally, and left ventricular failure does not occur. Therefore, few patients are symptomatic, and attention is often brought to this condition only by the murmur detected at a routine physical examination.

Physical growth is normal except in those children in whom maternal rubella was present. The peripheral pulses may be full, and the arterial pulse pressure is slightly increased unless the shunt is very small. Precordial activity usually is normal with no increased apical impulse. First and second heart sounds are normal, and the only significant abnormal auscultatory finding may be the presence of a murmur. In early infancy, before pulmonary vascular resistance has decreased completely, there may be a short period in which no murmur is heard. A short systolic murmur may then be heard, which may progress to the typical, continuous murmur heard in older children. This murmur is heard best in the second left intercostal space and often is accentuated when the patient is recumbent or during inspiration. Administration of a vasopressor agent such as phenylephrine raises systemic vascular resistance and increases left-to-right shunt, and the murmur will become longer and louder. The important features of the characteristic continuous murmur first described by Gibson (80) are the late systolic accentuation and continuation through the second sound into diastole. The murmur ordinarily starts shortly after the first sound, peaks at the second heart sound, and fades away, ending in the last third of diastole.

The ECG and chest roentgenogram are usually normal in these children; however, slight prominence of the main and peripheral pulmonary arteries may be seen on the roentgenogram (Fig. 33.5A). The two-dimensional echocardiogram Doppler study will delineate the PDA size and flow patterns as described before.

Moderate Ductus Arteriosus. In infants, a moderate left-to-right shunt may produce symptomatology related to left ventricular failure. Poor feeding, irritability, and tachypnea may

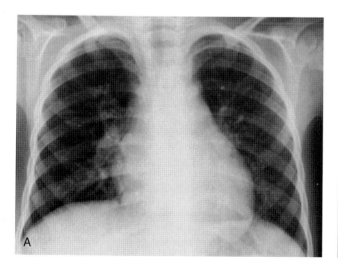
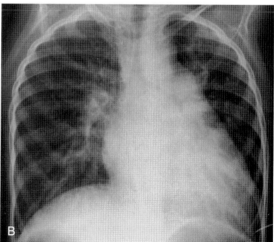

FIGURE 33.5 Posterior-anterior chest roentgenograms in two children each with a patent ductus arteriosus. **A:** A 4-year-old child with a small left-to-right shunt. Slight cardiomegaly and prominence of the pulmonary vascularity are present. **B:** A 4-year-old child with a very large left-to-right shunt. A double density and elevation of the left mainstem bronchus are present owing to left atrial enlargement. The left ventricle, main and peripheral pulmonary arteries, and ascending aorta are prominent. Pulmonary venous congestion is also present.

be present, and weight gain is often slow. The symptoms ordinarily increase until about the second to third month of age. If the left ventricular failure does not produce severe disease at this stage, compensatory myocardial hypertrophy occurs, and in many instances these infants improve considerably. Some, in fact, are detected only on subsequent routine physical examination, but close questioning will yield the previous abnormal history. General physical development is slightly retarded, and easy fatigability may be present in the older child. The pulse rate is often increased, with the peripheral pulses full and bounding. The systemic arterial pressure is widened with a low diastolic pressure. The precordium is hyperdynamic, and left ventricular enlargement produces a thrusting apical impulse. A systolic thrill may be palpable at the upper left sternal border. Both the first and second sounds may be difficult to hear, because they often are masked by a loud murmur. A third heart sound is often heard at the apex. The progression from a systolic murmur to a continuous murmur is considerably more rapid in these infants than in those with a small shunt. The continuous murmur is more intense, has more extensive radiation, and generally is well heard posteriorly. It has a much harsher quality with low-frequency components, and because of the large flow and great turbulence, eddy sounds that vary from beat to beat give the murmur a machinery quality.

If heart failure occurs, the murmur may lose its continuous character and occupy only systole. A middiastolic, low-frequency, rumbling murmur is ordinarily heard at the apex. Early pulmonic or aortic ejection sounds may occur. The increased left ventricular stroke may produce a functional systolic pressure difference across the aortic valve that may be manifested by a soft ejection systolic murmur. In early infancy, left ventricular failure with increased left atrial size and pressure often induces a left-to-right shunt through a stretched and incompetent foramen ovale (13). Depending on the magnitude of left-to-right atrial shunting, right ventricular hyperactivity may become evident and the right ventricular outflow murmur typical of atrial left-to-right shunting may be heard. In addition, a middiastolic flow rumble owing to the increased flow across the tricuspid valve may be audible at the lower left sternal border.

The ECG may be relatively normal during infancy, but left ventricular hypertrophy is usual in older infants and children. The mean frontal plane axis usually is normal. Left ventricular hypertrophy is manifested by a deep Q wave and a tall R wave in leads II, III, aVF, and the left precordial leads V5 and V6. The T waves in these leads ordinarily are upright and show increased amplitude. A pattern compatible with left bundle branch block also has been described in some children. A widened P wave indicating left atrial enlargement may be present. If there is a left-to-right atrial shunt as well as mild pulmonary hypertension, right ventricular hypertrophy may increase the amplitude of the R waves in the right precordial leads. Right atrial enlargement may increase the height of the P wave.

The chest roentgenogram shows an enlarged heart with prominence of the left ventricle and the typical signs of left atrial enlargement (Fig. 33.5B). The main pulmonary artery segment is prominent, and the pulmonary vascular markings in the peripheral lung fields are increased. The ascending aorta is often very prominent and may be associated with unfolding of the aortic arch. The two-dimensional echocardiogram demonstrates increased left atrial and ventricular diameters, hypertrophy if present, and the PDA itself. Doppler evaluation will demonstrate flow and velocity patterns and will allow for an estimate of pulmonary arterial pressure (38).

Large Ductus Arteriosus. Infants with a large PDA are invariably symptomatic. They are irritable, feed poorly, fail to gain weight normally, tire easily—particularly while feeding—and sweat excessively. They have increased respiratory effort and respiratory rates, also aggravated by feeding, and are prone to develop recurrent upper respiratory infections and pneumonia. These symptoms indicative of severe left ventricular failure with pulmonary edema may occur early in infancy.

Many of the typical physical signs may be absent when there is severe left ventricular failure. However, tachycardia and tachypnea are present, and if there is pulmonary edema, rales will be heard throughout the lung fields. The respiratory signs may be suggestive of bronchial pneumonia. The peripheral pulses are bounding with a rapid upstroke and a wide pulse pressure unless there is severe left ventricular failure when the pulse volume decreases. The precordium is markedly hyperdynamic, and clinical evidence of cardiac enlargement is present. The left ventricular apical impulse is thrusting and, if right ventricular enlargement occurs, may be accompanied by a left parasternal impulse. A systolic thrill is often palpable. The first and second heart sounds are accentuated, and a third sound ordinarily is heard at the apex. Occasionally no murmur is heard, especially with severe failure. When left ventricular failure is controlled, a moderately loud systolic murmur is heard best in the pulmonary area or occasionally in the third or fourth intercostal space. The murmur peaks late in systole, and the prolongation into diastole is variable; the murmur commonly ends within the first third of diastole. The typical continuous murmur heard with a small or moderate-sized PDA may be heard but is less usual. A prominent middiastolic mitral flow rumble commonly is audible at the apex.

The ECG shows more prominent left ventricular enlargement, with deep Q and taller R waves than in the previous group. The T waves may be diphasic or even inverted. Right ventricular hypertrophy may be evident, with upright T waves in the right precordial leads and increased R-wave amplitude in the right precordial leads. Left atrial enlargement, as demonstrated by a widened P wave, also will be seen. The chest roentgenogram shows striking enlargement of the heart with predominant left atrial and left ventricular enlargement. The main pulmonary artery segment usually is markedly enlarged, and the peripheral pulmonary vascular markings are markedly accentuated. Evidence of left ventricular failure with increased pulmonary venous markings and interstitial fluid also may be seen. With an enlarged left atrium or pulmonary arteries, lobar collapse or emphysema owing to bronchial compression may occur. The two-dimensional echocardiogram/Doppler study is as described for the previous group.

Infants with large left-to-right shunts through a PDA may not survive the resultant cardiac failure without treatment. However a certain proportion of those capable of compensating adequately survive the initial period. A moderate or large left-to-right shunt either undetected in infancy or treated but allowed to persist eventually leads to the development of obstructive pulmonary vascular disease. As pulmonary vascular resistance increases, pulmonary hypertension increases until systemic levels are reached. The left-to-right shunting decreases and this leads to improvement in the infant's symptomatology and signs, usually 8 to 15 months after birth. Feeding problems, poor weight gain, and the increased sweating previously present disappear, with far fewer episodes of respiratory infection. The murmur becomes shorter, and the diastolic component may be completely lost. The middiastolic rumble decreases and disappears, and the first heart sound becomes softer. The second heart sound remains markedly accentuated, but the third heart sound disappears. Precordial hyperactivity diminishes, and the pulses become less bounding. The chest roentgenogram shows decreasing pulmonary vascularity, and a decrease in heart size also may be noted. The period of time over which these changes occur varies and may last several years, but irreversible changes are common after 15 to 18 months of age.

As the increased pulmonary vascular resistance progresses to irreversible pulmonary vascular disease, the symptoms and clinical features change even further. The murmur continues to shorten until eventually it disappears. The second sound becomes single and progressively louder, an ejection systolic click occurs, and a faint blowing early-diastolic regurgitant murmur owing to pulmonary incompetence may be heard at the upper left sternal edge. Left ventricular hyperactivity disappears, and the right ventricular parasternal impulse increases. The ECG shows increasing right ventricular hypertrophy with dominant R waves in the right precordial leads. Peaked P waves indicative of right atrial enlargement also may occur. The chest roentgenogram shows increasing right ventricular enlargement with decreasing left ventricular size, a large main pulmonary artery, and progressive decrease in peripheral vascular markings.

Cyanosis, often more pronounced in the lower than in the upper limbs, begins to appear, initially only with exertion, but eventually becoming continuous as persistent right-to-left shunting across the ductus arteriosus occurs. The final picture, if allowed to progress, is one of irreversible pulmonary vascular disease with marked right-to-left shunting. The precordial activity is now dominantly right ventricular, and the pulses are either of normal or small volume. The second heart sound typically is palpable in the pulmonic area, and a diastolic thrill also may be felt. The first heart sound is slightly accentuated, and the pulmonic component of the second heart sound is markedly accentuated. A harsher and longer early diastolic blowing murmur caused by pulmonary incompetence is heard at the left sternal border. A blowing systolic murmur owing to secondary tricuspid insufficiency may be heard at the lower left sternal border. The ECG shows right axis deviation in the frontal plane with marked right ventricular hypertrophy and eventually T-wave inversion in older patients. The chest roentgenogram shows moderate cardiomegaly with predominant enlargement of the right ventricle and a markedly enlarged main pulmonary artery with prominence of the central vessels but no peripheral plethora. Right atrial enlargement may be evident.

CARDIAC CATHETERIZATION

Based on careful clinical evaluation—principally the characteristic continuous murmur, together with the ECG, chest roentgenogram, and two-dimensional echocardiogram Doppler study—diagnosis of PDA (and any associated defects) is usually possible without catheterization. Color Doppler flow mapping is generally as sensitive as cardiac catheterization for detecting even a small PDA. In children with pulmonary hypertension, determining the exact location of the shunt can be difficult. Contrast echocardiography can assist in the localization, but generally patients will require catheterization to determine the severity of pulmonary hypertension and determine if closure is indicated.

Right heart catheterization alone usually suffices to confirm the diagnosis. However, if an additional lesion such as ventricular septal defect is suspected, retrograde catheterization may be required if the interatrial septum is intact and the left ventricle cannot be entered prograde. The venous catheter usually can be passed from the main pulmonary artery through the ductus arteriosus into the descending aorta. If the venous catheter cannot be passed through the ductus arteriosus, retrograde aortic catheterization is indicated to define the anatomy with an aortic angiogram.

An increase of pulmonary arterial blood oxygen content of >0.5 mL/dL or a saturation increase of >4% to 5% from that in right ventricular blood indicates a significant left-to-right shunt at the pulmonary arterial level. Occasionally an increase in oxygen saturation is noted in blood just below the pulmonary valve owing to pulmonary regurgitation. Because preferential streaming of oxygenated blood from the PDA into one or another of the branch pulmonary arteries is common, a sample from either one does not reflect mixed pulmonary arterial blood oxygen saturation (13). Measuring pulmonary blood flow accurately from the blood oxygen data is therefore difficult, making an accurate calculation of the true magnitude of left-to-right shunting impossible. In the presence of left ventricular failure with pulmonary edema, pulmonary venous blood oxygen saturation may be reduced. If the foramen ovale is incompetent, a left-to-right atrial shunt may be detected by an increase in oxygen saturation in the right atrial blood. A large increase in oxygen saturation at the right atrial level may mask a smaller rise of saturation in the pulmonary artery, even though the increase represents a significant shunt at the pulmonary arterial level. With significant pulmonary hypertension and right-to-left shunting through the PDA, oxygen saturation of blood in the descending aorta will be lower than that obtained in the ascending aorta. Bidirectional shunting may be present until pulmonary vascular disease is severe, when right-to-left shunting alone occurs.

A small left-to-right shunt may not be detected by blood oxygen saturation data alone. An increase in oxygen saturation in pulmonary arterial blood is not diagnostic of a PDA, but may be present in lesions such as aortopulmonary window or a high ventricular septal defect (supracristal), in which streaming may direct the highly saturated blood into the pulmonary artery.

With a small communication, pulmonary arterial blood pressures are normal, but systemic arterial pulse pressure may be slightly widened owing to a low diastolic pressure. With a moderate-sized defect, pulmonary arterial systolic, diastolic, and mean blood pressures may be slightly elevated. Systemic arterial diastolic blood pressure falls, whereas systemic arterial pulse pressure increases. Both left and right atrial mean pressures are moderately elevated in the presence of a moderate shunt. With a large shunt, pulmonary and systemic arterial pressures are equal, left atrial mean pressure may be increased substantially, and a prominent V wave is seen. Left ventricular end-diastolic pressure may be elevated, and with a large flow, a diastolic pressure gradient between the left atrium and left ventricle is demonstrated. A small systolic pressure difference between the left ventricle and aorta is also encountered occasionally when there is a large shunt. Because calculation of pulmonary blood flow in PDA is often inaccurate, the calculation of pulmonary vascular resistance is also inaccurate (13).

ANGIOGRAPHY

Although angiography cannot accurately measure the magnitude of left-to-right shunting, it is the most effective test for defining the anatomy of the PDA. Contrast medium is injected into a catheter passed through the PDA into the aorta from the pulmonary artery (Fig. 33.6) or into the aorta retrogradely from the femoral artery. As shown in Figure 33.6, the aortic end of the

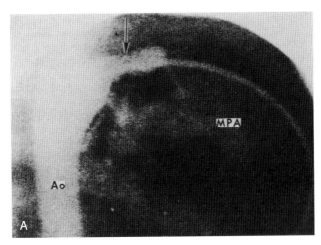 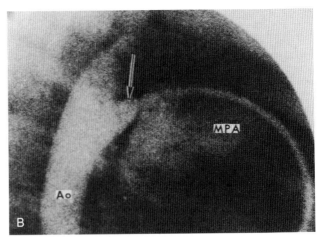

FIGURE 33.6 Angiograms in the lateral position in two children each with a patent ductus arteriosus. The variable anatomy in this lesion is demonstrated. Ao, aorta; MPA, main pulmonary artery.

PDA usually is widely dilated, and the ductus narrows down at the pulmonary arterial end. This is the usual shape in most children, but occasionally other shapes are observed, including tubular (long ductus arteriosus of similar diameter throughout), complex (narrowing at both the pulmonary artery and aortic end), and short (windowlike PDA) (81). In most instances the lateral projection, or occasionally the left anterior oblique projection, demonstrates the anatomy most clearly. The AP camera can be positioned in the right anterior oblique caudal position to demonstrate the PDA. One should remember that in infants with severe heart failure associated with a ventricular septal defect or interatrial communication, a PDA may coexist; selective descending aortography is essential in these infants to exclude a PDA if not defined clearly by echocardiography.

OTHER IMAGING TECHNIQUES

Magnetic Resonance Imaging or Computed Tomography Scan

Although simpler techniques such as two-dimensional echocardiography Doppler evaluation accurately define the anatomy and flow patterns of the ductus arteriosus, nuclear magnetic resonance imaging (MRI) or computed tomography (CT scan) can, except perhaps in very small infants, clearly delineate the anatomy (82,83). These studies can be of use in adolescents or adults with poor echo windows where the diagnosis is suspected but not anatomically confirmed. Velocity-encoded cine MRI imaging for estimation of left-to-right shunting may have additional clinical utility (84).

CLINICAL DIFFERENTIAL DIAGNOSIS

Venous Hum

The continuous bruit produced by flow through the large veins in the neck is often confused with the continuous murmur of a PDA. The venous hum varies in intensity with head and neck position as well as the phase of respiration and is usually obliterated by firm pressure over the neck, by turning the head to one side, or by lying flat.

Total Anomalous Pulmonary Venous Connection

Unobstructed total anomalous pulmonary venous connection to the innominate vein occasionally produces a continuous murmur very much like a venous hum. The other features of this lesion serve to differentiate it from a PDA.

Ruptured Sinus of Valsalva

Rupture of one of the sinuses of Valsalva into either the right atrium or right ventricle is accompanied by a continuous murmur. However, onset of symptoms and signs in this condition is usually abrupt and often follows trauma to the chest. The murmur is usually heard lower in the precordium.

Arteriovenous Communications

Arteriovenous fistulas involving one of the coronary arteries, an intercostal artery, or an internal mammary artery may be associated with continuous murmurs similar to those occurring in PDA. The murmurs typically are more superficial and sound extracardiac in origin. Origin of one of the pulmonary arteries from the aorta (hemitruncus arteriosus) also may produce a continuous murmur, as may lobar sequestration, in which an anomalous artery arising from the aorta supplies one or more pulmonary lobes. Pulmonary arteriovenous fistulas may produce a continuous murmur, but when large enough to do so are usually associated with cyanosis and classical radiographic findings.

Anomalous Origin of the Left Coronary Artery from the Pulmonary Artery

In this lesion, retrograde flow occurs from the right coronary artery and then the pulmonary artery. If this retrograde flow is sufficiently large, a continuous murmur may be heard, but this is rare. The clinical presentation and electrocardiogram are diagnostic of this condition.

Absent Pulmonary Valve

This lesion is associated invariably with massive dilation of the pulmonary arteries and almost always with a ventricular septal defect. The murmur has been described as "sawing wood" in character and is not really continuous, but has more of a to-and-fro character. The massively dilated pulmonary artery evident on chest roentgenogram ordinarily allows for accurate differentiation.

Aortic Insufficiency Associated with a Ventricular Septal Defect

Prolapse of one aortic sinus complicates ventricular septal defects, particularly supracristal defects. The murmur is not strictly continuous, and the systolic murmur produced by the ventricular septal defect and the blowing regurgitant diastolic murmur produced by the incompetence are usually separated. However, accurate clinical differentiation may be difficult.

Peripheral Pulmonary Stenosis

Although commonly associated with a PDA, peripheral pulmonary stenosis may occur as an isolated defect and give rise to a soft, continuous murmur heard best in the infraclavicular areas and conducted to the axillae. Stenosis may occur in only one pulmonary artery, producing a unilateral murmur. This lesion may be difficult to distinguish clinically from a PDA.

Truncus Arteriosus

Truncus arteriosus may not be accompanied by cyanosis in early infancy, and with a low pulmonary vascular resistance and increased pulmonary blood flow, there may be a continuous murmur. Absence of the pulmonary artery segment on the posterior-anterior chest roentgenogram suggests this diagnosis; furthermore, the relatively common occurrence of right aortic arch with truncus arteriosus excludes the diagnosis of isolated PDA.

Aortopulmonary Window

This defect may be extremely difficult to differentiate from a PDA. The murmur commonly is heard best lower down the left sternal border and is often mistaken for the murmur of a high ventricular septal defect.

Pulmonary Atresia

When pulmonary atresia is accompanied by markedly enlarged bronchial arteries supplying pulmonary blood flow, a continuous murmur may be heard. However, cyanosis is present, and the peripheral pulses are not bounding as in PDA. The chest roentgenogram also shows absence of the pulmonary artery segment.

COMPLICATIONS

Endarteritis

Bacterial endarteritis has become extremely uncommon in developed countries, although it remains a serious complication of PDA. Because of the advent of surgical correction of many congenital heart defects, the prevalence of endocarditis, particularly in defects associated with left-to-right shunts, has declined dramatically (85). In one survey of major congenital heart defects, PDA had the lowest frequency, which was attributed to early surgical closure (86). In undeveloped countries PDA accounts for ≤15% of all endocarditis cases and for 4.8 of 1,000 hospital admissions at a tertiary cardiac referral center (87). Organisms are typical with *Streptococcus viridans* and *Staphylococcus aureus* the most common. Vegetations occur in >80% and are always seen on the pulmonary artery end of the duct.

Aneurysm/Calcification Formation

Marked dilation of a PDA or of the ampulla of the closed ductus arteriosus has been described. The massive dilation that occurs may be diagnosed as a mediastinal mass. It also has been found as an incidental finding at autopsy. It occurs in ≤1.5% of normal births (88). In adults calcification of the PDA is frequent and may increase the surgical risk (89).

TREATMENT

Management in preterm infants has been described above. In older infants or children, the complications resulting from isolated PDA, including failure to grow, recurrent respiratory infections, cardiac enlargement and failure, lobar emphysema or collapse, bacterial endarteritis, and the eventual development of irreversible pulmonary vascular disease are all indications for early correction. Because treatment of an uncomplicated PDA is accompanied by minimal risk, closure should be recommended soon after the diagnosis is made. Treatment options currently include catheter coil or device closure or surgery. Indomethacin is ineffective in term infants and older children and therefore should not be used. If intractable cardiac failure is present, intravenous infusion of epinephrine or dopamine may be beneficial (90) prior to immediate catheter or surgical closure.

Catheter closure with occluding coils has become the treatment of choice for all children more than a few months of age with ducts <3 mm in diameter. This 3-hour outpatient procedure is performed using conscious sedation allowing the children to return to full activity by the next day. A catheter is advanced from the femoral artery or vein across the PDA. An occluding coil is placed in the PDA with a single coil loop on the pulmonary artery side and the remaining three to four loops in the ductal ampulla. Occasionally immediate placement of a second coil is needed to achieve complete closure. This procedure is >97% successful with zero mortality and no significant morbidity (91,92). For larger PDAs ≤12 mm in diameter, specialized devices, such as the Amplatzer duct occluder, are available for catheter-based repair. The procedure is similar in duration, risk, and recovery time to the coil closure procedure. The devices are implanted antegrade from the femoral vein using long sheaths sized 6 to 8 French. There is a

>98% complete closure rate at 6 months with minimal complications and no mortality (93,94). PDAs larger than 12 mm have been closed using septal closure devices (AGA septal occluder, VSD device, NMT CardioSEAL device) or covered stents in select cases (95).

Surgery remains the treatment of choice for premature infants and for children with very large PDAs. The traditional surgical approach to closure of the PDA involves division or transsection of the ductus through a lateral thoracotomy. Suture ligation without division has the potential for recanalization, particularly following single-suture ligation. Surgery is extremely safe with minimal mortality and morbidity. Hospital stays can be as short as 3 days, with return to full activity within 3 weeks. A recent surgical advance is thoracoscopic surgical closure. In this technique, three small 1.5-inch incisions are made in the lateral thorax through which a thoracoscope and several surgical tools are inserted. Several surgical clips are placed on the PDA under direct visualization through the scope. Obvious advantages of this technique include less operative lung manipulation, less chest wall pain, faster recovery, and a smaller scar. Some critics of this new technique have raised concerns regarding the potential for tearing and hemorrhage with clipping of large PDAs, particularly in adults in whom the ductus may be calcified. This technique remains in limited use, but the preliminary results are encouraging with similar efficacy and shorter hospital stay, but in at least one study a higher rate of laryngeal nerve injury compared with standard thoracotomy (96,97).

The decision to recommend closure of PDAs in children with moderately significantly elevated pulmonary vascular resistance is not simple. Catheterization is recommended in these patients to evaluate the pulmonary vascular bed's response to test occlusion with a balloon catheter and pulmonary vasodilators. If a good response to balloon occlusion or pulmonary vasodilators such as oxygen or nitric oxide has occurred, closure is advised. However, if the response is poor or equivocal, the decision is considerably more difficult. Device closure may be considered in this setting if the surgical risk is increased because of significant pulmonary hypertension (98). Some children respond extremely well and show significant improvement after closure, whereas others show a progressive increase in pulmonary vascular resistance after closure. Fortunately, the latter are encountered only rarely. The only contraindication to closure of an isolated PDA is severe pulmonary hypertension with irreversible pulmonary vascular disease. If the PDA is closed in these children, they are incapable of maintaining an adequate systemic output in response to stress, and rapid deterioration and death frequently occur.

ROLE OF THE DUCTUS ARTERIOSUS IN CONGENITAL CARDIAC MALFORMATIONS

In right ventricular outflow obstruction lesions such as pulmonary atresia, the normal flow patterns in fetal life are altered, and development of the ductus arteriosus is probably abnormal (1,99). The diameter is large and orientation is vertical from the underside of the aortic arch (Fig. 33.7). Because patency of a PDA is essential for maintenance of pulmonary blood flow, the constrictor response to an increase in pO_2 is undesirable. Despite the hypoxemia in these infants, the ductus arteriosus closes, resulting in cessation of pulmonary blood flow, progressive hypoxia, acidosis, and death. PGE_1 is currently used as pharmacologic prevention of this closure before the creation of a surgical aortopulmonary communica-

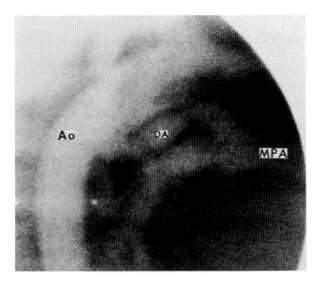

FIGURE 33.7 Angiogram in the lateral position in a newborn infant with pulmonary atresia. The typical anatomy associated with right ventricular outflow obstruction is demonstrated. The aorta is widely dilated, and the aortic isthmus is wider than the descending aorta. The typical narrow tortuous ductus arteriosus with an acute rather than the normal obtuse inferior angle with the aorta is present. This orientation is consistent with aortic-to-pulmonary arterial blood flow in fetal life. Ao, aorta; DA, ductus arteriosus; MPA, main pulmonary artery.

tion. PGE_1 produces dilation of the ductus arteriosus with a significant increase in systemic arterial pO_2 (100). Systemic oxygenation is markedly improved, acidemia reversed, and the infants ordinarily can be stabilized for days to weeks before palliative surgery. Maintenance of patency for a more prolonged period has been produced by placement of a metal intravascular stent in the PDA (101–103). The preliminary results are encouraging but may be limited to short straight ducts found most commonly in lesions such as pulmonary atresia with intact ventricular septum.

Maintenance of systemic blood flow in hypoplastic left heart lesions such as aortic or mitral atresia or in interrupted aortic arch depends on patency of the ductus arteriosus. PGE_1 has proved extremely valuable in improving lower body perfusion in these infants. Acidemia is often reversed and renal function markedly improved so that the infants can be stabilized and returned to electrolyte and hemodynamic balance before corrective surgery is undertaken (100). Recent developments in the initial palliative treatment of hypoplastic left heart syndrome have included the placement of a metal stent in the ductus arteriosus and banding of the pulmonary arteries (hybrid approach) to stabilize systemic and pulmonary blood flow until infants reach the age of 4 to 6 months at which time surgical Glenn shunt with arch reconstruction is performed. It has yet to be shown whether this new approach will have significant advantages, but preliminary data suggest a potential reduction in early mortality for high-risk patients (104).

It has been shown that the ductus arteriosus plays an important role in the presentation of infants with juxtaductal aortic coarctation. Localized coarctation ordinarily is produced by a well-circumscribed posterior shelf protruding into the aortic lumen at a point opposite the insertion of the ductus arteriosus (1). If the ductus arteriosus remains patent or if there is a well-formed ductus ampulla even when the ductus arteriosus is closed, obstruction by the juxtaductal coarctation may not occur. However, as the ductus arteriosus closes and the ampulla retracts, progressive interference with flow occurs, and clinical symptoms and signs will develop. The sudden occurrence of acute left ventricular failure in infants with juxtaductal coarctation of the aorta may be produced by rapid constriction of the ductus arteriosus in the postnatal period. PGE_2 has been of great benefit in the management of these infants as well (104).

AORTOPULMONARY WINDOW

Aortopulmonary window, or aortopulmonary septal defect, is a relatively rare cardiac malformation. Since first described by Elliotson (105) just over 300 cases have been reported (105–119). It accounts for 0.2% to 0.6% of all cases of congenital heart disease (115). Nearly half of all patients have associated cardiac lesions, including aortic origin of the right pulmonary artery (107,110,117,120), type A interruption of the aortic arch (108,110,115,118), tetralogy of Fallot (106,109,115), and anomalous origin of the right or left coronary artery from the pulmonary artery and right aortic arch (111,115,121). More rarely, it is associated with ventricular septal defect (107,119), pulmonary (119) or aortic atresia (118), d-transposition (122, 123), and tricuspid atresia (112).

The aortopulmonary septum is formed by the two opposing truncal cushions, which appear at the 9-mm stage, then rapidly enlarge and fuse, dividing the truncus arteriosus into separate aortic and pulmonary channels (124). This division is influenced by cells that migrate from the neural crest. Removal of neural crest tissue results in various arterial abnormalities including truncus arteriosus, transposition of the great arteries, and aortic interruption. However, aortopulmonary window is not seen when neural crest tissue is removed (125). In addition, unlike truncus arteriosus, aortopulmonary window has not been reported in association with DiGeorge syndrome (126). In contrast to other conotruncal abnormalities, there is no known association with monosomy 22Q11 (123,127,128). Finally, whereas type B aortic interruption is associated with truncus arteriosus, type A is seen more frequently with aortopulmonary window (110,115). Thus, although these anomalies involve the same region of the heart, they appear to be unrelated embryologically, not variants of the same disease.

In most cases there is a defect in the proximal portion of the aortopulmonary septum, midway between the semilunar valves and the pulmonary bifurcation. The defect is variable in size, but all defects result in a large, generally continuous left-to-right shunt when the pulmonary vascular resistance falls, similar to other interarterial communications such as patent ductus arteriosus or truncus arteriosus. Without corrective surgery, irreversible obstructive changes in the pulmonary vascular bed develop early, followed by death in the second decade, although patients surviving into the fourth decade have been reported (109).

Pathology

Following the immediate perinatal period, once hemodynamic changes have occurred, the heart is large, owing primarily to an enlarged, volume-loaded left atrium and left ventricle. The branch pulmonary arteries are usually enlarged because of the increased pulmonary flow. The ascending aorta is often small, particularly in cases with a very proximal defect or with associated aortic arch anomalies. The aortopulmonary defect is a discrete area, variable in size, usually positioned midway

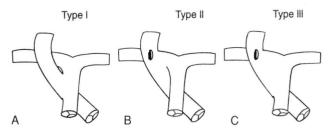

FIGURE 33.8 Classification of aortopulmonary window. **A:** Type I, proximal defect, midway between the semilunar valves and pulmonary bifurcation. **B:** Type II: distal defect, with posterior border absent and aortic origin of right pulmonary artery. **C:** Type III, total defect, incorporating defects present in both types I and II. (From Mori K, Ando M, Takao A, et al. Distal type of aortopulmonary window. Report of 4 cases. *Br Heart J* 1978;40:681–689, with permission.)

between the semilunar valves and the pulmonary bifurcation. It has a regular edge and is usually circular, although a form has been described with a border that is not continuous but describes slightly more than one turn of a spiral (115).

Although several classifications have been presented, the one proposed by Mori et al. (117) is most commonly used (Fig. 33.8). It describes three types of aortopulmonary connection. Type I is the most common type described earlier: A small defect midway between the semilunar valves and the pulmonary bifurcation. Type II is a more distal defect, the distal border of which is formed by the pulmonary bifurcation. This type is more commonly associated with aortic origin of the right pulmonary artery (107,110,117). Type III, a large, confluent defect involving essentially the entire aortopulmonary septum, is the rarest.

Manifestations

Clinical Features

The clinical features of aortopulmonary window are not specific but are those of a large left-to-right shunt, and clinically this lesion often mimics either a VSD or a PDA or both. Signs of congestive heart failure (tachypnea, diaphoresis, failure to thrive, and recurrent respiratory difficulty) usually begin in the first weeks of life (109,111,117). Cyanosis usually is not present, although large defects can produce desaturation owing to bidirectional shunting and mixing at the arterial level. When aortic arch anomalies are present, the presenting symptoms may be those of metabolic acidosis when the ductus arteriosus closes, and the aortopulmonary window may be masked.

Physical examination shows tachypnea, abdominal breathing, and overexpansion of the lungs with intercostal retractions. There may be a prominent right ventricular impulse at the left sternal border. The pulses may be bounding, indicating arterial runoff into the lungs. On auscultation, the second heart sound generally is accentuated and narrowly split, suggesting pulmonary hypertension. In some patients a prominent ejection click is heard in the pulmonic area (109,117). There is either a loud systolic ejection murmur at the left upper sternal border or a machinery-type murmur similar to that found with a patent ductus arteriosus (117). Often a mid-diastolic rumbling murmur is present at the apex, indicating increased flow across the mitral valve.

Patients with very small defects may be asymptomatic. In these patients, the second heart sound may be normal, with only a systolic ejection murmur and possibly a middiastolic murmur audible at the apex. The defect in these patients may be mistaken clinically for a small ventricular septal defect and may be diagnosed accurately only during routine echocardiography.

Electrocardiographic Features

There are no characteristic electrocardiographic findings in patients with aortopulmonary window. Evidence of right ventricular hypertrophy usually is present, although biventricular hypertrophy may be present when the defect is large or has been present for some time (111,117). Rarely, the electrocardiogram is normal or shows only a mild degree of right ventricular hypertrophy suggested by an rsR' pattern in the right precordial leads.

Radiologic Features

The chest roentgenogram is indicative of a large left-to-right shunt. A moderately enlarged heart with prominent pulmonary vascular markings is usually present. The main pulmonary artery segment is usually pronounced, as are the left atrial and left ventricular borders. The aortic knuckle usually is not prominent. The lung fields frequently show hyperinflation, and pulmonary edema may be present.

Echocardiographic Features

Two-dimensional echocardiography can accurately diagnose aortopulmonary window and generally describe any associated anomalies (Fig. 33.9). In addition, the lesion is readily diagnosed in utero using fetal echocardiography (129). The left atrium and ventricle are dilated owing to the large left-to-right shunt. The right ventricle may be hypertrophied,

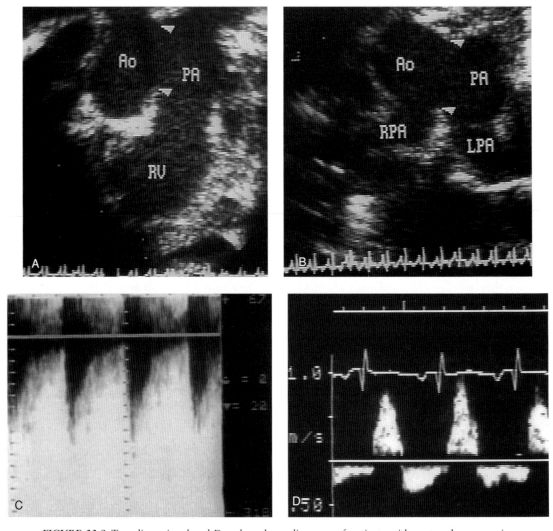

FIGURE 33.9 Two-dimensional and Doppler echocardiograms of patients with aortopulmonary window. **A:** Subcostal coronal view of type I defect shows a large defect (*arrows*) in midportion of aortopulmonary septum. Ao, aorta; PA, pulmonary artery; RV, right ventricle. **B:** Parasternal short-axis view of a type II defect (*arrows*) shows associated aortic origin of right pulmonary artery (RPA). LPA, left pulmonary artery. **C:** Doppler flow signal in pulmonary artery shows continuous forward flow indicating arterial communication. **D:** Doppler flow signal in abdominal aorta shows significant retrograde flow, indicating runoff into pulmonary arteries.

although not always. The semilunar valves usually are normal in both position and motion. The pulmonary arteries are significantly enlarged. The aortopulmonary window can usually be seen directly, but dropout is often seen in the aortopulmonary septal area of normal patients. Balaji et al. (106) described a "T" artifact at the edges of the defect to help distinguish it from normal dropout. In addition, color Doppler flow mapping demonstrates flow through the defect.

Doppler echocardiography is helpful in the diagnosis of aortopulmonary window (Fig. 33.9). Abnormal, continuous forward flow in the pulmonary arteries indicates the presence of an aortopulmonary communication (106). The forward direction of the flow in the distal main or in the branch pulmonary arteries distinguishes this defect from patent ductus arteriosus. Significant retrograde descending aortic diastolic flow is found in both the proximal aortic arch and the abdominal aorta; this is also in contrast to a patent ductus, where the proximal arch has diastolic prograde flow. Doppler echocardiography also demonstrates the presence of pulmonary hypertension when pulmonary or tricuspid insufficiency is present.

Cardiac Catheterization

With current echocardiographic techniques, cardiac catheterization usually is not required. The right ventricular and pulmonary arterial pressures usually are at systemic levels (111,117). The left atrial pressure may be elevated from the left-to-right shunt and increased pulmonary venous return, whereas the left ventricular pressure is usually normal. Aortic pressure usually is normal, but in the presence of large defects may have a decreased diastolic and widened pulse pressure owing to runoff into the pulmonary vascular bed. The catheter often can be manipulated directly from the main pulmonary artery through the defect into the ascending aorta.

Either an ascending aorta or main pulmonary angiogram will demonstrate the defect. An ascending aorta angiogram shows filling of the pulmonary arteries, including the pulmonary valve sinuses, and main and branch pulmonary arteries (117). It also will demonstrate associated aortic arch anomalies. A main pulmonary arterial angiogram shows filling of the ascending aorta, and when present, also can demonstrate anomalous origin of a coronary artery from the pulmonary artery (111).

Differential Diagnosis

Because aortopulmonary window is an extremely rare defect, the clinical features are often ascribed to a large ventricular septal defect, a large patent ductus arteriosus, or persistent truncus arteriosus. The bounding pulses, wide pulse pressure, and continuous murmur, if present, indicate the presence of an arterial communication (109). Distinguishing aortopulmonary window from either a large patent ductus arteriosus or from persistent truncus arteriosus often is extremely difficult by physical examination alone. A systolic ejection or continuous murmur is also present in patients with patent ductus arteriosus; however, significant clinical symptoms in the first weeks of life are very unusual. Patients with persistent truncus arteriosus usually have more arterial desaturation than patients with aortopulmonary window and the same degree of congestive failure, as the common ventricular outlet results in complete mixing. They often also have a diastolic murmur indicative of regurgitation of the truncal valve. The murmur of a ventricular septal defect usually is heard toward the base of the sternum, and the pulses are not bounding.

Treatment

Closure of the defect is indicated in essentially all patients with aortopulmonary window. The standard treatment is surgical closure of the defect. Since the first reported correction by Gross (113), several types of surgical correction have been attempted. Simple ligation (111) and division with suture closure of the defect (109) both have met with poor results. Although exposure and patch closure of the defect from the pulmonary artery is possible (111, 113), most authors recommend a transaortic approach using a median sternotomy and cardiopulmonary bypass (111,117,130). This approach provides optimal exposure of the defect and also allows access for correction of associated defects, particularly arch anomalies and anomalous origin or either the right pulmonary artery or right coronary artery. In patients with aortic origin of the right pulmonary artery, the patch closure can be tunneled to include the right pulmonary artery in the repair (110). Recent revisions have used a pulmonary artery flap to close the defect (131–133). This technique avoids the use of prosthetic material. More recently, several patients have had successful closure using various catheter-delivered devices (134–137).

The prognosis of patients with aortopulmonary window is excellent if surgical correction is performed early in life, before irreversible pulmonary vascular changes occur (130). Although long-term follow-up is limited, late complications of the defect in patients adequately repaired are unlikely to be significant. Patients with associated anomalies will likely be limited more by the associated anomaly than by the repaired aortopulmonary window.

References

1. Rudolph AM, Heymann MA, Spitznas U. Hemodynamic considerations in the development of narrowing of the aorta. *Am J Cardiol* 1972;30:514–525.
2. Fay FS, Cooke PH. Guinea pig ductus arteriosus. II. Irreversible closure after birth. *Am J Physiol* 1972;222:841–849.
3. Gittenberger-de Groot AC, Van Ertbruggen I, Moulaert AJMG, et al. The ductus arteriosus in the preterm infant: Histologic and clinical observations. *J Pediatr* 1980;96:88–93.
4. Heymann MA, Rudolph AM. Control of the ductus arteriosus. *Physiol Rev* 1975;55:62–78.
5. Clyman RI. Ontogeny of the ductus arteriosus response to prostaglandins and inhibitors of their synthesis. *Semin Perinatol* 1980;4:115–124.
6. Coceani F, Olley PM. Role of prostaglandins, prostacyclin, and thromboxanes in the control of prenatal patency and postnatal closure of the ductus arteriosus. *Semin Perinatol* 1980;4:109–113.
7. Clyman RI, Heymann MA. Pharmacology of the ductus arteriosus. *Pediatr Clin North Am* 1981;28:77–93.
8. Clyman RI. Ductus arteriosus: Current theories of prenatal and postnatal regulation. *Semin Perinatol* 1987;11:64–71.
9. Clyman RI. Developmental physiology of the ductus arteriosus. In: Long W, ed. *Fetal and Neonatal Cardiology*. Philadelphia: WB Saunders, 1990: 64–75.
10. Rudolph AM, Drorbraugh JE, Auld PAM, et al. Studies on the circulation in the neonatal period. The circulation in the respiratory distress syndrome. *Pediatrics* 1961;27:551–566.
11. McMurphy DM, Heymann MA, Rudolph AM, et al. Developmental changes in constriction of the ductus arteriosus: Responses to oxygen and vasoactive substances in the isolated ductus arteriosus of the fetal lamb. *Pediatr Res* 1972;6:231–238.

12. Rudolph AM. Congenital *Diseases of the Heart: Clinical-Physiologic Considerations in Diagnosis and Management*. Chicago: Year Book Medical, 1974.

13. Rudolph AM, Mayer FE, Nadas AS, et al. Patent ductus arteriosus. A clinical and hemodynamic study of patients in the first year of life. *Pediatrics* 1958;22:892–904.

14. Lister G, Walter TK, Versmold HT, et al. Oxygen delivery in lambs: Cardiovascular and hematologic development. *Am J Physiol* 1979;237: H668–H675.

15. Baylen BG, Ogata H, Oguchi K, et al. The contractility and performance of the pre-term left ventricle before and after early patent ductus arteriosus occlusion in surfactant-treated lambs. *Pediatr Res* 1985;19:1053–1058.

16. Lebowitz EA, Novick JS, Rudolph AM. Development of myocardial sympathetic innervation in the fetal lamb. *Pediatr Res* 1972;6:887–893.

17. Friedman WF. The intrinsic physiologic properties of the developing heart. In: Friedman WF, Lesch M, Sonnenblick EH, eds. *Neonatal Heart Disease*. New York: Grune & Stratton, 1973:21–49.

18. Tsang RC, Light IJ, Sutherland JM, et al. Possible pathogenetic factors in neonatal hypocalcemia of prematurity. *J Pediatr* 1973;82:423–429.

19. Hoffman JIE, Buckberg GD. Regional myocardial ischemia-causes, prediction and prevention. *Vasc Surg* 1974;8:115–131.

20. Delivoria-Papadopoulos M, Roncevic NP, Oski FA. Postnatal changes in oxygen transport of term, premature, and sick infants: The role of red cell 2,3-diphosphoglycerate and adult hemoglobin. *Pediatr Res* 1971;5:235–245.

21. Hoffman JIE, Rudolph AM, Heymann MA. Pulmonary vascular disease with congenital heart lesions: Pathologic features and causes. *Circulation* 1981;64:873–877.

22. Braudo M, Rowe RD. Auscultation of the heart: Early neonatal period. *Am J Dis Child* 1961;101:575–586.

23. Huhta JC, Cohen M, Gutgesell HP. Patency of the ductus arteriosus in normal neonates: Two dimensional echocardiography vs Doppler assessment. *J Am Coll Cardiol* 1984;4:561–564.

24. Silverman NH. Patent ductus arteriosus. In: *Pediatric Echocardiography*. Baltimore, MD: Williams & Wilkins, 1993:167–177.

25. Liao PK, Su WJ, Hung JS. Doppler echocardiographic flow characteristics of isolated patent ductus arteriosus: Better delineation by Doppler color flow mapping. *J Am Coll Cardiol* 1988;12:1285–1291.

26. Clyman RI, Brett C, Mauray F. Circulating prostaglandin E2 concentrations and incidence of patent ductus arteriosus in preterm infants with respiratory distress syndrome. *Pediatrics* 1980;66:725–729.

27. Moss AJ, Emmanouilides GC, Adams FH, et al. Response of ductus arteriosus and pulmonary and systemic arterial pressure to changes in oxygen environment in newborn infants. *Pediatrics* 1964;33:937–944.

28. Alzamora-Castro V, Battilana G, Abugattas R, et al. Patent ductus arteriosus and high altitude. *Am J Cardiol* 1960;5:761–763.

29. Baden M, Kirks DR. Transient dilation of the ductus arteriosus—the "ductus bump." *J Pediatr* 1974;84:858–860.

30. Danilowicz D, Rudolph AM, Hoffman JIE. Delayed closure of ductus arteriosus in premature infants. *Pediatrics* 1966;37:74–78.

31. Siassi B, Emmanouilides GC, Cleveland RJ, et al. Patent ductus arteriosus complicating prolonged assisted ventilation in respiratory distress syndrome. *J Pediatr* 1969;74:11–19.

32. Kitterman JA, Edmunds LH Jr, Gregory GA, et al. Patent ductus arteriosus in premature infants: Incidence, relation to pulmonary disease, and management. *N Engl J Med* 1972;287:473–477.

33. Clyman RI. The role of the patent ductus arteriosus in respiratory distress syndrome. *Semin Perinatol* 1984;8:293–299.

34. Strauss HW, Wagner HN Jr, Wesselhoeft H, et al. Radionuclide angiocardiography in pediatrics. In: James AE, Wagner HN, Cooke RE, eds. *Pediatric Nuclear Medicine*. Philadelphia: WB Saunders, 1974:219–231.

35. Clyman RI, Jobe A, Heymann MA, et al. Increased shunt through the patent ductus arteriosus after surfactant replacement therapy. *J Pediatr* 1982;100:101–107.

36. Serwer GA, Armstrong BE, Anderson PAW. Noninvasive detection of retrograde descending aortic flow in infants using continuous wave Doppler ultrasonography. *J Pediatr* 1980;97:394–400.

37. Smallhorn JF, Gow R, Olley PM, et al. Combined noninvasive assessment of the patent ductus arteriosus in the preterm infant before and after indomethacin treatment. *Am J Cardiol* 1984;54:1300–1304.

38. Houston AB, Lim MK, Doig WB, et al. Doppler flow characteristics in the assessment of pulmonary artery pressure in ductus arteriosus. *Br Heart J* 1989;62:284–290.

39. Fyhrquist F, Tikkanen I, Totterman KJ, et al. Plasma atrial natriuretic peptide in health and disease. *Eur Heart J* 1987;8(suppl B):117–122.

40. Doust JA, Glasziou PP, Pietrzak E, et al. A systematic review of the diagnostic accuracy of natriuretic peptides for heart failure. *Arch Intern Med* 2004;164:1978–1984.

41. Holmstrom H, Omland T. Natriuretic peptides as markers of patent ductus arteriosus in preterm infants. *Clin Sci (Lond)* 2002;103(1):79–80.

42. Puddy VF, Amirmansour C, Williams AF, et al. Plasma brain natriuretic peptide as a predictor of haemodynamically significant patent ductus arteriosus in preterm infants. *Clin Sci (Lond)* 2002;103(1):75–77.

43. Yoshibayashi M, Kamiya T, Saito Y, et al. Plasma brain natriuretic peptide concentrations in healthy children from birth to adolescence: Marked and rapid increase after birth. *Eur J Endocrinol* 1995;133(2):207–209.

44. da Graca RL, Hassinger DC, Flynn PA, et al. Longitudinal changes of brain-type natriuretic peptide in preterm neonates. *Pediatrics* 2006;117: 2183–2189.

45. Sanjeev S, Pettersen M, Lua J, et al. Role of plasma B-type natriuretic peptide in screening for hemodynamically significant patent ductus arteriosus in preterm neonates. *J Perinatol* 2005;25:709–713.

46. Eerola A, Jokinen E, Boldt T, et al. The influence of percutaneous closure of patent ductus arteriosus on left ventricular size and function: A prospective study using two- and three-dimensional echocardiography and measurements of serum natriuretic peptides. *J Am Coll Cardiol* 2006;47:1060–1066.

47. McGrath RL, McGuiness GA, Way GL, et al. The silent ductus arteriosus. *J Pediatr* 1978;93:110–113.

48. Thibeault DW, Emmanouilides GC, Nelson RJ, et al. Patent ductus arteriosus complicating the respiratory distress syndrome in preterm infants. *J Pediatr* 1975;86:120–126.

49. Clyman RI, Mauray F, Heymann MA, et al. Cardiovascular effects of a patent ductus arteriosus in preterm lambs with respiratory distress. *J Pediatr* 1987;111:579–587.

50. Martin CG, Snider AR, Katz SM, et al. Abnormal cerebral blood flow patterns in preterm infants with a large patent ductus arteriosus. *J Pediatr* 1982;101:587–593.

51. Gleason CA, Clyman RI, Heymann MA, et al. Indomethacin and patent ductus arteriosus: Effects on renal function in preterm lambs. *Am J Physiol* 1988;254:F38–F44.

52. Cotton RB, Stahlman MT, Berder HW, et al. Randomized trial of early closure of symptomatic patent ductus arteriosus in small preterm infants. *J Pediatr* 1978;93:647–651.

53. Heymann MA, Rudolph AM, Silverman NH. Closure of the ductus arteriosus in premature infants by inhibition of prostaglandin synthesis. *N Engl J Med* 1976;295:530–533.

54. Mahony L, Carnero V, Brett C, et al. Prophylactic indomethacin therapy for patent ductus arteriosus in very-low-birth-weight infants. *N Engl J Med* 1982;306:506–510.

55. Gersony WM, Peckham GJ, Ellison RC, et al. Effects of indomethacin in premature infants with patent ductus arteriosus: Results of a national collaborative study. *J Pediatr* 1983;102:895–906.

56. Way GL, Pierce JR, Wolf RR, et al. ST depression suggesting subendocardial ischemia in neonates with respiratory distress syndrome and patent ductus arteriosus. *J Pediatr* 1979;95:609–611.

57. Merritt TA, White CL, Jacob J, et al. Patent ductus arteriosus treated with ligation or indomethacin: A follow-up study. *J Pediatr* 1979;95:588–594.

58. Keller RL, Tacy TA, Fields S, et al. Combined treatment with a nonselective nitric oxide synthase inhibitor (l-NMMA) and indomethacin increases ductus constriction in extremely premature newborns. *Pediatr Res* 2005;58:1216–1221.

59. Lago P, Bettiol T, Salvadori S, et al. Safety and efficacy of ibuprofen versus indomethacin in preterm infants treated for patent ductus arteriosus: A randomised controlled trial. *Eur J Pediatr* 2002;161(4):202–207.

60. Mosca F, Bray M, Lattanzio M, et al. Comparative evaluation of the effects of indomethacin and ibuprofen on cerebral perfusion and oxygenation in preterm infants with patent ductus arteriosus. *J Pediatr* 1997; 131:549–554.

61. Patel J, Roberts I, Azzopardi D, et al. Randomized double-blind controlled trial comparing the effects of ibuprofen with indomethacin on cerebral hemodynamics in preterm infants with patent ductus arteriosus. *Pediatr Res* 2000;47(1):36–42.

62. Pezzati M, Vangi V, Biagiotti R, et al. Effects of indomethacin and ibuprofen on mesenteric and renal blood flow in preterm infants with patent ductus arteriosus. *J Pediatr* 1999;135:733–738.

63. Su PH, Chen JY, Su CM, et al. Comparison of ibuprofen and indomethacin therapy for patent ductus arteriosus in preterm infants. *Pediatr Int* 2003;45:665–670.

64. Van Overmeire B, Smets K, Lecoutere D, et al. A comparison of ibuprofen and indomethacin for closure of patent ductus arteriosus. *N Engl J Med* 2000;343:674–681.

65. Thomas RL, Parker GC, Van Overmeire B, et al. A meta-analysis of ibuprofen versus indomethacin for closure of patent ductus arteriosus. *Eur J Pediatr* 2005;164(3):135–140.

66. Aranda JV, Thomas R. Systematic review: Intravenous Ibuprofen in preterm newborns. *Semin Perinatol* 2006;30(3):114–120.

67. Ohlsson A, Walia R, Shah S. Ibuprofen for the treatment of patent ductus arteriosus in preterm and/or low birth weight infants. *Cochrane Database Syst Rev* 2005(4):CD003481.

68. Gournay V, Roze JC, Kuster A, et al. Prophylactic ibuprofen versus placebo in very premature infants: A randomised, double-blind, placebo-controlled trial. *Lancet* 2004;364:1939–1944.

69. McCurnin DC, Yoder BA, Coalson J, et al. Effect of ductus ligation on cardiopulmonary function in premature baboons. *Am J Respir Crit Care Med* 2005;172:1569–1574.

70. Szymankiewicz M, Hodgman JE, Siassi B, et al. Mechanics of breathing after surgical ligation of patent ductus arteriosus in newborns with respiratory distress syndrome. *Biol Neonate* 2004;85(1):32–36.

71. Brooks JM, Travadi JN, Patole SK, et al. Is surgical ligation of patent ductus arteriosus necessary? The Western Australian experience of conservative management. *Arch Dis Child Fetal Neonatal Ed* 2005;90(3):F235–239.

72. Wagner HR, Ellison RC, Zierler S, et al. Surgical closure of patent ductus arteriosus in 268 preterm infants. *J Thorac Cardiovasc Surg* 1984;87:870–875.

73. Hines MH, Raines KH, Payne RM, et al. Video-assisted ductal ligation in premature infants. *Ann Thorac Surg* 2003;76:1417–1420.

74. Fowlie PW, Davis PG. Prophylactic indomethacin for preterm infants: A systematic review and meta-analysis. *Arch Dis Child Fetal Neonatal Ed* 2003;88:F464–466.

75. Van Overmeire B, Allegaert K, Casaer A, et al. Prophylactic ibuprofen in premature infants: A multicentre, randomised, double-blind, placebo-controlled trial. *Lancet* 2004;364:1945–1949.

76. Mitchell SC, Korones SB, Berendes HW. Congenital heart disease in 56,109 births: Incidence and natural history. *Circulation* 1971;43:323–332.

77. Knight DH, Patterson DF, Melbin J. Constriction of the fetal ductus arteriosus induced by oxygen, acetylcholine and norepinephrine in normal dogs and those genetically predisposed to persistent patency. *Circulation* 1973;47:127–132.

78. Mani A, Meraji SM, Houshyar R, et al. Finding genetic contributions to sporadic disease: a recessive locus at 12q24 commonly contributes to patent ductus arteriosus. *Proc Nat Acad Sci USA* 2002;99:15054–15059.

79. Khau Van Kien P, Mathieu F, Zhu L, et al. Mapping of familial thoracic aortic aneurysm/dissection with patent ductus arteriosus to 16p12.2-p13.13. *Circulation* 2005;112:200–206.

80. Gibson GA. Persistence of the arterial duct and its diagnosis. *Edinburgh Med J* 1900;8:1–5.

81. Krichenko A, Benson LN, Burrows P, et al. Angiographic classification of the isolated, persistently patent ductus arteriosus and implications for percutaneous catheter occlusion. *Am J Cardiol* 1989;63:877–880.

82. Higgins CB, Silverman NH, Kersting-Sommerhoff BA, et al. Left-to-right shunt lesions. In: *Congenital Heart Disease: Echocardiography and Magnetic Resonance Imaging*. New York: Raven Press, 1990:99–133.

83. Morgan-Hughes GJ, Marshall AJ, Roobottom C. Morphologic assessment of patent ductus arteriosus in adults using retrospectively ECG-gated multidetector CT. *AJR Am J Roentgenol* 2003;181:749–754.

84. Brenner LD, Caputo GR, Mostbeck G, et al. Quantitation of left to right atrial shunts with velocity-encoded cine nuclear magnetic resonance imaging. *J Am Coll Cardiol* 1992;20:1246–1250.

85. Morris CD, Reller MD, Menashe VD. Thirty-year incidence of infective endocarditis after surgery for congenital heart defect. *JAMA* 1998;279:599–603.

86. Johnson DH, Rosenthal A, Nadas AS. A forty-year review of bacterial endocarditis in infancy and childhood. *Circulation* 1975;51:581–588.

87. Sadiq M, Latif F, Ur-Rehman A. Analysis of infective endarteritis in patent ductus arteriosus. *Am J Cardiol* 2004;93:513–515.

88. Jan SL, Hwang B, Fu YC, et al. Isolated neonatal ductus arteriosus aneurysm. *J Am Coll Cardiol* 2002;39:342–347.

89. Celermajer DS, Sholler GF, Hughes CF, et al. Persistent ductus arteriosus in adults. A review of surgical experience with 25 patients. *Med J Aust* 1991;155(4):233–236.

90. Rudolph AM, Mesel E, Levy JM. Epinephrine in the treatment of cardiac failure due to shunts. *Circulation* 1963;28:3–13.

91. Patel HT, Cao QL, Rhodes J, et al. Long-term outcome of transcatheter closure of small to large patent ductus arteriosus. *Catheter Cardiovasc Interv* 1999;47:457–461.

92. Alwi M, Kang LM, Samion H, et al. Transcatheter occlusion of native persistent ductus arteriosus using conventional Gianturco coils. *Am J Cardiol* 1997;79:1430–1432.

93. Masura J, Tittel P, Gavora P, et al. Long-term outcome of transcatheter patent ductus arteriosus closure using Amplatzer duct occluders. *Am Heart J* 2006;151:755.e7–755.e10.

94. Masura J, Walsh KP, Thanopoulous B, et al. Catheter closure of moderate- to large-sized patent ductus arteriosus using the new Amplatzer duct occluder: Immediate and short-term results. *J Am Coll Cardiol* 1998;31:878–882.

95. Hazama S, Sakamoto I, Yamachika S, et al. Endovascular surgery using an original occluder for patent ductus arteriosus in an adult patient. *Jpn J Thorac Cardiovasc Surg* 2005;53(1):58–61.

96. Laborde F, Folliguet TA, Etienne PY, et al. Video-thoracoscopic surgical interruption of patent ductus arteriosus. Routine experience in 332 pediatric cases. *Eur J Cardiothorac Surg* 1997;11:1052–1105.

97. Vanamo K, Berg E, Kokki H, et al. Video-assisted thoracoscopic versus open surgery for persistent ductus arteriosus. *J Pediatr Surg* 2006;41:1226–1229.

98. Roy A, Juneja R, Saxena A. Use of Amplatzer duct occluder to close severely hypertensive ducts: Utility of transient balloon occlusion. *Indian Heart J* 2005;57(4):332–336.

99. Santos MA, Moll JN, Drumond C, et al. Development of the ductus arteriosus in right ventricular outflow tract obstruction. *Circulation* 1980;62:818–822.

100. Freed MD, Heymann MA, Lewis AB, et al. Prostaglandin E1 in infants with ductus arteriosus-dependent congenital heart disease. *Circulation* 1981;64:899–905.

101. Gibbs JL, Uzun O, Blackburn ME, et al. Fate of the stented arterial duct. *Circulation* 1999;99:2621–2625.

102. Michel-Behnke I, Akintuerk H, Thul J, et al. Stent implantation in the ductus arteriosus for pulmonary blood supply in congenital heart disease. *Catheter Cardiovasc Interv* 2004;61(2):242–252.

103. Gewillig M, Boshoff DE, Dens J, et al. Stenting the neonatal arterial duct in duct-dependent pulmonary circulation: New techniques, better results. *J Am Coll Cardiol* 2004;43:107–112.

104. Lim DS, Peeler BB, Matherne GP, et al. Risk-stratified approach to hybrid transcatheter-surgical palliation of hypoplastic left heart syndrome. *Pediatr Cardiol* 2006;27(1):91–95.

105. Elliotson J. Case of malformation of the pulmonary artery and aorta. *Lancet* 1830;1:247.

106. Balaji S, Burch M, Sullivan ID. Accuracy of cross-sectional echocardiography in diagnosis of aortopulmonary window. *Am J Cardiol* 1991;67:650–653.

107. Berry TE, Bharati S, Muster AJ, et al. Distal aortopulmonary septal defect, aortic origin of the right pulmonary artery, intact ventricular septum, patent ductus arteriosus and hypoplasia of the aortic isthmus: A newly recognized syndrome. *Am J Cardiol* 1982;49:108–116.

108. Bertolini A, Dalmonte P, Bava GL, et al. Aortopulmonary septal defects. A review of the literature and report of ten cases. *J Cardiovasc Surg* 1994;35:207–213.

109. Blieden LC, Moller JH. Aorticopulmonary septal defect. An experience with 17 patients. *Br Heart J* 1974;36:630–635.

110. Boonstra PW, Talsma M, Ebels T. Interruption of the aortic arch, distal aortopulmonary window, arterial duct and aortic origin of the right pulmonary artery in a neonate: Report of a case successfully repaired in a one-stage operation. *Int J Cardiol* 1992;34(1):108–110.

111. Deverall PB, Lincoln JC, Aberdeen E, et al. Aortopulmonary window. *J Thorac Cardiovasc Surg* 1969;57:479–486.

112. Geva T, Ott DA, Ludomirsky A, et al. Tricuspid atresia associated with aortopulmonary window: Controlling pulmonary blood flow with a fenestrated patch. *Am Heart J* 1992;123:260–262.

113. Gross RE. Surgical closure of an aortic septal defect. *Circulation* 1952;5:858–863.

114. Johnasson L, Michaelsson M, Westerholm CH, et al. Aortopulmonary window: A new surgical approach. *Ann Thorac Surg* 1978;25:564–567.

115. Kutsche LM, Van Mierop LHS. Anatomy and pathogenesis of aorticopulmonary septal defect. *Am J Cardiol* 1987;59:443–447.

116. McElhinney DB, Reddy VM, Tworetzky W, et al. Early and late results after repair of aortopulmonary septal defect and associated anomalies in infants <6 months of age. *Am J Cardiol* 1998;81:195–201.

117. Mori K, Ando M, Takao A, et al. Distal type of aortopulmonary window. Report of 4 cases. *Br Heart J* 1978;40:681–689.

118. Redington AN, Rigby ML, Ho SY, et al. Aortic atresia with aortopulmonary window and interruption of the aortic arch. *Pediatr Cardiol* 1991;12(1):49–51.

119. Shore DF, Yen Ho S, Anderson RH, et al. Aortopulmonary septal defect coexisting with ventricular septal defect and pulmonary atresia. *Ann Thorac Surg* 1983;35:132–137.

120. Richardson JV, Doty DB, Rossi NP, et al. The spectrum of anomalies of aortopulmonary septation. *J Thorac Cardiovasc Surg* 1979;78:21–27.

121. McMahon CJ, DiBardino DJ, Undar A, et al. Anomalous origin of left coronary artery from the right pulmonary artery in association with type III aortopulmonary window and interrupted aortic arch. *Ann Thorac Surg* 2002;74:919–921.

122. Duca V, Sulliotti G, Maggio C, et al. Transposition of the great arteries and aortopulmonary window in the same patient: Clinical report and follow-up. *Pediatr Cardiol* 2002;23:474–475.

123. Takahashi K, Kido S, Hoshino K, et al. Frequency of a 22q11 deletion in patients with conotruncal cardiac malformations: A prospective study see comments. *Eur J Pediatr* 1995;154:878–881.

124. Van Mierop LHS, Kursche LM. Embryology of the heart. In: Hurst JW, ed. *The Heart*. 6th ed. New York: McGraw-Hill, 1986.

125. Kirby ML, Gale TF, Stewart DE. Neural crest cells contribute to normal aorticopulmonary septation. *Science* 1983;220:1059–1061.

126. Marmon LM, Balsara RK, Chen R, et al. Congenital cardiac anomalies associated with the DiGeorge syndrome: A neonatal experience. *Ann Thorac Surg* 1984;38:146–150.

127. Iserin L, de Lonlay P, Viot G, et al. Prevalence of the microdeletion 22q11 in newborn infants with congenital conotruncal cardiac anomalies. *Eur J Pediatr* 1998;157:881–884.

128. Webber SA, Hatchwell E, Barber JC, et al. Importance of microdeletions of chromosomal region 22q11 as a cause of selected malformations of the

ventricular outflow tracts and aortic arch: A three-year prospective study see comments. *J Pediatr* 1996;129(1):26–32.

129. Valsangiacomo ER, Smallhorn JF. Images in cardiovascular medicine. Prenatal diagnosis of aortopulmonary window by fetal echocardiography. *Circulation* 2002;105:E192.

130. Bagtharia R, Trivedi KR, Burkhart HM, et al. Outcomes for patients with an aortopulmonary window, and the impact of associated cardiovascular lesions. *Cardiol Young* 2004;14:473–480.

131. Di Bella I, Gladstone DJ. Surgical management of aortopulmonary window. *Ann Thorac Surg* 1998;65:768–770.

132. Matsuki O, Yagihara T, Yamamoto F, et al. New surgical technique for total-defect aortopulmonary window. *Ann Thorac Surg* 1992;54:991–992.

133. Messmer BJ. Pulmonary artery flap for closure of aortopulmonary window. *Ann Thorac Surg* 1994;57:498–501.

134. Atiq M, Rashid N, Kazmi KA, et al. Closure of aortopulmonary window with Amplatzer duct occluder device. *Pediatr Cardiol* 2003;24(3):298–299.

135. Jureidini SB, Spadaro JJ, Rao PS. Successful transcatheter closure with the buttoned device of aortopulmonary window in an adult. *Am J Cardiol* 1998;81(3):371–372.

136. Naik GD, Chandra VS, Shenoy A, et al. Transcatheter closure of aortopulmonary window using Amplatzer device. *Catheter Cardiovasc Interv* 2003;59(3):402–405.

137. Tulloh RM, Rigby ML. Transcatheter umbrella closure of aorto-pulmonary window. *Heart* 1997;77:479–480.

CHAPTER 34 ■ CONGENITAL ANOMALIES OF THE CORONARY VESSELS AND THE AORTIC ROOT

G. PAUL MATHERNE, MD, AND D. SCOTT LIM, MD

Coronary and aortic root anomalies represent a small but interesting group of malformations that may occur alone or in association with structural heart disease (1–3). Recognizing and identifying these anomalies has become an important part of the evaluation of complex congenital heart disease. In the absence of structural heart disease, coronary anomalies are also important in certain clinical situations such as dilated cardiomyopathy (4), hypertrophic cardiomyopathy (5), and sudden cardiac events in older children (6). This chapter will review coronary artery development and anatomy, coronary anomalies in the absence of structural heart disease, coronary anomalies in the presence of structural heart disease, and aortic root anomalies. Coronary arterial venous malformations will be covered in Chapter 35.

CORONARY VASCULAR ANOMALIES

Embryology

The cells of the developing myocardium initially receive nourishment directly from circulating blood in the ventricular cavity. As the myocardium thickens and develops, the presence of multiple trabeculations allows close proximity of the myocardial cells to the ventricular cavity. These trabeculations then develop into a sinusoidal system that continues to minimize diffusion distance between myocytes and the circulation. It was previously thought that these sinusoids were the forerunners of the coronary vascular system, but new data have provided evidence for an epicardial origin of the coronary vascular system (7).

The new model of coronary vascular development (7) begins with formation of a proepicardial protrusion by cells of the primordial liver. These cells establish the proepicardium

and epicardial cells and then migrate over the surface of the heart. The epicardial cells invade the forming subepicardial matrix and form the coronary vascular plexus. The epicardial cells then undergo epithelial mesenchymal transformation by an as yet undefined mechanism that probably involves multiple growth factors. Nascent capillaries then are associated with subepicardial mesenchymal cells to form mature vessels. It has now been shown that small vessels on the surface of the heart fuse and grow inward to penetrate the aorta rather than coronary buds from the aortic sinuses fusing with the coronary vessels (8).

The new experimental data on the development of the coronary system implicate multiple growth factors as well as adhesion molecules and chemotactic factors in this complicated coordinated migration and transformation of cells to form coronary vessels. The presence of congenital anomalies of coronary arteries suggests abnormalities in these signaling pathways or alterations in local factors that direct coronary vessel development.

Anatomy

Coronary Arteries

Normal coronary artery anatomy will be briefly reviewed, but for a complete discussion on this subject the reader is referred to Frank Netter's diagrams in the *CIBA Collection of Medical Illustrations* (9). The entire blood flow to the myocardium is derived from two main coronary arteries arising from the right and left aortic sinuses of Valsalva (Fig. 34.1). The left main coronary artery is about 13 mm long in adults (range 2 to 40 mm) and gives rise to the circumflex branch, which courses posteriorly in the atrioventricular groove; the left main coronary then continues as a left anterior descending branch. The right coronary artery gives rise to a small conal

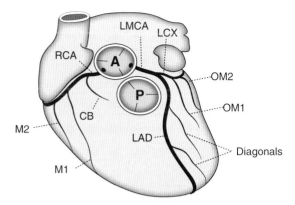

FIGURE 34.1 Normal anatomy of the coronary arteries. A, aortic valve; CB, conus branch of the right coronary artery; Diagonals, first and second diagonal branches of the left anterior descending coronary artery; LAD, anterior descending branch of left coronary artery; LCX, circumflex branch of the left coronary artery; LMCA, left main coronary artery; M1/2, first and second marginal branches of the right coronary artery; OM1/2, first and second obtuse marginal branches of the left coronary artery; P, pulmonic valve; RCA, right coronary artery.

branch and then courses posteriorly in the opposite direction along the atrioventricular groove. There is no separate septal branch, the septum being supplied by perforating branches that enter the septum from the anterior and posterior descending coronary arteries. In 69% of the population, the right coronary artery is dominant (10), giving rise to the posterior descending coronary artery, which extends to the apex and supplies the posterior part of the ventricular septum, the inferior wall of the left ventricle, and the atrioventricular node (11). In 11% the left coronary artery is dominant, thereby giving rise to the posterior descending coronary artery, and in 20% there is codominance (10). The left coronary artery supplies only the free wall of the left ventricle. Interestingly, a significant number of patients with bicuspid aortic valves or aortic stenosis (20% to 57%) have left-dominant systems and a short left main coronary artery (10,12,13).

Within the myocardium, small arteries branch repeatedly until they reach the endocardium. Normally, there are connections between coronary arterial branches that are 25 to 200 mm in diameter and are known as collaterals. They may be superficial or subendocardial, and they are capable of enlarging if pressure gradients develop between branches.

Cardiac Veins

The coronary sinus arises from the proximal portion of the left sinus horn and the common cardinal vein. The great cardiac vein begins at the apex and runs up the anterior interventricular groove to enter the coronary sinus just below the left lower pulmonary vein. The coronary sinus then runs around the left edge of the heart in the posterior atrioventricular groove until it enters the right atrium near the atrioventricular node. The middle cardiac vein runs up in the posterior atrioventricular groove to enter the coronary sinus. The posterior ventricular vein drains the free wall of the left ventricle up to the coronary sinus. The small cardiac vein runs with the right coronary artery in the right posterior part of the atrioventricular groove; it drains into the coronary sinus or directly into the right atrium, as do the small veins draining the right ventricular free wall (14,15).

ANOMALIES OF CORONARY ARTERIES IN THE ABSENCE OF STRUCTURAL HEART DISEASE

Normal Variations

The right and left coronary arteries arise from the right and left aortic sinuses of Valsalva (Fig. 34.1). Usually they come from the middle of the sinuses, but they may arise from the sinotubular junction or even above it. The position of the ostium does not appear to affect the flow through it. The ostia may be round, oval, or elliptical. The arteries are usually perpendicular to the aortic wall; that is, they are radially arranged relative to the center of the aorta.

Separate origin of the conus branch of the right coronary artery occurs commonly (11). The corresponding anomaly on the left side—separate origins of the left anterior descending and left circumflex coronary arteries—occurs in about 1% of people and is more frequent with bicuspid aortic valves (11). Neither of these anomalies appears to have any clinical consequences.

Abnormal Origin of Right or Left Coronary Artery from Inappropriate Sinus

Anomalous Origin of Left Coronary Arterial Branches from Right Sinus of Valsalva

The most common anomaly, accounting for about one third of all major coronary arterial anomalies, is origin of the left circumflex coronary artery from the right main coronary artery (Fig. 34.2A) (2,3,16,17). The left circumflex coronary artery passes behind the aorta to reach its normal territory of supply. This anomaly has no general clinical significance, but the artery may be compressed if both mitral and aortic prosthetic fixation rings are implanted. These anomalous arteries may have an unusually high incidence of coronary atheroma (2).

Much less common, accounting for 1% to 3% of major coronary arterial anomalies (2,16), but of greater clinical significance is origin of the left main coronary artery from the right sinus of Valsalva (1,16,18). There are four pathways that the left main coronary artery can take after leaving the sinus: Posterior to the aorta (Fig. 34.2B), anterior to the right ventricular outflow tract (Fig. 34.2C), within the ventricular septum beneath the right ventricular infundibulum (Fig. 34.2D, the most common variant), and between the aorta and the right ventricular outflow tract (Fig. 32.4E). With rare exceptions, the first three courses have not been associated with sudden death or premature myocardial ischemia. The course that passes between the two great arteries, however, has often been associated with sudden death in children during or just after vigorous exercise. Several of these patients had had episodes of syncope or chest pain during previous exercise. In most of these patients, the ostium of the left main coronary artery was slitlike, with an intramural course within the aortic root and adherent to it for about 1.5 cm (18).

In some patients, the left anterior descending coronary artery originates in the right sinus of Valsalva or from the right main coronary artery (Fig. 34.2F). This anomaly is rare in the absence of congenital heart disease (2,18) but is common in tetralogy of Fallot. The artery usually passes in

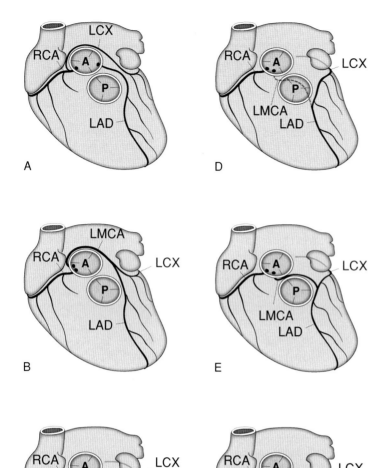

FIGURE 34.2 Anomalous origin of the left main coronary artery from the right sinus of Valsalva. **A:** Left circumflex coronary artery arising from the right coronary artery. **B:** Left main coronary artery arising from the right sinus of Valsalva (posterior course). **C:** Left main coronary artery arising from the right sinus of Valsalva (anterior course). **D:** Left main coronary artery arising from the right sinus of Valsalva (interventricular septal course). **E:** Left main coronary artery arising from the right sinus of Valsalva, and with a course between the two great arteries. Note the oblique origin of left main coronary artery (LMCA). **F:** Separate origin of the left anterior descending coronary artery from the right sinus of Valsalva. A, aorta; LAD, left anterior descending coronary artery; LCX, left circumflex coronary artery; LMCA, left main coronary artery; P, pulmonary outflow; RCA, right coronary artery.

front of the right ventricular outflow tract or through the interventricular septum but has rarely been seen to pass between the aorta and right ventricular outflow tract. Should there be atheroma near the ostium of the common arterial trunk, then most of the heart will become ischemic, so that the lesion is the equivalent of a left main coronary stenosis.

Anomalous Origin of Right Coronary Arterial Branches from the Left Sinus of Valsalva

Origin of the right main coronary artery from the left sinus of Valsalva, first described by White and Edwards in 1948 (19), is relatively common, making up about 30% of all major coronary arterial anomalies (2,18), and has a significantly higher incidence in Asians and Hispanics (20). The right coronary artery then runs between the aorta and the right ventricular outflow tract to reach the right side of the atrioventricular groove, after which it is distributed normally (Figs. 34.3 and 34.4). This anomaly was once thought to be benign, but there are now many reports of myocardial ischemia, infarction, or sudden death (21–23). In many of the autopsies, the origin of

the right main coronary artery was angulated and the ostium described as slitlike.

Single Coronary Artery

In 5% to 20% of major coronary arterial anomalies, a single coronary artery arises from the aorta and then branches (17,24). Sometimes an atretic cord connects part of the artery to a sinus of Valsalva that has no ostium. About 40% of these anomalies are associated with other cardiac malformations, including transposition of the great vessels, tetralogy of Fallot, truncus arteriosus, coronary-cameral fistulas, and bicuspid aortic valves. The single artery can arise from either the right (Fig. 34.5A–C) or the left sinus of Valsalva (Fig. 34.5D–F) with many variations (24). The single coronary artery on either side can follow its usual course and then continue on to supply the other side of the heart, or separate branches can arise from a main coronary artery and course posteriorly or anteriorly to supply the other side of the heart. Branches also can pass between the great vessels.

For the single coronary arteries arising from the right side, the right coronary can follow the course of the normal right coronary artery and continue as the left circumflex artery,

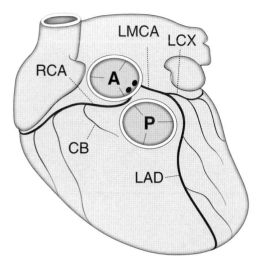

FIGURE 34.3 Anomalous origin of the right coronary artery from the left sinus of Valsalva, with oblique origin and course between the great arteries. A, aorta; CB, conal branch of the right coronary artery; LAD, left anterior descending coronary artery; LCX, left circumflex coronary artery; LMCA, left main coronary artery; P, pulmonary outflow, RCA, right coronary artery.

which then gives off the left anterior descending coronary artery (Fig. 34.5A). Alternatively, after the right coronary artery arises, a separate branch to the left side can arise that passes posterior to the aorta and gives rise to a circumflex vessel and a left anterior descending coronary artery (Fig. 34.5B),

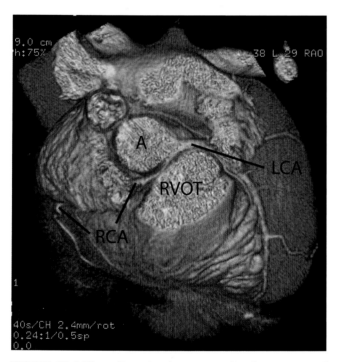

FIGURE 34.4 Three-dimensional reconstruction from computed tomographic imaging of the coronary arteries demonstrating anomalous origin of the right coronary artery from the left sinus of Valsalva, with oblique origin and course between the great arteries. Note the oblique origin of the right coronary artery, which then runs between the two great arteries. A, aorta; LCA, left coronary artery; RCA, right coronary artery; RVOT, right ventricular outflow tract.

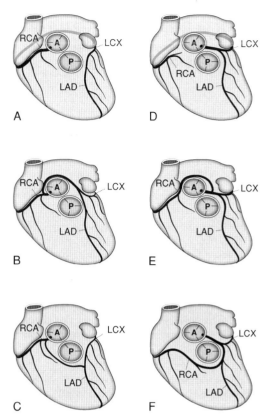

FIGURE 34.5 Single coronary artery variants. **A to C:** Single coronary artery originating from right sinus of Valsalva. **A:** Right coronary continuation to the left circumflex coronary artery (LCX) and left anterior descending coronary artery (LAD). **B:** Posterior course of separate LCX giving off the LAD. **C:** Anterior course of a separate LAD branch feeding back to the LCX. **D to F:** Single coronary artery originating from the left sinus of Valsalva. **D:** Left coronary artery giving rise to the LAD and the LCX, which then continues as the right coronary artery. **E:** Posterior course of separate right coronary branch off the left main coronary artery. **F:** Anterior course of separate right coronary artery coming off of the LAD. Variants passing between great vessels are not illustrated. A, aorta; P, pulmonary artery; RCA, right coronary artery.

or the separate branch can follow a course anterior to the right ventricular infundibulum, giving rise to the anterior descending coronary artery before continuing on as the circumflex (Fig. 34.5C).

A single left coronary artery can display branching patterns similar to those on the right. A single left coronary artery can branch into the left anterior descending and left circumflex coronary arteries with the circumflex continuing across the crux to form the right coronary artery (Fig. 34.5D). A separate right coronary vessel also can arise from the single left coronary artery and pass posterior to the aorta (Fig. 34.5E) to reach the opposite side of the heart, or the vessel can pass anterior to the right ventricular infundibulum (Fig. 34.5F). Most single coronary arteries produce no symptoms in the absence of severe atheroma (which is clearly more serious when there is only one main artery supplying the whole heart), but a small number of premature deaths have been reported with this anomaly (24). It is usually those variants in which a major branch passes between the aorta and the right ventricular infundibulum that are at greatest risk for sudden death (24), but other patterns can cause myocardial ischemia.

Left or Right Coronary Arterial Branches Arising from the Posterior Sinus of Valsalva

These are very rare (18) and have not been associated with premature or sudden death.

Pathology and Clinical Features of Abnormal Origin of Right or Left Coronary Artery from Inappropriate Sinus

Pathology

In about 20% of autopsies there are subendocardial scars, and occasionally a major myocardial infarct is reported. However, the suddenness of death in most of these patients prevents infarction from occurring. Occasionally, severe atherosclerosis has been seen in a segment of the abnormal vessels, even in children (25). In some of the anomalies, the initial few millimeters of artery may run within the aortic wall. Finally, the anomalous artery may arise tangentially from the aorta, and its ostium may be slitlike and partly covered by a valvelike flap.

Mechanisms of Death

Death is almost certainly due to myocardial ischemia, but the exact mechanism is unknown. The left ventricular myocardium has a huge demand for oxygen during strenuous exercise. Systolic pressure increases during strenuous exercise, and there is activation of the sympathetic nervous system. The root of the aorta therefore distends in systole. If part of the anomalous artery runs within the wall, it may be compressed, and if the artery runs adjacent to the wall, it may be stretched, compressed, or both. Presumably, the severe myocardial ischemia that occurs from any of these mechanisms produces either ventricular fibrillation or electromechanical dissociation. In those with previous syncope, the severe ischemia might have produced transient ventricular tachycardia or fibrillation, or else suddenly impaired ventricular function might have decreased cardiac output catastrophically. Why some patients with apparently identical anomalies survive without ischemia until their seventies and eighties is unknown.

Clinical Features

Most of these anomalous arteries do not cause myocardial ischemia, particularly if the anomalous branch does not pass between the aorta and the right ventricular infundibulum. Even those that do run between these structures do not always lead to sudden or premature death. However, this is the group that accounts for symptoms and sudden death in children, adolescents, and young adults. Although the first sign of the anomaly is sometimes sudden death or a fatal myocardial infarction, in many of these patients there may be a history of syncope or prolonged chest pain before the fatal event. These symptoms almost invariably come on during or just after strenuous exercise, and many of the victims have been athletes.

Diagnosis

Any episode of syncope or of severe chest pain during or after exercise calls for intensive investigation. The standard clinical examination usually shows no abnormalities. A resting elec-

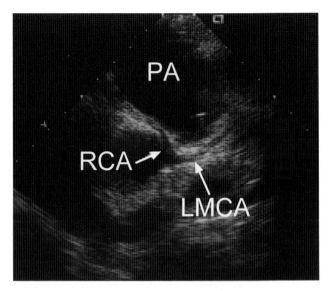

FIGURE 34.6 Echocardiogram demonstrating a single coronary artery with both the right coronary artery (RCA) and left main coronary artery (LMCA) arising from the left sinus. Note that the RCA passes between the aorta and pulmonary artery (PA), and originates at an oblique angle from the aorta.

trocardiogram should be performed to look for ventricular hypertrophy, evidence of prior infarction, and persistent arrhythmia; an echocardiogram should be performed to exclude intracardiac anomalies, hypertrophic cardiomyopathy, and proximal coronary anatomy. Careful attention should be directed to the origins of the coronary arteries because most of the anomalies affect the origins of the major arteries or their major branches and therefore may be detectable by echocardiography. Following the course of the coronary vessels is also important because the lesions with the highest risk of sudden death are associated with a major branch passing between the great vessels. Proving that a coronary artery passes between the great vessels can be difficult by angiography and may be easier by echocardiography (Fig. 34.6). Because most patients are older children or adults, the resolution of the transthoracic echocardiogram may be inadequate to show the anomalies, and transesophageal echocardiography (26), magnetic resonance imaging (27), or computed tomographic scans (28) (Fig. 34.4) may be more sensitive.

Evaluating blood pressure and the electrocardiogram or injecting thallium at near-maximal exercise can be useful. However, a normal near-maximal stress test result has been reported in patients who subsequently died suddenly and had an anomalous left main coronary artery (29). Because of this, exertional syncope or severe exertional chest pain in a child or young adult warrants further investigation if the echocardiogram is inconclusive.

Anomalous Left Coronary Artery from the Pulmonary Artery

In this anomaly the left coronary artery arises from the pulmonary artery, usually from the left posterior facing sinus (Fig. 34.7A). This anomaly was first described by pathologists in 1866 (30), and by 1962 Fontana and Edwards (31) had collected descriptions of 58 necropsies with this anomaly; most

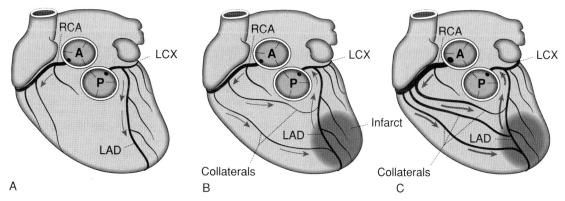

FIGURE 34.7 Anomalous origin of the left main coronary artery from the pulmonary artery. **A:** In the fetus, both right and left coronary arteries receive forward flow from the great arteries. **B:** Early after birth, before collaterals are well developed, there may be an anterolateral infarct and slight retrograde flow from the left coronary artery to the pulmonary artery. **C:** After collaterals have enlarged, there is high flow in the enlarged right coronary artery and the collaterals and significant retrograde flow into the pulmonary artery. *Arrows* indicate direction and approximate magnitude of flow in the right and left coronary arteries and the collaterals between them. A, aorta; LAD, left anterior descending coronary artery; LCX, left circumflex coronary artery; P, pulmonary artery; RCA, right coronary artery.

of these patients died at less than 13 months of age. The first report relating clinical and autopsy findings in a 3-month-old boy was by Bland et al. (32). The anomaly has thus been called the Bland–White–Garland syndrome.

Pathophysiology

In fetal life, this anomaly probably has no harmful effect: Pressures and oxygen saturations are similar in the aorta and pulmonary artery. Myocardial perfusion is presumably normal, and there is no stimulus to collateral formation (Fig. 34.7A). After birth, however, the pulmonary artery contains desaturated blood at pressures that rapidly fall below systemic pressures. Therefore, the left ventricle, with its huge demand for oxygen, is perfused with desaturated blood at low pressures. Collateral flow is initially low. The left ventricular myocardial vessels dilate to reduce their resistance and increase flow, but soon coronary vascular reserve becomes exhausted and myocardial ischemia ensues. At first, ischemia is transient and occurs only with exertion such as feeding or crying, but further increases in myocardial oxygen demand lead to infarction of the anterolateral left ventricular free wall (Fig. 34.7B), with resultant compromise of left ventricular function. This causes congestive heart failure, which is often made worse by mitral regurgitation secondary to a dilated mitral valve ring or infarction and dysfunction of the anterolateral papillary muscle. Collateral vessels between the normal right and abnormal left coronary artery enlarge, and with the increased flow so does the right coronary artery itself (Fig. 34.7C). However, because the left coronary artery is connected to the low-pressure pulmonary artery, the collateral flow tends to pass into the pulmonary artery rather than into the high-resistance myocardial blood vessels; there is a pulmonary–coronary steal with a left-to-right shunt. The shunt is usually relatively small in terms of cardiac output but relatively large in terms of coronary flow. In about 15% of these patients, myocardial blood flow can sustain myocardial function at rest or even during exercise. These are the patients who reach adult life (33).

Pathology

This anomaly is usually isolated but has been associated with patent ductus arteriosus (17,33), ventricular septal defect,

tetralogy of Fallot, or coarctation of the aorta (33). If there is pulmonary hypertension, as with a large ventricular septal defect, left ventricular perfusion may be adequate to prevent ischemia. Under these circumstances, closure of the defect with a decrease in pulmonary arterial pressure is catastrophic.

The right coronary artery is greatly dilated, and large collaterals may be visible on the surface of the heart. The left coronary artery is seen entering the main pulmonary artery, usually in the left pulmonary sinus, but rarely enters a branch pulmonary artery. It is usually only 2 to 5 mm long before it branches.

In infancy, the heart is large, the left ventricle and atrium in particular being dilated and hypertrophied. The anterolateral papillary muscle is atrophic and scarred, and the chordae attached to it may be shortened. In some studies, the posterior papillary muscle has been similarly affected (33). There may be diffuse endocardial fibroelastosis of the left ventricle, and the anterior mitral valve leaflet is often thickened. Thinning and scarring of the anterolateral left ventricular wall and apex owing to infarction are noted, and there are often mural thrombi.

In adults, the left coronary artery is thin-walled, resembling a vein. The heart is usually enlarged, but not as much as in infants, and there is usually no endocardial fibroelastosis. However, there is usually scarring and calcification of the anterolateral papillary muscle and occasionally even of the adjacent left ventricle (18,34).

Clinical Features

For infants, the description by Bland et al. (32) still applies:

> Nothing remarkable was noted about the patient until the tenth week; while nursing from the bottle, the onset of an unusual group of symptoms occurred which consisted of paroxysmal attacks of acute discomfort precipitated by the exertion of nursing. The infant appeared at first to be in obvious distress, as indicated by short expiratory grunts, followed immediately by marked pallor and cold sweat with a general appearance of severe shock. Occasionally, with unusually severe attacks, there appeared to be a transient loss of consciousness. The eructation of gas at times seemed to relieve the discomfort and to shorten the duration of the attack which usually lasted from 5 to 10 minutes, and following which the infant might proceed to nurse without

difficulty and remain free of symptoms for several days. . . . It seems probable that in this infant the curious attacks of paroxysmal discomfort . . . were those of angina pectoris. If this is true, it represents the earliest age at which this condition has been recorded.

Not all infants present in this way. Many present with the signs and symptoms of congestive heart failure. A few children have severe difficulties in infancy and then gradually improve until they are asymptomatic. Older children and adults may be asymptomatic or may have dyspnea, syncope, or angina pectoris on effort. Sudden death after exertion has been common (35). However, typical myocardial infarctions or congestive heart failure are rare in adults.

On physical examination, there may or may not be signs of congestive heart failure. In infants, the heart is usually enlarged, the left ventricle being the predominant ventricle affected. However, there may be right ventricular enlargement and a loud pulmonary component of the second heart sound if left ventricular failure has caused considerable pulmonary hypertension. The first heart sound may be soft or absent (if there is mitral regurgitation), and apical gallop rhythms are common. There may be no murmurs, or the murmur of mitral regurgitation, or at times a soft continuous murmur at the upper left sternal border that is similar to the murmur of a small patent ductus arteriosus, which is due to the continuous flow from the anomalous coronary artery into the pulmonary artery.

Electrocardiography

Classically, because there is an anterolateral infarct by the time the infant presents for diagnosis, there will be abnormal Q waves in leads I, aVL, and precordial leads V4 to V6. There also may be abnormal R waves or R-wave progression in the left precordial leads. Although this pattern is not pathognomonic for this anomaly (it is seen in myocardial infarcts from other causes or occasionally in cardiomyopathies), if found, the diagnosis of this anomaly should be considered and evaluated by other means. Even in asymptomatic adults, the resting electrocardiogram is abnormal, and abnormal ischemic responses occur with exercise (34).

Noninvasive Imaging

On the chest film in affected infants there is marked cardiomegaly, predominantly of the left atrium and ventricle, and evidence of pulmonary edema. These features are similar to those of many forms of cardiomyopathy, with which this anomaly is often confused.

Nuclear myocardial perfusion imaging is quite sensitive, showing reduced uptake in the anterolateral ischemic region. However, this finding is not specific because it has been seen in cardiomyopathies as well.

Echocardiography with Doppler color flow mapping has replaced cardiac catheterization as the standard method of diagnosis (36). The improved resolution of current echocardiographic equipment often allows the abnormal attachment of the origin of the left coronary artery to be seen. Color Doppler interrogation shows that flow passes from the coronary artery into the pulmonary artery (Fig. 34.8A). Therefore, even if the attachment of the coronary artery to the great artery is uncertain by two-dimensional imaging, the presence of diastolic flow in the pulmonary artery will be informative. An enlarged right coronary artery should also raise the suspicion of the diagnosis (Fig. 34.8B). The study also will show the size and function of the cardiac chambers, particularly the left ventricle, as well as regional left ventricular wall motion abnormalities and mitral regurgitation. There may be increased echogenicity of the papillary muscle and adjacent endocardium due to fibrosis and fibroelastosis.

Computed tomography scans have shown their high resolution in defining coronary artery anatomy and origination in most older patients. The main advantage of this technique is rapid acquisition times and, particularly with the 32- and 64-detector scanners, high resolution. However, ECG gating of the scans requires heart rates to be slow or, in the younger child, pharmacologically slowed. There remains a significant radiation exposure with this technique, but its ability to define coronary artery abnormalities is excellent (Fig 34.4).

Cardiac Catheterization and Angiography

Although previously cardiac catheterization and angiography were commonly used in the diagnosis of congenital coronary

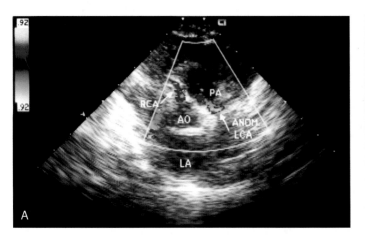
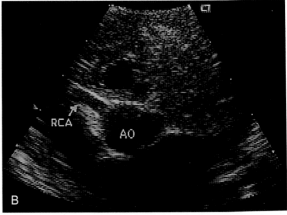

FIGURE 34.8 Echocardiographic images of anomalous left coronary artery. **A:** Color echocardiogram demonstrating retrograde flow of the anomalous left coronary artery (ANOM.LCA) into the pulmonary artery (PA). Note appropriate attachment of the right coronary artery (RCA) to the aorta (AO) and continuous flow into the pulmonary artery from the anomalous left coronary artery. LA, left atrium. **B:** Echocardiogram demonstrates the right coronary artery (RCA) attached to the aorta (AO), which is significantly dilated owing to the increased flow draining into collaterals.

abnormalities, currently they are used only if the results of noninvasive imaging are uncertain. In symptomatic infants, diagnostic cardiac catheterization demonstrates a low cardiac output and high filling pressures, and usually some degree of pulmonary hypertension. In asymptomatic older patients, output and pressures are usually normal except for a slight increase in left ventricular end-diastolic pressure. There may be a left-to-right shunt at the pulmonary arterial level, but because the shunt may be small, its absence does not rule out the diagnosis. Ventriculography demonstrates the dilated left ventricle and atrium with dysfunction of the anterolateral left ventricular free wall and the presence and severity of mitral regurgitation. Aortic root angiography will show the dilated right coronary artery and, if there are large collaterals, will show filling of the left coronary artery and passage of contrast material from the left coronary to the main pulmonary artery. Although main pulmonary arterial angiography may show reflux of contrast medium into the origin of the left coronary artery, neither this nor left ventriculography can reliably exclude the diagnosis.

Natural History

Of all children born with this rare anomaly, approximately 87% present in infancy (33) and of these, 65% to 85% die before 1 year of age from intractable congestive heart failure (37), usually after 2 months of age. A few children improve spontaneously (38). Others never have symptoms, perhaps because of extensive collaterals and even a restrictive opening between the origin of the left coronary artery and the pulmonary trunk. Nevertheless, even these people are at high risk of sudden death (35), especially during exercise. Some present as adults with exercise-induced angina (34) or with congestive heart failure owing to mitral regurgitation (18).

Treatment

The first effective surgical treatment was ligation of the left coronary artery at its origin from the pulmonary artery to prevent the steal. Most older children benefit from this procedure, especially if they have extensive coronary-to-pulmonary arterial shunting, but late sudden death can still occur (34,39).

Ligation of the origin of the left coronary artery and reconstitution of flow through it with a subclavian arterial or saphenous venous graft has been successful (40,41), although graft thrombosis and stenosis has occurred. Late obliterative changes in saphenous vein grafts have been seen (41), which can seriously complicate the patient's course because by approximately 3 years after successful revascularization, there is usually marked reduction of collaterals from the right coronary artery (16). Grafts using the internal mammary artery have a longer survival and may be desirable in older children.

Direct reimplantation of the origin of the left coronary artery into the aorta (with a button of pulmonary artery around the origin) has been proven successful and is considered the standard approach in many centers (42–45). An alternative approach is the Takeuchi procedure, in which an aortopulmonary window is created and then a tunnel fashioned that directs blood from the aorta to the left coronary ostium (46).

In the past it was recommended that, because surgical mortality is high in the sickest infants, surgery should be delayed until after 18 to 24 months of age (47). More recently, as surgical experience has accrued, early surgical intervention to establish a two-coronary system has been found to have significantly improved outcomes (45,48). However, because of papillary muscle infarction and dysfunction, significant preoperative mitral insufficiency has been found to be a risk factor for both mortality and need for late mitral valve surgery. Additionally, it has been reported that a two-vessel repair is feasible even in the sickest infants if postoperative support with a left ventricular assist device is used (49).

RARE CORONARY ANOMALIES

Coronary Atresia

Total absence of the extramural coronary arteries is rare and occurs most often with pulmonary atresia and aortic atresia. In both these anomalies, pressure in the small but hypertrophied right or left ventricle is at or above aortic pressure, and enlarged sinusoids carry blood from the ventricle to be distributed in the distal coronary arterial branches.

Stenosis or Atresia of a Coronary Ostium

Stenosis or atresia of the ostium or first few millimeters of the left main coronary artery is one of the rarest of the congenital coronary anomalies. The more distal branches are normal and develop multiple collaterals from the right coronary artery. Patients may present from 3 months to 60 years of age with sudden death, angina pectoris, myocardial infarction, or congestive heart failure.

All Coronary Arteries from Pulmonary Artery

Rarely both right and left coronary arteries, or a single coronary artery, come from the pulmonary trunk. Unless there is a cardiac lesion causing pulmonary hypertension, these children do not survive infancy without surgical intervention. More recently, these rare patients who have had dual coronary surgical reimplantation have survived (50).

Left Anterior Descending Coronary Artery from the Pulmonary Artery

This is a very rare anomaly (18), with few patients having been described. Apart from a 7-month-old child who died with an anterior myocardial infarct, all the others have been 18 to 55 years of age. Five had angina pectoris, one an anterior myocardial infarct, and one mitral regurgitation from papillary muscle dysfunction. Precordial murmurs were common, most had electrocardiographic evidence of ischemia, and chest radiographs were normal in three and showed cardiomegaly in three. Cardiac catheterization and angiography were diagnostic. Echocardiographic findings have not been reported. Surgical treatment by ligation of the anomalous artery or connecting it to the aorta has been recommended (18).

Left Circumflex Coronary Artery from the Pulmonary Artery or Branches

A few of these anomalies have been reported (18), and in many patients the circumflex coronary artery was attached to a branch pulmonary artery rather than to the main pulmonary trunk. All have been in children, and all but one had other congenital cardiac lesions.

Right Coronary Artery from the Pulmonary Artery

This anomaly is rare, only about one tenth as common as the left main coronary artery coming from the pulmonary artery (17,31,33). The anomaly was initially known only as an incidental finding at autopsy (18), but recently it has been associated with ischemia, syncope, cardiomyopathy, and sudden death (51,52).

Diagnosis

There may be a continuous murmur at the left sternal border. The electrocardiogram and chest radiograph are usually normal. Echocardiography with Doppler examination or cineangiography demonstrates the abnormal attachment of the right coronary artery to the pulmonary trunk and the retrograde flow from the right coronary artery to pulmonary artery. If echocardiography is nondiagnostic, definitive imaging of the anomalous right coronary artery origin can be obtained by computed tomography scan (28).

Treatment

Because most patients are asymptomatic and remain so, there is no way to determine which patients are at risk of dying without surgical correction of this defect. Nevertheless, because sudden death is a risk, many cardiologists recommend surgical correction, which has been done by reimplanting the right coronary artery into the aortic root (51).

MISCELLANEOUS ANOMALIES

Myocardial Bridges

The large epicardial coronary arteries run on the surface of the heart, with only their terminal branches penetrating the muscle, but it is very common for part of the epicardial artery to dip beneath the epicardial muscle for several millimeters so that there is a muscle bridge over the large artery (53). Most of these bridges are not functionally important, particularly if they are superficial. There are, however, documented examples of myocardial ischemia (54) or infarction associated with these bridges, including relief of ischemia after myotomy. During coronary angiography, a portion of the coronary artery appears to be narrowed in systole but widely patent in diastole, distinguishing it from a partially occlusive lesion of the artery (53).

Because myocardial bridges are so common and do not necessarily indicate present or future coronary arterial disease, the decision about myotomy to relieve anginal symptoms must be made carefully. Not only should there be a well-defined muscle bridge, but there should be ischemia, based on electrocardiography or documented on nuclear scan or stress echocardiography, in the region supplied by the artery with the bridge. Ischemia may be due to long, thick bridges that compress the artery and relax unusually slowly so that diastolic filling of the coronary artery beyond the bridge is impaired. Under these circumstances, disappearance of symptoms and of signs of ischemia may follow myotomy (54).

Although myocardial bridges causing ischemia are rare in children with normal hearts, they may represent a significant cause of morbidity and mortality in children with hypertrophic cardiomyopathy (55), although this is also debated. Myocardial bridges with hypertrophic cardiomyopathy have been associated with chest pain, exercise intolerance, ventricular arrhythmias, and cardiac arrest in some, but debated in other studies (5,56). Unroofing the myocardial bridge has been reported to reduce the incidence of sudden death and arrhythmias in these patients (55). Children with hypertrophic cardiomyopathy and the above symptoms should be evaluated for bridges by stress perfusion imaging and selective coronary arteriography, and consideration should be given for unroofing the bridges if detected and felt to be causative.

CORONARY ARTERY PATTERNS WITH CONGENITAL HEART DEFECTS

Complete Transposition of the Great Arteries

Anomalies of the coronary arteries in transposition of the great arteries are important to identify because some patterns have been more difficult to transfer with the arterial switch operation. Anomalies occur in both the origin and distribution, with further anomalies secondary to intramural coursing of some vessels. This topic will be briefly reviewed in this chapter, and a more complete review can be found in Chapter 51.

The terminology of the anomalies has been controversial because the aorta and main pulmonary artery are abnormally related in complete transposition of the great arteries, and the aortic sinuses do not have their normal positions. The two sinuses adjacent to the pulmonary artery are termed facing sinuses (57). The nomenclature of the facing sinuses depends on the relationship of the great vessels. If the vessels are side by side, then the sinuses are termed anterior or posterior. If the great vessels are oblique, the sinuses are left anterior or right posterior. If the vessels are anterior-posterior, the sinuses are right or left (57).

The presence of a ventricular septal defect or of side-by-side great vessels should alert the cardiologist to an increased likelihood of coronary anomalies. In almost all patients, the coronary arteries arise from the facing sinuses (57,58). In 60%, the coronary arteries come from their appropriate sinuses and branch normally, a pattern seen most often with the aorta anterior and to the right of the pulmonary artery. The coronary arteries usually take the shortest course to reach their distribution, and because the aorta is anterior, the left main and circumflex coronary arteries pass anterior to the right ventricular outflow tract (Fig. 34.9A). The next most common variation is the left circumflex arising from the right coronary artery and coursing posterior to the pulmonary artery, which is seen in about 20% of patients, usually with side-by-side great vessels (Fig. 34.9B). The coronary arteries also may be completely inverted, with the right coronary artery arising from a left anterior sinus and the left coronary artery arising from the right posterior sinus (Fig 34.9C). The coronary vessels also may be partially inverted, with the left circumflex arising from the right posterior sinus and the left anterior descending arising with the right coronary artery from the left anterior sinus (Fig. 34.9D).

Finally, various single coronary anomalies may occur, and intramural coursing of any of the variants may occur, usually with branches passing between the great vessels. These variations affect the planning and conduct of the arterial switch

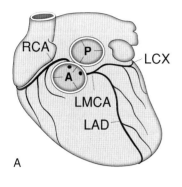

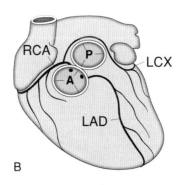

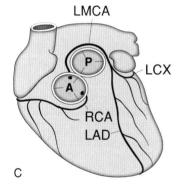

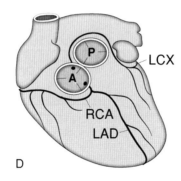

FIGURE 34.9 Coronary arteries in complete transposition of the great arteries. **A:** Most common variant (60%). **B:** Next most common variant, with left circumflex coronary artery (LCX) coming from the right coronary artery (RCA) (20%), which is seen most often with side-by-side great arteries. **C:** Inverted arteries coming from the inappropriate sinuses (4%). **D:** Inverted arteries with the left anterior descending coronary artery (LAD) coming from the right coronary artery (4%). Variants with single (8%) and intramural (5%) coronary arteries are not illustrated. A, aorta; LMCA, left main coronary artery P, pulmonary artery.

operation because they may make it difficult to move the coronary arterial origins to the neoaortic root without excessive tension.

Tetralogy of Fallot

About 40% of patients have an abnormally long, large conus artery that supplies a significant mass of myocardium. In 4% to 5%, the left anterior descending coronary artery arises from the right coronary artery and passes across the right ventricular outflow tract (Fig. 34.2F) (59). Occasionally, a single coronary artery comes from either the right or left sinus, and the major branch that crosses the heart may pass across the right ventricular outflow tract (Fig. 34.5C, F) or else pass behind the aorta and so avoid the outflow tract (Fig. 34.5B, E). Rarer variations also occur (33,59).

If major arteries cross the right ventricular outflow tract, it makes surgery with the traditional transannular incision more difficult. To avoid cutting the artery and infarcting part of the myocardium supplied by it (60), the surgeon may make incisions parallel to the artery, make incisions above and below the artery, tunnel underneath the artery, or bypass the stenotic region with a conduit (59). All these approaches interfere with the effectiveness of the surgery and in the small infant may lead to the decision to palliate rather than perform a total repair.

These anomalies may be detected by echocardiography, and if the anatomy is uncertain, then aortic root angiography or selective coronary arteriography is needed (59). Although the surgeon can usually see the anomalies, there are advantages in knowing about them in advance to plan the procedure more effectively. Furthermore, the anomalous arteries may not be visible if they are obscured by epicardial adhesions from previous surgery or if they run deep in the myocardium.

Corrected Transposition (l-Transposition) of the Great Arteries

The aorta is anterior and to the left of the pulmonary artery, and the two main coronary arteries come from the facing sinuses as seen with d-transposition of the great arteries. The anterior sinus is usually the noncoronary sinus. Because of this anatomy, there is some confusion about naming coronary arteries that appear to arise from incorrect sinuses (58,61). Some describe the vessels as right or left sided, based on their sinus of origin (61), whereas others (62) describe the arteries based on their territory of supply, and this terminology will be used here. The left coronary artery supplies the left ventricle but arises in the right facing sinus. It passes in front of the pulmonary annulus and divides into left anterior descending and circumflex branches, the latter passing in front of the right atrial appendage in the atrioventricular groove. The right coronary artery supplies the right ventricle. It arises from the left facing sinus and runs in the atrioventricular groove in front of the left atrial appendage to terminate as the posterior descending artery. The most common variant is a single coronary artery coming from the right facing sinus.

Double-Inlet Left Ventricle (Univentricular Heart)

Because there is no true ventricular septum, there is no typical interventricular groove, and the arterial branches that run along the borders of the rudimentary outlet chamber are referred to as delimiting arteries (33,63) rather than as anterior descending arteries.

When the outlet chamber is anterior and to the right, the aorta and pulmonary artery are related as in a complete transposition. The right coronary artery arises from the right facing aortic sinus and runs along the right atrioventricular sulcus. The left main coronary artery comes from the left facing sinus and continues around the left atrioventricular groove as the circumflex artery. The left and right coronary arteries give off the left and right delimiting arteries, respectively. When the outlet chamber is anterior and to the left, the great vessels are related like those in (corrected) l-transposition. The right and left main coronary arteries arise from their respective facing sinuses, and the "anterior descending" coronary artery may come from the left or the right coronary arteries, or there may be two delimiting arteries that border the rudimentary outlet chamber (63). With any of these variants, there may be several large diagonal arterial branches that run parallel to the delimiting branches and cross the outflow tract of the right ventricle, making septation difficult.

Double-Outlet Right Ventricle

The coronary artery origins are usually normal in most forms of this group of anomalies, except that because the aortic sinuses are rotated clockwise, the right coronary artery arises anteriorly and the left coronary artery arises posteriorly (58). When the aorta is anterior and to the right, the coronary pattern is similar to that in complete transposition of the great arteries, with the right coronary artery arising from the right facing sinus. In 15% there may be a single coronary artery arising anteriorly or posteriorly (64). Occasionally, the left anterior descending coronary artery comes from the right coronary artery and crosses the right ventricular outflow tract, as in tetralogy of Fallot (64). When the aorta is to the left, the right coronary artery passes to the right from the anterior sinus of the leftward aorta in front of the pulmonary artery to reach the atrioventricular groove.

Truncus Arteriosus

The right and left coronary arteries usually arise normally from their appropriate sinuses (65). If, however, the valve has more than three cusps, conventional descriptions must be abandoned. What is most consistent is that the left main coronary artery arises from the posterior sinus. Major variants include unusually high ostia, closely approximated ostia, or a single ostium (65). Large diagonal branches of the right coronary artery may cross over the anterior surface of the right ventricle and contribute to flow to the ventricular septum and even part of the left ventricular free wall (65).

CONGENITAL ANOMALIES OF THE AORTIC ROOT

Aortic-Left Ventricular Defect (Tunnel)

This rare lesion is a vascular connection between the aorta and the left ventricle (Fig. 34.10). Some describe it as a tunnel that begins above the right coronary ostium, usually separated from it by a ridge, and passes behind the right ventricular infundibulum and through the anterior upper part of the ventricular septum to enter the left ventricle just below the right and left aortic cusps (66). It is usually short and direct but may be aneurysmal. Levy et al. (66) attributed the tunnel to a congenital endothelialized connection between the aorta and the

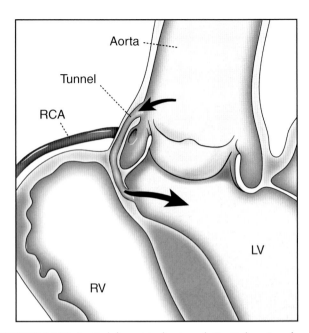

FIGURE 34.10 Aortic-left ventricular tunnel. Sagittal section showing the tunnel burrowing through the septal wall to enter the left ventricle. The proximal opening of the tunnel is superior to the right coronary ostium. LV, left ventricle; RCA, right coronary artery; RV, right ventricle.

left ventricle. Others (67) have considered the lesion to be a congenital defect associated with the thinned-out anterior wall of the left ventricular outflow tract where the right aortic sinus meets the membranous septum.

Many of these patients present in infancy with congestive heart failure. They have signs resembling marked aortic incompetence: A wide pulse pressure with a low diastolic blood pressure, a hyperactive dilated left ventricle and enlarged left atrium, and a loud to-and-fro murmur at the base. The electrocardiogram shows varying degrees of left ventricular and atrial hypertrophy. The chest radiograph shows variable cardiomegaly, possibly signs of congestive heart failure, but in all patients there is a dilated ascending aorta and in some a bulge of the enlarged right aortic sinus. Echocardiography with Doppler color flow mapping and aortography serve to separate this lesion from aortic incompetence by the absence of retrograde flow through the aortic valve; from a coronary artery–left ventricular fistula by the finding of normal right and left main coronary arteries; from an associated ventricular septal defect by the absence of a left-to-right shunt through the defect; and from a ruptured sinus of Valsalva by the anterior position of the tunnel and the absence of a dilated sinus of Valsalva (68). Treatment is surgical, but there is a high incidence of aortic incompetence after surgery.

Aneurysms of the Sinus of Valsalva

A localized weakness of the wall of a sinus of Valsalva, a relatively rare lesion reported in the nineteenth century (69), leads to aneurysmal bulging and even rupture. It is to be distinguished from diffuse dilation of all the sinuses in Marfan syndrome. The localized aneurysms are usually congenital, with thinning just above the annulus at the leaflet hinge owing to absence of normal elastic and muscular tissue (70). These aneurysms can follow infective endocarditis; at times, deciding if the endocarditis is the cause or the consequence of the aneurysm is impossible.

Pathologic Anatomy and Physiology

About 75% of the patients are male. Two thirds of the aneurysms are located in the right aortic sinus, one fourth in the noncoronary sinus, and the rest in the left aortic sinus (71). The aneurysms may be isolated, or in 30% to 50% may be associated with ventricular septal defects, especially defects of the outlet septum. The proportion of patients with ventricular septal defects is higher when the aneurysm arises from the right sinus. With an associated ventricular septal defect, particularly if subpulmonic, there is often prolapse of the aortic valve cusp and aortic incompetence. The aortic incompetence tends to be progressive as the valve prolapses farther and becomes fibrous and stiff. Coarctation of the aorta, atrial septal defect, tetralogy of Fallot, and patent ductus arteriosus also may be associated with these aneurysms. Because the aortic root is central, the aneurysms can rupture into any cardiac chambers, and virtually all combinations of sinus and chamber fistulas have been described. Rupture is most often of the right sinus aneurysm into the right ventricle, particularly if there is an outlet ventricular septal defect. The next most frequent site of rupture is into the right atrium from an aneurysm in the noncoronary sinus. Rupture into the pericardium is rare. At surgery, most fistulas resemble wind socks projecting from the sinus into the chamber of entry, with one or more openings near the end of the wind sock.

These aneurysms do not always rupture but may cause symptoms by obstructing the right ventricular outflow tract, distorting the aortic valve and causing aortic incompetence, compressing the left coronary artery and causing myocardial ischemia, or causing conduction disturbances or even complete heart block by compressing the conduction system. Because all complications of these aneurysms are functions of their size, and because they grow slowly, they seldom present in infancy and early childhood. The mean age for the onset of symptoms owing to sudden rupture of the aneurysms was 31 years (71). Rupture can follow acute chest trauma or severe exertion.

If the aneurysm ruptures, the size of the fistula determines how large the shunt will be, and its site of entry into the heart often determines the specific features. Thus, aneurysmal rupture into the left heart does not produce signs of a left-to-right shunt, whereas rupture into the right heart produces a left-to-right shunt of variable size.

Infective endocarditis is an important complication of the smaller fistulas; it may occur in 5% to 10% of patients with these congenital aneurysms (71).

Clinical and Laboratory Features

Before rupture, these aneurysms are diagnosed only incidentally during imaging for other lesions (72). Rupture may be accompanied by a tearing pain in the chest or upper abdomen.

If a huge shunt develops rapidly, the symptoms of congestive heart failure appear almost immediately, but with smaller fistulas it may take several months for heart failure to develop (71). About 20% of patients are asymptomatic.

With a small fistula, there may be only a continuous murmur like that of a ductus arteriosus, but with its maximal intensity in the third or fourth intercostal space near the sternal edge; if the fistula enters the right atrium, the murmur may be maximal to the right of the sternum. With larger fistulas, there will be a wide pulse pressure, a collapsing pulse, and left ventricular hyperactivity. If the fistula enters the right side, there will be right ventricular hyperactivity as well. A large fistula entering the left ventricle may display a to-and-fro murmur and simulate aortic incompetence. Occasionally, there is only a diastolic murmur in fistulas entering the left ventricle (71) or the high-pressure right ventricle in a neonate. If a ventricular septal defect is present, especially with infundibular obstruction, the combined murmurs can be confusing.

With a large chronic fistula, the electrocardiogram will show hypertrophy of the appropriate chambers. Occasionally, signs of myocardial ischemia or conduction defects occur because of compression of the coronary artery or the conduction system.

The chest roentgenogram will show enlargement of the appropriate chambers, as well as pulmonary overcirculation if there is a large left-to-right shunt. Evidence of congestive heart failure may be seen. The aortic root is not enlarged, although in the rare aneurysms of the left sinus of Valsalva there may be a bulge on the left aortic root border.

Two-dimensional echocardiography with Doppler color flow mapping shows the aneurysm dilation, even before rupture (73), but transesophageal echocardiography may give information not obtainable by routine transthoracic echocardiography (74), including information on degree and mechanism of associated aortic insufficiency. Further noninvasive imaging with computed tomography or magnetic resonance scans have been shown to provide excellent definition of the aneurysm and the tissue planes involved (75).

Cardiac Catheterization and Angiography

Previously, cardiac catheterization was used for diagnostic purposes in this entity, to define the magnitude of any left-to-right shunt, ventricular systolic and diastolic pressures, pulmonary hypertension, and any infundibular obstruction. However, its diagnostic use has been largely supplanted by noninvasive imaging with CT or MRI. More recently, in highly selected cases percutaneously delivered devices have been used to occlude the ruptured aneurysm (76); but caution must be advised so to not cause future aortic valvar insufficiency by the device.

Management

While previously, some authors have advocated treatment of congestive heart failure, with emphasis on afterload reduction to minimize runoff through the fistula, current definitive therapy is surgical anatomic correction.

References

1. Alexander RW, Griffith GC. Anomalies of the coronary arteries and their clinical significance. *Circulation* 1956;14:800–805.
2. Click RL, Holmes DR Jr, Vlietstra RE, et al. Anomalous coronary arteries: Location, degree of atherosclerosis and effect on survival–a report from the Coronary Artery Surgery Study. *J Am Coll Cardiol* 1989;13:531–537.
3. Liberthson RR, Zaman L, Weyman A, et al. Aberrant origin of the left coronary artery from the proximal right coronary artery: Diagnostic features and pre- and postoperative course. *Clin Cardiol* 1982;5:377–381.
4. Chang RR, Allada V. Electrocardiographic and echocardiographic features that distinguish anomalous origin of the left coronary artery from pulmonary artery from idiopathic dilated cardiomyopathy. *Pediatr Cardiol* 2001;22:3–10.
5. Mohiddin SA, Begley D, Shih J, et al. Myocardial bridging does not predict sudden death in children with hypertrophic cardiomyopathy but is associated with more severe cardiac disease. *J Am Coll Cardiol* 2000;36:2270–2278.

6. Davis JA, Cecchin F, Jones TK, et al. Major coronary artery anomalies in a pediatric population: Incidence and clinical importance. *J Am Coll Cardiol* 2001;37:593–597.

7. Tomanek RJ. Formation of the coronary vasculature: A brief review. *Cardiovasc Res* 1996;31 Spec No:E46–51.

8. Tomanek RJ. Formation of the coronary vasculature during development. *Angiogenesis* 2005;8:273–284.

9. Netter FJ. *A compilation of paintings on the normal and pathologic anatomy and physiology, embryology, and diseases of the heart. The CIBA collection of medical illustrations.* Caldwell, NJ: CIBA Pharmaceutical Company, 1978.

10. Hutchins GM, Nazarian IH, Bulkley BH. Association of left dominant coronary arterial system with congenital bicuspid aortic valve. *Am J Cardiol* 1978;42:57–59.

11. Baroldi G, Scomazzoni G. *Coronary circulation in the normal and the pathologic heart.* Washington, DC: Office of the Surgeon General, 1967.

12. Johnson AD, Detwiler JH, Higgins CB. Left coronary artery anatomy in patients with bicuspid aortic valves. *Br Heart J* 1978;40:489–493.

13. Scholz DG, Lynch JA, Willerscheidt AB, et al. Coronary arterial dominance associated with congenital bicuspid aortic valve. *Arch Pathol Lab Med* 1980;104:417–418.

14. Gensini GG, Giorgi S, Coskun O. Anatomy of the coronary circulation in living man: Coronary venography. *Circulation* 1965;31:778–784.

15. Gilard M, Mansourati J, Etienne Y, et al. Angiographic anatomy of the coronary sinus and its tributaries. *Pacing Clin Electrophysiol* 1998;21:2280–2284.

16. Donaldson RM, Raphael MJ, Yacoub MH, et al. Hemodynamically significant anomalies of the coronary arteries. Surgical aspects. *Thorac Cardiovasc Surg* 1982;30:7–13.

17. Ogden JA. Congenital anomalies of the coronary arteries. *Am J Cardiol* 1970;25:474–479.

18. Roberts WC. Major anomalies of coronary arterial origin seen in adulthood. *Am Heart J* 1986;111:941–963.

19. White NK, Edwards JE. Anomalies of the coronary arteries. Report of four cases. *Arch Pathol* 1948;45:766–771.

20. Ho JS, Strickman NE. Anomalous origin of the right coronary artery from the left coronary sinus: Case report and literature review. *Tex Heart Inst J* 2002;29:37–39.

21. Brandt B 3rd, Martins JB, Marcus ML. Anomalous origin of the right coronary artery from the left sinus of Valsalva. *N Engl J Med* 1983;309:596–598.

22. Taylor AJ, Byers JP, Cheitlin MD, et al. Anomalous right or left coronary artery from the contralateral coronary sinus: "High-risk" abnormalities in the initial coronary artery course and heterogeneous clinical outcomes. *Am Heart J* 1997;133:428–435.

23. Taylor AJ, Rogan KM, Virmani R. Sudden cardiac death associated with isolated congenital coronary artery anomalies. *J Am Coll Cardiol* 1992;20:640–647.

24. Shirani J, Roberts WC. Solitary coronary ostium in the aorta in the absence of other major congenital cardiovascular anomalies. *J Am Coll Cardiol* 1993;21:137–143.

25. Jim MH, Siu CW, Ho HH, et al. Anomalous origin of the right coronary artery from the left coronary sinus is associated with early development of coronary artery disease. *J Invasive Cardiol* 2004;16:466–468.

26. Dawn B, Talley JD, Prince CR, et al. Two-dimensional and Doppler transesophageal echocardiographic delineation and flow characterization of anomalous coronary arteries in adults. *J Am Soc Echocardiogr* 2003;16:1274–1286.

27. Casolo G, Del Meglio J, Rega L, et al. Detection and assessment of coronary artery anomalies by three-dimensional magnetic resonance coronary angiography. *Int J Cardiol* 2005;103:317–322.

28. Schmitt R, Froehner S, Brunn J, et al. Congenital anomalies of the coronary arteries: Imaging with contrast-enhanced, multidetector computed tomography. *Eur Radiol* 2005;15:1110–1121.

29. Barth CW 3rd, Roberts WC. Left main coronary artery originating from the right sinus of Valsalva and coursing between the aorta and pulmonary trunk. *J Am Coll Cardiol* 1986;7:366–373.

30. Brooks HSJ. Two cases of an abnormal coronary artery of the heart, arising from the pulmonary artery; with some remarks upon the effect of this anomaly in producing cirsoid dilatation of the vessels. *J Anat Physiol* 1885;20:26–29.

31. Fontana RS, Edwards JE. *Congenital Cardiac Disease: A Review of 357 Cases Studied Pathologically.* Philadelphia: WB Saunders, 1962.

32. Bland EF, White PD, Garland J. Congenital anomalies of the coronary arteries: Report of an unusual case associated with cardiac hypertrophy. *Am Heart J* 1933;8:787–801.

33. Neufeld HN, Schneeweiss A. *Coronary Artery Disease in Infants and Children.* Philadelphia: Lea & Febiger, 1983.

34. Moodie DS, Fyfe D, Gill CC, et al. Anomalous origin of the left coronary artery from the pulmonary artery (Bland-White-Garland syndrome) in adult patients: Long-term follow-up after surgery. *Am Heart J* 1983;106:381–388.

35. George JM, Knowlan DM. Anomalous origin of the left coronary artery from the pulmonary artery in an adult. *N Engl J Med* 1959;261:993–998.

36. King DH, Danford DA, Huhta JC, et al. Noninvasive detection of anomalous origin of the left main coronary artery from the pulmonary trunk by pulsed Doppler echocardiography. *Am J Cardiol* 1985;55:608–609.

37. Wesselhoeft H, Fawcett JS, Johnson AL. Anomalous origin of the left coronary artery from the pulmonary trunk. Its clinical spectrum, pathology, and pathophysiology, based on a review of 140 cases with seven further cases. *Circulation* 1968;38:403–425.

38. Liebman J, Hellerstein HK, Ankeney JL, et al. The problem of the anomalous left coronary artery arising from the pulmonary artery in older children. Report of three cases. *N Engl J Med* 1963;269:486–494.

39. Shrivastava S, Castaneda AR, Moller JH. Anomalous left coronary artery from pulmonary trunk. Long-term follow-up after ligation. *J Thorac Cardiovasc Surg* 1978;76:130–134.

40. Cooley DA, Hallman GL, Bloodwell RD. Definitive surgical treatment of anomalous origin of left coronary artery from pulmonary artery: Indications and results. *J Thorac Cardiovasc Surg* 1966;52:798–808.

41. El-Said GM, Ruzyllo W, Williams RL, et al. Early and late result of saphenous vein graft for anomalous origin of left coronary artery from pulmonary artery. *Circulation* 1973;48:III2–6.

42. Grace RR, Angelini P, Cooley DA. Aortic implantation of anomalous left coronary artery arising from pulmonary artery. *Am J Cardiol* 1977;39:609–613.

43. Huddleston CB, Balzer DT, Mendeloff EN. Repair of anomalous left main coronary artery arising from the pulmonary artery in infants: Long-term impact on the mitral valve. *Ann Thorac Surg* 2001;71:1985–1988; discussion 8–9.

44. Jin Z, Berger F, Uhlemann F, et al. Improvement in left ventricular dysfunction after aortic reimplantation in 11 consecutive paediatric patients with anomalous origin of the left coronary artery from the pulmonary artery. Early results of a serial echocardiographic follow-up. *Eur Heart J* 1994;15:1044–1049.

45. Schwartz ML, Jonas RA, Colan SD. Anomalous origin of left coronary artery from pulmonary artery: Recovery of left ventricular function after dual coronary repair. *J Am Coll Cardiol* 1997;30:547–553.

46. Takeuchi S, Imamura H, Katsumoto K, et al. New surgical method for repair of anomalous left coronary artery from pulmonary artery. *J Thorac Cardiovasc Surg* 1979;78:7–11.

47. Driscoll DJ, Nihill MR, Mullins CE, et al. Management of symptomatic infants with anomalous origin of the left coronary artery from the pulmonary artery. *Am J Cardiol* 1981;47:642–648.

48. Ando M, Mee RB, Duncan BW, et al. Creation of a dual-coronary system for anomalous origin of the left coronary artery from the pulmonary artery utilizing the trapdoor flap method. *Eur J Cardiothorac Surg* 2002;22:576–581.

49. Del Nido PJ, Duncan BW, Mayer JE Jr, et al. Left ventricular assist device improves survival in children with left ventricular dysfunction after repair of anomalous origin of the left coronary artery from the pulmonary artery. *Ann Thorac Surg* 1999;67:169–172.

50. Ochoa-Ramirez E, Valdez-Garza HE, Reyes-Gonzalez R, et al. Double anomalous coronary origin from the pulmonary artery: Successful surgical correction in an infant. *Tex Heart Inst J* 2005;32:348–350.

51. Coe JY, Radley-Smith R, Yacoub M. Clinical and hemodynamic significance of anomalous origin of the right coronary artery from the pulmonary artery. *Thorac Cardiovasc Surg* 1982;30:84–87.

52. Yao CT, Wang JN, Yeh CN, et al. Isolated anomalous origin of right coronary artery from the main pulmonary artery. *J Card Surg* 2005;20:487–489.

53. Angelini P, Trivellato M, Donis J, et al. Myocardial bridges: A review. *Prog Cardiovasc Dis* 1983;26:75–88.

54. Hill RC, Chitwood WR Jr, Bashore TM, et al. Coronary flow and regional function before and after supraarterial myotomy for myocardial bridging. *Ann Thorac Surg* 1981;31:176–181.

55. Yetman AT, McCrindle BW, MacDonald C, et al. Myocardial bridging in children with hypertrophic cardiomyopathy—a risk factor for sudden death. *N Engl J Med* 1998;339:1201–1209.

56. Sorajja P, Ommen SR, Nishimura RA, et al. Myocardial bridging in adult patients with hypertrophic cardiomyopathy. *J Am Coll Cardiol* 2003;42:889–894.

57. Wernovsky G, Sanders SP. Coronary artery anatomy and transposition of the great arteries. *Coron Artery Dis* 1993;4:148–157.

58. Elliott LP, Amplatz K, Edwards JE. Coronary arterial patterns in transposition complexes. Anatomic and angiocardiographic studies. *Am J Cardiol* 1966;17:362–378.

59. Fellows KE, Freed MD, Keane JF, et al. Results of routine preoperative coronary angiography in tetralogy of Fallot. *Circulation* 1975;51:561–566.

60. Berry BE, McGoon DC. Total correction for tetralogy of Fallot with anomalous coronary artery. *Surgery* 1973;74:894–898.

61. Lev M, Rowlatt UF. The pathologic anatomy of mixed levocardia. A review of thirteen cases of atrial or ventricular inversion with or without corrected transposition. *Am J Cardiol* 1961;8:216–263.

62. Kirklin JW, Barratt-Boyes BG. Congenitally corrected transposition of the great arteries. In: Barratt-Boyes B, Kirklin JW. *Cardiac Surgery.* New York: John Wiley and Sons, 1993.

63. Lev M, Liberthson RR, Kirkpatrick JR, et al. Single (primitive) ventricle. *Circulation* 1969;39:577–591.
64. Gomes MM, Weidman WH, McGoon DC, et al. Double-outlet right ventricle without pulmonic stenosis. Surgical considerations and results of operation. *Circulation* 1971;43:I31–136.
65. Anderson KR, McGoon DC, Lie JT. Surgical significance of the coronary arterial anatomy in truncus arteriosus communis. *Am J Cardiol* 1978;41:76–81.
66. Levy MJ, Lillehei CW, Anderson RC. Aortico-left ventricular tunnel. *Circulation* 1963;27:841–853.
67. Serino W, Andrade JL, Ross D, et al. Aorto-left ventricular communication after closure. Late postoperative problems. *Br Heart J* 1983;49:501–506.
68. Fripp RR, Werner JC, Whitman V, et al. Pulsed Doppler and two-dimensional echocardiographic findings in aortico-left ventricular tunnel. *J Am Coll Cardiol* 1984;4:1012–1014.
69. Hope J. *A Treatise of Diseases of the Heart and Great Vessels.* London: John Churchill, 1839.
70. Edwards JE, Burchell HB. The pathological anatomy of deficiencies between the aortic root and the heart, including aortic sinus aneurysms. *Thorax* 1957;12:125–139.
71. Norwicki ER, Aberdeen E, Friedman S, et al. Congenital left aortic sinus-left ventricle fistula and review of aortocardiac fistulas. *Ann Thorac Surg* 1977;23:378–388.
72. Mayer JH 3rd, Holder TM, Canent RV. Isolated, unruptured sinus of Valsalva aneurysm: Serendipitous detection and correction. *J Thorac Cardiovasc Surg* 1975;69:429–432.
73. Hands ME, Lloyd BL, Hung J. Cross-sectional echocardiographic diagnosis of unruptured right sinus of Valsalva aneurysm dissecting into the interventricular septum. *Int J Cardiol* 1985;9:380–383.
74. Abdelkhirane C, Roudaut R, Dallocchio M. Diagnosis of ruptured sinus of Valsalva aneurysms: Potential value of transesophageal echocardiography. *Echocardiography* 1990;7:555–560.
75. Noji Y, Hifumi S, Nagayoshi T, et al. Sixteen-slice computed tomography, transthoracic real-time 3-dimensional echocardiography and magnetic resonance imaging assessment of a long-term survivor of rupture of sinus of valsalva aneurysm. *Intern Med* 2005;44:513–515.
76. Abidin N, Clarke B, Khattar RS. Percutaneous closure of ruptured sinus of Valsalva aneurysm using an Amplatzer occluder device. *Heart* 2005; 91:244.

CHAPTER 35 ■ VASCULAR ANOMALIES

RONALD G. GRIFKA, MD, AND TAMAR J. PREMINGER, MD

The earliest description of a vascular anomaly was the legend of Medusa, whose hair was turned into a tangle of snakes by Athena, probably representing an arteriovenous malformation of the scalp. The first clinical description of a vascular anomaly was in the 16th century by Guido (AKA Vidius), physician to King Francis I; the patient had markedly dilated scalp veins, extending from the forehead to the neck. In 1676, Sennertus reported an aneurysm that probably was an arteriovenous malformation, for it had "a thrill like boiling water, both palpable and audible, as if the vital spirits were passing through a narrow orifice" (1). In 1757, Hunter associated clinical findings to a traumatic arteriovenous fistula, with a thrill and bruit over the lesion and enlargement of the artery proximal to the fistula. He demonstrated that occluding the fistula diminished the venous distension and eliminated the thrill and bruit (2). In 1815, Bell published the first clinical description of a congenital arteriovenous malformation (3). Subsequently, there were multiple congenital vascular anomalies reported, including their effect on heart size, blood pressure, skin temperature, and limb growth (4,5). As a result of the varied characterizations, a confusing body of nomenclature evolved. As the vascular embryology, histopathology, and physiology were elucidated, a more concise and practical biologic classification of vascular malformations was developed.

EMBRYOLOGY AND PATHOGENESIS

The vascular system develops from the third to the tenth week of fetal life. The embryonic vascular endothelium arises in situ from primitive mesenchymal cells that aggregate to form isolated masses and cords, known as blood islands. These undiffer-entiated blood-containing spaces coalesce, disappear by absorption, and separate from one another to form discrete channels that ultimately evolve into the capillary bed. The pericytes and smooth muscle cells that surround the endothelium are derived from neuroectoderm (neural crest), not from mesoderm (6–8). Differentiation of the vascular bed results in separate venous and arterial conduits on either side of the capillaries. Arterial stems make their way into the evolving vascular system.

Folkman and Haudenschild's studies (9) provide further insight into this process. Capillarylike tubules can form in vitro from cloned capillary endothelial cells cultured from adult tissues, demonstrating that all the information necessary to construct a capillary network can be expressed in culture by a single cell type, the capillary endothelial cell. The complex morphogenetic processes that follow are poorly understood; blood flow, multiple local physicochemical events, and genetic control are important. The inability of known teratogens, toxins, chemicals, or trauma to produce a human vascular malformation is remarkable, suggesting that simple aberrations in local physicochemical factors are not responsible. Other predisposing factors that could affect vascular system development have been postulated, including a primary biochemical defect in thrombosis and fibrinolysis, and aberrations of the autonomic nervous system (10).

Congenital vascular malformations are structural abnormalities that result from arrests in normal morphogenetic processes. However, no histologic, embryologic, or experimental data define how, or at exactly which stage, maldevelopments occur. The diverse clinical findings suggest that the causative influence can be present at any time during development, and because embryologic processes are closely integrated, abnormalities in one area influence the growth and morphogenesis of another area (i.e., adjacent mesenchymal tissues and neuroectodermal derivatives) (11–13).

Although most vascular anomalies are sporadic, a few are inherited. Hereditary hemorrhagic telangiectasia (HHT), the Osler–Weber–Rendu syndrome, is an autosomal-dominant trait; vascular development is embryologically normal, but over time the vessels become morphologically abnormal. HHT is a structural weakness of the wall of small arteries and precapillary sphincters. Thus, patients with congenital vascular anomalies may not have symptoms at birth but may develop symptoms years or decades later.

CLASSIFICATION

A diverse nosology of vascular anomalies developed, following the historical sequence of descriptive, histomorphologic, embryologic, and biologic schemata. The biologic classification system, proposed in 1982, provides a logical, clinically useful approach. It defines the cellular features of childhood vascular anomalies, correlated with the clinical behavior and therapeutic requirements (14). Two major types of vascular anomalies were defined: Hemangiomas and malformations. Hemangiomas are benign "tumors" of infancy that demonstrate endothelial cell hyperplasia during the postnatal period (proliferative phase) and that undergo spontaneous regression over a 5- to 8-year period (involutive phase), without metastasis. Vascular malformations result from errors of vascular morphogenesis; they grow commensurately with the child and exhibit a normal rate of endothelial cell turnover. Vascular malformations are subdivided anatomically into groups based on the predominant anomalous vascular tissue: Capillary, lymphatic, venous, arterial, or a combination of vessel types. Clinically, they are subcategorized as either fast flow (arteriovenous fistulas [AVFs] or arteriovenous malformations [AVMs]) or slow flow (capillary, venous, lymphatic, or combined forms). Vascular anomalies can occur in the systemic or pulmonary circulation, resulting in different hemodynamic effects. In this chapter, vascular anomalies will be discussed according to the following biologic classification:

1. Systemic arterial venous malformations (systemic AVMs)
2. Pulmonary arterial venous malformations (pulmonary AVMs)
3. Hemangiomas

Often, these lesions are confused with congenital heart defects.

SYSTEMIC ARTERIAL MALFORMATIONS

Systemic AVMs and AVFs occur in various locations, may be congenital or acquired, and have diverse clinical manifestations. In pediatric patients, most lesions are congenital in origin. Factors associated with acquired lesions are trauma, vascular puncture, arterial dysplasia (e.g., neurofibromatosis), atherosclerosis, syphilis, and Wilms' tumor (15,16).

Prevalence

Most lesions affect both sexes equally, except cerebral AVMs, which affect males more frequently than females (17). Arterial malformations rarely result in hemodynamic symptoms.

Pathology

Arterial malformations have two vascular patterns (18): AVMs and AVFs. AVMs (microfistulas) are multiple arterial feeders joined via a nidus to draining veins. AVFs (macrofistulas) are direct shunts between large arterial and venous channels.

Histopathologically, arterial malformations are distinct from hemangiomas. Arterial malformations have no potential for cellular proliferation or involution. Their endothelium is nonproliferating (flat, single layered) and contains normal numbers of mast cells (which play a role in neoangiogenesis). The arterial vessels in systemic AVMs are hardly recognizable as arteries. They are dilated, tortuous, and frequently dysplastic with hyperplastic and disorganized medial smooth muscle fibers. The internal elastic lamina is typically fragmented or may be absent, which may result in aneurysm formation and eventual rupture. The veins within the systemic AVMs appear arterialized, which may be due to a primary dysmorphogenesis or to increased intraluminal pressure. These anomalous veinlike channels show reactive muscular hyperplasia and later degenerative changes including fibrosis, smooth muscle atrophy, and multiple thrombi, which may be calcified (18).

Most AVMs are single or involve a single extremity. Some AVMs are multiple and may involve more than one organ system. Systemic AVMs with profound hemodynamic effects occur in the brain, liver, thorax, and extremities. Less common locations include the neck, placenta, and kidneys. In HHT, the primary lesion is a vascular malformation that may be diffusely disseminated, involving the skin, oral and nasal mucosa, lungs, central nervous system (CNS), gastrointestinal tract, kidney, or liver (19).

Central nervous system AVMs manifest symptoms according to their hemodynamic effects. Infants presenting with congestive heart failure (CHF) typically have large AVFs. The most common cerebral AVMs presenting with CHF are located deep (vein of Galen), superficial (pial), or dural (20–25). Because of the high flow state, there is marked dilation of the feeding arteries and draining veins (Fig. 35.1). If there is venous outflow obstruction, the proximal draining veins dilate massively, as in vein of Galen aneurysms. Venous obstruction restricts flow through the AVM, so patients may present with symptoms related to mass effect (venous hypertension) or cerebral ischemia (vascular steal). They may present later in infancy or early childhood with hydrocephalus, seizures, or focal or generalized neurologic signs and symptoms. Smaller AVMs within the brain parenchyma frequently present in childhood with signs of cerebral or subarachnoid hemorrhage, occurring from the AVM itself or from a coexisting arterial aneurysm (10%) (20).

Thoracic AVMs often involve the internal mammary artery, with anomalous channels communicating with the mammary veins and the ductus venosus (Fig. 35.2) (26). Other lesions have been reported, located between the subclavian artery and innominate vein, intercostal arteries and azygos vein, axillary artery and axillary vein, carotid artery and jugular vein, right subclavian artery and right iliac vein (via the paravertebral plexus), and descending aorta to the azygos vein and superior vena cava (29–32). When these lesions are large, they can present in infancy with cardiac failure, but more commonly are diagnosed during childhood when they produce signs of a hyperkinetic circulatory state.

Most hepatic AVFs are associated with hemangioendotheliomas. Rarely, high-flow hepatic AVMs may result in CHF. Hepatic AVMs draining into the portal vein may present with gastrointestinal bleeding and other signs of portal hypertension (27,28).

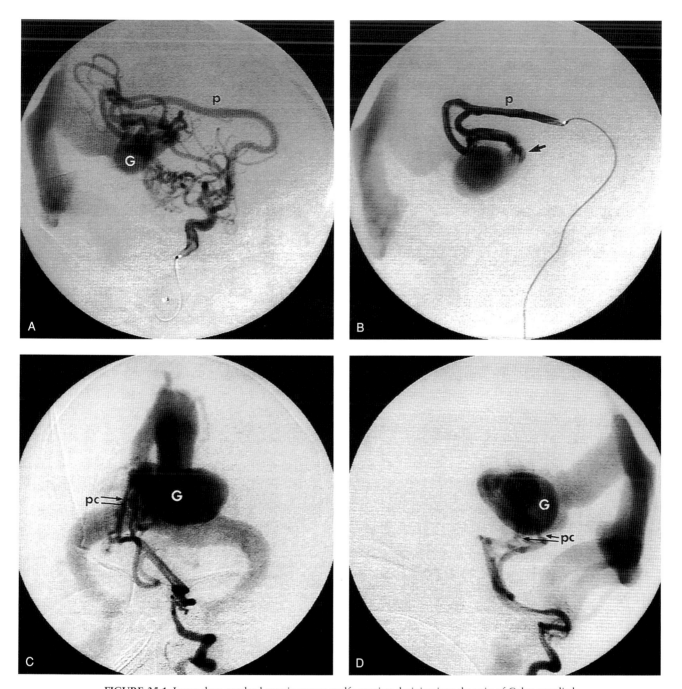

FIGURE 35.1 Large deep cerebral arteriovenous malformation draining into the vein of Galen supplied by the choroidal arteries and the pericallosal artery. Selective arteriography of the pericallosal artery demonstrates a direct arteriovenous fistula (*arrow*). **A:** Lateral projection of the right internal carotid artery. **B:** Lateral projection of a supraselective injection in the pericallosal artery prior to embolization. **C and D:** Frontal and lateral projections of the left vertebral angiogram. G, vein of Galen; p, pericallosal artery; pc, posterior choroidal artery.

In children, arterial malformations in the lower extremities and pelvis are more often congenital than traumatic, are usually diffuse, and may present with CHF during infancy. With high-flow AVMs, the affected limb has marked enlargement and is usually longer (rarely shorter) than the unaffected limb. Generalized extremity overgrowth including bone, muscle, and fat may be present. Low-flow vascular malformations of the overlying skin are frequently seen; they must be distinguished from vascular malformations that are predominantly venous and lymphatic in nature, as in Klippel–Trenaunay syndrome (12,33). Angiography demonstrates diffuse arteriovenous shunting, with focal areas of macroscopic AVFs. Transcatheter embolization of discrete fistulas may result in dramatic improvement; however, new fistulas may develop over time. Patients with diffuse extremity AVMs may present with extremity gigantism and trophic skin changes related to venous ischemia. They may have mild to moderate cardiac volume overload during childhood, becoming more severe in adult life.

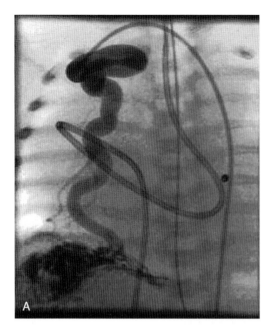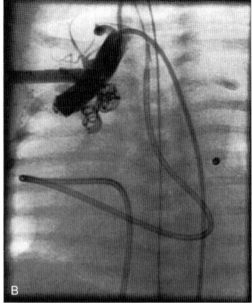

FIGURE 35.2 A 1-day-old child with cyanosis and congestive heart failure. Evaluation showed a large arteriovenous malformation arising from the right internal mammary artery, coursing through the diaphragm into the liver. Embolization coils were implanted, affording an excellent result. One week later, a small arterial feeder arising from the descending aorta was coil occluded.

Arterial malformations involving the face and neck are supplied predominantly by branches of the external carotid, subclavian, or vertebral arteries. Although most lesions present with bleeding (e.g., dental and nasal lesions) or facial deformity, large AVFs may lead to CHF in infancy (34,35). Lesions arising from vessels proximal to the aortic isthmus may be associated with preductal aortic coarctation, as in utero they divert blood flow from the aortic isthmus (36).

Rarely, placental arterial malformation or chorioangioma may result in fetal CHF (hydrops) owing to blood shunted from the caudal aorta through the malformation to the umbilical vein. Cardiac failure improves during the neonatal period (37). Intrarenal AVMs and AVFs are extremely rare, are usually acquired lesions, and may be associated with Wilms' tumor. Hematuria and systemic hypertension may be associated signs (16).

Physiology

In all systemic AVMs and AVFs, the primary physiologic disturbance is the left-to-right shunting from the artery to the vein, leading to a volume-overloaded circulation. Additionally, local tissue injury can occur from physiologic abnormalities owing to vascular insufficiency (steal phenomenon), compression or dilation of adjacent structures, and alterations in vascular autoregulation.

An AVM or AVF decreases the systemic vascular resistance. The heart rate and stroke volume increase, and plasma volume increases, resulting in an increased cardiac output and a widened pulse pressure. The increased venous return to the heart results in volume overload. The combination of increased venous pressure with increased cardiac output defines high-output heart failure (15). When the heart is no longer able to handle the volume overload, low-output cardiac failure develops.

The increased cardiac work results in increased myocardial oxygen consumption. There is some increased coronary blood flow owing to decreased resistance in the coronary circulation (15). However, myocardial dysfunction can occur because of the relative myocardial ischemia from the low diastolic blood pressure, shortened diastolic filling time (secondary to tachycardia), or vascular steal (38).

Clinical Manifestations

The signs and symptoms produced by systemic AVMs and AVFs are determined by their location, size, and the patient's age. Congenital lesions may present as intrauterine congestive heart failure (fetal hydrops), neonatal congestive heart failure, or beyond infancy as a hyperkinetic circulatory state with or without localized findings.

The neonate with a systemic AVM or AVF demonstrates unique cardiovascular hemodynamics owing to patency of the foramen ovale (PFO) and ductus arteriosus (PDA), elevated pulmonary vascular resistance, and the relative hypertrophy and diminished compliance of the right ventricle. The elevated pulmonary artery pressure and resistance, as well as the decreased systemic vascular resistance (produced by the lesion), promote right-to-left PDA shunting. The decreased pulmonary blood flow and left atrial volume contribute to right-to-left shunting across the PFO. The increased venous return to the right atrium elevates right atrial pressure, further augmenting right-to-left PFO shunting.

When the shunt is large, neonates present within the first days of life with profound CHF, often with cyanosis. The most common vascular lesions are located in the CNS, liver, or thorax (39–43). The delay in the postnatal onset of symptoms may be a reflection of the conversion from the *in utero* circulation where the malformation is in parallel with the low resistance placenta, limiting flow through the malformation to the extrauterine circulation where the increased systemic vascular resistance increases flow through the malformation. Cyanosis occurs in at least 70% of cases, reflecting decreased peripheral perfusion or right-to-left shunting through the PDA and PFO (43).

Arteries proximal to the anomaly may be enlarged and highly pulsatile, and demonstrate a thrill; arteries distal to the lesion have normal to diminished pulsations. Thus, in cerebral lesions, the carotid pulsations may be prominent and the femoral pulsations may be absent; this has led to diagnostic confusion with coarctation of the aorta. The heart is hyperdynamic and enlarged to palpation. Auscultation may demonstrate a prominent second heart sound, and a third or a fourth heart sound. Systolic murmurs may be present, secondary to tricuspid regurgitation or increased flow through the semilunar valves. Middiastolic murmurs of increased tricuspid or mitral flow may occur (36). Systolic or continuous murmurs may be heard in the area overlying the malformation because of non-laminar blood flow through the lesion (15). Cranial bruits have been reported in only 30% of vein of Galen malformations; bruits are heard less often with hepatic lesions. The liver and spleen are usually enlarged. Careful inspection of the scalp, skin, and eyes should be performed to assess for increased venous circulation and other vascular anomalies (24,41).

If a small volume of blood is shunted through the anomaly, clinical features develop later in childhood. The patient may be referred for evaluation of a murmur. He or she may present with a hyperkinetic circulatory state. Often, a pulsatile mass, thrill, and continuous or systolic murmur is detected over the malformation. Nicoladoni-Branham's sign may be present; with digital compression of the afferent vessel, the murmur diminishes or disappears, the heart rate slows, the arterial pressure increases, and the venous pressure decreases (44,45). Other localized signs and symptoms are due to spontaneous hemorrhage or to alterations in local physiologic function and vary according to the malformation location.

Electrocardiographic Features

The electrocardiographic (ECG) pattern is nonspecific. In neonates, the ECG may show right axis deviation, right atrial enlargement, and right or biventricular hypertrophy, depending on the *in utero* fetal blood flow. In neonates, isolated left ventricular hypertrophy is uncommon. In neonates with cerebral AVMs, variable ST-segment and T-wave changes occur, reflecting myocardial ischemia, occurring in ≤92% of such patients, with subendocardial myocyte necrosis involving mainly the right ventricle detected at autopsy (38). In older infants and children, the ECG may be normal or may display right ventricular conduction delay or left/biventricular hypertrophy.

Radiographic Features

In the neonate, chest roentgenograms may demonstrate generalized cardiomegaly, increased pulmonary arterial markings, and pulmonary edema. Neonates with large intracerebral malformations may show superior mediastinal widening (dilated ascending aorta, retrosternal fullness), and posterior displacement of the trachea (46). Dilation of the descending aorta has been described in infants with hepatic lesions (47). In older infants and children, the chest roentgenogram may be normal

or exhibit mild cardiomegaly, as well as prominence of the aortic or pulmonary arteries.

Echocardiography and Doppler

Neonates who are symptomatic due to an AVM are usually critically ill, making rapid diagnosis essential. Echocardiography is important to rule out congenital heart defects, evaluate intracardiac anatomy, abnormal blood flow patterns, cardiac chamber size, ventricular function, and possibly visualize the lesion. Increased blood flow to and from the low-resistance malformation leads to generalized enlargement of all cardiac chambers. Enlargement of the superior vena cava (diameter greater than the aortic arch) and innominate veins suggests a shunt in the upper part of the body; enlargement of the inferior vena cava and hepatic vessels suggests a hepatic or lower body lesion. The vena cava that drains the malformation has a turbulent, continuous Doppler venous flow pattern rather than the normal primarily diastolic flow pattern (48). Intracranial or thoracic lesions have dilation and tortuosity of the ascending aorta and brachiocephalic vessels. Doppler examination of the ascending aorta and carotid arteries shows low-velocity diastolic antegrade flow, whereas vessels distal to the lesion exhibit diastolic retrograde flow (dia-stolic runoff) (48,49). In the neonate, contrast echo and Doppler evaluation may reveal right-to-left shunting across the PFO and PDA.

The deep cerebral AVM appears as a large, fluid-filled structure, representing the dilated vein of Galen (50,51). Occasionally, the lesion's afferent and efferent vessels are displayed. Doppler or contrast echocardiography will distinguish the malformation from other nonvascular causes of an echolucent structure in the brain (cyst, enlarged ventricle, etc.). If there is persistent fetal circulation, contrast echocardiography performed from a peripheral venous injection demonstrates microcavitations passing from the right atrium across the PFO to the left atrium, to the ascending aorta, carotid arteries, and the AVM, bypassing filtration by the systemic capillary bed, appearing rapidly in the superior vena cava.

Cardiac Catheterization and Angiography

Diagnostic cardiac catheterization is usually unnecessary, as the diagnosis is suspected by clinical examination and confirmed by noninvasive imaging. When performed, catheterization demonstrates high cardiac output, elevated atrial and ventricular end-diastolic pressures, a widened systemic arterial pulse pressure, and a large difference in the oxygen saturation between the superior and inferior vena cava (higher saturation from the involved area). A small arteriovenous oxygen difference (i.e., high cardiac output) in the presence of congestive heart failure is paradoxical, suggesting a systemic arterial malformation. In neonates, the pulmonary artery pressure is increased (occasionally above systemic levels), whereas in children, it is usually normal (39,42).

Selective angiography provides definitive anatomic visualization of the lesion, its arterial blood supply, and venous drainage. Enlarged afferent and efferent vessels are displayed, with a rapid circulation time through the malformation (see Fig. 35.1). Digital subtraction angiography may be used. Occasionally in older children, cerebral AVMs may be angiographically occult owing to small lesion size, thrombosis of feeding vessels, compression by adjacent clot, or destruction from a hemorrhagic event.

Additional Noninvasive Imaging Techniques

Computerized tomography (CT) or magnetic resonance imaging (MRI) further characterizes the malformation, delineating both the extent and location of the lesion. The classification of vascular anomalies can be correlated with MRI. For hemangiomas, MRI detects both high-flow and solid tissue abnormalities on T2-weighted spin-echo images. For a systemic AVM, MRI detects the high flow but no solid tissue abnormality (52). For cerebral AVMs, coexistent abnormalities (hydrocephalus, parenchymal loss, calcifications, mass effect) may be identified (53). If transcatheter vessel embolization is performed, CT and MRI may be limited when reassessing the lesion. Stainless steel coils are ferromagnetic and should not be exposed to a magnetic field for several months after implant (if at all) because of the risk of migration and resultant hemorrhage, and they cause signal flow void. Newer embolization agents, such as platinum and other nonferromagnetic microcoils, are safer and produce minimal artifact on MRI. On CT, these coils produce artifact owing to their high density.

Differential Diagnosis

In the newborn period, congenital AVMs and AVFs may clinically resemble congenital heart defects (CHDs), leading to a delay in diagnosis. Diminished femoral pulses may mimic aortic coarctation. On occasion, CHDs may coexist, including hypoplastic left heart syndrome, total anomalous pulmonary venous return, myocardial ischemia, and cardiomyopathy. Noncardiac diseases (persistent fetal circulation, hypoglycemia, sepsis) may complicate the diagnosis. Intrathoracic AVMs may be confused with a PDA, coronary AVF, ruptured sinus of Valsalva aneurysm, or aortopulmonary window. Location of the murmur may help to localize the lesion. AVMs presenting later in childhood usually produce less diagnostic confusion with congenital heart defects because of other associated signs (abdominal mass, neurologic signs, cutaneous lesions).

Natural History and Management

The prognosis for most patients with large cerebral arterial malformations is grave. If untreated, most newborns (90%) die during the first week of life from intractable CHF or neurologic complications (seizures, intracranial hemorrhage). The minority of patients who survive the neonatal period often suffer profound neurologic morbidity, including hydrocephalus, intracranial hemorrhage, and mental retardation (24). In older patients with an intracranial malformation, 50% to 70% experience a hemorrhage. The peak age range for hemorrhage is 15 to 20 years. The hemorrhage is usually subarachnoid, but it may be intracerebral (54,55). If untreated, high-flow hepatic vascular lesions in neonates are associated with a high mortality rate (85%) (41,56).

For infants in severe CHF, the only treatment is to reduce the amount of shunting. Rapid diagnosis is crucial, followed by urgent therapeutic intervention. It is important to distinguish between hemangiomas and malformations. Ultrasonography can be used to establish the diagnosis. Further evaluation is necessary with MRI or CT to identify associated abnormalities (cerebral dysgenesis, extensive calcifications) that may be contraindications to intervention. Small calcifications may reflect ischemia, indicating the need for rapid intervention to minimize additional neurologic morbidity. Prior to surgical or transcatheter intervention to reduce or eliminate shunting, medical management of CHF is mandatory. It is difficult to compare the results among published series because of relatively small case numbers, different lesions and duration of follow-up, evolving technical advancements, and procedural expertise.

Surgical excision of systemic AVMs is not possible unless the lesion is both accessible and well circumscribed. Ligation or clipping of afferent arteries usually offers only short-term palliation, owing to recurrence of the malformation as other afferent arterial vessels enlarge. Morbidity and mortality may occur because of the elimination of blood flow to normal parenchyma. In a large series of cerebral AVMs, 45 of 128 patients presented during the neonatal period; 8 of 45 underwent surgery, resulting in 4 deaths and only 1 normal survivor (24).

Transcatheter embolization has emerged as the standard therapy for systemic arterial malformations. It offers the advantage of selectively occluding the involved vessels and reaching the nidus of the lesion, thus minimizing occlusion of vessels that perfuse normal tissue. AVFs that have a single connection between an artery and vein can be cured by placement of an occlusion device in the fistula. AVMs usually are not curable because of the complexity of their arterial supply and their tendency to develop new arterial supply after treatment. Embolization should be performed when symptoms occur, with the goal to occlude the nidus; if this is not possible, embolization of all of the feeding arteries may be palliative. Various embolic and occlusive agents have been developed, including mechanical devices, particles, and liquid or semisolid tissue adhesives. The choice of material depends on the location, type, and size of the malformation; vulnerability of surrounding tissues; and experience of the interventionalist. The ideal embolization agent is the most permanent material that can be delivered selectively and deeply into the lesion (57–66).

For neonates with a vein of Galen malformation, studies of initial transcatheter embolization procedures reported mortality rates up to 50%, while the survivors had a 41% incidence of seizures, a 37% risk of severe mental retardation, and an 82% prevalence of seizure disorders (67). These results were comparable with surgical treatment. Occasionally, the effluent veins are coil occluded to control the shunt and CHF symptoms; this has a high rate of perforation and hemorrhagic infarction, and they may recanalize, requiring repeated procedures (68). Because of more rapid noninvasive diagnosis and advancements in transcatheter embolization techniques and equipment, there is increased survival and reduced neurologic sequelae. In ten neonates who underwent embolization procedures, no mortality occurred, six patients were functionally normal up to 30 months follow-up) two patients had mild resolving neurologic deficits, and two patients had severe neurologic deficits and seizures; three had clinical neurologic abnormalities noted prior to embolization (69).

PULMONARY ARTERIAL MALFORMATIONS

Most pulmonary arterial malformations are congenital or associated with HHT (Fig. 35.3) (70). Acquired lesions have been associated with juvenile hepatic cirrhosis, portal vein thrombosis, trauma, schistosomiasis, and metastatic thyroid carcinoma (15). An "acquired" pulmonary artery malformation is becoming more common in patients who have been palliated with a cavopulmonary anastomoses (Glenn shunt, hemi-Fontan) (71,72). The cause of this pulmonary malformation appears to

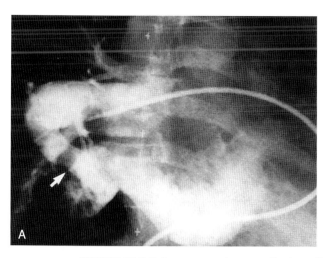 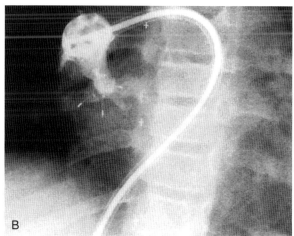

FIGURE 35.3 Pulmonary arteriovenous fistula, a direct communication between the right pulmonary artery (RPA) and the left atrium. **A:** Selective RPA angiogram illustrating the fistulous connection (*arrow*) with immediate opacification of the left atrium. **B:** Follow-up RPA angiogram after occlusion with a clamshell septal occluder (USCI Inc., Billerica, MA; NMT Inc., Boston, MA) demonstrates no residual flow via the fistula.

be exclusion of hepatic venous flow directly to the pulmonary circulation, analogous to AVMs associated with cirrhotic liver disease or the absence of pulsatile flow in the pulmonary arteries (Fig. 35.4) (73).

Pathology

Most lesions are AVMs. The vessel histopathology is similar to that of systemic malformations, with structural heterogeneity in the arterial and venous components. Degenerative changes and aneurysm formation may be associated with vessel wall rupture. Patients may have hemoptysis, hemothorax, and pulmonary hemosiderosis (18). Morphologically, pulmonary AVMs are divided into two types: (i) localized lesions commonly occurring in patients with HHT or isolated pulmonary AVMs, and (ii) diffuse lesions occurring in patients with CHD, liver disease, portal vein thrombosis, and Glenn shunts (Fig. 35.5). Pulmonary AVMs range from small pinpoint lesions (1 mm) to huge tubular or saccular multilobulated structures occupying most of a lobe

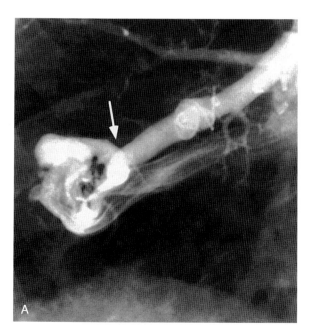 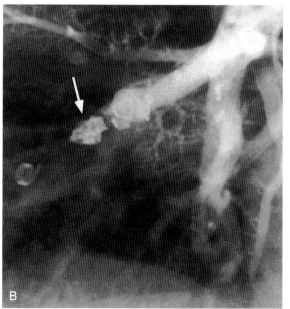

FIGURE 35.4 Large pulmonary arteriovenous fistula (AVF). **A:** A patient with multiple intrapulmonary AVFs. Several small AVFs were occluded with standard embolization coils. This large AVF measured 6.2 mm with prompt flow through the fistula into the pulmonary vein and left atrium. **B:** The AVF was occluded completely using a single 7-mm Gianturco-Grifka Vascular Occlusion Device (Cook Inc., Bloomington, IN) (*arrow*). (Angiograms provided by Martin O'Laughlin, M.D.)

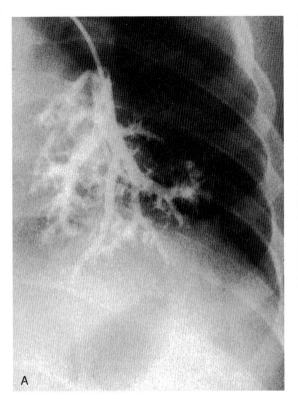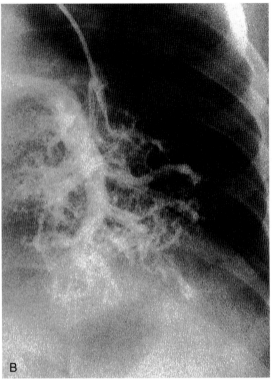

FIGURE 35.5 Selective left pulmonary arteriogram (**A**, arterial phase; **B**, venous phase) in a patient with a cavopulmonary anastomosis (bidirectional Glenn's) showing many large vessels extending distally into the left lower lobe with a generalized pattern of vasodilation, absence of the capillary phase, and early filling of the pulmonary veins.

or an entire lung. Lesions may be single or multiple, unilateral or bilateral. Small lesions tend to be multiple, diffuse, and located deep within the parenchyma. Larger malformations are usually isolated, involving the subpleural regions of the lower lobes (65%) (18,74). The airways and lung parenchyma surrounding the malformation are normal.

As with systemic AVMs, pulmonary AVMs enlarge as the child grows older. Approximately 30% to 50% of patients with pulmonary AVMs have HHT; the correlation is greater in patients with multiple lesions (88%) (75). Pulmonary AVMs are indistinguishable in patients with or without HHT. In patients with HHT, pulmonary AVMs are a significant cause of morbidity and possibly are the leading cause of death. HHT affects arteries of the brain, nose, and gastrointestinal tract, causing serious morbidity and mortality (10%) (75,76).

Physiology

The AVM or AVF creates a right-to-left shunt from the pulmonary arteries to the pulmonary veins, resulting in systemic arterial desaturation and secondary polycythemia (Fig. 35.6). If the channels through the malformation are small, they have high resistance, so there is no significant shunting.

Patients with pulmonary AVMs are hemodynamically stable. In contrast to systemic AVMs, cardiac output is not increased, plasma volume remains normal (polycythemia results in a small increase in the total blood volume), and the pulmonary blood flow and pressure are unchanged. The total pulmonary vascular resistance is normal; resistance within the AVM is low, whereas the resistance in the other lung segments

may be elevated twofold, although there is no histologic abnormality in these higher-resistance vessels (77,78). Because the normal pulmonary vasculature and the pulmonary AVM are in parallel, blood preferentially flows through the low-resistance AVM. However, since the normal pulmonary artery resistance is low, the AVM shunt does not significantly reduce the overall pulmonary vascular resistance. Because emboli and bacteria can pass directly through the AVM into the systemic circulation, stroke and brain abscess are well-known complications (79,80).

A high percentage of patients with pulmonary AVMs demonstrate orthodeoxia, the tendency for greater hypoxemia when assuming the sitting or standing position, attributable to the basal location of most pulmonary AVMs. This hypoxemia is most likely associated with gravitational shifts of pulmonary blood flow to the base of the lung when assuming erect posture (81).

The tendency for increased shunting and cyanosis with age is not well understood. Many factors have been implicated including an increasing number of intravascular communications, opening of previously unfilled channels, dilation of existing communications, or progressive polycythemia. Similarly, the mechanism by which pulmonary AVMs develop in children with hepatic cirrhosis remains enigmatic; there are reports of reversibility of the intrapulmonary shunts within several months following orthotopic liver transplant (82).

Clinical Manifestations

The clinical findings correlate with the amount of right-to-left shunting. The classic triad of cyanosis, clubbing, and polycythemia usually appears during early adult life. Cyanosis may

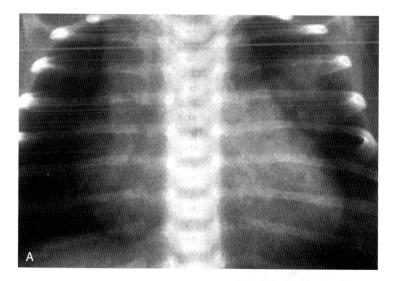

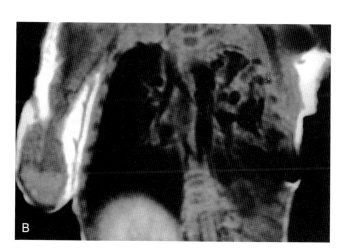

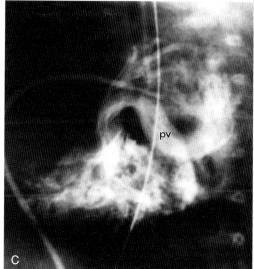

FIGURE 35.6 Pulmonary arteriovenous malformation (AVM) in a newborn. **A:** Chest roentgenogram in posteroanterior view with an opacity apparent in the left upper lobe. **B:** Coronal T1-weighted MRI demonstrates large flow voids within the pulmonary AVM. **C:** Corresponding selective left pulmonary angiogram in lateral projection. Venous phase demonstrates densely staining mass of abnormal vessels with rapid drainage to the left pulmonary veins (pv).

be evident from infancy, often occurring with CHF during the neonatal period (83,84). In older patients with HHT, these signs tend to be less obvious because of anemia, resulting from repeated blood loss (85). A few patients remain completely asymptomatic; in these cases, an abnormal chest roentgenogram or mild systemic desaturation noted by pulse oximetry may be the only findings.

Pulmonary symptoms include dyspnea on exertion (71%), hemoptysis (13%), and hemothorax (9%) (75). Hemoptysis is caused by lesions of the bronchial mucosa or by the rupture of a thin-walled AVM into the bronchus. Occasionally, chest pain occurs when a subpleural AVM ruptures, causing a hemothorax. Endarteritis may complicate the malformation.

In some patients, neurologic symptoms (headaches, seizures, speech disorders, ocular disturbances, transitory numbness, etc.) dominate the clinical picture; headaches are common (43%), typically migrainous in nature (80,81). Patients with

pulmonary AVMs are at risk for paradoxical embolization leading to transient ischemic attacks (37%) and stroke (18%). Their estimated annual risk of stroke is 1.5% per year (75). They are also at risk for cerebral abscess, often related to dental procedures, including cleaning (76). The cause of these complications may be multifactorial: Venous blood bypassing the pulmonary filter, hypoxemia, polycythemia, small vessel thrombosis, and recurrent cerebral AVM hemorrhage.

Symptoms related to HHT (nosebleeds, hemoptysis, hematuria, and vaginal or gastrointestinal hemorrhage) have been documented in 35% to 50% of patients (15,75,76). Often, the pattern of organ involvement is consistent among an affected family (85). In infants and young children with HHT, other organ systems may not have lesions.

On examination, the arterial pulse and precordial activity are normal, as are the heart sounds. In approximately 50% of patients, a faint systolic or continuous murmur is noted over the lesion; a murmur is not appreciated with small lesions, or with lesions deep within the lung parenchyma (15). These pulmonic bruits are accentuated by or may be detected during deep inspiration, which increases blood flow through the lesion.

Electrocardiographic Features

In most patients, the ECG is normal. In patients with huge fistulas or a direct communication between the right pulmonary artery and the left atrium, there may be left axis deviation, left atrial enlargement, and left ventricular hypertrophy (70,77). Occasionally, right axis deviation and right ventricular hypertrophy occur.

Radiographic Features

Usually, the cardiac size and configuration are normal. Cardiomegaly is seen only with very large lesions. In approximately 50% of cases, one or more round or lobulated opacities are apparent on frontal and lateral chest roentgenograms. They may be unilateral or bilateral and are usually peripheral, homogeneous, noncalcified, and well circumscribed. The dilated afferent and efferent vessels may resemble cordlike stalks connecting to the hilum and left atrium (15,77). In cases of direct communication between the right pulmonary artery and the left atrium, the communication appears as an opacity adjacent to the right posterior border of the cardiac silhouette (see Fig. 35.3) (70). A pleural effusion may be present. In cases with diffuse lesions, the chest roentgenogram may be unremarkable.

Echocardiography

To diagnose a pulmonary AVM with echocardiography, a high index of suspicion is required. In high-flow lesions, the pulmonary artery branches may be dilated and tortuous, with increased Doppler flow velocity in the pulmonary veins. Echocardiography can confirm the diagnosis. Following a peripheral venous injection of contrast agent, microcavitations opacify the right atrium and right ventricle, then several heart beats later, microcavitations appear in the left atrium and left ventricle. The contrast material bypasses filtration in the pulmonary capillary bed. The late appearance of contrast microcavitations in the left atrium differentiates a pulmonary AVM from an atrial right-to-left shunt (86).

Cardiac Catheterization

Oximetry samples should be obtained from every pulmonary vein. Affected lung segments show pulmonary venous desaturation that is unresponsive to supplemental oxygen administration (similar to intracardiac right-to-left shunts). It is important to identify all intrapulmonary shunts to determine the extent and location of involved lung segments; the shunt volume varies from 18% to 89% of the right ventricular output (78). Despite this amount of shunting, cardiac pressures and output are usually normal. The total pulmonary vascular resistance remains normal, even with polycythemia (77,78).

Angiography clearly defines the anatomic details of the AVM. Selective angiography into the affected pulmonary artery displays the lesion anatomy showing dilated and tortuous afferent and efferent vessels, early left atrium opacification, and scarce opacification of the uninvolved lung. Also, it may show smaller lesions that were not noted on chest

roentgenography. The angiographic appearance of small, diffuse lesions occurring in patients with congenital heart defects is different. During pulmonary angiography, there is a pattern of generalized vasodilation with rapid filling of the pulmonary veins (Fig. 35.6). Also, an AVM can be confirmed by echocardiography during catheterization by injecting echo contrast agent into the separate pulmonary artery branches and evaluating the pulmonary venous return for microcavitations.

Additional Noninvasive Imaging Techniques

Imaging studies have been performed including radionuclides, CT, and MRI (87,88). CT and MRI studies are superior owing to the tomographic views of the lung that identify the segmental location of lesions, delineate the lesion's relationship to adjacent structures, and are useful for monitoring both the effects of therapy and emergence of new lesions. Few studies have compared the diagnostic sensitivity, specificity, and accuracy of these imaging modalities. Following coil embolization procedures, CT and MRI imaging may be limited because of artifact from the coil. Recently, nonferromagnetic embolization coils have been introduced and may avoid these problems. Technetium-labeled albumin microspheres can detect and quantify shunting before and after transcatheter embolization procedures; the percentage of right-to-left shunt through the lungs is calculated from the fraction of the injected dose of microspheres reaching the kidneys (89). Rarely, lung biopsy is needed to confirm the diagnosis.

Differential Diagnosis

The clinical manifestations of pulmonary AVMs may resemble several cyanotic congenital heart defects, including various anomalous connections of the venae cavae with the left atrium (see Chapters 27–38).

Natural History and Management

Most patients with pulmonary AVMs are asymptomatic during infancy and childhood. Although rare, symptomatic infants are extremely difficult to treat. Their age, size, and the severe lung involvement, which allows diagnosis at such an early age, are poor prognostic indicators. Beyond infancy, the frequency of fatal complications (lesion rupture, massive hemorrhage, endocarditis, cerebral abscess, etc.) is high. Therefore, elective treatment is recommended. In one series, 27% of patients died in childhood or early adult life related to the pulmonary AVM, 12% were alive but symptomatic, 37% were alive and asymptomatic, and 24% died from unrelated causes (90).

Transcatheter embolization has become the treatment of choice. In 1977, Portsmann (91) used homemade metal coils, followed soon after by stainless steel coils and detachable balloons (91,92). Through refinements in interventional equipment and techniques, results have progressively improved. To avoid device embolization (through the AVM to the systemic circulation), transcatheter occlusion of the afferent artery or fistula is usually accomplished using a coil, umbrella, or sack device rather than liquid adhesive or beads (Figs. 35.3 and 35.4). The goal is to occlude all afferent arteries >3 mm in diameter and to raise the systemic arterial oxygen tension to 60 mm Hg. Excellent results have been achieved: In 76 adult patients, 276 pulmonary AVMs were occluded, providing persistent relief of hypoxemia, resolution of orthodeoxia, and minimal growth of small remaining AVMs. Some patients required multiple catheterizations. The embolization procedure was effective for preventing stroke and transient ischemic attacks but did not reduce the risk of brain abscess (66).

The surgical treatment for pulmonary AVMs is lobectomy or pneumonectomy. The first successful pneumonectomy was performed in 1940, and the first segmental resection was performed by Blalock in 1947 (90,93). Current surgical treatment is segmental resection or lobectomy, removing the smallest amount of lung to completely excise the AVM. The operative mortality rate is approximately 5%, with the cure rate up to 75% (93). In the infant or child, surgical lobectomy may result in chest wall deformities, causing alterations in pulmonary mechanics. There is the long-term risk of developing additional AVMs in the contralateral lung.

HEMANGIOMAS

Prevalence

Hemangiomas are lesions of infancy; approximately 40% are apparent at birth. They exhibit a growth phase of 6 to 12 months, invariably followed by slow involution over several years. Although hemangiomas are common, they rarely cause enough shunt to result in cardiac compromise. Hemangiomas have a female:male ratio of 3:1 (94).

Pathology

In marked contrast to arterial malformations, hemangiomas grow by cellular proliferation, establishing a large cellular mass, which necessitates the recruitment of new feeding and draining vascular channels (proliferative phase). Occasionally, these vascular tumors may mimic a fast-flow type of AVM.

Hemangiomas are composed of masses of endothelial cells, with or without vascular lumens. There is a histologic spectrum with respect to the size and density of the channels, the degree of endothelial cell proliferation versus involution, and the organ involved. During the proliferative phase, hemangiomas are composed of plump, rapidly dividing endothelial cells that demonstrate ^{3}H thymidine uptake and contain an increased number of mast cells that play a role in neoangiogenesis. A multilaminated basement membrane is the pathologic hallmark of the disorder (14). Involuting hemangiomas are less cellular, contain areas of progressive fibrofatty infiltration, incorporate little or no ^{3}H thymidine, and have normal numbers of mast cells. The basement membrane remains multilaminated. As the hemangioma matures, it becomes organized into lobular compartments separated by fibrous septa that contain large feeding and draining vessels. The end-stage involuted hemangioma is composed of thick or thin-walled vessels that resemble normal capillaries.

In tissue culture studies, capillary endothelium derived from infant hemangiomas forms capillary tubules and exhibits rapid outgrowth. Capillary endothelium from AVMs does not form tubules and is difficult to culture (95).

Fibroblast growth factor (b-FGF) may help to differentiate hemangiomas from arterial malformations. Urine b-FGF level may be useful to monitor treatment response. Markedly elevated b-FGF levels, reflective of cell proliferation, have been found in patients with hemangiomas; b-FGF levels were normal in patients with arterial malformations (96). Similarly, elevated serum levels of vascular endothelial growth factor were significantly higher in patients with proliferating heman-

giomas compared with that in patients with involuting hemangiomas and vascular malformations, and that in controls (97).

Hemangiomas are the most common hepatic vascular lesions. Commonly, they occur as hemangioendotheliomas, infantile cellular hemangiomas (98–100). Hemangioendotheliomas may be single or multiple nodules of tissue, lined by several layers of endothelium, and may be distributed throughout the liver (multinodular) in varying stages of proliferation and involution (Fig. 35.7). Lesions that manifest with CHF contain fistulous components and present almost exclusively within the first 6 months of life. They are perfused by enlarged branches of the hepatic arteries and portal veins, and drain into dilated hepatic veins. Hepatic hemangioendotheliomas display nodular hepatomegaly out of proportion to the degree of CHF, without signs of hepatic dysfunction. Cutaneous hemangiomas are present in 30% of cases (99).

Pulmonary hemangiomatosis is a rare, heterogenous disorder, characterized by diffuse microvascular proliferation. Involvement of the pleura, interlobular septa, bronchioles, parenchyma, and extrapulmonary structures (mediastinum, pericardium, thymus, and spleen) has been described. Infiltration and compression of pulmonary veins can result in secondary pulmonary veno-occlusive disease (101). The histologic findings in this disorder are not well characterized, and in fact may represent an AVM.

The physiology, clinical manifestations, and diagnostic evaluation of hemodynamically significant hemangiomatous lesions are analogous to those for AVMs, depending on their location in the systemic or pulmonary circulation. A rare complication of proliferating hemangiomas is Kasabach–Merritt's syndrome, a consumptive coagulopathy involving platelets and occasionally fibrinogen (102).

Cardiac Catheterization and Angiography

Hemangiomas and AVMs can be differentiated by their angiographic features. Burrows et. al. (103) angiographically characterized hemangiomas by the presence of a well-circumscribed mass that has intense, persistent tissue staining (tumor blush) and usually is organized in a lobular pattern (Fig. 35.7). AVMs are diffuse lesions, consisting entirely of numerous tortuous, enlarged, and irregular vessels without intervening tissue stain. Occasionally, hemangiomas have high blood flow and demonstrate direct arteriovenous shunting, making it difficult to distinguish angiographically between the two groups.

Hepatic lesions are unique. They may be difficult to differentiate from AVMs because of the presence of fistulous communications, cavernous dilations of the draining veins, and multiple sources of collateral supply (lumbar, intercostal, phrenic, or renal arteries), which are uncommon in hemangiomas in other parts of the body. Knowledge of such collateral arterial supply and portal vein involvement is essential prior to therapeutic embolization; survival after hepatic artery occlusion depends on the presence of normal portal or anomalous systemic flow to the liver (104).

Natural History and Management

Hemangiomas are lesions of infancy. Most are cutaneous and remain small and harmless. However, some grow to alarming size and proliferate simultaneously in various organs, causing life-threatening complications including CHF, hemorrhage, soft tissue destruction, deformation or obstruction of vital structures, and sepsis. By definition, hemangiomas regress with time. However, treatment may be necessary for hemangiomas

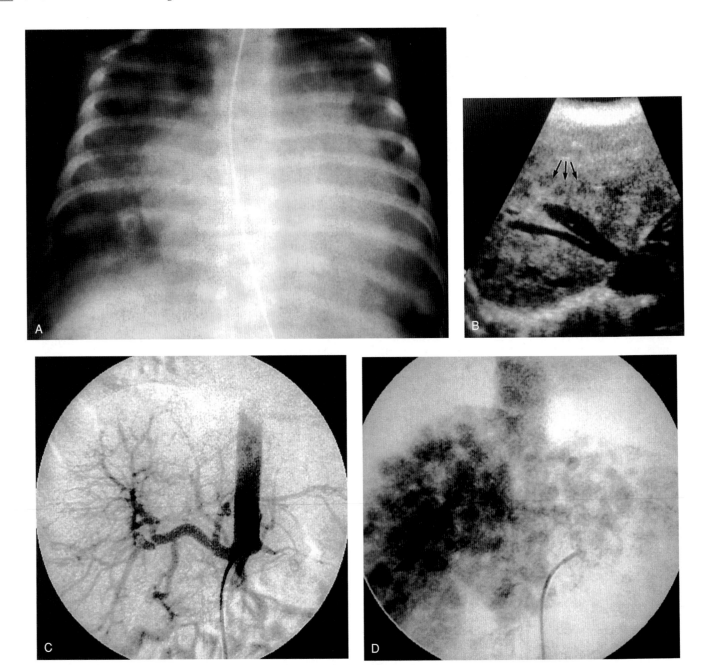

FIGURE 35.7 A: A posteroanterior chest roentgenogram of an infant with hepatic hemangiomas demonstrating generalized cardiomegaly and pulmonary edema. The coil apparent in the right lower lung field was placed externally as a size reference. **B:** Ultrasonogram through the liver shows hypoechoic nodules (*arrows*) and large hepatic vein draining the periphery of the hemangioma. **C:** Descending aortogram (arterial phase) of diffuse proliferating hepatic hemangioma, anteroposterior projection, shows hypervascularity with enlarged common hepatic artery and branches. **D:** Descending aortogram (capillary phase) demonstrating intense circumscribed tissue staining with discrete lesion margins and a lobular organization, characteristic of hemangiomas.

that cause life-threatening symptoms, affording the lesion time to regress. The importance of distinguishing between hemangiomas and arterial malformations lies in their differing responses to therapy.

Hemangiomas may be stimulated to begin involution by the systemic administration or intralesional injection of corticosteroids, cyclophosphamide, laser therapy, and embolization. Radiation therapy is not recommended (105–108). High-dose corticosteroids have been the primary pharmacologic treatment for palliating hemangiomas (107). The mechanism by which steroids affect vascular malformations is not known. Hypotheses include alterations of endothelial cell metabolism and the incitement of precapillary arterial constriction. However, only 30% respond to the systemic or intralesional administration of corticosteroids. The mortality rate may be as high as 65% for life-threatening visceral or hepatic hemangiomas and as high as 30% to 40% with platelet-consumptive coagulopathy despite the administration of steroids (109,110).

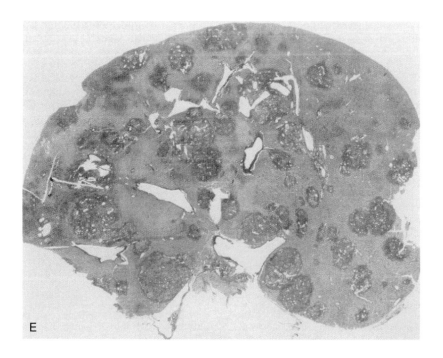

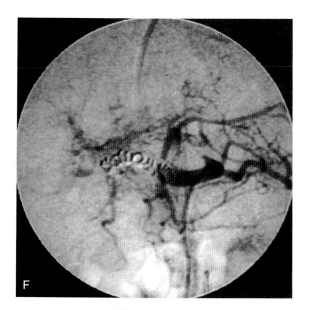

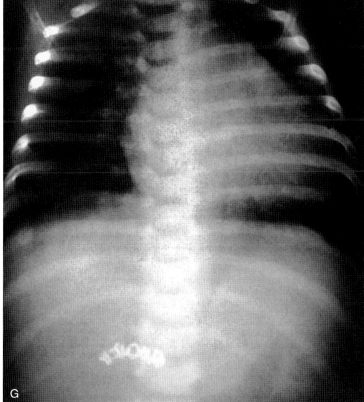

FIGURE 35.7 *(Continued)* **E:** Whole mount section of the entire liver stained with periodic acid-Schiff stain, showing multicentric hemangiomas as round nodules. The intervening hepatic parenchyma stains light pink. (Courtesy of Antonio Perez-Atayde, M.D., Department of Pathology, Children's Hospital, Boston, MA.) **F** and **G:** Follow-up hepatic angiogram and chest roentgenogram after successful coil embolization; the coils are apparent in the common hepatic artery. Chest roentgenogram demonstrates marked decrease in cardiac size and resolution of pulmonary edema; coils are evident corresponding to their angiographic position.

Favorable outcomes have been achieved with transcatheter embolization. In infants with CHF caused by hepatic hemangiomas, devascularization, including hepatic artery embolization, has improved cardiac failure in 78% of cases (108). Radiation and cyclophosphamide therapies are less effective and are fraught with side effects.

Interferon-a2a is a promising new therapy. In 90% of patients, it induced early regression of life-threatening steroid-resistant hemangiomas by at least 50%, including those with consumptive coagulopathies (108,109). Given subcutaneously, short-term side effects did not occur during an 8-month treatment course (range 9 to 14 months) (110).

Reported complications include leucopenia, granulocytopenia, and neurotoxicity (111). Interferon-a2a is thought to set off the message expression of b-FGF and may be effective in inhibiting the proliferation of endothelial cells, smooth muscle cells, or fibroblasts and decreasing the production of collagen or enhancing the production of endothelial prostacyclin (109,110). Initial therapy with interferon-a is more effective in rapidly reducing lesion size than when used after initial treatment with steroids. A proper diagnosis of hemangioma is crucial. Interferon-a may diminish the single endothelial layer of an AVM or AVF and thus induce secondary hemorrhage.

References

1. Osler W. Remarks on arteriovenous aneurysm. *Lancet* 1915;1:949.
2. Hunter W. The history of an aneurysm of the aorta with some remarks on aneurysms in general. *Med Obstet Soc Phys (Lond)* 1757;1:323.
3. Bell J. *The Principles of Surgery.* London: Longman, Hurst, Rees, 1815: 456–489.
4. Nicoladoni C. Phlebarteriectasie der rechten oberen extremitat. *Arch Klin Chir* 1875;18:252.
5. Holman E. *Arteriovenous Aneurysms: Abnormal Communications between the Arterial and Venous Circulations.* New York: Macmillan, 1957.
6. Sadler TW. Embryonic period (third through eighth week). In: *Langman's Medical Embryology.* 6th ed. Baltimore: Williams & Wilkins, 1989:71–73.
7. Sabin FR. Studies of the origin of blood vessels as seen in the living blastoderm. *Contrib Embryol* 1920;9:213.
8. Woollard HH. The development of the principal arterial system of the forelimb of the pig. *Contrib Embryol* 1922;14:139.
9. Folkman J, Haudenschild C. Angiogenesis in vitro. *Nature* 1980;288: 551–554.
10. Young AE. Pathogenesis of vascular malformations. In: Mulliken JB, Young AE, eds. *Vascular Birthmarks: Hemangiomas and Malformations.* Philadelphia: WB Saunders, 1988:107–113.
11. Woollard HH, Harpman JA. The relationship between the size of an artery and the capillary bed in the embryo. *J Anat* 1937;72:18–24.
12. Szilagyi DE, Smith RF, Elliott JP, et al. Congenital arteriovenous anomalies of the limbs. *Arch Surg* 1976;111:423–427.
13. Malan E, Puglionisi A. Congenital angiodysplasias of the extremities. *J Cardiovasc Surg (Torino)* 1964;5:87–92.
14. Mulliken JB, Glowacki J. Hemangiomas and vascular malformations in infants and children: A classification based on endothelial characteristics. *Plast Reconstr Surg* 1982;69:412–420.
15. Quero Jiménez M, Acerete Guillén F. Arteriovenous fistulas. In: Adams FH, Emmanouilides GC, Riemenshneider TA, eds. *Moss' Heart Disease in Infants, Children, and Adolescents.* 4th ed. Baltimore: Williams & Wilkins, 1989:617–626.
16. Sanyal SK, Saldivar V, Coburn TP, et al. Hyperdynamic heart failure due to A-V fistula associated with Wilms' tumor. *Pediatrics* 1976;57:564–568.
17. Olivecrona H, Riives J. Arteriovenous aneurysms of brain: Their diagnosis and treatment. *Arch Neurol Psychiatry* 1948;59:567–571.
18. Avery JB. Malformations of the systemic veins. In: Avery JB, ed. *Cardiovascular Pathology in Infants and Children.* Philadelphia: WB Saunders, 1984:277–281.
19. Esterly NB. Hereditary hemorrhagic telangiectasia. In: Nelson WE, Berman RE, Vaughan VC III, eds. *Textbook of Pediatrics.* Philadelphia: WB Saunders, 1987:1392.
20. Stein B. Arteriovenous malformations of the brain and spinal cord. In: Hoff J, ed. Neurosurgery, in *Goldsmith's Practice of Surgery.* New York: Harper & Row, 1979:1.
21. Amacher AL. Syndromes and surgical treatment of aneurysms of the great vein of Galen. *J Neurosurg* 1973;39:89–98.
22. Cronquist S. Hydrocephalus and congestive heart failure caused by intracranial arteriovenous malformation in infants. *J Pediatr* 1976;89:343–347.
23. Lasjaunias P, TerBrugge K, Lopez Ibor L, et al. The role of dural anomalies in vein of Galen aneurysms: Report of six cases and review of the literature. *AJNR Am J Neuroradiol* 1987;8:185–192.
24. Hoffman HJ, Chuang S, Hendricks EB. Aneurysms of the vein of Galen. *J Neurosurg* 1982;57:316–322.
25. Albright AL, Latchaw RE, Price RA. Posterior dural arteriovenous malformations in infancy. *Neurosurgery* 1983;13:129–135.
26. Glass IH, Rowe RD, Duckworth JWA. Congenital arteriovenous fistula between the left internal mammary artery and the ductus venosus: Unusual cause of congestive heart failure in the newborn infant. *Pediatrics* 1960;26:604–610.
27. Martin LW, Benzing G, Kaplan S. Congenital intrahepatic arteriovenous fistula. *Ann Surg* 1965;161:209–213.
28. Dehner LP, Ishak KG. Vascular tumors of the liver in infants and children. *Arch Pathol* 1971;92:101–111.
29. Sapire DW, Lobe TE, Swischuk LE, et al. Subclavian artery to innominate vein fistula with congestive heart failure in a newborn infant. *Pediatr Cardiol* 1983;4:155–157.
30. Atwood GF, King TD, Graham TP Jr, et al. Thoracic arteriovenous fistula. *Am J Dis Child* 1975;129:233–236.
31. Tollenaere P, Faidutti B, Fournet PC. Congenital arteriovenous fistula of the internal mammary vessels: Report of a case and review of the literature. *J Cardiovasc Surg* 1977;18:79–82.
32. Soler P, Mehta AV, Garcia OL, et al. Congenital systemic arteriovenous fistula between the descending aorta, azygous vein and superior vena cava. *Chest* 1981;80:647–648.
33. Wooley MM, Stanley P, Wesley JR. Peripherally located congenital arteriovenous fistulae in infancy and childhood. *J Pediatr Surg* 1977;12:165–176.
34. Burrows PE, Lasjaunias PL, Ter Brugge KG, et al. Urgent and emergent embolization of lesions of the head and neck in children: Indications and results. *Pediatrics* 1987;80:386–394.
35. Pearse LA, Sondheimer HM, Washington RL, et al. Congenital vertebral-jugular fistula in an infant. *Pediatr Cardiol* 1989;10:229–231.
36. Deverall PB, Taylor JFN, Sturrock GS, et al. Coarctation-like physiology with cerebral arteriovenous fistula. *Pediatrics* 1969;44:1024–1028.
37. Benson DF. Cardiomegaly in a newborn due to placental chorioangioma. *Br Med J* 1961;262:102–105.
38. Jedekin R, Rowe RD, Freedom RM, et al. Cerebral arteriovenous malformations in neonates: The role of myocardial ischemia. *Pediatr Cardiol* 1983;4:29–35.
39. Holden AM, Fyler DC, Shillito J, et al. Congestive heart failure from intracranial arteriovenous fistula in infancy. *Pediatrics* 1972;49:30–39.
40. Silverman BK, Breck T, Craig J, et al. Congestive heart failure in the newborn caused by cerebral arteriovenous fistula. *Am J Dis Child* 1955; 89:539–543.
41. Knudson RP, Alden ER. Symptomatic arteriovenous malformation in infants less than 6 months of age. *Pediatrics* 1979;64:238–241.
42. Watson DG, Smith RR, Brann AW Jr. Arteriovenous malformation of the vein of Galen: Treatment in a neonate. *Am J Dis Child* 1976;130:520–525.
43. Walker WJ, Mullins CE, Knovick GC. Cyanosis, cardiomegaly and weak pulses: A manifestation of massive congenital systemic arteriovenous fistula. *Circulation* 1964;29:777–781.
44. Branham HH. Aneurysmal varix of the femoral artery and vein following a gunshot wound. *Int J Surg* 1890;3:250–255.
45. Gupta PD, Singh M. Neural mechanism underlying tachycardia induced by nonhypotensive A-V shunt. *Am J Physiol* 1979;236:H35.
46. Swischuk LE, Crowe JE, Newborne EB Jr, et al. Large vein of Galen aneurysms in the neonate: A constellation of chest and neck radiologic findings. *Pediatr Radiol* 1977;6:4–9.
47. Sapire DW, Casta A, Donner RM, et al. Dilatation of the descending aorta: A radiologic and echocardiographic sign in arteriovenous malformations in neonates and young infants. *Am J Cardiol* 1979;44:493–497.
48. Starc TJ, Krongrad E, Bierman FZ. Two-dimensional echocardiography and Doppler findings in cerebral arteriovenous malformation. *Am J Cardiol* 1989;64:252–254.
49. Musewe NN, Smallhorn JF, Burrows PE, et al. Echocardiographic and Doppler evaluation of the aortic arch and brachiocephalic vessels in cerebral and systemic arteriovenous fistulas. *J Am Coll Cardiol* 1988;12:1529–1535.
50. Snider AR, Soifer SJ, Silverman NH. Detection of intracranial arteriovenous fistula by ultrasonography. *Circulation* 1981;63:1179–1185.
51. Stanbridge RDL, Westaby S, Smallhorn J, et al. Intracranial arteriovenous malformation with aneurysm of vein of Galen as a cause of heart failure in

infancy: Echocardiographic diagnosis and results of treatment. *Br Heart J* 1983;49:157–162.

52. Meyer JS, Hoffer FA, Barnes PD, et al. Biological classification of soft-tissue vascular anomalies: MR correlation. *AJR Am J Roentgenol* 1991; 157:559–564.

53. Leblanc R, Ethier R, Little JR. Computerized tomography findings in arteriovenous malformations of the brain. *J Neurosurg* 1979;51:765–769.

54. Henderson WR, Gomez R. Natural history of cerebral angiomas. *Br Med J* 1967;4:571–578.

55. Perret G, Nishioka H. Report on the cooperative study of intracranial aneurysms and subarachnoid hemorrhage. VI: Arteriovenous malformations. *J Neurosurg* 1966;25:467–475.

56. DeLorimier AA, Simpson EB, Baum RS, et al. Hepatic artery ligation for hepatic hemangiomatosis. *N Engl J Med* 1967;277:333–336.

57. Berenstein A, Lasjaunias P. Catheter and delivery systems. In: Berenstein A, Lasjaunias P, eds. *Surgical Neuroangiography.* New York: Springer-Verlag, 1987:5–18.

58. Berenstein A, Lasjaunias P. Embolic agents. In: Berenstein A, Lasjaunias P, eds. *Surgical Neuroangiography.* New York: Springer-Verlag, 1987:19–38.

59. Anderson JH, Wallace S, Gianturco C. Transcatheter intravascular coil occlusion of experimental arteriovenous fistulas. *AJR Am J Roentgenol* 1977;129:795–798.

60. Anderson JH, Wallace S, Gianturco C, et al. "Mini" Gianturco stainless steel coils for transcatheter vascular occlusion. *Radiology* 1979;132:301–303.

61. Forbess IW, O'Laughlin MP, Harrison JK. Partially anomalous pulmonary venous connection: Demonstration of dual drainage allowing nonsurgical correction. *Catheter Cardiovasc Diagn* 1998;44:330–335.

62. Preminger TJ, Lock JE, Perry SB. Transluminal vascular stenting using a Gore-Tex covered stent: An experimental study [Abstract]. *Cardiol Young* 1993;3(suppl 1):54.

63. White RI, Barth KH, Kaufman SL, et al. Therapeutic embolization with detachable balloons. *Cardiovasc Intervent Radiol* 1980;3:229–241.

64. Burrows PE, Lasjaunias P, TerBrugge KG. A 4-F coaxial catheter system for pediatric vascular occlusion with detachable balloons. *Radiology* 1989;170:1091–1094.

65. Bank WD, Kerber CW. Gelfoam embolization: A simplified technique. *AJR Am J Roentgenol* 1979;132:299–301.

66. Cromwell LD, Kerber CW. Modification of cyanoacrylate for therapeutic embolization: Preliminary experience. *AJR Am J Roentgenol* 1979;132: 799–804.

67. Friedman DM, Madrid M, Berenstein A, et al. Neonatal vein of Galen malformations: Experience in developing a multidisciplinary approach using an embolization treatment protocol. *Clin Pediatr (Phila)* 1991;30:621–629.

68. Mickle JP, Quisling RG. The transtorcular embolisation of vein of Galen aneurysms. *J Neurosurg* 1986;64:731–735.

69. Verma R, Friedman DM, Madrid M, et al. Recent improvement in outcome using transcatheter embolization techniques for neonatal aneurysmal malformations of the vein of Galen. *Pediatrics* 1993;91:583–586.

70. Jimenez M, Fournier A, Chossat A. Pulmonary artery to the left atrium fistula as an unusual cause of cyanosis in the newborn. *Pediatr Cardiol* 1989;10:216–220.

71. McFaul RC, Tajik AJ, Mair DD, et al. Development of pulmonary arteriovenous shunt after superior vena cava to right pulmonary artery (Glenn) anastomosis. *Circulation* 1977;55:212–216.

72. Cloutier A, Ash JM, Smallhorn JF, et al. Abnormal distribution of pulmonary blood after the Glenn shunt or Fontan procedure: Risk of development of pulmonary arteriovenous fistulae. *Circulation* 1985;72:471–479.

73. Srivastava D, Preminger TJ, Spevak PJ, et al. Development of pulmonary arteriovenous malformations following cavopulmonary anastomoses [Abstract]. *Circulation* 1993;8:I149.

74. Bosher LH, Blake A, Byrd BR. An analysis of the pathologic anatomy of pulmonary arteriovenous aneurysms with particular reference to the applicability of local excision. *Surgery* 1959;45:91–99.

75. White RI Jr, Lynch-Nyhan A, Terry P, et al. Pulmonary arteriovenous malformations: Techniques and long-term outcome of embolotherapy. *Radiology* 1988;169:663–669.

76. Kunahara O, Matumura A, Dohi H, et al. A clinical study on hereditary hemorrhagic telangiectasia (Osler's disease) and its relation to pulmonary arteriovenous fistula. *Nippon Kyobu Geka Gakkai Zasshi* 1987;35:804–809.

77. Chilvers ER. Clinical and physiologic aspects of pulmonary arteriovenous malformations. *Br J Hosp Med* 1988;39:188–192.

78. Friedlich A, Bing RJ, Blount SG. Physiological studies in congenital heart disease. IX: Circulatory dynamics in the anomalies of venous return to the heart, including pulmonary arteriovenous fistula. *Bull Johns Hopkins Hosp* 1950;86:20–57.

79. Roman G, Fisher M, Peri DP, et al. Neurologic manifestations of hereditary hemorrhagic telangiectasia (Osler-Weber-Rendu disease): Report of 2 cases and review of the literature. *Ann Neurol* 1978;4:130–144.

80. Gelfand MS, Stephen DS, Howell E, et al. Brain abscess: Association with pulmonary arteriovenous fistula and hereditary hemorrhagic telangiectasia—report of 3 cases. *Am J Med* 1988;85:718–720.

81. Robin ED, Laman D, Horn DR, et al. Platypnea related to orthodeoxia caused by true vascular lung shunts. *N Engl J Med* 1976;294:941–943.

82. Laberge JM, Brandt ML, Lebecque P, et al. Reversal of cirrhosis-related pulmonary shunting in two children by orthotopic liver transplantation. *Transplantation* 1992;53:1135–1138.

83. Clarke CP, Goh TH, Blackwood A, et al. Massive pulmonary AV fistula in the newborn. *Br Heart J* 1976;38:1092–1095.

84. Hall RJ, Nelson WP, Blake HA, et al. Massive pulmonary arteriovenous fistula in the newborn: A correctable form of "cyanotic heart disease"—an additional cause of polycythemia. *Circulation* 1965;31:762–764.

85. Hodgson CH, Burchell HB, Good CA, et al. Hereditary hemorrhagic telangiectasia and pulmonary arteriovenous fistula: Survey of a large family. *N Engl J Med* 1959;261:625–628.

86. Snider RA, Serwer GA. Abnormal vascular connections and structures. In: *Echocardiography in Pediatric Heart Disease.* Chicago: Yearbook Medical, 1990:273–274.

87. Remy J, Remy-Jardin M, Wattinne L, et al. Pulmonary arteriovenous malformations: Evaluation with CT of the chest before and after treatment. *Radiology* 1992;182:809–816.

88. Dinsmore BF, Gefter WB, Hatabu H, et al. Pulmonary arteriovenous malformations: Diagnosis by gradient refocused MR imaging. *J Comput Assist Tomogr* 1990;14:918–923.

89. Chilvers ER, Peters AM, George P. Quantification of right-to-left shunt through pulmonary arteriovenous malformations using Tc albumin microspheres. *Clin Radiol* 1988;39:611–614.

90. Sloan RD, Cooley RD. Congenital pulmonary arteriovenous aneurysm. *AJR Am J Roentgenol* 1953;70:183–210.

91. Portsmann W. Therapeutic embolization of arteriovenous pulmonary fistula by catheter technique. In: Kelop O, ed. *Current Concepts in Pediatric Radiology.* New York: Springer-Verlag, 1977:23–31.

92. Terry PB, Barth KH, Kaufman SL, et al. Balloon embolization for treatment of pulmonary arteriovenous fistulas. *N Engl J Med* 1980;302:1189–1190.

93. Steinberg I. Diagnosis and surgical treatment of pulmonary arteriovenous fistulas: A report of 3 cases and a review of nineteen consecutive cases. *Surg Clin North Am* 1961;41:523–535.

94. Mulliken JB. Classification of vascular birthmarks. In: Mulliken JB, Young AE, eds. *Vascular Birthmarks: Hemangiomas and Malformations.* Philadelphia: WB Saunders, 1988:3.

95. Mulliken JB, Zetter BR, Folkman J. In vitro characteristics of endothelium from hemangiomas and vascular malformations. *Surgery* 1982;92:348–353.

96. Folkman J. Clinical applications of research on angiogenesis. *N Engl J Med* 1995;333:1757–1763.

97. Zhang L, Lin X, Wang W, et al. Circulating levels of vascular endothelial growth factor in differentiating hemangioma from vascular malformation patients. *Plast Reconstr Surg* 2005:116:200–204.

98. Larcher VF, Howard ER, Mowat AP. Hepatic hemangiomata: Diagnosis and management. *Arch Dis Child* 1981;56:7–14.

99. Rocchini AP, Rosenthal A, Issenberg HG, et al. Hepatic hemangioendothelioma: Hemodynamic observations and treatment. *Pediatrics* 1976; 57:131–135.

100. McLean RH, Moller JH, Warwick WJ, et al. Multinodular hemangiomatosis of the liver in infancy. *Pediatrics* 1972;49:563–573.

101. Magee F, Wright JL, Kay JM, et al. Pulmonary capillary hemangiomatosis. *Am Rev Respir Dis* 1985;132:922–925.

102. Hagerman LJ, Czapek EE, Donnellan WL, et al. Giant hemangioma with consumption coagulopathy. *J Pediatr* 1975;87:766–768.

103. Burrows PE, Mulliken JB, Fellows KE, et al. Childhood hemangiomas and vascular malformations: Angiographic differentiation. *AJR Am J Roentgenol* 1983;141:143–147.

104. McHugh K, Burrows PE. Infantile hepatic hemangioendotheliomas: Significance of portal venous and systemic collateral arterial supply. *J Vasc Interv Radiol* 1992;3:337–344.

105. Brown SH Jr, Neerhout RC, Fonkalsrud EW. Prednisone therapy in the management of large hemangiomas in infants and children. *Surgery* 1972;71:168–173.

106. Matolo NM, Johnson DG. Surgical treatment of hepatic hemangioma in the newborn. *Arch Surg* 1973;106:725–727.

107. Rotman M, John M, Stowe S, et al. Radiation treatment of pediatric hepatic hemangiomatosis and coexisting cardiac failure. *N Engl J Med* 1980;10:852–853.

108. Burrows PE, Rosenberg HC, Chang HS. Diffuse hepatic hemangiomas: Percutaneous transcatheter embolization with detachable silicone balloons. *Radiology* 1985;156:85–88.

109. White CW, Sondheimer HM, Crouch EC, et al. Treatment of pulmonary hemangiomatosis with recombinant interferon alfa-2a. *N Engl J Med* 1989;320:1197–1200.

110. Ezekowitz RAB, Phil D, Mulliken JB, et al. Interferon alfa-2a therapy for life-threatening hemangiomas of infancy. *N Engl J Med* 1992;326:1456–1463.

111. Szymik-Kantorowicz S, Kobylarz K, Krysta M, et al. Interferon-alpha in the treatment of high-risk haemangiomas in infants. *Eur J Pediatr Surg* 2005;15:11–16.

CHAPTER 36 ■ AORTIC ARCH ANOMALIES

PAUL M. WEINBERG, MD

Congenital abnormalities of the aortic arch have been known at least since the anatomic reports of anomalous right subclavian artery by Hunauld in 1735 (1), double aortic arch by Hommel in 1737 (2), right aortic arch by Fioratti and Aglietti in 1763 (3), and interrupted aortic arch by Steidele in 1788 (4). Although the clinicopathologic correlation of swallowing difficulty with anomalous right subclavian artery was presented to the Medical Society of London by Bayford (5) in 1787, it was not until the 1930s and the use of barium esophagography that some arch anomalies were diagnosed during life. Since that time clinical interest has generally paralleled surgical capability. The first division of a vascular ring was performed by Gross in 1945 (6), and the first successful repair of interrupted aortic arch was accomplished by Merrill et al. in 1957 (7). In the current era with the advent of minimally invasive surgery (8,9) and more recently robotically assisted surgery (10), precise definition of aortic arch anatomy, preferably by noninvasive means, is essential.

ANATOMICAL CLASSIFICATION

Aortic arch anomalies can be thought of as falling into one or a combination of the following anatomic categories: Abnormalities of branching, abnormalities of arch position including right aortic arch and cervical aortic arch, supernumerary arches including double aortic arch and persistent fifth aortic arch, interrupted aortic arch, and anomalous origin of a pulmonary artery branch from the ascending aorta or from the contralateral pulmonary artery branch.

LEFT AND RIGHT ARCH DEFINITION

Left and right aortic arch refer to which bronchus is crossed by the arch, not to which side of the midline the aortic root ascends. This is particularly important to remember when looking at projection images from angiography where it may be difficult to make the determination directly without significant cranial angulation. Practically, the sidedness of the aortic arch is usually determined indirectly with echocardiography or angiography by the branching pattern of the brachiocephalic vessels. As a rule, the first arch vessel contains the carotid artery opposite the side of the arch. However, caution must be exercised in using this indirect method, particularly when surgical decisions, such as the approach to repair of esophageal atresia, hinge on this determination. The very rare cases of retroesophageal or isolated innominate artery are exceptions to this rule. But by far the more common source of error in the use of this rule is the difficulty in deciding which of two carotid arteries is the first. A more reliable rule but one that may be difficult to apply with ultrasound imaging is that retroesophageal vessels or isolated vessels, i.e., arising only from a ductus or ligamentum (without connection to the aorta), are always opposite the side of the aortic arch. Magnetic resonance imaging (MRI) or computed tomography (CT) show the relationship of the arch to the trachea and bronchi directly, thus eliminating ambiguity when atypical branching patterns are encountered.

Embryology

The specific anomalies can better be understood through an appreciation of their embryologic origins. Development of the aortic arch system can best be described as a sequential appearance and persistence or dissolution of six paired vessels connecting the truncoaortic sac of the embryonic heart tube with the paired dorsal aortae, which fuse to form the definitive descending aorta. Each arch corresponds to a branchial pouch derived from embryonic foregut. Although the mechanism for determining persistence or dissolution of aortic arch components is not completely known, migration of neural crest cells into the pharyngeal arches (11) may play a significant role. In addition, the association of various arch anomalies such as right aortic arch, cervical aortic arch, aberrant and isolated subclavian artery, and certain vascular rings with microdeletions of chromosome 22q11 (12) implies a genetic component to the derivation of at least some arch anomalies. The fact that neural crest cells are also involved in development of the conotruncus and that conotruncal anomalies also occur in chromosome 22q11–deleted patients provides a further etiologic link to aortic arch anomalies.

The normal left aortic arch as shown by Congdon (13) is derived from the aortic portion of the embryonic truncus arteriosus, the left branch of the truncoaortic sac, the left fourth arterial arch, the left dorsal aorta between the fourth and sixth embryonic arches, and the left dorsal aorta distal to the sixth arch. The three brachiocephalic branches of the arch are derived from the following: The innominate artery from the right branch of the truncoaortic sac with the right common carotid artery from right third embryonic arch and right subclavian from right fourth arch and (proximal) right dorsal aorta proximally and right seventh intersegmental artery distally; left carotid artery from left third aortic arch; and left subclavian artery from left seventh intersegmental artery. Whereas the appearance and loss of vessels as arches or portions of the brachiocephalic vasculature is sequential, Edwards (14) proposed the concept of a "hypothetical double aortic arch" which is, in essence, the potential contribution of nearly all embryonic arches to components of the definitive arch system. These diagrams are used extensively in the excellent monograph by Stewart, Kincaid, and Edwards (15). They are invaluable not only to demonstrate possible embryologic explanations for each arch anomaly but also to help the diagnostician determine possible and probable arch anomalies and their corresponding sequences of arch vessels. We have adopted a simplified schematic version of

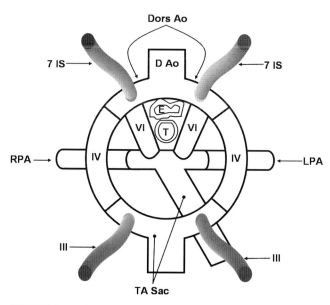

FIGURE 36.1 TOTIPOTENTIAL aortic and pulmonary components. D Ao, descending aorta; Dors Ao, dorsal aortae; E, esophagus, LPA; left pulmonary artery; RPA, right pulmonary artery; T, trachea; TA Sac, truncoaortic sac aortic and pulmonary artery components, III, IV, VI refer to third, fourth, sixth embryonic arches; 7 IS, seventh intersegmental artery. (Modified from hypothetical double aortic arch diagrams of Edwards [Edwards JE. Anomalies of the derivatives of the aortic arch system. *Med Clin North Am* 1948;32:925–949, with permission] as if viewed from overhead.)

the Edwards diagrams, which is feasible for those who are less artistically inclined, to provide similar information (Fig. 36.1). This can easily be drawn at the bedside or in the patient chart to diagram almost any arch anomaly and will be used throughout this chapter to illustrate many of the abnormalities.

Diagnostic Methods

Beginning in the 1930s, barium esophagography was the primary method for diagnosing arch anomalies. In the 1960s and 1970s, angiography became the gold standard and remained so even in the face of echocardiography. However, in the last 10 to 15 years, MRI and CT, where available, have supplanted angiography as the gold standard for definitive diagnosis of arch anomalies. Both modalities have the advantages of large fields of view and simultaneous visualization of vessels and airways, and both are minimally invasive. Although CT usually has shorter scan times, that advantage is disappearing as MRI sequences become faster. MRI has the advantage of no ionizing radiation—still a significant problem with CT even with the reduced dosage strategies used in some centers. Furthermore, MRI has capabilities for physiologic measurements, which are particularly helpful in patients with associated intracardiac disease.

There is still a role for ultrasonography in the diagnosis of arch anomalies and, in particular, vascular rings. That is in the fetus where the fluid-filled trachea does not preclude visualization the way the air-filled trachea does after birth. Furthermore, the ductus arteriosus is virtually always patent, so that nearly all rings can be seen completely encircling the trachea with blood-filled vessels. Specific strategies for recognizing

vascular rings in the fetus have been reported by several authors (16–18).

CLINICAL CLASSIFICATION

In addition to the anatomic categorization of aortic arch anomalies discussed above, one can subdivide arch anomalies according to clinical features as follows: Vascular rings; non-ring vascular compression of the trachea, bronchi, or esophagus; noncompressive arch malformations; and ductal-dependent arch anomalies including interrupted aortic arches and isolated subclavian, carotid, or innominate arteries. In addition, genetic syndromes represent an important group of patients from the standpoint of diagnostic criteria and associated abnormalities.

Chromosome 22q11.2 Deletion Syndromes

Chromosome 22q11.2 microdeletions are seen in >80% of patients with DiGeorge, velocardiofacial, and conotruncal anomaly face syndromes. The combination has been referred to collectively with the acronym CATCH 22 (cardiac defects, abnormal facies, thymic hypoplasia, cleft palate, and hypocalcemia together with microdeletion of chromosome 22) (19). Most of these patients have conotruncal anomalies: Either subaortic stenosis with posterior malalignment of the infundibular septum often associated with interrupted aortic arch, type B; truncus arteriosus communis; or tetralogy of Fallot, with or without pulmonary atresia. More than two thirds of these have aortic arch anomalies (20). What is more, nearly one fourth of patients with arch anomalies but without intracardiac defects have 22q11 deletion (21). Although a wide variety of arch anomalies has been noted in these patients, there is a predilection for anomalies involving absence of one or both embryonic fourth aortic arches, as seen most notably in abnormalities of the subclavian arteries: Aberrant, isolated, or cervical origin (20,22,23). When all three types of subclavian artery anomaly are included, >80% of patients with both conotruncal and arch anomalies involving the subclavian artery have 22q11 deletion compared with only 17% of patients with conotruncal anomaly and normal subclavians (23). Other fourth arch anomalies occurring in chromosome 22q11 deletion syndromes include type B interrupted aortic arch, cervical aortic arch with separate origins of internal and external carotid arteries from the arch (24), and possibly stenosis in the middle of the right aortic arch between right carotid and subclavian arteries along with a diverticulum of Kommerell (25).

Vascular Rings

A vascular ring is an aortic arch anomaly in which the trachea and esophagus are completely surrounded by vascular structures. The vascular structures need not be patent, e.g., a ligamentum arteriosum or atretic segment of aortic arch may complete a ring. The clinical picture typically includes stridor, though pneumonia, bronchitis, or cough may characterize the presentation. Infants may demonstrate a posture of hyperextension of the neck. Less commonly, patients exhibit reflex apnea associated with eating. A common history is that of a 1- to 3-month-old with "noisy breathing since birth" who develops more significant respiratory distress in association with an intercurrent upper respiratory infection. Less commonly and usually in toddlers or older children, the presentation will be swallowing difficulty or choking on food. These patients tend to have looser rings, but careful questioning of parents will sometimes reveal the presence of stridor in infancy, which was passed off as "recurrent bronchitis." Occasionally, in patients with associated intracardiac abnormalities, respiratory symptoms may mistakenly be attributed to the cardiac disease when, in fact, they are in part or completely due to the vascular ring. Older children and adults are occasionally followed for many years with a diagnosis of asthma only to have a vascular ring diagnosed and surgically treated with resolution of symptoms (26,27). However, respiratory symptoms may persist for months or years after surgical relief of the ring owing to the presence of tracheomalacia. Some asymptomatic patients will be discovered incidentally while imaging for another reason (28). The diagnosis may be suspected from the combination of history and plain chest film; however, if symptomatic, the patient should have definitive study.

When all elements of the ring are patent, visualization, especially by tomographic imaging, is straightforward. In cases where the ring is completed by an atretic segment of aorta or ligamentum arteriosum, those segments cannot be visualized with current imaging technologies. However, these rings are recognizable by the presence of one of three "d"s opposite the side of the aortic arch: diverticulum, dimple, or descending aorta (Table 36.1). A diverticulum is a large vessel arising from the descending aorta that gives rise to a smaller-caliber vessel with a sudden taper. A dimple is a tapered, blindly ending outpouching from the aorta. Descending aorta opposite the side of the aortic arch refers to the location of the descending aorta in the upper thorax. These three "d"s occur only when connected by a ligamentum arteriosum or an atretic segment of aortic arch.

TABLE 36.1

THREE "Ds" IS INDICATING VASCULAR RINGS WHEN NOT ALL VESSELS ARE PATENT

- Diverticulum
- Dimple   } Opposite the side of the arch
- Descending aorta

NORMAL LEFT AORTIC ARCH AND VARIANTS

The normal left aortic arch crosses the left mainstem bronchus at the level of thoracic vertebra T5 and descends left of the midline to the diaphragm and beyond in cases of visceral situs solitus. The normal branching pattern has the right innominate artery first. which, in turn, branches into the right common carotid and right subclavian arteries, the left carotid artery second, and the left subclavian artery third. Typically, the ductus arteriosus or the ligamentum arteriosum joins the aorta distal to the takeoff of the left subclavian artery but can insert more proximally, as in some cases of tetralogy of Fallot.

There are two frequent variants of the left aortic arch. One is common brachiocephalic trunk, in which the right innominate and left carotid arteries arise from a single origin. This is present in 10% of otherwise normal left arches (29) and usually is of no consequence, although some have suggested that innominate artery compression of the trachea (discussed below) is more frequent when common brachiocephalic trunk is present. The other variant is separate origin of the left vertebral artery from the aortic arch proximal to the takeoff of the left subclavian artery rather than from the subclavian artery (Fig. 36.2A).

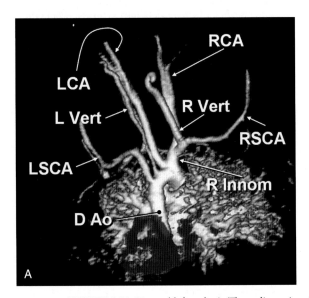

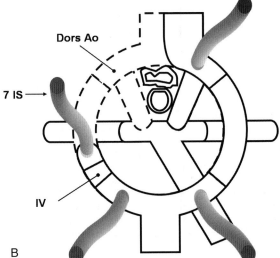

FIGURE 36.2 Normal left arch. **A:** Three-dimensional (3-D) surface display from MRI of normal variant with separate origin of left vertebral artery (L Vert) from the aortic arch., right posterior oblique view. Shows origin of right innominate artery (R Innom), which gives rise to right carotid (RCA) and right subclavian (RSCA) arteries, left carotid (LCA), L vert, and left subclavian (LSCA). Note the relatively short length of the R innom and the relatively distant division of RCA into internal and external carotid arteries. **B:** Presumptive embryonic arch diagram of normal left arch. *Dotted lines* indicate dissolution or disappearance of embryonic arches—right sixth arch and right dorsal aorta distal to right subclavian artery.

This too is seen in 10% of normal left arches (29) and is important only in the fact that it should not be confused angiographically or echocardiographically with anomalous right subclavian artery in which there are also four brachiocephalic vessels (see below). The distinguishing feature here is the normal appearance of the first arch vessel (right innominate artery), being larger than the second (left carotid), and the third (left vertebral) being smaller than the fourth (left subclavian). Again, no functional significance attends this common variant.

Embryology

Using the totipotential aortic arch diagram (Fig. 36.2B), one envisions the normal left arch resulting from dissolution of the right sixth aortic arch (ductus) and the right dorsal aorta distal to the origin of the seventh intersegmental artery (distal subclavian artery precursor). Thus the right fourth arch, rather than remaining an arch (connecting truncoaortic sac to descending aorta), becomes the proximal right subclavian artery as it arises from the innominate artery. The left fourth arch becomes the definitive aortic arch.

ABNORMAL LEFT AORTIC ARCH

Left Aortic Arch with Retroesophageal Right Subclavian Artery

This anomaly (also called anomalous or aberrant right subclavian artery) was first described anatomically by Hunauld in 1735. Bayford (5) linked the postmortem discovery of such a case with the history of swallowing difficulty during life and coined the term "dysphagia lusoria" (from the Latin, *lusus naturae*, trick of nature).

The branching pattern shows the first branch to be the right carotid artery, the second the left carotid, third the left subclavian, and fourth a retroesophageal right subclavian artery arising from the posteromedial aspect of the distal aortic arch (Fig. 36.3A). This is the most common arch anomaly, occurring in 0.5% of the general population, demonstrated in a large adult autopsy series (30). The incidence in Down syndrome patients with congenital heart disease is very high at 38% (31). Most cases of left aortic arch with retroesophageal right subclavian artery are asymptomatic, with the diagnosis made while imaging for another condition or at autopsy. Associated anomalies may include tetralogy of Fallot, various types of isolated ventricular septal defect (VSD), and a smattering of other intracardiac defects.

Embryology

This can be envisioned as a disappearance of the right fourth aortic arch (Fig. 36.3F). The distal right dorsal aorta (rather than the right fourth arch) becomes the proximal right subclavian artery forming its retroesophageal portion. The right sixth arch (ductus) also involutes.

Diagnosis and Management

Since there is no innominate artery, the first and second branches, the right and left carotid arteries, respectively, tend to be similar in size as are the last two branches, the left and right subclavian arteries. Barium esophagography is usually specific for the diagnosis with a fixed filling defect usually slanting upward to the right and best appreciated with fluoroscopy. The defect is relatively small (Fig. 36.3E) compared with that seen in other anomalies where an aortic arch, or

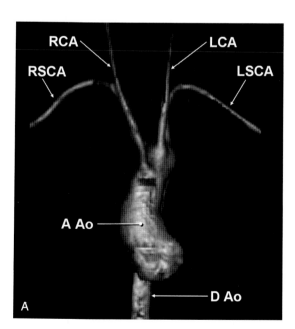
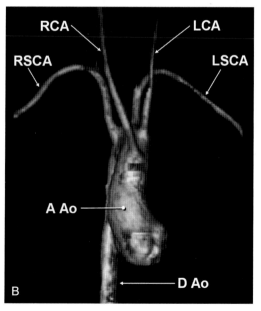

FIGURE 36.3 Left arch, retroesophageal right subclavian artery. **A:** Shaded surface display of 3-D reconstruction from MRI in straight anterior view. Note that RCA is superimposed on RSCA in this view. **B:** RCA and RSCA separated in slight right anterior oblique view showing sequence of arch vessels: RCA, LCA, LSCA, and RSCA. **C:.** Posterior view. Note virtually uniform caliber of RSCA from origin to peripheral extent. **D:** Overhead view showing proximity of RCA and RSCA. A Ao, ascending aorta, D Ao, descending aorta. Other abbreviations as previously defined. **E:** Barium esophagram showing small posterior indentation by retroesophageal subclavian artery. **F:** Presumptive embryonic arch diagram.

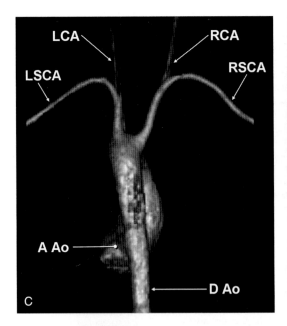

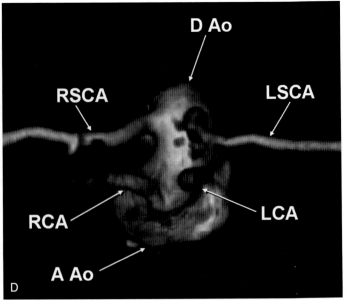

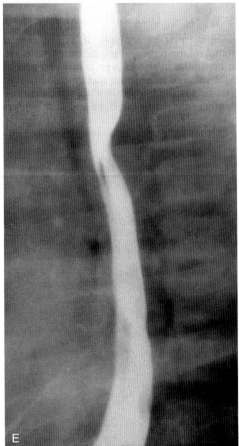

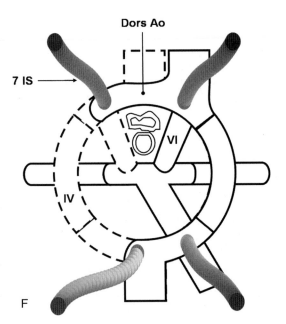

FIGURE 36.3 *(Continued)*

diverticulum, impinges on the esophagus (compare Fig. 36.11F). With angiography, the diagnosis may sometimes be missed in the anteroposterior projection since the right subclavian may be superimposed on the right carotid artery in the usual position. However, careful single-frame analysis will demonstrate the earlier filling of the right carotid on an aortic root injection or the earlier filling of the right subclavian on a descending aortic injection. This arch anomaly is usually recognized with echocardiography by the branching pattern discussed above, namely, a nonbifurcating first branch that ascends toward the right, followed by two successive left-sided vessels (left carotid and left subclavian arteries) followed by a fourth branch that heads toward the right but may disappear behind the trachea. The retroesophageal course of the subclavian artery is shown by MRI on transverse (axial) cuts, and the largest expanse from aortic origin to the thoracic apex is usually seen on coronal sections.

Left Aortic Arch with Retroesophageal Diverticulum of Kommerell

This very rare arch anomaly was actually the first vascular ring to be diagnosed in life with barium esophagography by Kommerell (32) whose name is associated with this diverticulum. Although the name is usually used in reference to the

much more common mirror image of this anomaly, viz., a diverticulum associated with a right aortic arch (discussed below). The branching pattern in left arch with retroesophageal diverticulum is identical to that of the more common left arch with retroesophageal right subclavian artery discussed above, which is not a vascular ring. The difference is in the caliber of the proximal subclavian artery (Fig. 36.4A, B). The significance of this is that the abrupt change of vessel size always indicates the presence of a ligamentum arteriosum, which completes a vascular ring.

Embryology

This anomaly exhibits embryology similar to that of left arch, retroesophageal right subclavian artery described

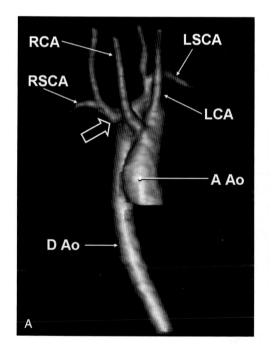

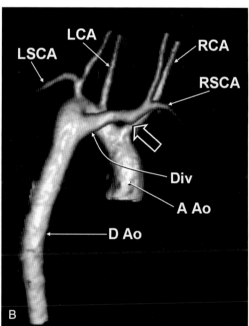

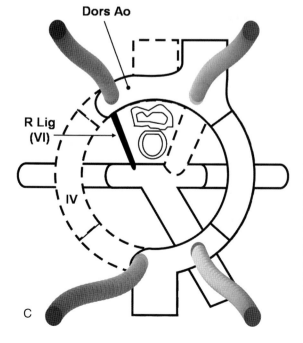

FIGURE 36.4 Left aortic arch, retroesophageal diverticulum of Kommerell. A: Anterior view of 3-D shaded surface display showing sequence of arch vessels arising from aorta: RCA, LCA, LSCA, and RSCA. Note that RSCA comes from diverticulum (Div) seen better in B. B: Right posterior oblique view. Note tapering of Div from aortic end to RSCA origin. Also note angulation of vessel at site of ligamentum arteriosum (*open arrow*). C: Presumptive embryonic arch diagram. Note similarity to Figure 36.3 above, but with addition of persistent arch VI (ductus arteriosus). Abbreviations as previously defined.

above, i.e., involution of the right fourth aortic arch. The difference is that unlike the aforementioned anomaly, the right sixth (ductal) arch persists and completes the ring (Fig. 36.4C).

Left Aortic Arch with Right Descending Aorta and Right Ductus (or Ligamentum)

This is a rare arch anomaly, also known as circumflex aortic arch, with a branching pattern similar to that of left arch with retroesophageal right subclavian artery. However, the arch itself is retroesophageal; hence the right subclavian artery, although it may arise as the last arch vessel, is not retroesophageal (Fig. 36.5). The descending aorta is connected by a ductus or ligamentum to the right pulmonary artery, forming a vascular ring.

Embryology

The embryology of this anomaly, also similar to left arch with retroesophageal subclavian artery, can be thought of as a disappearance of the right fourth aortic arch but with the distal left dorsal aorta forming the definitive distal aortic arch and passing retroesophageally to a descending aorta beginning to the right of the vertebral column (Fig. 36.5D). Thus the right seventh intersegmental artery arises from the right-sided descending aorta. There is also persistence of the right sixth (ductal) arch connecting the right pulmonary artery portion of the truncoaortic sac with the distal right dorsal aorta similar to the also rare left arch diverticulum of Kommerell (above).

Diagnosis and Management

This diagnosis can be suspected if a patient who presents with symptoms suggestive of a vascular ring has findings of a left

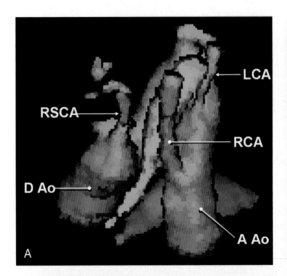
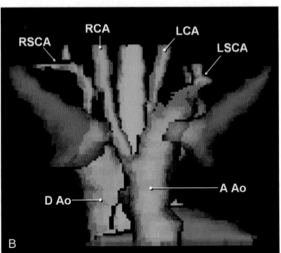
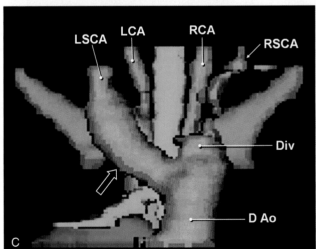
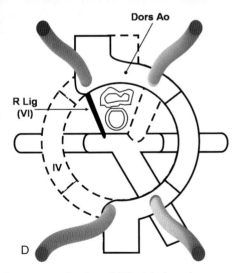

FIGURE 36.5 Cervical left arch, right descending aorta. **A:** 3-D reconstruction from MRI, right lateral view with slight cranial angulation. Trachea (*green*) trapped by ligamentum arteriosum (not visualized) between descending aorta (D Ao) and right pulmonary artery (*blue*). **B:** Anteroposterior (AP) view of same reconstruction showing arch extending above level of clavicles (*grey*). Hairpin appearance of cervical arch is seen through translucent rendering of left clavicle. **C:** Posterior view of same 3-D reconstruction. Circumflex aortic arch (*arrow*) connects to D Ao, from which arises a diverticulum (Div) that gives rise to RSCA and ligamentum arteriosum. **D:** Embryonic arch diagram showing dissolution of right fourth arch and left sixth arch and persistence of right sixth arch remnant, namely, right ligamentum (R Lig (VI)). Abbreviations as previously defined.

aortic arch without evidence of a right aortic arch. Plain chest roentgenogram can show the left-sided arch and the right-sided upper descending aorta, particularly in adults. The addition of barium esophagography can demonstrate the large posterior indentation from the retroesophageal aorta; however, the course of this vessel, upward to the left, is indistinguishable from the much more frequently occurring right aortic arch with retroesophageal diverticulum (see below). In both cases the upper descending aorta is right sided. Although the aortic knob on chest roentgenogram would be left sided, this is not always evident, especially in infants with a prominent thymus. Angiography will show the course of the aorta from left arch to retroesophageal segment to right upper descending. The subclavian artery can be seen arising from the descending aorta as it turns from its transverse to more nearly vertical course. This pattern can also be demonstrated by MRI with the addition of direct imaging of the aortic position relative to the trachea. Although most vascular rings can be divided through a left thoracotomy, this type and the rare diverticulum of Kommerell noted above are usually approached by a right thoracotomy (33), so that the ligamentum can be reached. A midline approach may also be used.

Left Aortic Arch with Isolated Subclavian Artery

Another rare anomaly, isolated subclavian artery, means that the subclavian artery arises only from the ductus arteriosus. While the ductus is patent, the subclavian and vertebral arteries are supplied from the pulmonary artery. When the ductus closes, the subclavian is supplied by retrograde flow from the vertebral artery via the circle of Willis.

Embryology

This occurs with dissolution of the right fourth arch and right dorsal aorta but persistence of the right sixth arch.

Diagnosis and Management

When this occurs in the absence of other anomalies, it may go unrecognized or may cause vertebrobasilar insufficiency with so-called congenital subclavian steal. In many cases there may be no symptoms or simply absence of the right arm pulse. This may be recognized with angiography by delayed filling of the subclavian artery after aortic root injection. With phase-encoded velocity mapping, retrograde flow in the vertebral artery can be detected on MRI. Symptomatic patients are treated by implantation of the subclavian artery into the aorta.

Left Aortic Arch with Cervical Origin of the Right Subclavian Artery

This rare anomaly was first reported by Kutsche and Van Mierop (34) in association with type B interrupted aortic arch. It was subsequently found in patients with tetralogy of Fallot, with or without pulmonary atresia, and has been seen only in patients with 22q11 deletion (22). This is an abnormality whose clinical significance appears to be that it is a marker for CATCH 22. Normally the right innominate artery bifurcates into a common carotid and subclavian artery near its origin from the aorta (see Fig. 36.2B). In this anomaly, the innominate trifurcates in the neck, giving rise to external and internal

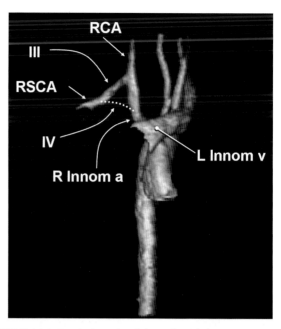

FIGURE 36.6 Cervical origin of the right subclavian artery. Slight right anterior oblique view of 3-D shaded-surface display from MRI. Note the high (i.e., cervical) origin of the RSCA from the right innominate artery (R Innom a) and the downward course into the thorax. Compare with Figure 36.2A. *Dotted line* shows expected location of absent embryonic fourth arch (IV). Note superior location of embryonic third arch (III) component of RSCA. L innom v = left innominate vein. Other abbreviations as previously defined.

carotids and the subclavian artery, which then travels caudally back to the thorax before heading out to the arm (Fig. 36.6).

Embryology

The presumptive embryology has been elegantly described by Kutsche and Van Mierop (34). This together with the observation of Rauch, et al. (22) that abnormalities of subclavian artery origin are frequently associated with 22q11 deletion sheds light on an important pathway in the pathogenesis of arch anomalies in CATCH 22 patients. There appears to be a predilection for unilateral or bilateral absence or atresia of the embryonic fourth arch. When this occurs on the side opposite the definitive arch, there are three main variations in the fate of the subclavian artery: (a) origin from the descending aorta, i.e., from the dorsal aorta distal to the seventh intersegmental artery—retroesophageal subclavian artery or circumflex aortic arch as described above; (b) origin from the sixth arch—isolated subclavian artery, also described above; and (c) origin from the third arch, which, being more cephalad than the fourth, gives origin to the subclavian artery in the neck rather than in the thorax.

When the fourth arch is absent or atretic ipsilateral to the definitive aortic arch, there are also three possibilities, which will be elaborated on below: (a) interrupted aortic arch, in which the sixth arch replaces the fourth; (b) persistent fifth aortic arch with atresia of the distal fourth; and (c) cervical aortic arch, in which the third arch replaces the fourth, analogous to cervical origin of the subclavian artery on the side opposite the arch. Of note is the fact that all of these have been seen in association with 22q11 deletion and collectively are more common than cases with normal origin of the subclavian arteries and well-developed fourth arches (20,23).

RIGHT AORTIC ARCH

Right aortic arches have in common (by definition) a single aortic arch that crosses over the right mainstem bronchus, passing to the right of the trachea. There are four major types of right arch: (a) with mirror image branching, (b) with retroesophageal left subclavian artery, (c) with retroesophageal diverticulum, and (d) with left descending aorta. There are also several infrequently occurring variations.

The incidence of right aortic arch among patients with tetralogy of Fallot has been reported to be anywhere from 13% to 34% (35); however, studies vary as to the source of the material (chest roentgenogram, angiography, surgery, or postmortem examination) and frequently do not distinguish between specific types of right arch. The incidence in truncus arteriosus is generally higher than in tetralogy. An overall incidence of 8% in patients with D-transposition of the great arteries, compared with 16% in those with transposition VSD and pulmonary stenosis, has been reported (36).

Right Aortic Arch with Mirror-Image Branching

Mirror-image right arch has the first branch as a left innominate artery, which, in turn, divides into left carotid and left subclavian arteries; the second as the right carotid; and the third a right subclavian (Fig. 36.7A, B). This is the left-right mirror of a normal left aortic arch. However, frequently that is the end of the symmetry, since the ductus arteriosus (or ligamentum arteriosum) is usually the left-sided one, arising from the base of the innominate artery rather than from the aortic arch. Therefore, typical mirror-image right aortic arch with left ductus or ligamentum does not form a vascular ring. This arch anomaly is almost always associated with congenital intracardiac disease. The most common association is with tetralogy of Fallot (48% in a series of 74 postmortem cases) (37), but truncus arteriosus communis, other conotruncal anomalies including transposition of the great arteries, double-outlet right ventricle, right ventricular aorta

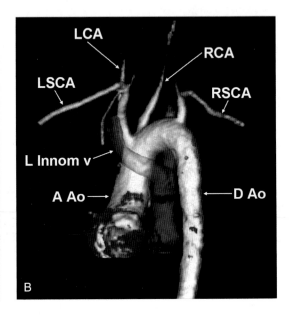

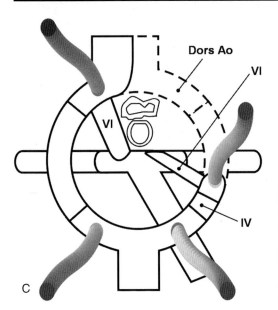

FIGURE 36.7 Right aortic arch, mirror-image type. **A:** Anterior view of 3-D shaded-surface display from MRI. Sequence of arch vessels is L Innom a, RCA, RSCA. **B:** Left posterior oblique view. Note incidental retroaortic L Innom v. There was no ductus arteriosus in this case. **C:** Embryonic arch diagram showing dissolution of left dorsal aorta after proximal migration of left subclavian artery. Note left fourth arch forms proximal left subclavian artery and left sixth (ductal) arch extends from underside of left innominate artery to left pulmonary artery. Abbreviations as previously defined.

with pulmonary atresia, and anatomically corrected malposition were also seen. In addition, lesions not usually considered being conotruncal anomalies such as pulmonary atresia with intact ventricular septum, conoventricular/perimembranous VSD with anomalous muscle bundle of the right ventricle, and isolated VSD are occasionally found to have mirror-image right arch.

A rare variation of mirror-image right aortic arch has a left ductus or ligamentum arising from a retroesophageal dimple from the right-sided descending aorta. This does form a vascular ring (Fig. 36.8). This is different from right arch with diverticulum of Kommerell in that no arch vessel arises from the dimple. Unlike other patients with mirror-image right aortic arch, the few reported cases with retroesophageal ductus dimple appear not to have associated congenital heart disease (38).

Embryology

The presumptive pattern of mirror-image right arch development includes dissolution of the left dorsal aorta distal to the

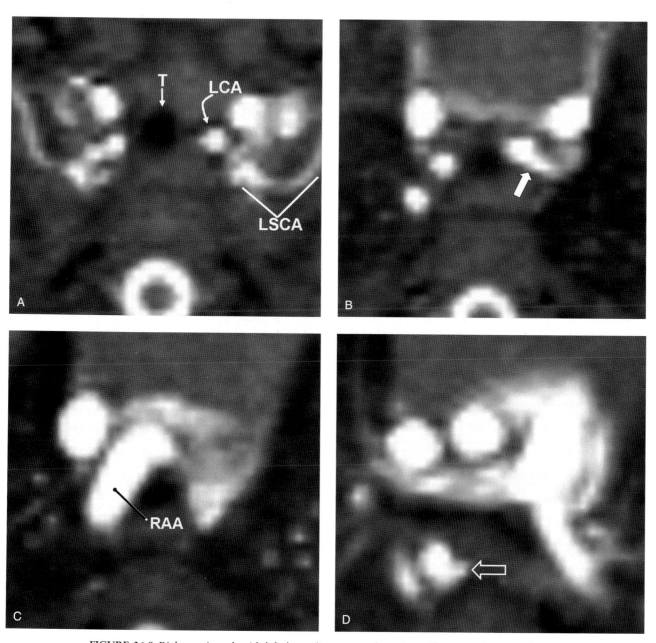

FIGURE 36.8 Right aortic arch with left ductus/ligamentum from descending aorta. **A–D:** Axial views from MRI. **A:** Superior image shows LSCA and LCA joining in **B** (*filled arrow*) and along with LCA and LSCA (not labeled) enter right aortic arch (RAA) shown in **C. D:** Inferior image shows dimple (*open arrow*) arising from left side of descending aorta. **E:** Coronal view shows dimple arising from left side of descending aorta. **F:** Embryonic arch diagram shows mirror-image right arch with left sixth arch connecting LPA to left dorsal aorta. Abbreviations as previously defined.

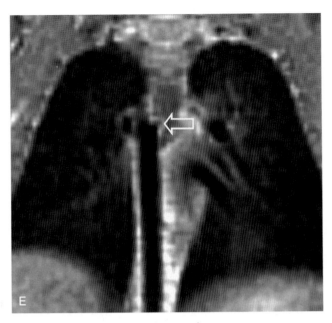

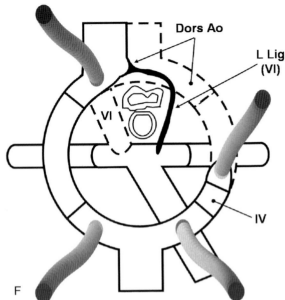

FIGURE 36.8 *(Continued)*

origin of the seventh intersegmental artery (distal subclavian artery precursor) so that the left fourth arch becomes the proximal subclavian artery rather than remaining as an aortic arch (Fig. 36.7C). Typically, the right sixth (ductal) arch involutes while the left sixth persists. However, with disappearance of the left dorsal aorta distal to the left seventh intersegmental artery, the sixth arch usually connects to the proximal or subclavian artery side of the disruption. Thus, in the definitive arch the left ductus arises from the underside of the left innominate artery and passes to the left pulmonary artery, appearing as a congenital modified left Blalock–Thomas–Taussig shunt. Alternatively, the left sixth arch will disappear and the right persist, giving a true mirror image of normal, that is, a ductus connecting the underside of the right-sided arch with the right pulmonary artery. Other cases, particularly when associated with tetralogy of Fallot, may have dissolution of both ductus. Finally, in those with retroesophageal ductus dimple, the left sixth arch connects the left pulmonary artery with the distal left dorsal aorta (Fig. 36.8F).

Diagnosis and Management

Since this type of right arch usually produces no retroesophageal compression or vascular ring, there are, with rare exception, no symptoms produced by the arch itself. Therefore, the diagnosis is usually made during imaging of the associated congenital intracardiac disease. The distinctive branching pattern can be used for echocardiographic and angiographic diagnosis, whereas the appearance of a right-sided indentation of trachea and esophagus on plain radiograph and barium esophagography, respectively, but without posterior impression on the esophagram, permits the diagnosis to be made with those modalities. The presence of a left innominate artery in a patient with symptoms suggestive of a vascular ring and in the absence of cyanotic congenital heart disease should suggest the differential diagnosis of the rare right arch, retroesophageal ductus or the more common right arch, left descending aorta or double aortic arch with atretic left arch distal to the subclavian artery (discussed below),

which is differentiated by presence of a left upper descending aorta.

No treatment of right aortic arch per se is required; however, it may be helpful for surgeons to know the sidedness of the aortic arch in certain circumstances. For systemic-to-pulmonary shunts, the classical Blalock–Thomas–Taussig (subclavian artery to pulmonary artery, direct end-to-side) anastomosis or the modified form (polytetrafluoroethylene [Gore-Tex] tube graft interposition side-to-side anastomosis of subclavian artery to pulmonary artery) are best carried out using the side with an innominate artery. With the classic form, the more nearly horizontal takeoff of the subclavian artery makes kinking of the vessel less likely when the cut end is brought down to the level of the pulmonary artery than with the subclavian artery arising directly from the arch. Even with Gore-Tex tube graft interposition, the innominate is a more favorable site of origin since the overall diameter of the innominate is greater, making the proximal anastomosis easier. Furthermore, the angle of takeoff is less acute, making kinking of the vessel of origin less likely even if there is some downward traction after completion of the anastomosis. Another situation in which knowledge of the side of the aortic arch may be useful is in the repair of esophageal atresia and tracheoesophageal fistula where it may be desirable to avoid having the arch obscure the view of the fistula.

Right Aortic Arch with Retroesophageal Diverticulum of Kommerell

Right arch with diverticulum of Kommerell is the second most common vascular ring after double aortic arch. It is far more common than its mirror image described above. It has as its first branch the left carotid artery, second the right carotid artery, third the right subclavian artery, and finally, a retroesophageal vessel from which the left subclavian artery arises and the left ductus arteriosus or ligamentum arteriosum connects (Fig. 36.9). This combination of vessels produces a

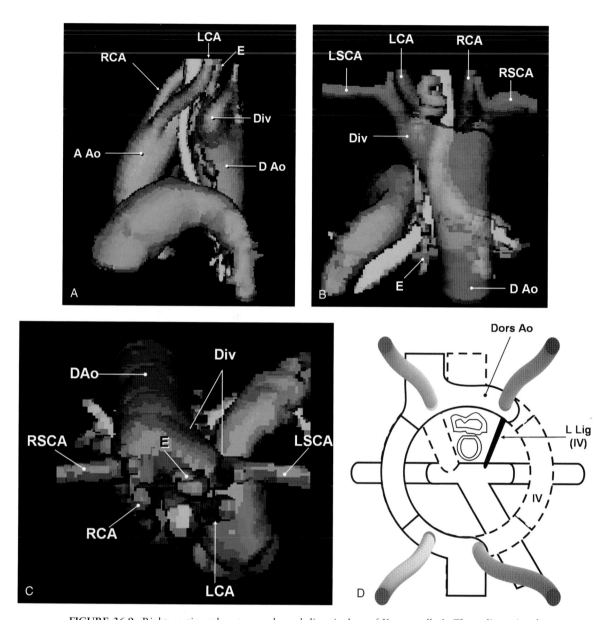

FIGURE 36.9. Right aortic arch, retroesophageal diverticulum of Kommerell. **A:** Three-dimensional reconstruction from MRI viewed in left anterior oblique. Trachea (*green*) and esophagus (E) are compressed by diverticulum (Div) tethered by ligamentum arteriosum (not visualized) to pulmonary artery (*blue*). **B:** Posterior view shows tapered Div behind esophagus giving rise to LSCA. The tracheal deviation to the left is seen through the translucent D Ao. Compare with Figure 36.10A. **C:** Cranial view shows trachea (*green*) and esophagus (E) compressed between Div and LCA and pulmonary artery (*blue*). **D:** Embryonic arch diagram showing formation of retroesophageal diverticulum from left dorsal aorta in the presence of a left ligamentum (L Lig [VI]). Abbreviations as previously defined.

vascular ring. The true incidence of this lesion is more difficult to obtain than that of mirror-image right arch where virtually all patients have associated intracardiac disease. However, of 26 consecutive patients undergoing surgical division of vascular rings at our institution, five (19%) had right arch, retroesophageal diverticulum, and most of them had no other heart defect. What is more, many people with this arch anomaly are asymptomatic and therefore go unrecognized except for incidental discovery.

If the ductus arteriosus is patent, it is easy to understand how one might visualize the complete ring formed by the aortic arch on the right, retroesophageal vessel supplying the left subclavian posteriorly, the ductus on the left and the pulmonary artery anteriorly. However, if the ductus is closed, it is not intuitive that one could distinguish this from the more benign right arch with retroesophageal subclavian artery (nonring) discussed below. The difference is the diverticulum of Kommerell, which is a much larger vessel than the subclavian artery itself. Typically, the origin of the diverticulum is equal in diameter to the descending aorta and tapers to the subclavian artery caliber at the site of juncture with the left ligamentum.

Embryology

Disappearance of the left fourth embryonic arch with persistence of the left sixth (ductal) arch between the truncoaortic sac (pulmonary artery precursor) and left dorsal aorta accounts for the findings in this arch anomaly (Fig. 36.9D). Note that the left dorsal aorta is not merely the proximal left subclavian artery but is also the continuation of the left sixth aortic arch leading to the fused dorsal aortae. Since the normal fetal ductus carries nearly the entire output of the right ventricle, the left dorsal aorta would also carry that amount and would become significantly larger than the subclavian artery. This size discrepancy persists after ductal closure, giving the diverticulum its characteristic appearance.

Diagnosis and Management

The presentation in symptomatic patients is usually that of a vascular ring. With that history, the appearance of a right aortic arch on a plain chest roentgenogram should raise the question of this anomaly and prompt further, more specific evaluation. Barium esophagram reveals a large posterior indentation on the esophagus similar to that seen in Figure 36.11E, in contrast to the smaller defect seen with simple retroesophageal subclavian artery (Fig. 36.3B). However, rare vascular rings such as left aortic arch with right descending aorta and right ligamentum can give similar findings on barium study, and since the surgical approach is different, this form of imaging should not be considered definitive. Although the ligamentum arteriosum is not visualized with any of the current imaging modalities, its presence is guaranteed by the characteristic appearance of the tapered diverticulum. Echocardiography will show the left carotid artery arising alone as the first arch vessel, but definitive diagnosis requires that the diverticulum be followed out to the point at which the caliber changes to that of the smaller subclavian artery. This is usually not possible since the trachea itself and nearby lung may thwart attempts to see this area. Angiography demonstrates the characteristic branching pattern, but more important, shows the abrupt change in caliber from diverticulum to subclavian artery. As mentioned previously in the section on left aortic arch with retroesophageal right subclavian artery, angiography in the straight anteroposterior (AP) view may produce superimposition of the posterior subclavian artery on the more anterior left carotid, giving the appearance of a left innominate artery as in mirror-image right aortic arch and therefore not a ring. However, careful single-frame viewing of cineangiography will confirm the separate origins. Contrast injection in the more distal portion of the arch will better delineate the plump aortic diverticulum giving rise to the noticeably smaller subclavian artery. Angiography, although definitive, showing both the characteristic branching pattern and the typical appearance of the aortic diverticulum requires arterial catheterization, less desirable in the young infant. Magnetic resonance imaging is ideal for making this diagnosis, being noninvasive and having the ability to display both vascular and airway structures. Axial or transverse imaging demonstrates the aortic arch to the right of the trachea and the diverticulum posterior to it. Coronal imaging shows the V-shaped juncture of the aortic diverticulum and the more right-sided descending aorta. However, computer-generated shaded-surface displays (three-dimensional representations) permit viewing of the entire aortic arch at once and in relationship to trachea and pulmonary artery (Fig. 36.9A–C), giving the surgeon a clear anatomic image with which to proceed.

Most people with this arch anomaly are asymptomatic. Treatment is surgical division of the ductus or ligamentum in those patients who are symptomatic. This is usually performed through a left thoracotomy, although a median sternotomy approach is preferred by some. Still others advocate not only division of the ligamentum but resection of the diverticulum and transfer of the left subclavian artery to the left carotid artery because of the recurrence of symptoms in some patients owing to compression from an aneurysmal diverticulum and traction by the subclavian artery (39).

In those patients undergoing surgery for another lesion such as an intracardiac abnormality or repair of tracheoesophageal fistula, even an asymptomatic ligamentum should be divided. With esophageal atresia, a symptomatic ring may be avoided when repairing the esophagus outside the ring.

Right Aortic Arch with Retroesophageal Left Subclavian Artery

Right aortic arch with retroesophageal (also called anomalous or aberrant) left subclavian artery consists of an arch passing to the right of the trachea with the following sequence of brachiocephalic arteries: Left carotid, right carotid, right subclavian, and retroesophageal left subclavian (Fig. 36.10A, B). This differs from the previous arch in that the proximal left subclavian artery is not significantly larger in caliber than its more distal portion (i.e., no aortic diverticulum). Therefore, there is no left-sided ductus arteriosus or ligamentum arteriosum and thus no vascular ring. Many of these patients have associated conotruncal anomalies. As has been noted previously, aberrant subclavian artery has a higher incidence of 22q11 deletion than does mirror-image right aortic arch (20).

Embryology

This is similar to the right arch with retroesophageal diverticulum with involution of the left fourth aortic arch but with loss of the left sixth (ductal) arch (Fig. 36.10C). In this way, the left dorsal aorta becomes only the proximal left subclavian artery and not the beginning of the descending aorta. A right sixth arch, if present, connects right pulmonary artery with right dorsal aorta, which is part of the definitive right arch.

Diagnosis and Management

The diagnosis may be suspected from barium esophagography with a relatively small posterior indentation on the esophagus passing upward to the left. Since there is no vascular ring, the trachea is unaffected except for the slight leftward deviation seen with virtually all right aortic arches. As noted above, echocardiography may be expected to identify the first branch of the aorta as a left carotid artery (since it does not bifurcate proximally as an innominate artery does and is similar in caliber to the second branch—right carotid artery), but appreciation of the size of the retroesophageal vessel itself may be difficult. Both magnetic resonance imaging and angiography can demonstrate the size of the left subclavian artery, which distinguishes this lesion from right aortic arch with retroesophageal diverticulum. Since there is no vascular ring, there is usually no need for treatment other than that of associated anomalies.

Right Aortic Arch with Left Descending Aorta and Left Ductus Arteriosus or Ligamentum Arteriosum

Right arch, left descending aorta, also known as right aortic arch with retroesophageal segment or circumflex right aortic

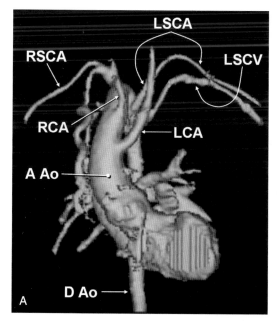

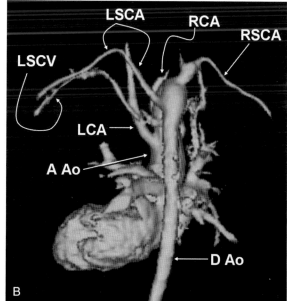

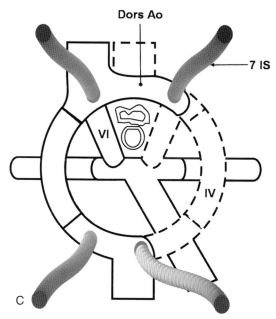

FIGURE 36.10 Right aortic arch with retroesophageal left subclavian artery. **A:** Three-dimensional reconstruction from MRI, left anterior oblique view. Note the constant caliber of the left subclavian artery, emerging from the aorta behind the trachea, compared with the marked tapering of a diverticulum of Kommerell (Fig. 36.9B). **B:** Embryonic arch diagram showing dissolution of left fourth and sixth arches. In the absence of a left ductus, the retroesophageal left dorsal aorta does not form a diverticulum. Abbreviations as previously defined.

arch, is similar in presentation to right arch with retroesophageal diverticulum (above), but it is less common. Unlike cases with retroesophageal diverticulum in which the aorta, after passing over the right mainstem bronchus, descends for some distance on the right, then gradually crosses to the left before reaching the level of the diaphragm, right arch left descending (aorta) has the aortic arch itself cross the midline to the left at the level of the T4 or T5 vertebral body, at which point it gives rise to the left ductus arteriosus or ligamentum arteriosum (Fig. 36.11). The first arch vessel may be the left innominate, followed by right carotid and right subclavian, or the left carotid artery alone, followed by the right carotid, right subclavian, and finally the left subclavian (Fig. 36.12). However, it is the aortic arch that is retroesophageal, not the subclavian artery or an aortic diverticulum.

Embryology

Two forms exist with dissolution of either the left dorsal aorta distal to the takeoff of the left subclavian artery (Fig. 36.11G) or the left fourth arch (Fig. 36.12E). The distal portion of the definitive arch is composed of the retroesophageal right-sided dorsal aorta. The persistent left sixth arch connects to the left-sided dorsal aorta, completing a vascular ring.

Diagnosis and Management

The findings on chest roentgenogram and barium esophagography (Fig. 36.11E) may be similar to those in right arch with retroesophageal diverticulum. Differences include a downward

(text continues on page 746)

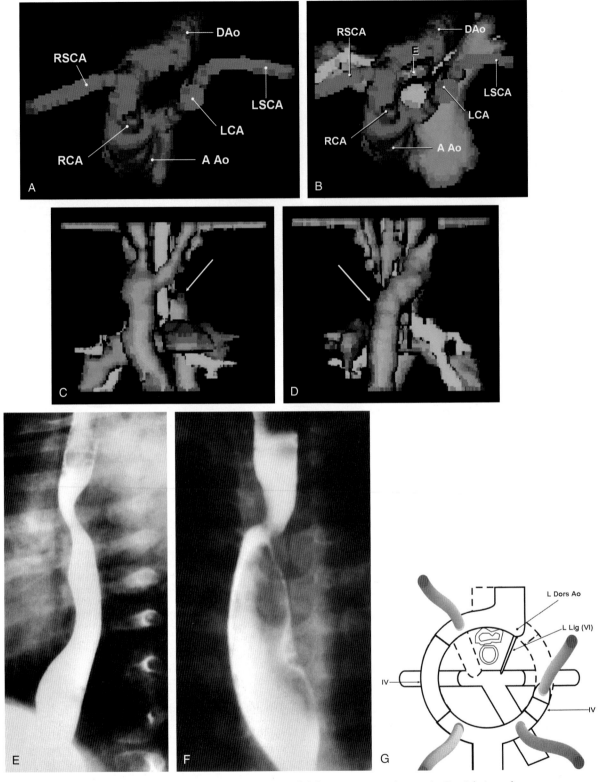

FIGURE 36.11 Right aortic arch, left descending aorta, left ligamentum arteriosum. **A:** Cranial view of 3-D reconstructed MRI showing takeoff of brachiocephalic arteries. **B:** Same view but with trachea (*green*), esophagus (E), and pulmonary artery (*blue*) showing further crowding. Anterior (**C**) and posterior (**D**) views of same reconstruction showing retroesophageal course of aortic arch with sharp turn inferiorly at point of attachment of ligamentum arteriosum to descending aorta (*arrow*). **E:** Barium esophagram in lateral view showing large posterior indentation. **F:** AP view showing bilateral indentations on the esophagus. Similar patterns are seen with double arch and right arch with diverticulum. **G:** Embryonic arch diagram showing left-sided descending aorta and dissolution of distal left dorsal aorta (L Dors Ao) with persistence of left ligamentum (L Lig [VI]). Abbreviations as previously defined.

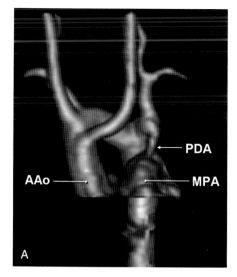

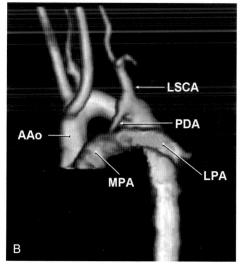

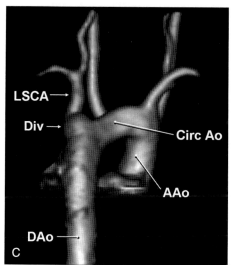

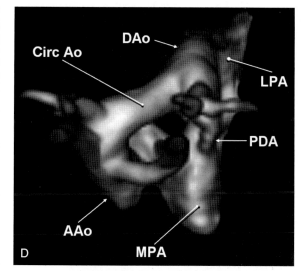

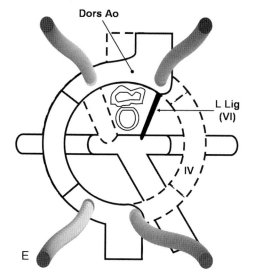

FIGURE 36.12 Right aortic arch with left descending aorta and aberrant left subclavian artery. 3-D shaded surface displays from MRI. **A:** Anterior view showing right-sided A Ao and left-sided descending aorta (labeled in **C** and **D**). First arch vessel is left carotid artery; last vessel is left subclavian artery. Patent ductus arteriosus (PDA) connects MPA to descending aorta. **B:** Left lateral view. **C:** Posterior view showing marked angulation between circumflex aortic arch and D Ao. **D:** Overhead view shows complete ring of vessels surrounding space occupied by trachea and esophagus (not displayed). Abbreviations as previously defined.

to the left instead of upward to the left orientation of the esophageal indentation (Fig. 36.11F). Furthermore, in some cases the descending aorta itself can be seen on the left of the spine instead of the right, but this is not a consistent finding. When associated with a hypoplastic arch, this anomaly can be mistaken for interrupted aortic arch (40).

With a projection image such as angiography, it may not be clear whether the aorta passes anterior to the trachea as it courses from right ascending to left descending, as is seen with a normal left aortic arch, or posterior to the trachea, i.e., a right aortic arch with left descending. A clue to which is the case (without attempting steep cranial angulation (usually more confusing than helpful because of overlapping shoulder, head, and liver) is the order of brachiocephalic artery branching. In the case of right aortic arch with left descending aorta, the first vessel contains the left carotid artery, whereas in normal left arches, a vessel containing a right carotid is first. Magnetic resonance imaging can avoid some of the pitfalls seen with projection images and can delineate the entire aorta, not only in its normal rightward ascending and leftward descending segments, but definitively in its relationship to the trachea (Fig. 36.11 A, B).

Division of the vascular ring is indicated when patients are symptomatic, although these are typically loose rings. However, an adult with dysphagia may require more than simple division of the ligamentum. Actual division of the aortic arch with mobilization of the retroesophageal portion and reanastomosis of ascending and descending aorta using a tube graft may be necessary to relieve the esophageal compression (41,42).

Right Aortic Arch with Retroesophageal Innominate Artery

Right aortic arch with retroesophageal (or aberrant) innominate artery is another rare abnormality of the aortic arch system.

Contrary to the general rule that the first arch vessel contains a carotid artery contralateral to the aortic arch, in these cases the sequence of brachiocephalic vessels is right carotid, right subclavian, retroesophageal left innominate artery (Fig. 36.13A). The ductus arteriosus or ligamentum arteriosum completes a vascular ring as it connects the left pulmonary artery with the base of the so-called innominate artery.

Embryology

The apparent site of arch dissolution is in the left branch of the truncoaortic sac (Fig. 36.13B). Thus the arch is formed by the right branch leading to the right fourth arch, which, in turn, connects to the right dorsal aorta. The left dorsal aorta supplies the left seventh intersegmental artery (distal left subclavian) and the left third arch (common carotid artery). It is not clear whether any remnant of the left fourth arch persists, although it may form the proximal left carotid artery.

Diagnosis and Management

With so few cases in the literature (43), it is difficult to draw conclusions about presentation and management. Tracheal compression seems to be the rule, although the degree of symptomatology varies considerably. The important anatomic clues to the diagnosis by any imaging modality are the presence of a single carotid artery arising from the proximal aorta. The other anomalies with that finding are also rare: Interrupted aortic arch with interruption between the two carotid arteries and isolated left carotid or innominate artery (see below). The differentiating feature is the presence of a normal-sized (right) aortic arch (missing in arch interruption) and the distal origin of the carotid artery from that arch (not present with isolated carotid or innominate). If symptomatic from the vascular ring, division of the ductus or ligamentum is in order. Conceivably in the adult, detachment of the innominate artery

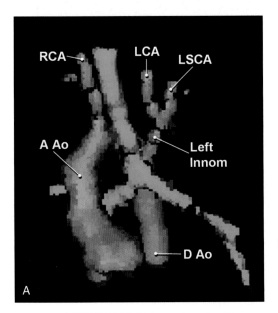

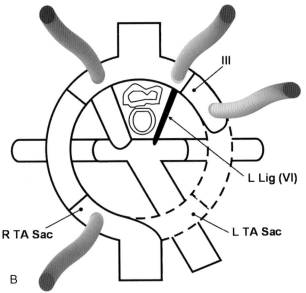

FIGURE 36.13 Right aortic arch with retroesophageal innominate artery. **A:** Left anterior oblique view of 3-D reconstruction from MRI showing LCA and LSCA arising from a single vessel, left innominate artery (Left Innom), from the D Ao. **B:** Diagram of embryonic arch contributions. Dissolution of left limb of truncoaortic sac (L TA Sac) with connection of left third arch to left dorsal aorta. R TA Sac, right limb of truncoaortic sac. Other abbreviations as previously defined.

from the distal arch and reimplantation in the ascending aorta might be necessary based on similar arch anomalies mentioned above in which the retroesophageal vessel continued to cause dysphagia even after relief of the ring by division of the ligamentum.

Right Aortic Arch with Isolation of Contralateral Arch Vessel

Isolation of brachiocephalic vessels is relatively uncommon. The term isolation means that the particular vessel arises exclusively from the pulmonary artery via the ductus arteriosus (or ligamentum) but without connection to the aorta. Three different forms have been noted: Isolation of the left subclavian artery (Fig. 36.14), isolation of the left carotid, and isolation of the left innominate artery. Isolated left subclavian is by far the most common of the three. Leutmer and Miller (44) reviewed the literature to 1990 describing 39 cases demonstrated by angiography or at postmortem examination. Congenital heart disease was found in more than half the cases with two thirds of those having tetralogy of Fallot. There are sporadic reports of isolated left innominate artery (45). A *forme fruste* is shown in Figure 36.15 with a small innominate artery and larger subclavian and carotid, suggesting that during fetal life they had been fed by a left ductus that had since closed.

Embryology

All cases of isolated arch vessels derive from two ipsilateral breaks in the aortic arch system (Fig. 36.14B). In isolated subclavian artery, the distal left dorsal aorta involutes after cephalad migration of the left seventh intersegmental (subclavian) artery to the level where left sixth (ductal) arch normally joins the proximal dorsal aorta. This together with involution of the left fourth arch leaves the subclavian isolated from the aortic arch but connected to the pulmonary artery via the ductus. In similar fashion, one could imagine disappearance of the left fourth arch and the left branch of the aortic sac with the sixth arch connecting the pulmonary artery portion of the truncoaortic sac to the third arch (common carotid artery precursor). With disruption of the left fourth arch, the left seventh intersegmental artery remains connected to the descending aorta via the left dorsal aorta, producing a retroesophageal left subclavian artery. It is postulated that isolated innominate artery derives from dissolution of the left branch of the aortic sac and the distal left dorsal aorta with the left sixth (ductal) arch connecting the pulmonary portion of the truncoaortic sac and the proximal dorsal aorta, which, in turn, feeds the left seventh intersegmental (subclavian) artery and the left third arch via the fourth. The resulting confluence of carotid and subclavian arteries is analogous to an innominate artery. An alternative mechanism based on identification of a pulmonary-to-brachiocephalic artery connection proximal to or upstream from the ductus in chick embryos is explained by an abnormal partition of the truncoaortic sac (46).

Diagnosis and Management

Cases of isolated brachiocephalic arteries may have diminished pulses or lower blood pressure in the affected artery. When the subclavian and vertebral arteries are involved, the possibility of subclavian steal syndrome exists in which blood flows down the vertebral artery into the subclavian, particularly when the arm is exercised. In 13% of cases reviewed by Leutmer and Miller (44), this produced cerebral insufficiency. Another 13% showed signs of left arm ischemia. If the ductus remains patent, pulmonary artery steal can occur with flow down the vertebral artery through the ductus into the low-resistance pulmonary artery (47). The diagnosis should be suspected in any patient with right aortic arch and diminished pulse amplitude or blood pressure in the left arm. Contrast injection in the aortic arch shows delayed filling of the subclavian artery via the vertebral and various collateral arteries (48).

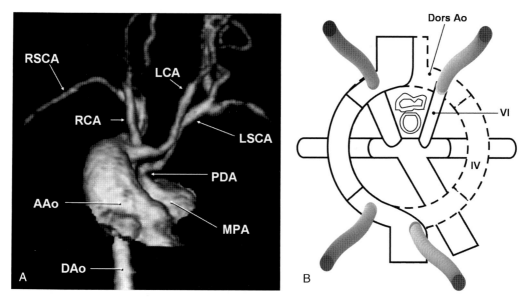

FIGURE 36.14 Right aortic arch with isolation of left subclavian artery. **A:** Anterior view of 3-D shaded-surface display from MRI shows exclusive origin of LSCA from left PDA. Sequence of arch vessels arising from aorta is LCA, RCA, RSCA. **B:** Embryonic arch diagram showing ipsilateral loss of fourth arch and distal dorsal aorta with persistence of ipsilateral sixth arch.

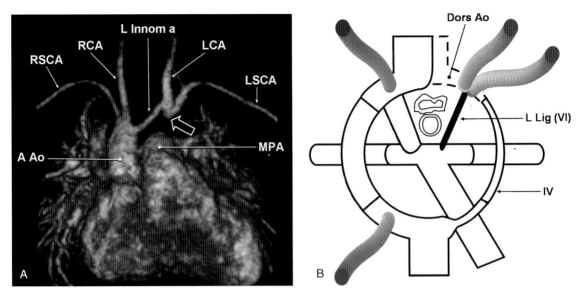

FIGURE 36.15 *Forme fruste* of isolated left innominate artery. Anterior view of 3-D shaded-surface display. Note small left innominate artery (LIA) giving rise to larger-caliber LSCA and LCA. These latter two appear to arise from a point consistent with a ligamentum arteriosum (*open arrow*) and apparently received more flow from that vessel than from the aorta during fetal development. Abbreviations as previously defined.

Barium esophagography is not helpful in making this diagnosis other than demonstration of the right aortic arch. Doppler echocardiography may be able to demonstrate the reversal of flow in the vertebral artery, which would corroborate this diagnosis, but phase-encoded velocity mapping on MRI can also be definitive.

Surgical management in children consists of repair of the accompanying heart disease and ligation of the ductus, if patent, to prevent pulmonary steal. Patients with central nervous system symptoms or claudication of the left arm may require surgical reimplantation of the subclavian artery into the carotid or aorta.

CERVICAL AORTIC ARCH

Cervical aortic arch is a rare anomaly in which the arch is found above the level of the clavicle (as high as the C2 vertebral body). There are two main subcategories of cervical arch: Those with anomalous subclavian artery and vascular ring, with either descending aorta contralateral to the arch (see Fig. 36.5) or retroesophageal diverticulum, and those with a virtual normal branching pattern. The first and larger group usually has a right aortic arch. This group is further subdivided into those with separate origins of the internal and external carotid arteries from the arch and those with a common carotid artery or a bicarotid trunk in which both common carotid arteries arise from a single vessel and the subclavian arteries both arise separately from the distal arch (49). Separate origin of the vertebral artery from the arch can be seen in each of the groups. Although most of the patients with contralateral descending aorta have an anatomic vascular ring from the aortic arch on the right, retroesophageal segment of aorta posteriorly, ligamentum arteriosum to the left, and pulmonary artery anteriorly, only about half are symptomatic from the ring. When a bicarotid trunk accompanies the contralateral descending aorta form of cervical arch, tracheal or esophageal compression

between the "V" of the bicarotid trunk and the retroesophageal aorta may occur without a complete vascular ring.

The second group (with ipsilateral descending aorta—nonring) typically has a left aortic arch. Aortic arch obstruction owing to a long, tortuous, hypoplastic retroesophageal segment is an uncommon but well-documented association (50). More discrete coarctations have been reported in both the ring and nonring groups (51). For reasons that are not clear, stenosis or atresia of the origin of the left subclavian artery is sometimes seen in either group (52).

Embryology

It would appear that the embryologic explanations for the various subgroups mentioned above are different. The normal common carotid artery comes about from the dissolution of the segment of dorsal aorta between the third and fourth embryonic arches, the so-called ductus caroticus. Both internal and external carotid arteries arise from the third arch. If the ductus caroticus were to persist while the embryonic fourth arch involutes, the embryonic third arch would become the definitive arch with separate internal and external carotid arteries arising from it (as they had when the third arch was, in part, the common carotid artery) (53). The third arch, being one branchial pouch higher than the fourth arch, would be expected to be more cephalad after completion of arch development. This type of cervical arch (i.e., with separate internal and external carotid arteries arising directly from the arch) owing to persistent ductus caroticus and absent fourth arch has been described in chromosome 22q11 deletion as previously mentioned (54).

An alternative explanation for this subgroup and more plausible for the other groups that have normal common carotid arteries, is a failure of the normal descent of the aortic arch system from its cephalic location at 3 weeks to its normal intrathoracic location by 7 weeks' gestation (55). The cause of this failure of caudal migration is not known.

Diagnosis and Management

Cervical arches may present as pulsatile masses in the supraclavicular fossa or in the neck. In infants, prior to the appearance of a mass, the presenting signs may be those of a vascular ring, namely, stridor, dyspnea, or repeated lower respiratory infections. In the adult, the most likely symptom from a vascular ring is dysphagia. In those patients with stenosis or atresia of the left subclavian artery and origin of the ipsilateral vertebral artery distal to the obstruction, a subclavian steal may exist with central nervous system symptomatology. In the presence of a pulsatile neck mass, a presumptive diagnosis can be made by notation of loss of femoral pulses during brief compression of the mass (52).

The diagnosis of cervical arch may be suspected on plain chest roentgenogram by the presence of a widened upper mediastinum and the absence of the aortic knob. Evidence of anterior deviation of the trachea is in favor of the diagnosis. In the past, angiography has been the standard diagnostic imaging tool, and in those cases with intracardiac anomalies, probably remains so. However, in those without congenital heart disease, the diagnosis of cervical aortic arch can by made by echocardiography. Treatment is necessary if the cervical arch is complicated by arch hypoplasia, symptomatic vascular ring, or rarely, aneurysm of the cervical arch itself (56). In these cases the surgical approach is dictated by the specific complicating feature. In some cases with cervical right aortic arch and a tortuous, hypoplastic retroesophageal segment, repair is accomplished by left-sided ascending-to-descending aorta anastomosis or tube graft interposition (57). Separate origin of external and internal carotid arteries from the arch warrants screening for 22q11 deletion.

DOUBLE AORTIC ARCH

Double aortic arch, as the name implies, is an anomaly in which both right and left aortic arches are present. Several variations on this basic theme occur: Both arches widely patent (Fig. 36.16A–D, G–K), hypoplasia of one arch (usually the left) (Fig. 36.16E, F), (occasionally the right) (Fig. 36.16L), and atresia of one arch, usually the left (Fig. 36.17). In addition, a ductus arteriosus or ligamentum may be present. Typically the right arch is the more superiorly located.

Although all double aortic arches technically form complete vascular rings around the trachea and esophagus, the branching pattern evident from various imaging modalities is determined by the patency of the various arch components and the side of the descending aorta. For example, whereas a double arch with both arches patent will show relatively symmetric origins of each of the four major brachiocephalic arteries from their respective arches (see Fig. 36.16K, L), double arch with atretic left arch distal to the origin of the left subclavian artery (see Fig. 36.17) will have a branching pattern similar to a mirror-image right aortic arch, that is, an apparent left innominate artery, followed by a right carotid and right subclavian, but with a left descending aorta. In fact, this pattern in conjunction with signs of tracheal compression may be indistinguishable (except at surgery) from the rare anomaly right aortic arch with left descending aorta, unless, as in Figure 36.17A, a distal left arch stump is present. Similarly, double arch with atretic left arch between left carotid and left subclavian can mimic right aortic arch with retroesophageal diverticulum of Kommerell. Atretic right arch is quite rare (58) but can simulate left arch variants. Of 17 patients at one institution undergoing division of the vascular ring, 11 had a left descending aorta, 6, a right (59). A review of 26 patients undergoing surgical division of vascular rings over an 8-year period at The Children's Hospital of Philadelphia showed 20 to have double aortic arches. Seventeen had both arches patent with the right arch larger in 16. The other three patients had an atretic left arch.

Double aortic arch is rarely associated with congenital heart disease, but when present, tetralogy of Fallot is most common (60), with transposition of the great arteries a distant second (60). Infrequent associated arch abnormalities including coarctation of the left (61) or both arches (62) and cervical left aortic arch (63) have been noted.

Embryology

Double aortic arch represents a persistence of both right and left embryonic fourth branchial arches joining the aortic portion of the truncoaortic sac to their respective dorsal aortae, both of which persist as well. Thus double aortic arch with both arches patent appears as persistence of the entire hypothetic double arch (Fig. 36.1) although usually with only one sixth (ductal) arch, whereas double arch with atretic left arch has patterns similar to either right arch with retroesophageal diverticulum (compare Fig. 36.17B with Fig. 36.9D) or right arch, left descending aorta (compare Fig. 36.17C with Fig. 36.11G). In keeping with the theme of absent or atretic fourth arches in 22q11 deletions, double arch with atretic left arch is more commonly associated with those syndromes than double arch with both widely patent.

Diagnosis and Management

The clinical manifestations of double aortic arches, as with the other vascular rings, are related to the tightness of the ring. With both arches widely patent, the rings are typically tight, and patients present with stridor in the first weeks of life, whereas with double arch and atretic left arch, the rings are usually looser with presentations at 3 to 6 months of age or later. Rarely, double aortic arches present in adulthood with swallowing or respiratory symptoms (64). The diagnosis of double arch with both arches patent can sometimes be made convincingly from the plain chest roentgenogram. The tracheal air column is indented by the more superior, right-sided arch and the more inferior left arch. In the lateral view, the right arch can be seen to indent the trachea posteriorly. These findings may be more obvious with barium esophagography. However confirmation by echocardiography, angiography, or magnetic resonance imaging is desirable because the two arches may be unequal in caliber, and it is important to identify the hypoplastic segment to divide it. In addition, a weblike coarctation of one arch may not be detectable by the surgeon from the external appearance of the vessel (65). Suprasternal imaging (66) permits the most extensive echocardiographic visualization of the two arches, whereas subcostal (67) and high parasternal imaging (68) rely more on deductive interpretation. Although statistically the left arch is much more likely to be hypoplastic than the right, numerous exceptions to that rule necessitate detailed evaluation of each case. Angiography has long been the standard for diagnosis but can be confusing because of overlapping structures. Digital

(text continues on page 752)

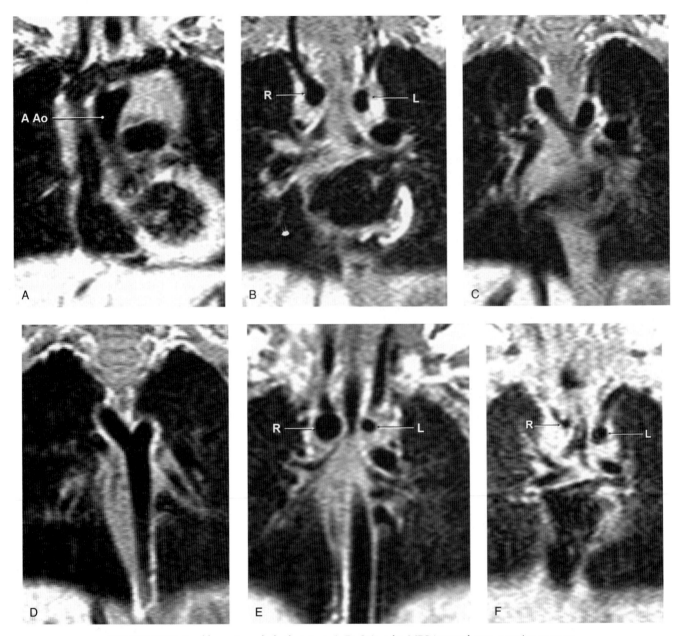

FIGURE 36.16 Double aortic arch, both patent. **A–D:** Spin echo MRI (coronal cuts, anterior to posterior) showing ascending aorta (A Ao) dividing into equal sized right (R) and left (L) aortic arches reuniting posteriorly as the descending aorta. **E–F:** Coronal images of patients with double arch, dominant right in **E** and rare case of dominant left in **F**. **G–J:** transverse cuts, cranial to caudal, from same patient as in **A–D.** Note marked decrease in caliber of trachea (T) from **G** to **H**, indicative of tracheal compression. **K:** 3-D shaded-surface display from MRI, left posterior oblique view with cranial angulation of same patient as in **A–D** and **G–J.** Note double aortic arch with nearly equal-sized right (R arch) and left (L arch) distal aortic arch components. **L:** 3-D shaded surface display from MRI, left posterior oblique view with cranial angulation showing large left and diminutive right arch surrounding trachea (green).

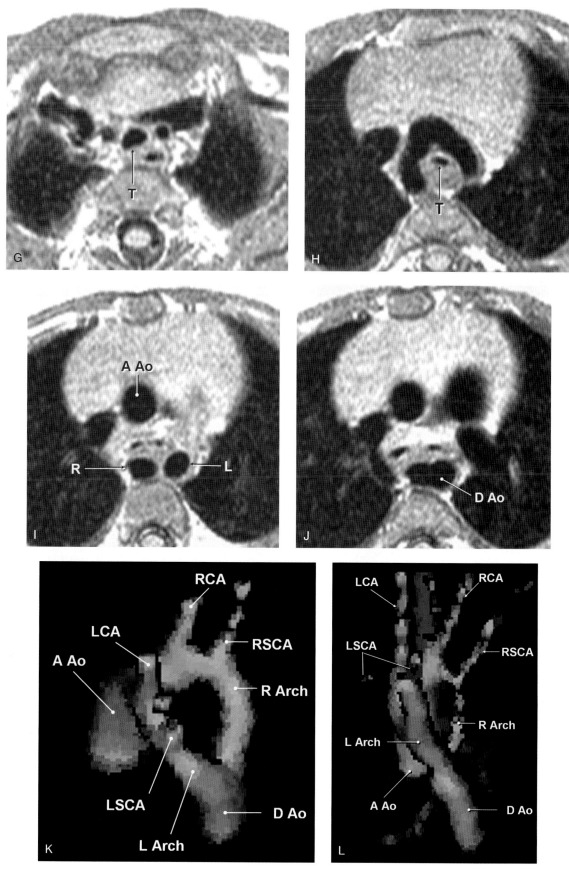

FIGURE 36.16 (*Continued*)

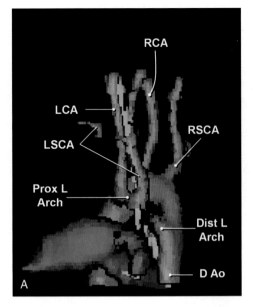

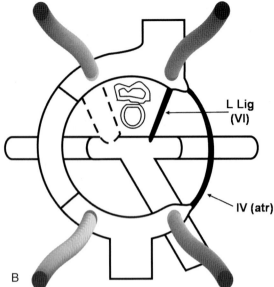

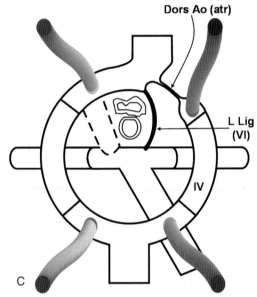

FIGURE 36.17 Double aortic arch with atretic left arch. **A:** 3-D shaded surface display from MRI of atretic left arch distal to left subclavian artery (LSCA) as in **C** (below). Patent proximal left aortic arch (Prox L Arch) connects LSCA with left carotid artery (LCA). Presence of a distal left arch (Dist L Arch) aimed at Prox L Arch and not at pulmonary artery (*blue*) ensures atretic left arch. **B:** Diagram of embryonic arches showing vascular ring formed by atretic left fourth arch (IV [atr]). **C:** Diagram of embryonic arches showing atretic distal portion of dorsal aorta (Dors Ao [atr]). Abbreviations as previously defined.

subtraction angiography (67) is less invasive but offers less sequential data. Magnetic resonance imaging provides information both noninvasively and together with the important spatial relationships of the vessels, trachea, and esophagus to better permit surgical planning (69).

Surgical division of the vascular ring is indicated in any patient who is symptomatic with airway or esophageal compression or in a patient undergoing surgery for intracardiac disease. The ring should be divided in its smaller limb, usually but not always the left. The decision to divide between left carotid and left subclavian or distal to the left subclavian is usually determined by accessibility and the length of the particular segment. In the absence of an accompanying conotruncal anomaly with a large ventricular septal defect, a ductus arteriosus must be present prenatally. Although the presence of a ductus or ligamentum does not appear to contribute to the severity of tracheal compression by the vascular ring, its

importance lies in the surgical management. If the arch is divided but the ligamentum remains intact, there may still be a vascular ring. Thus the surgeon must dissect down to the level of the trachea to be sure that all vascular contributors to a ring have been divided.

PERSISTENT FIFTH AORTIC ARCH

Persistent fifth aortic arch was first reported in man by Van Praagh and Van Praagh in 1969 (70) as a double-lumen aortic arch in which both arches appear on the same side of the trachea, as opposed to double aortic arch in which each arch is on the opposite side. Since the initial report, at least one other variation has been noted, resulting in the following subcategorization of this rare anomaly: Double-lumen aortic arch with both lumina patent and (Fig. 36.18C) atresia or

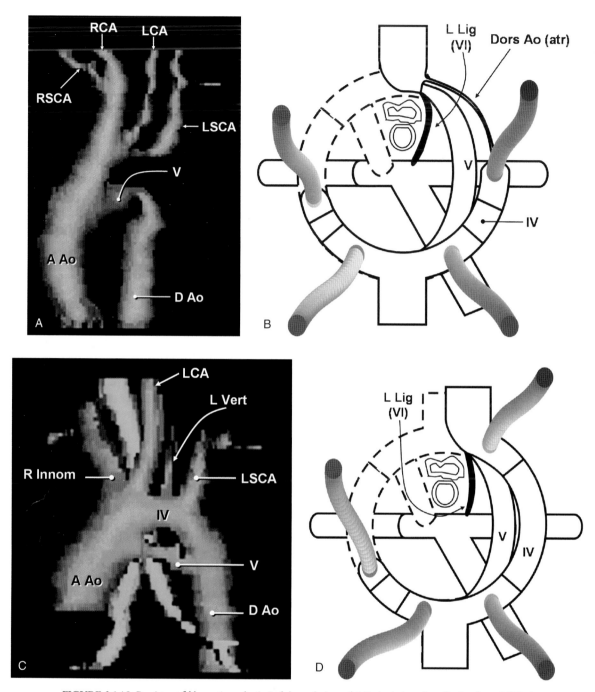

FIGURE 36.18 Persistent fifth aortic arch. **A:** Left lateral view of 3-D shaded-surface display from MRI of atretic fourth arch type. Note coarctation of fifth arch distally. At surgery, an atretic strand attaching the inferior aspect of the left subclavian artery (LSCA) to descending aorta (D Ao) beyond the coarctation was found. **B:** Embryonic arch diagram of case in **A**. **C:** Left lateral view of 3-D shaded-surface display from MRI of double-lumen type persistent fifth aortic arch. Note the trachea (T) behind both the embryonic fourth (IV) and fifth (V) arches. Incidentally, there is separate origin of the left vertebral artery (L Vert) from the normal fourth arch. **D:** Embryonic arch diagram of case in **C**. Abbreviations as previously defined.

interruption of the superior arch with patent inferior (persistent fifth) arch—common origin of all brachiocephalic vessels from the ascending aorta (Fig. 36.18A). Double-lumen aortic arch, in which a "subway" vessel occurs beneath the normal aortic (embryonic fourth) arch, appears to be the more common of the two types (71). This inferior arch extends from

the innominate artery to a point opposite the take-off of the left subclavian artery, just proximal to the ductus arteriosus or its remnant. Although frequently associated with major cardiac anomalies, it can be an incidental finding without clinical significance (72,73). Cases of atresia or interruption of the superior arch, with a single arterial trunk giving rise to all four brachiocephalic arteries, have had coarctation of the aorta as the cause for presentation (71).

Embryology

Although some animals have been noted to have all six pairs of branchial arches during embryonic development, the fifth pair is often seen as only incomplete arches in man (13), implying a brief appearance with no remnant in the definitive arch system. To understand the contribution of a persistent fifth arch to the development of the definitive arch, a modification to the hypothetic double arch is necessary (Fig. 36.18B, D). In cases of double-lumen aortic arch, the fourth arch persists as the superior arch connecting truncoaortic sac to dorsal aorta, and the fifth (inferior) arch does the same (Fig. 36.18D). With atresia or interruption of the superior arch, the fourth arch serves as the connection between carotid and subclavian artery, similar to an innominate artery, but ipsilateral to the definitive arch, which is the fifth arch. The portion of the dorsal aorta between the entrance of the fourth and fifth arches is atretic or disappears completely (Fig. 36.18B).

Diagnosis and Management

Double-lumen aortic arch has been recognized either by angiography or at postmortem examination, with the appearance of a subway vessel beneath the normal arch. This can also be seen with MRI as well, in coronal or off-axis sagittal (candy cane) sections, since axial slices have to be thin enough to resolve the small gap between the two arches (73). In atresia or interruption of the superior arch, there is the appearance of a truly common brachiocephalic trunk in which all four arch vessels, including the left subclavian artery, arise from a single vessel (Fig. 36.18A). In this situation, the branching pattern alone is the indication of a persistent fifth arch since the atretic dorsal aortic extension of the fourth arch cannot be visualized. However, at surgery for repair of coarctation of the aorta (distal to the fifth arch), an atretic strand connecting the left subclavian artery to the descending aorta may be seen. There appears to be no other plausible explanation for such a branching pattern. Without additional coarctation of the existing aorta, these two arch anomalies alone have no physiologic significance.

INTERRUPTED AORTIC ARCH

Interrupted, or congenitally absent, aortic arch is defined as a complete separation of ascending and descending aorta. It comprises several different anomalies, which generally relate to the pattern of branching of the brachiocephalic arteries. There are at least nine theoretically possible branching patterns. Celoria and Patton (74) classified these as type A if the interruption was distal to the left subclavian artery, type B if between carotid and subclavian arteries, and type C if between carotid arteries. However, these types may be further subcategorized (75) and definitions generalized to include both right and left arch patterns as follows:

A. Interruption distal to that subclavian artery that is ipsilateral to second carotid artery (i.e., if first carotid is right, interruption distal to left subclavian artery)
   1. Without retroesophageal or isolated subclavian artery
   2. With retroesophageal subclavian artery
   3. With isolated subclavian artery
B. Interruption between second carotid and ipsilateral subclavian artery
   1. Without retroesophageal or isolated subclavian artery
   2. With retroesophageal subclavian artery (i.e., both carotid arteries proximal, both subclavians distal) (Fig. 36.19A)
   3. With isolated subclavian artery
C. Interruption between carotid arteries
   1. Without retroesophageal or isolated subclavian artery
   2. With retroesophageal subclavian artery
   3. With isolated subclavian artery

The order of brachiocephalic artery branching suggests a right or left aortic arch pattern following the conventions of noninterrupted arches: In general, the first branch of the aorta proximal to the interruption contains the carotid artery opposite the side of the presumptive arch; a retroesophageal or isolated subclavian artery is always opposite the side of the presumptive arch. The significance of sidedness of the presumptive arch in cases of interruption is the finding that interrupted right aortic arch is apparently seen only in association with DiGeorge syndrome (76).

Type A interruptions tend to occur with aorticopulmonary septal defect and intact ventricular septum (77); they are seen in a disproportionately large subgroup of patients with transposition of the great arteries and interrupted aortic arch (75). Type B interruptions are much more common than type A and usually have a conotruncal anomaly with normally aligned great arteries in which there is a large malalignment-type ventricular septal defect associated with posterior displacement of the infundibular septum and subaortic obstruction. Those patients with DiGeorge syndrome and interruption have type B. Type C interruption is quite rare, permitting no general conclusions about associations.

Embryology

The etiology of interrupted aortic arches can be thought of in terms similar to those that describe the formation of the other arch anomalies discussed above. Type A interruptions show involution of both dorsal aortae distal to the fourth arches and proximal to the persistent sixth arch, which supplies the descending aorta in place of the fourth arch (Fig. 36.19C). Type B interruptions show involution of one fourth arch and one dorsal aorta between arches four and six (Fig. 36.19D) or, in the frequent variant with both subclavian arteries distal to the interruption, involution of both fourth arches and the sixth arch contralateral to the descending aorta (Fig. 36.19B). Type C interruption entails involution of one limb of the truncoaortic sac and its associated proximal third arch and entire fourth arch with persistence of the normally involuted dorsal aorta between arches three and four, the so-called ductus caroticus (Fig. 36.19E).

Virtually all cases of interruption between carotid and subclavian arteries (type B) are associated with a conotruncal anomaly in which hypoplasia of the subaortic region causes subaortic obstruction and a conal septal malalignment type of ventricular septal defect (78). The pathophysiology of the interruption is thought to be an absolute decrease in left ventricular output to the ascending aorta (owing to the combination of outflow obstruction and VSD) with maintenance of normal cerebral perfusion, resulting in a

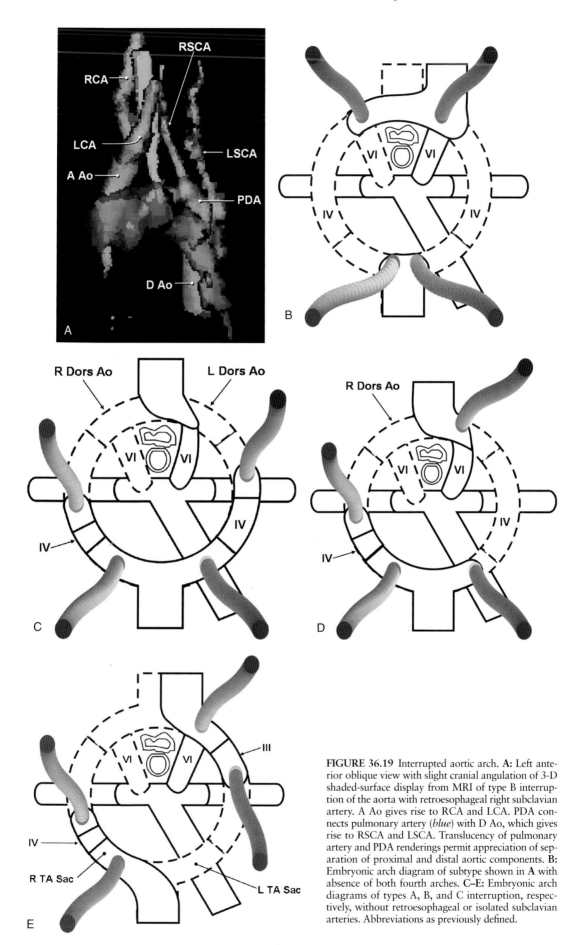

FIGURE 36.19 Interrupted aortic arch. **A:** Left anterior oblique view with slight cranial angulation of 3-D shaded-surface display from MRI of type B interruption of the aorta with retroesophageal right subclavian artery. A Ao gives rise to RCA and LCA. PDA connects pulmonary artery (*blue*) with D Ao, which gives rise to RSCA and LSCA. Translucency of pulmonary artery and PDA renderings permit appreciation of separation of proximal and distal aortic components. **B:** Embryonic arch diagram of subtype shown in **A** with absence of both fourth arches. **C–E:** Embryonic arch diagrams of types A, B, and C interruption, respectively, without retroesophageal or isolated subclavian arteries. Abbreviations as previously defined.

relatively large decrease in flow through the aortic arches beyond the takeoff of one or both carotid arteries. The contributing factors that determine precisely which combination of arch involutions occur in each case are not understood. In a large series of cases with DiGeorge syndrome (79), 43% were found to have type B interrupted aortic arch, and 68% of interrupted arch patients had DiGeorge syndrome. This contrasts with truncus arteriosus communis in which comparable figures were 34% and 33%, respectively. Again we see the predisposition to fourth arch abnormality in 22q11 patients. Cases in which subaortic obstruction is not present to explain arch involution are not well understood but may well relate to primary neural crest cell direct influence on the aortic arches themselves.

Diagnosis and Management

These patients typically present, similarly to patients with other ductal-dependent left heart obstructive lesions, with acute cardiovascular collapse or heart failure after spontaneous closure of the ductus arteriosus in the first days of life. Initial management entails fluid resuscitation, induction and maintenance of ductal patency with prostaglandin E_1, and establishment of stable hemodynamics, with inotropic support if necessary. Physical findings of pulse discrepancy, depending on branching pattern, are helpful only after restoration of satisfactory cardiac output. Absence of all limb pulses suggests interruption type B with anomalous subclavian artery, i.e., both carotid arteries proximal, both subclavians distal to the interruption. Strong carotid pulses help to differentiate interrupted arch from critical aortic stenosis in which all pulses are diminished. Differential cyanosis (pink upper body, blue lower body), although theoretically possible, is uncommonly seen since pulmonary arterial blood (hence ductal blood) is relatively highly saturated because of the large left-to-right shunt through the VSD. Currently, two-dimensional echocardiography is the most important tool for diagnostic imaging of interrupted arch. The diagnosis should be suspected from the marked discrepancy in size between ascending aorta and main pulmonary artery (80) with subcostal frontal imaging, in the presence of the typical malalignment type VSD with posterior deviation of the infundibular (conal) septum, best visualized in the parasternal long-axis view. Imaging of the arch entails determination of the branching pattern and notation of patency of the arch from suprasternal or high parasternal imaging (81). The smooth superior course of the carotid artery origins, especially in type B interruptions, in contrast to the usual posterior course of an intact aortic arch, is a further clue to the presence of interruption. Angiography is still used in many centers to confirm the diagnosis of interrupted aortic arch; however, torrential flow through a VSD makes it difficult to obtain high-quality imaging of the ascending aorta to distinguish between interruption and severe arch hypoplasia. Interruption can be diagnosed consistently by angiography when both carotid arteries arise proximal to, and both subclavian arteries distal to, the interruption (and ductus). The wide separation of carotid arteries from descending aorta unequivocally demonstrates interruption. Three-dimensional reconstruction from MRI can demonstrate the branching pattern and the separation between proximal and distal aorta (Fig. 36.19A).

The surgical approach to treatment depends on the degree of subaortic obstruction. Subaortic diameters of ≥5 to 6 mm seem to be compatible with primary intracardiac repair, namely patch closure of the VSD, plus aortic arch reconstruc-

tion. Subaortic regions of ≤3 mm are inadequate to support normal cardiac output in a full-term infant. In the case of normally aligned great arteries, the subaortic obstruction must be bypassed. The preferred method is to associate the proximal main pulmonary artery with ascending aorta using homograft augmentation to complete the aortic reconstruction, similar to that used for hypoplastic left heart syndrome (Norwood operation) (82). Pulmonary blood flow is provided by a Gore-Tex tube graft from the reconstructed aorta if the VSD is left open, or by a right ventricle–to–pulmonary artery confluence conduit if the ventricles are separated by a baffle from left ventricle to pulmonary valve via the VSD. When interrupted aortic arch is associated with transposition of the great arteries, arterial switch operation is combined with transannular patch across the neopulmonary outflow. Pulmonary artery banding is not a satisfactory palliation of VSD with interrupted aortic arch because it frequently results in biventricular hypertrophy with progressive subaortic stenosis, thus complicating definitive repair by any method at a later date.

The aortic arch itself can almost always be reconstructed by liberal dissection around the two arch components with direct anastomosis of the two ends (83) plus homograft augmentation of the reconstructed arch when necessary to achieve adequate arch size. Artificial tube grafts connecting proximal and distal aorta should be avoided in the initial operation in infancy, if possible, since they are rapidly outgrown, and with fibrous tissue encasement of the native aorta, complicate primary end-to-end anastomosis at a later date.

OTHER ANOMALIES OF THE AORTIC ARCH SYSTEM

Anomalous Origin of the Pulmonary Artery from the Ascending Aorta

Anomalous pulmonary artery branch arising from the ascending aorta in the presence of a main pulmonary artery arising separately from the heart is a rare anomaly. Although the term "hemitruncus" has been used, this lesion should be distinguished from true truncus arteriosus communis, with only one pulmonary artery branch arising in common with the ascending aorta and the other arising from a ductus or systemic collateral vessel from the descending aorta.

By far the more common form is anomalous origin of the right pulmonary artery, seen in 82% of 108 cases of an excellent review by Kutsche and Van Mierop (84). All had left aortic arch; many had patent ductus arteriosus; few had tetralogy of Fallot. Interrupted aortic arch distal to the left subclavian artery or coarctation of the aorta were present in 14% of those where the pulmonary artery arose just above the aortic valve, and 8 of 11 of those had an aorticopulmonary septal defect. In contrast, anomalous origin of the left pulmonary artery was associated with tetralogy of Fallot in 74%, and all cases had either tetralogy or right aortic arch or both. No cases of aorticopulmonary septal defect or interrupted aortic arch were present.

Embryology

The rather dramatic difference in associations between anomalous left and right pulmonary artery origins suggests different embryologic mechanisms. Kutsche and Van Mierop (84) propose that in anomalous origin of the right pulmonary artery, the embryonic branch pulmonary artery joins the truncoaortic sac (at its right side) but fails in leftward migration to reach the main pulmonary artery portion before septation occurs. They point out that this probably accounts for the significant incidence of aorticopulmonary septal defect. The mechanism of anomalous origin of the left pulmonary artery may be failure of the embryonic branch pulmonary artery to join the truncoaortic sac (or subsequent separation from it) in association with absence of the left sixth (ductal) arch and perhaps persistence of the left fifth arch, whereby the left pulmonary artery becomes associated with the ascending aorta.

Diagnosis and Management

The clinical presentation of anomalous origin of a pulmonary artery branch from the ascending aorta is predominantly that of congestive heart failure in infancy followed by the development of pulmonary vascular disease as early as 6 months of age, if unrepaired. In some patients, there may be an abbreviated (or no) period of clinical heart failure, in which case they may go on to develop pulmonary vascular obstructive disease without warning. Although many have a significant systolic murmur from turbulent, increased pulmonary blood flow, some have little or no murmur and only a loud, narrowly split or single second heart sound to suggest the abnormality. The above findings may be tempered by the relatively infrequent association with other major anomalies such as tetralogy of Fallot or interrupted aortic arch.

The chest roentgenogram may show differential pulmonary vascular markings, especially when superimposed on decreased flow in association with tetralogy of Fallot. Echocardiography is diagnostic, but one must be aware of the potential for mistaking right pulmonary artery merging posteriorly with aorta for normal confluence with main pulmonary artery when using a subcostal frontal sweep. Imaging in multiple views including parasternal short-axis permits differentiation of the pulmonary artery bifurcation from the juncture of right pulmonary artery with ascending aorta. In the case of the very uncommon origin of left pulmonary artery, the rule of thumb is to carefully search for all possible origins of both pulmonary artery branches in the face of tetralogy of Fallot. The more lateral origin of the left pulmonary artery from the ascending aorta also makes imaging of this abnormality easier. Cardiac catheterization usually shows pulmonary hypertension in both pulmonary arteries, although only one can be entered from the right ventricle via the main pulmonary artery. Angiographic demonstration is possible with a left ventriculogram but requires an ascending aortogram if there is a VSD. In patients with unexplained pulmonary hypertension, aortic root injection to rule out origin of a pulmonary artery branch from the ascending aorta or the physiologically similar aorticopulmonary septal defect should be considered. Although MRI can be diagnostic, at present it cannot be used to quantify pulmonary vascular resistance. Treatment consists of surgical division of the anomalously connected pulmonary artery branch and anastomosis directly, or with a graft, to the main pulmonary artery. This should be carried out as early as possible to avoid the development of pulmonary vascular disease.

Anomalous Origin of the Left Pulmonary Artery from the Right Pulmonary Artery

Origin of the left pulmonary artery from the right pulmonary artery, also known as anomalous left pulmonary artery, or pulmonary artery sling (85), is a rare anomaly in which the lower trachea is partially surrounded by vascular structures:

The left pulmonary artery arising as a very proximal branch of the right loops around the trachea. It is the only situation in which a major vascular structure passes between the trachea and esophagus. Pulmonary sling is frequently associated with complete cartilaginous rings in the distal trachea (86) resulting in tracheal stenosis, which may require direct surgical treatment in addition to relief from vascular compression. It usually appears as an isolated abnormality but can be associated with other congenital cardiac defects, including tetralogy of Fallot.

Embryology

The distal pulmonary arteries normally arise from their respective lung buds and join the pulmonary artery portion of the truncoaortic sac separately. If the two distal arteries join each other by incorporation of potential vascular islets from the splanchnic bed before becoming incorporated into the truncoaortic sac, one possibility is that the left pulmonary artery would pass behind the trachea before making this juncture. This would result in pulmonary artery sling. If it passed in front of the trachea, this would be indistinguishable from the normal situation.

Diagnosis and Management

These patients typically present with severe respiratory distress and stridor, although milder forms do exist and may be identified incidentally during imaging for another cardiovascular anomaly. Barium swallow when classic (Fig. 36.20A) is diagnostic if one can rule out mediastinal tumor. However, nondiagnostic barium swallows are common, and more definitive testing with either echocardiography, angiocardiography, MRI, or CT (Fig. 36.20C) is usually necessary to ensure the accuracy of the diagnosis. Symptomatic patients should be evaluated by bronchoscopy at the time of surgical repair because of the frequent association of complete cartilaginous rings. The usual surgical approach is division of the left pulmonary artery from the right and reanastomosis in front of the trachea. Alternatively, Jonas et al. (87) have recommended leaving the pulmonary artery and its branches intact while transecting the trachea, mobilizing it behind the pulmonary artery bifurcation and reanastomosing it. If complete cartilaginous tracheal rings are present, tracheal reconstruction may also be necessary. The latter approach is more amenable in that case since the trachea is already opened.

Innominate Artery Compression of the Trachea

Innominate artery compression of the trachea or so-called anomalous innominate artery is a poorly understood abnormality in which there is anterior compression of the trachea at the point where it is crossed by the innominate artery. Some have thought this due to a more distal, that is, leftward, takeoff of the innominate artery from the aortic arch; however three-dimensional reconstructions from MRI have not demonstrated any consistent abnormality of the aorta or its branching pattern. The presumed abnormality is tracheomalacia, whether idiopathic or in association with tracheoesophageal fistula (88), with the innominate artery in the vicinity of the malacic segment of trachea. The diagnosis is suspected when signs of severe inspiratory and expiratory stridor, usually in a 2- to 6-month-old child, are associated with anterior indentation of the tracheal air column on lateral chest roentgenogram.

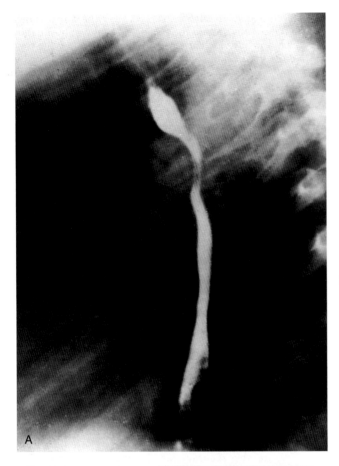

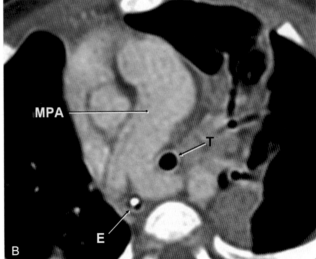

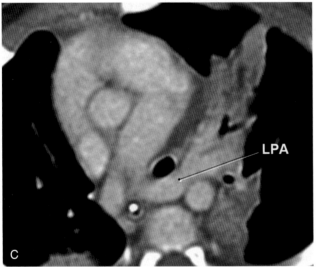

FIGURE 36.20 Anomalous origin of left pulmonary artery from right pulmonary artery (sling). **A:** Barium esophagram showing classic anterior indentation. **B** and **C:** Consecutive images from CT scan of another patient, showing left pulmonary artery (LPA) looping around a small distal trachea (T) but anterior to the esophagus (E) with high signal from a nasogastric tube. MPA, main pulmonary artery.

However, vascular rings should be ruled out with at least a barium esophagram. Simultaneous visualization of the innominate artery and the trachea is afforded by MRI and is shown dramatically with three-dimensional reconstruction (Fig. 36.21). Treatment usually entails waiting for the tracheomalacia to resolve, typically by age 2 years; however, in cases associated with apnea or repeated lower respiratory infections, surgical sectioning of the innominate artery and reimplantation more proximally, i.e., rightward in the aorta may be helpful. In limited cases suspension of the sternum has been used, but there is often little room behind the sternum to relieve pressure on the trachea.

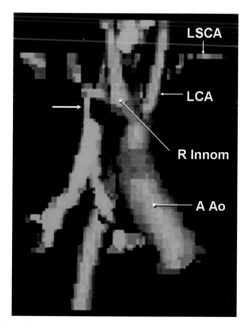

FIGURE 36.21. Innominate artery compression of the trachea. Right anterior oblique view of 3-D shaded-surface display from MRI showing severely compressed midtrachea (*arrow*) adjacent to innominate artery (Innom). Abbreviations as previously defined.

References

1. Hunauld. Examen de quelques parties d'un singe. *Hist Acad Roy Sci* 1735;2:516–523.
2. Hommel. Commercium literarium norimbergae. *Hebdom* 1737;21:162.
3. Fioratti G, Aglietti F. Osservazione anatomica. *Saggi Sci Litterari Acad Padova* 1763;1:69–72.
4. Steidele RJ. Sammlung verschiedener in der chirurgischen praktischen Lehrschule gemachten Boebachtungen. *Vienna* 1788;2:114–116.
5. Bayford D. An account of a singular case of obstructed deglutition. *Mem Med Soc London* 1794;2:275–286.
6. Gross RE. Surgical relief for tracheal obstruction from a vascular ring. *N Engl J Med* 1945;233:586–590.
7. Merrill DL, Webster CA, Samson PC. Congenital absence of the aortic isthmus. *J Thorac Surg* 1957;33:311–320.
8. Burke RP, Chang AC. Video-assisted thoracoscopic division of a vascular ring in an infant: A new operative technique.[see comment]. *J Card Surg* 1993;8:537–540.
9. Koontz CS, Bhatia A, Forbess J, et al. Video-assisted thoracoscopic division of vascular rings in pediatric patients. *Am Surg* 2005;71:289–291.
10. Mihaljevic T, Cannon JW, del Nido PJ. Robotically assisted division of a vascular ring in children. *J Thorac Cardiovasc Surg* 2003;125:1163–1164.
11. Kuratani S, Kirby ML. Initial migration and distribution of the cardiac neural crest in the avian embryo: An introduction to the concept of the circumpharyngeal crest. *Am J Anat* 1991;191:215–227.
12. Momma K, Matsuoka R, Takao A. Aortic arch anomalies associated with chromosome 22q11 deletion (CATCH 22). *Pediatr Cardiol* 1999;20:97–102.
13. Congdon ED. Transformation of the aortic-arch system during the development of the human embryo. *Contrib Embryol* 1922;14:47–110.
14. Edwards JE. Anomalies of the derivatives of the aortic arch system. *Med Clin North Am* 1948;32:925–949.
15. Stewart JR, Kincaid OW, Edwards JE. *An Atlas of Vascular Rings and Related Malformations of the Aortic Arch System.* Springfield: Charles C. Thomas Publisher, 1964.
16. Bronshtein M, Lorber A, Berant M, et al. Sonographic diagnosis of fetal vascular rings in early pregnancy. *Am J Cardiol* 1998;81:101–103.
17. Achiron R, Rotstein Z, Heggesh J, et al. Anomalies of the fetal aortic arch: A novel sonographic approach to in-utero diagnosis.[see comment]. *Ultrasound Obstet Gynecol* 2002;20:553–557.
18. Yoo SJ, Min JY, Lee YH, et al. Fetal sonographic diagnosis of aortic arch anomalies. *Ultrasound Obstet Gynecol* 2003;22:535–546.
19. Wilson DI, Burn J, Scambler P, et al. DiGeorge syndrome: Part of CATCH 22. *J Med Genet* 1993;30:852–856.
20. Goldmuntz E, Clark BJ, Mitchell LE, et al. Frequency of 22q11 deletions in patients with conotruncal defects.[see comment]. *J Am Coll Cardiol* 1998;32:492–498.
21. McElhinney DB, Clark BJ III, Weinberg PM, et al. Association of chromosome 22q11 deletion with isolated anomalies of aortic arch laterality and branching. *J Am Coll Cardiol* 2001;37:2114–2119.
22. Rauch R, Rauch A, Koch A, et al. Cervical origin of the subclavian artery as a specific marker for monosomy 22q11. *Am J Cardiol* 2002;89:481–484.
23. Rauch R, Rauch A, Koch A, et al. Laterality of the aortic arch and anomalies of the subclavian artery-reliable indicators for 22q11.2 deletion syndromes? *Eur J Pediatr* 2004;163:642–645.
24. Kazuma N, Murakami M, Suzuki Y, et al. Cervical aortic arch associated with 22q11.2 deletion. *Pediatr Cardiol* 1997;18:149–151.
25. Momma K, Kondo C, Matsuoka R, et al. Cardiac anomalies associated with a chromosome 22q11 deletion in patients with conotruncal anomaly face syndrome. *Am J Cardiol* 1996;78:591–594.
26. Payne DN, Lincoln C, Bush A, et al. Lesson of the week: Right sided aortic arch in children with persistent respiratory symptoms.[see comment]. *BMJ* 2000;321:687–688. Erratum in: *BMJ* 2000;321:1331.
27. Stoica SC, Lockowandt U, Coulden R, et al. Double aortic arch masquerading for thirty years. *Respiration* 2002;69:92–95.
28. Kindler H, Bagger JP, Tait P, et al. A vascular ring without compression: Double aortic arch presenting as a coincidental finding during cardiac catheterisation. *Heart* 2005;91:773.
29. Edwards JE. *An atlas of Acquired Diseases of the Heart and Great Vessels.* Philadelphia: WB Saunders, 1961.
30. Edwards JE. Malformations of the aortic arch system manifested as vascular rings. *Lab Invest* 1953;2:56–75.
31. Goldstein WB. Aberrant right subclavian artery in mongolism. *AJR Am J Roentgenol* 1965;95:131–134.
32. Kommerell B. Verlagerung der osophagus durch eine abnorm verlaufende arteria subclavia dextra (Arteria lusoria). *Fortschr Geb Rontgenstr* 1936;54:590–595.

33. Whitman G, Stephenson LW, Weinberg P. Vascular ring: Left cervical aortic arch, right descending aorta, and right ligamentum arteriosum. *J Thorac Cardiovasc Surg* 1982;83:311–315.

34. Kutsche LM, Van Mierop LH. Cervical origin of the right subclavian artery in aortic arch interruption: Pathogenesis and significance. *Am J Cardiol* 1984;53:892–895.

35. Hastreiter AR, DCruz IA, Cantez T, et al. Right-sided aorta. I. Occurrence of right aortic arch in various types of congenital heart disease. II. Right aortic arch, right descending aorta, and associated anomalies. *Br Heart J* 1966;28:722–739.

36. Mathew R, Rosenthal A, Fellows K. The significance of right aortic arch in D-transposition of the great arteries. *Am Heart J* 1974;87:314–317.

37. Knight L, Edwards JE. Right aortic arch: Types and associated cardiac anomalies. *Circulation* 1974;50:1047–1051.

38. Garti IJ, Aygen MM, Vidne B, et al. Right aortic arch with mirror-image branching causing vascular ring: A new classification of the right aortic arch patterns. *Br J Radiol* 1973;46:115–119.

39. Backer CL, Hillman N, Mavroudis C, et al. Resection of Kommerell's diverticulum and left subclavian artery transfer for recurrent symptoms after vascular ring division. [see comment]. *Eur J Cardiothorac Surg* 2002; 22:64–69.

40. Knight WB. Hypoplastic right retro-oesophageal aortic arch: Similarities to interrupted aortic arch. *Br Heart J* 1989;62:477–481.

41. Drucker MH, Symbas PN. Right aortic arch with aberrant left subclavian artery: Symptomatic in adulthood. *Am J Surg* 1980;139:432–435.

42. Konstantinov IE, Puga FJ, Konstantinov IE, et al. Surgical treatment of persistent esophageal compression by an unusual form of right aortic arch. *Ann Thorac Surg* 2001;72:2121–2123.

43. Garti IJ, Aygen MM. Right aortic arch with aberrant left innominate artery. *Pediatr Radiol* 1979;8:48–50.

44. Leutmer PH, Miller GM. Right aortic arch with isolation of the left subclavian artery: Case report and review of the literature. *Mayo Clin Proc* 1990;65:407–413.

45. Boren EL Jr, Matchett WJ, Gagne PJ, et al. Isolation of the left innominate artery in an elderly patient without congenital heart disease. *Cardiovasc Intervent Radiol* 2000;23:63–65.

46. Manner J, Seidl W, Steding G. The formal pathogenesis of isolated common carotid or innominate arteries: The concept of malseptation of the aortic sac. *Anat Embryol* 1997;196:435–445.

47. Killen DA, Battersby EJ, Klatte EC. Subclavian steal syndrome due to anomalous isolation of the left subclavian artery. *Arch Surg* 1972; 104:342–344.

48. Shuford WH, Sybers RG, Schlant RC. Subclavian steal syndrome in right aortic arch with isolation of the left subclavian artery. *Am Heart J* 1971;82:98–104.

49. Haughton VM, Fellows KE, Rosenbaum AE. The cervical aortic arches. *Radiology* 1975;114:675–681.

50. Kveselis DA, Snider AR, Dick M, et al. Echocardiographic diagnosis of right aortic arch with a retroesophageal segment and left descending aorta. *Am J Cardiol* 1986;57:1198–1199.

51. Tiraboschi R, Crupi G, Locatelli G, et al. Cervical aortic arch with aortic obstruction: Report of two cases. *Thorax* 1980;35:26–30.

52. Mullins CE, Gillette PC, McNamara DG. The complex of cervical aortic arch. *Pediatrics* 1973;51:210–215.

53. Harley HR. Development and anomalies of aortic arch and its branches with report of case of right cervical aortic arch and intrathoracic vascular ring. *Br J Surg* 1956;46:561–573.

54. Kumar A, McCombs JL, Sapire DW. Deletions in chromosome 22q11 region in cervical aortic arch. *Am J Cardiol* 1997;79:388–390.

55. Beaven TED, Fatti L. Ligature of aortic arch in the neck. *Br J Surg* 1947; 34:414–416.

56. Cooley DA, Mullins CE, Gooch JB. Aneurysm of right-sided cervical arch: Surgical Removal and graft replacement. *J Thorac Cardiovasc Surg* 1976; 72:106–108.

57. Hellenbrand WE, Kelley MJ, Talner NS, et al. Cervical aortic arch with retroesophageal aortic obstruction: Report of a case with successful surgical intervention. *Ann Thorac Surg* 1978;26:86–92.

58. Burrows PE, Moes CA, Freedom RM. Double aortic arch with atretic right dorsal segment. *Pediatr Cardiol* 1986;6:331–334.

59. Han MT, Hall DG, Manche A, et al. Double aortic arch causing tracheo-esophageal compression. *Am J Surg* 1993;165:628–631.

60. Higashino SM, Ruttenberg HD. Double aortic arch associated with complete transposition of the great vessels. *Br Heart J* 1968;30:579–581.

61. Ettedgui JA, Lorber A, Anderson D. Double aortic arch associated with coarctation. *Int J Cardiol* 1986;12:258–260.

62. Singer SJ, Fellows KE, Jonas RA. Double aortic arch with bilateral coarctations. *Am J Cardiol* 1988;61:196–197.

63. Cornali M, Reginato E, Azzolina G. Cervical aortic arch and a new type of double aortic arch: Report of a case. *Br Heart J* 1976;38:993–996.

64. Kron IL, Mappin G, Nolan SP, et al. Symptomatic double aortic arch causing tracheal and esophageal compression in the adult. *Ann Thorac Surg* 1987;43:105–106.

65. Raju S, Ratliff J, Timmis H, et al. "Internal coarctation" associated with double aortic arch. *J Thorac Cardiovasc Surg* 1973;66:192–195.

66. Enderlein MA, Silverman NH, Stanger P, et al. Usefulness of suprasternal notch echocardiography for diagnosis of double aortic arch. *Am J Cardiol* 1986;57:359–361.

67. Sahn DJ, Valdes Cruz LM, Ovitt TW, et al. Two-dimensional echocardiography and intravenous digital video subtraction angiography for diagnosis and evaluation of double aortic arch. *Am J Cardiol* 1982;50: 342–346.

68. Kan MN, Nanda NC, Stopa AR. Diagnosis of double aortic arch by cross sectional echocardiography with Doppler colour flow mapping. *Br Heart J* 1987;58:284–286.

69. Johnson TR, Goldmuntz E, McDonald-McGinn DM, et al. Cardiac magnetic resonance imaging for accurate diagnosis of aortic arch anomalies in patients with 22q11.2 deletion. *Am J Cardiol* 2005;96:1726–1730.

70. Van Praagh R, Van Praagh S. Persistent fifth arterial arch in man: Congenital double-lumen aortic arch. *Am J Cardiol* 1969;24:279–282.

71. Gerlis LM, Dickinson DF, Wilson N, et al. Persistent fifth aortic arch: A report of two new cases and a review of the literature. *Int J Cardiol* 1987; 16:185–192.

72. Geva T, Ray RA, Santini F, et al. Asymptomatic persistent fifth aortic arch (congenital double-lumen aortic arch) in an adult. *Am J Cardiol* 1990;65: 1406–1407.

73. Yang SG, Fogel MA, Stephens P Jr, et al. Noninvasive imaging of isolated persistent fifth aortic arch. *Pediatr Cardiol* 2003;24:179–181.

74. Celoria GC, Patton RB. Congenital absence of the aortic arch. *Am Heart J* 1959;58:407–413.

75. Oppenheimer Dekker A, Gittenberger de Groot AC, Roozendaal H. The ductus arterious and associated cardiac anomalies in interruption of the aortic arch. *Pediatr Cardiol* 1982;2:185–193.

76. Moerman P, Dumoulin M, Lauweryns J, et al. Interrupted right aortic arch in DiGeorge syndrome. *Br Heart J* 1987;58:274–278.

77. Braunlin E, Peoples WM, Freedom RM, et al. Interruption of the aortic arch with aorticopulmonary septal defect: An anatomic review. *Pediatr Cardiol* 1982;3:329–335.

78. Van Praagh R, Bernhard WF, Rosenthal A, et al. Interrupted aortic arch: Surgical treatment. *Am J Cardiol* 1971;27:200–211.

79. Van Mierop LH, Kutsche LM. Cardiovascular anomalies in DiGeorge syndrome and importance of neural crest as a possible pathogenetic factor. *Am J Cardiol* 1986;58:133–137.

80. Smallhorn JF, Anderson RH, Macartney FJ. Cross-sectional echocardiographic recognition of interruption of aortic arch between left carotid and subclavian arteries. *Br Heart J* 1982;48:229–235.

81. Riggs TW, Berry TE, Aziz KU, et al. Two-dimensional echocardiographic features of interruption of the aortic arch. *Am J Cardiol* 1982;50:1385–1390.

82. Rychik J, Murdison KA, Chin AJ, et al. Surgical management of severe aortic outflow obstruction in lesions other than the hypoplastic left heart syndrome: Use of a pulmonary artery to aorta anastomosis. *J Am Coll Cardiol* 1991;18:809–816.

83. Norwood WI, Lang P, Castaneda AR, et al. Reparative operations for interrupted aortic arch with ventricular septal defect. *J Thorac Cardiovasc Surg* 1983;86:832–837.

84. Kutsche LM, Van Mierop LH. Anomalous origin of a pulmonary artery from the ascending aorta: Associated anomalies and pathogenesis. *Am J Cardiol* 1988;61:850–856.

85. Contro S, Miller RA, White H, et al. Bronchial obstruction due to pulmonary artery anomalies. I. Vascular sling. *Circulation* 1958;17: 418–423.

86. Berdon WE, Baker DH, Wung JT, et al. Complete cartilage-ring tracheal stenosis associated with anomalous left pulmonary artery: The ring-sling complex. *Radiology* 1984;152:57–64.

87. Jonas RA, Spevak PJ, McGill T, et al. Pulmonary artery sling: Primary repair by tracheal resection in infancy. *J Thorac Cardiovasc Surg* 1989;97: 548–550.

88. Fearon B, Shortreed R. Tracheo-bronchial compression by congenital cardiovascular anomalies in children. *Ann Otol Rhinol Laryngol* 1963;72: 949–969.

Note: Page numbers followed by "f" refer to figures; page numbers followed by "t" refer to tables.